# Policy & Politics

### in Nursing and Health Care

# evolve

FIFTH EDITION

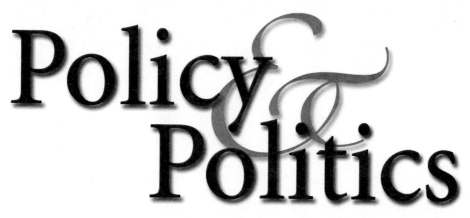

# Policy & Politics

## in Nursing and Health Care

**Diana J. Mason, RN, PhD, FAAN**
Editor-in-Chief
*American Journal of Nursing*
New York, New York

**Judith K. Leavitt, RN, MEd, FAAN**
Health Policy Consultant
Barnardsville, North Carolina

**Mary W. Chaffee, ScD(h), MS, RN,CNAA, FAAN**
Captain, Nurse Corps, U.S. Navy
Doctoral Student, School of Nursing
University of Maryland, Baltimore
Montgomery Village, Maryland

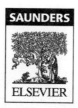

SAUNDERS

ELSEVIER

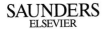

11830 Westline Industrial Drive
St. Louis, MO 63146

POLICY & POLITICS IN NURSING AND HEALTH CARE,
FIFTH EDITION

ISBN-13: 978-1-4160-2314-2
ISBN-10: 1-4160-2314-3

**The views expressed in this book are those of the authors and do not reflect the official policy or position of the Department of the Navy, the Department of Defense, or any other agency of the United States Government.**

Previous editions copyrighted 2002, 1998, 1993, and 1985.

**ISBN-13: 978-1-4160-2314-2**
**ISBN-10: 1-4160-2314-3**

*Senior Editor:* Yvonne Alexopoulos
*Senior Developmental Editor:* Lisa P. Newton
*Publishing Services Manager:* Jeff Patterson
*Senior Project Manager:* Clay S. Broeker
*Designer:* Andrea Lutes

Printed in the United States of America

Last digit is the print number: 9 8 7 6 5 4

**D**iana J. Mason, RN, PhD, FAAN, is Editor-in-Chief of the American Journal of Nursing, the dissemination leader among nursing journals. Under her leadership, *AJN* has received numerous awards from the Association from Women in Communication, Folio, the American Society of Healthcare Publishing Editors, the American Academy of Nursing, and Sigma Theta Tau International. Since 1985, she has been a producer and moderator of *Healthstyles,* an award-winning weekly radio program on health and health policy on WBAI-FM in New York City. For 5 years, she served as project director for *Youth Pulse,* a project to train New York City youth in radio production on health and social issues. Part of a larger national initiative called *Sound Partners for Community Health*; the project was funded by the Benton Foundation and Robert Wood Johnson Foundation. She is a noted speaker and writer on policy and politics in nursing and health care for local, national, and international audiences. Following two research fellowships, she conducted and published research on managed care arrangements with nurse practitioners, as well as other policy-relevant topics. Her involvement in nursing and health care organizations is extensive, including leadership positions on local, state, and national levels. Dr. Mason has received numerous awards, including fellowship in the American Academy of Nursing and the New York Academy of Medicine, the Pioneering Spirit Award from the American Association of Critical-Care Nurses, and media awards from the Public Health Association of New York City, the National Association of Childbirthing Centers, and the American Academy of Nursing. She holds an Honorary Doctorate of Humane Letters from Long Island University and earned her BSN at West Virginia University, MSN from St. Louis University (including graduate studies on medical care and public health in Norway at the University of Oslo), and PhD from New York University.

**J**udith K. Leavitt, RN, MEd, FAAN, is a health policy consultant. She retired as Associate Professor at the University of Mississippi Medical Center, School of Nursing, in 2005. She was formerly Executive Director of Generations United, a national organization dedicated to intergenerational policies and programs. She served on the National Advisory Council on Education and Practice for the Division of Nursing, U.S. Department of Health and Human Services. Ms. Leavitt was selected by President Clinton to serve on the Health Professional Advisory Group to the White House Task Force on Health Care Reform. She served as the upstate coordinator for Geraldine Ferraro's 1992 New York campaign for the U.S. Senate, was chairperson of the American Nurses Association Political Action Committee, was chairperson of New York State Nurses for Political Action, and was instrumental in the founding of the New York State Nurses Association's Political Action Committee. She is a noted speaker and author of extensive writings on policy and politics. Her many awards include the University of Mississippi Medical Center Nelson Award for Teaching Excellence, the Chancellor's Award for Teaching Excellence from the State of New York, the Health Policy Award from the Division of Nursing at New York University, the Legislative Award from the New York State Nurses Association, the Mississippi Nurses Association Nurse of the Year, and fellowship in the American Academy of Nursing. Ms. Leavitt earned her BSN from the University of Pennsylvania and her MEd from Teacher's College, Columbia University.

**M**ary W. Chaffee, ScD(h), MS, RN, CNAA, FAAN, is a Captain in the U.S. Navy Nurse Corps. She has served as Director of the Navy Medicine Office of Homeland Security, Bureau of Medicine and Surgery, in Washington, DC, and as a Senior Health Policy Analyst in the Office of the Assistant Secretary of Defense for Health Affairs.

She serves on the Executive Board of the International Nursing Coalition on Mass Casualty Education and the Editorial Board of *Disaster Management & Response*. She served as Vice President of the Federal Nurses Association, on the American Nurses Association Congress on Nursing Practice and Economics, and as an intern in the Office of Senator Daniel K. Inouye. She was the founding managing editor of the journal *Policy, Politics & Nursing Practice*. A Fellow of the American Academy of Nursing, she was awarded an honorary Doctor of Science degree by the University of Massachusetts. Her contributions to Navy Medicine and the Defense Health Program have been recognized with multiple individual awards. Captain Chaffee is an honors graduate of the University of Massachusetts at Amherst where she received bachelor's degrees in Nursing and Public Health and completed an internship at the Welsh National School of Medicine. She received her MS degrees in Nursing Health Policy and Nursing Administration from the University of Maryland, Baltimore, where she is currently a doctoral student in nursing.

# Contributors

**Linda H. Aiken, PhD, RN, FAAN, FRCN**
The Claire M. Fagin Leadership
   Professor of Nursing, Professor of Sociology
Director of the Center for Health Outcomes and
   Policy Research
University of Pennsylvania
Philadelphia, Pennsylvania

**Michael D. Aldridge, RN, MSN, CCRN, CNS**
Instructor in Clinical Nursing
The University of Texas at Austin
School of Nursing
Austin, Texas

**Linda Altizer, RN, MSN, ONC, CLNC**
Medical Legal Consultant
Forensic Investigator, Washington County
Johns Hopkins Medical Center
Hagerstown, Maryland

**Michelle Artz, MA**
Associate Director
Department of Government Affairs
American Nurses Association
Silver Spring, Maryland

**Frances E. Ashe-Goins, RN, MPH**
Affiliate Professor
University of South Carolina
College of Nursing
Columbia, South Carolina

**Elizabeth A. Ayello, PhD, RN, CWOCN, FAAN**
Faculty, Excelsior College
Senior Advisor, The John A. Hartford Institute for
   Geriatric Nursing
Albany, New York

**Sharon Baranoski, MSN, RN, CWOCN, APN,
   FAAN**
Director of Nursing
Provena St. Joseph Medical Center
Joliet, Illinois

**Connie Barden, MSN, RN, CCRN, CCNS**
Past President, American Association of Critical-
   Care Nurses
Clinical Nurse Specialist
Mercy Hospital
Miami, Florida

**Theresa L. Beck, RN, MPA**
Vice President, Community Initiatives
Visiting Nurse Association of Central Jersey
Red Bank, New Jersey

**Mary L. Behrens, RN, MSN, FNPC**
First Vice President of the American Nurses
Association
ANA/PAC Treasurer
Casper, Wyoming

**Kaye Bender, PhD, RN, FAAN**
Dean and Professor/Associate Vice Chancellor for
   Nursing
University of Mississippi Medical Center
School of Nursing
Jackson, Mississippi

**Kate Bent, RN, PhD, CNS**
Associate Chief, Nursing Service-Research
VA Eastern Colorado Health Care System
Denver, Colorado

**Virginia Trotter Betts, MSN, JD, RN, FAAN**
Commissioner of Mental Health and
   Developmental Disabilities
State of Tennessee
Nashville, Tennessee

**Thomas Blankenhorn, RN**
Captain, U.S. Air Force, Nurse Corps
David Grant Medical Center
Travis Air Force Base, California

**Linda Burnes Bolton, DrPH, RN, FAAN**
Vice President and Chief Nursing Officer
Cedars-Sinai Medical Center
Los Angeles, California

**Rebecca (Rice) Bowers-Lanier, EdD, RN**
Legislative Consultant
Macaulay & Burtch, PC
Richmond, Virginia

**Verena Briley-Hudson, MN, RN, CNA**
Chicago Director
Office of Healthcare Inspections
Office of the Inspector General
Department of Veterans Affairs
Hines, Illinois

**Charlotte Brody, RN**
Executive Director
Commonweal
Bolinas, California

**Dorothy Brooten, PhD, RN, FAAN**
Professor of Nursing
Florida International University
School of Nursing
Miami, Florida

**Patricia Burkhardt, CNM, DrPH**
Clinical Associate Professor and Coordinator,
  Midwifery Program
New York University
College of Nursing
New York, New York

**The Honorable Lois Capps, RN, MA**
Member of Congress (CA-23)
Washington, DC

**Laura Caramanica, RN, PhD**
Vice President of Nursing
Hartford Hospital
Hartford, Connecticut

**Tanisha Cariño, PhD**
Director Center for Evidence-Based Medicine
Avalere Health LLC
Washington, DC

**Anita J. Catlin, DNSc, FNP, FAAN**
Associate Professor of Nursing
Ethics Consultant
Sonoma State University
Rohnert Park, California

**Mary W. Chaffee, ScD(h), MS, RN,
  CNAA, FAAN**
Doctoral Student
University of Maryland, Baltimore
Montgomery Village, Maryland

**Shirley S. Chater, RN, PhD, FAAN**
Commissioner, U.S. Social Security
  Administration (1993-1997)
President Emerita, Texas Woman's University
University of California, San Francisco
San Francisco, California

**Mary Ann Christopher, MSN, RN, FAAN**
President and Chief Executive Officer
Visiting Nurse Association of Central Jersey
Red Bank, New Jersey

**Angela P. Clark, PhD, RN, CNS, FAAN, FAHA**
Associate Professor of Nursing
The University of Texas at Austin School
Austin, Texas

**James C. Cobey, MD, MPH, FACS**
Professor of Orthopaedic Surgery
Georgetown University
Senior Associate
Johns Hopkins School of Public Health
Washington, DC

**Laura B. Cobey, BSN, MPA**
Medecins Sans Frontieres, Holland, International
Rescue Committee
Washington, DC

**Elaine Cohen, EdD, RN, FAAN**
Corporate Director—Case Management
Methodist LeBonheur Healthcare
Memphis, Tennessee

**Sally S. Cohen, PhD, RN, FAAN**
Associate Professor
Director, Center for Health Policy and Ethics
Director, Nursing Management, Policy and
  Leadership Specialty
Yale University School of Nursing
New Haven, Connecticut

**Elizabeth B. Concordia, BA, MAS**
President, UPMC Presbyterian Shadyside
Senior Vice President, UPMC Academic
  and Community Hospitals
University of Pittsburgh Medical Center
Pittsburgh, Pennsylvania

**Colleen Conway-Welch, PhD, CNM, FAAN, FACNM**
Nancy & Hilliard Travis Professor of Nursing and Dean
Vanderbilt University School of Nursing
Nashville, Tennessee

**Johnny Sue Cooper, RN, MSN, FNP-BC**
Nursing Instructor
Holmes Community College
Grenada, Mississippi

**Mary M. Currier, MD, MPH**
Associate Professor
Department of Medicine
University of Mississippi Medical Center
Jackson, Mississippi

**Leah Curtin, RN, MS, MA, ScD(h), FAAN**
Editor, Journal of Clinical Systems Management
Cincinnati, Ohio

**Karen Daley, MS, MPH, RN**
Doctoral Student
Boston College
Connell School of Nursing
Chestnut Hill, Massachusetts

**Candy Dato, PhD, RN, NPP**
Associate Professor and Chairperson
Long Island University
School of Nursing
Brooklyn, New York

**Victoria J. Davey, RN, MPH**
Deputy Chief, Public Health
Department of Veterans Affairs
Washington, DC

**Shari Dexter, MA, BS**
ANA-PAC Administrator
American Nurses Association
Silver Spring, Maryland

**Betty R. Dickson, BS**
Contract Lobbyist
Jackson, Mississippi

**Donna Diers, RN, PhD, FAAN**
Annie W. Goodrich Professor Emerita
Yale University School of Nursing
New Haven, Connecticut

**Joanne Disch, PhD, RN, FAAN**
Professor and Director
Densford Center, University of Minnesota
School of Nursing
Minneapolis, Minnesota

**Alma Yearwood Dixon, EdD, MPH, RN**
Dean and Professor
Bethune-Cookman College
School of Nursing
Daytona Beach, Florida

**Catherine J. Dodd, RN, MS, FAAN**
Former District Chief of Staff
U.S. House Democratic Leader Nancy Pelosi
San Francisco, California

**Deborah Donahue, RNC, PhD**
Research Project Director
Florida International University
School of Nursing
Miami, Florida

**Donna M. Dorsey, MS, RN, FAAN**
Executive Director
Maryland Board of Nursing
Baltimore, Maryland

**Karen G. Duderstadt, RN, MS, CPNP**
Clinical Professor
University of California, San Francisco
School of Nursing
Department of Family Health Care
San Francisco, California

**Dezra Eichhorn, RN, MS, CNS, PMHNP-BC**
Family Psychiatric Mental Health Nurse Practitioner
Searcy Neuropsychiatry Clinic
Searcy, Arizona

**Nancy L. Falk, MBA, BSN**
John Heinz Senate Fellow (2004-2005)
Office of U.S. Senator Jeff Bingaman
Doctoral Student
George Mason University
College of Nursing and Health Science
Fairfax, Virginia

**Veronica D. Feeg, PhD, RN, FAAN**
Professor and Chair, Department of Women,
   Children & Family Nursing
AAN/ANF Institute of Medicine Scholar-
   in-Residence 2004-2005
University of Florida
College of Nursing
Gainesville, Florida

**Vernice Ferguson, RN, MA, FAAN, FRCN**
Senior Fellow Emeritus
School of Nursing
University of Pennsylvania
Philadelphia, Pennsylvania

**Mary Foley, MS, RN**
Associate Director, Center for Research and
Innovation in Patient Care
University of California, San Francisco
School of Nursing
San Francisco, California

**Eve Franklin, MSN, RN**
Representative, Montana House of Representatives
Great Falls, Montana
Executive Director, Montana Nurses Association
Helena, Montana

**Terry Fulmer, PhD, RN, FAAN**
Dean, College of Nursing
New York University
New York, New York

**Donna M. Gallagher, RNCS, MS, ANP, FAAN**
Principal Investigator/Director
New England AIDS Education and Training Center
University of Massachusetts Medical
Graduate School of Nursing
Boston, Massachusetts

**John F. Garde, CRNA, MS, FAAN**
Consultant
Park Ridge, Illinois

**Beth G. Gardner, BA**
New York University
New York, New York

**Deborah B. Gardner, RN, PhD**
Chief of Workforce Planning and
   Organizational Development
National Institutes of Health, Clinical Center
Bethesda, Maryland

**Richard Garfield, RN, DrPH**
Henrik H. Bendixen Professor of Clinical
   International Nursing
School of Nursing
Deputy Director for Public Health,
   Operation Assist
National Center for Disaster Preparedness
Mailman School of Public Health
Columbia University
New York, New York

**Kristine M. Gebbie, DrPH, RN**
Elizabeth Standish Gill Associate Professor of
Nursing and Director
Center for Health Policy
Columbia University School of Nursing
New York, New York

**Jill Gentry, BA**
Candidate for Master in Public Policy
Harvard University
Cambridge, Massachusetts

**Alicia Georges, EdD, RN, FAAN**
Associate Professor and Chairperson
Lehman College, City University of New York
Department of Nursing
Bronx, New York

**Greer Glazer, RN, CNP, PhD, FAAN**
Dean and Professor
University of Massachusetts, Boston
College of Nursing and Health Science
Boston, Massachusetts

**Cynthia M. Gonzalez, RN, MSN, ONC, APN**
President (2005-2006)
National Association of Orthopaedic Nurses
Chicago, Illinois

**Eric Goosman, RN, BSN**
Captain, U.S. Air Force, Nurse Corps
Student Registered Nurse Anesthetist
Uniformed Services University of the Health
   Sciences
Bethesda, Maryland

**Suzanne Gordon, BA**
Adjunct Assistant Professor
University of California, San Francisco
Journalist/Author
Arlington, Massachusetts

**Mary Margaret Gottesman, PhD, RN, CPNP**
Associate Professor of Clinical Nursing
PNP Specialty Program Director
Ohio State University
College of Nursing
Columbus, Ohio

**Deanna Gray-Miceli, DNSc, APRN, FAANP**
Adjunct Assistant Professor
University of Pennsylvania
School of Nursing
Philadelphia, Pennsylvania

**Rita Griffith, RN, MS, CRNFA**
Chief Executive Officer
First Assistants, Inc.
Indialantic, Florida

**Victoria H. Guisinger, MPH, MBA**
Associate Director of Programs, Lillian Carter
Center for International Nursing
Emory University

**Cathie E. Guzzetta, PhD, RN, AHN-BC, FAAN**
Director, Holistic Nursing Consultants
Washington, DC
Nursing Research Consultant
Children's Medical Center of Dallas
Dallas, Texas

**Kathryn V. Hall, RN, MS**
Executive Director
Maryland Nurses Association
Baltimore, Maryland

**Bethany Hall-Long, PhD, RNC, FAAN**
Associate Professor School of Nursing
University of Delaware
Delaware State Representative (District 8)
Newark, Delaware

**Barbara E. Hanley, PhD, RN**
Holistic Health Consultant, Educator
   and Provider
University of Maryland
School of Nursing
College Park, Maryland

**Charlene Harrington, PhD, RN, FAAN**
Professor, Sociology and Nursing
Department of Social and Behavioral Sciences
University of California, San Francisco
San Francisco, California

**Mary Ann Hart, RN, MSN**
Principal, Hart Government Relations
Cambridge, Massachusetts

**Susan B. Hassmiller, RN, PhD, FAAN**
Senior Program Officer
The Robert Wood Johnson Foundation
Princeton, New Jersey

**Barbara B. Hatfield, RN**
Delegate, West Virginia House of Delegates
West Virginia

**Pamela J. Haylock, MA, PhD, RN**
Oncology Consultant and Doctoral Student
University of Texas Medical Branch
School of Nursing
Galveston, Texas

**Sue Thomas Hegyvary, RN, PhD, FAAN**
Professor and Dean Emeritus
School of Nursing Adjunct Professor
School of Public Health and Community
   Medicine
University of Washington
Seattle, Washington

**Karrie C. Hendrickson, RN, MSN**
Doctoral Student and Research Assistant
Yale University
School of Nursing
New Haven, Connecticut

**R. Kyle Hodgen, MSN, RN, ACNP-BC**
Captain, U.S. Air Force, Nurse Corps
Student Registered Nurse Anesthetist
Uniformed Services University of the Health
   Sciences
Bethesda, Maryland

**Paula Colodny Hollinger, RN**
Maryland State Senator
Maryland General Assembly
Annapolis, Maryland

**Kim Welch Hoover, PhD, RN**
Professor & Associate Dean for Research
School of Nursing
University of Mississippi Medical Center
Jackson, Mississippi

**Becky Howard, MSN, RN, CS**
Psychiatric Clinical Specialist
Colorado Coalition for the Homeless
Denver, Colorado

**Ronda G. Hughes, PhD, MHS, RN**
Senior Health Scientist Administrator
Agency for Healthcare Research and Quality
Rockville, Maryland

**Veronica Hychalk, MS, BSN, CNA, BC**
Vice President, Professional Services
Northeastern Vermont Regional Hospital
St. Johnsbury, Vermont

**Jean Jenkins, PhD, RN, FAAN**
Senior Clinical Advisor
National Human Genome Research Institute
National Institutes of Health
Bethesda, Maryland

**Bonnie Mowinski Jennings, DNSc, RN, FAAN**
Colonel, U.S. Army Nurse Corps (Retired)
Health Care Consultant
Alexandria, Virginia

**The Honorable Eddie Bernice Johnson, RN**
Member of Congress (TX-30)
Washington, DC

**Katherine A. Kany, BS, RN**
Consultant
OOB Enterprises
Ashburn, Virginia

**David M. Keepnews, PhD, JD, RN, FAAN**
Associate Professor
Adelphi University
School of Nursing
Editor, Policy, Politics & Nursing Practice
Garden City, New York

**Karlene M. Kerfoot, PhD, RN, CNAA, FAAN**
Principal
Kerfoot & Associates, Inc.
Indianapolis, Indiana

**Judith B. Krauss, RN, MSN, FAAN**
Professor of Nursing & Health Policy
Yale University
New Haven, Connecticut

**Mary Jo Kreitzer, PhD, RN, FAAN**
Director, Center for Spirituality and Healing
Associate Professor, School of Nursing
University of Minnesota
Minneapolis, Minnesota

**Phyllis Beck Kritek, RN, PhD, FAAN**
Consultant, Trainer, Facilitator, and Coach,
    Conflict Transformation
Self-Employed Sole Proprietor
Courage: Conflict Transformation Services
Richmond, Virginia

**Kathleen Kuchta, BSN, RN**
American Nephrology Nurses Association
Pitman, New Jersey

**Corey C. LaLonde, BSN, RN**
Captain, U.S. Air Force, Nurse Corps
Student Registered Nurse Anesthetist
Uniformed Services University of the
    Health Sciences
Bethesda, Maryland

**Felissa R. Lashley, RN, PhD, FAAN, FACMG**
Dean and Professor
Rutgers, The State University of New Jersey
College of Nursing
Newark, New Jersey

**Ramón Lavandero, RN, MA, MSN, FAAN**
Director, Development and Strategic Alliances
American Association of Critical-Care Nurses
Aliso Viejo, California

**Dale Halsey Lea, RN, MPH, CGC, FAAN**
Director, Division of Genetics
Foundation for Blood Research
Scarborough, Maine

**Judith K. Leavitt, RN, MEd, FAAN**
Health Policy Consultant
Barnardsville, North Carolina

**Philip R. Lee, BS, MD, MS**
Professor of Social Medicine (Emeritus)
Department of Medicine, School of Medicine
University of California, San Francisco
San Francisco, California

**Tony Leiba, PhD, MPhil, MSc, BA, RN**
Professor—Educational Development
London South Bank University
Essex, England

**Sandra B. Lewenson, Ed.D, RN, FAAN**
Professor and Associate Dean for Academic Affairs
Lienhard School of Nursing
Pace University
Pleasantville, New York

**Carolyn K. Lewis, PhD, RN, CNAA, BC**
Assistant Dean
Bluegrass Community and Technical College
Magnet Consultant
The P.R.I.N.E. Group
Lexington, Kentucky

**Heather Lord, BS, MS**
Doctoral Student
Yale University
Department of Psychology
New Haven, Connecticut

**John R. Lumpkin, MD, MPH**
Senior Vice President & Director
Health Care Group
The Robert Wood Johnson Foundation
Princeton, New Jersey

**Courtney H. Lyder, ND**
Professor
University of Virginia
School of Nursing
Charlottesville, Virginia

**Patrick S. Malone, PhD**
Adjunct Professor
American University
Washington, DC

**Ruth E. Malone, RN, PhD, FAAN**
Associate Professor of Nursing and
    Health Policy
Department of Social and Behavioral Sciences
School of Nursing
University of California, San Francisco
San Francisco, California

**Tracy A. Malone, RN, MS, CMCN**
Executive Director
U.S. Family Health Plan Alliance
Washington, DC

**Pamela J. Maraldo, PhD, RN**
Managing Partner, PJM Associates
Pfizer Inc.
New York, New York

**Diana J. Mason, RN, PhD, FAAN**
Editor-in-Chief
American Journal of Nursing
New York, New York

**Mary Lynn Mathre, RN, MSN, CARN**
President and Co-Founder
Patients Out of Time
Howardsville, Virginia

**The Honorable Carolyn McCarthy, LPN**
Member of Congress (NY-4)
Washington, DC

**Kathleen M. McCauley, PhD, RN, BC, FAAN**
Past President, American Association of
    Critical-Care Nurses
Associate Professor of Cardiovascular Nursing
University of Pennsylvania
School of Nursing
Philadelphia, Pennsylvania

**Janice M. McCoy, MS, RN, CNAA, BC**
Vice President, Patient Care Services/Chief
    Nursing Officer
Cape Canaveral Hospital
Cocoa Beach, Florida

**Victoria Menzies, PhD, APRN, BC**
Florida International University
College of Health and Urban Affairs
School of Nursing
Miami, Florida

**Tamra E. Merryman, RN, MSN, FACHE**
Vice President Center for Quality Improvement
    and Innovation
University of Pittsburgh Medical Center
Pittsburgh, Pennsylvania

**Theresa A. Meyers, MS, BSN, RN, CEN**
Director, Emergency and Critical Care Services
Memorial Hospital
Colorado Springs, Colorado

**Mathy Mezey, EdD, RN, FAAN**
Independence Foundation Professor of Nursing
  Education and Director
The John A. Hartford Foundation Institute for
  Geriatric Nursing
New York University
College of Nursing
New York, New York

**Marie E. Michnich, DrPH**
Director
Health Policy Education Programs and
  Fellowships
Institute of Medicine
Washington, DC

**Helen M. Miramontes, MSN, RN,**
  **ACRN, FAAN**
HIV/AIDS Consultant
Clinical Professor Emerita
University of California, San Francisco
School of Nursing
San Francisco, California

**Patricia Montoya, RN, MPA**
Quality Improvement Project Manager
New Mexico Medical Review Association
Albuquerque, New Mexico

**Mary Margaret Mooney, DNSC, RN,**
  **CS, FAAN**
Professor and Chair
North Dakota State University
Fargo, North Dakota

**Patricia Mortiz, PhD, RN, FAAN**
Dean and Professor, School of Nursing
Director, Center for Children, Families and
  Communities
University of Colorado at Denver and Health
  Sciences Center
Denver, Colorado

**Thomas R. Oliver, PhD, MHA**
Associate Professor of Health Policy and
  Management
Bloomberg School of Public Health
Johns Hopkins University
Baltimore, Maryland

**Cynthia Kline O'Sullivan, RN, MSN**
Doctoral Student
Yale University
Yale School of Nursing
New Haven, Connecticut

**Judith A. Oulton, RN, BN MEd, DS(h)**
Chief Executive Officer
International Council of Nurses
Geneva, Switzerland

**Ryan W. Ozimek, MPP**
Chief Executive Officer
PICnet, Inc.
Washington, DC

**Bridgitte C. Patterson, RN, MSN, CRNP**
Clinical Faculty, Family Nurse Practitioner
University of Maryland
School of Nursing
College Park, Maryland

**Susan Pendergrass, DrPH**
Doctorate of Public Health
Director, Office of Strategic Initiatives
Department of Veterans Affairs Central Office
Washington, DC

**Sally Phillips, RN, PhD**
Director, Bioterrorism Preparedness Research
  Program
Agency for Healthcare Research and Quality
Rockville, Maryland

**Monika Piotrowska-Haugstetter, MHA**
Graduate Student
Yale University
School of Nursing
New Haven, Connecticut

**Virginia Plummer, PhD, RN, FACHSE, FRCNA**
Lecturer and Researcher
School of Nursing and Midwifery
Centre for Health Services Operations
  Management
Monash University
Victoria, Australia

**Patricia Reid Ponte, RN, DNSc, FAAN**
Senior Vice-President, Patient Care Services and
    Chief Nurse
Dana Farber Cancer Institute
Director, Oncology Nursing and Clinical Services
Brigham and Women's Hospital
Boston, Massachusetts

**Lynn Price, JD, MSN, MPH**
Associate Professor
Quinnipiac University
Hamden, Connecticut

**Joyce Pulcini, PhD, APRN, BC, PNP, FAAN**
Associate Professor
Boston College
William F. Connell School of Nursing
Chestnut Hill, Massachusetts

**Frank J. Purcell, Sr., BS**
Senior Director Federal Government Affairs
American Association of Nurse Anesthetists
Washington, DC

**Susan A. Randolph, MSN, RN, COHN-S,
    FAAOHN**
President, American Association of Occupational
    Health Nurses
Atlanta, Georgia
Clinical Instructor
Occupational Health Nursing Program
University of North Carolina at Chapel Hill
Chapel Hill, North Carolina

**Susan C. Reinhard, RN, PhD, FAAN**
Professor and Co-Director
Center for State Health Policy
Rutgers University
New Brunswick, New Jersey

**Richard Ricciardi, MS, CRNP**
Colonel, U.S. Army Nurse Corps
Doctoral Candidate
Uniformed Services University of the Health
    Sciences
Bethesda, Maryland

**Cathy Rick, RN, CNAA, FACHE**
Chief Nursing Officer
Department of Veterans Affairs
Washington, DC

**Kathy S. Robinson, RN, BS, FAEN**
Regional Coordinator
Lean Healthcare West
Missoula, Montana

**Rita M. Rupp, MA, RN**
Special Assistant, Office of the
    Executive Director
Executive Secretary, Council for Public
    Interest in Anesthesia
American Association of Nurse Anesthetists
    (Retired September 2005)
Park Ridge, Illinois

**Marla E. Salmon, ScD, RN, FAAN**
Dean and Professor
Nell Hodgson Woodruff School of Nursing
Director, Lillian Carter Center for International
    Nursing
Emory University
Atlanta, Georgia

**Christine W. Saltzberg, PhD, MS, APRN, BC**
Assistant Professor
Wayne State University
College of Nursing
Detroit, Michigan

**Yvonne Santa Anna, RN, BSN, MSG**
Director of Government Affairs
National Association for Home Care & Hospice
Washington, DC

**Alice Sardell, PhD**
Professor
Queens College, City University of New York
Queens, New York

**Jan Jones Schenk, MNA, RN, CNA, BC**
Principal Consultant, The PRINE Group
University of Utah College of Nursing
Park City, Utah

**Kristin Schmidt, RN, MBA, CHE**
Chief Operating/Nursing Officer
Arizona Spine and Joint Hospital
Phoenix, Arizona

**Nancy J. Sharp, MSN, RN, FAAN**
Health Policy Consultant
Bethesda, Maryland

**Rose O. Sherman, EdD, RN, CNAA**
Director of the Nursing Leadership Institute
Christine E. Lynn College of Nursing
Florida Atlantic University
Boca Raton, Florida

**Joanne Spetz, PhD**
Associate Professor
Department of Community Health Systems
University of California, San Francisco
San Francisco, California

**Susan McDonough Stackpoole, MSN, RN**
Director of Nursing Operations
Cape Canaveral Hospital
Cocoa Beach, Florida

**Christine Nordstrom Stainton, RN, BA, MSN**
Public Health Advocate
Planned Parenthood of Southeastern
Pennsylvania
Philadelphia, Pennsylvania

**Karen J. Stanley, RN, MSN, AOCN, FAAN**
President
Oncology Nursing Society
Pittsburgh, Pennsylvania

**Harry Jacobs Summers**
Senior Advisor
Center for Nursing Advocacy
Baltimore, Maryland

**Sandy Summers, RN, MSN, MPH**
Executive Director
Center for Nursing Advocacy
Baltimore, Maryland

**Keith Tarr-Whelan, BA**
Managing Partner
Tarr-Whelan & Associates, Inc.
St. Helena Island, South Carolina

**Linda Tarr-Whelan, BSN, MS**
Managing Partner
Tarr-Whelan & Associates, Inc
St. Helena Island, South Carolina

**Pamela Austin Thompson, MS, RN, FAAN**
Chief Executive Officer
American Organization of Nurse Executives
Washington, DC

**Eileen Toughill, RN, APN, C, PhD**
Director of Education, Quality & Compliance
Visiting Nurse Association of Central Jersey
Red Bank, New Jersey

**Patricia W. Underwood, PhD, RN, FAAN**
Associate Dean for Academic Programs
Frances Payne Bolton School of Nursing
Case Western Reserve University
Cleveland, Ohio

**Lynn Unruh, PhD, RN, LHRM**
Associate Professor
University of Central Florida
Orlando, Florida

**Karen Utterback, RN, MSN**
Vice President, Clinical Strategy
McKesson Extended Care Solutions Group
Springfield, Missouri

**Connie Vance, RN, EdD, FAAN**
Professor
College of New Rochelle
School of Nursing
New Rochelle, New York

**Antonia M. Villarruel, PhD, FAAN**
Professor and Nola J. Pender Collegiate Chair in
    Health Promotion
University of Michigan
School of Nursing
Ann Arbor, Michigan

**Wayne F. Voelmeck, PhD, RN**
Research Assistant
Cain Center for Nursing Research
University of Texas at Austin
School of Nursing
Austin, Texas

**Deborah von Zinkernagel, BSN, SM, MS**
Director, Clinical Systems and Program
Development
Pangaea Global AIDS Foundation
Consultant, Clinton Foundation HIV/AIDS
    Initiative
San Francisco, California

**Robin S. Voss, RN, MHA**
Director of Nursing: Emergency, Trauma &
    Orthopedic Services
Forsyth Medical Center
King, North Carolina

**Mary Wakefield, PhD, RN, FAAN**
Associate Dean for Rural Health
School of Medicine and Health Sciences
University of North Dakota
Grand Forks, North Dakota

**Ann Walker-Jenkins**
Legislative Associate
Association of Women's Health, Obstetric and
　Neonatal Nurses
Washington, DC

**Linda S. Warino, BSN, RN, CPAN**
Staff Nurse, Forum Health
Executive Director (District Three)
Ohio Nurses Association
Member, Board of Directors
American Nurses Association
Canfield, Ohio

**Joanne Rains Warner, DNS, RN**
Professor and Associate Dean
University of Portland
Portland, Oregon

**Kathleen M. White, PhD, RN, CNAA, BC**
Associate Professor
Johns Hopkins University
School of Nursing
Baltimore, Maryland

**Kristine Willingham, BSN, RN, CCRN**
Captain, U.S. Air Force, Nurse Corps
Student Registered Nurse Anesthetist
Uniformed Services University of the
　Health Sciences
Bethesda, Maryland

**Dana K. Woods, MBA**
Director, Marketing and Strategy Integration
American Association of Critical-Care Nurses
Aliso Viejo, California

**Steven J. Wyrsch, RN, BSN, MHA,
　CPHQ, CPUR, FAHM, FACHE**
Officer-in-Charge
Naval Branch Health Clinic
Portsmouth, New Hampshire

**JoAnne M. Youngblut, PhD, RN, FAAN**
Professor and Coordinator of Research
Florida International University
School of Nursing
Miami, Florida

# Reviewers

**Mary T. Boylston, RN, EdD(c), CCRN**
Chair and Associate Professor
Eastern University
St. Davids, Pennsylvannia

**Juliana C. Cartwright, RN, PhD**
Associate Professor
Oregon Health Sciences University School
  of Nursing
Ashland, Oregon

**Andrina (Tina) Lemos, MS, CNS, RN**
Assistant Professor
Dominican University of California
San Rafael, California

**P. Lea Monahan, PhD, RN**
Professor
Marian College
Division of Nursing
Fond du Lac, Wisconsin

*To the contributors to this book*
*&*
*All nurses who make a difference*

# Contents

# Foreword

As Democratic Leader in the United States House of Representatives, I know firsthand how important nurses are in working with policymakers to craft health policy. In my 18 years of serving in the U.S. Congress, nurses have significantly broadened my knowledge of health care issues. Their unique expertise provides essential perspectives in the debate on health policy and health care delivery. I trust the advice of registered nurses; they explain issues accurately and propose critical solutions to the problems we, as a nation, face. In fact, I selected a nurse to serve as the director of my home office in California. Catherine Dodd, a nurse-activist and former lobbyist, has been instrumental in my work on health and social issues.

America depends on citizen participation—including that of nurses—in the development and evaluation of public policy. During my tenure on the House Appropriations Subcommittee on Health and Human Services, Labor and Education, members relied upon input from nurses on crucial decisions about the allocation for scarce resources. Nurses involved in the care of people with HIV/AIDS emphasized the importance of drug therapies and advocated for support through all levels of care. Nurses working with children were vital in passing legislation that increased access to health insurance coverage for children through the State Children's Health Insurance Program (SCHIP). Nurses involved in occupational health have improved working conditions for workers across the country. Nurses have educated the public about environmental hazards and demonstrated the link between health and the environment.

Policy decisions are made by legislators, regulators, and leaders in many environments, but we depend on experts to educate us about specific issues. Nurses have significant knowledge about the health issues facing our nation. They must recognize how they can effectively use their expertise to improve health policy and, ultimately, the health of our citizens. By using this book, nurses will be able to identify how and where they can use their influence to address problems like the increasing number of uninsured and the quality of health care.

If health professionals want their perspectives on problems heard, they must bring information to those who make the decisions and the staff who advise them. There are many advocates on all sides of each issue, all competing for access to those who make the decisions. Therefore, nurses must not only understand their issues in great depth and be able to articulate a solution, but they should also know the weaknesses and strengths of the positions of other stakeholders.

Playing an active role in shaping policy can be a challenge. Fortunately, this book is an excellent resource to assist you in learning the policy process and the political forces that shape it. Whether you are running for office or are a novice in the world of policy and politics, this book will be an invaluable tool. The editors and more than 150 contributors have critical information and stories to share to enhance your learning. The public needs nurses to work with policymakers—and we need you now.

*Nancy Pelosi has represented California's 8th Congressional District since her election in 1987. In 2002, she was elected as Democratic leader of the U.S. House of Representatives, the first woman in history to lead a major party in Congress.*

# Foreword

Sheila Burke, RN, MPA, FAAN

In his foreword for the first edition of this book in 1985, Senator Edward M. Kennedy (D-MA) wrote that although nurses were America's largest group of health professionals, they had never played their proportionate role in helping to shape health policy. His cautionary note is as true today as when it was written.

In rereading Senator Kennedy's words, I thought of my path in policymaking, from serving as President of the National Student Nurses Association to serving on the Medicare Payment Advisory Commission. I considered why I had entered the world of policy and why many more nurses had not. Was it simply that I needed a job, or was it my belief in the importance of playing a role in the development of health policy? Though I needed the job, I rather liked the thought that I was being the altruistic "Cherry Ames, Nurse Politician." (Cherry Ames was the fictional character of a book series published in the 1940s through 1960s.) Cherry tried her hand at dozens of nursing roles including student nurse, army nurse, and chief nurse. Unfortunately, what she didn't become was a health policy expert!

Today, nurses have many real-life role models. Thousands of nurses have run for office, taken on challenging policy roles in the workplace and government, volunteered in political campaigns, and shaped how their organizations deal with policy issues. However, this is only a microcosm of what our leadership and expertise can bring to policy tables, and it shows why you should read this enlightening and instructive book.

Nurses have an obligation to care not only for the needs of patients, but to care about the health system. Increasingly, health policy in the public realm is being made by elected and appointed officials, many of whom have little or no experience in health care. As Mary Kelly Mullane noted in 1975, "The art of influencing policy, whether in government or in health care settings, can improve health care for all, if nurses recognize and use this valuable skill." Politics is simply a way to influence the changes that are made.

Members of Congress, the Administration, and state and local officials need our guidance and counsel and, most importantly, our views on what needs to be done to make the American health care system all that we want it to be. This fifth edition of *Policy & Politics in Nursing and Health Care* will give you the knowledge you need to help you assume this critical role. If Cherry Ames were with us today, I am certain she would choose to be a nurse leader in policy and politics.

*Sheila Burke is the Deputy Secretary and Chief Operating Officer of the Smithsonian Institution, Washington, DC. She was formerly the Executive Dean at the John F. Kennedy School of Government, Harvard University, and served as chief of staff to former Senate Majority Leader Bob Dole from 1986 to 1996. She is a member of the Medicare Payment Advisory Commission (MedPAC), a member of the Institute of Medicine (IOM), and a member of the board of the Kaiser Family Foundation.*

# *Preface*

This is the fifth edition of *Policy & Politics in Nursing and Health Care*. A lot has happened since the first edition of the book appeared in 1985:

- Three nurses have been elected to serve as Members of Congress.
- The Terri Schiavo case demonstrated the clash of health politics and values in the health system, in the courts, and within families.
- A nurse was elected President of the American Heart Association, nurses were appointed to key positions in the Federal government, and hundreds of nurses were elected to local and state government positions.
- Managed care and capitation were employed throughout the U.S. health system to control escalating costs, causing extensive financial restructuring.
- The Internet revolutionized how nurses learn, communicate, and find information to guide their practice, and it completely changed the political landscape through electronic campaigns, donations, and blogs.
- The National Center for Nursing Research (now the National Institute of Nursing Research) was established, and nursing research has expanded significantly, supporting a move to evidence-based professional practice.
- The emergence and spread of avian (bird) flu generated concern about the way in which mobile societies can spread a deadly infection very quickly, leaving entire nations vulnerable.
- A global shortage of nurses, and a significant shortage in the United States, led to the development of programs and strategies aimed at encouraging people to become nurses and remain in nursing.
- The terror attacks on the United States, as well as several catastrophic disasters, uncovered significant weaknesses in the public health infrastructure of the nation and exposed our lack of preparedness to handle disasters with large numbers of human casualties.
- The Woodhull study of nursing and the media, published in 1997, demonstrated that nursing was largely ignored in the American media.
- Therapies developed for HIV/AIDS changed it from being an always fatal condition into a chronic condition, sophisticated imaging now permits the identification of disease earlier, and robots can now be directed to perform surgery.
- The number of individuals in the United States who have no health insurance rose from 34 million in 1985 to 45 million in 2005; millions more are underinsured and are filing for bankruptcy due to the cost of health care.
- The United States remains the sole industrialized Western nation without universal access to health care for its citizens; health care has been an issue of debate in every presidential campaign since the first edition of this book appeared.

All of these points are evidence of the increasingly complex world in which nurses practice, the ongoing challenges nursing faces, and nursing's progress in policy and politics. We would like to think the previous editions of this book have helped prepare nurses to be effective in developing policy and influencing how health care is provided. Clearly, there is much work to do, because new challenges emerge regularly and past successes need to be reinforced and revised.

One of the premises of each edition of this book is that collective action is almost always essential for truly transformational change. Patient care is a political endeavor, and failure to recognize it as such will relegate nurses to playing the role of powerless discontents, a role we should not accept. However, individual effort is rarely sufficient for moving the profession forward and promoting the health of the nation. Nursing organizations have not had as much influence as would have been expected.

Association membership is down and nursing has yet to find a common voice.

So, we bring you the fifth edition of this book. We have no doubt about the value of nursing to this nation's health. We invite you to learn how you can be most effective in improving the health system, one policy or political activity at a time.

## WHAT'S NEW IN THE FIFTH EDITION?

This book has been developed to meet the needs of a diverse profession facing many challenges. We recognize nurses have varying levels of knowledge concerning policy and politics, so we have included content to meet the needs of nearly every nurse's background and level of knowledge and experience. We've included contributors who reflect the profession's diversity in terms of geography, gender, ethnicity, specialty, political affiliation, and practice setting.

The fifth edition contains four types of content: *Chapters*—overviews of foundational policy and political topics; *Vignettes*—first-person accounts of individual nurse's stories that illustrate political and policy concepts; *Policy Spotlights*—in-depth examinations of contemporary policy issues; and *Taking Action* sections—explorations of the strategies used by nurses to achieve specific policy goals.

The content of this edition reflects changes in society, in the economy, and within the health system. We've included new content on topics that include nurse staffing ratios, disaster policy, stem cell research, political philosophy, electronic political campaigns, regulating industrial chemicals, how nurses confronted the tobacco industry, the impact of war on health, and many others. We hope the stories of nurses' efforts, brilliant strategies, focused action, and persistence in these pages are truly inspiring for our readers.

## USING THE FIFTH EDITION

The book is organized using a framework of the four spheres in which nurses are politically active: the workplace, government, professional organizations, and community.

- Unit I, *Introduction to Policy and Politics in Nursing and Health Care,* provides the foundation for the remainder of the book. The content explores fundamentals of the policy process, political analysis, and strategy development.
- Unit II, *Health Care Delivery and Financing,* explores the larger health care delivery system, the basics of financing that system, and the economics of health care.
- Unit III, *Policy and Politics in the Workplace,* begins the application of concepts to the specific spheres of policy and political influence. The workplace is the first sphere discussed to emphasize the importance of nurses' recognizing the political nature of patient care.
- Unit IV, *Policy and Politics in the Government,* applies the concepts to the sphere of government. Contemporary issues, how to advocate on issues, and the paths that nurse-politicians pursue are examined.
- Unit V, *Policy and Politics in Organizations,* examines the important role that professional nursing organizations play in shaping policy that influences nursing practice and health care.
- Unit VI, *Policy and Politics in the Community,* describes nursing's opportunity to influence health in communities, current community health challenges, and the influence of the international community.

## USING THE BOOK AS A COURSE TEXT

As a textbook in undergraduate, masters-level, or doctoral courses, the organization of the book can serve as an outline for a course on policy and politics. The book also can be used in courses on trends and issues, foundations of nursing, leadership, research, advanced nursing practice, and population health. Perhaps the best use of the book by schools of nursing is as a foundational text that is used by the student throughout the curriculum, with readings assigned even in clinical courses. Consider, for example, the unit *Policy and Politics in the Workplace.* Nursing students in their first medical-surgical nursing course could study select readings from this unit, then identify and analyze a clinical issue that nurses on their assigned clinical unit have been instrumental in changing. The book can assist students to discern the political context of the care they provide, the influence of external policy on how they provide care, and opportunities to influence care on many levels.

## USING THE BOOK IN PROFESSIONAL ORGANIZATIONS

We encourage professional nursing organizations, including members of legislative committees and political action committees, to use the book as a guide for how to expand their influence. Furthermore, we challenge nurses working in a hospital or other health care organization to use the book to develop strategies to transform their immediate work environment for themselves and their patients.

## USE BY INDIVIDUAL NURSES

The book provides a wealth of rich learning opportunities for nurses who wish to prepare themselves to be more effective in influencing policy. The content provides both the 'how-to' and has inspiring stories of how other nurses have advanced important initiatives.

# Acknowledgments

As with previous editions, one of the remarkable features of this book is the large number of contributors who have donated their time, energy, and expertise to further nurses' political development. Over 150 nurses and other professionals participated in writing this edition. We're indebted to them for their commitment to this project. The book is also a reflection of the work of original co-editor Susan Talbott and the contributors to previous editions who helped establish the book's preeminence in the field. We remain grateful for their contributions.

It takes a village to produce a book. Our deepest gratitude goes to Michael Gardner, retired Navy Chief Hospital Corpsman, for his superb attention to detail and phenomenal managerial skill. As our Editorial Manager, he kept us on track and on time. We are indebted to our publisher, Elsevier, and Michael Ledbetter, our editor on the previous edition of the book and during the early development of this one. Our thanks also go to Yvonne Alexopoulos and Lisa Newton, who took the editorial reigns from Michael Ledbetter upon his promotion to another position, for their dedication to excellence. We are grateful for the expert editing provided by our Project Manager Clay Broeker and for the creative design work of the Elsevier team.

Our families and friends sustained us while this book was in development, so we have personal acknowledgments to add:

James Ware has been my partner, my daily support, and the nurturer of both me and my work. I am grateful for his understanding of the special perspectives that nurses and women have on life and living. Also, my apologies to Billy for walks deferred and bones forgotten.

I have been fortunate to work with a talented and creative editorial staff at the *American Journal of Nursing* who were incredibly supportive when my workload brought me perilously close to unraveling. They have taught me a great deal about excellence in writing and bringing laughter into one's work.

**Diana J. Mason**
**New York, New York**

As in previous editions, it has been my family and dear friends who have sustained me, nurtured me, and believed in the vision that this book conveys. Extra special gratitude goes to my sons Noah and David, my daughter Helen, my sister Joan Podkul and her wonderful family, and my Dad, who was my first mentor in policy and politics. Particular acknowledgment goes to my best buddy, Betty Dickson, one of the finest lobbyists for nursing anywhere.

**Judith K. Leavitt**
**Barnardsville, North Carolina**

Editing a book like this is like running a marathon. The stories of the nurses in these pages, who have done so much to improve health and health care through influencing policy, are the fuel that keeps us heading to the finish line. Helping me get to the finish line were a lot of people who kept a smile on my face. My warmest thanks to my daughter Sandra and friends Dr. George Zangaro, Dr. Nancy Valentine, Dr. John Murray, Kathleen Smith, Karolyn Klepacki Ryan, Joan Bold, Peggy McNeill, and Cherri' Shireman.

**Mary W. Chaffee**
**Montgomery Village, Maryland and**
**Brewster, Massachusetts**

# chapter 1

# Policy and Politics: A Framework for Action

Diana J. Mason, Judith K. Leavitt, & Mary W. Chaffee

*"You must become the change you want to see."*

MAHATMA GANDHI

Within 2 years, three unrelated events occurred that had significant implications for nurses practicing in the United States.

■ How could Hurricane Katrina affect a nurse practitioner in Atlanta, Georgia?

■ How might the war in Iraq have implications for school nurses in Worcester, Massachusetts?

■ How can cuts in health benefits by automobile manufacturers affect emergency nurses in Albuquerque, New Mexico?

Hurricane Katrina devastated economies, communities, families, and individuals along the U.S. Gulf coast in 2005. Although the levees in New Orleans were known to be vulnerable (Fischetti, 2001), policymakers chose *not* to invest the resources needed to strengthen them. The failure of the levees and the flooding that followed have led to the most expensive urban recovery and rebuilding effort in U.S. history. Federal dollars that now must rebuild the shattered coast are no longer available to fund daycare centers, school lunch programs, Medicaid, or nursing research. People fleeing from the Gulf coast evacuated to communities throughout the United States. On arrival in places such as Atlanta and Houston, they needed health services and replacement of essential prescription drugs—and most had no health records or insurance information and some had no identification. So, policies were rapidly needed to direct how nurse practitioners in Atlanta would manage the care for the patients who did not possess the documents that would normally be essential.

The war in Iraq, as all wars do, has required major expenditures from the federal budget. U.S. troops have better body armor now than in past wars; their torsos and vital organs are insulated from lethal injury, but troops remain at risk for head and extremity trauma. More soldiers are surviving war injuries but return home with significant mental health problems, mild traumatic brain injury, and limb amputations. These clinical problems will require extensive care in the U.S. health system for many years. Occupational health services will be needed, and the families of those adapting to a life without a limb will need support and guidance. The school nurse in Worcester will be caring for the children of deployed parents and may have a heavier workload because colleagues serving in the military reserves have been sent to Iraq.

Health care in the United States has traditionally been financed by insurance provided by employers. The U.S. automobile industry has set the standard for the type of health benefits an employer provides for its employees. General Motors recently slashed health care costs by cutting benefits for active and retired employees and their families. The cuts will save the world's largest automaker at least $1 billion (Isadore, 2005). The affected employees are faced with accepting the reduced benefits or searching in a troubled economy for a new job with good health benefits. The evaporation of health insurance benefits increases the amount that employees must pay for their own and their families' health care. If the employee can no longer afford a colonoscopy, a patient with cancer that could have been treated early if identified may come to the emergency department with symptoms of advanced disease. The emergency

**1**

nurse will see these sicker patients who have avoided preventive measures. The hospital will not be reimbursed for care provided to uninsured or underinsured patients and may then cut nursing staff as a cost-saving measure.

## THE BREEZE FROM A BUTTERFLY'S WINGS

A meteorologist named Edward Lorenz proposed in 1962 that the flapping of a seagull's wings in Brazil could cause a tornado in Texas (though in a speech at a 1972 meeting of the American Association for the Advancement of Science in Washington, DC the seagull became a butterfly) (Steele, 2004). The point was that an event seemingly far away can stir an environment, starting a chain reaction, and may cause unexpected results—like ripples on the surface of a pond when a stone is dropped into it. This concept grew into an emerging area of science known as *complex adaptive systems theory*. It is concerned with the constant adaptation within systems that occurs in order for the system, or elements of the system, to survive. In complex systems (like the health system or nursing) diverse parts of the system affect other parts. Complex systems demonstrate unpredictable behavior, broad change can result from a localized event, there is constant tension and balancing within systems, and order within the system is maintained without central control (Plsek & Greenhalgh, 2001; McDaniel, Jordan & Fleeman, 2003). The cases of Hurricane Katrina, the Iraq War, and eroded employee health benefits are examples of events that may ultimately influence nursing practice. The ripple effects of the event cascade outward—and when they affect another entity, like a nurse, that entity can in turn act in a way that has an influence on other parts of the system.

## NURSING WITHIN THE CONTEXT OF A COMPLEX HEALTH CARE SYSTEM

The health system is one example of a complex system. For most of the time humans have existed on earth, health care has been fairly simple. Until recently there were few effective strategies to deal with the diverse maladies and traumas that befall human beings. In the past, care was provided to the patient in the home. Family members served as care providers. Fast-forward to the present—past the development of anesthetic techniques, the discovery of the microbe, the flourishing of surgical procedures, and the transition from general practitioner or private duty nurse to board-certified specialist. Recall the effect of the growth of urban centers in America, the introduction of vaccinations and public health measures, and growth of visiting nurses. Consider the birth and growth of the hospital—the buildings that became the womb of sophisticated clinical and technologic advances. As clinical treatment options expanded, requiring diverse care providers and expensive equipment, patient care moved into the hospital from the home. The machinery of the hospital-based health system demanded trained workers—especially nurses.

As the possibilities for help, health, and healing expanded, patients demanded the best the system had to offer. In the twentieth century, the government entered the health care arena through the direct delivery of care, the financing of patient care, health care provider education, and health research. However, as circumstances conspired to cause health care costs to escalate in the late twentieth century, care changed. It was nipped, tucked, and moved back out of hospitals into ambulatory care centers, hospices, dialysis centers, and birthing centers and returned to the home. Financial and organizational restructuring measures were enacted as control mechanisms. Federal and state laws were passed in an attempt to regulate behavior in the increasingly complicated environment. It is this complex system that provides the context for the practice of nursing today.

The U.S. Health Resources and Services Administration (2005) reported that there were slightly over 2.9 million registered nurses living and working in the United States in 2004. These nurses conduct their practice in diverse organizations and at varying points in the process of health care. Nursing roles have expanded; over 100 specialty nursing associations serve their members, and multiple entry points to practice exist. Modern nursing practice, grounded in nursing science, has evolved significantly since its birth in the late nineteenth century.

## THE POLITICAL CONTEXT OF PATIENT CARE

Patient care is a highly political endeavor. Politics determines who gets what kind of care from whom and when. Patients are not well served when nurses fail to recognize the political context of care. For example, nurses who believe the work they do is "apolitical" are seldom able to marshal the resources they need to provide high-quality patient care or to seize the authority for important clinical decision-making. Nursing is concerned with health; therefore every action and decision that influences health and the health system should be important to nurses. Nursing does not exist in a vacuum. It is engaged in a continuous competition for scarce resources on behalf of patients. Policy and politics are the ways and means that nurses can use to influence the quality, safety, and accessibility of patient care.

Politics and policy may seem like remote, abstract concepts for extremely busy nurses in their workplaces. But patient care reflects policies within an organization and those developed externally. For example, when health care financing policies cause shortened hospital stays, an incontinent stroke patient may be catheterized because it is quicker than teaching bladder control. When the hospital's Medicare reimbursement is cut by Congress, the hospital may hire fewer staff, leading to clinical actions that may be more efficient for staff but less helpful and sometimes dangerous for patients. For example, an elderly patient is unable to feed himself, and his food intake drops precipitously. The staff do not feel they can spend the time required to feed the patient, so a nasogastric tube is inserted. Time is a precious political resource, and how nurses spend it has consequences for patients.

There is increasing recognition that nurses must have power and authority commensurate with their responsibility to promote and protect the health and well-being of patients. For example, why can't a nurse temporarily close a unit to new admissions if staffing levels and patient acuity jeopardize the ability of nurses to ensure adequate care of patients? In many hospitals, nurses have not had the power to make these decisions and have not developed a political strategy for acquiring this authority. But powerless nurses jeopardize the quality of care and well-being of patients—something that has been recognized by the best hospitals and by organizations such as the Institute for Healthcare Improvement, which are pushing to position nurses as key change agents.

Politics shape institutional and public policies at every point in their design and application. Understanding the policymaking process permits nurses to determine when and how to intervene to shape the policy to benefit the patient. By developing political skills, nurses are able to select and use the right tools to influence policy.

## DEFINING POLICY AND POLITICS

"Policy" often seems like an ethereal concept, and "politics" has taken on inaccurate connotations. Defining these terms is central to understanding their relevance to nursing.

### DEFINITION OF POLICY

Policy has been defined as "the principles that govern action directed towards given ends" (Titmus, 1974, p. 23) and as "a consciously chosen course of action (or inaction) directed toward some end" (Kalisch & Kalisch, 1982, p. 61). Stimpson and Hanley (1991, p. 12) define it simply as "authoritative decision making." Policy encompasses the choices that a society, segment of society, or organization makes regarding its goals and priorities and the ways it allocates its resources to attain those goals. Policy choices reflect the values, beliefs, and attitudes of those designing the policy.

Consider the example of policies related to tobacco use. In the twentieth century, the federal government subsidized tobacco farming and the nation watched the Marlboro Man riding across television screens. The Marlboro ads sent the implicit message that smoking was manly, "cool," good for social interaction, and sexy. To attract women to smoking, advertisements portrayed smoking as an attractive, independent choice, as in "You've come a long way, baby." But the 1990s brought a policy shift. By then, the actor who portrayed the Marlboro Man had died of lung cancer, tobacco ads were banned from television and radio, states' attorneys general were carving up tobacco settlement funds to pay for health care services needed for the millions who spent their lives smoking, and tobacco companies shifted their marketing plans to youth and developing nations (Annas, 1997). In 2004, nurses concerned about tobacco use as a continuing threat to the public's health formed the Nightingales, an activist organization that aims to educate the public about the strategies of the tobacco industry to perpetuate the addiction of smoking (see *The Nightingales Take on Big Tobacco* following Chapter 6).

## TYPES OF POLICY

- *Public policy* is policy formed by governmental bodies—for example, legislation passed by Congress and the regulations written from that legislation. Public policy related to tobacco use includes laws that ban selling cigarettes near schools and that require health warning labels on cigarette packaging.
- *Social policy* pertains to the policy decisions that promote the welfare of the public. For example, a local ordinance might set an age limit on the purchase of tobacco products. This policy would promote the welfare of children.
- *Health policy* includes the decision made to promote the health of individual citizens. For example, the federal government could decide to pay for smoking prevention programs for all persons in the military and their families. A state government might require coverage for smoking cessation programs by Medicaid managed care plans.
- *Institutional policies* are those governing workplaces: what the institution's goals are and how it will operate, how the institution will treat its employees, and how employees will work. For example, a hospital can institute a no-smoking policy that prohibits both patients and staff from smoking anywhere in the building.
- *Organizational policies* are the positions taken by organizations, such as state nurses' associations or specialty nursing organizations. For example, a state nurses' association may develop policy banning smoking at its meetings, a member might put forth a resolution calling on the association to offer free continuing education programs for nurses on smoking cessation, or the association might decide to join the Nightingales.

## DEFINITION OF POLITICS

Few words elicit the emotional response that the word *politics* does. Some people spit the word out like an epithet. It has come to be associated with negative images: smoke-filled rooms and shady deals made by power brokers, the corruption of Tammany Hall and Teapot Dome, bribes, unethical compromises, "pork barrel spending," payoffs, and vote buying, to name only a few. These images arise from media headlines of scandals and ethical breeches by elected officials.

Yet *politics* is actually a neutral term. It means simply the process of influencing the allocation of scarce resources. Examining this definition provides insight into what politics really is. *Influencing* implies that opportunities exist to alter the outcome of a process. *Allocation* means that decisions are being made about how to divide resources among competing groups or individuals. *Scarce* implies that there are limits to the amount of resources available—that all parties cannot have everything they want. *Resources* are commonly thought of in financial terms but may also be time, staff, or other entities in a process.

Nurses may contemptuously say "She plays politics" to describe someone who achieved a goal. However, ask the same nurses if they want a nurse executive who is politically astute, and they will usually say, "Absolutely!" *Politics* is therefore a term associated with conflicting values. The perception of politics as negative or positive depends largely on these factors:

- An individual's own biases, experiences, and knowledge of politics
- How the "game" of politics is played—that is, the system in which politics is operating and the rules that have been established as acceptable within that system
- Whether the goals or ends are important
- Whether one is in a position to change the rules of the system

## POLITICS, POLICY, AND VALUES

Making policy is a complex, multidimensional, dynamic process that reflects the values of those who are setting the policy agenda, determining policy goals and alternatives, formulating policy, and implementing and evaluating policy. John McDonough (2001), former health committee chair in the Massachusetts House of Representatives, notes that "much of the policy process involves debates about values masquerading as debates about facts and ideas" (p. 210). He writes from his own experience as a legislator listening to people tell compelling, sometimes inaccurate, anecdotes or using selective or unsubstantiated data to make a case for their own positions and values to shape policy decisions. When values are in conflict, as they often are in policy arenas with diverse constituencies, politics comes into play as participants attempt to influence the outcome of the policy process. Figure 1-1 illustrates the relationships among values, politics, and policy.

The values underlying policymaking activities related to tobacco and smoking illustrate this conflict. Should government be concerned about the economy of tobacco-growing states or the health of the public? Should the federal government support tobacco growers' businesses, or should it discourage smoking through laws that limit the age for purchasing tobacco products and that restrict where one can smoke? Should state or federal governments, or both, engage in legal action against tobacco companies to recover the costs of health care of smokers whose care is paid for by Medicare or Medicaid, even if it means that the tobacco companies' viability and their workers' jobs are threatened? Should public funds be used to help people to stop smoking, or is smoking a private issue?

Although nurses are educated to understand the biomedical model of disease management, many recognize its limitations: Caring is not part of the biomedical model. When the biomedical model dominates policy development in and out of institutions, the health and well-being of individuals, families, and communities are limited by policies that fail to reflect nurses' values, concerns, and priorities.

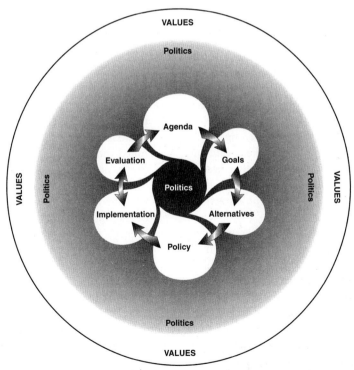

**Figure 1-1** A values framework for politics and the policy process. The figure illustrates the steps in the policy process. Politics can influence the process at any step. Both the politics of policy development and the policy itself are grounded in and influenced by values.

Support for nursing perspectives can be found in the work of those who value feminism and humanism.

## NURSING VALUES

American society is diverse, but policymaking bodies at local, state, and federal levels seldom reflect this diversity. The presence of sufficient numbers of ethnic minorities, women, and nurses at policy tables often shifts the nature of policies that are developed. Consider, for example, the impact of more women participating in public life. Caiazza (2005) studied how women of various religions made the transition from involvement in religious organizations to civic and political activism. She reported that whereas men tend to focus on individual rights, women contextualize this focus with values of connectedness, community, and collective responsibility. Indeed, analyses of the effect of women legislators on policy development has demonstrated that these policymakers are promoting agendas that were not a priority to their male counterparts, regardless of the women's political party affiliation (Ayres, 1997; Brenner, 1997). Women have been more likely to promote policies related to maternity leave, divorce, domestic violence, social safety nets, and family support (Dodson, 1997; Caiazza, 2002). In a qualitative study of nurses active in health policy in government and organizations, Gebbie, Wakefield, and Kerfoot (2000, p. 309) found a similar theme of consistency in values that shaped their policy agendas: "Some participants said nurses' strong beliefs in the capacity and importance of people to care for themselves distinguishes nurses from other health professions that share many of the same skills. This belief becomes an orientation toward policy action to enable people to help themselves."

Caring is a concept that is central to nursing (Benner & Wrubel, 1989). But as a profession that continues to be composed primarily of women, nursing embraces this value in a society that does not value caring (Reverby, 1987). And yet, there are other groups that share the value of caring and can serve as partners to nurses—most notably, feminists and humanists. For these three groups, a caring model encompasses the values of wholeness, interconnectedness, equality, process, support, diversity, and collaboration (Gilligan, 1982; Kurtz, 2000; Mason,

Backer, & Georges, 1991). It is not just women who hold these values. As some feminists and nurses are quick to point out (Gilligan, 1982; Pinch, 1996), caring is not gender based: Women do not "own" nurturing, compassion, and caring. To view caring as "female" trivializes the concept and precludes it from being integral to policymaking.

Nursing's values of caring, collaboration, collectivity, and high-touch care often conflict with the dominant values of society: competition, individuality, high-tech care, and profit (MacPherson, 1987). Consider the following examples:

- Because access to prenatal care is not guaranteed in the United States, some women receive little or no prenatal care and deliver very-low-birth-weight infants who require immediate and prolonged care in neonatal intensive care units. Yet prenatal care in the United States costs relatively little compared with the high cost of neonatal intensive care, which for the lowest-birth-weight infants is an average of $250,596 (Cuevas, Silver, Brooten, Youngblut, Bobo, 2005). Once stabilized, the infant will be sent home without a guarantee that the mother will receive the support she needs to provide for the infant or that the infant will receive any developmental support and special education that may be needed.

- In a thorough review of research and demonstration projects aimed at improving the odds for high-risk children and families, Schorr (1989, p. xxii) noted that successful programs have repeatedly shown that risk can be reduced through comprehensive, intensive, and responsive services by "staffs with the time and skill to establish relationships based upon mutual respect and trust." Since Schorr's review, Olds and colleagues (1997; Izzo et al., 2005; Kitzman et al., 2000) have reported that prenatal and postnatal home visits by nurses to low-income families were shown to reduce the risk of child abuse and neglect on evaluation 15 years later. In addition, the families that had the visits by nurses had fewer negative responses to stressful life events than those that had not received the visits. Such humanistic approaches to health and social problems are too seldom embraced by policymakers. A disease-oriented value system is predominant in the public policy arena, rather than a holistic wellness model.

- Mandatory overtime is used by hospitals to ensure adequate nurse staffing for patient care, but it's a policy that fails to reflect caring about patients or nurses. First, it's been shown to be harmful to patients. Rogers, Hwang, Scott, Aiken, and Dinges (2004) found that nurses working mandatory overtime reported more errors. Second, consider the potential impact of this policy on nurses who are parents and who could be forced to choose between commitment to their patients and commitment to their children. What does a single parent do if he's told he has to work another shift or lose his job, yet his young children will be arriving home from school and will be alone?

- Many hospitals cite financial constraints in their argument against improving nurse-patient ratios. Yet a study by Rothberg, Abraham, Lindenauer, and Rose (2005) looked at the cost of nurse staffing as a safety intervention and found that the "cost per death averted" of staffing at a 1:4 ratio was not as expensive as the use of the Pap test or the use of thrombolytics after a myocardial infarction—two procedures that are viewed as essential standards of care and are reimbursed accordingly.

If nurses want institutions and government to develop policies that reflect nursing's values, then nurses must be a part of the decision-making process—the *political* process.

## VALUES AND POLITICS

The values that nursing embodies can shape not just policies, but how those policies are developed. In the classic work *Toward a New Psychology for Women*, Miller (1976) noted that women and men often view power very differently. Whereas men tend to embrace hierarchic models of power embodied in the concept of "power grabbing" and inherent in terms such as *power over*, women tend to be more comfortable with power sharing, or *power with*. In the 1970s this view seemed both insightful and inspiring. In the years that followed, women's success in leading organizations, governments, workplaces, and communities was analyzed and found to be consistent with Miller's theory (Rosener, 1990). Transformational leadership

became popular, and leaders of both sexes espoused it as a style that embraced collaboration, creativity, and empowerment.

The concept of empowerment extended the values associated with a model of caring to a wide range of arenas. Mason and colleagues (1991) identified three components for the political empowerment of nurses:

- Consciousness raising about the sociopolitical realities of a nurse's life and work within society
- A sense of self-efficacy or self-esteem regarding nurses' ability to participate in the policymaking process
- Development of skills to influence the policymaking process: knowing how to use the traditional methods as well as new methods of relating to power and politics

Unfortunately the word *empowerment* came to be used in nursing and throughout society in ways that belied its true meaning, trivializing both the concept and its application. For example, too many nurse managers spoke of "empowering staff" when what they really meant was getting staff to do what the manager wanted. Nonetheless, the idea of empowerment is one that remains important to nursing's political development, because it "requires a commitment to connection between self and others, enabling individuals or groups to recognize their own strengths, resources, and abilities to make changes in their personal and professional lives" (Mason et al., 1991, p. 73). Nurses will not be effective in politics and policymaking until they value their voices, develop policy agendas that embrace their core values, and learn the skills of policy making and influencing. Nurses who are involved in shaping health policy reinforce this perspective. Gebbie and colleagues (2000, p. 310) found that nurses experienced in policy and politics used consensus-building skills that included "mobilizing and communicating with diverse groups," which the nurses saw as arising from their ability to "work with others, regardless of differences."

One can extend the concept of empowerment to societal approaches to problem solving. U.S. society functions primarily with a model of limited resources, whereby groups must compete to get their share. However, Smith (1997) has argued that it is possible to embrace a resource-sharing framework instead of a resource-limited one. A resource-sharing framework requires embracing values of empowerment, community collaboration, and partnerships. It assumes such partnerships can discover previously unknown resources and develop new ones to meet the needs of individuals, families, and communities.

Such a framework embraces the need for a global perspective on policymaking. Although most citizen action occurs on a local level, the decisions made there increasingly have a global impact. Promoting the health of local communities requires a focus on what is good for the world community, and vice versa. As a global perspective proliferates, the potential conflict in culture-bound values will need to be addressed. Nurses can be a leading voice in advocating for the values needed to integrate global perspectives on public policies and political action, and the International Council of Nurses has encouraged nurses to do so (Box 1-1).

Public and private policies are a result of choices. These choices are based on values that come into play in the political dynamics of policymaking. When individuals and groups with disparate values enter into the policymaking process, consensus around policies can be difficult to attain unless values are clarified and agreement is reached on how to proceed despite any differences. Although groups with markedly different values sometimes agree to the same solution, they may do so because the solution manages to reflect their value sets. In addition, individuals and groups, including nurses, should clarify which values they will embrace to guide their political behavior and strategies for advancing a policy agenda.

## THE FOUR SPHERES OF POLITICAL ACTION IN NURSING

Although political action and policymaking are usually associated with the government, there are three other spheres in which nurses are politically active: the workplace, professional organizations, and the community. Figure 1-2 illustrates the spheres of the government, workplace, and organizations contained in the broader sphere of the community. These four spheres are interconnected and overlapping. The political effectiveness of nurses in one sphere will be influenced by nurses' involvement in the other spheres. Although this book is structured to address each of these spheres separately, the interaction and interdependence are evident throughout.

---

**BOX 1-1    The International Council of Nurses and Public Policy**

In 2000, the International Council of Nurses (ICN) published a position statement, "Participation of Nurses in Health Services Decision Making and Policy Development" (available at *www.icn.ch/pspolicydev00.htm)*. The statement identifies the role individual nurses can play in health services planning and public policy, as well as the responsibility professional nursing organizations have to promote and advocate for nursing participation in policymaking. The ICN also published "Guidelines on Shaping Effective Health Policy" (2001) to encourage participation in policy and politics regardless of geographic setting (available at *www.icn.ch//Guideslines_shaping.pdf)*.

---

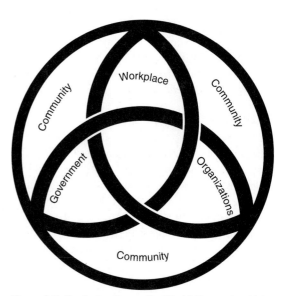

**Figure 1-2** The four spheres of political influence in which nurses can effect change. These are workplace, government, professional organizations, and community (the encompassing sphere).

Readers should look for this interaction and integrate it into their own plan for political activism.

## THE FIRST SPHERE: THE WORKPLACE

Nurses' workplaces can be any setting in which nurses practice, including acute care, home care, nursing homes, school-based health clinics, occupational health, and myriad other places. Nurses have not always recognized or been comfortable with the important role they have to play in creating workplace policies that will ensure supportive work environments and excellent outcomes for patients.

Most nurses are familiar with "policies and procedures" manuals. These manuals list workplace policies, but other policies also exist that determine what kind of care is provided and by whom—whether those policies are written or unwritten. Following are examples of policies found in many workplaces:

- Designation of no-smoking areas, or a ban on smoking in the entire facility
- Requirement for nurses to work overtime (mandatory overtime)
- Authority to delay a patient's discharge or refuse to admit a patient to the intensive care unit based on a nurse's professional assessment
- Decisions concerning the use of unlicensed personnel as substitutes for RNs
- A policy to permit family members to be present with their loved ones during emergency or invasive procedures (see *Family Presence at the Bedside: Changing Hospital Policy* following Chapter 17)

A hallmark of a "magnet" institution is nurses' involvement in decision-making at all levels of the organization and inclusion as an important voice in the development of its policies. Magnet status is conferred by the American Nurses Credentialing Center to applying institutions that can demonstrate high-quality nursing care and environments that support excellence in professional nursing practice (see the Policy Spotlight following Chapter 16). As of December 2005, fewer than 190 of the approximately 5000 hospitals in the United States held the Magnet designation.

The Robert Wood Johnson Foundation (RWJF) has responded to this need for improving the places in which nurses work. It has developed a multi-pronged strategy for reducing the shortage in nursing staff and improving the quality of nursing care by changing the way care is delivered at the bedside. Concerned about the lack of nursing representation in groups deliberating about patient safety, the RWJF has been advocating that nursing is the key to quality. One major initiative in their portfolio is Transforming Care At the Bedside (TCAB), a joint project with the Institute for Healthcare Improvement aimed at changing the work environment of hospitals to support bedside nurses as *the* key change agent (see *Transforming Care at the Bedside: Shadyside Hospital's Code Red* following Chapter 17).

Workplace policies are also shaped by the policies of government, professional organizations, and the community. For example, occupational and health standards established by the federal government may drive a workplace to develop policies on the handling of hazardous wastes. A professional nurses' association may keep this issue visible and, through a resolution of its own, decide to pressure nurses' workplaces to use particular protective equipment in high-risk areas. Indeed, nurses have led Health Care Without Harm, an international coalition whose mission is to "transform the health care industry worldwide, without compromising patient safety or care, so that it is ecologically sustainable and no longer a source of harm to public health and the environment" (see *Regulating Industrial Chemicals to Protect the Environment and Human Health* following Chapter 33). As of December 2005, 27 nursing organizations were members of this coalition.

## THE SECOND SPHERE: GOVERNMENT

The actions of government touch nearly every part of our lives, from laws requiring records documenting births; to mandatory childhood immunizations; to the legal establishment of the age at which people may drink alcohol, cast a vote, or join the military; to the laws determining what health services people are eligible for in old age and how assets are distributed on a person's death. Government determines whether children receive services that contribute to health and education, what drugs may be used, how business relationships are conducted, and to what extent a country uses diplomacy and military approaches in managing world conflicts.

We live in a society in which we are all connected; the welfare and safety of each one of us depends on the health and welfare of a cooperative and collective enterprise. Government has grown bigger and more centralized, not because we have become careless about freedoms or less committed to individual values, but because the important tasks that need to be done in our nation today are beyond the reach of individuals. Making our society work—and civilization flourish—is everyone's business. It's what *we* do. Individual freedom depends on full participation in democracy.

Government plays an enormously important role in nursing and health care. It provides society with a legal definition of what nursing is, and it defines what a nurse may do. It influences reimbursement systems for health care and nursing services, and to a great extent, it determines who receives what type of health services.

Throughout the last part of the twentieth century, federal, state, and local governments made decisions about some major issues for our society:

- Whether women could receive full information about reproductive rights and who could provide that information
- Where smoking is permitted, and where alcohol and tobacco products may be advertised
- The health services that are available in schools and whether schools may distribute condoms to prevent the spread of HIV and AIDS
- The resources available to communities for low-income housing development and maintenance
- Whether violence is treated solely as a crime or as a public health issue

The sphere of government is extensive. The interplay between the public and private sectors means that public policy may become policy in the private sector as well. For example, a local ordinance banning smoking in public buildings would result in a ban on workplace smoking for many workers when their employers try to comply with or follow the trend. Government policy often drives the policies and programs in health care organizations. The government's actions are, in turn, shaped by the public and organizations, including nursing. The Institute

of Medicine (IOM) (1988) argued that although not all efforts to improve and promote the health of the public must be made by government, the government does have the responsibility for providing guidance in the policy process:

Policy formulation takes place as the result of interactions among a wide range of public and private organizations and individuals. Although it joins with the private sector to arrive at decisions, government has a special obligation to ensure that the public interest is served by whatever measures are adopted. (p. 44)

In some cases, government provides leadership in defining a problem for both public and private sectors to address. For example, the IOM's report, *To Err is Human: Building a Safer Health System*, defined health care error, described the prevalence of error as a cause of death, identified the contributing factors, and recommended policy responses in both public and private sectors (IOM, 1999). This report stimulated a host of studies and actions aimed at making health care safer. Despite this flurry of activity, Lucian Leape and Donald Berwick (2005), two leaders in the movement for high-quality health care and patient safety, evaluated the progress that had been made 5 years after the report was released and concluded that not much improvement could be found, particularly in the private sector. However, they also concluded that the IOM report had "changed the conversation" about patient safety and that the rate of change is expected to accelerate.

## THE THIRD SPHERE: PROFESSIONAL ORGANIZATIONS

Professional organizations have been instrumental in shaping the practice of nursing—for example, in developing standards of practice, advocating for change in the scope of nursing practice, and playing a role in collective action in the workplace. Organizations can also be a significant force in the development of broader health and social policies to address issues such as the use of seat belts or motorcycle and bicycle helmets to prevent more trauma and mortality from vehicular accidents.

Although potentially powerful, nursing organizations could increase their influence if more nurses participated in them. The American Nurses

Association (ANA) represents the interests of all American nurses, yet only about 5% of nurses in the United States are members. Some specialty nursing organizations include a greater percentage of members but rarely exceed 30%. Yet these organizations are essential for advocating for nurses and for values of caring and health promotion.

A strong professional organization should be a visible force within its community: A national organization should have a national presence, and a local organization should be known in the local community. Organizations can and should identify issues of concern to nursing and health care, bring them to the attention of the public, and take a leadership role in calling for the development of policies that can improve the health of communities and ensure the provision of quality nursing care. To achieve this goal, organizations need the collective participation and support of nurses who will develop and use their political savvy to promote progressive policies.

At the same time, nursing organizations need to work together to advocate for patients, nursing, and health care. Formed in 2001, the Nursing Organization Alliance (NOA) is a coalition of more than 65 national nursing organizations. NOA's stated mission is "to increase nursing's visibility and impact on health through communication, collaboration and advocacy" (see *www.nursing-alliance.org*). Despite this promising mission, it has yet to use its collective power to influence national policy debates, get nurses appointed to key commissions and advisory groups, or ensure that nurses are available to journalists covering health-related stories. The fear of fragmentation arising from differences in the agendas among the various organizations may be outweighing the need for finding common ground for action. But what other venue does the profession have for multiple nursing organizations to push a policy agenda grounded in common values and goals?

## THE FOURTH SPHERE: THE COMMUNITY

In years past, nurse leaders such as Lillian Wald viewed the community as more than a practice site. It was seen as a social unit with a variety of special interest groups, community activities, health and social problems, and resources for solving those problems. A community can be one's neighborhood, or it can be the international online group with a common interest. The other three spheres of influence exist within the sphere of the community. As members of a community, nurses have a responsibility to promote the welfare of the community and its members. In turn, the community's resources can be invaluable assets for nurses' work in health promotion and health care delivery. Government officials, health care administrators, patients, corporate managers, presidents of private and public organizations—all players who can effect change in health policy—are affiliated with at least one community: the one in which they live. When nurses become visible in their communities, they represent the entire profession. Community networks can be called on to support nursing agendas.

Likewise, nursing should be called on to support the agendas of communities that are trying to develop a better place for citizens to live. Nurses can be and are involved in parent-teacher associations, senior citizens' councils, community planning boards, advocacy and civic organizations, and business groups. They can be instrumental in organizing and mobilizing communities on issues such as recycling, environmental cleanup, and safety. Although such activism may arise out of the private concerns of nurses for their own well-being and that of their families, it can also affect nurses' professional lives if, for example, they care for the victims of toxic waste disposal, pollution, or crime.

The interrelationships among nursing's four spheres of political activity become more distinct as nurses develop and use political skills. Ignoring one sphere can endanger one's effectiveness as a change agent.

## THE POLITICAL DEVELOPMENT OF NURSING

Where does nursing stand today with regard to its ability to influence policy? Cohen and colleagues (1996) developed a conceptual model that describes the political development of the profession. The model's stages mirror the stages that individual nurses navigate to become key players in policy arenas. The stages are buy-in, self-interest, political sophistication, and leadership.

## STAGE ONE: BUY-IN

Buy-in is a reactive stage in which the profession recognizes the importance of political involvement and encourages nurses to recognize the importance of policy development to their daily lives as professionals and citizens. From the perspectives of history and the profession, the late 1970s and the 1980s were a time when nurses recognized they were excluded from important policy developments. Decisions were being made that influenced their practice, but not with their input. Leaders began to identify ways in which nurses could become politically active. Nursing's first political action committee (PAC), Nurses Coalition for Action in Politics, was formed by a small group of savvy nurse leaders in New York. It later became the PAC for the ANA. Articles on political action began to appear with regularity in nursing journals in the 1980s and often called for enhanced efforts to educate nurses about policy and politics.

From the perspective of individual nurses, political action inevitably starts with buy-in. Each nurse must recognize the relevance of politics and policy to his or her work as a nurse and personal life as a citizen. It is not uncommon for nurses to be active in politics in their own communities but continue to believe that politics is irrelevant to their professional work. But the profession has a responsibility for shaping nurses' perceptions of the political context of their professional work.

Certainly, this is a major responsibility of nursing education at all levels. Although accrediting bodies for nursing education have pushed for a focus on policy and politics in nursing curricula, two controversial new educational pathways for nurses, spearheaded by the American Association of Colleges of Nursing (AACN), promise to strengthen this emphasis: the clinical nurse leader (CNL), prepared at the master's level, and the doctorate of nursing practice (DNP) for advanced practice nurses. As noted in a description of "Essential #5, Health Care Policy for Advocacy in Health Care," for the DNP role and curriculum:

Political activism and political commitment must become part of the definition of the nursing as a profession....

Nurses witness daily the consequences of policies and need to work for justice and equity in the health care system. These powerful clinical experiences can become potent influencers in policy formation for the advanced nursing practitioner who integrates these experiences with two additional skill sets: the ability to analyze the policy process and the ability to engage in politically competent action.... (AACN, 2005, p. 11)

The essentials of the CNL curriculum also include content on the political context of care. In addition, the CNL graduate is expected to demonstrate the following competency: "Is knowledgeable and active in the political and regulatory process." (AACN, 2004, p. 27)

These developments suggest that the profession is recognizing its responsibility for educating individual nurses about the political context of care and their social responsibility for shaping the policies that affect that care.

## STAGE TWO: SELF-INTEREST

Self-interest occurs when the nursing profession develops its identity as a special interest and crystallizes its political voice. In the last half of the twentieth century, nursing began to focus on issues associated with education and research and became involved in crafting legislation for expanded practice. Nursing coalitions began to garner political support for their issues in Congress and state legislatures. The ANA-PAC became the third largest federal health care special interest group as individual nurses came to realize the collective power of their individual donations.

If nurses can see the connections between their own personal circumstances and the political context of their lives, they are more likely to engage in political activism to advance their personal interests. Similarly, if nurses can see the connection to politics and policy in their professional lives, they are often moved to action. Therefore appealing to self-interest can be an important step in engaging nurses to participate in shaping workplace or public policies.

## STAGE THREE: POLITICAL SOPHISTICATION

In the mid-1990s, nurses began to be recognized by policymakers and health care leaders as having valuable perspectives and expertise in health policy. The ANA developed *Nursing's Agenda for Healthcare*

*Reform* in 1992 and brought together most national nursing organizations to speak with one voice about desired reforms in the health care system. Nurses were appointed to federal panels, agencies, and commissions. Increasing numbers of nurses campaigned for local, state, and national political offices and found support, not only among their peers, but also from the public. These advances arose from the profession's being ready to respond to opportunities presented by the administration of President Clinton. His mother was a nurse, and he often spoke about the importance of nurses to the nation's health. His vice president, Al Gore, had developed close connections with then ANA president Virginia Trotter Betts, who had served as a Robert Wood Johnson (RWJ) Health Policy Fellow in Gore's office. These personal experiences positioned the profession to seize opportunities for being at policy tables that had previously not sought nursing's presence.

But this example also illustrates the importance of individual nurses positioning themselves for such appointments. Trotter Betts had to seek the RWJ fellowship; it was not simply handed to her. She went on to hold the position of Special Assistant to U.S. Department of Health and Human Services Secretary Donna Shalala and then to be the first nurse Commissioner of Mental Health in Tennessee. This stage requires synergy between policymakers who recognize the importance of nursing perspectives and nurses who are ready to respond by adding their voices to policy debates and decision-making.

Although there was evidence in the 1990s that policymakers were recognizing the importance of nurses' participation in advisory committees and policy decisions, by the turn of the century nursing was not consistently responding to requests for its presence at these tables. For example, the National Health Council, founded in 1929, describes itself as "…a dynamic forum for policy development—the place where all segments of the health care community meet for reasoned discussion and persuasive advocacy." Its membership includes over 110 voluntary health agencies, nonprofit organizations with an interest in health, business and industry members, and professional and membership organizations (including the American Academy of Family Physicians, the American Thoracic Society, and the Association of Schools of Allied Health Professions). Any organization may become a member. Despite the organization's attempts to attract nursing organizations to participate, not one was a member as of the end of 2005.

## STAGE FOUR: LEADERSHIP

When nursing embraces a political identity exemplified by "setting the agenda" for change, it is functioning at the highest level of political involvement. Here nursing becomes the initiator of crucial policy change. Achieving appointments to positions outside of nursing, such as to university presidencies or as agency heads in federal and state government, characterizes stage four. Nurses are recognized for their unique expertise and perspectives and are supported by multiple constituencies. In some instances since the 1970s, nursing has been able to achieve this level; at other times the political status of nursing vacillates between stages three and four. The longer nursing functions in stage four, the more the public will benefit from nurses' knowledge and leadership in solving issues related to the well-being of society.

Nurses such as Rosalind Kurita are recognizing that the skills and vision they possess are valuable in public policy. In 2005, Kurita was raising money for a serious campaign for the U.S. Senate seat held by Senate Majority Leader, and physician, Bill Frist (R-TN) who was stepping down. Serving in her second term as the only RN in Tennessee's state senate, Kurita developed a record of action that focused on education, jobs, fiscal responsibility, and health care. Whether she wins or loses her race for the U.S. Senate, she has demonstrated one way for individual nurses to reach the fourth stage of political development.

Although Kurita is a contemporary example of a successful nurse activist, others in the past established a mandate for political activity.

## NURSING'S HISTORIC MANDATE

### FLORENCE NIGHTINGALE

It's important for today's nurses to learn from the bold actions of those who shaped nursing in this country. Though not an American nurse, Florence Nightingale was a consummate politician and visionary. She transformed the British and Indian health care systems and military health care, as well. She knew the value of data in influencing policy and came to be recognized as the first statistician. Reflecting on her first administrative position in nursing, Nightingale wrote the following:

When I entered into service here, I determined that, happen what would, I never would intrigue among the Committee. Now I perceive that I do all my business by intrigue. I propose in private to A, B, or C the resolution I think A, B, or C most capable of carrying in Committee, and then leave it to them, and I always win. (Huxley, 1975, p. 53)

Nightingale oversaw the development of British health policy from her bed; she became frail after the Crimean War and took to her bed for much of the remainder of her life. Policymakers visited her. She sent flowers to new graduates of nursing schools, invited them to tea, and then sent them on difficult assignments they rarely protested. She was a leader who knew how to garner the support of her followers, colleagues, and policymakers and used her skills to change her environment (Dossey, Selanders, & Beck, 2005).

## SOJOURNER TRUTH

Born into slavery, Sojourner Truth provided nursing care to Union soldiers and civilians during the Civil War. She became an ardent and eloquent advocate for abolishing slavery and a supporter of women's rights. An accomplished orator, through her words she helped to transform the racist and sexist policies that limited the health and well-being of African Americans and women. She worked to free slaves through the Underground Railroad, fought for human rights, and lobbied for federal funds to train nurses and physicians (Carnegie, 1986; Hine, 1989).

## LILLIAN WALD

Wald's political activism and vision reflected a set of values that varied from those of the dominant society at the turn of the twentieth century. She recognized the connections between health and social conditions as she established the Henry Street Settlement House on the Lower East Side of New York City. The settlement house was a "safe place" where Wald and a group of nurse and non-nurse colleagues used consensus building to establish programs for the largely poor immigrant population living—and dying—in squalid conditions. She was a driving force behind the federal government's development of the Children's Bureau, arguing that it was shameful for a nation to have policies and departments protecting animals but not children, since there were not yet child labor laws. An ardent peace activist, she was called on by the White House on frequent occasions to participate in the development of national and international policy. A suffragette, she campaigned for presidents even when she herself could not vote (Backer, 1993; Coss, 1989; Daniels, 1989).

## MARGARET SANGER

Finally, Margaret Sanger transformed a nation's attitudes and approaches to family planning, enduring jail and risking her own life to do so. Having seen firsthand the health effects of multiple unplanned pregnancies, she distributed literature on birth control at a time when such distribution was illegal. Sanger knew the power of information and civil disobedience (Chesler, 1992).

## CONTEMPORARY PIONEERS

Nurses in the twenty-first century are demonstrating similar bold activism. One example is Ruth Watson Lubic, a certified nurse midwife whose vision and politically astute activism resulted in the establishment of family-centered childbirthing centers in the United States. She led the first demonstration project of a freestanding birthing center in Manhattan at the Maternity Center Association and successfully fought for public and private payment for childbirthing services provided by nurse midwives. She was one of the founders of the National Association of Childbirthing Centers and led the movement to help women and families reclaim birthing as a "normal" process, rather than a disease as defined by the biomedical model. For this work she received a MacArthur Foundation "genius" award—the first to be bestowed on a nurse—and used the substantial cash award to support an expanded vision for birthing centers, one that acknowledged the social dimensions of childbirthing and healthy families. She founded the District of Columbia Developing Families Center in Washington, DC, a family-centered birthing, social services, and health center for people living in one of the neediest communities in our nation's capitol. Ruth Watson Lubic continues the rich legacy of nurses transforming health care and health through their visionary leadership, understanding of policy, and politically astute activism.

These nurse pioneers had vision that reflected an understanding of the connections between health and the broader social issues of their times. Their vision was grounded in values that reflected caring for the well-being of individuals, families, and communities. They were not silenced when they realized that policymakers did not share their values. Instead, they developed and used their political skills to transform neighborhoods, cities, states, nations, and the world. The work of these nurses can be used as exemplars for today's nurses who are embarking on challenging odysseys to improve the health of individuals, families, and communities. If we are successful, our actions will serve to ignite the efforts of nurses of tomorrow.

## *Key Points*

- Providing nursing care to patients is a highly political endeavor affected by social and health policies; it requires politically astute thinking and action.
- Nurses can improve the health of people by developing influence in four interconnected spheres: the workplace, government, professional organizations, and community.
- Values undergird policy and politics; therefore nurses need to be clear about the values they hold and how these values shape the policies and political strategies they will embrace, including how power is conceptualized and approached.
- There are four stages of nursing's political development: buy-in, self-interest, political sophistication, and leadership. Nursing is best served when it holds the fourth stage and assumes a leadership role in developing the health and social policies that promote the health of individuals, families, and communities.

- Today's nurses have a rich legacy of astute political activism that has been embodied by nurses including Florence Nightingale, Sojourner Truth, Lillian Wald, Margaret Sanger, and Ruth Watson Lubic.

## *Web Resources*

**American Nurses Credentialing Center Magnet Program**
*www.ana.org/ancc/magnet/index.html*
**Health Care Without Harm**
*www.noharm.org*
**National Sample Survey of Registered Nurses**
*www.bhpr.hrsa.gov/healthworkforce/reports/ rnpopulation/preliminaryfindings.htm*
**Nightingales**
*www.nightingalesnurses.org*
**Policy, Politics, & Nursing Practice**—a quarterly, peer-reviewed journal that explores the multiple relationships between nursing and health policy
*http://ppn.sagepub.com*
**Robert Wood Johnson Foundation**
*www.rwjf.org*
**Transforming Care at the Bedside, Institute for Healthcare Improvement**
*www.ihi.org/IHI/Topics/MedicalSurgicalCare/ TransformingCare*

### REFERENCES

American Association of Colleges of Nursing (AACN). (2004). Preparing graduates for practice as a clinical nurse leader: Draft curriculum framework. Retrieved December 19, 2005, from *www.aacn.nche.edu/cnl/pdf/DraftCurriculumFramework 12-04.pdf*.

American Association of Colleges of Nursing [AACN]. (2005). DNP essentials. Retrieved December 19, 2005, from *www. aacn.nche.edu/DNP/pdf/Essentials8-18.pdf*.

Annas, G. J. (1997). Tobacco litigation as cancer prevention: Dealing with the devil. *New England Journal of Medicine, 336*(4), 304-308.

Ayres, B. D. (1997, April 14). Women in Washington statehouse lead U.S. tide. *New York Times*, A1.

Backer, B. A. (1993). Lillian Wald: Connecting caring with activism. *Nursing and Health Care, 114*(3), 122-129.

Benner, P., & Wrubel, J. (1989). *The primacy of caring: Stress and coping in health and illness.* Menlo Park, CA: Addison-Wesley.

Brenner, E. (1997, January 19). The power women share as lobbyists. *New York Times*, 13:1.

Caiazza, A. (2002). *Does women's representation in elected office lead to women-friendly policy?* (Research-in-Brief #1910). Washington, DC: Institute for Women's Policy Research.

Caiazza, A. (2005). *The ties that bind: Women's public vision for politics, religion, and civil society.* Washington, DC: Institute for Women's Policy Research.

Carnegie, E. M. (1986). *The path we tread: Blacks in nursing worldwide, 1854-1994.* (3rd ed.). Boston: Jones and Bartlett.

Chesler, E. (1992). *Woman of valor: Margaret Sanger and the birth control movement in America.* New York: Simon & Schuster.

Cohen, S. S., Mason, J. M., Kovner, C., Leavitt, J. K., Pulcini, J., & Sochalski, J. (1996). Stages of nursing's political development: Where we've been and where we ought to go. *Nursing Outlook, 44*(6), 259-266.

Coss, C. (Ed.). (1989). *Lillian Wald: Progressive activist.* New York: The Feminist Press.

Cuevas, K., Silver, D., Brooten, D., Youngblut, J., & Bobo, C. (2005). The cost of prematurity. *American Journal of Nursing, 105*(7), 56-64.

Daniels, D. G. (1989). *Always a sister: The feminism of Lillian Wald.* New York: The Feminist Press.

Dodson, D. L. O. (1997). Women voters and the gender gap. In W. Crotty & J. Mileur (Eds.), *America's choice: The election of 1996.* New York: McGraw-Hill.

Dossey, B., Selanders, L., & Beck, D. (2005). *Florence Nightingale today: Healing, leadership, global action.* Washington, DC: American Nurses Publishing.

Fischetti, M. (2001). Drowning New Orleans. *Scientific American,* October. Retrieved December 20, 2005, from *www.sciam.com.*

Gebbie, K. M., Wakefield, M., & Kerfoot, K. (2000). Nursing and health policy. *Journal of Nursing Scholarship, 32*(3), 307-315.

Gilligan, C. (1982). *In a different voice: Psychological theory and women's development.* Boston: Harvard University Press.

Hine, D. C. (1989). *Black women in white.* Indianapolis: Indiana University Press.

Huxley, E. (1975). *Florence Nightingale.* New York: Putnam's Sons.

Institute of Medicine. (1988). *The future of public health.* Washington, DC: National Academy Press.

Institute of Medicine. (1999). *To err is human: Building a safer health system.* Washington, DC: National Academy Press.

International Council of Nurses. (2000). Position statement: Participation of nurses in health services decision making and policy development. Retrieved December 21, 2005 from *www.icn.ch/ pspolicydev00.htm.*

International Council of Nurses. (2001). *Guidelines on shaping effective health policy.* Geneva, Switzerland: International Council of Nurses.

Isadore, C. (2005). Doctor's orders: GM, UAW cut deal. *CNN Money.* Retrieved December 20, 2005, from *http://money.cnn.com/2005/10/17/news/fortune500/gm_wagoner.*

Izzo, C. V., Eckenrode J., Smith E. G., Henderson, C. R. Jr., Cole, R., Kitzman, H., & Olds, D. L. (2005). Reducing the impact of uncontrollable stressful life events through a program of nurse home visitation for new parents. *Prevention Science.* Retrieved December 20, 2005, from *www.springerlink.com/media/g275munuqjcjvnaged4t/contributions/t/7/0/v/t70v628636071708.pdf.*

Kalisch, B. J., & Kalisch, P. A. (1982). *Politics of nursing.* Philadelphia: Lippincott.

Kitzman, H., et al. (2000). Enduring effects of nurse home visitation on maternal life course: A 3-year follow-up of a randomized

trial. *Journal of the American Medical Association, 283*(15), 1983-1989.

Kurtz, P. (2000). *Humanist manifesto: A call for new planetary humanism.* New York: Prometheus.

Leape, L., & Berwick, D. (2005). Five years after *To Err Is Human:* What have we learned? *Journal of the American Medical Association, 293*(19), 2384-2390.

MacPherson, K. (1987). Health care policy, values and nursing. *Advances in Nursing Science, 9,* 1-11.

Mason, D. J., Backer, C., & Georges, C. A. (1991). Toward a feminist model for the political empowerment of nurses. *Image: Journal of Nursing Scholarship, 23*(2), 72-77.

McDaniel, R. R., Jordan M. E., & Fleeman, B. F. (2003). Surprise, Surprise, Surprise! A complexity science view of the unexpected. *Health Care Management Review, 28*(3), 266-278.

McDonough, J. (2001). Using and misusing anecdote in policy making. *Health Affairs, 20*(1), 208-212.

Miller, J. B. (1976). *Toward a new psychology for women.* Boston: Beacon.

*Nursing's agenda for health care reform.* (1992). Washington, DC: American Nurses Publishing.

Olds, D., Eckenrode, J., Henderson, C. R. Jr., Kitzman, H., Powers, J., Cole, R., Sidora, K., Morris, P., Pettitt, L. M., & Luckey, D. (1997). Long-term effects of home visitation on maternal life course and child abuse and neglect: Fifteen-year follow-up of a randomized trial. *Journal of the American Medical Association, 278*(8), 637-643.

Pinch, W. J. (1996). Is caring a moral trap? *Nursing Outlook, 44*(22), 84-88.

Plsek P. E., & Greenhalgh, T. (2001). Complexity science: The challenge of complexity in health care. *British Medical Journal, 323*(7313), 625-628.

Reverby, S. (1987). *Ordered to care: The dilemma of American nursing.* New York: Cambridge University Press.

Rogers, A., Hwang, W., Scott, L., Aiken, L., & Dinges, D. (2004). The working hours of nurses and patient safety. *Health Affairs, 23*(4), 202-212.

Rosener, J. B. (1990, November-December). The ways women lead. *Harvard Business Review, 68*(6), 119-134.

Rothberg, M. B., Abraham, I., Lindenauer, P. K., & Rose, D. N. (2005). Improving nurse-to-patient staffing ratios as a cost-effective safety intervention. *Medical Care, 43*(8), 785-791.

Schorr, L. (1989). *Within our reach: Breaking the cycle of disadvantage.* Garden City, NY: Doubleday.

Smith, G. (1997, June 18). *Shaping the future health system through community-based approaches* (keynote address). Vancouver, British Columbia, Canada: International Council of Nurses' Congress.

Steele, B. (2004). From butterfly wings to single e-mail, if one action can cause a torrent, Cornell researchers find the best place to start. *Cornell News.* Retrieved December 20, 2005, from *www.news.cornell.edu/releases/Feb04/AAAS.Kleinberg.ws.html.*

Stimpson, M., & Hanley, B. (1991). Nurse policy analysts. *Nursing and Health Care, 12*(1), 10-15.

Titmus, R. M. (1974). *Social policy: An introduction.* New York: Pantheon.

U.S. Health Resources and Services Administration. (2005). National Sample Survey of Registered Nurses. Retrieved December 20, 2005, from *http://bhpr.hrsa.gov/healthworkforce/reports/rnpopulation/preliminaryfindings.htm.*

## The Influence of Values on a Policy Agenda: The Quaker Perspective

*"Let your life speak."*

OLD QUAKER SAYING

War Is Not The Answer proclaims a bold banner on the side of a building that faces the Senate Hart office building in Washington, DC. That building houses the Friends Committee on National Legislation (FCNL), the organization that allows my Quaker beliefs and my public health nursing values to merge in the context of political advocacy. For the past 17 years I have served on FCNL's General Committee, including 6 years on the Policy Committee and 4 leadership years as clerk or assistant clerk (the Quaker term for *chair*) of the Executive and General Committee. Policy issues and political players changed over the years, but the constant was my passionate advocacy for peaceful alternatives to violence and war, as well as just ways to meet human needs at home and abroad (Figure 1-3).

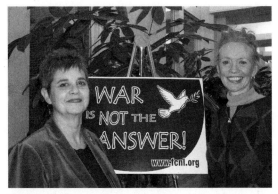

**Figure 1-3** Joanne Warner (right) at the 2005 annual meeting of Friends Committee on National Legislation (FCNL) with Kathy Guthrie, FCNL's Legislative Secretary.

If I had chosen traditional expressions of community service that my colleagues understood as "health related," I would have required less explaining over the years. If I had provided leadership in a nursing or health organization, such as ANA or APHA, my faculty colleagues would have readily understood. As it was, I have frequently had to clarify and defend my faith-based work, providing descriptions like those that follow.

The FCNL is described as a Quaker lobby in the public interest. "Friends" is short for the Religious Society of Friends, also called *Quakers*. The Committee is a group of about 250 individuals appointed by 26 Friends organizations across the United States. National legislation implies a focus on issues affecting the nation as a whole (at home and abroad) that can be addressed through policy, laws, executive action, and so on. FCNL is the Quaker witness on Capitol Hill. It is powered by a small DC staff of lobbyists, interns, and support staff, plus a rich grassroots network of activists across the nation. It was formed in 1943 partially as a response and in opposition to World War II.

My early years with FCNL overlapped with my doctoral study in health policy, and I appreciated the fit between the values. Although Quaker beliefs and public health nursing values may have had different beginnings, they share an emphasis on social justice, activism, and peace. The Quaker emphasis on equality relates to public health's egalitarian tradition. Quakers emphasize community and integrity, as does public health. As a Quaker I strive to see "that of God" in all persons and live as though all life is sacramental; those beliefs guide my nursing care and policy advocacy. Over the years I wove a tapestry of service that was equally faith based and professionally motivated.

FCNL's vision statement presents a broad and positive perspective, envisioning the world that could be.

---

### Friends Committee on National Legislation: Vision Statement

"We seek a world free of war and the threat of war; we seek a society with equity and justice for all; we seek a community where every person's potential may be fulfilled; we seek an earth restored."

---

These four areas provide the organizing structure for FCNL's Statement of Legislative Policy, the 20+-page document that gives direction to our lobbying effort and explicates the spiritual values behind our work.

FCNL's legislative priorities have been passionate concerns for me personally and professionally. We have sought to control arms and promote disarmament; we've worked to shift budget priorities away from military spending and toward human needs and a healthy environment at home and abroad; we've addressed economic, social, and racial disparity through a variety of legislative avenues. These efforts and many more promote community health and respect the inherent worth of each individual. They aim at building a more profound and lasting homeland security beyond the brute force of bombs and missiles.

One pervasive focus throughout FCNL's history has been promoting a culture of peace and nonviolent conflict resolution. The events of September 11, 2001, our nation's response in Afghanistan, and the threat of expanded war have torn at my pacifist heart and renewed my belief that war is not the answer. FCNL reframed the legislative priorities that had been adopted for the 107th Congress because of the urgency of war. Our simple yet comprehensive focus became the "peaceful prevention of deadly conflict." There seemed a window of opportunity to educate citizens and decision-makers about alternatives. "If not war, then what?" people asked, and FCNL responded with a tool kit of activities that could

support global stability and peaceful resolution of conflict. We worked to create a space for public debate that allowed respectful dissent from the enthusiasm for war without the accusation of anti-patriotism.

As a public health nurse, I believe war is one of the most counterproductive acts in relation to health, community building, and realization of human potential. Levy and Sidel (1997) present the most comprehensive analysis of the relationship of war and public health, noting that the human and environmental consequences of war are staggering (see *Conflict and War: Impact on the Health of Societies* following Chapter 34). Efforts toward arms control, education for peace, prevention of nuclear war, and conflict resolution are all valid nursing activities for a public health nurse with a global perspective.

When I began service on the Policy Committee in 1992, I began what would be 12 years as a frequent DC flyer—approximately five or six trips per year. The Policy Committee gives guidance to lobbyists in interpreting legislative policy in light of current issues, reviews and revises legislative policy, and facilitates the process of determining legislative priorities for each 2-year cycle of Congress. The priority-setting process made use of my qualitative research background, again incorporating my nursing skills. In the process of seeking input from Friends across the nation and determining the most pressing concerns, letters were mailed to all Friends churches (sometimes called *meetings*) nationally, inviting groups or individuals to respond to the central questions. Where should FCNL focus our attention? Where could we make a difference? How should FCNL speak for you in Washington? Stacks of responses would provide the prevailing wisdom from across the country. The Policy Committee would weigh this feedback in the context of anticipated legislation, the coalitions and relationships established by FCNL staff that could result in legislative outcomes, and the discernment of the Spirit's guiding. During the annual meeting business sessions the General Committee would consider, revise, and ultimately approve the priorities within the Quaker consensus process, nothing short of a miracle with almost 250 participants.

Attempted health care reform occurred on the national level during my 6 years on the Policy

Committee. I participated in a small working group to create our talking points and lobbying strategies and lobbied on behalf of accessible, available, and locally accountable services that would result in improved public health. Given the plethora of bills and ideas on health reform, I embraced our lobbying strategy as profoundly educational. When I made visits to congressional offices, I presented the key criteria that we wanted included in the negotiation and amending of legislative proposals. Points emphasized by FCNL corresponded to the platforms of ANA, APHA, and other health and nursing organizations.

My FCNL experiences have shaped me into the policy advocate I am today and have provided many examples and stories as I've taught nursing students the art and science of political activism. Some of the lessons I've learned are as follows:

- My involvement and leadership with a value-based national advocacy group is admittedly not the choice to make if you seek to be a rising star in academe. Safer choices would be traditional roles within the academy, a health organization, or a value-neutral agency. I would choose FCNL again today, however, because the rich opportunities to act and speak from explicit values and to interact in interdisciplinary arenas from my nursing perspective outweigh the safety of predictable choices. My FCNL work provided an arena for spiritual and professional growth, as well as a place to be authentically "me." Because politics is inherently a value-laden process, deep engagement for me meant daring to go public with my personal and professional values.

- The "cost" of involvement in value-based advocacy is a public label. This label will open some doors and close others. When I managed partisan political campaigns in my hometown, I lost the possibility of an identity as a neutral policy analyst whose interests were strictly academic. Access to Republican conversations ceased, but opportunities for Democratic conversations emerged. Another example comes from my Quaker policy work. In a recent interview for a prestigious health policy fellowship, my FCNL work was mentioned and the interviewee asked if

I had considered whether I would appear "too moral" for an appointment on Capitol Hill. Too moral? As I searched for an answer, I recognized the irony of this question, coming less than 3 months after the 2004 presidential election was considered won and lost based on values. I was not chosen for the fellowship; I'm left to speculate on whether the interviewer disagreed with my values or preferred a value-neutral scholar, or whether some other factors determined the final selection. The "cost" of making values explicit will not always be known.

- As an educator, I prod students toward the clarification of their personal values while they are in the process of socialization into professional values. Into the personal and professional equation I add "the political" and suggest that the integration of all into a cohesive and coherent tapestry produces a synergistic and powerful framework for action. This is the ideal within my life and an admitted bias and preference for my students. Faculty can serve as models of this integration and action—something I do with the explicit caveat and caution that I am not the "right" example with the "correct" values. When I reveal my story to students, the point is clarity, integration, and action, not the particular values that drive my life and my work.

- When one chooses a nontraditional role, one must expect that peers and administrators will require explanations. I learned to be more skilled in "connecting the dots" within professional frameworks so nurses, students, and other professionals could see the linkages. The classic article by Cohen and colleagues (1996) that describes nursing's political development (see Chapter 1) helped me defend a leadership role outside of nursing in a context where broad policy issues affecting health were shaped. I was personally encouraged by their recognition that this level of involvement benefited the public's health and made nursing visible. I also valued and used the conceptual model by Fawcett and Russell (2001) that described five levels of health policy work. My FCNL work belongs to level 5, where humankind is the unit of analysis, the global community is the environment, health is understood as global, and the nursing and health policy outcome is social justice. These models helped my colleagues link FCNL and nursing work.

Policymaking is value laden; values cannot be explicated from policies or the process. Nursing is also value driven, and we are well positioned to be effective players in this complex and interesting work.

## Lessons Learned

- Nurses can effectively lead value-driven organizations advocating for broad-based policy affecting the health of society.
- Powerful synergy can come from the integration of personal, professional, and political values.
- There are costs and benefits to value-laden advocacy work for nurses.

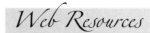

## Web Resources

**Friends Committee on National Legislation**
*www.fcnl.org*
**Religious Society of Friends**
*www.quaker.org*
**Quaker Information Center**
*www.quakerinfo.org*

### REFERENCES

Cohen, S. S., Mason, J. M., Kovner, C., Leavitt, J. K., Pulcini, J., & Sochalski, J. (1996). Stages of nursing's political development: Where we've been and where we ought to go. *Nursing Outlook, 44*(6), 259-266.

Fawcett, J., & Russell, G. (2001). A conceptual model of nursing and health policy. *Policy, Politics, & Nursing Practice, 2*(2), 108-115.

Levy, B. S., & Sidel, V. W. (1997). *War and public health.* New York: Oxford University and the American Public Health Association (APHA).

# chapter 2

# A Historical Perspective on Policy, Politics, and Nursing

Sandra B. Lewenson

*"… what's past is prologue …"*

WILLIAM SHAKESPEARE

The history of the modern nursing movement, which began in 1873, tells the story of a pioneering group of women who responded to the changing role of women in society. They advocated a new profession for women and better health care for the public. In forging the nursing profession in this modern period, nurses had to enter the political arena to gain legitimate authority over their education and practice. Over time, however, the history has blurred and often obscured from view the rich tapestry of nursing's political past. Nursing's political role and historical activism have been buried in the popular image of the nurse. When its political past is remembered at all, nursing has suffered accusations of conservatism and noninvolvement in the political arena and has been omitted from most women's histories. This can be explained in part by the fact that women are perceived by society to have historically played a small role in the political arena. Nursing, long considered "women's work," shares with the overall women's movement the many negative, devalued perceptions of the worth of its role (Reverby, 1987; Vance, Talbott, McBride, & Mason, 1985). As a result of such a perception, nursing suffers from "nursism," which has been defined as "a form of sexism that specifically maligns the caring role in society" (Lewenson, 1996, p. 226).

Public perception of nursing often depicts nurses as handmaidens to physicians and as subservient members of the health care team. The notion that "nurses are born, not made" persists in the twenty-first century and provides the rationale for hiring less-educated workers to perform professional nursing roles. To cut costs, hospitals downsize by firing nurses with experience and advanced degrees and cross-train uneducated health care workers to do jobs once done by registered nurses. This acceptance of less-qualified nurses reflects the decreased value society continues to place on professional nursing care. Buresh and Gordon (2000) write about the invisibility of nurses' contribution to health care and the lack of recognition for their work. This invisibility and the assumption that women's work is somehow free and expected perpetuate the negative aspects of nursism.

The historical research of Rogge (1987) and others has begun to provide the needed evidence that shows how nursing's use of political power is neither new nor confined to the twentieth and twenty-first centuries. Pioneers in nursing honed their political expertise when they persuaded various members of the status quo (e.g., hospital administrators, physicians, members of community boards of health, state legislators, politicians) to open nurse-training schools, organize professional associations, and participate in social issues such as woman suffrage, public health, birth control, and integration. The history of the four national professional nursing groups, beginning in the United States in 1893, documents nursing's political activism. The creation of the American Society of Superintendents of Training Schools for Nurses in 1893 (forerunner of the National League for Nursing [NLN]), the Nurses' Associated Alumnae of the United States and Canada in 1896 (forerunner of the American Nurses Association [ANA]), the National Association of Colored Graduate Nurses (NACGN) in 1908, and the National Organization of Public Health Nursing (NOPHN) in 1912 provided a forum for nurses to be politically active. The history of these organizations illustrates nursing's efforts to control its own education and practice and its strong interest in the Woman Movement.*

These four nursing organizations embody nursing's passage through the stages of political development as defined by Cohen and co-workers (1996). In the early years of each organization, nursing educators and practitioners joined forces to gain control and focus on professional development. Both the self-absorption with professional development and the beginning interest in the larger issues fit the "buy in" stage described by Cohen and colleagues (1996). Nursing activists educated other nurses on the need for woman suffrage for personal and professional reasons (e.g., to obtain nurse registration laws). Once established as professional groups, these organizations formed strong coalitions with other nursing organizations (both in the United States and abroad) to make their voices heard on social issues such as woman suffrage, public health, and women's rights. In this second stage, according to Cohen and colleagues (1996, p. 261), nursing moves toward political activism and "develops its own sense of uniqueness." As these organizations matured, they showed interest in issues aside from those that solely affected the profession.

To address the misconceptions about nursing's active political past, this chapter provides examples where nurses have been politically active and have made a significant difference in health care. Examples

include the influence of Florence Nightingale, the opening of nurse training schools, the founding of professional nursing organizations, the support of woman suffrage, the work of Lillian Wald in public health and Margaret Sanger in birth control, and the efforts of the NACGN, led by Mabel Staupers, to integrate African-American nurses into the U.S. armed forces. Because political activism in nursing parallels similar efforts of other women's groups in the same period, this overview examines the nursing profession's close ties with the Woman Movement of the nineteenth and early twentieth centuries, as well as its relationship with the more-recent women's movement of the mid-twentieth century.

## BEGINNING WITH THE WOMAN MOVEMENT

The profession of nursing rose out of the political efforts of women during what is known as the *Woman Movement* of the middle nineteenth and early twentieth centuries (1848 to 1920). During this period, women sought political control of their personal lives. They looked to change the laws that regulated their families, their education, and their political freedom. Because of these efforts, women's work came under scrutiny both by those who wanted to preserve the status quo and by those who wanted reform.

During the middle of the nineteenth century, men represented the family to the outside world, and women remained in the home, caring for the family. For some women the status quo sufficed, but for many the subordinate role they were expected to play did not, especially for women who did not marry and who did not accept the limitations of women's roles. By the 1830s, schools for women had opened, and women began to challenge their confined, set role in society. Society conceived women as the "natural born" caretakers for their families, responsible for the moral upbringing of its members. Some women, however, wanted to branch out of their allotted "separate sphere" and into the more "active sphere" of the world outside the home. For many women (especially middle-class women), this meant obtaining an education, finding a career, and financially supporting themselves. During the nineteenth century these women sought opportunity for

---

*Woman Movement* is the term used for the movement in the late nineteenth and early twentieth centuries to change society's ideas about women. *Women's movement* is the term that describes women's efforts of the 1960s and 1970s.

meaningful work, questioned the idea of marriage, and organized to bring about change in the social order (Cott, 1977; Daniels, 1987; Lerner, 1977).

## POLITICAL AWAKENING AND THE MODERN NURSING MOVEMENT

The modern nursing movement began when Florence Nightingale opened the nurse-training program at St. Thomas Hospital in England in 1860. This landmark event signaled to the world that nurses required schooling for the work they did. It also provided one of the first opportunities for women to work outside the home and be self-supportive. In turn, the rise of modern nursing served as the catalyst for political activities of nurses.

Nursing was one of the first professions that women sought to control and organize. It is taken for granted that, because women provided care to their own families, they would automatically control the profession. However, historically this was not the case; nursing's roots in the church and military fostered patriarchal control. Nurses had to maneuver politically to control their professional education, work, and lives. Nightingale's writing supports a feminist stance on who should control the education and work of nurses (Lewenson, 1996). Nightingale believed that nursing should be controlled by nurses. A 1908 editorial comment published in the *American Journal of Nursing (AJN)* acknowledged that her "brilliant essence lay in her taking from men's hands a power which did not logically or rightly belong to them, but which they had usurped, and seizing it firmly in her own, from whence she passed it on to her pupils and disciples" (Progress and reaction, 1908, pp. 333-334). Like women's education, education for nurses was considered unnecessary. The general attitude held that women were natural-born nurses and therefore did not require an education. Yet, after the extraordinary success of Nightingale's ideas about sanitation and nurses' education, an "educated" nurse was sought to reform the deplorable conditions found in hospitals throughout the United States.

In an 1872 letter, Nightingale sent her ideas about separating nursing and medicine to the founders of the nurse-training school at Bellevue Hospital in New York City. Nightingale advised that "discipline and internal management" of nurses should be "entirely under a woman, a *trained* superintendent, whose whole business is to see that the nursing duties are performed according to this standard" (Florence Nightingale's letter of advice to Bellevue, 1911, p. 362). Bellevue and many other schools used Nightingale's concept as a model.

Nightingale, the reformer, emerges as a complex individual who often achieved her goals "by behind-the-scenes management of the committees and doctors" (Vicinus & Nergaard, 1989, p. 159). It was her letter-writing to influential people that helped Nightingale revolutionize health care and nursing education. Moreover, it was the acceptance, around the world, of her ideas about sanitation, education, and separation of nursing and medicine that contributed to her ability to facilitate change.

## PROFESSIONAL EDUCATION AND THE OPENING OF NURSE-TRAINING SCHOOLS

Political activism of the early nursing pioneers took the form of creating the models for professional education. The year 1873 heralded the opening of Nightingale-influenced nurse-training schools and the beginning of the modern nursing movement in the United States. The first three schools credited with this distinction were at Bellevue Hospital in New York City; New Haven Hospital in New Haven, Connecticut; and Massachusetts General Hospital in Boston. Early nursing leaders implemented many of Nightingale's ideas about nursing. They skillfully demonstrated to hospital administrators that using nursing students improved sanitary conditions on wards and led to better patient outcomes. This success created a safer environment for the newly formed medical profession, consequently creating great financial incentives for hospitals to open such schools (Dock & Stewart, 1931). Between 1873 and 1893, nurse-training schools proliferated in the United States, and by 1910 the number of schools had risen to more than 1129 (Burgess, 1928).

The schools opened between 1873 and 1893, but they were not regulated by any professional group.

Hospital administrators wanted these schools because it was cheaper to use student labor than to employ the graduates. Exploitation of students took various forms. Education was secondary to work expected of the students. Often the students' education was limited by the size of the hospital. Many hospitals had too few beds to provide appropriate and sufficient learning opportunities.

Once a nurse's training was over, the school provided no support. Graduate nurses found themselves working in the only jobs they could find, such as private duty nursing or public health nursing. Physicians or pharmacists, as opposed to nurses, often controlled the private duty nursing directories, which distributed private duty work. This meant that the fee schedule rested outside the nurses' control, which often led to further exploitation of an already exploited group. The misuse of both the students and the graduate nurses contributed greatly to the strong political stance that early nursing leaders took when they formed professional nursing organizations.

## POLITICAL ACTION AND THE RISE OF PROFESSIONAL ORGANIZATIONS

Professional nursing organizations began to form between 1893 and 1912. Their interest first revolved around the issues confronting the profession but later expanded to include social and political reforms affecting society. As each organization formed and matured, political power bases grew and expanded. They moved away from their initial purpose of "the protection and education of one class of women workers" (Palmer, 1909, p. 956) toward interest in more-global concerns affecting the health care of the public.

### NATIONAL LEAGUE FOR NURSING

The first national nursing organization to form was the American Society of Superintendents for Training Schools, founded in 1893 and renamed the National League of Nursing Education in 1912 and the NLN in 1952. This organization originated at the nurses' congress that convened at the World's Columbian Exposition in Chicago in 1893. Superintendents, chief administrators, and hospital nursing staff sought uniformity in nursing curricula and standards of nursing practice. Alone in their work, they felt isolated and powerless to go before the entrenched powers, such as the hospital boards and medical groups, that sought to control the developing profession. By joining together as other women's groups of the day had, superintendents created an opportunity to work toward change. Leaders such as Isabel Hampton Robb, Lavinia Dock, and Sophia Palmer spoke out in favor of collective action. Their early speeches at the first few professional meetings reflected the political tone and progressive nature of the newly founded organization (Birnbach & Lewenson, 1993).

### AMERICAN NURSES ASSOCIATION

Mindful of the needs of the majority of "trained" or "graduate" nurses, superintendents in the newly formed society urged training schools to form alumnae associations that would provide the basic structure for a second national nursing organization. In doing so, the superintendents spearheaded the founding of the Nurses' Associated Alumnae of the United States and Canada in 1896 (renamed the ANA in 1911). Sophia Palmer, first editor-in-chief of the *American Journal of Nursing,* called for a grass-roots movement that would unite alumnae associations around the country for the purpose of political action and social reform (Figure 2-1). She urged small and large schools to form alumnae associations that would be able to come together in state associations and form a vital national professional organization. The state societies would form "for the definite and separate purpose of promoting legislation for state registration of nurses" (Palmer, 1909, p. 956). She recognized the inherent power that nurses would wield, given organization. Palmer (1897) said, "Organization is the power of the age. Without it nothing great is accomplished. All questions having ultimate advancement of the profession are dependent upon united action for success" (p. 55). It was clear to the early pioneer leaders that organizing was the only way to remove the obstacles that nursing experienced on its way to becoming a recognized profession.

The state alumnae associations organized around the highly political issue of state registration. This

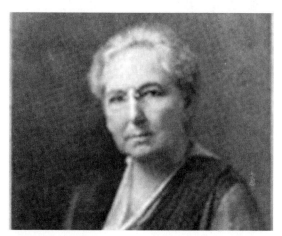

**Figure 2-1** Sophia Palmer was the founding editor of the *American Journal of Nursing* and used the journal to stimulate discussion among nurses about the important policy and political issues of the day, such as nurse registration. She challenged nurses' alumnae associations to use their collective power to influence legislation of importance to the profession and to public health.

issue galvanized the nursing membership and forced nurses to develop their political skills. Until 1903 anyone could call herself a nurse. It was not until 1903 that the first state nurse registration acts (in North Carolina, New York, New Jersey, and Virginia) were passed and the title *nurse* was protected by law. Although the early registration acts varied in their protection of the public from inadequate nursing education, they signified the political efforts of nurses and organized nursing. Nursing leaders in each of these states sought support for this legislation from legislators, politicians, other professionals, and the public through letter-writing campaigns, personal visits to the legislatures, use of the professional journals, and support of the public press (Birnbach, 1985).

Twenty-three nurse alumnae associations joined forces to form the Nurses' Associated Alumnae and met in New York in April 1898. At their first meeting, they learned firsthand how important it was for them to use their collective strength for political action. Just before the meeting, the United States entered the Spanish-American War. Isabel Hampton Robb, president of the new organization, led the group's

effort to serve as gatekeeper for the nurses who served during the war. After a long battle on the home front against Anita Newcomb McGee, a physician and Washington socialite, on who should screen the applicants, organized nursing failed to reach its goal. McGee, as history shows, held on to this pivotal role. Robb believed that this outcome was due to the lack of professional organization. The ANA had organized too late to win this issue, but its leaders learned from this experience (Armeny, 1983; Robb, 1900). Robb and other nursing leaders recognized their potential political power as an organization and continued to lobby successfully in the years to come.

## NATIONAL ASSOCIATION OF COLORED GRADUATE NURSES

Although the first two national organizations, the NLN and the ANA, addressed the needs of nurses, they primarily focused on issues within the mainstream culture. Discriminatory practices in parts of the United States barred many African-American nurses from membership in their state associations. This practice in turn prevented them from belonging to the ANA. Moreover, segregation and discriminatory practices throughout the country banned African-American nurses from attending most nurse-training schools and, in some states, prohibited them from taking state nurse registration examinations. In keeping with other women's organizations and the need for political activism, African-American nurses organized the NACGN in 1908. It was an organization created to overcome racial hostility and address professional issues. Along with issues of blatant racial discrimination, the NACGN focused on education, standards of practice, and the passage of state nurse registration acts (Figure 2-2) (Hine, 1989; Hine, 1990; Johns, 1925; Staupers, 1937).

To determine the need for such an organization, Martha Franklin, nursing leader and founder of the NACGN, had undertaken a study on African-American nurses in 1906 and 1907. Franklin sent more than 1500 surveys to African-American graduates of nurse-training schools, most of which had opened in historically African-American hospital settings (Thoms, 1929). From the survey results, Franklin learned that African-American nurses

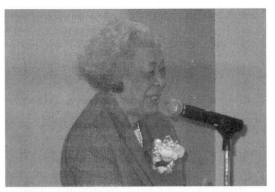

**Figure 2-2** While President of the Florida Association of Colored Graduate Nurses, Dr. Mary Elizabeth Carnegie, noted nurse educator, historian, and civil rights activist, actively sought the integration of African-American nurses in the American Nurses Association and the dissolution of the National Association of Colored Graduate Nurses in 1951. The National Black Nurses Association was founded after this integration was accomplished and has provided African-American Nurses with a venue for deeper explorations and actions regarding the issues confronting nurses of color and their communities.

needed an organization to address issues pertaining to their particular needs. Here, too, Franklin recognized that only in the collective would they gain enough power to change discriminatory practices and affect conditions in nursing and in health care (Lewenson, 1996).

At the early meetings, the NACGN members sought to raise professional standards, provide a collegial atmosphere for the graduate nurse, discuss community health nursing, and address issues of racial discrimination. Members of the NACGN constantly faced the double-edged sword of sexism and racism, which led to their political activism. A primary concern for the NACGN was the nurse registration acts that the profession as a whole sought. Not only did the organization support the passage of such acts, but its members also fought to ensure that nurses of color could sit for the state examination and be given the same examination as their white counterparts.

The collective action of the NACGN around the issue of racial discrimination toward African-American nurses in the military during World War II

serves as another example of political activism in nursing. Not until after the armistice in World War I were African-American nurses accepted into the Army Nurse Corps. Furthermore, it wasn't until after a great political campaign waged by the NACGN during World War II that they were integrated into the armed services, albeit in limited numbers. Mabel Staupers, considered one of the people instrumental in the integration of African-American nurses into the military, prepared the NACGN to engage in the political effort needed to effect change (Hine, 1993). Staupers not only mobilized the NACGN but also sought the "allegiance of sympathetic white nurses within the profession" (Hine, 1989, p. 170). The NACGN used letter-writing campaigns, alliances with the other professional nursing organizations, membership in the newly established National Nursing Council for War Service, meetings with politically significant people, and collective action to change the course of events forever.

## NATIONAL ORGANIZATION FOR PUBLIC HEALTH NURSING

At the beginning of the twentieth century the need for public health nurses increased as the United States experienced the outcomes of urbanization, industrialization, and immigration. Cities filled with people who wanted to find jobs in these growing industrialized centers. This change in demographics contributed to severely overcrowded housing, unsafe work conditions, inadequate sanitation, epidemics, and poor access to health care, causing progressive reformers to respond. The public health movement used trained nurses in public health departments and visiting nurse service agencies to bring their ideas about sanitation, immunization, and health care to the public. Between 1895 and 1905, 171 visiting nurse associations opened in more than 110 cities and towns. In 1902, there were only 200 public health nurses; by 1912, there were more than 3000 (Fitzpatrick, 1975; Gardner, 1933). With this steady proliferation of visiting nurse associations came unscrupulous home health care agencies that offered substandard visiting nurse services. To overcome poor and inferior nursing practices, the ANA and the NLN exerted their political expertise and in 1912 formed the NOPHN. This organization's members joined with other civic-minded citizens to improve the health of the American public.

To create the NOPHN, in 1911 nursing leaders of the ANA and the NLN developed a plan to organize public health nurses. Letters sent to organizations that employed public health nurses requested that they send a representative to the annual nursing convention of the ANA and the NLN who could vote on the issue of starting a new organization. Most of the agencies responded favorably, and 1 year later, in 1912, the NOPHN organized. The NOPHN objectives were to "stimulate responsibility for the health of the community by the establishment and the extension of public health nursing" and "to develop standards and techniques in public health nursing service" (Gardner, 1933, p. 27). From the outset, the NOPHN recognized the political expediency of forming coalitions with other health professionals and lay people and included these other individuals as members. This provided strong affiliations with other groups and a broader political base from which to advocate change.

## ORGANIZED NURSING AND WOMAN SUFFRAGE

While the four nursing organizations were forming, the campaign for suffrage was under way. Suffrage meant personal and political freedom and the means to control the laws that governed women. For nurses, suffrage meant gaining a political voice in the laws that regulated practice, education, and health. Professional nursing organizations provided the medium for nurses to share common experiences and thus find a collective voice. Once these organizations established themselves as viable associations, nurses expanded their horizons to include broader women's issues, including suffrage, in their political agenda (Lewenson, 1996). This period of political activism in nursing fits the description by Cohen and colleagues (1996) of the early stages of political development. Nursing, through the four organizations, had developed its identity, formed coalitions, built on its political base, and used the language needed for changing legislation. By advocating for patient rights, nurses began to shape policy. As nursing struggled to come to consensus over the issue

of woman suffrage, they published a journal, formed coalitions among themselves and with non-nursing groups, and discussed the political ramifications of both sides of the suffrage question.

In 1900 the ANA and NLN used an important political strategy when they founded the publication *AJN* for the purpose of communicating and sharing ideas. So imperative was the need to find a public forum in which to exchange their views that members funded the journal. The nursing membership raised money to start the journal by buying shares in the journal company. They invested their money, time, and ideas in the professional journal and, in the process, formed a strong coalition from which to carry on their political activities.

The *AJN* provided a public forum for nurses to present ideas about nursing care interventions, public health, social issues, and other professional issues. Within the pages of the *AJN*, nurses had the opportunity to express their views on nursing's support of woman suffrage. Although many nurses wanted to maintain the status quo and sought to avoid confrontational political battles, a sufficient number of nurses ardently believed that the survival of the profession rested on gaining suffrage.

Organized nursing's efforts to support the political agenda of the international nursing community led to the formation of the American Federation of Nurses (AFN) between 1901 and 1912. This newly created federation, a coalition forged between the ANA and the NLN, enabled organized nurses in the United States to join the National Council of Women and thus become members of the International Council of Women and later the International Council of Nurses (ICN) (Lewenson, 1994). It is significant to note that by 1901, nursing in the United States was ready to form strong coalitions with other nursing groups both domestically and abroad. Nurse organizations gained a political voice in international health issues affecting women and were specifically interested in supporting suffrage (Figure 2-3).

Interest in suffrage and connections with women's groups first appeared in *AJN* in 1906. *AJN* published letters from the National American Woman Suffrage Association asking nurses to support the Nineteenth Amendment, giving women the right to vote (Gordon, Myers, & Kelley, 1906). Nursing's staunchest

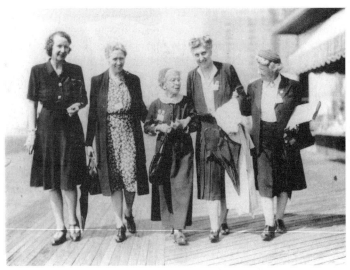

**Figure 2-3** The International Council of Nurses (ICN) provided a venue for nurse activists throughout the world to develop a collective voice and policies on nursing and important health care issues. Lavinia Lloyd Dock *(center)*, and other nurses are shown on the Atlantic City boardwalk during the 1947 ICN meeting.

suffragist, Lavinia Dock (1907), argued for nursing's involvement in the suffrage movement and wrote that the national associations would fall short of their mission if they did not get politically involved. She warned against following "the narrow path of purely professional questions" (p. 895), and strongly advocated nursing's understanding and support of this movement.

The argument that nurses used to oppose participation in the political suffrage campaign centered on fear that it would harm political efforts to obtain state nursing registration legislation. In 1908, at the ANA's eleventh annual convention, held in San Francisco, the membership opposed a resolution in favor of the organization's support of woman suffrage. Although this event is often used as an example of nursing's conservatism and lack of political activism, this very defeat served as a catalyst for organized nursing to join forces with other women suffragists. Palmer (1908) noted that "the action in San Francisco has brought the matter of suffrage sharply before the nurses of the country"

(p. 50). Within 4 years, nursing had responded to the efforts of nursing leaders to support the political franchise. By 1912, nursing organizations had voted to support women's right to vote (Chinn, 1985; Christy, 1984; Lewenson, 1996).

Proponents of nurses' support of woman suffrage linked health issues with the right to vote. Nurses could easily see the relationship between gaining the vote and improving the lives of their patients, families, and communities. Dock urged nurses to examine how the franchise would improve social conditions that led to illness. Using tuberculosis as an example, Dock (1908) said, "... take the present question of the underfed school children in New York. How many of them will have tuberculosis? If mothers and nurses had votes there might be school lunches for all those children" (p. 926).

The NACGN, although not invited to participate in the ANA and NLN resolution to support woman suffrage, did express grave concern for social issues that affected health. The NACGN became an invited member of the international nursing community through its membership in the International Council of Women. This affiliation reflects the NACGN's involvement in woman suffrage. Active discussions about woman suffrage, membership in the international women and nursing councils, and support for the ICN resolution to attain suffrage by 1912 indicated strong political activism among African-American nurses.

## SHAPING HEALTH AND PUBLIC POLICY

Several visionary leaders emerged during this initial period of organization. Some worked with the support of organized nursing, and others did not. Each leader who championed ideas about health care, equal rights, and professional opportunity had to be politically astute to attain the goals. As nursing moved into the stage that Cohen and co-workers (1996) describe as "self-interest," many of the leaders were paving the way into the next two stages, characterized as "political sophistication" and "leading the way" (p. 260). Women such as Lillian Wald and Margaret Sanger learned to speak the political language that enabled them to succeed in their respective missions. They spoke to a large audience, served on various national boards and commissions, and built strong coalitions around broad health concerns that went well beyond nursing.

### PUBLIC HEALTH: LILLIAN WALD

Before the formation of the NOPHN, trained nurses such as Lillian Wald and her friend from training school, Mary Brewster, understood the ramifications of economic, political, social, and cultural factors in regard to health. In 1893, Wald and Brewster opened the Henry Street Nurses' Settlement in New York City, providing nursing care, health education, social services, and cultural experiences to the residents of the Lower East Side (Fitzpatrick, 1975). Wald and the nurses at Henry Street lived within the community they served and became internationally noted for their success at addressing public health issues.

The work of the nurses at Henry Street reflected their ability to provide care in the home and to lobby for change in the body politic. Backer (1993) noted that Wald "connected her caring with activism by initiating practice and policy changes via administrative and organizational skills, persuasiveness, coalitions, delivering testimony and political power" (p. 128). Wald promoted public health nursing education and the formation of the NOPHN. Moreover, Wald's astute political awareness led to many social changes affecting the health and well-being of the Lower East Side residents.

Children's health and well-being struck a chord with Wald. Concerned for the welfare of children, Wald turned the backyard at Henry Street into a playground. Recognizing that too many children played in the overcrowded streets of the Lower East Side, Wald argued for the opening of city parks and in 1898 successfully formed the Outdoor Recreation League. This group obtained land in New York City and turned it into municipal parks (Siegel, 1983).

Wald's nursing knowledge, social concern, and political savvy joined forces when she maneuvered the board of health into hiring a school nurse in 1902. Wald writes her account in her 1915 book, *The House on Henry Street*, about how she and Brewster recognized a community health problem and kept records on those children excluded from school because of medical problems. After collecting these data, Wald convinced the president of the department of health of the need for nursing services in the public schools. Although the department of health decided to use physicians to inspect the children at schools, when the time was right, Wald encouraged the president to hire a public health nurse as well:

The time had come when it seemed right to urge the addition of the nurse's service to that of the doctor. My colleagues and I offered to show that with her assistance few children would lose their valuable school time and that it would be possible to bring under treatment those who needed it. Reluctant lest the democracy of the school should be invaded by even the most socially minded philanthropy, I exacted a promise from several of the city officials that if the experiment were successful they would use their influence to have the nurse, like the doctor, paid from public funds. (Wald, 1915, p. 51)

To Wald's credit, the experiment was successful, and in October 1902 the city of New York paid for the services of a school nurse. The board of estimates had allotted more than $30,000 for the employment of trained nurses who were, in Wald's words, the "first municipalized school nurses in the world" (Wald, 1915, p. 53). New York City's Bureau of Child Hygiene was an outgrowth of this service (Siegel, 1983; Wald, 1915).

## BIRTH CONTROL: MARGARET SANGER

At different points during the twentieth century, professional organizations and individuals engaged in political activism that attempted to address social ills. While organized nursing was seeking social change, Margaret Sanger, a nurse and noted political activist in the twentieth century, led the struggle for birth control.

Sanger, like Wald and Dock, understood the importance of political activism for effecting social change but sought support outside of organized nursing. She formed coalitions with other women's groups, labor organizers, and philosophers of the period. Sanger's political strength emanated from her outrage over society's control of women's reproductive process and her belief in reproductive autonomy. This one political issue led Sanger to argue for legalizing family planning and making it accessible and acceptable in the United States (Chesler, 1992; Cott, 1987).

Sanger, a visiting nurse at the beginning of the twentieth century, politically challenged America's restrictive laws about birth control (and literature on the subject) and personally experienced the untoward effect of defying the government. For example, in 1912 Sanger wrote an article about syphilis for the socialist weekly *The Call*. The United States Post Office declared that issue unmailable because of the nature of the material, invoking the Comstock Act of 1873, which deliberately prohibited the distribution of information about contraception and abortion (Reed, 1980). Sanger's crusade to disseminate contraception began in 1914, when she traveled to Europe to seek out safe contraception measures. After returning to the United States, she claimed that women could separate procreation from the sexual act and published her ideas in *Woman Rebel*. Again the Comstock Act thwarted Sanger's efforts. Because of her writings, Sanger was indicted and fled the country in October of 1914. When she returned in 1915, after the death of her daughter, public sympathy led the government to drop the charges against her.

In 1916, Sanger, along with her sister, Ethel Byrne, opened the first birth control clinic in the Brownsville section of Brooklyn, New York. These two women provided mothers in Brooklyn with advice about birth control until the police closed the clinic's doors. Sanger again faced arrest, prosecution, and imprisonment. Sanger challenged the legal restriction to distribute information about contraception. Her strong belief and determination led to changes in interpretation of the law and eventually to the founding of the organization known today as Planned Parenthood of America.

## ALLIANCE WITH THE WOMEN'S MOVEMENT: 1960 TO THE PRESENT DAY

Dock, Wald, and Sanger's political action set the stage for nurses' activism half a century later. In the 1960s the latest women's movement spread throughout the United States. Interest in the rights of women had continued after women gained the right to vote in 1920. This second wave of activists could conceivably harness the vote and gain equal status for women in the law, at work, and in the home. Although nursing in the latter half of the twentieth century remained essentially a profession dominated by women and shared a similar heritage of sexism and oppression, it took time to develop an acceptance of the ideas of the feminism espoused in this movement. In the early 1960s, nursing's presence in the women's movement was "obscure" or "notably absent" (Chinn & Wheeler, 1985, p. 74). The political activism frequently associated with feminist groups was not reported to have carried over into nursing. An "uneasy" relationship existed between those in the traditional female profession of nursing and those engaged in feminist activities (Allen, 1985).

By the 1970s some nursing leaders had enumerated the value of developing ties with the women's movement. Wilma Scott Heide (1973), a nurse and leader in the feminist movement who served as president of the National Organization for Women (NOW) between 1970 and 1974, called for nurses to embrace the ideas of the feminist movement. Heide (1973) believed that nurses and all women shared the similar dilemma of being characterized as caring, nurturing, compassionate, tender, submissive, passive, subjective, and emotional. Whereas some of the traits enhanced the professional role, others served to suppress proactive, empowering behaviors. Heide believed that nursing needed to join with the feminist movement in addressing the inequalities that women faced in society.

Another nurse and feminist, JoAnn Ashley (1976), argued that nurses could no longer be pacifists if they were to lead the health care changes that consumers needed. Ashley (1976, p. 133) recognized that "powerful, male-dominated groups, economically motivated, will not be reasonable with their interests and status threatened." Ashley challenged nurses to reflect on who they were and what their role was as nurses.

In the 1980s nursing became a metaphor for the "struggle of women for equality" (Diers, 1984, p. 23). Personal and professional empowerment served as essential qualities for gaining political power, and nurse leaders recognized that public policy would not change without advocates who could successfully use persuasive, political strategies. Feminism gave nurses "a world view that values women and that confronts systematic injustices based on gender" (Chinn & Wheeler, 1985, p. 74). Nursing's acceptance of this definition of feminism has assisted nursing's struggle for equality and can be traced to the early 1970s with the ANA's support of the Equal Rights Amendment; the formation of a group called Nurses-NOW; and the establishment of the Nurses Coalition for Action in Politics, nursing's first political action committee.

Changes in women's roles mirror society's perceptions of nursing roles. As women in the second half of the twentieth century challenged inequality and sought political power, nurses did so as well. Yet the political savvy of early pioneer leaders was lost to later generations of nurses. Too often nurses are not included in policy decisions, not involved in policy-making, or just not recognized at all (Gordon, 1997). Nurses have had to relearn political strategies and use them like Talbott and Vance (1981) even to be placed on the agenda of a women's conference on leadership. The nursism that exists within the broader society and at times within the women's movement has lessened, but nursing needs to be vigilant.

At the close of the twentieth century, three nurses served in the United States House of Representatives, but as of January 2005, no nurse serves or has served in the Senate. In 1998, 32 states benefited from having nurses as legislators, either elected or appointed (Feldman & Lewenson, 2000). At the end of the century, just over 100 nurses could be found to hold a political office, or fewer than 0.005% of the more than two million registered nurses (Findings from the national sample survey of registered nurses, 1997; Summers, 1996). Mary Wakefield, Director of the Center for Rural Health at the School of Medicine and Health Sciences at the University of North Dakota, notes that "the profession has fielded a strong class of individuals who are influencing public policy through an array of positions and activities" (Wakefield, 1999, p. 205), but argues that still too few are taking advantage of the opportunities.

Lois Capps, a U.S. Congresswoman from California, commented in an interview that people trust nurses (Feldman & Lewenson, 2000). Trust is something that nurses can capitalize on and use when advocating for health care reforms such as gun control, Medicare reimbursement for medication, and other important consumer health care advocacy issues. Nurses know from their experience and education what constitutes high-quality health care and what a healthy society needs. But nurses must learn to recognize that their tremendous power lies in their knowledge of people, their ability to communicate, and their role to advocate for a healthier population. To do this, Wakefield (1999, p. 205) suggests that political advocacy become a larger part of the educational experience and that students be given "first-hand exposure to the links between health care and health policy." Slowly, as the profession builds on the political activism learned in Cohen and colleagues' third stage of political development (1996), it needs to move into stage four, which is characterized as "leading the way" (p. 262). Nursing will use important strategic political skills such as coalition building, grassroots mobilization, issue-based collaboration, and media expertise to help set the future agenda for health care. Nurses will learn that their extensive knowledge base and experience lend themselves to political activism. In preparation, nurses may benefit by reflecting on their past, understanding what the health care consumer needs, and politically activating their profession for change.

## WHAT THE FUTURE HOLDS

Nurses need to know the history of the profession in order to understand the outcomes generated by nursing leaders from the past and impart this knowledge to new generations of nurses and the public. Nurses cannot just read what they believe to be the "latest" in published evidence and ignore historical evidence. To do so we risk what Nelson and Gordon (2004) describe as the "rhetoric of rupture" or the loss of knowledge because nurses constantly look for a "newer" way to advance and "reinvent" ourselves. Although using current data to support practice helps us provide better and safer care, without knowledge of past clinical practice or understanding of political efforts of past leaders to improve the health of the public, we miss the opportunity to understand what we can do now and in the future to assure a healthier society. Therefore we must assure a continuity of understanding by integrating history into our nursing education and ultimately into our nursing practice (Lewenson, 2004). Nurses need to learn about their past and value it so that they can avoid the constant reinvention that takes place and dilutes the strength that we could use to make changes.

## *Key Points*

- Nursing's legacy of political activism altered the course of events for the profession and for health care in this country.
- Forgetting this legacy has been detrimental to the profession because it denies the opportunity to learn from nursing's visionaries and leaders.
- Nursing leaders have used such strategies as persuasion, cultivation of political friendships, education, letter-writing campaigns, defiance of the law, and organization to harness the collective voice of nurses.
- History lessons from the architects of the profession can provide a road map for political action today and help address the adverse effects of "nursism."

## *Web Resources*

**American Association for the History of Nursing**
*www.aahn.org*
**Center for the Study of Nursing History, University of Pennsylvania**
*www.nursing.upenn.edu/history*

## REFERENCES

Allen, M. (1985). Women, nursing and feminism: An interview with Alice J. Baumgart, RN, PhD. *Canadian Nurse, 81*(1), 20-22.

Armeny, S. (1983). Organized nurses, women philanthropists, and the intellectual bases for cooperation among women, 1898-1920. In E. Condliffe Lagemann (Ed.), *Nursing history: New perspectives, new possibilities.* New York: Teachers College Press.

Ashley, J. (1976). *Hospitals, paternalism and the role of the nurse.* New York: Teachers College Press.

Backer, B. (1993). Lillian Wald: Connecting caring with actions. *Nursing and Health Care, 14*(3), 122-129.

Birnbach, N. (1985). Vignette: Political activism and the registration movement. In D. Mason & S. W. Talbott (Eds.), *Political action handbook for nurses: Changing the workplace, government, organizations, and community.* Menlo Park, CA: Addison-Wesley.

Birnbach, N., & Lewenson, S. B. (1993). *Legacy of leadership: Presidential addresses from the Superintendents' Society and the National League of Nursing Education, 1894-1952.* New York: NLN Press.

Buresh, B., & Gordon, S. (2000). *From silence to voice: What nurses know and must communicate to the public.* Ottawa: Canadian Nurses Association.

Burgess, M. A. (1928). *Nurses, patients, and pocketbooks.* New York: Committee on the Grading of Nursing Schools.

Chesler, E. (1992). *Woman of valor: Margaret Sanger and the birth control movement in America.* New York: Simon & Schuster.

Chinn, P. (1985). Historical roots: Female nurses and political action. *Journal of the New York State Nurses Association, 16*(2), 29-37.

Chinn, P. L., & Wheeler, C. E. (1985). Feminism and nursing: Can nursing afford to remain aloof from the women's movement? *Nursing Outlook, 33*(2), 74-76.

Christy, T. (1984). Equal rights for women: Voice from the past. In *Pages from nursing history: A collection of original articles from the pages of* Nursing Outlook, The American Journal of Nursing and Nursing Research. New York: American Journal of Nursing.

Cohen, S. S., Mason, J. M., Kovner, C., Leavitt, J. K., Pulcini, J., & Sochalski, J. (1996). Stages of nursing's political development: Where we've been and where we ought to go. *Nursing Outlook, 44*(6), 259-266.

Cott, N. (1977). *The bonds of womanhood: "Woman's sphere" in New England, 1780-1930.* New Haven, CT: Yale University Press.

Cott, N. F. (1987). *The grounding of modern feminism.* New Haven, CT: Yale University Press.

Daniels, L. (1987). *American women in the 20th century: The festival of life.* San Diego: Harcourt Brace Jovanovich.

Diers, D. (1984). To profess—To be a professional. *Journal of the New York State Nurses Association, 15*(4), 23.

Dock, L. (1907). Some urgent social claims. *American Journal of Nursing, 7*(10), 895-901.

Dock, L. (1908). The suffrage question. *American Journal of Nursing, 8*(11), 925-927.

Dock, L., & Stewart, I. (1931). *A short history of nursing.* (3rd ed., revised). New York: Putnam's Sons.

Feldman, H. R., & Lewenson, S. B. (2000). *Nurses in the political arena: The public face of nursing.* New York: Springer.

Findings from the national sample survey of registered nurses, March 1996. (1997). United States Department of Health and Human Services Health Resources and Services Administration Bureau of Health Professions Division on Nursing. Retrieved January 7, 2006, from *http://bhpr.hrsa.gov/healthworkforce/ reports/rnsurvey/rnss1.htm.*

Fitzpatrick, L. (1975). *The National Organization for Public Health Nursing, 1912-1952: Development of a practice field.* New York: NLN Press.

Florence Nightingale's letter of advice to Bellevue. (1911). *American Journal of Nursing, 11*(5), 361-364.

Gardner, M. S. (1933). *Public health nursing.* (2nd ed., revised). New York: Macmillan.

Gordon, K. M., Myers, A. J., & Kelley, F. (1906). Equal suffrage movement. *American Journal of Nursing, 7*(1), 47-48.

Gordon, S. (1997). *Life support: Three nurses on the front lines.* Boston: Little, Brown.

Heide, W. S. (1973). Nursing and women's liberation a parallel. *American Journal of Nursing, 73*(5), 824-827.

Hine, D. C. (1989). *Black women in white: Racial conflict and cooperation in the nursing profession. 1890-1950.* Bloomington, IN: Indiana University Press.

Hine, D. C. (1990). The Ethel Johns Report: Black women in the nursing profession, 1925; From hospital to college: Black nurse leaders and the rise of collegiate nursing schools. In D.C. Hine (Ed.), *Black women in United States history: Vol. 2. Black women in American history: The twentieth century.* Brooklyn, NY: Carlson.

Hine, D. C. (1993). Staupers, Mabel Keaton (1890-1989). In D. C. Hine (Ed.), *Black women in America: An historical encyclopedia* (Vol. 2). Brooklyn, NY: Carlson.

Johns, E. (1925). *A study of the present status of the Negro woman in nursing* (1.1, Series 200, Box 122, Folder 1507, pp. 1-43, Exhibits A-P, Appendixes I and II). New York: Rockefeller Archive Center.

Lerner, G. (1977). *The female experience: An American documentary.* Indianapolis: Bobbs-Merrill.

Lewenson, S. (1994). "Of logical necessity—they hang together": Nursing and the woman's movement, 1901-1912. *Nursing History Review, 2,* 99-117.

Lewenson, S. B. (1996). *Taking charge: Nursing, suffrage and feminism in America, 1873-1920.* New York: NLN Press.

Lewenson, S. B. (2004). Integrating nursing history in the curriculum. *Journal of Professional Nursing, 20*(6), 374-380.

Nelson, S., & Gordon, S. (2004). The rhetoric of rupture: Nursing as practice with a history. *Nursing Outlook, 52,* 255-261.

Palmer, S. (1897). *First and second annual conventions of the American Society of Superintendents of Training Schools for Nurses,* Harrisburg, PA. (Also found in Birnbach, N., & Lewenson, S. [1991]. *First words: Selected addresses from the National League for Nurses 1894-1933.* New York: NLN Press; and in Reverby, S. [1985]. *Annual conventions 1893-1899: The American Society of Superintendents of Training Schools for Nurses.* New York: Garland.)

Palmer, S. (1908). Editorial policy explained. *American Journal of Nursing, 9*(1), 49-50.

Palmer, S. (1909). State societies: Their organization and place in nursing education. *American Journal of Nursing, 9*(12), 956-957.

Progress and reaction. (1908). *American Journal of Nursing, 8*(5), 334-335.

Reed, J. (1980). Sanger, Margaret. In B. Sicherman & C. Hurd Green (Eds.), *Notable American women: The modern period.* Cambridge, MA: The Belknap Press of Harvard University Press.

Reverby, S. (1987). *Ordered to care: The dilemma of American nursing, 1850-1945.* New York: Cambridge University Press.

Robb, I. H. (1900). Original communications [address of the president]. *American Journal of Nursing, 1*(2).

Rogge, M. M. (1987). Nursing and politics: A forgotten legacy. *Nursing Research, 36*(1), 26-30.

Siegel, B. (1983). *Lillian Wald of Henry Street.* New York: Macmillan.

Staupers, M. (1937). The Negro nurse in America. *Opportunity: Journal of Negro Life, 15,* 339-341. (Also reprinted in Hine, D. C. [1985]. *Black women in the nursing profession: A documentary history.* New York: Garland.)

Summers, B. J. (1996). Nurses and politics: What can we gain? *Tennessee Nurse, 59*(5), 36-37.

Talbott, S. W., & Vance, C. (1981). Involving nursing in a feminist group—NOW. *Nursing Outlook, 29*(10), 592-595.

Thoms, A. (1929). *Pathfinders: A history of progress of the colored graduate nurses.* New York: Kay Printing House.

Vance, C., Talbott, S. W., McBride, A., & Mason, D. J. (1985). Coming of age: The women's movement and nursing. In D. Mason & S. Talbott (Eds.), *Political action handbook for nurses.* Menlo Park, CA: Addison-Wesley.

Vicinus, M., & Nergaard, B. (Eds.). (1989). *Ever yours, Florence Nightingale: Selected letters.* London: Virago.

Wakefield, M. (1999). Public policy: Canaries in the mine. *Journal of Professional Nursing, 15*(4), 205.

Wald, L. (1915). *The house on Henry Street.* New York: Henry Holt.

# chapter 3

# Learning the Ropes of Policy, Politics, and Advocacy

Judith K. Leavitt, Mary W. Chaffee, & Connie Vance

*"I am not afraid of storms for I am learning how to sail my ship."*

LOUISA MAY ALCOTT

Every politically active person, from presidents of the United States to organizational leaders, *learned* the political and policy skills that catapulted them into positions of power and responsibility. Nurses are no different. As others do, nurses learn the skills of politics and policy through mentoring, role modeling, and practice. The most important catalyst to becoming involved is to find mentors—colleagues and friends who are politically savvy—to teach us, to believe in and support us, and to celebrate our successes and help us build on our failures.

In this chapter the reader will explore how to develop political skills through mentoring, education, and direct experience. Students new to politics as well as experienced nurses have unlimited ways to expand their knowledge and involvement. Whatever our experience, we improve our skills as we engage in the process. There are infinite causes and issues to stimulate our interest if we want to become involved. We need only decide how much energy, time, and interest we have to advocate for our patients or advance the profession. Success in the world of policy and politics demands the strengths and skills that nurses possess. Working in the policy arena will open doors to opportunities where nurses can be equal players and leaders. Stories of some of these nurses are the essence of this book.

## POLITICAL CONSCIOUSNESS-RAISING AND AWARENESS: THE "AHA" MOMENT

How does one get started? Many find that there is a defining moment when the old ways of reacting to issues of injustice, inequality, or powerlessness no longer work. It is the moment when the person realizes that an issue or problem is due to problems in the larger health care system, such as an insensitive workplace, or to public policies that have to be changed. It might be the denial of needed care for a patient eligible to receive Medicaid or Medicare. It could be the urgent sense of concern when seeing small children riding in a car without a seatbelt or appropriate booster seat. It could be the frustration of the home health nurse who is unable to continue caring for her patient because insurance will not cover the cost. When the nurse knows that the solution is to confront the policies that create these inequities and decides to so, that is political consciousness-raising and an "aha" moment. It happens when one's consciousness is raised and one recognizes that change is necessary. It is the validity of one's personal experience as it relates to similar experiences of others. It is the adrenaline rush that urges, "Something must be done—and I need to become involved."

Until that defining moment, nurses may feel frustrated, angry, or hopeless. When the "aha" hits, we begin to see that it is some aspect of the *system* that is the problem and that we must do something to change it. We understand that we can influence those who make the decisions to right the wrong, change the law, or create a new policy. We see that an injustice is no longer seen as someone else's problem but rather has personal meaning to the individual. That is the meaning of the phrase "the personal is political." The problem in question requires political solutions, more than personal solutions, and it requires skills that can be learned.

When nurses accept that they are not at fault for the inadequacies of the health care system and instead believe that nursing can provide many of the solutions, the profession itself becomes political. Nurses then become proactive rather than reactive. The result is that the individual nurse, as well as the profession, become empowered to act. Feeling empowered is essential to true advocacy.

## GETTING STARTED

Through interviews with 27 American nurses involved in health policy at the national, state, and local levels, Gebbie, Wakefield, and Kerfoot (2000) set out to discover how and why these activist nurses became involved. Their results corroborated what we knew anecdotally:

- The majority of respondents had parents, most often fathers, who were active in policy and politics and who created a mentoring, supportive environment.
- Many were raised to be independent and to believe in their capacity to accomplish what they wanted.
- High school provided a training ground in political socialization.
- Nursing education provided role modeling and mentoring by faculty, deans, and alumni as well as the opportunity to increase political awareness through courses in policy, political science, and economics.
- Clinical practice often provided strong role models, and experiences in public health and community health provided opportunities for political insights.

- Graduate education opened doors for many, through such avenues as the study of law, health economics, and health policy.
- Some had their consciousness raised gradually through work experiences that exposed them to public policy and the need to understand how to influence the process.

The nurses who were interviewed confirmed that there are multiple points of entry into the policy arena. Whether this chapter, this book, a course in policy and politics, or a conversation with a colleague is your first exposure, you have already started.

The skills of politics—how to be persuasive, how to identify and use power effectively, how to analyze obstructions to goal attainment, and how to mobilize people to work collectively—are all learned. Nurses bring skills to the political arena that are learned through education and further refined in clinical practice. Politics requires the kind of communication skills that nurses use to persuade an unwilling patient to get out of bed after abdominal surgery or a child to swallow an unpleasant-tasting medication. All competent political experts possess effective communication skills. Nurses possess many of these skills. In addition, nurses, whether they realize it or not, are health care experts. Nurses can speak knowledgeably about what patients and communities need because they experience it firsthand.

## THE POLITICAL DEVELOPMENT OF NURSING AND HOW IT RELATES TO THE INDIVIDUAL

Cohen and colleagues (1996) developed a conceptual model describing the political development of the profession. It is interesting to note that it mirrors the stages that individual nurses go through to learn the ropes (see *Policy and Politics: A Framework for Action* in Chapter 1 for a more detailed description of the model). The four stages are buy-in, self-interest, political sophistication, and leading the way.

### STAGE ONE: BUY-IN

Buy-in is a reactive stage. For nursing it occurred when the profession began to promote the political awareness of nurses to injustices or changes needed in the policy arena. For the individual, this is the "aha" moment. One begins to decide how to become involved.

## STAGE TWO: SELF-INTEREST

At this stage the nursing profession began to develop its identity as a special interest and crystallized its uniqueness as a political voice. For the individual, this could be the time when one becomes most focused on specific issues related to one's practice rather than on the larger issues of health care and the profession. It is learning about the nuts and bolts of political activism and policy development. It is moving from recognition of a problem to developing a plan to deal with the problem. It could involve using political skills, such as enlisting support of colleagues and planning strategies to resolve the issue, or it could be volunteering to create a taskforce in the workplace to recommend policy changes of concern to the staff.

## STAGE THREE: POLITICAL SOPHISTICATION

Political sophistication is the stage in which policymakers and health care leaders view nurses as having valuable expertise in health policy. For the individual this is the time when legislators and other policymakers turn to nurse experts to be on their health advisory committees, when nurses testify before state legislatures and local health-related boards and commissions, and when nurses get appointed to policy-making bodies.

## STAGE FOUR: LEADING THE WAY

This stage is the highest level of political involvement, when nursing "sets the agenda" for change. Instead of just contributing knowledge, nursing becomes the initiator of crucial policy development. For the individual this is the point when individuals direct the dialogue and policy development of organizations and institutions whose mission is broader than health. This includes appointments to positions outside of nursing, to posts such as university president or department head in federal and state government. Nurses are recognized for their unique expertise and perspective and are seen by multiple constituencies as bringing solutions to issues related to the well-being of society as a whole.

Wherever one is in political development, there are higher stages to reach, if desired. Start somewhere. If you are a new graduate, pay attention to the work environment and let yourself be ready for the awakening, the "aha" moment. If you are an experienced nurse, think of whether you are ready and how you want to share your expertise and knowledge with policymakers. You may even decide to become the policymaker.

## ADVOCACY AND ACTIVISM

Nurses are considered to be powerful advocates— but what exactly does this mean? Patients are vulnerable, because of their illness as well as the organizational and financial complexities of navigating the health system. Curtin (1979) describes the end purpose of nursing as the welfare of other human beings. Because of the nurse's close relationship with the patient, a unique knowledge is developed. Curtin indicates that this "common humanity" leads to the development of "human advocacy"—the foundation of the nurse-patient relationship.

Florence Nightingale saw nursing in all of its forms as advocacy—a "calling" that required nurses to look for and act on ways to be world citizens for the sake of human health (Dossey, Slanders, Beck, & Attewell, 2005). The legacy of Nightingale's local and global advocacy and activism calls nurses to active involvement on behalf of people wherever they are.

Advocacy is increasingly presented as a component of professional nursing practice. The nurse as patient advocate is described in the *Revised Code of Ethics for Nurses with Interpretive Statements* (American Nurses Association [ANA], 2001), as promoting, advocating for, and striving to protect the health, safety, and rights of the patient. Furthermore, the nurse is expected to collaborate with "other health professionals and the public in promoting community, national, and international efforts to meeting health needs" and to shape social policy (p. 12). Nursing education at the baccalaureate level is expected to produce nurses who "advocate for health care that is sensitive to the needs of patients" and who "advocate for professional standards of practice using organizational and political processes" (American Association of Colleges of Nursing [AACN], 1998, pp. 15-17.) Nurses who have been educated at the master's degree level are charged with assuming the role of advocate for consumers and for the nursing profession and the role of change agent within the health care system (AACN, 1996).

How do nurses learn advocacy? "Standing up for others" is learned through family values, education, and work experiences, as well as by watching nurses interact with patients as role models for advocacy. "Nurses will have a stronger foundation in advocacy when nurse educators consciously teach advocacy skills and when nurse administrators consciously support nurses' advocacy in the work environment" (Foley, Minick, & Kee, 2002, p. 186).

In the workplace, nurses work with patients to achieve mutual goals by advocating for the patient or for the resources the patient needs. The placement of nurses throughout the health system permits them to act as "natural mediators" (Mallik, 1997). Outside the health system, nurses can be equally influential advocates—again because of their unique position. In the government, in professional associations, and in the community, nurses can use their political skills to advocate for policies and changes that will improve the health of populations. For example, the National Association of Pediatric Nurse Practitioners (NAPNAP) advocates for children by supporting federal legislation on child gun safety, prevention of youth suicide, expansion of access to health services to reduce unintended pregnancy, and increasing access to care for children with special needs (Duderstadt, 2004). While individual nurse practitioners serve as advocates for individual patients, NAPNAP uses the power of its membership to advocate on a larger scale for the needs of children.

Nurses may serve as advocates in a variety of roles. Kubsch, Sternard, Hovarter, and Matzke (2004) described five types of nurse advocacy:

1. Legal advocate: The nurse guards the patient's rights.
2. Moral-ethical advocate: The nurse upholds the patient's values.

3. Spiritual advocate: The nurse provides access to spiritual support.
4. Substitutive advocate: The nurse protects the interests of patients unable to do so themselves.
5. Political advocate: The nurse facilitates equal access to health care.

Several of these roles are used by nurses in providing direct care for patients; others are roles nurses assume in the political and policy arenas.

The end point of all advocacy is the health and welfare of the public. When we advocate for nurses and the profession, for healthy practice environments, and for the improvement of social and health care policies, then we are truly advocating for our patients (Smith, 2004). Every nurse, within the framework of his or her practice and position, should become empowered to practice advocacy in its broadest sense. Like Nightingale, we should be citizen-activists, as envisioned by Chinn (2002), who believes that nurses' unique backgrounds in health promotion and health care advocacy prepare us for true global citizen advocacy.

## THE ROLE OF MENTORING

At every stage of a nursing career—from student to novice to expert—mentor relationships are an essential element for professional success, socialization, and leadership development. This is particularly true in political and policy arenas, in which nurses' involvement is relatively recent and the majority of nurses receive no formal training in their educational programs. In the traditional world of politics, the "old boys' network" consisted of strong mentoring components. Gaining entry into the inner circle of policy and politics required the mentorship of political party leaders who served as sponsors, role models, and door-openers to aspiring "politicians." Nurses are discovering the necessity of receiving mentoring from a variety of leaders and peers at every career stage, particularly as they expand their influence from the bedside to wider spheres of policy and political involvement. Nurses' mentor connections will take them beyond traditional nursing boundaries, where they can influence decisions and policies that affect their patients and their professional practice.

A mentor or role model provides inspiration and encouragement to get involved, as well as coaching and tutoring in the nuts and bolts of political involvement. As with any other nursing skill, learning the political or policy process requires both theoretic and experiential knowledge. Political mentors can be found in classrooms, clinical settings, professional associations, political parties, government, and community settings. Politically active nurses in one study (Winter & Lockhart, 1997) identified their nursing colleagues in various settings as important policy mentors. These mentors facilitated political involvement by modeling their expertise and inspiring those in their formative years. Nursing political leaders in another study stated that they had found traditional mentors or peer mentors who believed in their abilities, guided their learning, and nourished their self-worth (Leavitt & Barry, 1993). The nationwide "nurse-influentials" studied by Vance (1977) reported that their mentors were crucial "role models for change and risk-taking and for political and diplomatic action." These leaders claimed the mentoring support of nursing colleagues as well as those in administrative, political, and corporate circles.

Mentoring relationships among students, teachers, and colleagues are developmental and empowering. Mentors inspire, guide, advise, and model behavior as they interact with novices and peers (Vance & Olson, 1998). In both formal and informal teaching situations, teacher and learner grow and mature together through a developmental process, and the same learning process occurs between mentor and protégé. There is also mutual empowerment as all persons in the relationship gain confidence, motivation, and strength (Cohen & Milone-Nuzzo, 2001).

In the nursing profession, the mentor model consists of both expert-novice and peer-peer mentor connections. The developmental and empowering aspects of mentoring relationships are necessary aspects of learning the policy and political ropes. One example of developmental mentoring is the modeling of political behavior at lobby days in Congress or in state legislatures that are sponsored by nursing associations. At these events, nurse lobbyists and nurse activists serve as mentor-guides and role models to nurses and students who are less experienced in the political process. They provide information and strategies and model effective behaviors while lobbying policymakers on specific legislation. These activists also provide the inspiration and vision of what can be done if nurses join together on behalf of shared goals. This is real-life experiential learning between mentor-experts and protégé-novices, and it is a highly effective and practical way of developing political awareness and know-how. Check your state nurses association for lobby days (Figure 3-1).

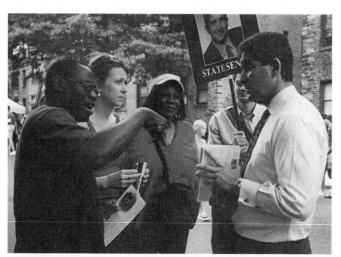

**Figure 3-1** Nursing students from College of New Rochelle, New York, with New York State Senator Jeff Klein.

Mentors can empower others by drawing them into the process and inspiring them with their commitment to making change and a "can-do" attitude that "we can indeed make a difference." Empowerment, as a model for political action, has been described as development in three dimensions:

- Consciousness raising about the sociopolitical realities of nursing
- Strong and positive self-esteem
- Political skills for changing the system (Mason, Backer, & Georges, 1991)

Political nurses demonstrate that there is power in numbers and in the collective strength of nursing. Association with optimistic mentors who are committed to their profession and who are not afraid to take risks on behalf of creating change through the political process is empowering to others, particularly those new to political activism. Nurses whose consciousness is raised by empowerment experiences with mentors often report that their professional pride, confidence, and motivation are strengthened. They come to believe that they, too, can improve nursing and health care by engaging in change activities.

Anecdotal and research data continue to demonstrate that mentoring activities and relationships are essential to the ongoing development of policy knowledge and expertise. This is a particular challenge in the formal education and professional socialization of most nurses. Studies continue to point to the lack of formal course work and the scarcity of formal mentors on policy and politics in nurses' education. In the political study by Gebbie and colleagues (2000), nurse activists reported that they were not encouraged to seek mentoring or other developmental experiences and training. There still may not be adequate numbers of politically engaged nurses and faculty who can inspire and inform others as to the value of this involvement. One nurse in the Gebbie study noted that there are three "hooks" that pull nurses into health policy: personal experience, mentors, and dramatic interventions (p. 311). Clearly, mentors, whether they are experts, teachers, or peers, are a critical element in learning the ropes in political policy involvement. As greater numbers of nurses begin to value and engage in the political dimensions of their profession, they will mentor others in the how-to's of this crucial aspect of nursing.

## FINDING A MENTOR

If you want to become involved in policy and politics, you can find a mentor, even if you don't know someone personally. Start with a list of what you would like to learn, who you would like to mentor you, people you know who might know the individual, and how to gain access to that person. You can contact the person directly, via e-mail, by phone, or with a note, or you can ask someone who knows the individual to make the first contact. It helps to be able to state what you want to learn from the individual and why you selected that person. For instance, one author went to the campaign manager of the local congressman to learn how to organize nurses for his campaign. The campaign manager saw a motivated, committed volunteer in the author and was thrilled to be able to show her the "ins and outs" of organizing. That was the start of many such organizing campaigns that culminated in the author's achieving a major staff position with a U.S. Senate campaign. Remember that the mentor need not be a nurse, and often the mentor is not. The important criteria for a mentor are knowledge and an interest in you. Sometimes the mentor need only get you started; in other situations a mentor becomes a lifelong friend and role model.

## COLLECTIVE MENTORING

Because the majority of nurses are newcomers to political and policy activism, every nurse should possess the mentality of being both a mentor and a protégé in the political process. Learning politics is not a solitary activity. This means that nurses should be on the lookout for mentors who can serve as their teachers and guides as they hone political and policy skills. Likewise, every nurse should assume responsibility for actively mentoring others as they refine their repertoire of skills and deepen their involvement. This reciprocal collective mentoring is extremely effective in expanding the political and power base of the profession and its members. Collective mentoring can occur in nursing schools, clinical agencies, and professional associations. This means that wherever we practice nursing, we can each refine our skills by seeking mentors and serving as mentors to others.

Leavitt and Mason (1998) wrote a case study of the principles and activities associated with collective mentoring in a fledgling political action committee for nurses in New York. This small group of nurses used peer mentoring to develop their political knowledge and influence. They in turn reached out to coach novices in the skills of political organizing, fund raising, and public speaking.

Collective mentoring is about the process of working together to extend nursing's solidarity of activists. It also is about recognizing that new, even inexperienced, voices can contribute to the development of the most seasoned mentors. Finally, collective mentoring is about moving a vision in creative ways and being committed to the development of people who can move that vision (Leavitt and Mason, 1998).

Joining with others to expand our political influence is a necessary strategy. Each nurse can learn with and from others, regardless of current level of knowledge.

Inherent in this form of mentoring is the development of networks of persons who are active in policy and who take responsibility for expanding these networks. The nurses in these networks should develop intentional strategies for mentoring political neophytes and for "claiming" nurses who may not be in traditional career paths (Gebbie et al., 2000). Organizational networks, including those in academic, clinical, and association settings, are a natural place to establish developmental mentoring activities. For example, politically active faculty members can network with political leaders in professional associations in order to provide undergraduate and graduate students with lobbying and leadership opportunities. Many state nursing associations are successfully reaching out to collectively mentor hundreds of nursing students through lobby days in national and state capitols. Nursing students and practicing nurses also have many opportunities to experience collective mentoring in learning the political ropes through relationships with leaders and peers in organizations such as the National Student Nurses Association, the ANA, specialty and state nursing associations, and volunteer health-related organizations. In addition, local political parties, community organizations, and the offices of elected officials offer nurses opportunities to learn through mentored experiences. These organizations can offer numerous mentoring opportunities for involvement in lobbying, policy development, media contacts, fundraising, and the political process in various venues (Figure 3-2).

Mentoring in policy development in any of the spheres also requires connections to knowledgeable leaders. In the workplace one can learn from health professionals who serve as leaders on

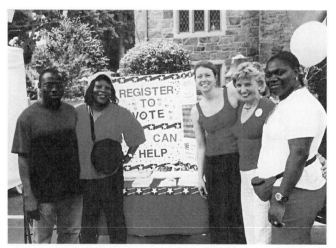

**Figure 3-2** BSN students with faculty member Dr. Connie Vance (second from right), participating in voter registration.

policy committees. For example, if one wants to work on improving staffing systems, the nurse would need to know the cost of staffing, the cost of bringing in temporary staff, the budget allocation for staffing on the unit. The unit manager might have that information and can help the nurse gather that information. In addition, one would need to know how much Medicare and Medicaid allocates to particular types of patients (outside the control of the institution) or the acuity level of patients. By working with experienced and knowledgeable staff, one can learn how to put this information together, how to influence colleagues to support the policy, and how to gain access to and acceptance of organizational leaders.

## EDUCATIONAL OPPORTUNITIES

There are many ways to learn how to influence health policy; some will depend on your own learning style, where you live, and your interests. Whatever your educational and political goals, there is something for everyone—from continuing education programs to graduate programs in political science and policy. With a little effort and some help getting started, an exciting world of educational possibilities is available. These educational opportunities often lead down paths many nurses did not realize existed when they completed their initial nursing studies.

Is it really worth putting the time and energy into learning new skills? Can nurses make a difference? Absolutely—many nurses and professional nursing associations have profoundly influenced health policy through their political efforts. Nursing's successful work is now being recognized by other professions as an example of how to be politically effective. The great success of nurse practitioners has been described as a model for how pharmacists can move their practices forward (O'Brien, 2003).

### PROGRAMS AND COURSES IN SCHOOLS OF NURSING

A few degree programs in policy have been established in schools of nursing. More commonly, nursing programs offer courses, either as core requirements or electives, related to health policy or with health policy content embedded. Many of these can be taken as continuing education credits even if you are not enrolled as a part-time or full-time student. Examples include the following:

- The University of California, San Francisco, offers Health Policy Nursing as a master's specialty area and a Nursing PhD in Health Policy (University of California, San Francisco, 2005).
- The University of Pennsylvania School of Nursing offers a Health Leadership minor that includes a course on "History, Health and Social Policy" (University of Pennsylvania, 2005).
- The University of Rhode Island offers a 3-credit course on "Advanced Leadership in the Health Policy Process" (University of Rhode Island, 2005).

### DEGREE PROGRAMS AND COURSES IN PUBLIC HEALTH, PUBLIC ADMINISTRATION, AND PUBLIC POLICY

College and university departments of public health, political science, policy science, and others are a rich source of policy content in academic programs. Programs in these areas take a little more effort to find because they reside under many different names. Programs leading to degrees that include health policy content are widely available at the baccalaureate, master, and doctoral levels. Numerous programs exist at all academic levels (associates, baccalaureate, masters, and doctorate). For courses in your area, examine the online listings for local colleges.

### CONTINUING EDUCATION PROGRAMS

Annual conferences on health policy topics are conducted by academic institutions and professional associations. Specialty nursing associations and state nursing associations often offer legislative workshops. Check websites and publications for the most current offerings, and monitor your state nursing association's meeting announcements. Search the Internet using *health policy meeting, health policy conference,* or *health care meeting* as search terms.

### EXPERIENTIAL LEARNING

There are many ways to obtain valuable practical experience, from internships to self-study programs.

**Internships and Fellowships.** Internships and fellowships provide great learning opportunities. In addition to teaching nurses the ropes, these practical experiences offer valuable mentoring and networking opportunities and may lead to employment options. Internships may be arranged for credit in academic programs. Summer or year-long internships are available on Capitol Hill, in some federal agencies, and through professional associations. See the Appendix for a list of formal internships and fellowships.

**Volunteer Service.** A great way to learn politics is to volunteer to work on a political campaign. Volunteer time and energy are welcomed by candidates for elective office at all levels of government—local, state, and federal. First-time candidates with tight budgets are especially appreciative of volunteer assistance. Building relationships through volunteer service is a critical part of learning the ropes. Also consider contacting Democratic or Republican national party headquarters for training and information about volunteer activities. (See *Anatomy of a Political Campaign* following Chapter 27.)

**Professional Association Activities.** Many professional nursing associations offer opportunities for volunteer service that lead to rich educational, mentoring, and networking experiences. Members of the ANA may participate in Nurses Strategic Action Team (N-STAT), a national grassroots political activity program. N-STAT members are alerted about critical health care issues, are encouraged to contact their members of Congress, and are provided examples of how to write effective letters to legislators. Some N-STAT members who serve as statewide leaders interview and evaluate candidates for federal office (Congress) and make recommendations to ANA's Political Action Committee (ANA-PAC) about endorsement.

Many specialty nursing associations and other health professional associations such as the American Public Health Association, the American Cancer Society, and the American Heart Association have strong advocacy and legislative programs. Contact your specialty association or explore its website for learning and volunteer opportunities.

**Self-Study.** The value of reading and self-directed learning cannot be underestimated in learning about policy and politics. There is something for everyone—from scholarly peer-reviewed journals to *Politics for Dummies*.

*Professional Journals.* Many professional nursing, health care, and social sciences journals include updates on current political issues. Some are wholly focused on policy and politics; others publish regular political content.

PROFESSIONAL JOURNALS WITH POLICY AND POLITICAL FOCUS

- *American Journal of Nursing,* a monthly publication that includes commentary on current political issues affecting nursing
- *Health Affairs,* a bimonthly journal published by Project HOPE that is known for thought-provoking articles that inform and influence discussion of health policy issues
- *Journal of the American Medical Association (JAMA),* the weekly publication of the American Medical Association, which covers health policy issues of interest to physicians
- *Journal of Health Politics, Policy and Law,* a bimonthly peer-reviewed publication of Duke University Press
- *Journal of Professional Nursing,* the official journal of the American Association of Colleges of Nursing, which includes a regular column on public policy
- *New England Journal of Medicine,* published weekly by the Massachusetts Medical Society; a journal that publishes innovative perspectives and background on health policy issues
- *Nursing Economic$:* a bimonthly publication that includes "Capitol Commentary," a regular feature that examines health care policy issues
- *Policy, Politics, & Nursing Practice,* a peer-reviewed quarterly journal that publishes articles on legislation affecting nursing practice, case studies in policy and political action, interviews with policymakers and policy experts, and articles on trends and issues
- *Yale Journal of Health Policy, Law, and Ethics,* a biannual publication that provides a forum for interdisciplinary discussion of topics in health policy, health law, and biomedical ethics

***Books.*** Browse through the political science, government, or current events sections of your favorite bookstore and you are likely to find a goldmine. You can also browse an online bookseller such as *www.amazon.com* or *www.barnesandnoble.com*. Search for the words *politics, policy,* or *health policy* and see what piques your interest. (Many booksellers sell used books at discounted prices.)

## POLICY AND POLITICS BOOKS TO GET STARTED

- *Politics for Dummies* (2nd ed.) by Ann DeLaney (For Dummies, 2002). This is a great book for anyone who slept through civics class in high school. Related reading: *Congress for Dummies* and *The Complete Idiot's Guide to American Government.*
- *The One-Hour Activist: The 15 Most Powerful Actions You Can Take to Fight for the Issues and Candidates You Care About* by Christopher Kush (Jossey-Bass, 2004). Practical guidance on how to influence policymakers.
- *MoveOn's 50 Ways to Love Your Country: How to Find Your Political Voice and Become a Catalyst for Change* by MoveOn (Inner Ocean Publishing, 2004). MoveOn, an Internet advocacy group, provides tips on taking political action.
- *The House and Senate Explained: The People's Guide to Congress* by Ellen Greenberg (WW Norton, 1996). Greenberg provides an excellent guide to understanding what happens on Capitol Hill.

## POLICY BOOKS FOR READERS WHO WANT TO DIG A LITTLE DEEPER

- *The Politics of Health Legislation: An Economic Perspective* (2nd ed.) by Paul Feldstein (Health Administration Press, 1996). An economist explores how individuals, groups, and legislators act in their own self-interest.
- *Governing Health: The Politics of Health Policy* by Carol Weissert and William Weissert (Johns Hopkins University Press, 2002). Excellent overview of health policy and how politics shapes policy.
- *Don't Think of an Elephant! Know Your Values and Frame the Debate* by George Lakoff (Chelsea Green Publishing Company, 2004). An examination of how conservatives and liberals think differently.

- *Agendas, Alternatives, and Public Policies* by John Kingdon (Longman, 2002). Kingdon is highly revered and constantly quoted by policy experts.
- *The New Politics of State Health Policy* by Robert Hackey and David Rochefort (University Press of Kansas, 2001). Essays on health care issues with which the states have had to struggle.

***Newspapers.*** Major metropolitan newspapers offer political analysis of national, regional, and local politics. Those recognized for their in-depth political reporting on health issues include the *Washington Post (www.washingtonpost.com)*, the *New York Times (www.nytimes.com)*, the *Los Angeles Times (www.latimes.com)*, and the *Wall Street Journal (www.wsj.com)*.

***Television.***  Network and cable news programs and television news-magazines address political issues and government activities. The ultimate viewing experience for true political voyeurs is C-SPAN. This channel is available as a public service created by the U.S. cable television industry to provide access to the live gavel-to-gavel proceedings of the U.S. House of Representatives and the U.S. Senate and to other forums in which public policy is discussed, debated, and decided. C-SPAN provides a wealth of information about the democratic process, without editing, commentary, or analysis.

***Radio.*** Radio continues to be a rich source of political information and debate.

- National Public Radio. Founded in 1970, National Public Radio (NPR) serves an audience of more than 15 million Americans each week via 620 public radio stations and the Internet *(www.npr.org)*. NPR provides carefully researched in-depth reporting.
- C-SPAN Radio. C-SPAN Radio offers public affairs commercial-free programming 24 hours a day. Listeners may listen through the radio or Internet. The broadcast schedule is available at *www.c-span.org*.
- Liberal and conservative political talkfests. Many political "talking heads" such as G. Gordon Liddy, Rush Limbaugh, Martha Zoller, and Al Franken have radio programs that serve as forums to debate

hot political topics. Check your local newspaper and the radio program Website for air time and station.

**Blogs.** *Blog* is short for *weblog*—one of the communication strategies made possible by the Internet. A blog is an interactive online journal that shares postings from individuals, usually with the most recent entry on top. Many types of blogs have evolved, including personal, advice, political, sports, and corporate blogs. Blogs went mainstream in 2004, when political candidates and news services began to use them. Some examples of political blogs are:

- Blog for America *(www.blogforamerica.com)*. Blog for America (BFA) is the weblog of Democracy for America. It was initiated on March 15, 2003 as a communication tool of the former "Dean for America" campaign. BFA was the first official blog of a presidential candidate.
- Republican National Committee 2008 Presidential Blog *(http://blog.4president.org/2008/)*. Thoughts on the next presidential election.
- South Dakota Politics Blog *(http://southdako-tapolitics.blogs.com)*. Self-described as "a little blog on the prairie."
- Science and Politics. *(http://sciencepolitics.blogspot.com)*. A blog focused on the intersection of politics and science with about 250 postings per day.

What can you learn from a blog? The value of participating in political blogs may be in gaining a "gestalt" of views about certain topics. Offering well thought-out opinions may help others consider issues from your point of view. Keep in mind that there are few controls about what is written on the Internet, so let the blogger beware.

## APPLICATION OF LEARNED SKILLS

Once a nurse learns the basics of influencing policy and politics it is time to decide how and where to apply those skills. Everyday, political decisions are made in hospitals, schools, legislatures, corporations, insurance companies, and professional associations that influence the practice of nursing. Nurses have a choice—to let others make decisions that affect nursing practice or to participate in shaping their own practice. Nurses who desire to have a voice can opt to be engaged at any of three levels described by Leavitt and Trotter Betts (2005). These levels of involvement in politics are identified as the nurse-citizen, the nurse-activist, and the nurse-politician.

## THE NURSE-CITIZEN

Are you a nurse-citizen? The nurse-citizen is a nurse who takes part in fundamental civic responsibilities (Box 3-1). A nurse-citizen brings the perspective of health care to the voting booth, to public forums, and to community activities. The individual keeps current on local, state, and national news related to health and social issues and speaks out in the workplace or in public arenas about issues of concern to residents. For example, the nurse may speak at a school board meeting about the need for health prevention services for children or the necessity of implementing tobacco prevention programs in the school system; or the nurse citizen may work with colleagues at a hospital to establish day care services for employees. The nurse citizen is a committed professional who applies the skills of being an involved citizen with health expertise.

## THE NURSE-ACTIVIST

A nurse-activist takes a more active role in the policy arena than a nurse-citizen, often focusing on issues related to providing expert care to patients (Box 3-2). These may be practice issues related to working conditions that require legislation or collective action to bring about policy change. An example might be challenging limits on advanced

---

**BOX 3-1** The Nurse-Citizen

- Registers to vote
- Votes in every election
- Keeps informed about health care issues
- Speaks out when services or working conditions are inadequate
- Participates in public forums
- interacts regularly with local, state, and federal elected officials
- Joins politically active nursing organizations

Adapted from Chitty, K. (Ed.). (2005). *Professional nursing: Concepts and challenges* (4th ed.). Philadelphia: Saunders.

**BOX 3-2** The Nurse-Activist

- Contacts public officials through letters, email or telephone
- Registers people to vote
- Contributes money to a political campaign
- Works on a political campaign
- Lobbies decision-makers by providing pertinent statistical and anecdotal information
- Forms or joins coalitions that support an issue of concern
- Writes letters to the editors of local papers
- Invites legislators to visit the workplace
- Holds a media event to publicize an issue
- Provides testimony

Adapted from Chitty, K. (Ed.). (2005). *Professional nursing: Concepts and challenges* (4th ed.). Philadelphia: Saunders.

**BOX 3-3** The Nurse Politician

- Runs for elected office
- Seeks appointment to a regulatory agency
- Seeks appointment to governing boards in the public or private sector
- Uses nursing expertise as a policymaker in public or private sector

Adapted from Chitty, K. (Ed.). (2005). *Professional nursing: Concepts and challenges* (4th ed.). Philadelphia: Saunders.

practice, such as those by nurse anesthetists (see *Reimbursement Issues for Nurse Anesthetists: A Continuing Challenge* following Chapter 19), as well as issues such as eliminating mandatory overtime, which creates unsafe conditions for the nurse and patient. The nurse-activist applies political skills to challenge the stakeholders who attempt to restrict practice. Nurse-activists understand the necessity of collective political activity and collective political mentoring to advance the political skills of all nurses.

## THE NURSE-POLITICIAN

The nurse-politician seeks elective office or an appointment to a policy position (Box 3-3). Many examples of nurse-politicians are included in this book. This level of involvement reflects stage four of nursing's political development, in which nursing has attained the power and position to set the agenda and guide the process of policy development and implementation. Although it is often challenging and difficult, more and more nurses are willing to take this giant leap in political activism.

Nurses have made great leaps forward as political candidates. Three nurses have been elected to Congress (see *A Nurse in Congress, I Believed I Could Make a Difference,* and *My Path to Congress,* all of which follow Chapter 24). In 2004 and 2005 there were 79 nurses serving as state legislators (ANA, 2005). These nurses are making a difference

in creating laws and regulations that affect nurses everywhere. They are role models who are leading the way toward more enlightened health policies at the local, state, and federal levels.

## *Key Points*

- All nurses have the opportunity and ability to engage in policy and politics. One needs only the desire to start learning.
- Mentoring and networking are vital parts of learning how to advocate effectively in the political arena.
- There are many ways to learn the ropes of politics and policy; all nurses can design their own learning activities based on personal preference and political goals.

## *Web Resources*

**C-SPAN**
*www.c-span.org*
**GEM-Nursing**—an online mentoring program
*www.gem-nursing.org*
**Mentoring: The Experience of a Lifetime**—
video from the National Student Nurses Association
*www.nsna.org*
**American Nurses Association (Government Affairs)**
*http://nursingworld.org/gova/*

*Continued*

## *Web Resources — cont'd*

**American Nurses Association political newsletter**
*www.capitolupdate.org.newsletter/*
**Roll Call**—Congressional news source
*www.rollcall.com*
**Daily summary of health issues and commentary**
*www.healthleaders.com*
**Resource on multiple policy issues**
*http://hippo.findlaw.com/hippohome.html*
**Synopses of national political news**
*http://politicalinsider.com*
**Policy analysis site**
*www.hschange.org*
**Policy resources**
*http://hippo.findlaw.com/hippohome.html*

## REFERENCES

American Association of Colleges of Nursing (AACN). (1996). *The essentials of master's education for advanced practice nursing.* Washington, DC: AACN.

American Association of Colleges of Nursing (AACN). (1998). *The essentials of baccalaureate education for professional nursing practice.* Washington, DC: AACN.

American Nurses Association (ANA). (2001). Revised code of ethics for nurses with interpretative statements. Retrieved September 19, 2005, from *www.nursingworld.org/ethics/code/protected_nwcoe303.htm.*

American Nurses Association (ANA). (2005). 2004-05 Nurse state legislators and state administrative leaders. Retrieved September 19, 2005, from *www.nursingworld.org/gova/state/nursleg2.htm.*

Chinn, P. (2002). Living in a post–September 11 world. *Advances in Nursing Science, 24*(3).

Cohen, S., Mason, D., Kovner, C., Leavitt, J., Pulcini, J., & Sochalski, J. (1996). Stages of nursing's political development: Where we've been and where we ought to go. *Nursing Outlook, 44*(1), 20-23.

Cohen, S., & Milone-Nuzzo, P. (2001). Advancing health policy in nursing education through service learning. *Advances in Nursing Science, 23*(3), 28-40.

Curtin, L. L. (1979). The nurse as advocate: A philosophical foundation for nursing. *Advances in Nursing Science, 1*(3), 1-10.

Dossey, B., Slanders, L., Beck, D. M., & Attewell, A. (2005). *Florence Nightingale today: Healing, leadership, global action.* Silver Spring, MD: ANA.

Duderstadt, K. G. (2004). Advocacy for children through activism. *Journal of Pediatric Health Care, 18*(5), 217-218.

Foley, B. J., Minick, M. P., & Kee, C. (2002). How nurses learn advocacy. *Journal of Nursing Scholarship, 34*(2), 181-186.

Gebbie, K. M., Wakefield, M., & Kerfoot, K. (2000). Nursing and health policy. *Journal of Nursing Scholarship, 32*(3), 307-315.

Kubsch, S. M., Sternard, M. J., Hovarter, R., & Matzke, V. (2004). A holistic model of advocacy: Factors that influence its use. *Complementary Therapies in Nursing & Midwifery, 10*, 37-45.

Leavitt, J. K., & Barry, C. T. (1993). Learning the ropes. In D. J. Mason, S. W. Talbott, & J. K. Leavitt (Eds.), *Policy and politics for nurses.* Philadelphia: Saunders.

Leavitt, J. K., & Mason, D. J. (1998). The good ol' girls and collective mentoring. In C. Vance & R. K. Olson (Eds.), *The mentor connection in nursing.* New York: Springer.

Leavitt, J. K., & Trotter Betts, V. (2005). Nurses and political action. In K. Chitty (Ed.), *Professional nursing: Concepts and challenges* (4th ed.). Philadelphia: Saunders.

Mallik, M. (1997). Advocacy in nursing—A review of the literature. *Journal of Advanced Nursing, 25*, 130-138.

Mason, D. J., Backer, B. A., & Georges, C. A. (1991). Toward a feminist model for the political empowerment of nurses. *Image: Journal of Nursing Scholarship, 23*(2), 72-77.

O'Brien, J. M. (2003). How nurse practitioners obtained provider status: Lessons for pharmacists. *American Journal of Health System Pharmacy, 60*(22), 2301-2307.

Smith, A. (2004). Patient advocacy: Roles for nurses and leaders. *Nursing Economics, 22*(2), 88-90.

University of California, San Francisco. (2005). Health policy nursing. Retrieved April 28, 2005, from *http://nurseweb.ucsf.edu/www/spec-hpl.htm.*

University of Pennsylvania. (2005). Health leadership minor. Retrieved April 28, 2005, from *www.nursing.upenn.edu/academic_programs/grad/masters.*

University of Rhode Island. (2005). Core courses—Masters program in nursing. Retrieved April 28, 2005, from *www.uri.edu/nursing/msn.html.*

Vance, C. (1977). A group profile of contemporary influentials in American nursing (Doctoral dissertation, Teachers College, Columbia University, 1977). *Dissertation Abstracts International, 38*, 4734B.

Vance, C., & Olson, R. K. (Eds.). (1998). *The mentor connection in nursing.* New York: Springer.

Winter, M. K., & Lockhart, J. S. (1997). From motivation to action: Understanding nurses' political involvement. *Nursing and Health Care Perspectives, 18*(5), 244-250.

# *Vignette*　Sally Phillips

## *Learning to Be the Lead Goose: Making the Leap into Policy*

Canada geese fly in a V-shaped formation, with the lead goose at the point of the V. The V formation is used for flying efficiently; it conserves energy, reduces the workload by decreasing wind resistance, and makes it easy to keep track of each bird in the flock (Library of Congress, 2005). Although fighter pilots use this formation too, I have not found this behavior in nurses since I've been involved in health policy.

### A NOVICE IN THE HOT SEAT

As a young clinician and new faculty member, I joined my professional association, the Colorado Nurses Association, to stay informed about professional and health care issues. Political activism was fairly intimidating, but I knew I could contribute at a basic level: be informed, show up, and listen. At a monthly Colorado Nurses Association meeting, a call went out to the members to come down to the Colorado General Assembly the next morning to demonstrate nursing support for a bill to amend state insurance statutes to include third-party reimbursement for nursing services. We each received a copy of the testimony to be delivered by our association spokesperson. At the time, I was a hospital-based nurse. I knew the significance of such a state law change, but I knew little about the substantive nature of the issue. I felt it would be a good learning experience for me, because I had never been to a committee hearing before—so I decided to go.

### The Memorable Policy Moment

I showed up at the designated room and found a packed hearing room with many familiar faces. The hearing was under way, and the chair called for the association spokesperson to deliver her testimony. No one responded. The chair turned to the audience and asked if anyone was prepared to deliver the testimony before the vote. I looked around the room and saw about 30 faces gazing at the floor. I decided that I could definitely read, so I stepped up and read the prepared testimony on behalf of our association. I was peppered with questions from the committee, and I turned to the audience for support and guidance—but they were gone! The room had cleared! I sat in the hot seat and answered questions for 45 minutes on behalf of nursing and the people we serve. Fortunately, I had paid attention at meetings, read our association publications, and listened to my colleagues at the university lament their inability to be reimbursed.

### THE LESSON LEARNED: BE PREPARED

In a policy forum, you are never a casual observer; be prepared for any opportunity. It is easier and more effective to provide testimony if you are passionate about the subject, immediately affected by the outcome of the issue being considered, and have support lined up.

This early experience in my career was empowering. I learned a lot about myself and about the process. The power we hold as private citizens to influence the legislature is significant, but it pales in comparison with the power nurses have as credible and highly respected health care providers. An unanticipated outcome of this experience was that my colleagues determined that I had skills in lobbying and providing testimony, and they did not hesitate to quickly give that role to me as often as possible. That was all right, though, because, surprisingly, I enjoyed it! Suddenly, I was the lead goose!

### Be Prepared for Opportunity

Soon after my testimony experience, I was approached by the university where I taught about being nominated to serve on the state board of nursing. The nurse educator position on the board was being vacated by a respected educator and colleague. I knew little about the work of the board, but felt it would be a good way to provide a service to my profession. My credentials were submitted to the governor, and I requested endorsement from my state senator (from a different political party than the governor). I had little hope that I would be appointed by the governor—but I was. The first board meeting I attended was overwhelming, and I was awed by the hard work this volunteer board contributed. The regulatory role was impressive but at times inconsistent with the advocacy role I had begun to assume. It was going to be a challenge to align the two. I missed the second meeting of the board while completing my doctoral dissertation defense. On my return, I was notified that I had been elected president of the board!

### LESSON LEARNED: NEVER, EVER MISS A MEETING

Lead goose again, I was assured that the position of president was mostly a "figurehead" position and that my primary role was to facilitate the monthly board meetings. However, that's not what happened. Usually, the state Nurse Practice Act comes before the state legislature for reauthorization every 10 years. Major changes to the legal and regulatory authorities for nursing practice rarely take place in the intervening years. The Nurse Practice Act would be under review for reauthorization by the legislature at the end of my second term, if I was reappointed. So I did not anticipate having to be involved with legislative activity as president. Well, I served two terms, and the Nurse Practice Act was revised *six* times during this period—requiring extensive testimony from the state board of nursing representative.

Before my service, the board's executive director, a paid employee, provided all testimony on behalf of the board. The first revision of the Nurse Practice Act during my tenure was the creation of a Peer Health Assistance Program for nurses with substance abuse problems. I was asked to accompany the executive director and the assistant attorney general to the committee hearing at which the Peer Health Assistance Program was being discussed. I was told, "Just be there, you won't have to say anything." However, after the executive director provided the initial testimony, the committee turned to me with questions. An hour later we were dismissed. Remember the caution, "You are never a casual observer"? After this day, the Nurse Practice Act was revised five more time to address nurses selecting medications from protocols and standing orders, nurse aid certification, advanced practice registration, prescriptive authority for advanced practice nurses, and continuing education for relicensure. Each revision required board testimony, and I was the point person on it each time.

### Memorable Policy Moment: "Touch" Becomes Touchy

The state board of nursing had been challenged with the issue of whether to permit nurses to receive credit for continuing education units in the practice of therapeutic touch. On review of the Nurse Practice Act and the relevant statute and the rules and regulations for continuing education, it was found by the board that education in therapeutic touch was acceptable. Therefore the board ruled that it would continue to accept this training, as it did for other practices, for nursing continuing education credits. However, the issue became controversial—stimulated by a very conservative and political religious group. They mounted a campaign to expose the practice of therapeutic healing touch as "mysticism" and asserted that public safety was at risk and that it was inappropriate for the state to recognize such education programs.

An expert panel was convened several months later to review the scientific and therapeutic validity of this healing modality. The board found once more that it was acceptable for nursing continuing education. As a result of media frenzy and calls to legislators, the state board of nursing members were mandated to participate in a hearing with a senate committee "to attest to their conduct." A call went out to all 11 board members to attend. Two members showed up—I was one and was lead goose again. At the end of the hearing, the authority of the board to interpret and implement the Nurse Practice Act was upheld, and the decision of the board to allow continuing education credits to be earned by nurses in therapeutic touch was supported and sustained.

### Challenge the Status Quo

Nursing college and university faculty members have some unique challenges and opportunities for professional development and career growth. One benefit many faculty members enjoy is the sabbatical. The typical purpose of a sabbatical is to allow a faculty member time to enhance research and publication activities with a temporary break from academic activities. The desired outcome of a sabbatical is a reenergized professional, with new skills and a greater opportunity to generate funding through research grants or prestigious publishing projects. I decided to challenge the status quo and pursue health policy as the focus for a sabbatical. This was highly unusual and had never been done before at the university where I worked. I realized I had to interpret this activity in terms of how it would benefit the university in order to have it approved. I encouraged the university to have a "leap of faith" and give me the chance to turn this sabbatical into a funding opportunity. They tentatively supported the sabbatical proposal. I was lead goose again, but the other geese were no longer with me—I was on my own.

My educational sabbatical proposal was a logical next step in my transformation into "policy wonk." Until this time, my policy activities had been on one side of the legislative hearing table. I had honed my skills in providing expert testimony to committee members on issues related to the professional and legal scope of nursing practice. I had also testified and advocated for support for health care issues as we moved into a managed care environment. My sabbatical was designed to give me a chance to

explore what it was like to be on the "other side of the table." I spent the 120-day legislative session working with the Senate Health, Education, Welfare and Institution Committee of the Colorado State Legislature. This was an opportunity to analyze how policy decisions are made. What were the most influential and effective strategies? What was compelling testimony that influenced a decision? What were the elements of effective testimony and other influential strategies before and after the hearing? What influences were more motivating than the issue itself and the advocacy provided through lobbying efforts?

I learned about all of these policymaking activities and much, much more. The results of my sabbatical were never published, because there were no journals or books interested in such findings at the time. I shared my lessons learned with whoever would listen and used what I learned within my professional association.

## LESSON LEARNED: LOOK OUT FOR UNFUNDED MANDATES

State revenues are finite. Therefore policy decisions must always be made in a fiscally responsible context. An excellent policy proposal that offers good things for the public may be in jeopardy or, at a minimum, in competition with all of the other good policy proposals in light of competing budgetary demands. These budgetary demands are also affected by the unfunded mandates from Washington—federal laws requiring the state to take action but without any funds provided to enact the law. The concept of unfunded mandates intrigued me, and I'd have the chance to see the impact of it.

### Memorable Policy Moment

My clinical background was in neonatal, obstetric, and pediatric nursing. During my sabbatical, a bill was introduced that would codify (make into law) a change to the public indecency statutes. Breastfeeding women in some communities had been arrested for public indecency when breastfeeding in public. I attended a hearing on the issue and expected that the predominantly female committee would not vote the bill out. I was wrong.

I sat in the hearing and was amazed at what I heard. A female legislator with a new granddaughter was the sponsor of the bill. As I listened to her introduction of the bill, my face must have revealed all. Shortly into the testimony phase of the hearing, the chairwoman called for a break. She asked me to join her for a "personal" break. I had been with the committee two months and she had been quite generous with opportunities to engage her in dialogue. She asked my opinion on the bill and why I had problems with it. Remember lesson #1: Be prepared; you are never just an observer. This was my chance to influence the chair on an issue about which she already had made up her mind. She was supporting the bill in concert with her party's conservative agenda. She always voted with the sponsor of the bill. After I spoke with her, though, she voted against the bill and it failed. Lead goose, again on my own.

## MAKING THE LEAP INTO POLICY

The lessons I learned during my sabbatical prepared me for the next step in my evolution. I saw an opportunity not only to address the issue of unfunded mandates from Washington, but also to complete the requirements of my sabbatical (obtain funding and gain prestige for the university). I requested that the chancellor of my university nominate me for the prestigious Robert Wood Johnson Health Policy Fellowship. I was selected. The fellowship would take me to Washington, DC—a new world completely outside of my comfort zone. It was a complete immersion into the world of health policy.

I arrived in Washington, DC in 1999 with five other fellows. The federal health policy agenda at the time was complex. The high-priority issues were Medicare reform and a prescription drug benefit, organ donation, health privacy, health insurance for children, and the Patient's Bill of Rights. A number of important programs were up for reauthorization (provision of ongoing funding), such as the Ryan White Care Act and the Older Americans Act. Although these were the main focus of our early work in the Capitol Hill fellowship, I gravitated toward the issues of terrorism and public health. Before I started the fellowship, a federal multisite exercise had been conducted to test our national response to major disasters—TOPOFF (so named because it was an exercise of Top Officials). I was intrigued by the after-action reports and the work of the Institute of Medicine (IOM) related to terrorism and bioterrorism. I pursued this interest through my early fellowship, building a large file of information and contacts. I served in the office of Senator Tom Harkin (D-IA) during my fellowship year. I worked issues with the Senate Health, Education, Labor, and Pensions committee and the Senate Labor, Health, and Human Service Appropriations Subcommittee. The experience I brought to this work from my nursing education years, and my advocacy on health and regulatory issues, served me well (Figure 3-3).

### Memorable Policy Moment

The IOM is a sponsor of the Robert Wood Johnson Fellowship. The fellows in my group had 3 months of preparation before beginning Capitol Hill experiences. We were aware of an IOM study on health care errors during our fellowship that was soon to be released. The final report—titled "To Err Is Human"—was released in January 2000, my first week in Senator Harkin's office. I was assigned to read the report, synthesize it into one page, and recommend to the Senator what key elements he

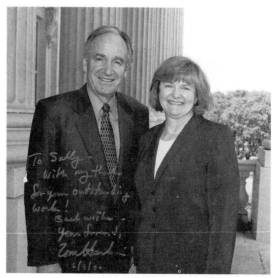

**Figure 3-3** Senator Tom Harkin and Sally Phillips.

should attend to and what his position should be. I was directed to write his floor statements. Within days, I was on the floor of the senate with Senator Harkin as he read the remarks, and that evening I worked with his staff to craft his bill. The bill was not taken up in committee, but the provisions for the proposed program were incorporated into the senate appropriations bill later in the session, supporting research at the Agency for Healthcare Research and Quality (AHRQ) to implement the initiative.

The fellowship covered my university salary for 1 year. On completion of the year, I was expected to return to my university position. However, Senator Harkin asked me to remain on his staff to continue to work on some important issues. My university supported this, and I taught through the online distance education program. I had not made the leap to Washington fully yet. This second year I served on the senate staff as a policy analyst, which positioned me for the future. The lessons learned from the TOPOFF disaster response exercise were published during this period, and a series of other problems got the attention of legislators: the Rajneeshi contamination of restaurant salad bars in Oregon with salmonella and the sarin gas attack in Tokyo, Japan. Senators Edward Kennedy (D-MA) and William Frist (R-TN) introduced a bill intended to bring awareness to the erosion of the public health infrastructure and our vulnerability to a terrorist attack. I aggressively pursued this initiative and encouraged Senator Harkin's support. The bill was not passed that session, but funds were appropriated for AHRQ to begin to address bioterrorism preparedness. Lesson learned: Take advantage of being in the right place at the right time.

## DIAGNOSIS: POTOMAC FEVER

When I finished my second year on Capitol Hill, it was time for the return to my university responsibilities in Colorado. I needed to choose between a fulfilling career as a nurse educator and continuing involvement with policy at the state and association level, or the pursuit of work in health policy at the national level. I interviewed with Dr. John Eisenberg at AHRQ to discuss career options. His analysis was very insightful; he suggested that I had an incurable disease—"Potomac Fever." The only "fix" for my problem was the excitement of policy work "on the Hill." He suggested that I, a new policy wonk, belonged in Washington, DC, and he offered me an opportunity to join his staff. After several months of interviews, and examining my career and life goals, I decided to take him up on his offer. I entered into negotiations for a 1-year nurse scholar position that permitted AHRQ to contract with my university. The position I was offered would allow me to work on issues including nursing workforce, patient safety, and interprofessional education. These were initiatives I had worked on in Colorado, so it was a good fit. I also expressed interest in bioterrorism and public health preparedness and requested to work on this area if anything should develop. AHRQ had received $5 million to do preliminary bioterrorism preparedness research in fiscal year 2000, and the projects were coming to completion. I was offered the opportunity to oversee these final projects. My start date was set for September 12, 2001 but was delayed because of air travel problems after 9/11. I joined AHRQ 1 week before the anthrax attacks in the United States.

### Memorable Policy Moment

A major project at Weill Medical College at Cornell University, funded by AHRQ, was underway in 2001. This research team developed a model for mass prophylaxis and vaccination in collaboration with the New York Mayor's Office of Emergency Management and the New York Department of Health and Mental Hygiene. The model was scheduled to be tested in an exercise on September 12, 2001. The test was postponed, but the model was used to conduct mass prophylaxis for the anthrax attacks in early October in New York City. This simulation model was only one example of the exemplary work that had been done by AHRQ in the area of preparedness and laid the groundwork and visibility for the agency to expand its research capabilities in the development of models and tools for state and local planners to address this new threat environment.

From this point forward, I was hooked. I developed a portfolio of research that would closely partner with the newly created Office of Public Health Emergency Preparedness and the Health Resources Services Administration Bioterrorism Hospital Preparedness Program. In 2002, I resigned from my university teaching position and accepted a full-time position as Director of the Bioterrorism and Public Health Emergency Preparedness Research Program at AHRQ. The portfolio has grown to nearly $30 million—producing over 60 projects and 50 tools and reports for emergency preparedness and response planning. It is a policy wonk's dream job. I serve as the senior advisor for the Agency for Bioterrorism and Public Health Emergency Preparedness Research initiatives, reporting directly to the Director of the Center for Primary Care, Prevention, and Clinical Partnerships. In this position, I respond to all requests for internal or external information and I am the lead project officer on all new extramural grants and contracts on bioterrorism and public health emergency preparedness research. I work collaboratively with other project officers providing oversight and monitoring of projects. I represent AHRQ within the U.S. Department of Health and Human Services. I respond to congressional requests for information, testimony, or other appropriate communications and oversee AHRQ publications for professional journals. I'm also involved in the preparation of budget requests and strategy on funding and dissemination of information.

### LESSON LEARNED: SEIZE THE DAY ... AND NEW OPPORTUNITIES

In my new role, I find opportunities to improve health services, work with the public, and capitalize on my previous experiences. I speak to nursing groups frequently and, when possible, teach classes. Health policy is at the nexus of change, and it is a privilege to work in the field. In my new role, sometimes I'm lead goose and sometimes I'm back in the V. Wherever I am in the formation, I know I'm making a difference.

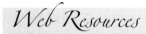

*Lessons Learned*

- I, a nurse educator, successfully made the leap to working in policy.
- Opportunities exist in a variety of government agencies for nurses to influence health policy.
- Nurses are encouraged to take advantage of all opportunities to use their professional knowledge in policy and political activities.

*Web Resources*

> **Agency for Healthcare Quality and Research**
> *www.ahrq.gov*

**REFERENCES**

Library of Congress. (2005). Why do geese fly in a V? *Mysteries of Science.* Retrieved August 30, 2205, from *www.loc.gov/rr/ scitech/mysteries/geese.html.*

---

*Vignette*    Marie Michnich

## The Robert Wood Johnson Health Policy Fellowship

*"Education is for improving the lives of others and for leaving your community and world better than you found it."*

MARIAN WRIGHT EDELMAN

Like most faculty at academic medical centers, I learned that the path to a successful career is built on teaching, research, and community service. As a junior faculty member at the University of

Washington in Seattle, I spent most of my time preparing for classes, juggling grants, advising students, serving on community boards, and keeping abreast of the burgeoning literature in my field of health services research. My career provided me with more than enough opportunities and challenges. Naïve though it now sounds, public policy seemed peripheral to both patient care and academic life, and getting involved in politics sounded like an unrelated, even undesirable diversion. What little I did know about politics and the political process seemed neither compatible nor congruent with professional advancement in my academic career. The notion that a role in national health policy formation and the political process was attainable or even appropriate never occurred to me.

As chance would have it, a classmate of mine from graduate school who was working in Washington told me about the Robert Wood Johnson Health Policy Fellowships (RWJ/HPF) and persuaded me that this was a fantastic opportunity. Why not at least "toss my hat into the ring"? He explained that the fellowship brings mid-career health professionals to Washington, DC to experience a year-long immersion in national health policy, primarily through working assignments in Congress. He even sent me the program brochure to get me started. I was skeptical at first, particularly after noting the prominence of prior awardees, many of whom were tenured medical school faculty. But I needed to find a sabbatical, and this fellowship was well funded, so it became one of several possibilities I decided to pursue. With the support of my dean, I submitted the application in November and tried not to think about my chances.

Two months later, in January, I was notified that I had been selected as a finalist. In February, I headed to Washington, DC for a series of interviews as one of 14 candidates for the fellowship. Admittedly, although the interviews were daunting, I decided that all I could do was give it my best shot, enjoy a side visit to a few museums, and keep my hopes in check. I was surprised when within a day my name appeared on the list of the six awardees invited to start the fellowship the following September. This marked the beginning of a life-transforming adventure.

## BECOMING A ROBERT WOOD JOHNSON FELLOW

My class of fellows included two nurses, three physicians, and a PhD, MBA operations researcher. We began our experience together in an intense and exhaustive orientation to federal health policy-making that spanned 3 full months. We met with the Secretary of Health and Human Services, the Surgeon General, and leaders of the Veterans Administration, the Department of Defense, the National Institutes of Health, the Food and Drug Administration, the Centers for Disease Control, the Health Care Financing Administration (now the Centers for Medicare and Medicaid Services), and the Health Resources and Services Administration. We also visited with influential think tanks, professional societies, trade associations, voluntary health organizations, lobbyists, and law firms. We traveled on foot, in cabs, and by Metro rail to every corner of the District of Columbia, with side trips to Maryland and Virginia. The orientation alone was well worth the move across country and all the challenges associated with taking a year's leave of absence.

After the orientation, we began another new experience—the "job search," or what is euphemistically called "negotiating a work assignment." It had been several years since I had had to look for a job, and I found this anxiety provoking. However, when you don't need to ask for a salary, it was easy to find excellent options, especially since the reputation of this health policy fellowship program is unsurpassed, with congressional offices actually competing to attract a fellow. I interviewed with, among others, the budget office of the White House—called the *Office of Management and Budget,* better known as the OMB; the office of then Congressman Richard Gephardt (D-MO); and the U.S. Senate Finance Committee, under the Chairmanship of Senator Bob Dole (R-KS). All three offered me a placement. The Senate Finance Committee won out, primarily because the principle health staffer on the Committee at that time was Sheila Burke, one of the most respected and talented Hill staffers, with extensive health legislative experience. She was also a nurse and an enthusiastic mentor. In November, I began my assignment with the Committee.

During my first few weeks at the Senate Finance Committee, Senator Dole was elected Majority Leader of the U.S. Senate. Although it was possible to remain with the Finance Committee under the incoming Chair, I was invited by Sheila to join her on Senator Dole's Leadership staff. Truthfully, I did not have a clue what this change meant to my ability to work on health issues; however, I took a chance and stayed with my first preference—to continue working with Sheila and Senator Dole. Within a few months, I was able to see, first hand, what author Eric Redman called "The Dance of Legislation" from the best catbird seat in the U.S. Senate. I worked on bills that reformed physician reimbursement, changed the formula for graduate medical education funding, revised payments for rural hospitals, and fashioned the ill-fated catastrophic health insurance proposal for Medicare beneficiaries that was later repealed. The most thrilling experience in those early days, though, was meeting with just about every major player in the arena of health policy. Given the hearings, conferences, and meetings with myriad lobbying groups and coalitions, the opportunities to both learn and contribute were limitless.

Equally thrilling, but more accurately reflecting the role of the fly on the wall, were the times when I found myself in the same room as England's Prime Minister, Margaret Thatcher, or when I turned a corner and found myself face to face with President Ronald Reagan or took a shortcut through the press office and bumped into news anchor Tom Brokaw. Attending the State of the Union Address, walking to the floor of the U.S. Senate, delivering a message to the Senate Cloak Room and watching the 4th of July fireworks with senators and congressmen from the West front of the Capitol will always stand out as my fondest memories.

My own experience was mirrored by that of my colleagues. Three of them also worked in Congress; we even found opportunities to work together on particular pieces of legislation. One fellow worked on a congressional advisory body, and another accepted an assignment with the Department of Defense. Subsequent to the fellowship year, three fellows went on to become deans of medical schools and a school of nursing, one became chair of a department in a school of public health and one added a significant health policy research component to his career in academic medicine. I remained in Washington, DC, initially as a U.S. Senate health staffer, then in an executive position with a medical professional

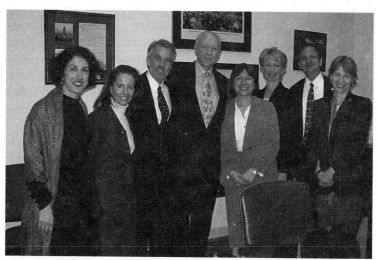

RWJ Fellows Class of 2003-2004. *Left to right*, Rita Redberg, MS, MD; Ellen-Marie Whelan, RN, PhD; Michael Painter, JD, MD; Senator Orrin Hatch (R-UT); Susan Sacvo-Gallagher, MPH; Pam Bataillon, RN, MBA; Vipul Mankad, MD; Debra Haire-Joshu, RN, PhD.

society; later I held a directorship at the Institute of Medicine of the National Academies.

The experiences and outcomes of my cohort were typical of others who came before, and those who followed. In formal and informal evaluations of the fellowship, program alumni routinely report that the experience they gained with the RWJ/HPF accelerated the rate of leadership advancement, added a new dimension to their previous careers, or, as in my case, created an entirely new career path.

## A CHOICE FOR NURSING

I am concerned that many talented, capable, and experienced nursing leaders share my earlier and erroneous perceptions about the nature, value, and attainability of a role in national health policy. In conversations with my colleagues at conferences and meetings, as well as in talking with those who make inquiries about this particular fellowship, it is common to hear doubts about successfully adding health policy formation to the list of one's professional accomplishments. Others identify the daunting logistics associated with taking time out of busy and complicated lives to become active in Washington, DC.

Nurses have well-established track records and have been highly successful players in shaping health policy at the federal level. Of the nurses who have been Robert Wood Johnson Health Policy Fellows, most remain, to this day, highly regarded members of the policy community. Unfortunately, over the last 32 years and 200 fellows and alumni, only 18 recipients of the award have been nurses.

My two decades of work experience as a health policy analyst in Washington, DC alongside a wide range of health professionals confirm that the experience and skills that we acquire as nurses, including our additional capabilities as administrators, educators, and researchers, make us well suited to policy roles at the federal level. Our clinical training, skills as team players, observation abilities, and role as patient advocates combine to make us legitimate assets in the policymaking process. The experience in DC enables a different but complimentary capability. I frequently point out that we now see the world through a different lens. One alumnus has described the transition as moving from "playing checkers to playing chess."

## HOW NURSES CAN GET INVOLVED

For more than three decades, mid-career health professionals, including behavioral and social scientists, have competed for the nationally prestigious Robert Wood Johnson Health Policy Fellowships. Over the years, the program has gained wide recognition as the premiere health policy fellowship in Washington, DC, if not the entire nation. Established academicians and health professionals have come to Washington, DC to take on the challenge of working at the nexus of health science, policy, and politics in our nation's capital. The fellowship has a proven track record of success with several of our most prominent health policy leaders. It has always welcomed nurses with well-developed careers and leadership potential. However, for nurses to take advantage of this special experience, they need to apply.

## NURSES WHO HAVE COMPLETED THE FELLOWSHIP

Among the 18 nursing alumni of this program, three have become deans of schools of nursing. More than half have taken appointments as state and federal health officials or served on advisory commissions. One became a president of the American Nurses Association. Most who returned to academia have been promoted to the rank of full professor. Two accepted professional staff positions in Congress, and two are currently working in the U.S. Senate, one as a fellow in the personal office of the Majority Leader of the Senate, and one as a professional Staff Director to a senator. Most of the nursing alumni who continue to teach have retained a health policy component in their teaching and their community service (Table 3-1).

## Professions of Robert Wood Johnson Health Policy Fellows: 1974-2005

| | | |
|---|---|---|
| Internal Medicine or Family Practice | 58 | (30%) |
| Pediatrics | 21 | (10%) |
| Other Physician Practices | 37 | (19%) |
| Social Science | 25 | (12%) |
| Nursing | 18 | (8%) |
| Dentistry | 12 | (6%) |
| Public Health | 10 | (5%) |
| Other | 18 | (9%) |

**TABLE 3-1** Robert Wood Johnson Fellowship Listing

| NURSE AND YEAR OF FELLOWSHIP | CURRENT POSITION |
|---|---|
| Marion D'Lugoff, RN, MA 1976-1977 | Formerly Clinical Director, Lillian D. Wald Community Housing Center, Assistant Professor of Community Health<br>The Johns Hopkins University School of Nursing |
| Sister Rosemary Donley, RN, C-ANP, PhD 1977-1978 | Ordinary Professor and Director of Community, Public Health Nursing<br>The Catholic University of America |
| Diane O. McGivern, PhD, RN, FAAN 1981-1982 | Professor, College of Nursing<br>New York University |
| Judith B. Collins, RNC, MS, OGNP, FAAN 1982-1983 | Associate Professor Emeritus<br>Virginia Commonwealth University Schools of Nursing and Medicine |
| Marie E. Michnich, RN, DrPH 1984-1985 | Director, Health Policy Educational Programs and Fellowships<br>The National Academies—Institute of Medicine |
| Mary O. Mundinger, RN, DrPH 1984-1985 | Dean, School of Nursing, Centennial Professor in Health Policy<br>Columbia University School of Nursing |
| Hurdis Griffith, PhD, RN 1986-1987 | Emeritus Dean and Professor<br>Rutgers, The State University of New Jersey College of Nursing |
| Virginia Trotter Betts, MSN, JD, RN 1987-1988 | Commissioner<br>Tennessee Department of Mental Health and Developmental Disabilities |
| Barbara E. Langner, PhD, RN 1988-1989 | Policy Advisor<br>University of Kansas School of Nursing |
| Debra R. Wirth, RN, MSN 1994-1995 | Executive Director, The Consortium for Southeastern Hypertension Control<br>Wake Forest University Baptist Medical Center |
| Wendy B. Young, RN, PhD 1995-1996 | Retired |
| Sally Phillips, RN, PhD 1999-2000 | Director of Bioterrorism Preparedness Research Program<br>Agency for Health Care Research and Quality |
| Pamela Bataillon, RN, MSN, MBA 2003-2004 | Assistant Dean for Administration<br>University of Nebraska Medical Center, College of Nursing |
| Debra Haire-Joshu, RN, PhD 2003-2004 | Professor of Behavioral Science and Director Obesity Prevention and Policy Center<br>St. Louis University School of Public Health |
| Ellen-Marie Whelan, RN, NP, PhD 2003-2004 | Staff Director<br>Senator Barbra Mikulski (D-MD) |
| Nancy Short, DrPH, MBA, RN 2004-2005 | Assistant Dean<br>Duke University School of Nursing |

## Program Overview

The stated goals of the fellowship are:
- To develop leaders in academic medicine, nursing, pharmacy, dentistry, public health, and the social and behavioral sciences who will contribute more effectively to the health of the public and the professions and institutions that contribute significantly to the nation's health by virtue of their experience in the RWJ Health Policy Fellowships program
- To enable outstanding and experienced professionals to obtain first-hand experience in the development of health policy and programs in the Congress or the executive branch of the federal government
- To assist Congress in its legislative and oversight responsibilities through the provision of staff with expertise in the health professions or the behavioral and social sciences applied to health

The program is unique among fellowships in a number of ways. First, unlike many fellowships targeted to entry-level "post-docs," this one is aimed at exceptional academics and seasoned health professionals. The program seeks those who have an established track record of outstanding achievement and evidence of increasing levels of responsibility and leadership in their home communities, institutions, or organizations. The selection process favors individuals who are quick learners, team players, and personable. These traits are essential for the fast-paced orientation and the eventual work assignments in high-powered federal offices.

Fellows typically take on the role of congressional staff and fully participate in the responsibilities of deliberating and crafting most aspects of health legislation and/or other elements of the policy formation process. They bring valuable and real-world experience and knowledge about health and health care to the negotiating table, substance that might otherwise not be found in traditional federal legislative and regulatory policy formulations. They meet with constituents, lobbyists, and nationally prominent opinion leaders. They staff committee hearings, and some even participate in negotiations among the House, the Senate, and the Administration on health legislative initiatives.

Finally, this fellowship is well funded. The stipend is $155,000 for up to 3 years. Up to $84,000 is available for the salary offset for the year in Washington, plus fringe benefits. The remaining funds may be used either to extend the fellow's stay in Congress or to fund post fellowship leadership development activities, such as attending conferences or seminars or dedicating a portion of time to health policy projects. The award may be made only to nonprofit institutions and organizations, and not to individuals. More recent updates on application deadlines and selection criteria may be found on the program website at *www.iom.edu/rwj.*

## *Lessons Learned*

- Too few nurses participate in policy debates and deliberations, which have a profound impact on our profession and our patients.
- We need to be sure that our brightest and most accomplished are ready to become full partners in the policymaking process.
- The Robert Wood Johnson Health Policy Fellowship is an excellent option for those nurses ready to learn how to shape the solutions.

## *Web Resources*

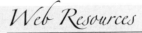

**Information about the Robert Wood Johnson Health Policy Fellowships**
*www.healthpolicyfellows.org*

## How a Nurse Learned to Advance Geriatric Nursing Issues

*"Any time you have an opportunity to make a difference in this world and you don't, then you are wasting your time on Earth."*

ROBERTO CLEMENTE

In 1968, when I first considered focusing my professional efforts in geriatrics, the field was very young. Medicare and Medicaid had just been enacted in 1965, and people aged 65 and over constituted only 9% of the nation's population. In nursing, students were not yet learning to do physical assessments, and the nurse practitioner movement was in its infancy. While completing my masters and doctorate at Teachers College, Columbia University, I was influenced by one of the strongest gerontology faculty in the country, led by Ruth Bennett, a renowned social gerontologist. Their perspective on aging, and specifically their focus on family systems and on healthy aging, has colored my thinking about geriatric nursing throughout my career. Over the past 37 years, I have been privileged to help shape geriatric nursing. In this essay, I emphasize a few lessons learned that I hope are helpful to others embarking on careers in which they too hope to influence policy.

### TAKE ADVANTAGE OF SERENDIPITY IN MOVING A POLICY AGENDA FORWARD

Early in my career I was lucky to be in the right place at the right time. The first teaching position I accepted, in 1973, was in the nursing program at Lehman College, City University of New York. In working with Dr. Claire Fagin, Department Chair, and Dr. Diane McGivern, Director of Medical-Surgical Nursing, I was exposed to some of the most creative thinking in nursing. The program at Lehman was very young, and senior faculty were open to new ideas.

With my newly minted doctorate, I asked for and was encouraged to shape the junior year Medical Surgical course at Lehman to focus on care of older patients. Course content and clinical experiences were developed that provided a perspective on aging—for example, content on geriatric assessment and syndromes was added to existing content on pathophysiology of hip fractures. This was my first experience in trying to "turn students on" to geriatrics, and we soon realized that clinical faculty knowledge, experience, and enthusiasm were key to successful student evaluations. I continue to encounter Lehman graduates who directed their clinical and academic careers toward geriatrics as a result of our initial experiments in geriatric undergraduate education.

My initial position in academia taught me several things that have stayed with me throughout my career. It confirmed my love for my chosen field of geriatrics. I learned that situations of ambiguity or flux often offer enormous opportunity for change and for creativity. I tasted what it felt like to develop and publish about a new program area, and I found that I liked the challenge. I also became acutely aware of the benefits that came from working with outstanding professionals who are willing to serve as mentors in moving one's career forward.

### APPRECIATE THE DIFFERENCE BETWEEN A "JOB" AND A "CAREER"

My experience at Lehman had changed me. I no longer saw teaching as a "job," but rather envisioned myself has having a "career" in academic geriatric nursing. In the late 1970s, when Drs. Fagin and McGivern accepted positions as Dean and Associate Dean at the University of Pennsylvania School Of Nursing, I had to weigh their offers to recruit me to Penn against the needs of a husband and four

**58**

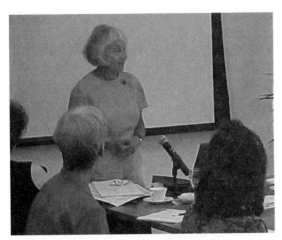

Mathy Mezey has prepared nurses from across the country to conduct important research on nursing care of older adults, disseminate best practices, and influence policymakers on important older adult issues confronting our nation and communities.

teenage daughters. The opportunity to start and to lead the geriatric nursing initiative at Penn eventually won out, and, with my family's encouragement, in 1981 I began 10 years of commuting, most often daily, between New York and Philadelphia.

From the beginning of my tenure at Penn, I recognized that developing and leading a clinical program in geriatric nursing at a Research I university was no small undertaking. In my first 5 years at Penn, we recruited geriatric faculty, started a geriatric nurse practitioner program, integrated geriatrics into the undergraduate nursing program, markedly expanded a university-wide geriatrics initiative, and wrote, sometimes successfully, numerous federal and foundation research and education grants. My position required long hours at the university, travel, and work on weekends. None of this, obviously, could be accomplished without the active support and involvement of my family, who both took pride in my work and picked up the pieces left by my chaotic work schedule.

## ACCOMMODATE TO THE NOTION THAT YOU ARE NEVER READY FOR THE NEXT STEP

In 1982, Claire Fagin told me about a new program of the Robert Wood Johnson Foundation (RWJ),

the Teaching Nursing Home (TNH). Modeled on medical school relationships with Veterans Administration hospitals, the TNH was a 5-year initiative that linked schools of nursing with nursing homes for the expressed purpose of improving care in the nursing homes and strengthening geriatrics in undergraduate and graduate nursing programs. The TNH would be RWJ's first, and highly visible, national clinical nursing initiative, and the foundation wanted to establish the coordinating center for the TNH at Penn. I thought that my lack of experience in nursing homes and in leading national programs left me ill equipped to lead such an initiative, but when Claire indicated that if not me she would find someone else, I immediately agreed to the position.

The TNH thrust me, and Joan Lynaugh, PhD, RN, FAAN, the TNH Co-Director, into a totally new arena of health policy and politics. I participated with the nation's best and the brightest minds in health care at quarterly meetings held at the RWJ Foundation. The TNH required us to identify, convene, and travel with an advisory board made up of, in addition to nurses of national renown, leaders in health policy, regulation, academic medicine, and geriatrics. At the 11 schools of nursing and nursing homes selected to participate in the TNH, we worked with some of the most prestigious deans of nursing and administrators in long-term care. Finally, as leaders of a major initiative of the major foundation in health care, we were expected to act as national spokespersons for the TNH program. The TNH evaluation showed significant improvements in resident care as a result of the involvement of schools of nursing and more faculty involvement and stronger geriatric experiences for nursing students (Mezey & Lynaugh, 1989; Shaughnessy, Kramer, Hittle, & Steiner, 1995). An important, unanticipated outcome was the development of a cadre of nursing faculty who have sustained a commitment to practice and research in long-term care.

The TNH allowed me to gain confidence in my ability to "speak" for geriatric nursing. Critical to honing my skill in advancing a policy agenda was the ongoing mentoring of Claire Fagin and others who advised me with regard to how to:

■ Think strategically about how to "behave" in groups (e.g., speaking up and posing key questions)

- Maximize the input of an advisory board (e.g., educating non-nurse board members about the importance of geriatric nursing and asking for their consultation in specific aspects of the TNH initiative such as policy and reimbursement)
- Take hold of and shape site visits (e.g., using site visits to further an agenda by engaging key stakeholders in the TNH project)
- Seek out and develop lasting relationships with leaders

These lessons were especially important in my sustained relationships with policymakers and geriatric leaders, including Bruce Vladeck, who headed the Health Care Financing Administration (now CMS), and Robert Butler, who at the time was Director of the National Institute on Aging. Under their tutelage I came to appreciate that every meeting and social event should be approached as "work" and as an opportunity to advance an agenda.

I acquired confidence in my "ownership" of geriatrics and geriatric nursing and my ability to frame arguments, skills critical to influencing nurses, policymakers, and health care professionals other than nurses. I became comfortable writing and speaking about geriatrics and geriatric nursing and to their broad effect on health care in general. I came to know the "best and brightest" in geriatric care, a network that I continue to call on. I developed a point of view regarding how change occurs, becoming more enamored of incremental change as opposed to dramatic change. I came to appreciate the benefits of persistence (which was not hard for me) and patience (which *was* hard).

## CAPITALIZE ON THE "PULSE" OF THE HEALTH CARE ENVIRONMENT

In the 35 or so years since I attained my masters degree, the world has seen a revolution in the population aged 65 and over. The declining birth rate and the increased actual longevity of populations, primarily in the developed world but now increasingly in the developing world, have dramatically changed our views on aging. In the United States today, over 12% of people are 65 years of age; this number will increase to 20% of the population by 2030. On average, people who live to age 65 can anticipate living an additional 19 years. The number of people aged 85

and over has grown from just over 100,000 in 1990 to 4.2 million in 2000.

With the rising number of older people with chronic physical illnesses and who experience the cognitive declines of dementia, and with Medicare as a major payer for care, geriatrics is now the core business of hospitals, home care, and nursing homes, and this will become even more true in the years to come.

At the same time, we have seen a revolution in how information is disseminated to and communication occurs among health care professionals and the public. The emergence of the Internet as a vehicle for communicating knowledge and as a teaching tool, unknown obviously when I began my academic career, continues to shape our thinking with regard to how to reach students, faculty, practicing nurses, and health care institutions where nurses work.

The lessons I learned in the TNH stood me in good stead when in 1993, soon after I accepted a faculty position at New York University, I was asked by the John A. Hartford Foundation to develop and then head the John A. Hartford Foundation Institute for Geriatric Nursing (the Hartford Institute; *www.hartfordign.org*). The Hartford Institute was the first national program in nursing undertaken by the Hartford Foundation. Since the initial $5 million investment in the Hartford Institute, the Hartford Foundation has committed $35 million in support of geriatric nursing (*www.hgni.org*). The Hartford Institute remains the only nurse-led organization seeking to shape the quality of the nation's health care for older Americans by promoting geriatric nursing excellence to the nursing profession and to the larger health care community. The Hartford Institute accomplishes its mission through work in nursing education, practice, research, and policy.

Capitalizing on the evolving health care and information environment has shaped the Hartford Institute's policy agenda in nursing and aging. The Hartford Institute has sought to take advantage of this demographic imperative on several fronts:

- We are targeted and focused (a "Johnny one-note") in determining Institute priorities and programs. As one example, our singular focus was useful in engaging the American Association of Colleges of Nursing (AACN) to examine their involvement in promoting geriatrics in baccalaureate education, an initiative that has led to substantial funding to AACN from the Hartford Foundation for a multi-pronged initiative in geriatric nursing.

■ We direct our programs to the level of the individual nurse and the environments (hospitals, home care, nursing homes) in which nurses work.

■ We seek out alliances with nationally recognized organizations. Our alliances with AACN, the American Nurses Association (ANA), the American Organization of Nurse Executives, and the Alzheimer's Disease Association have been instrumental in the broad adoption of Hartford Institute products in academia and practice.

■ We create coalitions and use the "bully pulpit" to arrive at and disseminate policy statements. We are publishing guidelines on caseloads for advanced practice nurses in nursing homes that resulted from a Hartford Institute initiated Consensus Conference. At the Hartford Institute, we have developed a diverse number of initiatives that address our strategic approach to policy in nursing and aging *(www. hartfordign.org)*.

■ We shape public policy on aging and care of older adults. Responding to national and state legislative concerns about care of residents in nursing homes, we proposed and disseminated higher standards for nurse staffing in nursing homes than current Medicare requirements, standards that have been adopted by some states and have influenced legislation and regulations such that they are now the mandated levels of staffing in those states' nursing homes.

■ We influence educational policy. In nursing education, we have taken advantage of the changing demographics to engage national nursing associations in setting standards and competencies for geriatric nursing education. Partnering with the AACN, the Institute has developed competencies for geriatric nursing care for baccalaureate and for masters programs that influence nursing education now and potentially for years to come.

■ We support the development of organizational policy on competence. Recognizing the needs of practicing nurses for help in caring for their older patients, the Institute has produced and partnered with the ANA to widely disseminate print and online information sources about best practices in geriatric care that are shaping practice for specialty nurses and geriatric policies throughout the health care system *(www.geronurseonline.org)*.

■ We advocate institutional policies that support excellence in the care of older adults. Anticipating the need of hospitals to address their increasing case load of older patients, the Institute developed NICHE (*N*urses *I*mproving *C*are for *H*ealthsystem *E*lders) (Mezey et al. 2004). Currently NICHE provides technical assistance on how to improve care to older patients to 160 hospitals nationwide *(www.NICHE.org)*.

■ We seek to build one voice for nursing on geriatric care. The Institute has convened a Coalition of Geriatric Nursing Organizations representing five nursing associations whose sole focus is the care of older adults, to speak with "one voice" on issues of concern to nursing and older adults.

■ We actively create opportunities to disseminate information on caring for older adults. The Institute publication, *Nursing Counts*, provides data related to nursing care of older adults and is distributed through the *American Journal of Nursing* and through mailings to local, state, and national legislatures and their staffs.

## LEARN, AS A LEADER, TO USE YOURSELF AS AN "INSTRUMENT FOR CHANGE"

As my career has evolved, I have come to appreciate the potential of the opinions and observations of leaders to influence policy; to support, mentor, and advance the careers of the next generation of nurses; and to act as a spokesperson and promoter for the field as a whole. My goal is to position myself, but more importantly the next generation of talented nurses working in academic nursing and in practice, at the major tables where health care for older adults is being debated and decisions are framed. My message regarding the role of nurses in shaping health care for older adults has become clearer, sharper, and more consistent. For example, in my speeches and writing, my message is consistent, e.g. that care of older adults is *the* core business of health care and that with few exceptions every nurse is a geriatric nurse. Increasingly I take advantage of writing editorials and white papers, convening consensus conferences, and accepting speaking engagements, almost always in collaboration with others, as vehicles to drive an agenda in nursing and aging. A key strategy is to seek out opportunities to introduce myself and other nurses to policymakers, federal and state legislatures, regulators and funding bodies, foundation staff, and other key decision-makers in health care. Finally, through nominations for awards and fellowships and prestigious positions in professional associations, I seek to celebrate and advance the careers of the nurses who will carry the torch of geriatric nursing into the next generation.

## *Lessons Learned*

- Take advantage of serendipity in advancing a policy agenda.
- Appreciate the difference between a "job" and a "career."
- Accommodate to the notion that you are never ready for the next step.
- Capitalize on the "pulse" of the health care environment.
- Learn, as a leader, to use yourself as an "instrument for change."

## *Web Resources*

**Federal Interagency Forum on Aging-Related Statistics, National Center for Health Statistics**
*www.agingstats.gov*
**John A. Hartford Foundation Institute for Geriatric Nursing**
*www.hartfordign.org*
**John A. Hartford Foundation Geriatric Nursing Initiatives**
*www.hgni.org*
**Nurse Competence in Aging**
*www.geronurseonline.org*

## REFERENCES

Mezey, M., Kobayashi, M., Grossman, S., Firpo, A., Fulmer, T., & Mitty, E. (2004). Nurses Improving Care for Healthsystem Elders (NICHE): Implementation of best practice models. *Journal of Nursing Administration, 34*(10), 451-457.

Mezey, M., & Lynaugh, J. (1989). The Teaching Nursing Home Program: Outcomes of care. *Nursing Clinics of North America, 24*(3), 769-780.

Shaughnessy, P., Kramer, A., Hittle, D., & Steiner, J. (1995). Quality of care in teaching nursing homes: Findings and implications. *Health Care Financing Review, 16*(4), 55-83.

*chapter*

4

# A Primer on Political Philosophy

Sally S. Cohen & Monika Piotrowska-Haugstetter

*"If I were to attempt to put my political philosophy tonight into a single phrase, it would be this: Trust the people."*

ADLAI STEVENSON

All of the politics and policies discussed in this book have underlying issues that are infused with some basic understanding of political philosophy. Although most people engaged in health policymaking focus primarily on the strategies used in advocating for a particular issue, it is also important to understand the fundamental themes that structure debates, limit options, and motivate many of those in positions of power. Most of these themes are derived from political philosophy and have historical roots that have evolved over time and assume slightly different meaning in contemporary health policy deliberations

In this chapter, we present major concepts from political philosophy so that nurses will be mindful of the ideologic, philosophic, and political themes that structure contemporary health policy debates.* Such knowledge can enhance the ability of nurses to develop strategies that take into account political and ideologic perspectives, many of which are not always evident but nonetheless often drive political deliberations. After an introduction to political philosophy, we present an overview of the state and

---

*This chapter provides a cursory overview of political philosophy, but in no means is meant to be a comprehensive discussion. Readers interested in more detail are encouraged to pursue items on the reference list or consult the *Internet Encyclopedia of Philosophy*, available online at *www.iep.utm.edu*.

its relationship with individuals. Next, major political ideologies and their evolution are explained. This leads to a discussion of what policy analysts often refer to as the "welfare state" and its differences across nations in terms of public and private roles and responsibilities. We conclude with a discussion of the implications of political philosophy for nurses involved in health politics and policy.

## POLITICAL PHILOSOPHY

Political philosophy examines, analyzes, and searches for answers to fundamental questions about the state (discussed later) and its moral and ethical responsibilities. It asks questions such as, "What constitutes the state?" "What rights and privileges should the state protect?" "What laws and regulations should be implemented?" "To what extent should government control people's lives?" Political philosophy encompasses the goals, rules, or behaviors that citizens, states, and societies ought to pursue. It provides generalizations about proper conduct in political life and the legitimate uses of power (Hacker, 1960). Political philosophers take into account the capabilities of people and societies. Therefore philosophers' moral assumptions and the realities of their times shape their perceptions and writings. Today's political philosophers build on the classic works of the past and apply them to contemporary issues, including health policy. From another perspective, political philosophy addresses two issues. The first is about the distribution of material goods, rights, and liberties. It encompasses the rights and responsibilities of residents of a specific geographic locale and how people can exercise those privileges and duties to meet their personal and social needs. The second issue pertains to the possession and determination of political power. It includes questions such as, "Why do others have rights over me?" "Why do I have to obey laws that other people developed and with which I disagree?" "Why do the wealthy often have more power than the majority?" (Wolff, 1996).

Political philosophy is a normative discipline, meaning that it tries to establish how people ought to be, as expressed through rules or laws. It involves making judgments about the world, rather than simply describing or observing people and society. Political philosophers attempt to explain what is right, just, or morally correct. It is a constantly evolving discipline, prompting us to think about how the concerns and questions just described, although as ancient as society, affect us today.

For nurses, political philosophy offers ways of analyzing and handling situations that arise in practice, policy, organizational, and community settings. For example, it helps determine how far government authorities may go in regulating nursing practice. It offers ways of understanding complex ethical situations—such as end-of-life care, the use of technology in clinical settings, and reproductive health—when there is no clear answer regarding what constitutes the rights of individuals, clinicians, government officials, or society at large. Political philosophy offers normative ways of addressing such situations by focusing on the relationships among individuals, government, and society. Finally, political philosophy enables nurses to think about their roles as members of society, organizations, and health care delivery facilities in attempting to attain important health policy goals, such as reducing the number of people without health care coverage and eliminating disparities among ethnic groups. To achieve these goals, nurses also need to address larger issues of poverty, income distribution, and allocation of resources, all of which entail the balance among the rights and responsibilities of individuals, health care professionals, and the state.

## THE STATE

The "state" in political philosophy (and political science) does not pertain to the 50 U.S. states. Rather,

it is a "particular kind of social group" (Shively, 2005, p. 13). Centuries ago government as we know it today did not exist. Rather, kings and their soldiers held power. Over time, states developed control over war, peace, governance, and industry. The nineteenth century Industrial Revolution greatly contributed to the growth of the modern state. Commerce and industry relied on states to support the expansion of transportation and communication through laws and other policy venues. Conversely, commerce and industry enhanced the development of the state as the latter sought ways to levy taxes, build their defense apparatuses, and develop internal operations.

The state arose from the notion that people cannot rule at their will. As Andrew Levine (2002) explained, "Few, if any, human groupings have persisted for very long without authority relations of some kind" (p. 6). Concentration of power in a "single, centrally controlled mechanism of administration and coercion" characterizes the origins of the modern state (Levine, 2002, p. 6). This coercion or, more precisely, the ability to influence people's compliance with rules is necessary for sustaining peace and orderly conduct and for advancing the good of individuals and society as a whole. Political ideologies, described later, provide ways of discerning the best way to achieve those ends.

Today's modern state is a highly organized government entity that influences many aspects of our lives (Shively, 2005). It typically refers to the "governing apparatus that makes and enforces rules" (Shively, 2005, p. 56). Therefore the terms *state* and *government* may be interchangeable. It is the role of the state (or government) in health policy issues—such as licensure of health professionals and institutions, financing care, ensuring adequate environmental quality, protecting against bioterrorist attacks, and subsiding care—that affects nurses in their professional practice and personal lives. Usually people think of national governments as the modern state. However, local and state governments also assume important roles in protecting individuals, regulating trade, and ensuring individual rights and well-being. In distinguishing between a nation and a state, note that a state is a *political entity* "with sovereignty," meaning it has responsibility for the conduct of its own affairs. In contrast, a nation is "a large *group of people* who are bound together, and recognize a similarity among themselves, because of a common culture" (emphasis added) (Shively, 2005, p. 51).

Despite these distinctions, the terms *state* and *nation* often overlap in common parlance because government leaders often appeal to the "emotional attachment of people in their nation" in building support for the more legal entity, a state (Shively, 2005, p. 52). Furthermore, our global society, with the cultural diversity of most countries, makes claims of common cultural ties as the distinguishing feature of any nation increasingly difficult to uphold. That said, few would dispute that the political culture of the United States is different from that of other countries. We pride ourselves on individualism, a laissez-faire approach to government and economics, and a strong belief in the rights of individuals. Policy analysts often point to our unique political culture as an explanation for why U.S. social policy deviates from that of other countries. Two examples are our lack of a universal health insurance policy and our being one of two nations (out of 192) that have not ratified the United Nations Convention on the Rights of the Child. (The other is Somalia.) These policies follow a strong American tradition of a carefully delineated relationship between individuals and the state.

## INDIVIDUALS AND THE STATE

**Thomas Hobbes.** One of the major political philosophers to describe the relationship between individuals and the state was Thomas Hobbes (1588-1679). (See Table 4-1 for a summary of the contributions of Hobbes and other major philosophers discussed in this chapter.) Hobbes developed the concept of the "social contract," which basically claims that "individuals in a hypothetical state of nature would choose to organize... their political affairs" (Levine, 2002, p. 18). As Shively succinctly explained, "Of their free will, by a cooperative decision, the people set up a power to dominate them for the common good" (Shively, 2005, p. 38). Hobbes's theory was intended to defend the rights of kings, but one can use it to justify other forms of government and authority. His thinking was important in establishing governance and authority,

**TABLE 4-1** Major Political Philosophers*

| POLITICAL PHILOSOPHER | MAJOR CONTRIBUTIONS |
| --- | --- |
| Thomas Hobbes (1588-1679) | Social contract; individuals will voluntarily form governments to provide for common good |
| Thomas Locke (1632-1704) | Individual inalienable rights; different from legal rights |
| Jeremy Bentham (1748-1832) | Utilitarianism—individuals are utility maximizers; government exists to maximize happiness for greater good |
| John Stuart Mill (1806-1873) | Liberalism, but not to the extent that it might harm others |
| Karl Marx (1818-1883) | Socialism—reliance on state policies to protect working class and ensure equity; common ownership of resources |

*An excellent resource for reading about these and other major philosophers is the *Internet Encyclopedia of Philosophy* (www.iep.utm.edu).

without which people would live in a natural state of chaos. To avoid such situations, according to Hobbes, people living in communities voluntarily establish rules by which they abide.

Nurses can view the social contract as a rationale for government intervention in aspects of practice, public health, and delivery of care. We turn to government to protect us from situations such as unregulated care and unlicensed practice, which might cause harm to patients if professionals and administrators were left to their own devices. We voluntarily adhere to these rules to prevent danger and minimize the consequences of unmonitored care.

**John Locke.** Despite its advantages, the social contract doesn't adequately address the importance of individual rights. British political philosopher John Locke (1632-1704) greatly influenced liberal thinkers, including the writers of the U.S. Constitution, by emphasizing the importance of individual rights in relationship to the state. His defense of individual rights was fundamental to liberalism (discussed later) and the development of democracies around the world. For Locke, individual rights were more important than state power. States exist to protect the "inalienable" rights afforded mankind. One of the premises of Locke's theories is that people should be free from coercive state institutions. Moreover, the rights inherent in such freedom are different from the legal rights established by governmental authority under a Hobbesian contract. They are basic to the nature of humanity.

**Jeremy Bentham.** Jeremy Bentham (1748-1832), heralded as the father of classic utilitarianism, rejected the natural law tradition. His utilitarianism theory basically asserted that individuals and governments strive to attain pleasure over pain. When applying this "happiness principle" to governments, "it requires us to maximize the greatest happiness of the greatest number in the community" (Shapiro, 2003, p. 19). Instead of relying on natural law, Bentham favored the establishment of legal systems, "enforced by the sovereign" (Shapiro, 2003, p. 19). Acknowledging that people are "individual utility-maximizers who care nothing for the overall good of society," Bentham called for a "robust role for government in computing people's utilitarian interests and enacting policies to further them" (Shapiro, 2003, pp. 22-23). Therefore quantitative reasoning and cost-benefit calculations to "determine the best course for society" were central to his thinking (Shapiro, 2003, p. 24). Bentham's utilitarianism has become foundational to many contemporary theories in economics, political science, bioethics, and other disciplines.

The tension between individual rights and the role of the state is inherent in many health policy discussions. Consider, for example, substance abuse. On one hand, individuals have the right to smoke tobacco and drink alcohol. One might even argue that the state should protect individuals' rights to do so. On the other hand, such freedoms may interfere with others' rights to fresh air and freedom from harm (e.g., from second-hand smoke inhalation or from incidents related to alcohol use). In such cases, the state has a legitimate role to intervene and protect the rights of others—the greater good. The challenge lies in finding the right balance between the rights of individuals on both sides of the issue and balancing them with the rights of the state.

Hobbes, Locke, and Bentham are among the classic philosophers whose work set the stage for subsequent moral, political, and ethical discourse. Locke's concepts of liberty, in particular, are basic to other versions of liberalism, a description of which is beyond the scope of this chapter. Liberalism has also been the underlying premise of many contemporary political ideologies.

## POLITICAL IDEOLOGIES

A political ideology is a "set of ideas about politics, all of which are related to one another and that modify and support each other" (Shively, 2005, p. 19). Political ideologies are characterized by distinctive views on the organization and functioning of the state. Ideologies give people a way of analyzing and making decisions about complex issues on the political agenda. They also provide a way for policy-makers to convince others that their position on an issue will advance the public good. Three major political ideologies—liberalism, socialism, and conservatism—originated with eighteenth and nineteenth century European philosophers and are the basis of political deliberations and policies throughout the world (Shively, 2005). Each is described in the following sections, followed by an overview of contemporary American ideologies, which are variations of traditional liberalism and conservatism. It is important to remember that terms and definitions of liberalism and conservatism as they have evolved over time are not necessarily consistent with these two ideologies as they exist today. Nonetheless, without appreciating their origins, the nuances in their rhetoric and their role in health policy cannot be fully understood.

### LIBERALISM

American political thought was greatly influenced by eighteenth century European liberalism and the political thinking of Hobbes, Locke, and others. To fully grasp the impetus for such intellectual revival, one must recall that medieval Europe was a repressive agricultural society with wealthy nobility, monarchs, and clergy (especially the Roman Catholic Church) holding power. The seventeenth and eighteenth centuries brought industrialists, who sought to move goods across land and sea; scientists, who sparked innovation in work and family life; and artists, whose creativity freed the mind from parochialism. Thus, eighteenth century liberalism meshed well with political, economic, scientific, and cultural trends of the time—all of which sought to free people from confining and parochial values. Liberalism relies on the notion that members of a society should be able to "*develop their individual capacities to the fullest extent*" (emphasis in original) (Shively, 2005, p. 24). People also must be responsible for their actions and must not be dependent on others.

**John Stuart Mill.** John Stuart Mill (1806-1873), a British political philosopher, is considered a major force behind contemporary liberalism. His essay *On Liberty* (1859) is foundational to modern liberal thinking. Mill was committed to individual rights and freedom of thought and expression, but not unconditionally. He based his work on Locke's philosophies, tempered by Bentham's utilitarian philosophy.

Mill contended that individuals were sovereign over their own bodies and minds but could not exert such sovereignty if it harmed others. In a sense, Mill provides a way of reconciling Locke's emphasis on individual rights with Hobbes' focus on the importance of an authoritarian state. A leading contemporary political philosopher, Ian Shapiro, applied Mill's balancing of individual rights with his "harm principle" as follows:

. . . although sanitary regulations, workplace safety rules, and the prevention of fraud coerce people and interfere with their liberty, such policies are acceptable because the legitimacy of the ends they serve is "undeniable" (Shapiro, 2003, p. 60).

The best form of government under liberal ideology is a democracy, in which individuals participate in political decision-making and express their views freely. The right to vote confers an important privilege to members of a democracy in that it is a form of political expression free from domination by others.

In sum, liberal ideology is based on the importance of democracy; intellectual freedom (e.g., freedom of speech and religion); limited government involvement in economic activities and personal life; government protections against abuse of power by one person or group; and placing as many choices as possible in the private realm (Shively, 2005). In many ways, liberalism lies at the center of American political thought. Our early settlers came here seeking a new life, free from the old, more-rigid order in Europe. Centuries later the liberal tenets that motivated our founders and those who followed endure.

## CONSERVATISM

In response to liberals' calls for changing the existing social and political order, conservatives countered with a preference for stability and structure. They preferred patterns of domination and power that had the benefit of being predictable and gave people familiar political terrain. Under conservative thought, those in power had the "awesome responsibility" to "help the weak." In contrast, liberals preferred to give such individuals "responsibility for their own affairs" (Shively, 2005, p. 26). Liberals wanted people to be free of government intrusion in their lives; conservatives favored a strong government role in helping those in need of assistance.

Guided by the notion that government had a responsibility to provide structured assistance to others, nineteenth century European conservatives, especially in Great Britain and Germany, developed many programs that featured government support to the disadvantaged (e.g., unemployment assistance and income subsidies). They accepted welfare policies (discussed later) that were foundational to the revival of Europe after World War II. Despite the upheavals of the war, which destroyed the status quo, conservatives have found their place in European politics today. They have been major players in contemporary European politics, especially in Great Britain, offering a synergy with American conservatism (discussed later).

## SOCIALISM

Socialism grew out of dissatisfaction with liberalism from many in the working class. Unable to prosper under liberalism, which relied on individual capacities, socialists looked to the state for policies to protect workers from sickness, unemployment, unsafe working conditions, and other situations.

**Karl Marx.** Karl Marx (1818-1883), a German philosopher, is widely considered the father of socialism. For Marx, individuals could improve their situation only by identifying with their economic class. The nineteenth century Industrial Revolution had created a new class—the working class—which, according to Marx, was oppressed by capitalists who used workers for their profits. According to Marx, only revolution could relieve workers of their oppression.

As a political ideology, socialism encompasses many ideas. Among them are equality regardless of professional and/or private roles; the importance of a classless society; an economy that contributes equally to the welfare of a majority of citizens; the concept of a common good; lack of individual ownership; and lack of any type of privatization. Therefore socialism is also an economic concept under which "the production and distribution of goods is owned collectively or by a centralized government that often plans and controls the economy" (Socialism, 2005). The collective nature of socialism is in contrast to the primacy of private property that characterizes capitalism.

Socialism originated and proliferated in Europe toward the end of the nineteenth and in the early twentieth centuries. Then it split into two parties: Communist and Democratic Socialist. In 1917, Communists, under the leadership of V. I. Lenin, took over the Russian Empire and formed a socialist state, the Union of Soviet Socialist Republics (USSR). Lenin and his Communist followers believed in revolution as the only way to advance socialism and achieve total improvement in workers' conditions. Democratic Socialists, in contrast, were more willing to work with government institutions, participate in democracies, and "settle for partial improvements for workers, rather than holding out for total change" (Shively, 2005, p. 33). Communism prevailed in most Eastern Europe countries until the late 1980s. Between 1989 and 1991, communist regimes in Eastern Germany, in the USSR, and throughout Eastern Europe collapsed. In their quest for economic and political change, the new Eastern European governments have turned to democracy, democratic socialism, capitalism, and other economic and political models.

Today, only a handful of countries (e.g., Cuba, China, North Korea, and Vietnam) are under communist rule. Socialists, especially Democratic Socialists, have prevailed in Scandinavia and Western Europe. They have been instrumental in advancing the modern welfare state in those countries and elsewhere around the world (Shively, 2005).

## CONTEMPORARY CONSERVATISM AND LIBERALISM

Contemporary political conservatism, which grew in popularity in the late twentieth century, is similar to classic conservatism (described previously) but differs from it in several ways. In particular, conservatives oppose a strong government role in assisting the disadvantaged. Recall that the conservative political philosophers of the eighteenth and nineteenth centuries supported the state's role in helping individuals through social policies. Now, liberals are the ones who generally favor a strong government role in social policies such as health, welfare, education, and labor, whereas conservatives prefer minimal government intervention and reliance on privatization and individual choice.

As proponents of earlier models of conservatism did, contemporary conservatives oppose rapid and fundamental change. They call for devolution of federal responsibility for health and other social issues to state governments, a diminished presence of government in all aspects of policy, reduced tax burden, and the importance of traditional social values. Many political observers point to the 1980 election of President Ronald Reagan as a turning point for the rise of American conservatism. Reagan had a strong conservative constituency, and once in office he promoted policies that were in keeping with its views. For health care this meant a decrease in federal spending on public health initiatives such as maternal and child health, mental health, and reproductive health services, especially abortions. The 1980s and the rise of conservatism diminished the influence of liberal voices on the American political and health care scene.

In contrast to conservatives' calls for a decreased federal presence in health care policy, liberals today support an expanded government role to help people who need income support, health care coverage, child care assistance, vocational guidance, tuition, and other aspects of social policy. They follow their liberal predecessors, who in the 1930s and 1940s supported President Franklin D. Roosevelt's New Deal policies, which aimed to help the disadvantaged in the wake of the Great Depression. The Great Society programs of President John F. Kennedy and Lyndon B. Johnson in the 1960s and early 1970s further boosted American liberal policies. Among the highlights of the Great Society initiatives were the enactment of Medicare, Medicaid, and Head Start. These federal government programs are founded on the importance of the state helping the disadvantaged through government-sponsored programs. These initiatives are in line with traditional liberal philosophies, described previously, which support the notion that individuals should be given equal opportunities to pursue their inalienable rights. Such rights include their health and welfare, broadly defined, even though the right to health care is not a legal one under our Constitution.

Since the mid 1990s, conservatives and liberals have found themselves in a somewhat ironic situation. Conservatives have deviated from their preference for the status quo by favoring rampant changes in certain aspects of social policy. Among them are privatizing Social Security and inserting the federal government into the public education domain under the No Child Left Behind (NCLB) law. Liberals, on the other hand, often find themselves as the defenders of the status quo as they fight to sustain public programs, such as Medicaid. Each of these stances also reflects ideologies of their respective camps. In calling for the privatization of Social Security, for example, conservatives are staking their claim for a diminished federal role and for a stronger market orientation. In wanting to preserve and increase funding for Medicaid and other social policy programs, liberals retain their position that the federal government has an important role in helping the disadvantaged.

George Lakoff, a well-known linguist and political scientist, has developed an interesting way of explaining the differences between contemporary liberals and conservatives by designating each as a particular type of parent. For Lakoff, conservatism revolves around the so-called "Strict Father" model. It is an authoritarian structure that emphasizes the traditional nuclear family in which the father plays the essential role in supporting and protecting the family as well as in establishing rules for the behavior of children and strictly reinforcing these policies. Parental authority is expressed through "tough love" (Lakoff, 2002, p. 33).

According to Lakoff, liberalism favors an entirely different approach to family life, the so-called "Nurturant Parent." "Love, empathy, and nurturance are primary" (Lakoff, 2002, p. 33). "Children become responsible ... and self-reliant through being cared for, respected, and caring for others, both in their family and in their community" (Lakoff, 2002, p. 34). This metaphor of caring for children applies to liberals who support policies for other dependents, such as welfare recipients and the disabled. These liberals want to make sure that basic needs such as food, shelter, health care, and education of members of society are met. They focus on investing in social programs as a form of social support. Conservatives oppose this approach because it fails to sustain self-discipline and reinforces moral weakness.

These differences between conservatives and liberals can be seen with many issues, such as health care. Conservatives think that government regulation interferes with individual choice and "the pursuit of self-interest" (Lakoff, 2002). They prefer policies that increase coverage of the uninsured through tax credits. The latter would give money to individuals and families in the form of a credit on taxes owed. The recipients could then use the money to purchase health care of their choice.

Liberals regard governmental regulations as a protection. Citizens must be protected against those who pollute the natural environment, jeopardize workers' safety and health, deceive customers, and manufacture danger products. Their approach to covering the uninsured is typically to extend existing government entitlement programs, such as Medicaid and Medicare, and the State Children's Insurance Program (SCHIP), to those who are ineligible under existing law.

This description places liberals and conservatives at two extremes of an ideological continuum. Most people's views, however, lie between these two extremes. Nonetheless, it is clear that conservatives have succeeded in framing their issues in ways that have attracted voters and increased their political strength. Lakoff (2002) and other political observers have noted how conservatives have successfully framed their positions so as to attract popular support and appeal to voters' emotions. Since 1980, they have linked their moral politics with public policy. In contrast, liberals have struggled to reframe their message and find a comparably strong approach that will elevate their status among American voters and policymakers. The question is, can liberals regain their position or is the conservative ascendancy a sign of a large political and social shift in American society? Lastly, it should be noted that although conservatives are usually Republicans and liberals are usually Democrats, this is not always the case. Many moderate Republicans side with Democrats on issues such as covering the uninsured, abortion, and women's rights. Similarly, many conservative Democrats side with Republicans when voting in their legislative bodies or in considering the role of the modern welfare state.

Many organizations are aligned with a liberal or conservative ideology (Table 4-2). They often take policy positions on health care and other issues that are in concert with an ideological perspective. However, similar to elected officials, they may deviate from these positions on any given issue. Nursing organizations welcome members of all political persuasions and strive to foster tolerance among different ideological and partisan points of view.

## THE WELFARE STATE

The welfare state refers to the "share of the economy devoted to government social expenditures" (Hacker, 2002, pp. 12-13). Health policy analysts often compare aspects of the welfare state among developed countries. In such comparisons the United States typically ranks lowest for public social

**TABLE 4-2** Organizations and Think Tanks That Are Aligned with a Political Ideology on Health Policy Issues

| ORGANIZATION | WEBSITE |
|---|---|
| **CONSERVATIVE** | |
| American Enterprise Institute | *www.aei.org* |
| American Council on Science and Health | *www.acsh.org* |
| American Family Association Foundation | *www.afa.net* |
| Concerned Women of America | *www.cwfa.org/main.asp* |
| Family Research Council | *www.frc.org* |
| Heritage Foundation | *www.heritage.org* |
| Hudson Institute | *www.hudson.org* |
| National Center for Public Policy Research | *www.nationalcenter.org* |
| **LIBERAL** | |
| Americans for Democratic Action | *www.adaction.org* |
| Center for Public Policy Priorities | *www.cppp.org* |
| Center for Law and Social Policy | *www.clasp.org* |
| Center for the Study of Social Policy | *www.cssp.org* |
| Children and Family Futures | *www.cffutures.org* |
| Choice USA | *www.choiceusa.org* |
| Families USA | *www.familiesusa.org* |
| Institute for Women's Policy Research | *www.iwpr.org* |
| National Health Law Program | *www.healthlaw.org* |
| New America Foundation | *www.newamerica.net* |
| People for the American Way | *www.pfaw.org/pfaw/general* |

expenditures as a percentage of the gross domestic product (GDP). Explanations for this "American exceptionalism" include the philosophical traditions inherent in American culture, as discussed previously. However, if one adjusts for tax burdens, such as income taxes, and other public subsidies, then the United States ranks closer to the middle (Hacker, 2002).

Social policies have many different components. When health care expenditures alone are considered, the United States ranks highest among industrialized nations for health care spending as a percentage of GDP. Another unique aspect of the American welfare state is that most health care spending comes from the private sector. Nonetheless, escalating public expenditures, primarily for Medicare and Medicaid, are a main cause of concern to federal and state policymakers and are an important aspect of the American welfare state.

The origins for much of the modern welfare state in Europe and the United States can be traced to the post–World War II period, when, after the war's devastation, government leaders wanted to provide health and other social services to rebuild their economies and their people. One of the best examples of such activities was the establishment of the British National Health Service (NHS), a government-administered and government-financed health insurance and delivery system to which all U.K. residents are entitled (see *The National Health Service in the United Kingdom* following Chapter 13). In the late 1930s the United States also expanded its welfare state to ameliorate the devastation of the Depression. The 1935 Social Security Act, which established the Social Security program, welfare, federal maternal and child health programs, and other important initiatives, is the cornerstone of our welfare state. As described above, it was expanded in the 1960s and early 1970s, when activist government again prevailed.

Since the 1980s the welfare state has been in a state of flux in the United States and across Europe. Government budgetary constraints and a wave of conservatism put a brake on the expansion of the welfare state and made policy analysts question its future direction. One response to the constraints on the welfare state in countries such as the United States

and Canada, the United Kingdom, and Germany has been the infusion of competition, accountability, and requirements for increasing private sector responsibility in the provision of health care. This was exemplified by the growth of managed care in the United States, the increased accountability of physicians and the infusion of market-oriented practices in the United Kingdom, and tightening of rules regarding physician income in Canada.

## TYPES OF WELFARE STATES

There are many different types of welfare states, based on the division of responsibilities for social services between public and private sectors and the role of a central government authority. The most well-known categorization is Esping-Andersen's (1990) description of three types of welfare states: social-democratic, corporatist, and liberal. Remember that this categorization encompasses all aspects of social policy. Health care as a specific component of welfare policy is discussed later.

*Social-democratic* welfare states refer to the Scandinavian countries, where most social programs are publicly administered and relatively few privately sponsored social benefits are offered. In these countries, social democratic regimes, as described previously, "were the dominant force behind social reform." These countries have "pursued a welfare state that would promote an equality of the highest standards…." This means that services are generally all on a par with those provided to the "new middle classes" and that workers are guaranteed "equality of rights enjoyed by the better-off" (Esping-Andersen, 1990, p. 27).

*Corporatist* welfare states are typically the Western European nations (e.g., France, Italy, and Germany), where social rights and status differentials have endured and affected social policies. These countries grant social rights to many but primarily provide state interventions when family capacities fail. They lack the universal tendencies of social-democratic states. Because of the strong influence of the church, especially the Catholic Church, in these nations, they tend to preserve traditional values.

*Liberal welfare states* stand apart from the more socially stratified corporatist welfare states and include the United States, Canada, and Australia, where privately sponsored benefits dominate. Among liberal-welfare states, the United States is distinctive for its large percentage of social spending in the form of privately sponsored benefits (Hacker, 2002). In liberal welfare states the "traditional, liberal, work ethic norms" prevail. Welfare and other social benefits are highly stigmatized, and the state encourages market involvement as much as possible (Esping-Andersen, 1990, p. 26).

## HEALTH CARE AND THE WELFARE STATE

Moran distinguishes between the "welfare state" and the "health-care state." The latter is part of the welfare state but needs to be analyzed separately. "Health care institutions are influenced by, and of course influence, the wider welfare state; but they are also shaped by dynamics of their own—some of which are internal to, and some of which are external to, the health care system" (Moran, 2000, p. 139). The concept of "health care state" is important because states and health care institutions... are joined symbiotically" (Moran, 2000, p. 147). As Moran explained:

[H]ealth care is the biggest single consumer of resources in the modern welfare states and states are either directly the dominant financiers of health care or are central to the regulation of institutions that provide the money... Health care looms large in the modern welfare state, and states loom large in modern health-care systems" (Moran, 2000, pp. 138-139).

Moran proposed three "governing areas" of the health care state: health care consumption, provision of care, and the development and use of technology. Each involves a particular role for the state and its own "system of politics" (Moran, 2000, p. 146).

**Consumption.** Regarding consumption, many schemes exist for a package of services to the whole population or a subgroup, each involving a key role for the state. They may be the "only third party payer who matters (United Kingdom and Scandinavia); the biggest single third party payer (United States); they may be centrally involved in struggling with the inadequacies of existing systems of third-party payment (United States, again)"; or they may "provide a public law framework for the institutions

that dominate third-party payment" as in Germany and other countries (Moran, 2000, p. 142).

**Provision of Care.** Moran identifies two major aspects of the provision of care: hospital government and professional government. Arrangements for hospital government vary from the NHS, where the "central state" owns and controls hospital care, to the United States, where most hospitals are privately operated with large public subsidies. As for professional government, analyses typically focus on physicians, who are perceived as the mainstay of most important providers. This provides an excellent opportunity for nurse researchers to examine how nursing care varies in its governance and arrangements across countries as part of welfare and health care policy analysis. Nonetheless, regarding physicians, variations across nations persist—for example, in Scandinavian nations, physicians are salaried state employees, and in the United Kingdom, physicians are "self-employed contractor[s]... with little freedom to generate discretionary income" (Moran, 2000, p. 143).

**Development and Use of Technology.** States have been crucial for the development of technology, especially regarding its funding. States also regulate technology by "promoting drug safety" or "classifying medical devices" (Moran, 2000, p. 145). It is also important to recognize that much technology is produced by private corporations. Even though the state regulates their commerce and development, entrepreneurs from the private sector own the technology and have a huge deal of discretion over property rights, marketing strategies, and other aspects of technology production (Moran, 2000, p. 146).

## POLITICAL PHILOSOPHY AND THE WELFARE STATE: IMPLICATIONS FOR NURSES

How might nurses apply these concepts of political philosophy to their involvement in health politics and policy? Rather than sitting on the sidelines, nurses—regardless of partisan preference—can participate in the ideological and political debates that shape health policies. Each of us has perspectives on the role of government and the rights of individuals with regard to certain health policies. They form our own ideology and political positions. Figure out where you stand on an issue and the underlying ideology that informs your views. Then use that knowledge as the basis for advocating for policies that have the potential to improve health policy and patient outcomes. In so doing, be mindful of the philosophical traditions that shape your views.

When engaging in political deliberations, listen to the rhetoric that others use and identify the underlying political and philosophical threads. Use similar language, as long as it is based on sound knowledge, when you meet with policymakers or use written texts to advance your positions. Two cases, covering the uninsured and motor-cycle helmet use, make these points more clearly.

First, consider the issue of reducing the number of uninsured Americans. If one believes that the government's role should be minimal and individuals should largely be accountable for health care purchasing and costs, then tax credits and other types of individual health care accounts would be the policy of choice. If, on the other hand, one believes that the state is largely responsible for ensuring a basic minimum of health care, then one would prefer the expansion of government-sponsored programs, such as Medicare, Medicaid, and SCHIP, to cover those presently lacking insurance. People in this camp might also lean toward a single-payer option, with the state or federal government being the designated payer. The same model can be used for the issue of health care quality—that is, one would rest responsibility with the private sector or the state, depending on one's ideology.

Similar issues arise when considering issues of public health, such as motorcyclists' use of helmets. For example, one view, taken predominantly by traditional liberals, might be that motorcyclists have the right to decide for themselves whether or not they wear helmets. Others, using a Hobbesian or social contract framework, might argue that it is in the best interest of society at large for riders to wear helmets and abide by laws requiring them to do so. This is partly because of the cost to society, but mostly because the state has a responsibility to protect individuals, which in turn promotes a peaceful and orderly society. Individuals, in turn, have a responsibility to yield to the state in its attempts to maintain order. There are some cases in which the state may need to limit individual freedoms in order to protect the state at large. Variations among the American states in helmet laws depict the different approaches to the balance of power among individuals, the state, and the community at large. The relationship between nursing and the state has yet to be carefully explored. Connolly (2004) states, "Undertaking political history...requires an understanding of how government works, in both theory and practice" (p. 16). Yet, there are many aspects of nursing's political history that remain untapped and that warrant a close examination of how the profession has interacted with state structures in the policy process. Recent examples that come to mind are the 2002 Nursing Reinvestment Act and the role of nursing under health care reform.

Whether working with public officials, strategizing to create links between policy and practice, or studying the role of the state in public policies that pertain to nursing, political philosophy is the foundation of thought and action. It can be a lively aspect of nurses' strategic thinking in linking policy, politics, and practice.

## Key Points

- Philosophers have developed concepts for explaining the relationships between individuals and the state.
- Modern conservative and liberal ideologies are based on past political philosophies but are adapted to the realities of today's welfare state.
- Issues such as covering the uninsured and motorcycle helmet laws demonstrate the legacies of past philosophers, the endurance of the role of the state, and the conflicts over exactly what that role might be.
- Nurses have many opportunities to be involved in such deliberations and to research the role of the state in nursing issues.

## REFERENCES

Connolly, C. A. (2004). Beyond social history: New approaches to understanding the state of and the state in nursing history. *Nursing History Review, 12,* 5-24.

Esping-Andersen, G. (1990). *The three worlds of welfare capitalism.* Princeton, NJ: Princeton University Press.

Hacker, A. (1960). *Political theory: Philosophy, ideology, science.* New York: MacMillan.

Hacker, J. S. (2002). *The divided welfare state: The battle over public and private social benefits in the United States.* New York: Cambridge University Press.

Lakoff, G. (2002). *Moral politics: How liberals and conservatives think.* Chicago: University of Chicago Press.

Levine, A. (2002). *Engaging political philosophy from Hobbes to Rawls.* Malden, MA: Blackwell Publishers.

Moran, M. (2000). Understanding the welfare state: The case of health care. *British Journal of Politics & International Relations, 2*(2), 135-160.

Shapiro, I. (2003). *The moral foundations of politics.* New Haven: Yale University Press.

Shively, W. P. (2005). *Power and choice: An introduction to political science* (9th ed.). Boston: McGraw-Hill.

Socialism. (2005). Online encyclopedia, thesaurus, dictionary definitions and more. Retrieved August 8, 2005, from *www.answers.com/topic/socialism.*

Wolff, J. (1996). *An introduction to political philosophy.* Oxford, UK: Oxford University Press.

# chapter 5

# Policy Development and Analysis: Understanding the Process

Barbara Hanley & Nancy L. Falk

*"A problem clearly stated is a problem half solved."*
DOROTHEA BRANDE

Nursing's progress toward reaching full professional status are largely due to nurses' active involvement in state and federal policymaking. Accomplishments for nurses, such as direct insurance reimbursement, prescriptive authority, obtaining major funding for the National Institute for Nursing Research, and obtaining higher levels of autonomy for nurses in practice, are a direct result of the nursing community's active political and policy involvement. The purpose of this chapter is to provide a theoretic and rational approach to the study of broad policy development and analysis and a primer on identifying and analyzing policy issues. Through this chapter, nurses will have a greater theoretic and practical knowledge of both the policy-making process and issue analysis as they seek to resolve policy problems in either the institutional or public policy sphere.

A major thrust of the chapter is the current and projected nursing shortage. What has been perceived as a "nursing issue" is now identified as a public policy problem because of its implications for access to health care services. Recent findings depict a growing shortage of nurses compounded by a lack of qualified nursing faculty. This situation portends the policy problem of how to ensure public access to nursing services in light of growing demand as the "Baby Boomer" generation ages. Concurrently, escalation in the frequency of health system change continues to create power vacuums, offering new opportunities for nursing—usually outside the hospital setting. Meaningful contribution to the debates on workplace issues concerning staffing, mandatory overtime and safety concerns, access to health care services, new models for insurance coverage, and Medicaid and Medicare reform necessitates nurses' understanding of how the policymaking system works, including development and analysis of proposals.

Although nurses are increasingly employed or participating in policy-related positions, their influence on institutional as well as governmental policy requires integration of policymaking knowledge and skills into all nursing roles. Understanding the concepts, approaches, and strategies in policymaking and having basic skills in issue analysis are essential to nurses' meaningful contribution to policy development in both the private and the public sectors.

## DEFINITIONS

### POLICY

Policy encompasses the authoritative guidelines that direct human behavior toward specific goals, in either the private or the public sector. It includes the broad range of activities through which authority figures make decisions directed toward a goal and levy sanctions that affect the conduct of affairs. Such courses of action may be termed *policy proposals, alternatives,* or *options* (Anderson, 1997). Health care agencies or institutions make *private* policy, including directives governing conditions of employment and guidelines for service provision. *Public* policy refers to local, state, and federal legislation, regulation, and court rulings that affect individual and institutional behaviors under the respective government's jurisdiction, such as state licensure for professional practice, insurance reimbursement policy, and Medicare and Medicaid legislation. However, the two are closely linked because institutional policy frequently reflects implementation of or compliance with public policy.

## HEALTH POLICY

*Health policy* refers to public and private policies directly related to health care service delivery and reimbursement.

## POLICY ANALYSIS

*Policy analysis* is the systematic study of the background, purpose, content, and anticipated or actual effects of standing or proposed policies and the study of relevant social, economic, and political factors (Dye, 1992). It is a process that is extremely valuable to researchers, practitioners, and educators and is applicable within any discipline.

## PUBLIC POLICYMAKING

All public policy definitions refer to policy made on behalf of the public, developed or initiated by government, and interpreted and implemented by public and private bodies (Birkland, 2001). Public policy applies to all members of society and prescribes sanctions for failure to comply. Although Anderson (1990) describes public policy as a purposive course of governmental action to deal with an issue of public concern, Dye's succinct definition (1992), "Whatever a government chooses to do or not to do," is directly to the point. The *failure* to take

action is as important as a decision *for* action. For example, Congressional failure to enact some form of the Clinton Health Security Act in 1994 left a policy vacuum rapidly filled by the for-profit restructuring of the health care system into managed care, and the continued prevalence of the uninsured. In a broader social policy context, during an interview regarding the failure of governmental response after hurricane Katrina in 2005, which had devastating effects on the poor and African Americans, Senator Barack Obama (D-IL) stated that "passive indifference is as bad as active malice" (Page, 2005, p. 15A).

Processes to create public policy include the enactment of legislation and its accompanying rules and regulations, which hold the weight of law; administrative decisions in interagency and intraagency activities, including interpretative guidelines for rules and regulations; and judicial decisions that interpret the law. Schneider and Ingram (1997) extend this list to include more subtle indicators such as texts, practices, symbols, and discourses that define the value-laden delivery of goods and services. Interaction between the public and private health policymaking sectors is increasing because of the complexity of policy implementation and the increasing role of corporate structures in health care finance and delivery.

## POLICY SUBSYSTEMS AND STAKEHOLDERS

**Policy Subsystem.** A policy subsystem includes a network of elected or appointed officials, legislative subcommittees, and interest group representatives and individuals directly involved in shaping a particular policy. The term *stakeholder is* applied to actors that may be directly affected by its outcome. Stakeholders are also relevant in private sector policymaking, although they may not be as highly visible. To address specific policy decisions over time, analysts must also consider the substantive input from researchers, specialist reporters, professional associations, and institutional policy specialists (Sabatier, 1991).

**Health Services Research.** The growing role of policy subsystems underscores the importance of research. Health services research is a powerful tool for interest groups and other stakeholders in influencing the policy process and is therefore a fertile field for nurse researchers. It can be used throughout the policy cycle in supporting one's case, particularly in problem and issue identification and evaluation. Findings can support policy stipulations or the shaping of programs through identification of effective approaches to solving the policy problem. Research is also a key component in policy evaluation; findings may then serve to support the given program or support revision if necessary. For example, Lambrew (2004) describes finding the research data answering the question "Does health insurance matter for children?" as essential for justifying the Clinton proposal to establish the State Child Health Insurance Program (SCHIP). For maximum effectiveness, health services researchers should maintain open communication with legislative staff who address problem areas in their expertise so that they can design studies to produce data relevant to major issues.

Nurses' subsystem roles include interest group activity. To ensure a unified and forceful voice, coalition-building is essential at local, state, and national levels. The Tri-Council for Nursing (American Nurses Association, National League for Nursing [NLN], American Association of Colleges of Nursing [AACN], and Association of Nurse Executives) ensures a unified nursing approach in key policy debates for general nursing issues, and nurse practitioner coalitions such as the National Organization for Nurse Practitioner Faculty address advanced practice issues. The Nursing Organizations Alliance is a more general network of specialty organizations. It supports political education of nursing leaders through the annual Nurses in Washington Internship. Governmentally, the Division of Nursing (DON) in the Health Resources Services Administration sponsors the National Advisory Council for Nursing Education and Practice, which makes policy recommendations to the DON. This creates a mutually beneficial link between this federal agency and the nursing community. Other essential subsystem roles for which nurses are strongly suited and increasingly prepared include elected office and legislative and regulatory staff roles.

True, Jones, and Baumgartner (1999) observe that the American political system is designed to protect the status quo; change requires major mobilization efforts to destabilize the institutionalized gridlock created by policy subsystems. While incrementalism is the primary model for policy change, crises may stimulate major policy change. Cynicism of the system ignores the reality that citizens in a democracy hold the power and entrust authority for decision-making to the three branches of government—the executive branch, the legislature, and the judiciary. Because the judicial process is usually reserved for resolution of dispute, in practice the basic policy loop includes the "Iron Triangle" of the executive branch, the legislature, and interest groups. Policymaking therefore has many points of access, enabling citizens, constituents, legislators, agency officials, interest groups, researchers, and media representatives to exert influence at local, state, and federal levels. The input of substantive experts on behalf of these players is also increasing. Interest group strategies include data gathering, mass marketing, and Internet mobilization of fund raising and lobbying. Finally, Barker (1996) observes that historical, geographic, and technologic contexts play into development of health policy.

Another example of a policy subsystem is the relationship among federal, state, and local governments in the context of health programs (Sabatier, 1991). All three levels function interdependently, creating subgovernments to resolve complex policy issues such as the problem of the underinsured, the uninsured, and the medically indigent. *Federalism* refers to shared power between federal and state governments based on the Constitution; all powers not specifically granted to the federal government reside with the state. The federal role in health and social policy was enhanced during the Great Depression, when states were unable to provide for the basic needs of citizens. The next spurt occurred in the 1960s with President Lyndon Johnson's "Great Society," including the enactment of Medicare and Medicaid to ensure health care for elderly and poor persons. Enactment of the Medicare prescription drug benefit in 2004 is the first major expansion of the program since its inception. However, as health care costs consume an increasingly greater proportion of the gross domestic product, both federal and state policymakers have sought ways to reduce costs and balance budgets.

Changes in Medicaid policy over the past decade, such as the movement of Medicaid into managed care and SCHIP, reflect this budgeting dilemma. Medicaid is a federal program administered by the state with joint federal-state funding. State Medicaid costs rose sharply in the early 1990s because of an increase in federally mandated program benefits and the loss of private health insurance as people lost jobs during the recession. Since 1994, encouraged by the Clinton administration and bolstered by an expanding economy, nearly all states have moved their Medicaid populations into managed care. Enactment of SCHIP in 1997 through the Balanced Budget Act addressed the need for states to provide health insurance for the increasing number of uninsured children when welfare reform eliminated long-term Medicaid eligibility. States expanded coverage of children under Medicaid or special state programs, thereby saving money and in some cases expanding the number of beneficiaries. However, as the federal deficit is increasing as a result of the Bush administration tax cuts and the costs of the war in Iraq and homeland security, the federal government is shifting more of Medicaid costs to the states. This creates strong competition among state programs for scarce dollars, increasing the burden on those in society with the fewest resources.

## FOUR APPROACHES TO PUBLIC POLICYMAKING

Classic conceptual models developed by political scientists provide varying perspectives on public policymaking. Models such as the rational approach, incrementalism, the policy stream model, and the stage-sequential model enable one to consider policy dynamics. Adherents of each model may therefore identify different variables or view the same variables differently in conceptualizing the way in which specific policy decisions are made. All models have merit, although each may have some limitation in its application depending on the policy in question (Sabatier, 1999).

## THE RATIONAL APPROACH

The rational approach to policy decisions reflects the goals of an ideal world. Here, policymakers define the problem; identify and rank social values in policy goals; examine each policy alternative for positive and negative consequences, costs, and benefits; compare and contrast these factors among all options; and select the policy that most closely achieves the policy goals (Anderson, 1997; Dye, 1992). However, because the rational model holds the possibility of sweeping policy change, except for times of national crisis such as the Great Depression when major initiatives are essential, it is an unrealistic approach to general policymaking. Its importance lies in its striving for the ideal solutions in the face of political pressures. The failed Clinton Health Security Act of 1994 provides an example. The Clinton plan proposed a total revision of the health care industry through a blend of market competition and regulation. However, the magnitude of the proposed change enabled those with a vested interest in the status quo to target numerous components, mobilize public fear, and ultimately defeat the proposal. Health care reform was relegated to the state level, where small changes have been made, primarily in insurance law, to increase citizens' access to private insurance. However, state experimentation with different models of health care reform may provide data for future national debate.

## INCREMENTALISM

Policy changes in the United States are most often made incrementally, with small changes at the margins as opposed to radical restructuring of ineffective or dysfunctional systems. Proposals begin with the status quo, and the limited changes reflect the turf, goals, and politics of policy subsystems. The political dynamics among these subsystems are so important that policy options developed without addressing them would have little or no chance for success. Lindblom (1987, 1995) terms this approach "the science of muddling through." Consider the legislative success of the bipartisan Health Insurance Portability and Accountability Act (HIPAA) in 1996 in contrast to the rational and liberal Clinton Health Security Act. As an incremental step in increasing access to health insurance, HIPAA directly addresses the problem of "job lock," the inability to leave a job because a preexisting health problem would prevent a person from obtaining health insurance elsewhere. However, its effectiveness is limited by its failure to limit the amount individuals would have to pay for continued coverage. Furthermore, HIPAA's vague language left to regulators the problem of specifying the complex system necessary for its implementation. Resultant problems continue to plague both state and federal bodies.

Incremental health care reform efforts continue at the state level, where experimentation is occurring with different models such as managed competition and universal access, and both private and public health care financing systems are being overhauled. *Nursing's Agenda for Health Care Reform* (1992), established during the Clinton initiative, provides criteria that are still useful for nurses to evaluate health care reform legislation (Box 5-1).

Similarly, as federal legislation does not mandate reimbursement or prescription authority for advanced practice nurses, power struggles over nurses' roles as primary care providers and managed care network panel members, as well as disputes over prescriptive authority, continue to be fought in many state venues. States continue to take small steps to develop strategies for resolution of the growing nursing shortage.

---

**BOX 5-1   Nursing's Agenda for Health Care Reform**

American nursing became involved with the movement to reform health care in the early 1990s. Several professional nursing associations joined forces to develop *Nursing's Agenda for Health Care Reform* and promote their plan for controlling cost, improving quality, and increasing access. Endorsed by nearly all nursing organizations, it became a visible component of the health care reform debate and produced significant visibility for the nursing profession. Ultimately, however, legislative efforts to comprehensively reform health care in the 103rd Congress failed.

The full text may be viewed at *www.nursingworld.org/readroom/rnagenda.htm*.

---

## THE POLICY PROCESS

Two additional approaches to policymaking use a stepwise process through which a policy moves from problem to working program. Here we look at two models that illustrate how this has been conceptualized. A brief discussion of Kingdon's model (1995) is followed by a detailed description of the stage-sequential model as described by Ripley (1996) and Anderson (1990). The stage-sequential model—the classic chronologic nuts-and-bolts approach—may be more helpful to those new to public policy.*

**Kingdon's Policy Streams Model.** Kingdon's model is based on Cohen, March, and Olsen's "garbage can" model (1972), which describes the process as a series of options floating around seeking a problem. Kingdon likens the situation to a "soup" that contains three streams of activities:

1. *Problem stream.* The problem stream describes the complexities in getting policymakers to focus on one problem out of many problems facing constituents, such as the high out-of-pocket costs of prescription drugs for elders.
2. *Policy stream.* The policy stream describes policy goals and ideas of those in policy subsystems, such as researchers, congressional committee members and staff, agency officials, and interest groups. Ideas in the policy stream float around policy circles in search of problems.
3. *Political stream.* The political stream describes factors in the political environment that influence the policy agenda, such as an economic recession, special interest media or Internet campaigns, or a pivotal political power shift, such as the 2000 presidential election shift of power from Democrat to Republican that intensified when the Republican party gained control of both the House and the Senate in 2004.

---

*Sabatier's Advocacy Coalition Framework (1991, 1999) is another newer model that analyzes political development over at least 10 years. It addresses the dynamics of interacting within policy subsystems based on participants' values and beliefs and the role of policy learning over time. Readers who wish to delve more deeply into policy analysis may find this a very helpful approach.

Kingdon sees these streams as floating around and waiting for a "window of opportunity" to open through "couplings" of any two streams (particularly in the political stream), creating new opportunities for policy change. However, such opportunities are time limited; if change does not occur while the window is open, the problems and options return to the soup and continue floating. An example of this phenomenon is enactment of the Medicare Prescription Drug Improvement and Modernization Act of 2003. The rate of increase in prescription drug costs for aging Americans has kept the problem before legislators over the past decade. However, the window of opportunity opened in 2003 when the problem and political streams came together, allowing enactment of a law that would assist most Medicare beneficiaries.

**The Stage-Sequential Model.** This classic systems-based model views the policy process as a sequential series of stages in which a number of functional activities occur (Anderson, 1990; Anderson, Brady, Bullock, & Stewart, 1984; Ripley, 1985; Ripley, 1996). In this model a policy problem is identified and placed on the policy agenda, then a policy is developed, adopted, implemented, evaluated, and terminated (Figure 5-1). The process is dynamic and cyclical, with policy evaluation and oversight, to identify either a well-functioning program or new problems, thereby restarting the cycle. However, in reality, the stages are often not clear-cut, implementation and evaluation are often done in tandem, and proposals may move back and forth among the stages. Once established, programs are rarely terminated. Figure 5-1 provides Ripley's (1996) model, demonstrating stages of the policy process, activities

inherent in each stage, and resultant policy products. *Stages* refer to the functional activities of policy actors, and *Products* indicate the outcomes or results from each stage. The arrows on the right indicate the theoretic flow of activities with their Products, which allow the next stage to begin. Arrows on the left reflect the activities possible after program evaluation as policymakers determine the future of the policy or program, where new problems may be identified, restarting or reentering the cycle at various points.

*Stage One: Policy Agenda Setting.* The first step in setting a policy agenda is the identification of a policy problem, a "situation that produces needs or dissatisfaction among people for which relief is sought through governmental action" (Anderson, 1997, p. 94). There are many public problems, but only those that gain policymakers' attention for action qualify as policy problems. Anderson and colleagues (1984) term this *getting the government to consider action on the problem.* Ripley (1985) cautions that there may be competition here among groups trying to attract governmental attention to their problems, and competition over the definition of specific problems.

Next, the problem is refined to a policy issue, a problem with societal ramifications of concern to a number of people and for which there are conflicting opinions for resolution. Values of the involved stakeholders play a large role here and determine the amount of political interest the issue will generate, the identification of policy options, and the analysis that should follow. Operationally, it is useful to frame the issue as a question: What could or should be done about this problem? In practice, Wildavsky (1979) cautions, it is only through analysis that the true

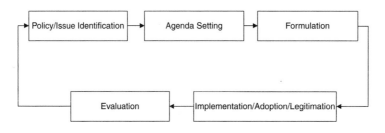

**Figure 5-1** The policy process stage-sequential model.

underlying issue is identified. For example, at the institutional level, hospitals have been developing policies to increase salaries to reduce the hemorrhaging of registered nurse staff rather than addressing the negative workplace environment issues such as mandatory overtime and low staffing that have created the exodus. As a result, both state and federal policymakers are proposing legislation that addresses the underlying issue: "How should hospitals create a positive work environment to increase nurse retention?"

Problem and issue definition and mobilization of support move the issue to the governmental policy agenda—the list of issues being addressed by public policymakers. When seeking policy change, one must identify the policymaking body holding jurisdiction over the matter, as well as the individuals and groups that might support the position and be willing to work to achieve policy change. Policy agendas convey the notion of issue prioritization by policymakers, particularly in the first two stages (policy agenda setting and policy formulation). The discussion agenda includes issues that merit policymakers' attention based on input from involved interest groups, consumers, or policy elites in stage one.

The action agenda designates those issues actively moving through the formulation stage. Media coverage and Internet activism from both liberal and conservative political organizations play a major role in broadening public interest, enlisting group support, and alerting policymakers to the issue. They remain a vital force throughout the policy process.

Finally, the decision agenda reflects policy issues in the last stages of legitimization by policymakers during the legislative or regulatory processes (Kingdon, 1995; Nelson, 1978). Political activity and negotiation are major forces in moving issues onto the decision agenda and through to final enactment. To illustrate, despite enactment of the Medicare prescription drug law, which moved between discussion and decision agendas during two administrations, costs remain high for many beneficiaries and state Medicaid programs. Although Congress postponed action, individuals and state Medicaid programs recognized that drugs cost far less in Canada and overseas and found creative ways to purchase them. Legislative proposals to address prescription drug importation are now on the discussion agenda.

***Stage Two: Policy Formulation.*** Here policymakers determine policy options to resolve questions such as, "What could or should be done to deal with X?" Formulation is a technical phase in which information on the issue is collected, analyzed, and disseminated, and legislative or regulatory language is drafted. Various interest groups and policymakers may develop alternative proposals, each of which must be evaluated in terms of its costs and benefits to the target group and the "spillover" effects on those external to it.

Policy proposals now move through the legislative or regulatory process, and the policy decision is made. A critical component here is the development of a program budget and the funding appropriation process. This phase is characterized by input from all those holding a stake in the issue: interest groups, policymakers, and target groups. However, the legitimate authority will make the final decision. Public pressure must be continued or increased to move the issue forward on the action agenda until resolution is achieved in the form of a policy document such as a statute or regulation. Ripley (1985) stresses the importance of compromise and negotiation to reach a decision. As a result, policy and program design may be vague and sketchy; details for legislation will be defined in the less-contentious regulatory process. Jones (1977) describes this as the "action in government" stage.

***Stage Three: Program Implementation.*** This stage reflects the government's formal response to the initial problem. The executive or regulatory body charged with implementing the program develops the guidelines and regulations necessary for a functioning program. In effect, the implementing body translates the authorizing policy into a workable program. Although less contentious than the legislative process, implementation activities of legislative interpretation, planning, and organizing are still very political (Ripley, 1985). Anderson (1990) cautions that interest groups and those to be regulated frequently seek loopholes when implementation begins. Here, analysts identify criteria for program evaluation to determine whether it meets policy goals and objectives.

Nursing organizations should communicate with regulatory agency staff as soon as possible after enactment of policy affecting nursing practice to ensure that initial regulatory drafts reflect their position and legislative intent. Interested nursing groups must monitor the *Federal Register* and corresponding state publications for notices of proposed rule making and publication of rules, regulations, standards, and guidelines to ensure that these reflect the original intent of the legitimating body and to assess their impact on health care delivery and professional practice. Interest groups frequently use the regulatory process to include program elements they were unable to put into legislation, thereby undermining legislative intent. Furthermore, interest groups often try to bypass legislative scrutiny by persuading regulatory bodies to initiate program changes favorable to their interest. Continuous monitoring of proposed state and federal regulations is a tedious but essential nursing organization responsibility.

**Stage Four: Policy Evaluation.** The policy evaluation phase addresses the question "Did the policy work?" (Anderson et al., 1984). The program's implementation, performance, and impact are evaluated to determine how well the program has met its goals and objectives. Evaluation should identify whether a program has satisfactorily met the original concerns and should be continued, whether segments of the original policy goals remain unmet, and whether new issues have surfaced, thereby restarting the cycle. A program that has met its objectives or is superseded by a newer policy and is no longer necessary may be terminated. An example is the policy of deinstitutionalization of mentally ill persons and the subsequent closure of state mental institutions. The policy may have met its initial goal of reducing excessive institutionalization of the mentally ill; however, the problem of adequate community mental health services, especially for the homeless, remains unresolved.

Although the stages model offers a rational and systematic schema for policymaking, it has many shortcomings. Dye (1992) argues that it fails to explicate who gets what and why in policy decisions, and Sabatier (1999) raises the concern that it fails to address the role of stakeholders' ideas and their underlying values during policy debate and evaluation. Plans for evaluation are usually developed in the formulation phase. In their bill or program analysis, nurses should therefore assess whether the evaluation criteria identified adequately address the desired outcome and potential for secondary problems. Staff preparing for evaluation may lack the background for understanding potential negative outcomes or have an ideologic predisposition.

Nevertheless, the stages model is useful in simplifying the "how" of a frequently confusing and complex process. Confusion in the process may be due to the mix of political factors ingrained in each of the analytic phases of the process. Stone (1997) observes that analysis is inherently political because the decisions on what to analyze and how to analyze it are based on one's political stance or world view.

## POLICY AND ISSUE ANALYSIS

Policy analysis is a systematic approach to describing and explaining the causes and consequences of government action and inaction. The consequences of inaction may be as important as those of action because they, too, constitute policy (Dye, 1992). Historically, many social science disciplines and professions have focused their research activities on government policies as system outputs. More recently the study of policy science theory and methodology has become an interdisciplinary subspecialty with programs in most major universities. Formally, policy analysis is conducted in universities, policy research firms, legislatures and governmental agencies, or organizations. It uses principles and analytic tools from economics, probability theory, and statistics. Based on the sponsoring organization's purpose and function, the analyst's role may vary from the academically oriented "objective technician," to the more politically oriented "issue advocate" who promotes societal welfare, to the "client advocate," whose role is to develop the best case for the employer (Jenkins-Smith, 1982). Nurses tend to function as issue advocates.

Nurses have a unique perspective for policy decision-making because of their clinical knowledge and advocacy orientation. They are increasingly visible as stakeholders in health policy debates through policy positions in both legislative and executive branches of government and as members of special interest groups. The role of the nurse policy analyst is a distinct advanced-practice role because it includes components of research, leadership, and change agency (Stimpson & Hanley, 1991). To this end, nurses in master's degree and doctoral programs receive formal preparation in policy development, analysis, action, and research.

However, registered professional nurses in entry level positions also participate in policy issue debate and need a format to analyze policy issues and take action regarding policy change in both clinical and governmental settings. Inclusion of content on policymaking and politics is therefore essential in baccalaureate nursing curricula. This is reflected in the criteria for accreditation of baccalaureate nursing programs developed by the major accrediting bodies: the Commission on Collegiate Nursing Education, the accrediting body of the AACN, and the NLN.

## ANALYST VALUES AND INHERENT BIAS

Any issue or policy analysis holds the inherent bias of the originating group based on the group's values, frame of reference, and ideology. Although the analyst strives for objectivity, the truth will be filtered through the stakeholder's values, ideology, perspective, and goals (Dunn, 1981). Consequently, the same data may be used to support opposing points of view; only the perspective in viewing the data changes. Nevertheless, analysts within the legislature and administrative agencies sometimes develop proposals not supported by data. Throgmorton (1991, p. 174) addresses the persuasive quality inherent in all policy analyses and suggests that "analysis should stimulate and maintain a conversation among scientists, politicians and lay advocates" to mediate rather than polarize their communication and perspectives. Awareness of one's biases in crafting or evaluating policy will assist nurses, like other interest groups, in developing an effective strategy for success.

## ISSUE ANALYSIS

Policy analysis involves a structured approach to problem solving and decision-making that is useful in any setting. Stokey and Zeckhauser (1978) offer this useful five-point framework:

1. Establish the context, including definition of the problem and specific objectives.
2. Identify alternatives for resolving the issue.
3. Project consequences for the identified alternatives.
4. Specify criteria for evaluating an alternative's ability to meet objectives.
5. Recommend the optimal solution.

The policy issue paper, the first step in the policy analysis process, serves as a valuable tool in these situations. Figure 5-2 outlines a useful model for issue analysis.

## POLICY ISSUE PAPERS

Policy issue papers provide a mechanism to structure the problem at hand and identify the underlying issue. This step is essential in identifying stakeholders and specifying alternatives with their positive and negative consequences. It also identifies variables to be included in full analysis models such as cost-effectiveness or cost-benefit analyses (Hatry, Blair, Fisk, & Kimmel, 1976). Issue papers help one to clarify arguments in support of one's cause, to recognize the arguments of opposing stakeholders, and to develop strategies to advance the issue through the policy cycle (Box 5-2).

## POLICY ISSUE PAPER ORGANIZATION

The following list describes the sections of the policy issue paper. A sample paper on the federal financing of nursing education is included at the end of this chapter. Figure 5-3 divides the sections for issue paper development into four categories: A, Context (Definition); B, Policy Goals/Options; C, Evaluation of Options; and D, Recommended Solution.

### A. Context

1. *Problem identification.* Problem identification clarifies the underlying problem. It specifies problem causes, current and future effects on the community, those who raised the issue and those now interested in it, and how the problem moved to the public agenda (Hatry et al., 1976).

*Text continued on p. 90*

Stages (Functional Activities)

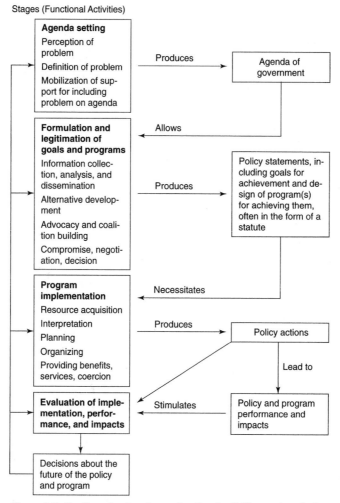

**Figure 5-2** The flow of policy stages, functional activities, and products.

| Context (Definition) | Policy Goals/ Options | Evaluation of Options | Recommended Solution |
|---|---|---|---|
| Policy problem | Identify policy goals/objectives | Set criteria to meet objectives | |
| Background:<br>  Social<br>  Economic<br>  Ethical<br>  Political/legal | Specify policy options (including "do nothing") | Evaluate each option on criteria | |
| | | Compare options (using scorecard) | |
| Stakeholders | | | |
| Issue statement | | | |

**Figure 5-3** Issue analysis for decision-making.

**BOX 5-2**   Policy Issue Paper Example: Federal Financing for Nursing Education

### POLICY PROBLEM

The United States faces an increase in demand for nursing services, an aging nursing workforce, and a shortage of nurses. To ensure an adequate number of registered nurses (RNs), federal policymakers must actively examine and implement solutions that address current and future funding challenges related to nursing education. Federal funding for nursing education is not adequate to address current and future nursing shortages.

The U.S. Department of Labor projects a shortage of over 1 million nurses by 2012 (Employment by occupation, 2004). Because nursing shortages jeopardize both quality of service and access to care, it is essential to examine new options that help to build and educate an adequate supply of nurses.

### A Brief History of Funding for Nurse Education

Historically, the federal government has played a major role in funding and supporting nursing education. Federal funding for nursing education began in 1935 with provisions in the Social Security Act that provided financial assistance for nurses studying public health. Similarly, the government supported psychiatric nursing, another shortage nursing practice area, with scholarship assistance from 1947 to 1955 (Kalisch & Kalisch, 1986).

Additional measures were taken to help curb the nursing shortage when Congress enacted provisions in Title II of the Health Amendment Act of 1956 to provide traineeships for RNs to embark on full-time study in administration and education. These funds covered travel, tuition, fees, and allowances (Kalisch & Kalisch, 1986).

In 1963 the U.S. Surgeon General's Consultant Group on Nursing identified nursing shortage concerns that closely mirror today's problems. Their recommendations led to the 1964 enactment of the Nurse Training Act in the Public Health Service Act (Public Law [PL] 88-581), the first comprehensive federal legislation to consolidate a number of nurse education and training programs. The act also provided funds for construction grants to nursing schools, student loans, education grants, and traineeships (Reyes-Akinbileje & Coleman, 2005). This program was a major stimulus to enhancing the quality of nursing education, moving it from student-labor training to a professional model.

### Nurse Education Funding on a Capitation Basis

PL 92-158 provided capitation funding, a set sum per student, to schools of nursing, enabling them to increase enrollment. Enacted in 1971, it provided capitation only until 1978 (Expand the reach, 2001). Capitation was repealed in the Nurse Education Amendments of 1985 (PL 99-92) (Reyes-Akinbileje & Coleman, 2005).

In 2004 a House bill (HR 5324), the Nurse Education, Expansion, and Development (NEED) Act, was introduced. Like the Nurse Training Act of 1971, the bill is intended to ease the nursing shortage by assisting nursing education programs. The bill makes provisions for funding to nursing schools on a per student basis, with assistance ranging from $966 for each associate degree student to $1405 per bachelor's degree nursing student, and $1800 for each master's degree or doctoral student. The funds could be used to hire and retain faculty, enhance clinical laboratories, purchase educational equipment, repair and expand infrastructure, or recruit students. The bill would cost a projected $85 million in fiscal year (FY) 2006. (Nurse Education, 2004).

### Funding through Title VIII of the Public Health Service Act

Since 1964 Title VIII of the Public Health Service Act has been the key federal initiative in the United States that provides funds in support of nursing education. Title VIII has been amended or reauthorized 14 times, the latest in 2002 (Reyes-Akinbileje & Coleman, 2005). It is interesting to note that Title VIII has been given various names with reauthorization: the Nurse Training Act, the Nursing Education Act, and most recently the Nurse Reinvestment Act. Title VIII programs are administered by the Bureau of Health Professions of the Health Resource and Services Administration (HRSA) of the Department of Health and Human Services (HHS). The breadth and scope of Title VIII is broad, with provisions for programs in health disparities, advanced education nursing, nursing workforce diversity, nursing education, practice and retention, loan repayment and scholarships, nursing faculty loans, public service announcements, and geriatric education (Reyes-Akinbileje & Coleman, 2005).

Federal nursing education funding provides support for programs such as advanced practice nursing education, expansion of minority nurse enrollments, and expansion of and enrollment in baccalaureate nursing programs. The funding provides grants, loans, and scholarships. In FY 2005, Title VIII of the Public Health Service Act provided about $150 million for Nursing Workforce Development programs (Historical appropriations, 2005).

*Continued*

**BOX 5-2**   Policy Issue Paper Example: Federal Financing for Nursing Education—cont'd

### Funding Nursing Education through Medicare

Since 1965, Medicare has reimbursed hospitals for a portion of the educational costs of training nurses, physicians, and other health personnel. The intent of PL 89-97, the Social Security Amendments of 1965, was to promote high-quality inpatient care for beneficiaries of Medicare (Aiken & Gwyther, 1995). In medicine the funds are used to pay salaries of interns and residents who in turn teach medical students and provide patient care (Thies & Harper, 2004). In nursing these Medicare funds have been used to support hospital-based diploma nursing education programs. However, the nursing education model is now academically based in associate, bachelor's, and higher degree programs. The dramatic decrease in the percentage of nurses prepared in hospital diploma programs, from 80% to 7%, demonstrates the need for revision in Medicare funding for nursing education. Hence, it is important to revisit the use of Medicare funds in supporting nursing education, the total funds being paid toward nursing education in relation to other professions, and the resultant decrease in federal support of nursing education in face of a nursing shortage. Change is necessary to ensure that nursing continues to benefit from Medicare funds to the maximum extent possible. It is therefore important to reexamine relevant federal law to ensure that Medicare language reflects the changes in nursing education and current and future trends in health care delivery.

Health policy analysts, nurse researchers, and others periodically reexamine the feasibility of using Medicare payments for training nonphysician health professionals. Although the concept shows promise, the issue is complex. The varying perspectives of these groups, as well as the Commissioners on the Medicare Payment Advisory Commission (MedPAC) reflect this complexity (Report to Congress, 2001).

The role of the federal government in the financing of nursing education, needs to be examined in light of history, but also in regard to current and future social, economic, ethical, political, and legal factors.

### Background

*Social Factors*

The population of the United States is aging. Demographics show that the 85-years-and-older age group is projected to grow from 4.2 million in 2000 to 21 million in 2050. From 2010 to 2030, the population aged 65 years and older is projected to be two times as large as the same group in 2000 and will represent about 20% of the population (Older Americans, 2004).

As the population ages, there will continue to be an increased demand for health care services.

In parallel, there is an aging nurse workforce both clinically and academically. The problem is multifaceted. Women have far more career options available today and as a result nursing does not attract as many young people as in prior years. In addition, nurses seeking advanced practice degrees often opt for higher-paying clinical opportunities instead of lower-paying academic positions. This has contributed to the current shortage of nurse educators. Furthermore, the average age of nurses and nurse educators continues to rise. In 2000 the average age of working RNs was 41.9 years; expectations are that this will increase to 45.4 years by 2010 (Buerhaus, Staiger, & Auerbach, 2000). The number of nurses reaching retirement age will continue to increase, as 40% of the RN workforce will be over age 50 by 2010 (Buerhaus et al., 2000). With the overall shift in demographics, nursing will face competition to attract the diminishing proportion of younger workers.

*Economic Factors*

Hospitals, health care systems, and students face mounting economic challenges. Historically, hospitals received graduate medical education (GME) funding, which included support for diploma nursing education, and they had a ready source of staff through hospital diploma programs. In addition to the continuing shift in nursing education away from diploma programs toward associate-, baccalaureate-, and graduate-degree levels, hospitals and health care systems face new economic pressures and staffing challenges. Increasing staff shortages force hospitals to close units, thereby decreasing services available in a given community, or hire temporary nurses, which increases operating costs and the financial burden.

The economic impact on students is also sizeable. A shorter education pathway at a diploma or community college program means fewer student loans and expedited entry into the workforce. Bachelor's degree or master's level advanced practice options provide valuable skills necessary in the nursing and health care world. Additional education comes at a price, in terms of increased tuition payments and delayed entry into the workforce.

Salary structure also contributes to attracting and retaining nurse educators. Overall trends show that, on average, nurse educators have lower earning potential than nurses in clinical practice, yet the cost of obtaining the master's degree or PhD needed to teach is high.

**BOX 5-2** Policy Issue Paper Example: Federal Financing for Nursing Education—cont'd

## POLICY PROBLEM—cont'd

In contrast, clinical nurses can practice with a minimum of a diploma, associate, or baccalaureate degree. Hence, nurses often choose clinical practice over nurse education. This contributes greatly to the lack of nursing educators. In addition, the aging of both faculty and facilities, the need for a sizeable qualified faculty to meet the required faculty-to-student ratios, and the overall economic challenges of operating a nursing program continue to be problematic (Greene, Allan, & Henderson, 2003). Furthermore, tighter state budgets have led to cuts in funds for higher education. States, educators, and employers are therefore looking at a variety of financing opportunities that include state and local workforce investment boards and employer-matched state funding. Medicaid funding is available for nursing education in some states (Greene et al., 2003).

### Ethical Factors

Two ethical factors are of primary concern. As the nursing shortage increases, there is a growing dependence on foreign-trained nurses. Opportunities for higher pay, better working and living conditions, political and economic stability, and travel pull foreign nurses to the United States. However, although dependence on foreign nurses may help solve U.S. workforce challenges, it also contributes to the "brain drain" from poor, underdeveloped countries with a limited number of trained health care professionals (Kline, 2003). Furthermore, there is the tension and challenge of building solutions that resolve today's problems while establishing programs and policies that provide a solid foundation for meeting the health care needs of future generations.

### Political and Legal Factors

Identification of problems and possible solutions for funding nursing education are not new endeavors. For years, there has been discussion that nursing education should be financed by GME dollars. Although institutions currently receiving little or no funding have a strong incentive to support policy change, the current federal political and fiscal climate will be problematic for changing GME. Spending for military operations and homeland security will continue to be high for the foreseeable future. With the government facing fiscal deficits and curtailed domestic spending, costly new programs face strong scrutiny. Furthermore, Medicare costs are already increasing because of an aging and needy population

and the addition of the new Medicare prescription drug plan.

Yet the looming crisis in the nurse workforce may lead the drive for policy change in funding for nursing education. As the nursing shortage becomes more acute, the crisis mode will increase the visibility of the problem. At this critical juncture, the growing body of research and evidence related to workforce challenges and patient care may take on new visibility and meaning. Market and legal issues also serve as drivers. For example, immigration laws are already under review; loosening or tightening of laws will affect the supply of available nurses. Political factors internal to nursing will affect development and enactment of this legislation.

Historically, the nursing community's weak lobbying presence, internal divisions, and inconsistent message have lead to a lack of support on Capitol Hill. These factors may limit ability to make substantive policy changes in federal funding for nursing education. In fact, recent federal monies have focused on programs for increasing nurses in advanced practice roles, to the detriment of baccalaureate programs preparing entry-level nurses. Finally, the physician education and hospital lobbies may oppose this change in GME if they perceive any expansion in the law as a threat to their funding stream.

### Issue Statement

How should the federal government finance nursing education to ensure the necessary supply of entry level and advanced practice nurses to meet future health care demand?

### Stakeholders

There exists a wide variety of stakeholders, including hospitals, academic programs, patients, nurses, and foreign-trained nurses. Staff shortages hinder both access to and quality of care. New streams of funding have the potential to enhance education and staffing, thereby having a positive effect on patients' access to high-quality care. However, hospitals have much at stake, as is evidenced by their history. In the 1960s, approximately 80% of RNs were trained in hospital-based diploma programs, strongly supported by Medicare funding (Coffman, Mertz, & O'Neil, 1999), and compared with approximately 7% today. Data tracking of GME funding for nursing and allied health workers' education in hospitals has been problematic. Improved tracking is necessary for fully understanding this issue (Report to Congress, 2001).

*Continued*

**BOX 5-2** Policy Issue Paper Example: Federal Financing for Nursing Education—cont'd

Data show that in 1996 almost 70% of the $149 million of GME funding for RN education was paid to hospital diploma programs producing less than 10% of the RN nursing workforce and that more than half of the diploma programs were in three states (Pennsylvania, New Jersey, Ohio) (Thies & Harper, 2004). Hospitals and states that have diploma programs will be hit harder than others if changes are made to the GME funding stream.

Academic programs and their related institutions could benefit from an increase in funding through GME dollars. Depending on the program specifics, nurses and other employees would directly benefit. These changes, coupled with other institutional policy improvements, could create a more positive work environment and improve retention of nurses. Ultimately, increased education and training will enhance patient care.

If more students from the United States enrolled in nursing programs and dependence on foreign nurses declined, there would be a mixed impact on other countries. Fewer nurses would be sending earnings back to their homelands to help support families, yet more would stay in their homelands to provide valuable health care human resources. Anecdotal evidence suggests that some foreign nurses are brought to the United States under false circumstances and are subjected to lower wages and poorer living conditions than promised.

**POLICY GOALS AND OBJECTIVES**

The goal of federal nursing education legislation is to ensure adequate recruiting, education, and retention of RNs and nursing faculty in order to meet patient care and health care service demands. Policy objectives include the following:

1. Establish funding policies that are consistent with the demands of the current and future health care systems.
2. Acknowledge that the structure of nursing education has changed and policies must be updated to reflect current and future demand.
3. Develop policies, legislation, and regulations that provide steady funding to establish and support a solid foundation for nursing education at all levels.
4. Establish and develop programs that address both short- and long-term attraction, education, and retention of high-quality students from traditional and nontraditional backgrounds.
5. Build funding and recruitment policies based on sound ethics, and strive to ensure positive national and international outcomes.

**POLICY OPTIONS AND ALTERNATIVES**

Policy alternatives for resolving the issue of federal financing of nursing education include the following:

1. *Do Nothing Option: Title VIII of the Public Health Service Act.* Continue primary federal support of nursing education as in current practice.
2. *Incremental Change Option: Capitation Payments in Addition to Title VIII.* Enact legislation to increase financial support for nursing education institutions based on the number of students.
3. *Major Change Option: Medicare Funding of Nursing Education.* Although the GME program has traditionally supported hospital-based nursing programs, it is only one possibility for funding through Medicare.

Note: For the purposes of this analysis, we have assumed that, as in the past, the government will continue to support funding of nurse education. One could make the argument that a fourth option or alternative should be added, indicating that the federal government should not be supporting education for nursing or any of the health professions.

**Criteria for Evaluation**

1. Likelihood of ongoing funding
2. Size and availability of funding stream
3. Ability to meet current and future demand
4. Political feasibility

**ANALYSIS OF OPTION 3**

Because this is a sample paper, only one option, Medicare Financing, will be analyzed using the four criteria listed above. In an actual analysis, the process that follows would be repeated for each option.

**Criterion 1: Likelihood of Ongoing Funding**
*Pro*

Whereas other options, such as Title VIII, are funded through *discretionary* spending and are made available through Congressional appropriations, Medicare is an *entitlement* program funded through mandatory spending. If a law is passed to authorize spending for nurse education through the Medicare entitlement program, the federal government is obligated to make payments to those persons, institutions, or governments that meet the legal criteria delineated in the law. Therefore the funding stream will be ongoing, unless the law is changed.

**BOX 5-2** Policy Issue Paper Example: Federal Financing for Nursing Education—cont'd

### ANALYSIS OF OPTION 3—cont'd

Discretionary funds are made available through the Congressional appropriations process and may fluctuate significantly depending on politics and the priorities of the country at any given point in time.

*Con*

The cost of health care continues to increase each year. Changing demographics, increased health care needs, and the addition of new benefits to Medicare (e.g., drug coverage) contribute to higher health care costs. The rate of cost increases will be unsustainable over time, and Medicare will continue to fall under increasing scrutiny. Major policy changes that raise costs will have a lower likelihood of acceptance. Trends toward pay-for-performance, quality outcomes, and evidence-based medicine will have an impact on federal expenditures.

### Criterion 2: Size and Availability of Funding Stream

This criterion looks at the total dollars available through the major change option.

*Pro*

By comparison, the funds available to support education through Medicare have been significantly higher than discretionary funds through Title VIII. Total Medicare medical education payments were over $6 billion in 1996 in contrast to about $149 million for nursing education (Aiken, Anderson, & Zhang, 1999). In fiscal year 2005, $150 million was available to nursing through Title VIII funding (Historical appropriations, 2005). Information on current payments to nursing education through GME is difficult to obtain. Overall, the potential dollars at stake are substantially higher through Medicare than through Title VIII.

*Con*

It is difficult to fully analyze the funding availability and use of GME support for diploma nursing education because data are incomplete. However, we do know that with the decline in the number of diploma programs, few nursing programs are benefiting from GME funds. With the shift away from diploma programs and toward associate and baccalaureate programs, it is critical to revisit federal, state, and local funding policies, now and on an ongoing basis, to ensure that nursing programs remain adequately funded as shifts take place.

### Criterion 3: Ability to Meet Current and Future Demand

*Pro*

The good news is that hospitals with diploma nursing education programs are currently benefiting from GME funding. Physicians and hospitals reap benefits from GME funding and will continue to lobby to ensure that GME funding is not cut.

*Con*

Although nursing has received some benefit from GME funding, the benefit continues to trend downward as diploma programs close. Medicare funding for nursing education has supported primarily preprofessional education (Aiken & Gwyther, 1995). Current federal law has not kept pace with the nursing education models in place today. To be most effective, laws need to be updated to account for changes in nurse education and practice models, as well as current and future nurse and nurse educator supply and demand.

### Criterion 4: Political Feasibility

*Pro*

An aging nursing workforce and a shortage of new nurses will grow increasingly visible as the baby boomers age and our overall population faces increased health care needs. As the shortage heightens, legislators, health care systems, regulatory agencies, academic institutions, and both public and private health care institutions will be open to new and creative solutions to meet society's nursing needs. There are over 2.7 million RNs in the United States (Spratley, Johnson, Sochalski, Fritz, & Spencer, 2002). A feasible strategy is for the RN community to develop a consistent message and exercise a concerted lobbying effort to educate legislative and regulatory bodies in support of nursing education funding in Medicare to alleviate the nursing shortage.

*Con*

Medicare funding is sizeable. Significant funds flow from Medicare to physician education in GME. In addition, a small number of diploma programs receive critical funds to support nursing education. Those who benefit from GME funds, such as hospitals and physicians, will use their formidable power to protect their turf by lobbying and influencing legislators to maintain the status quo.

### COMPARISON OF ALTERNATIVES AND RESULTS OF ANALYSIS

Analysis and comparison of the three policy alternatives on the criteria and alternatives matrix as

*Continued*

---

**BOX 5-2** Policy Issue Paper Example: Federal Financing for Nursing Education—cont'd

outlined on the scorecard (Figure 5-4) reveal a tie score between Alternative 2, the Capitation and Title VIII combination for federal nurse education funding, and Alternative 3, Expansion of Medicare funding for nursing education, similar to the program for medicine. The Capitation and Title VIII alternative scores positively on each of the four criteria, but not strongly on any individual one. Alternative 3, Medicare funding, strongly meets three of the criteria (substantive funding, likelihood of ongoing funding, meeting current and future demand for nursing education), but it has a major weakness in the area of political feasibility. Amendment of the Medicare Professional Education section is likely to stimulate strong opposition from the medical, professional, and hospital lobbies, as they fear competition for scarce dollars.

Option 1, continuation of Title VIII funding, fails on the criterion of meeting current and future demand. However, it is politically the most feasible, as it would have the least direct political opposition.

In using an Alternatives and Criteria matrix, a "tie score" is not unusual. On the matrix, as in life, alternatives and decisions are not always black and white. There are shades of gray. The key is to look beyond the tie to complete the analysis. In our example, the tie represents two potentially viable alternatives, each with different challenges. Given the current political climate and fiscal challenges, particularly with regard to Medicare, a two-pronged approach would be feasible. Capitation funding could be pursued through legislation immediately. This is a solution that would fit well with the current political climate and concern for improving the nursing supply through federal support of education.

At the same time, the nursing community could ramp up educational efforts, develop the political base, and mobilize for broad professional, congressional, and agency support. With this concerted effort, the nursing community could then push to examine the potential for increased Medicare funding of nurse education, as a solution that goes well beyond Title VIII and capitation.

---

2. *Background.* Exploration of the background of the problem puts the problem in context and facilitates specification of the policy issue. It should include an examination of social, economic, ethical, legal, and political factors.

3. *Stakeholders.* Stakeholders are the parties who have a stake in the outcome of the policy debate, such as policymakers with specific proposals related to the issue, those who would be potentially affected by the policy, special interest groups (who may or may not be included with the previous group), and those with a position on the issue.

4. *Issue statement.* The issue statement, which is actually usually a question, should be phrased in a way that recognizes the underlying problem and conflicting values and seeks to identify options. Questions such as "How could or should X be addressed?" shift focus from a specific policy proposal to an objective analysis of the issue. The analyst maintains focus by keeping the issue statement in mind through each stage of the analysis.

### B. Policy Goals and Options

5. *Policy objectives.* The policy goal should be stated succinctly. It is useful to keep the policy goal and objectives in mind when developing policy options to ensure that they have the potential to resolve the underlying issue.

6. *Policy options and alternatives.* Wildavsky (1979) defines policy alternatives as hypotheses: If X is done, then Y will be the result. Resources necessary for programs should be considered, along with program objectives and criteria. Policy alternatives could include any current proposals, as well as one developed by the analysis sponsor. It is also useful to analyze the "do nothing" option because there may be strong pressure to preserve the status quo.

### C. Evaluation of Policy Options and Alternatives

7. *Evaluation criteria.* Criteria must reflect the policy's potential to achieve policy goals and objectives, such as quality, access, fairness, cost, and administrative and political feasibility.

Analysts may identify other criteria relevant for the policy or the sponsoring group (e.g., inclusion of reimbursement for nonphysician).

8. *Analysis of policy alternatives.* Alternatives are analyzed with regard to each criterion, addressing both positive and negative potential.

9. *Comparison* of alternatives by scorecard. It is useful to summarize the analysis findings using a scorecard format (Figure 5-4). This is a two-dimensional grid, with the evaluation criteria on the vertical axis and the alternative policies on the horizontal. A summarizing notation is made for each alternative on the criteria, facilitating comparison of their strengths and weaknesses. Examples of scoring systems are the plus-minus system used in Figure 5-4 (an example of an alternatives matrix for federal nursing education financing options), designation of "high," "medium," and "low," and brief verbal descriptions. In Figure 5-4, hypothetical scores are included for the other alternatives for illustrative purposes.

### D. Recommended Solution(s)

10. *Summary and recommended policy.* The closing section includes an analytic summary of the comparison of policy options and alternatives, and identification of the most effective or feasible policy. Failure of one option to score significantly

high on most criteria, particularly political feasibility, indicates that tradeoffs among the costs and benefits of option components will have to be negotiated. Furthermore, the score on each criterion provides information useful in planning a strategy to reach one's political or policy goals. An illustration of this is seen in the sample issue scorecard analysis.

## SUMMARY

Nurses' participation in the policy process through their primary roles as analysts or their secondary roles as professional advocates in institutions or organizations will ensure the inclusion of their unique perspective in private sector and governmental policy decisions. The definitions, sequential model of the policy cycle, and outline of a policy issue paper as described here offer tools to facilitate nurses' participation. This analytic approach is particularly valuable for nurses and nursing organizations because it allows nurses to anticipate the arguments they will face when seeking or supporting policy change. Such information is essential in developing an effective political strategy and in communicating with legislators and legislative or regulatory staff. Nurse involvement in the policy process is necessary for enactment and implementation of federal proposals to financially support a nursing education

| | Alternatives | | |
|---|---|---|---|
| | Title VIII, Public Health Service Act | Capitation Funding PLUS Title VIII | Medicare Funding of Nursing Education |
| **Criteria** | | | |
| Substantive Funding Stream | + | + | ++ |
| Likelihood of Ongoing Funding | + | + | ++ |
| Ability to Meet Current/Future Demands | − | + | ++ |
| Political Feasibility | ++ | + | − − |
| | 4+/1− | 4+/0− | 6+/2− |
| Score for Each Alternative | 3 | 4 | 4 |

**Figure 5-4** Policy analysis scorecard example: comparison of policy alternatives for federal financing of nursing education.

system and workforce adequate to meet the health care needs of the future. Furthermore, nurse participation in the debate of broad health care issues such as Medicaid funding enlightens the debate and enhances nurses' image as patient advocates. Finally, decision-making in any professional situation requires clear, systematic thinking; the analytic approach described here is directly applicable.

## Key Points

- The stage-sequential model of the policy process includes problem or issue identification, policy formulation, program implementation, and program evaluation.
- Issue analysis clarifies the issue and provides a baseline for developing a strategy to advance a policy proposal; it is useful in the organizational or public policy setting.
- Issue analysis includes clarifying the problem and issue; gathering social, economic, ethical, political, and legal background information; identifying policy goals, alternatives, and evaluation criteria; and evaluating each alternative based on the criteria.
- A scorecard format summarizes and clarifies findings to support a strategy for moving your proposal forward.
- The analytic approach of this chapter facilitates the clear systematic thinking required in decision-making for any professional situation.

## Web Resources

**Academy Health**
*www.academyhealth.org*
**American Association of Colleges of Nursing**
*www.aacn.nche.edu*
**American Association of Community Colleges**
*www.aacc.nche.edu*
**KaiserEdu.org—Issue Module: Addressing the Nursing Shortage**
*www.kaiseredu.org/issue_index.asp*

**National Advisory Council on Nursing Education and Practice (NACNEP)**
*www.bhpr.hrsa.gov/nursing/nacnep.htm*
**National League for Nursing, Public Policy Action Center Current Federal Nursing Legislation Updates**
*www.nln.org*

## REFERENCES

Aiken, L. H., Anderson, G. F., & Zhang, N. (1999). *Medicare funding of nursing education.* Unpublished manuscript.

Aiken, L. H., & Gwyther, M. E. (1995). Medicare funding of nursing education: The case for policy change. *Journal of the American Medical Association, 273*(19), 1528-1532.

Anderson, J. E. (1990). *Public policymaking.* Boston: Houghton-Mifflin.

Anderson, J. E. (1997). *Public policymaking* (3rd ed). Boston: Houghton-Mifflin.

Anderson, J. E., Brady, D. W., Bullock III, C. S., & Stewart, J. J. (1984). *Public policy and politics in America.* Monterey, CA: Brooks/Cole.

Barker, C. (1996). *The health care policy process.* Thousand Oaks, CA: Sage.

Birkland, A. (2001). *An introduction to the policy process: Theories, concepts and models of public policy making.* Armonk, NY: M. E. Sharpe.

Buerhaus, P. I., Staiger, D. O., & Auerbach, D. I. (2000). Policy responses to an aging registered nurse workforce. *Nursing Economics, 18*(6), 278-284.

Coffman, J., Mertz, B., & O'Neil, E. (1999). Medicare funding of nursing education: Policy options. San Francisco, UCSF Center for Health Professions, April 26.

Cohen, M. D., March, J. G., & Olsen, J. P. (1972). A garbage can model of organizational choice. *Administrative Science Quarterly, 17*, 1-25.

Dunn, W. N. (1981). *Public policy analysis.* Englewood Cliffs, NJ: Prentice-Hall.

Dye, T. R. (1992). *Understanding public policy* (7th ed.). Englewood Cliffs, NJ: Prentice Hall.

Employment by occupation, 2002 and projected 2012. (2004). Retrieved April 18, 2005, from *www.bls.gov/emp/emptab21.htm*.

Expand the reach of the Nurse Education Act with new initiatives—AACN recommendations to address the nursing shortage. (2001). Retrieved April 18, 2005, from *www.aacn.nche.edu/Government/nea2.htm*.

Greene, D. L., Allan, J. D., & Henderson, T. (2003). *The role of states in financing of nursing education.* Washington, DC: National Conference of State Legislatures, The Nursing Workforce Institute for Primary Care and Workforce Analysis.

Hatry, H., Blair, L., Fisk, D., & Kimmel, W. (1976). *Program analysis for state and local governments.* Washington, DC: Urban Institute.

Historical appropriations fiscal year 2001-2005. (2005). Retrieved April 18, 2005, from *www.aacn.nche.edu/Government/pdf/HistoricFY01-05.pdf*.

Jenkins-Smith, S. (1982). Professional roles for policy analysts: A critical assessment. *Journal of Policy Analysis and Management, 2*, 88-93.

Jones, C. O. (1977). *An introduction to the study of public policy.* North Scituate, MA: Duxbury.

Kalisch, P. A., & Kalisch, B. J. (1986). *Advance of American nursing.* Boston: Little, Brown.

Kingdon, J. W. (1995). *Agendas, alternatives, and public policies.* Boston: Little, Brown.

Kline, D. S. (2003). Push and pull factors in international nurse migration. *Journal of Nursing Scholarship, 35*(2), 107-111.

Lambrew, J., in Folz, C. E. (2004). Health policy roundtable discussion: Translating health insurance studies into policy proposals. *Health Services Research 39,* 3433-3444.

Lindblom, C. E. (1987). Still muddling, not yet through. In D. L. Yarwood (Ed.), *Public administration politics and the people.* New York: Longman.

Lindblom, C. E. (1995). The science of "muddling though." In D. C. McCool (Ed.), *Public policy theories, models and concepts: An anthology.* Englewood Cliffs, NJ: Prentice-Hall.

Nelson, B. J. (1978). Setting the policy agenda. In J. May & A. Wildavsky (Eds.), *The policy cycle.* Beverly Hills, CA: Sage.

Nurse Education, Expansion, and Development (NEED) Act summary (108th Congress) H.R. 5324. (2004). Retrieved April 18, 2005, from *http://frwebgate.access.gpo.gov/cgi-bin/getdoc.cgi?dbname=108_cong_bills&docid=f:h5324ih.txt.pdf.*

*Nursing's Agenda for Health Care Reform.* (1992). Washington, DC: American Nurses Publishing.

*Older Americans 2004 Key indicators of well-being.* (2004). Hyattsville, MD: Federal Interagency Forum on Aging-Related Statistics.

Page, C. (2005, September 16). Reporting on televised interview with Sen. Barack Obama: Obama points to danger of 'passive indifference'. *Baltimore Sun,* A15.

*Report to Congress: Medicare payment for nursing and allied health education.* (2001). Washington, DC: Medicare Payment Advisory Commission.

Reyes-Akinbileje, B., & Coleman, S. K. (2005). *Nursing workforce programs in Title VIII of the Public Health Services Act.* Washington, DC: Congressional Research Service.

Ripley, R. B. (1985). *Policy analysis in political science.* Chicago: Nelson-Hall.

Ripley, R. B. (1996). Public policy theories, models and concepts: An anthology. In D. C. McCool (Ed.), *Stages of the policy process.* Englewood Cliffs, NJ: Prentice-Hall.

Sabatier, P. A. (1991). Toward better theories of the policy process. *PS: Political Science & Politics, 24*(2), 147-156.

Sabatier, P. A. (Ed.). (1999). *Theories of the policy process.* Boulder, CO: Westview.

Schneider, A. L., & Ingram, H. (1997). *Policy design for democracy.* Lawrence: University Press of Kansas.

Spratley, E., Johnson, A., Sochalski, J., Fritz, M., & Spencer, W. (2002). *The registered nurse population: Findings from the 2000 National Sample Survey of Registered Nurses.* Rockville, MD: U.S. Department of Health and Human Services, Health Resources and Service Administration, Bureau of Health Professions, Division of Nursing.

Stimpson, M., & Hanley, B. E. (1991). Nurse policy analyst: Advanced practice role. *Nursing and Health Care, 12*(1), 10-15.

Stokey, E., & Zeckhauser, R. (1978). *A primer for policy analysis.* New York: W.W. Norton.

Stone, D. (1997). *The policy paradox: The art of political decision-making.* New York: W.W. Norton.

Thies, K. M., & Harper, D. (2004). Medicare funding for nursing education: Proposal for a coherent policy agenda. *Nursing Outlook, 52,* 297-303.

Throgmorton, J. A. (1991). The rhetoric of policy analysis. *Policy Sciences, 24*(2), 153-179.

True, J. L., Jones, B. D., & Baumgartner, F. R. (1999). Punctuated equilibrium theory: Explaining stability and change in American policymaking. In P. A. Sabatier (Ed.), *Theories of the policy process.* Boulder, CO: Westview.

Wildavsky, A. (1979). *Speaking truth to power.* Boston: Little, Brown.

*chapter*

6

# Political Analysis and Strategies

Judith K. Leavitt, Sally S. Cohen, & Diana J. Mason

*"The wind and the waves are always on the side of the ablest navigators."*

EDWARD GIBBON

Nursing and politics are a good match. First, nurses understand people. Success in any political situation depends on one's ability to establish and sustain strong interpersonal relationships. Second, nurses appreciate the importance of systematic assessments. Nurses engaged in the politics of the policy process will find that their efforts are most effective when they systematically analyze their issues and develop strategies for advancing their agendas. Finally, nurses bring to the deliberations of any health policy issue an appreciation of how such policies affect clinical care and patient well-being. Few policymakers have such an ability. Thus nurses have much to offer public and private sector discussions and actions around health policy issues.

## GENDER ISSUES AND CONFLICT

"Gender politics" affects every political scenario that involves nurses. Working in a predominantly female profession means that nurses are accustomed to certain norms of social interactions (Tanner, 2001). They are most familiar with discourse among women and nursing colleagues. In contrast, the power and politics of public policymaking typically are male dominated, although women are steadily increasing their ranks as elected and appointed government officials. Moreover, many male and female public officials have stereotypic images of nurses as women who lack political savvy. This may limit officials' ability to view nurses as potential political partners. Therefore nurses need to be sensitive to gender issues that may affect, but certainly not prevent, their political success (see the stories of nurse legislators in Chapters 24 and 27, as well as Chapter 35).

Many nurses find political work unsavory because of the inevitability of conflict. Conflicts between political parties, between those with different ideologic values, and between nurses and other stakeholders are inherent to the political process. Conflict is unavoidable, and it is also necessary for identifying the different viewpoints that will structure subsequent negotiations. Unlike other situations in which conflict may be unwelcome, in politics it is necessary for establishing the parameters of discourse and the terms of compromise. This holds true for any setting in which nurses are involved with politics, whether it is the workplace, the community, or organizational or governmental arenas.

Stone (2002) notes that policymaking in any arena involves a struggle over ideas. Conflict occurs whenever:

- An individual's or group's ideas are opposed by another
- There are limited resources or rewards, so that one individual or group gains at the expense of another
- There is a scarcity of goods or services, which almost all societies confront

The ubiquitous nature of conflict should help nurses realize that, like power, conflict is unavoidable and something to be addressed rather than sidestepped.

A renowned political scientist, E.E. Schattschneider (1960), developed a useful framework for understanding the role of conflict in political situations. He described how expanding the scope of a conflict, or what he called the "contagiousness of conflict," could affect the outcome of political deliberations. As he explained, "competitiveness is the mechanism for the expansion of the scope of conflict" (pp. 17-18). The loser may call in outside groups to shift the balance of power. New scope and balance can make possible many things and can also make many things impossible. According to Schattschneider, every conflict has two parts: the individuals engaged and the audience attracted to the conflict. The audience is never neutral. Once people become involved, they take a side and influence the outcome. The larger the audience, the more likely there will be conflict. Therefore, the "most important strategy of politics is concerned with the scope of the conflict" (Schattschneider, 1960, p. 3).

Schattschneider also pointed out the importance of visibility. One can't expand scope without making issues visible to one's constituency and outside audiences. As he explained, "a democratic government lives by publicity" (p. 16). According to Schattschneider, "politics is the socialization of conflict." Moreover, as long as the conflict remains private, the political process is limited, if it is initiated at all. "Conflicts become political only when an attempt is made to involve the wider public" (p. 39).

These words are significant to nurses looking to exert political influence. First, expanding the scope of conflict can be a strategy for achieving political change, used by one's friends and foes alike. Second, when the scope of conflict is expanded, it is important to engage the media and other avenues of publicity (see Chapter 9 on the media). Of course, this doesn't ensure that the outcome will be what one wants. The outcome depends on many other factors, including "which of a multitude of possible conflicts gains the dominant position" (Schattschneider, 1960, p. 62). Success in the political arena means knowing the environment, potential stakeholders, and the

> **BOX 6-1** Steps of a Political Analysis
>
> 1. Identifying and analyzing the problem
> 2. Outlining and analyzing proposed solutions
> 3. Understanding the background of the issue: its history and previous attempts to address the problem
> 4. Locating the political setting and structures involved
> 5. Evaluating the stakeholders
> 6. Conducting a values assessment
> 7. Recognizing the resources, both financial and human, needed to reach the intended goals
> 8. Analyzing power bases

misperceptions policymakers may have, recognizing the lack of sufficient information, and creating strategies to meet the challenges.

## COMPONENTS OF POLITICAL ANALYSIS

The best approach to accomplish change must include a thoughtful analysis of the politics of the problem and proposed solutions. Although this chapter explores the *political* analysis of a problem and proposed solutions, Chapter 5 provides an in-depth discussion of *policy* analysis. These two analytic processes should actually be done simultaneously. (See Box 6-1 for an overview of this process.)

### THE PROBLEM

The first step in conducting a political analysis is to identify the problem. Answering several questions is useful for framing the problem:

- What are its scope, duration, and history, and whom does it affect?
- What data are available to describe the issue and its ramifications?
- What are the gaps in existing data?
- What types of additional research might be useful?

Not all serious conditions are problems that warrant government attention. The challenge for those seeking to get public policymakers to address particular problems, such as poverty, the uninsured, or unacceptable working conditions, is to define the problem in ways that will prompt lawmakers to take action. This requires careful crafting of messages so that calls for public, as opposed to private sector, solutions are clearly justified. This is known as "framing" the issue. In the workplace, framing may entail linking the problem to one of the institution's priorities or to a potential threat to its reputation or financial standing. For example, inadequate nurse staffing could be linked to increases in rates of infection, morbidity, and morality—outcomes that can increase institutional costs and jeopardize an institution's reputation and future business.

Sometimes what appears to be a problem is not. For example, proposed mandatory continuing education for nurses is not a problem. Rather, it is a possible solution to the challenge of ensuring competency of nurses. After an analysis of the issue of clinician competence, one might review the policy outcomes and establish a goal that includes legislating mandatory continuing education. The danger of framing solutions as problems is the possibility that it can limit creative thinking about the underlying issue and leave the best solutions uncovered.

## PROPOSED SOLUTIONS

Typically, there is more than one solution to an identified problem, and each option differs with regard to cost, practicality, and duration. These are the *policy* options. The *political* analysis revolves around what is politically feasible. What support or opposition (as well as resources) can be mobilized to create more power than that of the competition? By identifying and analyzing possible solutions, nurses will acquire further understanding of their issue and what is feasible for government or the workplace to undertake. For example, if nurses want the federal government to provide substantial support for nursing education, they need to understand the constraints of federal budgets and the demands to invest in other programs, including those that benefit nurses. Moreover, support for nursing education can take the form of scholarships, loans, tax credits, aid to nursing schools, or incentives for building partnerships between nursing schools and health care delivery systems. Each option presents different types of support, and nurses would need to understand

the implications of the alternatives before asking for federal intervention.

The amount of money and time needed to address a particular problem also needs to be taken into account. Are there short-term and long-term alternatives that nurses want to pursue simultaneously? How might one prioritize various solutions? What are the tradeoffs that nurses are willing to make to obtain stated political goals? Such questions need to be considered in developing the political strategy.

## BACKGROUND

When striving to affect policy formation, one must know about previous attempts to move an issue. This will provide insight into the *feasibility* of a particular approach. For example, many child care advocates view federal child care standards as vital for protecting the health and safety of children in child care settings and for minimizing variation among states. However, a review of child care policymaking over the past few decades would reveal that federal child care standards were always contentious and that by 1990 most child care policymakers considered them politically impractical (Cohen, 2001).

Knowledge of past history will also provide insight into the *position* of key public officials so that communications with those individuals and strategies for advancing an issue can be developed accordingly. For example, if one knows that a particular legislator has always questioned the ability of advanced practice nurses (APNs) to practice independently, then that individual would need special coaxing to support legislation allowing direct billing of APNs under Medicare.

*Historical precedent* for one issue can affect the politics of another. For example, in the United States today, one would not expect to be successful in moving social welfare legislation that was associated with high taxes because of the predominant value of "get government out of our lives." This was not always the case. Social Security, Medicare, and Medicaid were all passed because at that time the public understood the need for government support to help those lacking adequate resources. In a classic work, Fox-Piven and Cloward (1993) documented that societies go through cycles of expanding and contracting social policies and programs aimed at supporting vulnerable citizens. As the size and need of the vulnerable population increases, social policies for safety nets are more likely to be put into place as a response to escalating social unrest and upheaval. This work reminds us that historical precedent does not mean that what happened in the past will remain the same. In fact, it suggests that we should be cognizant of cycles of change, seek to support a shift in political climate that will support our agendas, and be prepared to act when the time is right.

## POLITICAL SETTING

Once the problems and solutions have been clearly identified and described, the appropriate political arenas for influencing the issue need to be analyzed. Usually this begins by identifying the entities with jurisdiction over the problem. Is the issue primarily within the public domain or does it also entail the private sector? Many issues require a mix of public and private sector players, but responsibility for decision-making will ultimately rest with one sector more than the other. For example, nurses interested in improving workplace conditions would first turn to their employers and other local stakeholders. It is seldom prudent to turn to public officials until other efforts in the private sector have failed.

With regard to public policy, nurses need to clarify which level of government (federal, state, or local) is responsible for a particular issue. When one communicates with legislators and developing strategies, it is critical to understand the level of government responsible for a particular issue and how the levels interrelate. (See Chapter 23 for a full discussion of how government works.)

In addition to the level of government, nurses need to know which branch of government (legislative, executive, or judicial) has primary jurisdiction over the issue at a given time. Although there is often overlap among these branches, nurses will find that a particular issue falls predominantly within one branch (see Chapter 24, which discusses the legislative and regulatory processes).

If the issue is in the problem definition and policy formation stage, then nurses will focus on the legislative branch. If an issue entails the implementation of a program, including promulgating regulations, then nurses will focus on the executive branch.

Issues that are within the courts call for knowledge of the judicial system.

Nurses can apply a political analysis to settings beyond government, in the workplace or community organization. Regardless of the setting, nurses will want to identify who has responsibility for decision-making for a particular issue; which committees, boards, or panels have addressed the issue in the past; the organizational structure; and the chain of command.

At an institutional level, once the relevant political arenas are identified, the formal and informal structures and functioning of that arena need to be analyzed. The formal dimensions of the entity can often be assessed through documents related to the organization's mission, goals, objectives, organizational structure, constitution and bylaws, annual report (including financial statement), long-range plans, governing body, committees, departments, and individuals with jurisdiction.

Does the entity use parliamentary procedure? Parliamentary procedure provides a democratic process that carefully balances the rights of individuals, subgroups within an organization, and the membership of an assembly. The basic rules are outlined in *Robert's Rules of Order Newly Revised* (Robert, 2000). Whether in a legislative session or the policymaking body of large organizations, such as the American Nurses Association (ANA) House of Delegates, one must know parliamentary procedure as a political strategy to get an issue passed or rejected. Countless issues have failed or passed because of insufficient knowledge of rule making.

It is also vital to know the informal processes and methods of communication. A well-known example of the power of informal processes and communication is the case of the business lunch or the golf game that in the past excluded women.

## STAKEHOLDERS

Stakeholders are those parties who have influence over the issue or who could be mobilized to care about the issue. In some cases, stakeholders are obvious. These are the overt stakeholders. For example, nurses are stakeholders in issues like staffing ratios (see *California Nurse Staffing Ratios* and *Mandatory Staffing Ratios: Australia's Experience* following

Chapter 18). In other situations, one can develop potential stakeholders by helping them to see the connections between the issue and their interests. Many individuals and organizations can be considered stakeholders when it comes to staffing ratios. Among them are employers (hospitals, nursing homes) payers (insurance companies), legislators, other professionals, and, of course, consumers.

Who could be turned into stakeholders by virtue of their interests and values? Nursing has increasingly realized the potential of consumer power in moving nursing and health care issues. For example, nurses have worked with AARP on long-term care, with the National Alliance for Mental Illness on mental health parity, and with the American Cancer Society on tobacco issues. Who brings a powerful voice or presence to the issue? For example, before running for office, Congresswoman Carolyn McCarthy became a respected and powerful spokesperson for gun control through the media coverage of the fatal shooting of her husband (see *I Believed I Could Make a Difference: The Honorable Carolyn McCarthy* following Chapter 24). Certainly she was able to mobilize other stakeholders, such as victims of gun violence, during her campaigns for gun control and for election to Congress. But one of the most significant stakeholders she identified was the American Academy of Pediatrics, which brought significant clout and resources to the table.

What kind of relationships do you or others have with key stakeholders? Look at your connections with possible stakeholders through your schools, places of worship, or business. Which of these stakeholders are potential supporters or opponents? Can any of the opponents be converted to supporters? What are the values, priorities, and concerns of the stakeholders? How can these be tapped in planning political strategy? For example, as nurses determine how to increase recruitment and retention, it is obvious that some of the most important stakeholders will be organizations that need to hire nurses, such as hospitals, home health agencies, and nursing homes, all of which have trade organizations that represent their interests. In addition, consumer groups, especially senior citizens, have a stake in whether nursing care will be

available as they age. Do the supportive stakeholders reflect the constituency that will be affected by the issue? For example, as states expand coverage of health services through each state's Children's Health Insurance Program (SCHIP), it is vital to have parents of enrolled children lobby policymakers. These parents can share the personal stories of how the program has made a difference for their children. Yet stakeholders who are recipients of the services are too often *not* identified as vital for moving an issue. Nurses as direct caregivers have an important role in ensuring that recipients of services are included as stakeholders.

A thorough political analysis of an issue includes identification of policy entrepreneurs. Similar to entrepreneurs in business, policy entrepreneurs are individuals who are pivotal in "bringing issues to the fore and moving them from incubation to enactment" (Weissert, 1991, p. 262). Or, as stated by Feeley (2002), " A successful policy entrepreneur is able to correctly assess which goals will be most attractive to the constituency groups she is targeting and will adjust her tactics accordingly to maximize her chances for success and minimize political failure" (p. 126). Policy entrepreneurs can be elected or appointed government officials; representatives of advocacy, professional, or research organizations; legislators; legislative staff; or any other individual within a policy community. Policy entrepreneurs are characterized by a willingness to invest time, money, or other resources in an issue, in anticipation of some type of policy change. They are intensely committed to the issue or cause and have an ability to broker and move an issue to implementation. This policy change can be for personal interest, for promotion of certain values, for advancement of issues, or simply for the love of political strategizing and gamesmanship (Kingdon, 2003). Kingdon discusses how policy entrepreneurs use the "open window" provided by the merging of policy, political, and problem streams to advance an issue.

The terms *policy* and *political entrepreneur* are sometimes used interchangeably. Nurses seeking to influence policy outcomes are wise to identify and work with policy entrepreneurs on both sides of their issue. They use their connections, their political and policy expertise, and their passion to move issues. It is vital for nurses to step up to the plate and be willing to work as policy entrepreneurs.

## VALUES ASSESSMENT

Every political issue, especially those issues that entail "morality policies," could prompt discussions about values. Morality policies are those that primarily revolve around ideology and values, rather than costs and distribution of resources. Among the most well-publicized morality issues are abortion, stem cell research, and the death penalty (Mooney, 2001). But even issues that are not classified as morality policies require that stakeholders assess their values and those of their opponents.

Values underlie the responsibility of public policymakers to be involved in the regulation of health care. In particular, calls for extending the reach of government in the regulation of health care facilities implies that one accepts this as a proper role for public officials, rather than as a role of market forces and the private sector. Thus, electoral politics affect the policies that may be implemented. An analysis that acknowledges how congruent nurses' values are with those of individuals in power can affect the success of advancing an issue.

Although nurses may value a range of health and social programs, legislators will hear their calls for increased funding for nursing research and education within the context of demands from other constituencies. Any call for government support of health care programs implies a certain prioritization of values: is health more important than education, or jobs, or the war in Iraq? Elected officials must always make choices among competing demands. And their choices reflect their values, the needs and interests of their constituents, and their financial supporters such as large corporations. Similarly, nurses' choice of issues on the political agenda reflects the profession's values and political priorities.

## RESOURCES

An effective political strategy must take into account the resources that will be needed to move an issue successfully. Resources include money, time, connections, and intangible resources, such as creative ideas. Analyzing the resources requires both short-term and long-term views.

The most obvious resource is money, which must be considered in relation to both the proposed solution or policy and the campaign to champion it. The proposed solution needs to include an analysis of the resources needed for the solution to be successful. Thus, before launching a campaign for a particular bill or program, campaign leaders must know how much the proposed solution will cost, who will be bearing those costs, and the source of the money. In addition, it is helpful to know how budgets are formulated for a given government agency or institution. What is the budget process? How much money is allocated to a particular cost center or budget line? Who decides how the funds will be used? How is the use of funds evaluated? How might an individual or group influence the budget process?

Money is not the only resource. Sharing available resources, such as space, people, and expertise, may be best accomplished through a coalition (see Chapter 8). It may require a mechanism for each entity to contribute a specific amount or to tally their in-kind contributions. In-kind contributions can include office space for meetings; use of a photocopier, telephone, or other equipment; or use of staff to assist with production of brochures and other communications. Other cost considerations include accessing the media or other publicity efforts; printing brochures and other educational materials; paying for postage; and establishing access to electronic communications.

When nurses and other volunteers are recruited for a political issue, project, or campaign, a common response is lack of time for involvement. Nurses need to figure how to get volunteers while simultaneously protecting one of their most precious commodities, time. One must find creative ways to use available resources. For instance, an option for limited volunteer time might be contracting for specific services, such as writing testimony or other communications. In other cases, time and money may both be scarce. This requires delegating and sharing of responsibilities and setting realistic goals about what can be achieved in a given time. Alternatively, creating a diversified coalition can enhance achievement of the goals.

Creativity is a precious resource that enables nurses and others to develop strategies that will be inspiring and captivating to one's audience. How much creativity is evident among the stakeholders? How can one stimulate and channel creativity? Allocating enough time for brainstorming and planning strategically will pay off in the end if well-designed and creative approaches emerge from such sessions.

## POWER

In the workplace, government, professional organizations, and community, effective political strategy requires an analysis of the power of proponents and opponents of a particular solution. Power is one of the most complex political and sociologic concepts to define and measure. It is also a term that politicians and policy analysts use freely, without necessarily giving thought to what it means.

Power can be a means to an end, or an end in itself. Power also can be actual or potential. The latter implies power as undeveloped but a "force to be reckoned with" (Joel & Kelly, 2002). Many in political circles depict the nursing profession as a potential political force, given the millions of nurses in this country and the power we could wield if most nurses participated in politics and policy formation.

There are no absolute or definitive models of power, and, at times, aspects of power can seem contradictory—that is, power may be considered a prerequisite for social or political action, or it may be an indicator of behavior or a result of a certain action. Sometimes power is asymmetric, as when one person or group has more control than another. In other circumstances, power is more symmetric, involving reciprocal influences between two parties, such as between leaders and followers (Duke, 1976). Power can also be considered a zero-sum entity in which one person's or group's possession of power precludes possession by another. In other cases, power is a less-restricted and more "sharable commodity," with its benefits being distributed among many parties (Duke, 1976, p. 42). All these perspectives illustrate the dynamic nature of power and ways in which nurses can analyze and use power to their advantage.

For example, when power bases among parties are determined to be asymmetric, consensus building and shared decision-making may be unlikely unless the dominant party values these methods of conflict resolution (see Chapter 11 for a discussion of conflict management).

Although individuals develop political skill and expertise, it is the influence of large organizations, coalitions, or like-minded groups that wield power most effectively. Too often nurses become concerned about a particular issue and try to change it without help from others. Although the individual may hold expert power, it will be limited if one attempts to "go it alone." In the public arena particularly, an individual is rarely able to exert adequate influence to create long-term policy change. For instance, many APNs have tried to change state Nurse Practice Acts to expand their authority. As well intentioned and knowledgeable as the policy solutions may be, they will likely fail unless nurses who support them can garner the support of other powerful stakeholders such as members of the state board of nursing, a state nurses' organization, and physicians, either through the medical association or the state board of medicine. Such stakeholders hold the power to either support or oppose the policy change.

Any power analysis must include reflection on one's own power base. Power can be obtained through a variety of sources (Ferguson, 1993; French & Raven, 1959; Joel & Kelly, 2002; Mason, Backer, & Georges, 1991):

1. *Coercive power* is rooted in real or perceived fear of one person by another. For example, the supervisor who threatens to fire those nurses who speak out is relying on coercive power, as is a state commissioner of health who threatens to develop regulations requiring physician supervision of nurse practitioners.

2. *Reward power* is based on the perception of the potential for rewards or favors as a result of honoring the wishes of a powerful person. A clear example is the supervisor who has the power to determine promotions and pay increases.

3. *Legitimate (or positional) power* is derived from an organizational position rather than personal qualities, whether from a person's role as the chief nurse officer or the state's governor.

4. *Expert power* is based on knowledge, special talents, or skills, in contrast to positional power. Benner (1984) argues that nurses can tap this power source as they move from novice to expert practitioner. It is a power source that nurses must recognize is available to them and tap. Policymakers are seldom experts in health care; rather, nurses are.

5. *Referent power* emanates from associating with a powerful person or organization. This power source is used when a nurse selects a mentor who is a powerful person, such as the chief nurse officer of the organization or the head of the state's dominant political party. It can also emerge when a nursing organization enlists a highly regarded public personality as an advocate for an issue it is championing.

6. *Information power* results when one individual has (or is perceived to have) special information that another individual desires. This power source underscores the need for nurses to stay abreast of information on a variety of levels: in one's personal and professional networks, immediate work situation, employing institution, community, and the public sector, as well as in society and the world. Use of information power requires strategic consideration of how and with whom to share the information.

7. *Connection power* is granted to those perceived to have important and sometimes extensive connections with individuals or organizations. For example, the nurse who attends the same church or synagogue as the president of the home health care agency, knows the appointments secretary for the mayor, or is a member of the hospital credentialing committee will be accorded power by those who want access to these individuals or groups.

8. *Empowerment* arises from shared power. This power source requires those who have power to recognize that they can build the power of colleagues or others by sharing authority and decision-making. Empowerment can happen when the nurse manager on a unit uses consensus building when possible instead of issuing authoritative directives to staff or when a coalition is formed and adopts consensus building and shared decision-making to guide its process.

An analysis of the extent of one's power using these sources can also provide direction on how to enhance that power. This analysis can be done both for short-term and long-term purposes. For example, consider the nursing organization that finds itself unable to secure legislative support for a key piece of legislation. It can develop a short-term plan for enhancing its power by finding a highly regarded, high-profile individual to be its spokesperson with the media (referent power), by making it known to legislators that their vote on this issue will be a major consideration in the next election's endorsement decisions (reward or coercive power), or by getting nurses to tell the media their stories that highlight the problem the legislation addresses (expert power). Its long-term plan might include extending its connections with other organizations by signing onto coalitions that address broader health care issues and expanding connections with policymakers by attending fundraisers for key legislators (connection power); getting nurses into policymaking positions (legitimate power); hiring a government affairs director to help inform the group about the nuances of the legislature (information power); and using consensus building within the organization to enhance nurses' participation and activities (empowerment).

There is ample evidence that nurses have succeeded in flexing their political muscles and have demonstrated the power behind their political effectiveness. Examples include direct Medicare reimbursement for APNs as part of the 1997 Balanced Budget Act and breakthrough enactment of legislation establishing the National Center for Nursing Research in 1985 and its subsequent legislated designation as the National Institute of Nursing Research in June 1993. More recently nurses have successfully worked to get passage of legislation for staffing ratios, prohibition of mandatory overtime, and whistleblower protections. (See the ANA Website at *www.nursingworld.org/gova/state.*)

## POLITICAL STRATEGIES

### THE PLAN

Once a political analysis is completed, it is necessary to develop a plan of action that identifies strategies for action. Political strategies are the methods and guidelines used in the formulation of a plan to achieve desired goals, including policy goals. They are the means to the goal. Well-planned and practiced strategies can make the difference between success or failure of a plan.

No single strategy works in all situations. However, an important guideline in selecting any strategy is to choose one that shows respect and consideration for policymakers. At no time should one threaten or be disrespectful. Sometimes that can happen in the "heat of battle." For women, particularly, it may be difficult to depersonalize the conflict in tense negotiations. Yet it is the successful advocate who understands that as passionate as one may feel about an issue, the opposition feels just as strongly. Remaining calm, showing respect, and listening well are qualities that make for success. "Do unto others as you would have others do unto you" is one of the most important principles for engaging in politics.

Politics, particularly to the novice, may have a negative connotation because of the long history of policymakers who used Machiavellian strategies in which political expediency takes precedence over morality to win issues. However, most policymakers who are effective are individuals with reputations for honesty, fair play, and commitment. Certainly, nurses have a trustworthy reputation in the public's eye and are seen as credible stakeholders. A Gallup poll from December 2005 indicates that for the sixth year out of seven, the public places nurses at the top of all other groups in honesty and ethical behavior (Jones, 2005). This is where the ethics of politics becomes most critical. Will nurses be successful if they take the high road in politics? Should they sacrifice the public's trust and use Machiavellian tactics, reasoning that the ends are more important than the means? As more women enter politics, the approach for resolving conflicts through consensus building and principled negotiating has become increasingly common and provides nurses with options for political strategy development that can be both ethical and effective.

## PERSISTENCE

Another consideration regarding the development of political strategies is the importance of persistence. Rarely does change happen overnight. Because of the conflict inherent in most policy initiatives, resolution often occurs after discussion, wrangling, delays, regrouping, and shifting of power bases. Securing changes in policy or establishing new public policies requires a commitment to a long-term process. But persistence can pay off.

Legislation can take a long time to be passed. It took 10 years for all APNs to receive Medicare reimbursement. It took 18 years to pass the Family and Medical Leave Act that gave parents and family members 12 weeks of unpaid leave from their jobs for the birth or adoption of a child or care of a sick family member. During those intervening 18 years, much changed except the continuing effort to lobby legislators. More women entered the workforce, and employers recognized that they could not lose critical workers because of the birth or adoption of children. By the time the bill was passed, the public and policymakers realized that act was necessary to maintain a stable workforce and enable workers to provide care for family members. In addition, a president was elected (Clinton) who supported the issue. Political work requires patience, perseverance, and an exquisite sense of timing.

## INCREMENTAL VERSUS REVOLUTIONARY CHANGE

Policy implementation almost always happens through incremental change. Incremental changes or actions may have a better chance of success than a change of major proportions. Resistance to change can often be overcome if a pilot or demonstration project is created to test an idea on a small scale.

Many times we are confronted with situations in which we may not get all we want. One must be clear about what are acceptable solutions or alternatives and what are not. Identification of alternatives represents a good way to test one's convictions and to consider what the long- and short-term goals are. The initial failure to get reimbursement for all APNs had to be accepted in order to get reimbursement for some. The failure of President Clinton's health care reform legislation, which would have overhauled health care in the United States, was partly attributed to the fact that policymaking in this country is usually incremental rather than revolutionary. Although his package failed, Congress did pass the Health Insurance Portability and Accountability Act (HIPAA), an incremental policy to ensure that employees could maintain their health insurance when they leave or lose a job, so that individuals with "preexisting health conditions" could not be denied health insurance.

Failure to recognize the importance of timing and the primacy of incremental change can cause nurses to become discouraged and feel inadequate as political operatives. The following are helpful ways to minimize the frustrations that can accompany political work:

- Have a well-defined political plan with both long-term and short-term objectives
- Evaluate one's progress, and modify the plan as needed
- Seize opportunities that arise from unforeseen social changes
- Identify how to turn seeming defeats into victories
- Celebrate the small gains
- Thank, keep informed, and actively support collaborating stakeholders

Persistence and use of multiple political strategies are needed for a successful outcome to political action.

## THE "PILOT" APPROACH

Change is difficult for people, particularly major policy change. Proposing even modest changes in an organization or to a public policy can be met with skepticism and outright opposition by key decision-makers and those who will be affected by the change. Even when the change is dictated by executive administration, change at the local or unit level may be half-hearted, sabotaged, or dismissed. Demonstration or pilot projects can make the change more palatable by suggesting that it be tested before being implemented on a full scale, whether in one hospital or in society, particularly when the idea is seen as radical or risky (Roberts, 1998).

Demonstration projects are planned implementation and evaluation of models or ideas to determine their merits, problems, and costs before adopting them for a larger population. They test the effects of new ideas, develop solutions to barriers that arise, explore costs, and provide justification for future policies. An example of piloting ideas before

spreading them to a broader audience can be seen with Transforming Care At the Bedside (TCAB), an initiative sponsored by the Institute for Healthcare Improvement and the Robert Wood Johnson Foundation. TCAB targets change on medical-surgical nursing units in participating hospitals, to identify ways to improve care, empower multidisciplinary teams, and position staff nurses as the key change agents on these units. Staff use "rapid-cycle feedback," a specific quality improvement methodology, to do the following:

- Identify innovations that can improve the quality and efficiency of care
- Plan, implement, and evaluate the pilot
- Modify the innovation as needed
- If the pilot shows the innovation to be effective, help other units to adopt the innovation

If the innovation were to be proposed hospital-wide before piloting, the resistance to adoption would be difficult to surmount. By piloting the innovation, the originators of the idea are able to provide the data to support or refute its appropriateness for widespread dissemination.

When the innovation requires cooperation from other departments or key decision-makers, the pilot or demonstration project can provide them with firsthand experience with the change and turn them into supporters. Consulting key stakeholders early on during a pilot project can be instrumental in reducing the risk of opposition because of "wounded egos." In public policy, this translates into building the political support for the demonstration project from legislators if legislation is needed to authorize it, executive branch support for signing such legislation, and public employees who will be responsible for government oversight of the project.

In other cases, demonstration or pilot projects can provide the impetus for people to experience changes that they would otherwise oppose. "Family presence" is the idea of permitting family members to be present during codes and when invasive procedures are being conducted on their loved ones. The idea of family presence is anathema to providers who are accustomed to excluding family members from the patient's bedside. In *Family Presence at the Bedside: Changing Hospital Policy* (following Chapter 17), Clark and colleagues show how they have used the idea of "piloting" family presence to quell the fears of nurses, physicians, administrators, and others and demonstrate that most family members and patients value the experience. Piloting a family presence procedure is part of a comprehensive plan for instituting organizational policies to enable the practice.

Such buy-in can help with subsequent full-scale adoption of the policy but is not fool-proof. It used to be thought that securing legislation for a demonstration project to test a policy initiative or innovation would lead to widespread adoption of the desired policy even before the project had sufficient data to warrant this leap. But today's environment of evidence-based practice, cost control, and government accountability has made this quick adoption the exception rather than the rule. Therefore it is important to plan well for the evaluation of the demonstration project. What are the expected outcomes of the project? What data are needed to demonstrate the efficacy and cost impact of the idea? Who will design and who will conduct the evaluation of the demonstration project? What biases does the evaluator bring to the evaluation? What are the potential problems expected during the demonstration project? Is there sufficient time for achieving the stated aims in utilization rates, clinical outcomes, or costs? Is there enough funding for undertaking a well-designed evaluation of the project?

There is a danger in small, underfunded demonstration projects to test the cost-effectiveness and utility of potential changes in programs and policies intended for large populations. Gold, Lake, Black, and Smith (2005) point out that demonstration projects involving high-risk elders often fail because of problems in the conceptualization, design, and implementation of the project that make it difficult to show the intended outcomes. "We speculate that part of the reason for this is that organizational and political processes lead to fundamentally conservative demonstrations that assume that small amounts of resources directed at incremental change can be effective in generating substantial change in organizations and can do so rapidly." In addition, when such projects depend on voluntary participation by the targeted population, selection bias can be introduced and lead to a group

that is substantively different from the population as a whole. Box 6-2 describes the problems associated with a Medicare demonstration project for community nursing organizations, an approach to care highly touted by the nursing community; the project, however, was terminated because its

---

**BOX 6-2**  The Demise of the Community Nursing Organization Demonstration Projects

The Community Nursing Organizations (CNOs) were funded as a Medicare demonstration project from 1994 to 1996 through a mandate included in the 1987 Omnibus Budget Reconciliation Act and subsequent reauthorizations to extend the projects through 2001. CNOs used capitated payment and a nurse case management model of prevention, health promotion, community nursing, and ambulatory care to reduce use of acute care services and be more cost effective than the traditional Medicare program. Four CNOs contracted with the federal government to participate in the demonstration project: Carle Clinic (Urbana, IL); Carondelet Health Care (Tucson, AZ); Living at Home/Block Nurse Program (Minneapolis, MN); and the Visiting Nurse Service (New York). The capitation to the CNOs was partial—if an enrollee was hospitalized, the CNO would continue to receive the capitated payment for the CNO services available to that enrollee, but the cost of the hospitalization and physician services would be shifted to the traditional fee-for-service (FFS) Medicare program.

The CNOs were initially required to randomly assign interested beneficiaries into a control (traditional FFS Medicare) or treatment group (capitated CNO case management model), but the pressure to enroll sufficient numbers of beneficiaries in the treatment group in a specific time frame resulted in changes in the sampling procedures. This in turn led to voluntary enrollment and selection bias. Frakt, Pizer, Schmitz, and Mattke (2005) evaluated the CNO demonstration project and explained this deviation in random assignment:

To accommodate the program's need to build up enrollment quickly, two applicants were assigned to the treatment group for every applicant assigned to the control group. The fact that the control group was smaller than the treatment group reduced the statistical power of the evaluation, increasing the size of the minimum impact that could be detected reliably.

evaluation suggested it was not living up to its promise of cost savings.

## STRATEGIES FOR SUCCESS*

### LOOK AT THE BIG PICTURE

It is human nature to view the world from a personal standpoint, focusing on the people and events that influence one's daily life. However, this strategy requires that one step back and take stock of the larger environment. It can provide a more objective perspective and increase nurses' credibility as broad-minded visionaries, looking beyond personal needs. It also means that one should not get bogged down in details that may seem important at the time but that in the larger schema may not be critical to the success of the issue. For example, legislation to address "patients' rights" under managed care plans was sidetracked by issues around medical liability and the high cost of malpractice insurance for physicians. The intent of the legislation was to give patients more choices for care under managed care plans. The original intent of the legislation became lost because certain stakeholders were more concerned with liability than with patients' rights.

In the heat of legislative battles and negotiations, it is easy to get distracted. However, the successful advocate is the one who does not lose sight of the big picture and is willing to compromise for the larger goal.

### DO YOUR HOMEWORK

We can never have all the information about an issue, but we need to be sufficiently prepared before we advocate. Usually one does not know beforehand when a particular policy will be acted on. It is not sufficient to claim ignorance when confronted with questions that should be answered. It diminishes policymakers' respect of nurses. However, if one has done everything possible to prepare and is asked to supply information that is not anticipated, it is reasonable and preferable to indicate that one does not know the answer. It does mean that one

must get the information as soon as possible and distribute it to the policymaker who requested it.

There are numerous ways to be adequately prepared:

- Clarify your position on the problem and possible solutions.
- Gather data, and search the clinical literature.
- Prepare documents to describe and support the issue.
- Assess the power dynamics of the players.
- Assess your own power base and ability to maneuver in the political arena.
- Plan a strategy, and assess its strengths and weaknesses.
- Prepare for the conflict.
- Line up support.
- Know the opposition and their rationale.

### IT'S NOT WHAT YOU SAY, IT'S HOW YOU SAY IT

The content of an issue is important, but it may be secondary to the way the message is framed and conveyed to stakeholders. Know the context of the issue (as described earlier). Learn to use strong, affirmative language to describe nursing practice. Use the rhetoric that incorporates lawmakers' lingo and the "buzz words" of key proponents. This requires having a sense of the values of the target audiences, be they policymakers, the public, hospital administrators, or community leaders.

Appealing to a variety of stakeholders often requires developing rhetoric or a message to frame your issue that is succinct and appealing to the values and concerns of those you want to mobilize or defeat. For example, "Cut Medicare" was an ineffective political message that the Republicans used in 1997 to try to gain public support for decreasing spending on Medicare. When the message was changed to "Preserve and Protect Medicare," the public was more supportive, even though the policy goals were the same. In the earlier example of reimbursement of APNs under the BBA, APNs framed their issue in terms of quality of care and cost savings. At a time when Congress was concerned about the amount of money spent on Medicare, the message of reducing costs without compromising quality resonated with the members. How you convey your message

---

*We are grateful to Susan Talbot for the original rendition of these political adages in the first edition of this book.

involves developing rhetoric or catchy phrases that the media might pick up and perpetuate (see Chapter 9, which discusses the media). Nurses need to develop their effectiveness in accessing and using the media, an essential component of getting the issue on the public's agenda.

## READ BETWEEN THE LINES

Often issues are not what they seem. It is just as important to be aware of the way one conveys information as it is to provide the facts. Communication theory notes that the overt message is not always the real message (Gerston, 1997). Some people say a lot by what they choose not to disclose. When legislators say they think your issue is important, it does not necessarily mean that they will vote to support it. The real question that needs to be asked is, "Will you vote in support of our bill?" What are the hidden agendas of the stakeholders concerned with the issue? What is not being said? When framing an issue, be aware of the covert messages. Be careful to make the issue as clear as possible and test it on others to be certain that reading between the lines conveys the same message as the overt rhetoric.

## IT'S NOT JUST WHAT YOU KNOW, IT'S WHO YOU KNOW

Using the power that results from personal connections is often the most important strategy in moving a critical issue. Sometimes it comes down to one important personal connection. In the example of APN reimbursement, the original legislation that gave some APNs Medicare reimbursement was greatly facilitated because the chief of staff for the senate majority leader was a nurse. Or consider the nurse who is the neighbor and friend of the secretary to the chief executive officer (CEO) in the medical center. This nurse is more likely to gain access to the CEO than will someone who is unknown to either the secretary or the CEO. Networking is an important long-term strategy for building influence; however, it can be a deliberate short-term strategy as well.

## QUID PRO QUO

Developing networks involves keeping track of what one has done for you and not being afraid to ask a favor in return. Often known as *quid pro quo* (literally, "something for something"), it is the way political arenas work in both public and private sectors. Networking is an important skill for achieving personal and political goals. Leaders expect to be asked for help and know the favor will be returned. It makes the one doing the favor feel good to be asked. Because nurses interface with the public all the time, they are in excellent positions to assist, facilitate, or otherwise do favors for people. Too often, nurses forget to ask for help from those whom they have helped and who would be more than willing to return a favor. Consider the lobbyist for a state nurses association who knew that the chair of the Senate public health and welfare committee had a grandson who was critically injured in a car accident. She visited the child several times in the hospital, spoke with the nurses on the unit, and kept the legislator informed about his grandson's progress and assured him that the boy was well cared for. When the boy recovered, the legislator was grateful and asked the lobbyist what he could do to move her issue. Interchanges like this occur every day and create the basis for quid pro quo.

## STRIKE WHILE THE IRON IS HOT

The timing of an issue is often the strategy that makes the difference in a successful outcome. A well-planned strategy may fail because the timing is off. An issue may languish for some period because of a mismatch in values, concerns, or resources. Yet suddenly, something can change to make an issue ripe for consideration. Before September 11, 2001, the issue of bioterrorism was of limited concern to the public and a low priority for most health care professionals. Yet warnings and preparations had actually begun. In response to the first bombing of the World Trade Center in 1993, President Clinton had convened a group of experts to develop a national strategy for responding to a bioterrorist attack. However, the effort received limited resources. After the attacks of September 11 on the World Trade Center and the Pentagon, the issue moved to the top of the congressional and presidential agenda. President Bush asked for and got billions of dollars to prevent and respond to bioterrorism.

Certainly hurricane Katrina elucidated the problems of the poor condition of the levees around New Orleans. Despite numerous requests by the Army Corps of Engineers to fix the levees, Congress never appropriated adequate funding to fix them. Katrina not only forced a reconsideration of the need to rebuild the levees, but it made clear that much of the funding for bioterrorism should have been used for communication links with emergency responders and hospitals. The timing of the hurricane provided the impetus to increase funding for both projects.

## UNITED WE STAND, DIVIDED WE FALL

The successful achievement of policy goals can be accomplished only if supporters demonstrate a united front. Collective action is almost always more effective than individual action. Collaboration through coalitions (see Chapter 8 on coalitions) demonstrates broad support for the issue. Besides having your own group organized and ready to be mobilized, what other networks do you have or can you develop?

Sometimes diverse groups can work together on an issue of mutual support, even though they are opponents on other issues. Public and private interest groups that identify with nursing's issues can be invaluable resources for nurses. They often have influential supporters or may have research information that can help nurses move an issue. Rallies, letter-writing campaigns, and grassroots efforts by such groups can turn up the volume on nursing's issues and create the necessary groundswell of support to overcome opposition.

It is in nursing's best political interest to end the divisiveness among nurses and professional nursing organizations and to foster ways for nurses to become flexible and politically responsive. On the other hand, nurses are so diverse that perhaps we should not expect to agree on everything. Instead, we should look for opportunities to reach consensus or remain silent in the public arena on an issue that is not of paramount concern.

## NOTHING VENTURED, NOTHING GAINED

Nurses have always been risk takers. Margaret Sanger fled to England after she was sentenced to jail for providing women with information about birth control (Chesler, 1992). Clara Maas lost her life while participating in research on malaria (Kalisch & Kalisch, 1995). Harriet Tubman risked her life to transport and care for more than 300 slaves who sought freedom in the North before and during the Civil War (Carnegie, 1986). Such thoughtful risk takers weigh the costs and benefits of their actions. They consider possible outcomes in relation to the expenditure of available resources. For example, a nurse may decide to run for Congress, knowing that she has little chance of winning. She risks losing, but running will give her the opportunity to bring important health issues to the public's attention and will help her gain name recognition for her next race.

Risk taking requires analyzing both the risks and the benefits of an action. This can be much easier for an individual than for an organization, but nonetheless it warrants open and thoughtful discussion by those taking the risk. The strongest case for risk taking comes when the core values of an individual or organization are at stake.

## THE BEST DEFENSE IS A GOOD OFFENSE

A successful political strategy is one that tries to accommodate the concerns of the opposition. It requires disassociating the emotional context of working with opponents—the first step in principled negotiating. The person who is skillful at managing conflict will be successful in politics. The saying that "politics makes strange bedfellows" arose out of the recognition that long-standing opponents can sometimes come together around issues of mutual concern, but it often requires creative thinking and a commitment to fairness to develop an acceptable approach to resolving an issue.

One must also anticipate problems and areas for disagreement and be prepared to counter them: When the opposition is gaining momentum and support, it can be helpful to develop a strategy that can distract attention from the opposition's issue or that can delay action. For example, one nurses association continually battled the state medical society's efforts to amend the nurse practice act in ways that would restrict nurses' practice and provide for physician supervision. Nurses became particularly concerned about the possibility of passage during a year when the medical society's influence with the legislature was high. Working with other nonphysician provider organizations engaged in similar battles (e.g., optometrists, pharmacists), the nurses proposed a bill that would go after the medical practice act by removing all oversight authority. The physicians knew that there would be a large coalition supporting such a bill. As a result they agreed to drop efforts to amend the Nurse Practice Act.

The other dimension of this axiom is creating opportunities for your opposition and power holders to gain firsthand experience with your issue. The many "walk a mile with a nurse" campaigns, when legislators or others spend time trailing a nurse, have provided hospital executives and public officials with the opportunity to understand the complexities of a nurse's daily work and the barriers that nurses confront (McEachen, Mason, & Jabara, 1992). Once they have seen issues through the nurse's lens, they may be more willing to find satisfactory policy solutions. Media coverage of your issue can also help to accomplish this end, particularly when personal stories are used to illustrate the conflicts or concerns raised by an issue.

## SUMMARY

The future of nursing and health care may well depend on nurses' skills in moving a vision. Without a vision, politics becomes an end in itself—a game that is often corrupt and empty. Instead, nurses can use the vision to define the goals.

## *Key Points*

- A systematic analysis of moving a defined policy to implementation is critical to understand the political dimensions of particular issues.
- Once that is achieved, a plan can be created that should incorporate issues such as gender politics, power dynamics, and the specific strategies that would be most appropriate to achieve the goals and the vision.

- Similar strategies can be used in the workplace, government, organizations, and the community to assure that nurses use their power, through their expertise and numbers, to protect and improve the health of all Americans.

## *Web Resources*

**American Nurses Association**
*www.nursingworld.org/gova*
**American Political Science Association policy section**
*http://apsapolicysection.org/currents.html*
**Cook Political Report**
*www.cookpolitical.com*

## REFERENCES

Benner, P. (1984). *From novice to expert*. Menlo Park, CA: Addison-Wesley.

Carnegie, M. E. (1986). *The path we tread: Blacks in nursing, 1854-1984*. Philadelphia: Lippincott.

Chesler, E. (1992). *Woman of valor: Margaret Sanger and the birth control movement in America*. New York: Anchor Books.

Cohen, S. S. (2001). *Championing child care*. New York: Columbia University Press.

Duke, J. T. (1976). *Conflict and power in social life*. Provo, UT: Brigham Young University Press.

Feeley, T. J. (2002). The multiple goals of science and technology policy. In F. Baumgartner & B. Jones (Eds.), *Policy dynamics*. Chicago: University of Chicago Press.

Ferguson, V. D. (1993). Perspectives on power. In D. J. Mason, S. W. Talbott, & J. K. Leavitt (Eds.), *Policy and politics for nurses: Action and change in the workplace, government, organizations, and community* (2nd ed.). Philadelphia: Saunders.

Fox-Piven, F., & Cloward, R. (1993). *Regulating the poor: The functions of public welfare*. New York: Vintage Press.

Frakt, A. B., Pizer, S. D., Schmitz, R. J., & Mattke, S. (2005). Voluntary partial capitation: The Community Nursing Organization Medicare demonstration. *Health Care Financing Review, 26*(4). Retrieved November 25, 2005, from *www.cms.hhs.gov/review/05summer/05summerpg21.pdf*.

French, J. R. P., & Raven, B. (1959). The basis of social power. In D. Cartwright (Ed.), *Studies in social power*. Ann Arbor, MI: University of Michigan Press.

Gerston, L. N. (1997). *Public policy making: Process and principles*. Armonk, NY: M.E. Sharper.

Gold, M., Lake, T., Black, W. E., & Smith, M. (2005). Challenges in improving care for high-risk seniors in Medicare. *Health Affairs (Millwood)*. Retrieved November 25, 2005, from *http://content.healthaffairs.org/cgi/content/full/hlthaff.w5.199/DC1*.

Joel, L., & Kelly, L. (2002). *The nursing experience: Trends, challenges, and transitions* (4th ed.). New York: McGraw-Hill.

Jones, J. (2005). Nurses remain atop ethics and honesty lists. Retrieved December 7, 2005, from *http://poll.gallup.com/content/?ci=20254*.

Kalisch, P. A., & Kalisch, B. J. (1995). *The advance of American nursing* (3rd ed.). Philadelphia: Lippincott.

Kingdon, J. W. (2003). *Agendas, alternatives and public policies.* New York: Longman.

Mason, D. J., Backer, B. A., & Georges, C. A. (1991). Towards a feminist model for the political empowerment of nurses. *Image: Journal of Nursing Scholarship, 23*(2), 72-77.

McEachen, I., Mason, D. J., & Jabara, I. (1992). Walk a mile with a nurse. *Nursing Spectrum, 4*(3), 5.

Mooney, C. Z. (Ed.). (2001). *The public clash of private values: The politics of morality policy.* New York: Chatham House.

Robert, H. M. (2000). *Robert's rules of order newly revised.* Reading, MA: Addison-Wesley.

Roberts, N. (1998). Radical change by entrepreneurial design. *Acquisitions Review Quarterly.* Retrieved November 25, 2005, from *www.au.af.mil/au/awc/awcgate/dau/roberts.pdf.*

Schattschneider, E. E. (1960). *The semi-sovereign people.* New York: Holt, Rhinehart & Winston.

Stone, D. (2002). *Policy paradox: The art of political decision making.* New York: W.W. Norton.

Tanner, D. (2001). *Talking from 9 to 5: Women and men in the workplace—Language, sex, power.* New York: Quill.

Weissert, C. (1991). Policy entrepreneurs, policy opportunists, and legislative effectiveness. *American Politics Quarterly, 19*(2), 262-273.

# *Taking Action*   Ruth E. Malone

## The Nightingales Take on Big Tobacco

*"Neglecting to discuss the industry's role as the disease vector in the tobacco epidemic is like refusing to discuss the role of mosquitoes in a malaria epidemic or rats in an outbreak of bubonic plague."*
ROB CUSHMAN, MD, MEDICAL OFFICER OF HEALTH, OTTAWA

I smoked all the way through nursing school, and I smoked for the first 10 years of my career as a registered nurse. I'd smoke my cigarettes in the utility room or the nurses' lounge and emerge, feeling guilty, to care for patients who were suffering from emphysema or lung cancer or heart disease. I tried to quit so many times, but it was incredibly difficult. I felt so alone.

I also used the cigarette as a way to feel "tough," to show that I wasn't afraid of death—after all, I was an emergency nurse. I could take it. I had seen it all. I used the cigarette as solace when I felt lonely. I used it as a badge of independence. I was very, very addicted, and I had my first cigarette as soon as I got out of bed, even before I had coffee, and my last just before I turned out the light.

That was more than 20 years ago, but I vividly remember reading newspaper and magazine articles at the time about new studies showing that actually, smoking was not really so bad, and interviews with academics who compared smoking with eating chocolate or having a glass of wine: something pleasurable. Smoking, they said, was actually helpful because it helped one relax, relieved stress. Although rationally I knew better, I wanted to believe, because I worried about smoking. I also wanted to believe it was true that many other things caused lung cancer besides smoking, because then it would seem like it was only one among so many "risk factors"—rather than being the cause of more than 80% of lung cancers.

What I didn't know then would fill a book. Mainly, though, I didn't realize that the tobacco industry had set up front groups, hired scientists, and organized massive campaigns to promote bogus ideas, had sponsored "distracting" scientific studies selected by industry lawyers to be sure they would result in findings favorable to the industry, and had promoted their intentionally deceptive ideas through an astonishingly large and varied assortment of paid "consultants" and front groups (Bero, 2003; Bero, 2005; Glantz, Slade, Bero, Hanauer, & Barnes, 1996). I had no idea that the tobacco companies had special marketing plans developed to reassure those, like me, who worried even as we lit up another cigarette (Brown and Williamson Tobacco Company, 1971) and that they were working on a global scale to fight tobacco control policies and ensure that smoking remained socially acceptable (Zeltner, Kessler, Martiny, & Randera, 2000).

## THE PERSONAL BECOMES POLITICAL: GRASPING THE NATURE OF THE PROBLEM

I finally got free. It probably took me 20 tries to do it, but I finally did quit smoking for good. Living in California, a state with a strong tobacco control program, helped me, because the state developed strong laws for smoke-free public places and workplaces, and that made me think more about it every time I lit up. I think now that going back to school also helped me, because it built my confidence and helped me realize that my addiction was holding me back. And once I went back to school, I just kept going. I was an associate degree nurse who returned for a baccalaureate after practicing for 10 years and continued all the way through a postdoc, where I began working on tobacco control policy research and learning more about tobacco than I ever learned in nursing school.

For example, I learned that until the advent of the machine-rolled cigarette in the late 1800s, almost nobody ever died from lung cancer. It was such a rare disease that most physicians would never see a case of it in their lifetimes. Although individuals used tobacco at the time, it was mostly in pipes or cigars, and there was no massive advertising campaign aimed at getting people to use them. In fact, the same entrepreneurs who made tobacco into machine-rolled cigarettes also introduced aggressive, innovative advertising techniques that linked cigarettes with glamour, freedom, sexuality, and status (Kluger, 1997). I realized for the first time that we were facing an *industrially produced* disease epidemic from tobacco.

As a bit of a history buff, then, I was thrilled when more than 7 million internal tobacco company

documents became publicly available as the result of multiple state attorneys general lawsuits in the late 1990s. These documents, which are now accessible online *(http://legacy.library.ucsf.edu)*, offered an amazing window into how this incredibly destructive industry came to be so powerful. They include business plans, budgets, scientific research, public relations and marketing plans, memos, letters, and much more. Reading them was fascinating work, and I began to develop a whole program of research drawing on them; many a night I would call my husband at 10 PM to tell him I still couldn't quite tear myself away from an especially compelling batch of materials.

## COMPELLING VOICES

It was one of those late nights when I found the first of the letters that expanded my career path into activism. It was one among several hundred (there are probably thousands; I just found these files quite by accident amid the 7 million poorly indexed documents) written to tobacco companies by suffering customers and their families. These searing, gut-wrenching letters changed my life forever.

"My father died last October at the age of 50 due to lung cancer," I read. "He purchased many of your items in your 'Marlboro Country Store Catalog' with his cigarette coupons...Now myself and my 16 year old sister are left fatherless...The only thing I have to say to you is that smoking does cause cancer, smoking does kill and destroy families. You don't need to be a scientist or conduct a study to figure that out, just visit my Dad's grave if you want proof." The words were written in the fat, round script of a teenage girl, but the file I had stumbled onto contained letter after letter like this, written by every sort of human hand. Most of them were written on the backs of or in response to slick mailers that the tobacco companies had sent out: catalogs, birthday cards, offers of coupons for discounted cigarettes, surveys. There were letters from grieving mothers, widows, sons and daughters; letters from friends and family; and letters from dying smokers and those struggling to escape tobacco addiction. They had been sent from all over the country, from large cities and small towns. They were testimony.

"When will the greed in your industry stop?" asked a man from Colorado whose parents had died prematurely from tobacco-caused disease, noting that his two boys would grow up without knowing their grandparents. "I know that we all have to work to put food on the table and pay bills. But are there no other choices?"

The letters weren't asking for money; they were asking for their human pain and loss to be acknowledged and asking the company to stop promoting cigarettes and get into other businesses. A woman, grieving over her mother's death at 57 from lung cancer, wrote, "I realize you don't force people to smoke, but…smoking is an addiction, people cannot help themselves. My mother wanted to quit so badly…When I close my eyes at night, all I can see is my mother's face as she lay dying, and all the hell that she went through…that will haunt our family forever. It was such a waste." Another printed out in bold black letters: "Cancer of the lungs due to smoking. Painful, wasteful, sorrowful. It's on your hands, Philip Morris."

I sat at my computer and cried, because as a nurse I could so easily fill in the terrible subtext that accompanied every anguished word. I knew that behind each letter were family members who had used every economic and emotional resource they had trying to cope with the suffering and loss of a loved one; orphaned children who would never have the guidance of a father or mother; aging parents who helplessly watched their children die before them. I knew that the suffering from tobacco-related illnesses such as emphysema and lung cancer was often terrible to witness, much less to experience. I knew that these stories were repeated 440,000 times every year—the estimate of the Centers for Disease Control and Prevention (CDC) for annual deaths from tobacco—year after year, in the United States alone (CDC, 2005).

I also knew, from having spent months digging into and reviewing the industry's own documents, that the products that had killed all these people had been engineered for addictiveness and that the industry had discussed internally the addictive nature of its products for decades, in some cases comparing themselves favorably with the pharmaceutical industry. I knew that companies had targeted their aggressive marketing and outreach efforts to the most vulnerable groups: the poor, less educated, and minority groups (Apollonio & Malone, 2005; Balbach, Gasior, & Barbeau, 2003; Cook, Wayne, Keithly, & Connolly, 2004; Hackbarth, Silvestri, & Cosper, 1995; Landrine et al., 2005; Muggli, Pollay, Lew, & Joseph, 2002; Smith & Malone, 2003; Yerger & Malone, 2002). I knew that tobacco companies had joined together in public relations efforts aimed at creating doubt about the scientific evidence that cigarettes caused disease, and later, that secondhand smoke caused disease (U.S. Tobacco Companies, 1954). I knew the tobacco companies had obstructed public health efforts, including trying to undermine the work of the World Health Organization (WHO) and other public health bodies. For example, they hired consultants who then "volunteered" (without revealing their industry ties) to help WHO pesticide regulatory bodies with their work and who influenced the outcome by writing reports that minimized the harmfulness of pesticides used by the tobacco industry (McDaniel, Solomon, & Malone, 2005; Zeltner et al., 2000). I knew that the industry's huge political and philanthropic contributions bought silence from policymakers and groups that should have been protecting the public (Yerger & Malone, 2002). I didn't really think the tobacco industry was particularly benign. After all, pushing something that kills millions every year isn't exactly a benevolent endeavor. But somehow, I had never once considered the idea that these companies had been getting letters like these for decades and filing them away, year after deadly year.

## CONSIDERING ACTIONS

At first, I didn't know what to do. I shared the letters with family and friends, who were horrified, equally astonished to think that any human being could read them and yet continue to promote use of such dangerous and destructive products. I thought about writing a scholarly ethics paper about them, but that didn't seem enough. Besides, seeing or hearing just one didn't have the same effect. That was part of the problem, I began to see: The industrially produced epidemic of tobacco-caused disease and death comes one by one by one, slowly. None of us realizes quite how big it really has become, and how many people are hurt—not only smokers, but their families and friends, their communities. That's why we can't solve this problem one by one: We have to do it collectively, by acting to affect the policies and politics that allow it to continue.

After I turned out the light at night I was haunted by the letter from the elderly widower who wrote, as though speaking in the voice of his dead wife, "The latest news from me is that I died May 9, 1990 of lung cancer. Maybe my widower would like your free trip. Although I doubt it very much. You see, he has been mourning my death for 4 years. I was all he had left—me and my Benson & Hedges. Wish you were here" (Halpin, 1994). I could see him, sitting alone under the lamp at the kitchen table where they had eaten so many meals together, writing the letter in his trembling hand on the back of a glossy Benson & Hedges cigarette brand mailer. I found myself revisiting the letters, reading them over one by one, and crying again. They would not let me rest. Although I tried to continue with my research projects, which had nothing to do with the letters, the suffering those letters bespoke was palpable: It simply wasn't right for them to remain forever mute, filed away.

There was no evidence that any top tobacco executive ever read the letters. I found a handwritten note on one, suggesting that the letter writer be added to the company's "no-mail" list and sent the "we'll take your comments seriously form letter." It was hard to decide which was more chilling: the idea that top tobacco industry executives never read them at all, and ordered them filed away, or the notion that they *did* read them, and filed them all away, year after year, decade after deadly decade. But I felt that these letters needed to see the light of day, and that other families like this should know they were not alone.

## DOING *SOMETHING*

Inspired by some youth activists who had attended the Altria/Philip Morris shareholders' meeting to speak out about the industry's targeting of youth, I decided to buy one share of stock and go to the shareholders' meeting as a nurse, taking some of the letters with me. But I knew that a single nurse

**NIGHTINGALES**

The Nightingales is a group of nurses who use advocacy, activism, and education to focus public attention on the role of the tobacco industry in creating the epidemic of tobacco-caused suffering, disease, and death. For more information or to join, visit the Nightingales website at *www.nightingalesnurses.org.*

would not have much impact and could be easily dismissed. By e-mailing networks of students, friends, and colleagues and just asking for help, I managed to gather together 11 other nurses from around the country who would agree to buy one share of Altria stock (only shareholders could attend the meeting) and travel with me to the meeting in New Jersey. Other nurses sent contributions to help pay for airfares for those who went to the meeting. We picked the Altria/Philip Morris meeting because Philip Morris is the largest U.S. tobacco company.

We worked together via e-mail and telephone to craft our key message and goals for the meeting. We decided that our strength as activists lay in our deep grounding in the clinical experience of caring for those who suffered from tobacco, and therefore our theme was "nurses bearing witness." We also sought to point out the contradictions inherent in the company's claims to be "changed" and "socially responsible" while continuing the aggressive promotion of the most deadly consumer products ever made, products that were killing 440,000 Americans annually and were responsible for the premature deaths of millions more worldwide. Our key message was, "A socially responsible company would not continue to promote products that it admits addict and kill." We also decided that initially our focus would be on trying to get coverage in nursing media, which would help us spread the word about our group, so we contacted the *American Journal of Nursing*, which agreed to send a reporter to cover us "making history" as the first group of nurses ever to confront Big Tobacco on its own turf (Schwarz, 2004; Schwarz, 2005).

Lots of groups are working on tobacco, including many major health organizations. We didn't want to duplicate their efforts, but instead to make a unique contribution as nurses, through a relatively decentralized activist network that could watch for local opportunities to challenge the industry's messages. Our aim was to be "guerrilla nurses" (but highly professional ones!) rather than to develop a big bureaucratic structure that would impede our ability to be creative and fast on our feet.

We discussed names for our group. I think I suggested the Nightingales, because of the immediate link of the name with nursing in the public eye, the image of the lamp, which I thought resonated with shining the light of day on these secret letters, and the bird, which sings a particularly clear, true song. We had considerable discussion about this, including the concerns of some that it might be interpreted as gender-exclusionary; the men in the founding group were some of the strongest defenders of the name. We also sought counsel from other tobacco control advocates, who were excited to hear that nurses were prepared to be activists and loved the name, saying it was memorable and meaningful. So, as the newly minted Nightingales, we prepared to meet in person (many of us for the first time) one late April 2004 day in suburban New Jersey as Altria/Philip Morris shareholders.

## STRATEGIC PLANNING

Through my tobacco control e-mail networks, I located a nurse in New Jersey, Elizabeth Wilson, who scoped out the site for us, as we had no idea what to expect or how difficult it might be logistically. She sent us digital photos of the location, reassuring us that parking would not be a problem and that the neighborhood was residential and safe. Other activists invited us to be part of a press conference outside after the meeting. Some of my students helped me assemble a selection of the letters into a 30-foot banner which we would display at the press conference, since we were not allowed to bring anything into the meeting itself. We also made up packets of materials about our efforts, including some of the letters and a press release (Box 6-3).

The night before the meeting, we met in a hotel room, swapped stories about what drew us to undertake such a mission, and formulated our questions. We had learned from other activists how the meeting was structured: a business report followed by a

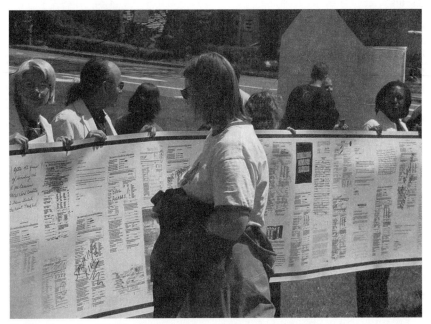

Nightingales at the 2004 shareholders meeting displaying banner. *Left to right, behind banner:* D. Hackbarth, IL; Terry Sayre, CA; C. Southard, IL (head turned); P. Jones, CA.

**BOX 6-3**   Nightingales' Press Release

**www.nightingalesnurses.org**
**PRESS RELEASE: FOR IMMEDIATE RELEASE**
INFORMATION: Ruth Malone, RN, PhD,
   rmalone@itsa.ucsf.edu

**PRESS RELEASE**
**Embargo until 12:00 Noon Eastern Time Thursday
April 29, 2004**
EAST HANOVER, NJ: Nurses from across America
will attend the annual shareholders meeting of Philip
Morris (now under the parentage of Altria) today in
East Hanover, NJ to call on the company to
voluntarily end active promotion of cigarettes.
This will be the first time in the history of Philip Morris
that nurses have attended the meeting. After the
meeting, the nurses will hold a reading and share a
display of letters from the secret tobacco industry
documents, sent to the company by its dying
customers and their families and never before
exposed.

   "We're here to say that this can't go on," said
Nightingales organizer Ruth Malone, RN, Associate
Professor of Nursing at the University of California,
San Francisco School of Nursing. "The tobacco industry
spends more than $1 million an hour, 24/7, on making
their deadly, addictive products look fun, cool, and
glamorous—but these letters show the terrifying,
painful reality of what cigarettes do."

As the largest group of health care providers, the
nation's 2.5 million nurses are in a unique position at
the bedside and in the community to witness firsthand
the deadly effects of tobacco products. "A socially
responsible company would not continue to promote
a product that they themselves admit addicts and
kills," said Diana Hackbarth, RN, Professor of Nursing
at Loyola University in Chicago and a Fellow of the
American Academy of Nursing.

   Nurses are attending the shareholders meeting
as a group to tell their patients' stories, giving voice to
those who can no longer speak because tobacco
addiction has robbed them of breath and life. "Tobacco
products cause devastation to so many families,"
noted Lee S. Clay, RN, CNM, a nurse midwife from
New Jersey who is attending to call attention to the
tobacco industry's aggressive marketing to young
women of childbearing age. Wearing black armbands
to honor the memories of their patients who have
suffered and died from cigarette-caused disease;
nurses will call on Philip Morris to show genuine
corporate social responsibility by voluntarily ending
the active promotion and marketing of tobacco
products. *Press Conference starting about 12 noon
near company entrance at 188 Rover Road.*

**Contact Information**
Ruth Malone, RN, (415) 123-4567;
Diana Hackbarth, RN, PhD, FAAN (773) 123-4567

question-and-answer period, then discussion of shareholder resolutions, several of which concerned health-related topics. We laid out ground rules: everyone would wear a white lab coat and black armband, indicating solidarity with those who suffered from tobacco; we would be professional in all respects; we would wear outer coats over our lab coats, and all would take off their overcoats when the first nurse spoke.

   Some worried that the company might try to have us removed from the meeting when we revealed our lab coats. We decided that the tobacco company was not likely to do this, as it would certainly attract press attention, something companies assiduously try to avoid unless the attention is on their own terms and favorable. We agreed that we would follow the rules of the meeting.

## THE NIGHTINGALES' FIRST FLIGHT

The day of the meeting, we met very early and drove in our rented van through a security gauntlet to get to the meeting buildings, our vehicle stopped repeatedly by large, dark-suited men in dark glasses who examined our meeting passes as though we were trying to penetrate the inner sanctum of the FBI. Once at the building, we went through more intensive screening, including x-ray searches and examination of our bags. No cameras or other electronic devices are permitted.

   After locating the meeting room, one of our nurses asked a security person where the microphones would be set up, and we secured seats on the aisles nearby to assure that we would have a chance to speak, as we had been told by other activists that time for questions was limited.

The meeting began with a video showcasing all the corporation's products. It was strange to see Oreo cookies and Parliament cigarettes practically side by side; I found that a favorite tea of mine was a corporate product, and quietly resolved not to buy it again. The video included old TV footage of the Marlboro Man, with the stirring theme so many of us remember from childhood. I hadn't realized until that moment how Marlboro cigarettes had hijacked the very image of the American West: merely seeing a desert landscape evokes that brand, to the point that now the company need only show a boot by a campfire and we immediately know it is a Marlboro ad.

After the video, there was a business report, delivered by CEO Louis Camilleri, highlighting how successful the company had been in increasing cigarette sales worldwide and how profitable an investment the stock was. Then it was time for the shareholder "question-and-answer" period. I jumped from my seat to stand before the microphone.

As it turned out, I was the first to speak, and I was shaking as I read from the letters and asked the CEO, Louis Camilleri, whether the board of directors had an ethics committee that actually read these letters and decided how to respond, and what ethical criteria were used in deciding whether to continue promoting products that caused such harm. Camilleri looked a little startled when I said I was going to read from letters found in the company's documents. He never answered my question, saying he was "sorry to hear about those people" and resorting instead to talking about how the company was changing and being "responsible." The company now admits, after decades of denying that cigarettes were harmful (and even making health claims for them), that "there is no safe cigarette." But saying that is small comfort to those who receive conflicting messages from tobacco marketers that smoking is glamorous, cool, sexy, and fun and are addicted by the time they figure out it isn't.

Another nurse, Sharon Brown from Pennsylvania, rose and asked for a moment of silence before asking her question, in honor of her father, whose birthday was that very day. After what seemed an excruciatingly long moment of utter stillness, she informed the room that her father had died prematurely,

killed by cigarettes. It was a powerful feeling, for a nurse to basically shut down the meeting for even one minute, a meeting where some of the richest and most powerful men (and they did seem to be mostly men, although there are women tobacco executives) in the world were gathered. Other nurses rose, one by one, and spoke about the suffering they had witnessed: a nurse practitioner spoke about the harm tobacco does to pregnant women and children; a burn nurse about caring for burn victims from cigarette-caused fires. Each time, the room fell silent as we spoke; I felt the symbolic power of our white lab coats and our nursing presence as we asked the company to do the socially responsible thing and stop marketing these deadly products.

## EXTENDING THE MESSAGE

After the meeting, we joined other groups outside for a press conference. We held a public reading of the letters, taking turns reading them, tears in all our eyes. We congratulated the youth activists, who were thrilled that "the nurses" had joined their fight. We got great coverage in the nursing press, an interview on public radio, and some attention from newspapers, and after a Nightingales' partner helped us develop a Website, we began to get lots of interest from nurses. As of August, 2005, just a little more than a year after we started, we have Nightingales in more than half the states and in Canada. We have attended the shareholders meeting a second time with more Nightingales, who spoke with equal dignity and passion. We've also challenged the company's claims of "responsibility" at Philip Morris public relations events in California and Kentucky and have spoken at several other events.

Our efforts (see *www.nightingalesnurses.org*) are attracting more attention, including from the industry itself. For example, at a recent national tobacco conference we were invited to include some of our printed materials at a national nursing organization's table. The organization's staffer reported that a woman claiming to work for Philip Morris stopped by to collect copies of all our materials and complained that there were not enough company representatives there to report on all the sessions. The industry regularly sends spies to

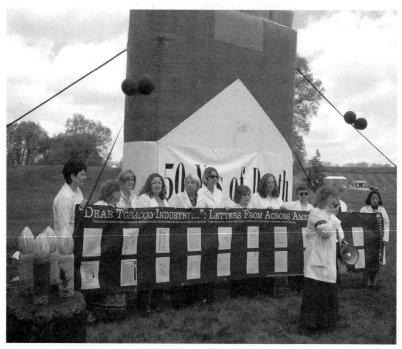

Nightingales conducting press conference after the 2005 shareholders meeting. Left to right, holding banner: S. Toner, MO; D. Tasso. WV; L. Greathouse, KY; S. Brown, PA; D. Hackbarth, IL; J. Buss, CA; C. Southard, IL; M. Wertz, CA; E. Wilson, NJ; MJ Schymeinsky, CA (partially hidden); A. Apacible, CA; and Ruth Malone (speaking), CA.

cover major national health meetings (Malone, 2002).

Our work has all been done with volunteer effort, by the seat of our pants.

Of course, Altria/Philip Morris and the other tobacco companies are still promoting tobacco products. Although, as Mr. Camilleri reported this year, sales are dropping in the United States, the company plans for aggressive expansion into Asia and Africa, into countries with little public health infrastructure and historically low smoking rates among women. The U.S. tobacco companies, according to the Federal Trade Commission's 2003 figures, spend more than $1.7 million an hour, 24/7, promoting these deadly products. We still have a long way to go, and we will need to develop new and innovative strategies to get there.

But our efforts have borne fruit in several respects. First, and perhaps most powerfully, we have sent a message to the tobacco industry. Nurses are trusted and respected by the public, and we simply owe it to our patients to speak out and tell the whole truth about Big Tobacco. Sustaining a discussion about the tobacco industry is important because the public must begin to understand that this is not just "business as usual," that pushing these highly engineered, deadly products for profit just can't continue forever, luring generation after generation to early deaths. Nurses need to be promoting public dialogue on how to phase out the industrial production and promotion of tobacco—perhaps, as suggested in a recent article, by converting the tobacco market to a nonprofit entity with a public health mandate (Callard, Thompson, & Collishaw, 2005).

The context within which nurses' clients are taking up or trying to quit smoking includes receiving constant messages from the tobacco industry, straight into their homes, and increasingly through much more subtle marketing methods, such as experiential programs, viral marketing, and music events. Philip Morris has a database of more than 20 million smokers, which it uses to establish personalized relationships and targeted communications (Philip Morris USA, 2003). We need to educate clients so they understand how the industry has studied their every psychologic weakness, segmenting the market to reach everyone from the starter "replacement smokers," as the industry called youth, to the worried older smokers like me, whom they seek to reassure. We would not continue to treat malaria victims without ever mentioning the mosquito that transmits the disease. If we are true advocates for our patients, we must likewise name, discuss, and find ways to combat the industry vector of the tobacco disease epidemic.

Second, our efforts have inspired others. The youths who saw us join them are still talking at meetings about "the nurses" and how our presence helped them feel part of something larger. Who knows? Perhaps some of those young people will decide to become nurses. We need them; we need their passion and political awareness, and nursing will give them great opportunities to put those attributes into practice.

Third, these efforts are empowering us as nurses in a way I would never have envisioned. I'll never forget coming back after the first trip, when one of my students observed thoughtfully that "this experience has changed the whole way I feel about being a nurse." Another said to me this year, "now I feel that I can say anything, to anyone, with confidence."

## WHAT NURSES CAN DO

There is perhaps no other health issue on which nurses—if we really took it on in a major way—could have so much impact. Tobacco affects almost every body system and every demographic group across the lifespan. It affects individuals, families, and communities; there is no nurse for whom tobacco could not be relevant. But there is something about attending the shareholders' meeting and "speaking truth to power" that takes the deadly politics of tobacco out of the realm of the abstract and makes it as real as the suffering we witness.

The tobacco industry has worried about this prospect for years. Among the industry documents,

I had earlier found a list of organizations the industry viewed as its opponents, with each one's strengths appraised. The list included the American Medical Association, the American Public Health Association, and specific tobacco control activist groups. I was intrigued to see that the American Nurses Association was included. "Nurses, as a group, feel strongly and negatively about tobacco use," the report read. "As they become more active in politics…at all levels, they could easily become formidable opponents for the tobacco industry" (Osmon, 1990). *Formidable opponents.* I wasn't used to thinking of nurses in those terms. But when it came to the tobacco industry, I really liked how that sounded. I started to consciously *think* of myself as a "formidable opponent."

Now I talk about tobacco all the time, to whomever will listen, and each time I am more confident. Repetition is our friend. For people to begin to see this issue differently, they need to hear it more than once, and we need to say it more than once to get it right. The industry spent decades and billions of dollars convincing us that putting these toxic chemical cocktails in our mouths and lighting them is normal. It will take time to help the public understand that there's nothing normal about smoking cigarettes and that, although people have used tobacco for centuries, it is only with the corporate production and promotion of cigarettes that we face suffering and disease on this scale. We need to educate the public—not only about tobacco use, but about the industry that promotes it.

My part of this work has extended into other arenas now. I've worked within health-related organizations to develop policies on holding future meetings and conventions only in cities that are smoke free, because no one should have to breathe carcinogens to hold a job and because convention business is important to cities. I've developed, and teach, a graduate course on tobacco control policy issues. The Nightingales challenged a Philip Morris executive giving a talk on corporate social responsibility at a major California university, did educational outreach on World No-Tobacco Day, and traveled to the California state capitol for a rally to support the victims of tobacco disease.

Our Nightingales listserve provides opportunities for nurses working on tobacco to hear about the work of others, problem solve together, and exchange good ideas. The Nightingales build on the great work of many nurses all over the country—in many cases, important work they've been doing for years with little recognition or support from colleagues. Here are some other examples of work nurses are doing: Linda Sarna, Stella Bialous, and Erika Froelicher are doing the Tobacco Free Nurses project (www.tobaccofreenurses.org), aimed at helping nurses quit smoking. At UCLA, Professor Sarna convinced her fellow nurse faculty members to pass a policy against accepting tobacco industry research funding, and although the policy is still being disputed at the university level, the dialogue helps educate others about how providing funding allows the tobacco industry to benefit from the association with respected institutions, lending it legitimacy it does not deserve.

In Lexington, Kentucky, Nightingale and nursing professor Ellen Hahn spearheaded the Smokefree Lexington policy, a strong smoke-free ordinance, and Nightingale Lisa Greathouse organized a World No-Tobacco Day display of our banner showing the letters at the University of Kentucky—right in the heart of tobacco country. But it's not only more-senior nurses doing good work. Nightingale Cheryl Bisping, a nursing student in Minnesota, chairs two coalitions working on secondhand smoke, smoke-free restaurants, and tobacco-free youth recreation policies.

Internationally, Nightingale and nursing professor Sophia Chan developed the first smoking cessation counseling training program in Hong Kong since 2000 and created a new role for nurses (Chan, 2002). She also influenced the government to fund 10 smoking cessation health clinics in the formal health care system and launched the first youth quitline in Hong Kong.

Nightingales founding member Diana Hackbarth, another professor of nursing from Chicago, is chair of the statewide Illinois Coalition Against Tobacco, the oldest anti-tobacco coalition in the United States, and for decades has worked on statewide, county, and local legislation, including clean indoor air legislation, getting rid of tobacco billboards,

and raising tobacco taxes. She has picketed against the Virginia Slims Tennis Tournament, Joe Camel, and Philip Morris's sponsorship of a major art exhibit.

Carol Southard, a tobacco cessation specialist in Illinois and another Nightingales founding member, is managing a major smoking cessation initiative working with the American Dental Hygienists' Association, provides smoking cessation services for Chicago city employees, and is a sought-after speaker for media, educational and outreach efforts for youth, and smoke-free campaigns. Nightingale Colleen Hughes of Nevada served as president of the Nevada Tobacco Prevention Coalition, which obtained more than 65,000 signatures in favor of a smoke-free public places ballot initiative.

Doctoral student and cardiac nurse Gina Intinarelli in California is using her organizing skills to secure smoke-free campus policies for our medical center and to ensure that current tobacco content (including content about the role of the tobacco industry) is incorporated into the curriculum of all health professions programs. Nightingale Pamela Jones, another doctoral student, is studying ways to help encourage African-American leaders in tobacco control. Nightingale Lucia Migrditchian, a psychiatric nurse, is challenging practices at the mental health hospital where she works that include providing cigarettes for patients and having nurses light them. Other nurses are organizing letter-writing campaigns, developing cessation services for special populations, conducting tobacco-related research, and working on a wide range of policy efforts to reduce tobacco's deadly toll. The Nightingales are always looking for more nurses to help—even writing a letter to the editor once a year can make a difference, if enough letters appear at the right time.

Some nurses are a little afraid of being "political." But let's face it: *health* and *disease* are political; resources, education, and care are not distributed evenly in our society, and tobacco is a social justice issue. Just *caring* about those beyond ourselves and our immediate families is itself a deeply political act. Our most powerful nursing roots, after all, lie in our concern for those who feel voiceless and powerless, as exemplified by the early leaders in public health nursing. We can use our voices to ensure that the voices of those harmed by Big Tobacco do not remain forever filed away—and in so doing, we can find a way to strengthen nursing's voice in the world.

## Lessons Learned

- *Don't* think you have to have a big organization and money to do *something* political. We started with just a few committed nurses and a loosely organized network. We are still growing.
- *Do* try to get consensus on what you want to achieve and what kind of effort will be required, recognizing that this will need to be revisited as events change. For example, one of our group's aims is to get media coverage of our activism in order to change perspectives about the tobacco industry. When we started, however, we focused our efforts mostly on the nursing press, in order to build our network.
- *Don't* assume you need a lot of money to be effective. Most of our efforts have used volunteers or been covered by donations. If you have a good idea, the money often follows—if you're willing to ask for it.
- *Do* coordinate your efforts with other groups working on the same issues, recognizing that you may not always agree on everything. Build on common ground and share resources when possible. For example, we coordinated our press conference with Essential Action, a youth-focused tobacco control group.
- *Do* work to find ways to build on the strengths of all members. If doing activism, realize that not everyone is comfortable with public speaking or confrontation; however, they may contribute in other ways, such as preparing press releases or banners, managing logistics, working on a Website, or facilitating productive dialogue.

## Future Directions

- Expand our numbers
- Develop the listserve and Website into resources for nurses all over the world who are working to end the tobacco epidemic
- Develop creative activities that could be used to attract free media attention to our efforts
- Explore international partnerships

## Web Resources

> **The Nightingales**
> *www.nightingalesnurses.org*
> **Tobacco Free Nurses**
> *www.tobaccofreenurses.org*
> **Americans for Nonsmokers' Rights**
> *www.no-smoke.org*
> **Legacy Tobacco Documents Library**
> *http://legacy.library.ucsf.edu*
> **Essential Action**
> *www.essentialaction.org*
> **American Lung Association**
> *www.lungusa.org*
> **American Cancer Society**
> *www.cancer.org*
> **American Heart Association**
> *www.americanheart.org*
> **Campaign for Tobacco Free Kids**
> *www.tobaccofreekids.org*

### REFERENCES

Apollonio, D., & Malone, R. E. (2005). Marketing to the marginalized: Tobacco industry targeting of the homeless and mentally ill. *Tobacco Control, 14*(6), 409-415.

Balbach E. D., Gasior R. J., & Barbeau E. M. (2003). R.J. Reynolds' targeting of African Americans: 1988-2000. *American Journal of Public Health, 93*(5), 822-827.

Bero, L. (2003). Implications of the tobacco industry documents for public health and policy. *Annual Review of Public Health, 24,* 267-288.

Bero, L. A. (2005). Tobacco industry manipulation of research. *Public Health Reports, 120*(March-April), 200-208.

Brown and Williamson Tobacco Company. (1971). If you are worried about cigarettes—may we confuse you with some facts? [advertisement]. Retrieved January 12, 2006, from *http://legacy.library.ucsf.edu/tid/mgw93f00.*

Callard, C., Thompson, D., & Collishaw, N. (2005). Transforming the tobacco market: Why the supply of cigarettes should be transferred from for-profit corporations to non-profit enterprises with a public health mandate. *Tobacco Control, 14,* 278-283.

Centers for Disease Control and Prevention. (2005). Annual smoking-attributable mortality, years of potential life lost, and productivity losses—United States, 1997-2001. *Morbidity and Mortality Weekly Report, 54,* 625-628.

Chan, S. (2002). Nurses' initiatives in smoking cessation in Hong Kong. *Progress in Cardiovascular Nursing, Winter 17*(1), 47-48.

Cook, B. L., Wayne, G. F., Keithly, L., & Connolly, G. (2004). One size does not fit all: How the tobacco industry has altered cigarette design to target consumer groups with specific psychological and psychosocial needs. *Addiction, 98*(11), 1547-1561.

Glantz, S., Slade, J., Bero, L., Hanauer, P., & Barnes, D. (1996). *The cigarette papers.* Berkeley: University of California Press.

Hackbarth, D. P., Silvestri, B., & Cosper, W. (1995). Tobacco and alcohol billboards in 50 Chicago neighborhoods: Market segmentation to sell dangerous products to the poor. *Journal of Public Health Policy, 16*(2), 213-230.

Halpin, P. E. (1994). Letter to Benson and Hedges in response to mailed survey. In Legacy Tobacco Documents Library. Retrieved January 12, 2006, from *http://legacy.library.ucsf.edu/tid/usc62e00.*

Kluger, R. (1997). Ashes to ashes: America's hundred-year cigarette war, the public health, and the unabashed triumph of Philip Morris. New York: Vintage Books.

Landrine, H., Klonoff, E. A., Fernandez, S., Hickman, N., Kashima, K., Parekh, B., et al. (2005). Cigarette advertising in Black, Latino, and White magazines, 1998-2002: An exploratory investigation. *Ethnicity and Disease, 15*(1), 63-67.

Malone, R. E. (2002). Tobacco industry surveillance of public health groups: The case of STAT and INFACT. *American Journal of Public Health, 92*(6), 955-960.

McDaniel, P. A., Solomon, G., & Malone, R. E. (2005). The tobacco industry and pesticide regulations: Case studies. *Environmental Health Perspectives 113(12) December.* Retrieved January 12, 2006, from *http://ehp.niehs.nih.gov/docs/2005/7452/abstract.html.*

Muggli, M. E., Pollay, R. W., Lew, R., & Joseph, A. M. (2002). Targeting of Asian Americans and Pacific Islanders by the tobacco industry: Results from the Minnesota Tobacco Document Depository. *Tob Control, 11*(3), 201-209.

Osmon, H. E. (1990). Letter to T. C. Harris and others: Attached is the updated overview of anti-smoking organizations. In Legacy Tobacco Documents Library. Retrieved January 12, 2006 from *http://legacy.library.ucsf.edu/tid/dkf24d00.*

Philip Morris USA. (2003). PM USA Adult Smoker Database Marketing Past, Present and Future. In Legacy Tobacco Documents Library. Retrieved January 12, 2006, from *http://legacy.library.ucsf.edu/tid/msh95a00.*

Schwarz, T. (2004). Nightingales vs. Big Tobacco: Nurses confront the nation's biggest public health threat. *American Journal of Nursing 104*(6), 27.

Schwarz, T. (2005). Nightingales confront tobacco company, redux: Nurses from around the country gather to clear the smoke. *American Journal of Nursing, 105*(6), 35.

Smith, E. A., & Malone, R. E. (2003). The outing of Philip Morris: Advertising tobacco to gay men. *American Journal of Public Health, 93,* 988-993.

U.S. Tobacco Companies. (1954). A frank statement (advertisement). Retrieved January 12, 2006, from *www.tobacco.neu.edu/litigation/cases/supportdocs/frank_ad.htm.*

Yerger, V. B., & Malone, R. E. (2002). African American leadership groups: Smoking with the enemy. *Tobacco Control, 11,* 336-345.

Zeltner, T., Kessler, D. A., Martiny, A., & Randera, F. (2000). Tobacco company strategies to undermine tobacco control activities at the World Health Organization. Geneva: World Health Organization. Retrieved January 12, 2006, from *www.who.int/genevahearings/inquiry.html.*

# chapter 7

# Communication Skills for Political Success

Mary W. Chaffee

*"Good communication is as stimulating as black coffee, and just as hard to sleep after."*

ANNE MORROW LINDBERGH

In nursing school we find that many professional skills can be learned in the classroom, in a learning lab, or on the computer. We practice our skills on mannequins before approaching a real patient. As we progress through our nursing careers, many of us find ourselves in situations for which we were not prepared in the relative comfort of the classroom: participating in executive-level board meetings; attending fund-raisers, receptions, and black tie social events; and being interviewed. We may find we are more comfortable responding to a complex clinical emergency than making small talk with a stranger at a reception. It may be less terrifying to perform cardiopulmonary resuscitation than to stand at a podium and address an audience. Scary or not, communicating effectively in a wide variety of environments and situations is critical to achieving professional, political, and policy objectives.

## WHAT'S DIFFERENT ABOUT COMMUNICATION SKILLS FOR POLITICAL SUCCESS?

Politics is the process of influencing the allocation of scarce resources—figuratively, influencing who gets a slice of the pie, how big it is, and whether they get ice cream too. The action, *influencing*, occurs because people *communicate*. The process of influencing through communication can occur anywhere: in one-to-one conversations while scooping up shrimp

from a buffet, in testimony provided to congressional committees, in e-mail, and in meetings. Daniel Goleman, author of *Emotional Intelligence* and *Working with Emotional Intelligence* (1998), defines emotional intelligence as the skills that distinguish star performers in every field. He identifies the ability to communicate and influence as a critical emotional intelligence competency. When nurses participate in political and policymaking activities, a whole range of communication and social skills becomes important in successfully achieving political and policy goals.

## ENGAGING IN CONVERSATION

### WHY CHAT?

Communication is simply the transfer of information. That may sound boring, but communication is anything but boring! Did you ever try to *not* communicate? To not gasp at a shocking situation, to not comfort a frightened pediatric patient? Humans are designed to communicate with one another. As a species, we instinctively join together and form connections. Life is better when we share it with others—when we're adding new people and friends to our circle of colleagues. We link to each other in friendships, groups, and communities, and our link to one another is communication. It was the case when Neanderthals joined together to plan a mastodon hunt, and it is the same today when a group of nurses visits a policymaker to influence legislation being drafted.

We communicate for specific reasons: to gather information, to direct, to educate, to provide feedback, to question, and to understand. The tools we use are spoken words and written symbols as well as nonverbal movements including eye contact and body position and movement. It sounds simple, but frequently it isn't. If it were, no one would hesitate when entering a reception full of strangers, no one would fear standing behind a podium to address a large audience, no one would feel uncomfortable pulling a colleague aside in the hallway to discuss a problem, and no one would feel rejected when a hoped-for conversation evaporates into silence.

An important aspect of communicating is that we can learn to do it better and we can learn new communication skills. Excellent communication skills set you apart as a polished and practiced professional (Sabath, 1993). In the world of politics and policy, in which influencing others, making connections, and getting one's views understood are absolutely critical to advancing issues, finely tuned communication skills are as necessary as oxygen. Becoming active in policy and politics can open up a whole new world of opportunities to influence health care. These opportunities may include new business and social activities. With practice, knowledge, and guidance from colleagues, you can develop all the skills you need to be effective in policy and politics.

## ARRIVING AT AN EVENT

Gary just began a new job and is walking into his first meeting with hospital executives. Caroline has just given her car keys to a hotel valet and is approaching an evening reception honoring a nursing leader. Juanita is attending a political fund-raiser at a museum. What do they have in common? They are all entering social situations where they must tackle sometimes daunting tasks: mingling and making conversation. Many people find the first few minutes of mingling to be most awkward. Walking into a room full of strangers is the social equivalent of skiing down the Black Diamond Trail—a ski run that is a challenge even to experts! To ease your entry into an event, find something to do while you get your bearings.

- If the event is hosted, find the hosts and greet them. If they are experienced and thoughtful hosts, they will introduce you to others.
- If there is a registration table, register, pick up brochures, and chat with the staff working at the event.

- Take a few minutes to survey the room. Are people talking in groups of twos? Larger groups? Who looks engaged? Who looks bored?
- Get a beverage or help yourself to offered food.
- If you're at a private party, offer to assist the host in food preparation.
- Really panicked? Visit the bathroom, take a deep breath, and head back in.
- Not a great idea: Consuming several alcoholic drinks. Embarrassing yourself is not career enhancing.

## MEET AND GREET, GRIP AND GRIN

If you've run out of things to do on your own and no one has approached you, it's time to be brave: Introduce yourself to someone or commit a "B&E" ("break and enter" a conversation). The words you choose for a greeting will depend on the relationship and will vary if you have met the individual before. In a business setting or in meeting a senior colleague, you may need to be more formal ("Good morning, Senator Phillips, I'm Tina Gunderson. It's a pleasure to meet you."). If it's a social situation and you are greeting a stranger, less formality is fine ("Hi, I'm Warren Jones. It's good to meet you.").

If you don't see anyone standing alone, you could wait for someone to find you and offer an introduction. Chances are, it won't happen, because approaching a stranger is as difficult for others as it is for you. Be brave and approach people who are already engaged in conversation. Look for a group of three or more who look like they are enjoying themselves (avoid groups of two who are leaning in toward each other and intently involved in conversation). Position yourself near the group. Most likely, members of the group will make eye contact and acknowledge you, thereby opening the group conversation to you. Feel free at this point to join the conversation. Be open to others who appear to want to join the group. When you see someone on the periphery, step back to make room and include the newcomer.

## FIRST IMPRESSIONS

When we meet another person we instinctively assess, appraise, and form opinions within about 30 seconds (Boothman, 2000). It is important to recognize this instinct, especially if you are greeting someone with whom you need to connect to advance an issue. To make a good first impression, remember that words and body language play a role in how you are perceived by others.

- Make your first words count. Introduce yourself clearly. Repeat the name of the person you are meeting (this will help you remember the name, and people like to hear their own names).
- Smile and make eye contact. Let your smile reflect that you are glad to be meeting the other person.
- Face the person you are meeting. If you are seated, stand up for the introduction.
- If you've made a name tag, make sure your name is written clearly.

## SHAKE IT UP

A handshake is the expected business greeting in the United States. Greet a stranger with an extended hand. How firm and how long should you shake? Grip the offered hand firmly—midway between wimpy and causing orthopedic trauma. Shake hands only for as long as it takes to greet someone (Sabath, 1993). At social events and meetings where introductions are likely, keep your right hand free in order to greet others quickly. Make sure to stand up or come out from behind a desk when greeting someone.

## FUELING THE CONVERSATIONAL FIRES

You've made it past the greeting; now what? If you have just met someone about whom you know something, acknowledge it:

- "Dr. Bold, congratulations on the award you received from the governor."
- "I read the article you published last month on ethics in practice, and I enjoyed reading it. How did you come to write about that topic?"
- "I understand you're conducting research on pain management in amputees. How's the project going?"

With these comments, you've made it easy for someone to talk with you—you've offered several topics for discussion and made it clear that the other person won't have to do all the conversational work.

If you are speaking with a stranger, comment on any potentially shared experience:

- "Are you a member of the association?"
- "Have you heard this speaker before?"
- "What do you think of the proposed legislation?"

If you are comfortable with humor, try a joke or something like, "I don't know a single person here. What about you?"

These are all lead-ins to *small talk*, a form of conversation that has a bad reputation but serves an important purpose. Small talk leads to developing rapport and can lead to the discovery of common interests. Rapport is the establishment of common ground, a comfort zone where two or more people can mentally join together (Boothman, 2000). To keep conversation going, respond to questions and add your own:

- "No, I'm not a member of the association, but I thought the meeting agenda looked great. What about you?"
- "I think this proposal offers a number of advantages to nurses. What do you think?"

Mandell (1996) points out the importance of being prepared for conversation by being familiar with the meeting agenda, organizational background, and leaders; by reading current journals and being conversant with current events; and by reading newspapers and other matter. Box 7-1 lists a few other tips for drawing people in. Although these tips will help, don't think you are a failure if you don't establish rapport. The person with whom you're speaking may have just learned disturbing news, or he or she may have a splitting headache. If conversation is not flowing, politely excuse yourself and chat with someone else.

---

**BOX 7-1 Behaviors and Attitudes That Draw People In**

- Sense of humor
- Good manners
- Confidence
- Nonthreatening appearance
- Smiling and eye contact
- Starting a conversation rather than waiting for someone else to do it
- Knowledge of the subjects at hand
- Not taking oneself too seriously
- Fearlessness
- Respect for cultural differences

From Mandell, T. (1996). *Power schmoozing: The new etiquette for social and business success.* New York: McGraw-Hill.

## THE POWER OF LISTENING

A colleague of mine once referred to someone else as "being set on transmit and not on receive." Good conversationalists are not those who talk a lot. A good conversationalist does as much listening as speaking, and possibly more (Sabath, 1993). Active listening means *hearing* what people say, concentrating on their words, and responding appropriately. When listening, maintain eye contact; nod, smile, or laugh when appropriate; and make statements that reflect your interest.

Nurses tend to be very effective listeners. The skills that permit us to gather and process information from patients can be successfully applied in business and social situations too. Conversation can be a wonderful adventure when you listen carefully and encourage the individual with whom you are speaking to speak freely.

## CONVERSATION STOPPERS

Just as there are ways to encourage comfortable conversation, there are many ways to bring it to a grinding halt. Avoid these errors if you want to keep things going:

■ Being unprepared, or being unaware of topics of interest to the group you are with

■ Complaining about the food, the room temperature, your tight shoes, the price of parking (you get the picture)

■ Interrupting and not listening to others or competing and trying to "one-up" others (RoAne, 2000)

# MORE COMMUNICATION SKILLS FOR SUCCESS

## NETWORKING

Meeting new people and renewing relationships with previous acquaintances is the heart of networking. Networking can be defined as making contacts that may be valuable to you in some aspect of your professional activities. Networking is critical for nurses involved in policy and politics because most issues are advanced with the support and power of allies, colleagues, and those interested in attaining the same goal. Advocates of networking laud its benefits: information, feedback, referrals,

and a sense of collegiality with others (Puetz & Shinn, 1998).

Sharing information is seen as a valuable benefit derived from developing a healthy network of professional contacts. Everyone needs information—to learn about employment opportunities, to track the status of a legislative issue, to identify colleagues who share a common interest, or to influence a policy. Effective networking is based on developing relationships with "contacts," or individuals from whom you may obtain information, advice, or business. Always carry business cards, and keep the ones you collect organized and accessible. Jot down notes about conversations on the back of a card to jog your memory.

Developing a wide range of contacts can be extremely enlightening. Puetz and Shinn (1998) recommend developing a network of colleagues who have less experience, equal experience, and more experience than you do. The social role of networking cannot be minimized. It is much more enjoyable to tackle a problem, write a press release, or plan a campaign when working with a team of friends and colleagues than to do it alone.

## "WORKING A ROOM"

Does the phrase "working a room" conjure up a mental image of a cigar-smoking, overweight politician slapping backs and "pressing the flesh" at a fund-raiser? That's not what it is now. RoAne (2000, p. xxviii) defines working a room today:

The ability to circulate comfortably and graciously through a gathering of people; meeting, greeting and talking with as many of them as you wish; creating communication that is warm and sincere; establishing an honest rapport on which you can build a professional or personal relationship; and knowing how to start, how to continue, and how to end lively and interesting conversations.

Working a room isn't a cold, calculated process, but it does involve some thought and care. Before attending an event, think about what it is you'd like to accomplish. Do you want to learn about a Medicare funding proposal? Do you want to meet people in your professional association? Do you need to find colleagues to work on a grassroots campaign? Do you just want to have fun?

To survive mingling, and have fun, you should recognize the real benefits to working a room. Identifying these benefits gets easier with practice. As you make connections that turn into ongoing professional relationships, or even friendships, you'll feel better about tackling the next event or meeting on your schedule. Working a room is a new skill for many professionals. Learn from others who are experienced. Watch what they do to move effortlessly between conversations and what they do to make people feel comfortable.

Working a room is an exercise in strategic planning and an investment in the future. As you lose touch with some colleagues and develop new interests, it's one way to refresh your professional contacts. It can feel risky, but extending ourselves to others is almost always worth the risk, and it gets easier with practice. It can't hurt to try. RoAne points out that, "No one ever died from eating spinach or from going to a charity fund-raiser" (2000, p. xxix).

## THE FINE ART OF ASKING FOR WHAT YOU WANT

Making things happen is what leaders do. And to make things happen—whether you are at a reception, a congressional hearing, or a meeting with your boss—you often have to ask for things. Whether you are asking for a budget increase for your unit, the support of a legislator, or a letter of reference, there are several key points to keep in mind. Your chances of success will increase if you do the following:

- Say exactly what you want
- Say exactly when you want it
- Say exactly whom you want it from (Krisco, 1997)

The key word is *exactly*. The less precise you are in your request, the more chance there is for a less-than-desirable response. Another key is to make it as easy as possible for the person you are making a request of to comply with your request. If you are asking someone to provide a letter of reference, bring a draft that you have prepared. If you want your chief executive officer to meet with a group of nurse executives, offer to provide a briefing in advance. If you want policymakers to support specific legislative language in a pending bill, make sure they see what the benefits are. If you are asking someone

to be the keynote speaker at a meeting, let him or her see that you will make the appearance effortless by providing all the meeting information in advance.

Making the request is only the beginning. Next, you need to discern what the response is. If you've made a distinct request, there are several replies possible from the person you have approached. They may do any of the following:

- *Accept.* Your request is accepted as is.
- *Decline.* Your request is turned down; a reason may or may not be provided.
- *Make a counteroffer.* Some aspect of your request is modified.
- *Promise to reply later.* The response is on hold. If you are met with this delaying tactic, agree on when you can expect a decision.
- *Make a referral.* You may be referred to another individual for assistance.

Even when you make a clear request, you may receive a nonresponse. Nonresponses include "I'll think about it," "That's a great idea," "I'll see what my boss thinks," and "I'll look into it." These are all dodges or avoidance techniques. If you find yourself dealing with one, be respectfully persistent. "Does that mean you will do it?" or "I'd like to call you tomorrow to follow up on this issue." These comments send a message that you want an answer one way or another.

## BODY LANGUAGE

Body language—the wide range of conscious and unconscious physical movements we make—can either strengthen your verbal messages or sabotage you. Because of the range of movements and subtlety, body language can sometimes be tough to interpret—and to control (Heller, 1998). However, in a business or social situation it's extremely important to monitor your body language and to monitor the nonverbal cues you receive from those who are speaking with you. Pay attention to the following:

- *Your signals.* You signal interest in others by maintaining eye contact, by holding a comfortable body position, and by not doing anything that signals your mind is wandering. If you want to continue a conversation, try to avoid fidgeting with jewelry, checking your watch, scanning the room, or constantly shifting position—these all indicate you are trying to break contact.

- *Reading body language in others.* Be alert to physical cues that are being sent to you while you are engaged in conversation. If the person you are speaking with is maintaining eye contact and remains facing you, she is probably comfortably engaged and interested in continuing to speak with you. If you are speaking with someone who is looking behind you, checking the food table, picking lint off his sleeve or backing up, you're being told that he is ready to move on and speak with someone else.
- *Sexual messages.* Sexual body language excludes others from conversation. Nonsexual body language keeps conversation open and keeps you a part of the group rather than in a private, exclusive huddle. In business and professional situations, sexual body language is inappropriate. It can include the following:
  - Leaning in closely to the person with whom you're speaking, which excludes others from conversation
  - Speaking in soft, intimate tones that discourage others from joining the conversation
  - Touching the other person or touching your own body, hair, or clothes (Mandell, 1996)

## ESCAPING UNWANTED CONVERSATION

There are few social situations as tricky—or as uncomfortable—as being trapped in conversation that you desire to end. If you are seated at a dinner, you are probably stuck, so try to make the best of the situation. If you are at a meeting or "stand-up" social event and find yourself in an extended conversation that you would like to politely wrap up, there are several strategies you may employ. Mandell (1996) encourages telling the truth as the first choice, as should be the case with all communicating. After making a comment, extend your hand and say, "It was nice to speak with you." You may want to add a concluding comment like, "It was nice to see the pictures of your family" or "I'm glad you told me about your work with the association." If you say you are going to get another drink or food as a segue to escape, you risk finding yourself with company. If you are having a conversation

that is unpleasant, merely say as you shake hands, "I hope you enjoy the rest of the meeting/party/conference." When you extricate yourself from a conversation, move at least one quarter of the room away (RoAne, 2000).

If you are attending an event with a friend or partner, you may want to plan a subtle "help" signal that will alert your friend that you need assistance. The person responding to a signal for help could join your conversation by saying, "Excuse me, could I borrow Linda? There is someone I want to introduce her to."

## CULTURAL DIFFERENCES

Recognizing cultural differences is vital in communicating effectively. In today's "global village," there is one universally recognized gesture: the smile. From that point on, things get a little more complex (Sabath, 1993). When you interact with others from cultural backgrounds different from your own, whether you are in the United States or traveling internationally, the key to success is respecting differences.

Physical gestures and language that are acceptable in one culture may be vague or even offensive in another. Not recognizing or respecting cultural differences can lead to disaster in business and social communications. The Ford Motor Company was puzzled by poor sales of the Ford Pinto in Brazil. Ford had not recognized that in Portuguese—spoken in Brazil—the word *pinto* means "small penis." Few Brazilian men wanted to be associated with a Ford Pinto (Morrison, Conaway, & Borden, 1994). It is important to avoid communication errors like that.

These general caveats may be helpful in navigating the slippery slope of intercultural communication:

- *Gestures.* Recognize that gestures and other nonverbal language mean different things in different cultures. The traditional North American thumb and forefinger symbol for "okay" may be offensive to someone from Denmark. Pointing a finger is considered rude by the Chinese, hugging in public is not acceptable in Singapore, and shaking your head "no" may mean "yes" in some cultures (Heller, 1998). Take time to learn about the etiquette and behavior codes of other cultures if you will be working with or socializing with people from a background unfamiliar to you.

- *Handshakes.* In some cultures, touching is a sensitive issue. In Europe and North America the handshake is a welcome gesture, but that may not be the case in the Middle East, especially if you are a woman greeting a man. If you are traveling in unfamiliar territory, find out in advance what is acceptable and what is considered rude.
- *Personal space.* The British and North Americans tend to require more personal space and are more likely to move away from others if their space is "invaded."
- *Jokes.* Be careful in using jokes to communicate with people from other cultures, especially if you are dealing with a language barrier. Jokes may not translate well and could be embarrassing.

## A MILLION THANKS! EXPRESSING GRATITUDE

One simple act can set you apart from others and demonstrate your exceptional social expertise: saying thank you. As you advocate for action on issues, request help from others, and lead others, it is vital to recognize the contributions and support you receive. Never pass up an opportunity to show your appreciation. When people extend themselves, they always appreciate knowing that their efforts were recognized, whether the person is a U.S. Senator or one of your neighbors who helped stuff envelopes for a candidate. When you receive any type of significant assistance, send a brief thank-you note. A phone call or e-mail note will suffice for other efforts to assist you or help you advance a project. When you are writing a note to express gratitude, describe in some detail exactly what you are grateful for. Comment on why you are appreciative, and close with one or two sentences unrelated to the thank you. Try to avoid general remarks such as "Thanks for your help" (Maggio, 1990).

## CHALLENGING SITUATIONS AND HOW TO SURVIVE THEM

### PUBLIC SPEAKING

Polls suggest that some people are more frightened of public speaking than of dying. Speaking publicly may be frightening (at first), but it can be a powerful tool in advocating for a specific issue or moving a project forward. You may not recall the first steps you took as a toddler, but odds are, you fell down. After some practice, walking becomes effortless. Public speaking may never be effortless, but with practice you can become comfortable and effective. You may not recognize it, but you have been speaking publicly all your life—from reading a paragraph aloud in your sixth grade class to talking about the work schedule at a staff meeting. Public speaking, in a broad sense, is making a presentation to three or more people who are sitting still to listen to what you have to say (Figler, 1999).

To develop comfort and skill in speaking to audiences, start with some "low-risk" situations, such as speaking at your place of worship, presenting to a small group of colleagues in your workplace, teaching a class in your community, or even practicing in front of family or friends. Hone your skills every chance you get, then take advantage of speaking to more-challenging groups. Some suggestions for success include the following:

- *Practice.* Plan your comments to fit the allotted time, and practice, whether it's in front of your mirror or with a tape recorder. Ask for feedback from a trusted friend. Consider learning the ropes with a group like Toastmasters International.
- *Keep focused.* Be clear about your objective and why you are speaking to a specific group.
- *Know your audience.* What is the background of the people in the audience, and what do they expect from you? How many will be present? If you are speaking to an organized group, do your homework. Learn about them through their Website or by talking to members.
- *Meet and greet your audience.* If you have the chance to speak with members of your audience in advance, it will be less frightening to merely continue your conversation with them from the podium.
- *Observe the experts.* Watch expert public speakers, and note what they do that works.
- *Watch the clock.* Do not go beyond your allotted time period.

### CONDUCTING A BRIEFING

Providing a briefing can be a powerful method of influencing how someone views an issue or a course of action. You may have the opportunity to brief a leader in your organization, a policymaker, or a community leader about a health care topic. These factors will contribute to successful briefings:

■ Know your topic. *Really* know your topic. Do not brief at "the fringe of the topic."
■ Present the topic in a concise and logical manner. (It is called a *brief* for a reason.)
■ Be prepared for questions, but able to say "I don't know."
■ Make yourself available for follow-up.

Your organization may use a standard briefing format. It might be referred to as a position paper, a decision brief, or simply a "one-pager." You may want to prepare a one-page paper if you are meeting with a policymaker or the policymaker's staff. It will reinforce your verbal comments and leave your listeners with a document to refer to. A standard briefing paper usually includes the following:

■ Summary of the issue
■ Background information
■ Analysis of alternatives
■ Your recommendation for action
■ Your contact information

Box 7-2 gives an example of a briefing paper.

## WORKING WITH JOURNALISTS AND THE MEDIA

The media offer diverse opportunities to get your message out. You may have the opportunity to influence an issue's progress by writing a press release, by writing a letter to the editor, or by participating in an interview., The American Nurses Association (ANA) has developed tools to help nurses build skills so they may serve as experts in media interviews. A tool kit of information and other resources are available at the ANA Website *(www.nursingworld.org)*. ANA and some nursing specialty associations offer training for nurses to develop media skills. ANA also offers a guidebook and video titled "ANA Media Relations & You," which provides guidance on effective communication and how to participate in print, radio, and television interviews and related activities (ANA, 1999).

---

**BOX 7-2** Example of a Policy Decision Brief: The Issue of Importation of Prescription Drugs to the United States from Canada

To: Congressman John Murray
From: Legislative Analysts Corey Lalonde, Kris Willingham, Kyle Hodgen, Eric Goosman, and Thomas Blakenhorn
Re: Importation of Prescription Drugs to the United States from Canada

**THE ISSUE**

Escalating prescription drug prices have caused U.S. consumers to search for ways to control their out-of-pocket medication expenses. Some U.S. citizens are illegally purchasing prescription medications from Canada to decrease their out-of-pocket costs. Current U.S. law lacks enforcement and regulatory capability and therefore undermines the ability of the U.S. Food and Drug Administration to protect American consumer health and safety. The issue has domestic economic consequences also.

**BACKGROUND**

■ In 2004, 2 million U.S. consumers spent $800 million on medications from Canadian pharmacies via fax, phone, or Website, an increase of 33% from 2003.
■ U.S. consumers saved between $7 to $31 per prescription utilizing generic medications in recent years.
■ Nearly all prescription drugs imported for personal use into the United States from Canada violate 21 U.S.C. due to their unapproved status, inadequate labeling, and unapproved prescription distribution.
■ Electronic, telephone, and mail order prescriptions from Canada violate the U.S. Food, Drug, and Cosmetic Act; however, enforcement efforts have focused only on those who commercialize drug imports.
■ Several U.S. cities have instituted programs to assist residents and employees to obtain Canadian pharmaceuticals to save constituents an average of 25% to 50% as compared with those on the U.S. market.

---

**BOX 7-2** Example of a Policy Decision Brief: The Issue of Importation of Prescription Drugs to the United States from Canada—cont'd

- Former federal officials have voiced concern regarding illegal importation of prescription drugs from Canada; the current HHS secretary refuses to endorse medication importation due to issues of drug safety.
- FDA maintains that many drugs obtained from foreign sources appear to be comparable to U.S. approved prescription drugs but in fact are of unknown quality.
- In 2005 the Canadian Health Minister proposed legislation under the Food and Drugs Act to allow the government of Canada to restrict the bulk export of prescription drugs when necessary to protect Canada's drug supply.
- A U.S. Government Accountability Office (GAO) report in June 2004 noted prescription drugs ordered from Canadian Internet pharmacies contained proper chemical compositions, were shipped in accordance with special handling requirements, and arrived undamaged.
- Canadian pharmacies saved U.S. consumers $72 to $226 per prescription in recent years in a comparison of five brand-name medications.
- A 2004 study on pharmaceutical price controls by the U.S. Department of Commerce found U.S. consumers would benefit from the elimination of foreign price controls by free market competition.
- Canada's Patented Medicine Pricing Review Board undermines the goals of the North American Free Trade Agreement and shifts the entire burden of funding future research and development costs onto U.S. consumers.

**ALTERNATIVES**

1. *Legalize Importation of Prescription Medications from Canada.*
   *Advantages:* About 42% of uninsured Americans report an inability to fill prescriptions based on financial limitations. Obtaining Canadian prescription drugs could result in significant savings and improve access to critical treatment regimens. Less expensive Canadian prescription medications may translate to Medicare cost containment, allowing for additional allocations to other needed medical interventions. Legalization and regulation would result in safer product delivery to U.S. consumers.
   *Disadvantages:* Short-term savings may lead to much higher long-term costs in both the United States and Canada, resulting in a loss of research funding and possibly the introduction of 4 to 18 fewer drugs per decade. Standardization and monitoring of legitimate and illegitimate online prescriptions may prove difficult and costly for both nations.
2. *Do Not Legalize Importation from Canada.*
   *Advantages:* The HHS Secretary's unwillingness to support importation of Canadian pharmaceuticals indicates the federal government's inability to guarantee foreign drug safety and efficacy. According to research conducted by the Congressional Budget Office in 2004, allowing importation of Canadian medications produces negligible reductions in drug spending. Preventing the legalization of imported medications ensures the proper prescriptive control through the physician-patient-pharmacy interface, maintaining pharmacist and provider supervision of the prescribing, dispensing, and monitoring of medications. Maintaining FDA domestic control of drug manufacturing certifies standardization of chemical composition and preserves consumer safety.
   *Disadvantages:* Enforcement of 21 U.S.C. and the U. S. Food, Drug and Cosmetic Act will exhaust federal, state, and local resources. No provisions are in place for implementation and enforcement of the current law in addition, there is a lack of clearly identifiable federal agency oversight. The prevention of drug importation does not address the absence of programs to offset the high cost of prescription medications within the United States.
3. *Develop Additional Data.* Direct the Government Accountability Office (GAO) to conduct a study on the feasibility of alternatives pertaining to the legalization of importation, specifically addressing safety, cost, regulation, prescription validity, third-party payment, and Canadian government participation. Study alternatives for decreasing U.S. medication costs through utilization of FDA-approved sources.

**RECOMMENDATION**

Direct a study to determine the feasibility of the above alternatives. The illegal importation of prescription drugs undermines safety regulations that are in place for the U.S. consumer. It is imperative that the best alternative from the data be enacted. Explore the development of a partnership with Canada after both countries examine the feasibility of alternatives.

## ENCOUNTERING WELL-KNOWN PEOPLE AND CELEBRITIES

The world of politics is replete with well-known policymakers and officials, famous journalists who cover politics, and internationally recognized business leaders. Politically active celebrities (such as Michael J. Fox advocating for Parkinson's research, Nancy Reagan advocating for Alzheimer's disease research, and Heather French Henry [Miss America 2000] advocating for prostate cancer research) provide testimony and make appearances to draw attention to causes. You may find yourself at an event at which a celebrity is present. Mingling with a "star" can be intimidating and can bring out strange behavior. If you feel you *must* meet a celebrity, make a brief introduction, compliment the star's most-recent film, book, or show, and make a graceful exit. Martinet (1996) advises the following for meeting with celebrities:

- Take a deep breath and stay relaxed.
- Be respectful and admiring, but not worshipful and gushing.
- Project an attitude of not wanting anything from the celebrity.

If you do have a specific reason for wanting to meet someone famous, be careful about making a pitch. Recognize that your request for an interview, support for your cause, or other activity is probably one of dozens the celebrity receives each day. You may be referred to one of the celebrity's staff members. Make a connection with that person and obtain a business card for follow-up.

Celebrity presence can help you draw attention to a political cause or health care issue. If you are hosting an event where a celebrity will appear, make careful preparations with the person's staff. Be prepared to handle security, to provide a private space, and to handle excitable fans. Baldridge (1993) recommends not permitting autograph signing unless it is agreed to in advance. Make arrangements for photographs as the celebrity's staff directs. Find out the celebrity's preferences for meeting fans, signing books, and dining (for example, any special food requirements). Also keep in mind that questions are being raised about the appropriateness of celebrity involvement in political advocacy (Curiel, 2005).

## PROTOCOL

If you have the opportunity to attend an event at the White House or another venue with high-level government representatives in attendance, you will be faced with the rules of protocol. Good manners are the rules that guide behavior in everyday contacts, but protocol is the set of rules prescribing good manners in official life and ceremonies involving governments, nations, and their representatives. Protocol includes the observance of the order of precedence at all functions at which officials of a government are present. Precedence drives seating of individuals at public or private events. Failure to recognize proper rank and precedence is considered an insult (McCaffree & Innes, 1997).

The order of precedence begins with the President of the United States and winds down through cabinet secretaries, ministers of foreign powers, Supreme Court justices, senators, governors, members of the House of Representatives, directors of federal agencies, undersecretaries of executive departments, flag and general officers of the military, and many others. Protocol also includes rules for using the correct titles and forms of address for all officials, extending and responding to invitations, arranging table seating, and parading the U.S. flag.

## COMMUNICATION NIGHTMARES

Have you ever asked a woman with a roundly protruding belly when her baby is due, only to receive a cool look as she informs you she's not pregnant? Have you ever greeted a well-known individual by the wrong name? Have you ever introduced a keynote speaker and used the wrong title? Even the most socially adept among us have made faux pas that defy understanding. Sooner or later, you may join the ranks of those who have survived "foot-in-mouth disease." When a communication disaster happens, what is the best way to handle it? We can learn from those who have been down the "path of disaster" before us. One health care professional who was attending a small meeting of very senior officials in his organization spilled a 32-ounce drink into the center of the table as the meeting began. As he mopped up the lake of iced tea spreading out before him, he apologized and smiled at all of the participants. "People have trouble being annoyed at you when you're smiling at them," he reports.

A nurse, newly elected as a leader in a specialty association, tripped as she approached the podium to address the association members. Recovering her footing, she greeted the group and said "I guess you all will remember me!" She revisited the event 3 years later when she addressed the meeting again. In her opening comments, she talked about her growth as a professional, saying "Three years ago I tripped on my way up here; last year, I shook the whole time I spoke; this year, I stand in front of you full of confidence." Her words were very well received, and she used her ability to not take herself too seriously to make the best of the situation.

If you find something has slipped out of your mouth inadvertently, acknowledge your error. Don't pretend it didn't happen. If you can use humor to defuse the situation, humor can make people comfortable again quickly. A self-deprecating comment can go a long way toward getting a conversation back on track.

# ELECTRONIC COMMUNICATION: BEEP, BUZZ, RING, VIBRATE

Technology has transformed how, when, and where we communicate with one another. Just as with face-to-face communication, there are steps you can take that demonstrate how professional and thoughtful you are, and they will help you be as effective as possible.

## SMART MESSAGES BY PHONE

The telephone can be a vital communication tool or an instrument of torture. Remember those phone manners mom drilled into you when you were a child? They still work today. A few phone basics will help make your interaction a success:

- Answer your business line with a cheerful greeting and your full name ("Good morning. This is Brad Hill."). If you answer calls directly (without first being referred by another staff member), greet callers with both your name and organization ("Good afternoon, West Side Health Center, this is Mr. Austin.").

- When you place a call, identify yourself and the purpose for your call ("Hello, Mr. Thompson. This is Hannah Davis. I'm calling about the organ donation legislation you are sponsoring.")
- Return every phone call—quickly. Returning calls promptly demonstrates your respect for the caller and is always appreciated.
- If you find yourself in a game of "telephone tag," leave very specific information about where and when you may be reached, or try another means of communication.
- If you must put a caller on hold, ask permission ("Excuse me, may I put you on hold for a moment?"). Use this feature only when it is absolutely essential. Don't leave a caller on hold for more than 30 to 60 seconds. When you return, thank the person that you put on hold.
- If you are speaking with someone and are using your phone's speaker feature or your car's Bluetooth wireless system, alert the caller—especially if there are other people with you who are listening to the conversation.

## SMART MESSAGES BY VOICEMAIL

If you use voicemail to greet callers and record messages when you are not available, record a clear and coherent outgoing message that lets callers know when they can expect to hear from you. You may want to write out your outgoing message to callers and practice it before recording. The words you use and your inflection project an image to callers. Your outgoing message should include your name, title, and location, as well as a brief message to inform the caller when he or she may receive a call back from you: "Hello, you've reached Ann Ryan, Legislative Director for Congressman Owens. I'll be out of the office on August 12 but will return calls on August 13. Please leave a message and I'll contact you when I return." Change your outgoing message whenever your circumstances change.

When you leave a voicemail message for someone, summarize the reason for your call in a few sentences and be brief. A lengthy message can be tedious, and the recipient may hit the delete button before getting to the most important part. Make it easy for someone to return your call by speaking clearly when you leave your name and phone number. If you are a first-time caller, consider repeating your name and number.

## JUST THE FAX

The key to success with sending a fax is to ensure that you use a cover sheet that provides your contact information so the recipient may reach you. Make sure you include your name, title, phone and fax numbers, and e-mail addresses. When you send faxes, check the transmission record to determine if the fax was sent successfully. A phone call made to a wrong number will usually give you immediate feedback that you misdialed, but the same is not so with a fax. A fax sent to the wrong number will end up in fax Never Never land. Make sure you send your fax to the correct number. If you are faxing to an individual who shares a fax machine in a work-place, you may want to send a courtesy e-mail to let the person know that a fax has been sent.

## MOBILE (CELL) PHONES AND PAGERS

Mobile phones, nearly ubiquitous in contemporary society, can be problematic as well as useful. Many situations call for turning off a cell phone (or setting it to silently vibrate) so that it does not disturb others. Also, there are social considerations when using a mobile phone in public. Wisegeek.com (2005) recommends that mobile users modulate their voices, keep approximately 10 feet away from others when using a mobile phone in public, and keep the conversation short.

## NETIQUETTE—GETTING THE MOST OUT OF THE INTERNET

Electronic mail (e-mail) is a quick, easy, and direct means of communication that has proven to be a social phenomenon as well as a technologic one. The Internet is a major thoroughfare for communications, carrying millions of messages a day. It is viewed by some as the most politically potent technology ever invented (Carr, 1998). Like other means, it can be used with finesse or employed in a manner that is annoying and frustrating to others. "Netiquette" is an informal code for behavior in "cyberspace." It lets you communicate effectively and avoid gaffes. Etiquette permits you to display good manners at the dinner table; netiquette lets

you do the same at your computer terminal. Keep these suggestions in mind so you can be a good "netizen" (Internet citizen):

- Keep it short and spell it right. Many Internet users are inundated with e-mail, so keep your messages concise and use appropriate spelling and grammar.

- Use a signature line. Set up your e-mail account so that each e-mail message contains your contact information, including your address, phone, and fax numbers and alternate e-mail addresses. This will be extremely helpful to those who need to contact you and don't have your business card. Keep the e-mail signature about four lines long.

- Avoid fatal errors. If you are writing an emotional message, pause and carefully review what you are writing and exactly who you are sending it to before hitting the send button. You can't take your words back, and once they are sent, they can be forwarded to others. Don't assume any e-mail will remain completely private.

- DON'T SCREAM IN ALL CAPS! Words typed in all upper case are "heard" by most Internet users as shouting.

- Always reply. If someone contacts you asking for something, let the person know you received the message even if you don't have an answer yet. No response leaves the writer unsure if the message got to the right place.

- Cool your enthusiastic forwarding. Don't assume everyone in your e-mail address book wants to read all the jokes, urban myths, sermons, poems, virus alerts, and other junk mail that people send you. Be selective in forwarding mass e-mail; not everyone appreciates it.

- Hide the addresses. If you are sending an e-mail to many recipients, consider using the BCC (blind copy) feature to hide all of the recipients' names and e-mail addresses. Your colleagues may greatly appreciate your discretion.

- Clean up e-mails that have been forwarded multiple times. When forwarding e-mail (if you must), remove headers from previous mailing, including the e-mail addresses, and delete the >>> symbols on the left margin that indicate a message has been forwarded.

# COMMUNICATION TOOLS

## BRIEF BIOGRAPHY

Numerous situations may arise where it is valuable to have a brief biography prepared. It serves as a quick introduction to you and your professional activities. Begin with your current position, then provide a brief summary of your career, specific professional highlights, and educational background. Consider embedding a current photo and your business or organization logo for a professional look. Make sure to update it as needed.

## CURRICULUM VITAE AND RESUME

As with a brief biography, you will probably find many uses for your curriculum vitae (CV) and resume outside of the traditional use in job hunting. A CV is a document that contains extensive details of your professional life: education, employment, publications, presentations, association contributions, academic activities, research activities, honors, and awards. A CV can be quite long and provides the reader with global view of your professional contributions. A resume, on the other hand, is a shorter version of the CV. It should be no more than two pages in length and should summarize your work and educational history and other professional activities. There are many resources available that offer guidance and examples of both effective CVs and effective resumes. The critical factor in successfully managing both is to update them frequently to keep them current.

## BUSINESS CARDS

Your card is a vital networking tool: Don't leave home without it! Business cards can be your link to important new professional relationships. You won't dazzle anybody by tearing a napkin in half and writing your name and number on it. As you collect business cards from colleagues, you may want to jot notes about the acquaintance on the card so you don't forget an important connection. Keep the cards you collect in a file so you can access a needed card quickly. Most e-mail systems permit the creation of an electronic business card that can be attached to your outgoing e-mail traffic.

## WEBSITES

Your organization may post information about you on the company Website (another use for that brief biography you wrote), or you may choose to create your own Website. If you do, accuracy of information is critical. Review it carefully or have a colleague with a sharp eye review it for you to catch mistakes. Make sure you periodically review Website content to ensure that it is current and accurate. It is not recommended to include personal contact information, such as home address and phone number, in a forum that is open to the public.

# CONCLUSION

## ETIQUETTE

Etiquette has taken on a whole new life as professionals and leaders recognize the immense impact of personal relationships on the outcomes of business and political initiatives. If you bite off a carrot and dip it back into the ranch dip at a reception, pick broccoli out of your teeth with a toothpick at a formal dinner, or blow your nose into someone's expensive white linen napkins, even if you are the most brilliant thinker in the Western hemisphere, your manners will probably limit your success.

Business etiquette means using good manners in interacting with people and putting them at ease (Andrica, 1999). Purchasing a book on manners and etiquette will serve you well; two such books are the *New Complete Guide to Executive Manners* by Letitia Baldridge (1993) or *Business Etiquette for Dummies* by Sue Fox (2000). Etiquette has become so important that consultants, resources, and training programs abound. Personal coaches can be hired to provide one-on-one etiquette coaching. Courses are available on how to outclass the competition, effective business entertaining, the art of working a room, and basic manners and office politics.

## ATTIRE

Are you any less knowledgeable or committed if you wear comfortable old jeans and sandals to a meeting with a policymaker? No. Will you be taken as seriously as if you had on a business suit? Probably not. In contemporary society, a professional image is important. Take care with your attire and how you present yourself, just as you do with your language and nonverbal communication. Whether we like it or not, opinions are formed about us initially based on our appearance. When you are attending a social event, check the invitation or speak with the host to determine appropriate attire.

## COMMUNICATION AND LEADERSHIP

Communication is the heart of leadership (Tappen, 2001). Leaders lead by *communicating* a vision so that others may move toward it. Without clear, effective communication, leadership crumbles, and goals can't be achieved. But look what leaders can do with effective communication:

- Take positions
- Present evidence to back up their positions
- Speak simply
- Propose a course of action
- Address objections before they are raised
- Press their case with conviction (Toogood, 1996)

Exceptional communication skills enhance all leadership actions, including those in the arenas of policy and politics. Taking risks, learning new skills, and fine-tuning those skills you possess will make you more effective and will ultimately benefit the people for whom you are advocating.

## Key Points

- The ability to communicate effectively is critical to exercising influence.
- Nursing education often does not prepare nurses to communicate effectively in some social situations such as high-level meetings, political engagements, and formal affairs.
- Social skills, including etiquette, can be learned and will increase an individual's level of comfort and confidence in unfamiliar social situations.

## Web Resources

**Polished Professionals**
*www.polishedprofessionals.com*
**The Etiquette Company**
*www.theetiquettecompany.com*
**The Lett Group**—international business protocol and business etiquette
*www.lettgroup.com*

### REFERENCES

American Nurses Association (ANA). (1999). *ANA media relations and you.* Washington DC: ANA.

Andrica, D. C. (1999). Business etiquette. *Nursing Economic$, 17*(1), 63.

Baldridge, L. (1993). *Letitia Baldridge's new complete guide to executive manners.* New York: Rawson Associates.

Boothman, N. (2000, March/April). *How to make people like you in 90 seconds or less.* New York: Workman.

Carr, N. (1998). The politics of e-mail. *Harvard Business Review,* 12-13.

Curiel, J. (2005, June 5). Star power—When celebrities support causes, who really winds up benefiting? *San Francisco Chronicle.* Retrieved August 8, 2005, from *www.sfgate.com.*

Figler, H. (1999). *The complete job search handbook.* New York: Henry Holt and Company.

Fox, S. (2000). *Business etiquette for dummies.* New York: Hungry Minds.

Goleman, D. (1998). *Working with emotional intelligence.* New York: Bantam Books.

Heller, R. (1998). *Communicate clearly.* New York: DK Publishing.

Krisco, K. H. (1997). *Leadership and the art of conversation.* Rocklin, CA: Prima.

Maggio, R. (1990). *How to say it: Choice words, phrases, sentences and paragraphs for every situation.* Paramus, NJ: Prentice-Hall.

Mandell, T. (1996). *Power schmoozing: The new etiquette for social and business success.* New York: McGraw-Hill.

Martinet, J. (1996). *Getting beyond "hello."* New York: Citadel Press.

McCaffree, M. J., & Innis, P. (1997). *Protocol: The complete handbook of diplomatic, official and social usage.* Washington, DC: Devon.

Morrison, T., Conaway, W. A., & Borden, G. A. (1994). *Kiss, bow or shake hands: How to do business in sixty countries.* Holbrook, MA: Adams Media.

Puetz, B. E., & Shinn, L. J. (1998). Networking. In D. J. Mason & J. K. Leavitt (Eds.), *Policy and politics in nursing and health care* (4th ed.). Philadelphia: Saunders.

RoAne, S. (2000). *How to work a room.* New York: HarperCollins.

Sabath, A. M. (1993). *Business etiquette in brief.* Holbrook, MA: Bob Adams.

Tappen, R. M. (2001). *Nursing leadership and management: Concepts and practice.* Philadelphia: F.A. Davis.

Toogood, G. N. (1996). *The articulate executive—Learn to look, act, and sound like a leader.* New York: McGraw-Hill.

Wisegeek.com. (2005). What is cell phone etiquette? Retrieved August 8, 2005, from *www.wisegeek.com.*

# chapter 8

# Coalitions: A Powerful Political Strategy

Rebecca (Rice) Bowers-Lanier

*"When spider webs unite, they can tie up a lion."*
ETHIOPIAN PROVERB

In 2002 a regional health care foundation in a southern state awarded close to $500,000 toward the development of a regional nursing workforce coalition (Regional Coalition) of service providers to expand and improve the nursing workforce in the region. By 2005 the coalition had fallen apart, even with ample funding and other support provided by the foundation. How and why did the coalition fail?

In 2002 a statewide coalition of nurses and nursing stakeholders [Statewide Coalition] in a northern Midwestern state was formed to work on nursing workforce issues. The aim of the coalition was to secure state funding, in a recession, for expanding nursing education capacity in the state and for developing a state nursing workforce center. The coalition secured the passage of three bills—one to increase nurse re-licensure fees to fund the nursing workforce center, one to expand enrollment in the state public associate degree and baccalaureate nursing programs, and one to provide loan forgiveness to nurses who practice for 2 years in the state after graduation. How and why did the coalition succeed?

The first example illustrates that, even with ample funding, coalitions can fail. The second example demonstrates that coalitions with the right ingredients can achieve spectacular success in changing policies. The power of coalitions lies in their ability to bring people together from diverse perspectives around clearly defined purposes to achieve common goals. Strength lies in numbers: in working together and in strategizing for success. This chapter illustrates the ingredients for successful coalition building, maintenance, and success, using these two coalitions as the primary examples. The ingredients presented in this chapter work in small sizes for local and regional coalitions and are equally effective in creating and participating in larger coalitions at the organizational, national, and international levels.

## BIRTH AND LIFE CYCLE OF COALITIONS

In simplest terms a coalition is a group of individuals and/or organizations with a common interest that agree to work together toward a common goal (Berkowitz & Wolff, 2000). Coalitions almost always arise out of a challenge or opportunity. For example, the challenges of a decreasing supply of nurses in the face of increasing demands over the next 15 years create endless opportunities for nursing leaders. Other pressing health care issues such as universal health care, tobacco cessation activities, environmental concerns, and malpractice insurance reform create additional opportunities for nurses and nursing organizations to participate in coalitions.

Around the country nurses are participating in coalitions on nursing workforce issues in unprecedented numbers. For example, given the forecast for the increasing gap between the supply of and demand for nurses, many coalitions began in the mid 1990s as part of the national program of The Robert Wood Johnson Foundation (RWJF), Colleagues in Caring: Regional Collaboratives for Nursing Workforce Development. The original intent of the Colleagues program was to establish coalitions to assess the capacity of the nursing workforce to meet the needs of the citizens of the states or regions as defined by the grantees. RWJF funded 20 coalitions in 1996; by 2003, when Foundation funding ended, approximately 41 states had coalitions involved in nursing workforce assessment and development work. RWJF initially served as the catalyst for the development of the coalitions; however, as predictions about the rising demand and falling supply of nurses increased, other states galvanized without RWJF support into using the coalition approach toward nursing workforce issues (Rice, 2005) (Table 8-1).

Like the regional coalition mentioned in the introduction, some coalitions are short-lived and either achieve their goal or wither away shortly after formation. Those that are deliberately short-lived join together diverse groups of stakeholders around issues that resonate with people across the political spectrum. Once the goal is achieved, the coalition disbands. Other coalitions last for many years if

**TABLE 8-1** State Nurse Workforce Coalition Websites

| STATE | INITIATIVE NAME | WEBSITE |
|---|---|---|
| Alaska | Alaska Nursing Workforce Initiative | www.dced.state.ak.us/occ/pnur.htm |
| California | California Institute for Nursing and Health Care | www.cinhc.org |
| Colorado | Colorado Center for Nursing Excellence | www.coloradonursingcenter.org |
| Connecticut | Nursing Career Center of Connecticut | www.nursingcareercenterct.com |
| Florida | Florida Center for Nursing | www.FLCenterForNursing.org |
| Hawaii | Hawaii State Center for Nursing | www.nursing.hawaii.edu/nursing_shortage.html |
| Illinois | Illinois Coalition for Nursing Resources | www.ic4nr.org |
| Indiana | Indiana Nursing Workforce Development | www.indiananursingworkforce.org |
| Iowa | The Iowa Center for Health Workforce Planning | www.idph.state.ia.us/hpcdp/workforce_planning.asp |
| Massachusetts | Massachusetts Center for Nursing | www.nursema.org |
| Michigan | Michigan Center for Nursing | www.michigancenterfornursing.org |
| Mississippi | Mississippi Office of Nursing Workforce | www.monw.org |
| Nebraska | Nebraska Center for Nursing | www.center4nursing.org |
| Nevada | Nursing Institute of Nevada | www.nursinginstituteofnevada.org |
| New Jersey | New Jersey Collaborating Center for Nursing | www.njccn.org |
| New Mexico | New Mexico Center for Nursing Excellence | www.nmnursingexcellence.com |
| North Carolina | The North Carolina Center for Nursing | www.nurseNC.org |
| North Dakota | North Dakota Nursing Needs Study | www.med.und.nodak.edu/depts/rural/ |
| Oregon | Oregon Center for Nursing | www.oregoncenterfornursing.org |
| Pennsylvania | Pennsylvania Center for Health Careers | www.hcwp.org |
| South Dakota | South Dakota Center for Nursing | www.sdcenterfornursing.org/ |
| Tennessee | Tennessee Center for Nursing | www.centerfornursing.org/ |
| Texas | Center for Health Statistics: Texas Nursing Workforce Data Section | www.tdh.state.tx.us/chs/nwds/Ncoverpg.htm |
| Vermont | Office of Nursing Workforce Research Planning and Development | www.choosenursingvermont.org |
| Virginia | Virginia Partnership for Nursing | www.virginiapartnershipfornursing.org |
| Washington | Washington Center for Nursing | www.WACenterforNursing.org |
| Wisconsin | Wisconsin Nursing Redesign Consortium | www.marquette.edu/nursing/wnrc/ |

their mission and goals remain consistent with those of the coalition members. The key for coalitions is to maintain their existence until the goal is achieved and not to die before succeeding.

## BUILDING AND MAINTAINING A COALITION: THE PRIMER

### ESSENTIAL INGREDIENTS

To build and maintain an effective coalition requires four ingredients. They are leadership, membership, resources, and serendipity. First and foremost is leadership. Coalitions cannot exist without outstanding leadership. Leaders may exist a priori or may emerge early from the membership of the coalition, but without leaders, coalitions will falter and fade away.

Two types of leadership are critical to coalition work, and rarely are the two types found within one person. No coalition can exist without an inspiring or passionate leader—one who possesses the inner qualities critical for coalition success, such as passion for the coalition's mission and energy to achieve coalition goals. This leader uses personal strengths and power to constructively and ethically influence others to an endpoint or goal. The inspiring leader motivates others to participate and meet their obligations. The leader balances a personal inner drive to move forward while assisting coalition members to solve problems and make decisions, knowing when to steer forward, when to idle, and when to back up if necessary. The leader intuits the sense of the coalition members while continually urging them to remain on target. The leader also works to build leadership capacity in other coalition members. Finally, the leader has a sense of humor and knows when to use it, to defuse situations and help put weighty issues into perspective (Bleich, 2003; Bolton & Guion, 2002a).

The second type of coalition leader is the organizational leader. This person possesses the skills to keep members on track between meetings, ensures that communication methods are in place, and follows through on coalition assignments. Depending on the fiscal resources of the coalition, this leader may be compensated for his or her work, whereas other leaders and members may be

volunteers (Berkowitz & Wolff, 2000; Community Tool Box, 2005).

In the examples given above, the Regional Coalition disbanded within 3 years without achieving its primary goals; however, the Statewide Coalition was extremely successful. The unsuccessful coalition suffered from a lack of leadership. A well-meaning nurse executive from a small rural hospital led that coalition's board. Because the coalition was well funded, it hired an executive director who was a retired military officer and therefore should have possessed excellent organizational leadership skills. However, neither the volunteer nor the paid leader possessed either the inspiring or organizational leadership skills necessary to help the coalition execute its mission, tactically achieve initiatives, or engage coalition members and other stakeholders in coalition work. On the other hand, the successful Statewide Coalition was led by two leaders, both of whom had visionary skills, but who also shared tactical responsibilities, organizational prowess, and competencies to engage coalition members in the advocacy activities they needed to achieve legislative successes.

As important as leaders are, they are no more important than the coalition members, without whom the coalition would not exist. Members can increase the productivity of the coalition as well as increasing the potential for conflict. Members also increase the visibility of the coalition, because they represent diverse constituencies and networks. Members learn new skills as part of their membership roles, and these skills can be transferred to their constituent organizations. Thus membership is mutually beneficial for the coalition and the individual (Berkowitz & Wolff, 2000; Community Tool Box, 2005).

Coalitions need adequate resources to accomplish their work. Resources include money and in-kind donations from members and others, such as support for developing marketing materials, purchasing supplies, putting on educational sessions, and the like. Resources are the tools for the leaders and members to accomplish the goals of the coalition. A coalition can be most effective with adequate resources, but adequate resources in and of themselves cannot make successful coalitions, as in the example of the Regional Coalition that was adequately funded but floundered.

Finally, an essential ingredient for coalition success is serendipity—the happy occurrence of an opportunity not specifically sought—so long as coalition members take advantage of the serendipitous event or opportunity. Successful coalitions use resources at hand, devise innovative ways to sustain their work, seize opportunities that come along unexpectedly, and are willing to take risks. In order to effectively use serendipity, leaders and members must obligate themselves to conduct continual environmental scans, such as tracking current events, connecting with many different kinds of people, and spending time thinking creatively. The successful Statewide Coalition was informed early in its life cycle by the work of Joseph Jaworski (Jaworski & Flowers, 1998), who described the role of scenario planning in helping stakeholders develop future-oriented strategies designed to meet possible trends. Scenario planning is a decision-making tool in which coalition members envision certain futures depending on changes in a set of circumstances that are derived from environmental scanning. The Coalition members determined that scenario planning for the nursing workforce in their state might assist them in meeting workforce demands. Seizing the moment, they obtained a scenario planner who had worked with Jaworski and who assisted them in crafting scenarios that eventually led in part to their legislative initiatives. They created three possible future scenarios based on demographic, sociocultural, and economic predictions about their state. From these scenarios they were able to derive a set of actions that would help position nurses and nursing for future growth and population needs.

## COALITION STRUCTURE

*Structure* refers to the organization of the coalition, and it defines the procedures by which the coalition operates. The structure serves the members, not the other way around. It also includes how members are accepted, how leadership is chosen, how decisions are made, and how differences are mediated. Coalitions operate using group process, meaning that they go through a life cycle that involves "norming and storming" (creating group behavioral

norms and settling disagreements) before working together. Having a structure helps to provide a framework for the processing that must take place in order for the coalition to be active and successful.

Coalition structure, while necessary, is difficult to determine. Some structures will be tight, with formal committees, task forces, or work groups and communication mechanisms; others will be more loosely structured, with shared leadership and work done by ad hoc groups. Moreover, the structure may change over time, depending on the lifespan and work of the coalition. Highly structured coalitions may be necessary if the coalition work is complex, is multifaceted, and involves more than one goal. Committees and/or task forces can be established around the goals. For instance, the unsuccessful Regional Coalition established initiatives around enhancing the image of nurses and nursing in the region through a public relations campaign, recruiting young people into nursing through school presentations and health careers fairs, enhancing the development of the existing nurses through continuing education programs, and retaining students in schools of nursing through mentoring programs. Unfortunately, the Coalition failed to form committees around these initiatives, leaving the implementation work of all its initiatives to chance and, by default, to the Coalition's executive director. Hence, some work was completed, but most of the Coalition's plans lay dormant.

Coalition structure should make provisions for a governance group. This is especially true if the size exceeds 15 people. Beyond this number, the group becomes too large for effective, efficient decision-making. The governance structure should, at the very least, include all committee and work group chairs to facilitate communication among the various parts of the coalition. The governing committee should represent the diversity of the coalition members (Bolton & Guion, 2002a).

No matter what coalitions call themselves or how they structure themselves to accomplish their work, an important factor to achievement of goals is to have appropriate support systems. Someone must agree to do a task, and that someone should have the means to get the task done. The work may be done by volunteers, as it is in many coalitions.

However, there may be consequences to all-volunteer efforts. Volunteer compensation is always zero, and that, unfortunately, may also be the outcome. On the other hand, a paid support system can deliver on the tasks and move the coalition along more effectively, but as seen in the example of the Regional Coalition, one paid person doing the work of everyone may not be sufficient either.

## DECISION-MAKING

Decision-making is a source of great concern, usually in the beginning of a coalition's life. Because people joining a coalition represent different constituencies, they will most likely not trust one another. Everyone wants to protect his or her own interests. As the coalition decides on its mission and goals, it also has to figure out how it will make its decisions. Almost always within coalitions, decisions are made without votes (Berkowitz & Wolff, 2000). It is more common for the members to simply agree or disagree. However, here's a word of caution on close "polls" of agreement or disagreement. If the decision is "close," then the coalition should step back and discuss the situation again. When one is operating on consensus, the coalition members must come to a decision with which all are comfortable. In the discussion to get to comfort, what frequently happens is that alternative solutions are offered until one is made to which all can agree. Consensus building is by nature time-consuming, but it fosters involvement and buy-in from all the coalition members, and coming to consensus requires leadership skill and finesse.

On the other hand, voting connotes a formal rigid structure that rarely exists in coalitions. Therefore, a coalition should refrain from using voting as an operating norm. One proviso on voting occurs in coalitions that have corporate status, such as tax-exempt organizations. In decisions involving finances and board elections, votes must be recorded.

## MEETINGS

Coalitions have to meet; otherwise, the work doesn't get done. People come to coalition meetings for at least two reasons—to get work done and to make social connections. The meetings must combine both, in just the right combination, to keep people coming back.

From the work angle, the leader should create an agenda and circulate it before the meeting. Agenda items should be assigned time slots, and the leader should stick to the schedule. The leader should also make certain that all members know about the disposition of decisions made: what they were, who is in charge of accomplishing them, the timeframe for accomplishment, and the expected outcome.

From the social angle, the leader should build in time for mingling either before or after the meeting. Having food is good. The leader should greet members enthusiastically and allow opportunities for laughing and sharing.

The interval between meetings and the time of meetings are very important. The time interval should be long enough that work can be accomplished between meetings, with reports on accomplishments made at the meetings. If the interval between meetings is too long, little interim work will get done, as the human response is to wait until right before a meeting to get one's work done. Furthermore, meetings should occur on days and times when members can attend. For example, the unsuccessful Regional Coalition met monthly midweek from 8:30 to 11:00 AM. A nurse executive of the largest health care facility in the region stated that he stopped going to the meetings because they were scheduled inconveniently during the mornings, did not accomplish business, and were too long. The coalition should be sensitive and sensible about timing of the meetings.

The content of the meeting should be focused on problem solving and decision-making. There should be a sense among members that work is being done and decisions made at meetings; otherwise, results-oriented members will soon stop attending meetings. A good meeting has energy. If the meeting is primarily conducted to exchange information, some members will see this as a waste of their time, and they may choose to drop out. Alternatives such as e-mail exist for disseminating information. Consequently, coalition leaders and members should regularly assess the content of the meetings to see what works and what doesn't work and to make necessary adjustments.

## PROMOTING THE COALITION

What good is a coalition if no one knows it exists? Coalitions are formed to advance a common agenda, and communication is the vehicle with which that agenda is advanced. Early on in the coalition's life, members must develop and implement a communications plan aimed at getting the coalition's message out to the broader community of interest.

The advantages of publicizing the work of the coalition are twofold, both internal and external to the coalition. Internally, publicity attracts members. When others hear about the work that the coalition is doing, they may join because they want to be associated with an active group. Publicity also attracts resources, such as financial support. Furthermore, publicity is needed for growth. If no information about the coalition is disseminated, the coalition will languish.

Externally, publicity achieves its most vital purpose, and that is to reach the people whom the coalition needs to reach in order to get its work done. For example, the successful Statewide Coalition developed two types of information. One was based on credible data about the nursing workforce needs in the state. The briefing materials contained graphs and statistics from several recognized, objective sources. The other materials were "stories" about the effects of the nursing shortage on nurses, institutions, and patients. These stories told of the dire consequences of having too few nurses. They put a face on the problem. Finally, this Coalition developed a "tagline" for its work, which was "Quality [health] care depends on experienced RNs" (Hegge, 2005).

## FUNDING

Coalition work takes money. Some coalitions run on little or no money, using the time and talent of their members. These coalitions may be unable to sustain their work over the long haul because of lack of resources. Most coalitions require funds to pay for staff and buy the necessary resources to achieve coalition goals. Where does the money come from?

Membership dues help to fund the coalition. Dues may be modest and on a sliding scale, depending on the resources of the representative constituencies.

Requiring dues helps to get buy-in from the members: "If I'm paying for it, I'd better be there."

Generally speaking, however, coalitions will need to look for additional sources of funds to stay solvent and accomplish their work. How much money is needed depends on several factors. First are the mission and aims of the coalition. Second, the strategic plan will point to the resources needed, then members can decide how to best obtain the funds they need. Third, accompanying the strategic plan, the members should develop a fund-raising plan that would include tailoring the message to prospective funding sources, assigning people to make the contacts, communicating the mission and aims of the coalition, and seeking funding.

Where are the sources of funds for coalition work? If the coalition or a member organization has charitable tax-exempt status, obtaining contributions is easier to achieve because of the tax write-off. Coalition members may also look for grant opportunities, through either the public or the private sector. This means that resources must be freed up for the writing of proposals for grants. It takes money to get money.

As mentioned earlier, the donation of ample funds to the coalition in and of itself does not guarantee success of the coalition. However, having funds makes life much easier for members to achieve coalition goals.

## EVALUATING COALITION EFFECTIVENESS

Evaluation should be both formative (assessing the progress of the coalition on a continual and regular basis such as after each meeting) and summative (assessing the status of coalition deliverables after a defined period of time such as annually) and should occur at regular intervals. The coalition is created to bring diverse groups of people together around a common cause. From a formative perspective the coalition should assess whether the right members are at the table. Who is missing? Are all equal players? Why or why not? Members should look at the work of the coalition. How is it being accomplished? Is there a better way? What is it? How would we know? Where are the barriers and facilitators?

Having a quarterly calendar with benchmarks may be useful for the coalition to assess its effectiveness. Making goal assessment part of each coalition meeting is a useful exercise for the leader and members. If not on track, members can revisit the barriers to and facilitators of goal achievement and make the necessary adjustments.

From a summative perspective, annually the coalition should evaluate whether it has achieved its goals set out for the year. Which have been achieved? Why? Why not? Are the goals still relevant to the mission of the coalition? What needs to be changed?

## PITFALLS AND CHALLENGES

Coalitions usually start out with a flurry of excitement and activity. Leadership plays a critical role in sustaining the excitement and guiding the activity. Nevertheless, coalition work is difficult and complex, with lots of challenges. Following are some common pitfalls and challenges, with suggestions for overcoming them.

### FAILURE TO GET THE RIGHT PEOPLE TO PARTICIPATE

Coalitions should attract those who are most interested in seeing that the work gets done, and these members will commit to participating in the coalition. At regular intervals coalitions should assess who is "at the table" and who is not. Three common membership errors exist.

First is the error of selective exclusion of an entire group of stakeholders. For example, the unsuccessful Regional Coalition in the chapter introduction chose early on to represent the interests of nursing service and limited its membership to the nurse executives of hospitals, long-term care facilities, and home health organizations. Schools of nursing were excluded from membership, because coalition members thought that the major barriers to nursing workforce development in the region were related to the competitive nature of the employers and problems with the major educational provider of nurses in the region. The assumption was that if the coalition members were to learn to trust one another, they might begin to collaborate on areas such as continuing education, which in turn would help to decrease competition for nurses and make the region a better place for nursing in general. Also, if they were to become "united," they might be able to exert pressure to make needed changes in the educational program from the outside. In the course of the Coalition's work, two activities affected the schools— the establishment of a mentoring program and recruitment-into-nursing activities. Having the schools at the table could have produced more cooperation from the educational providers, even though bringing the schools into the coalition would have made the process of forming a working coalition more complex. In the end, all the stakeholders lost.

The second error in coalition membership is not achieving buy-in from major players, like the "800-pound gorillas." For example, in most nursing-related coalitions, the major employers and research universities with schools of nursing are the 800-pound gorillas. Coalition leaders must continually involve these major players by whatever means are at their disposal, including finesse, flattery, a seat on the board, holding special one-on-one meetings with them, and so on. Even when all means fail, the coalition should on occasion revisit how to get the 800-pounders to the table and should continue to try to accomplish this feat.

Finally, the coalition must recognize the existence of the broad array of other stakeholders who may be interested in the coalition's mission but will not become members. These may include constituencies related to nursing such as insurers, hospital executive officers, consumers, and business leaders. These people want nursing to be the best it can be because the health of the population depends on good nursing care. To engage these stakeholders, the coalition must develop a plan that includes regular communication with these individuals. The coalition should also assign members to present the coalition's work face-to-face with the broad community.

### CULTURAL AND LANGUAGE DIFFERENCES AMONG COALITION MEMBERS

Because coalition members represent different perspectives on the goals and mission of the coalition, all must learn the meaning of significant words used by coalition members. The words are actually proxies for the different cultures represented on the coalition. For example, *time* as perceived by nursing service administrators usually connotes a self-limited frame of perhaps today, yesterday, or at the maximum 6 months. Nursing service administrators are concerned with staffing on the next shift. They worry about the financials perhaps out to 6 months, given the trends of occupancy for the last 6 months. Nurse educators, on the other hand, visualize "time" as semesters. So nurse educators speak of curriculum change in perhaps a semester or maybe a year. Coalitions that will be working over an extended period of time should identify the words that may challenge the work of the members, such as *time*.

## PERSISTENT DISTRUST AMONG COALITION MEMBERS

Distrust is perhaps one of the thorniest challenges that coalition leaders face, because much of the success of coalitions comes from the ongoing interaction among members that allays misperceptions and builds trust. Two examples of sources of distrust include member disengagement and perceived member inequality or unworthiness. When members become disengaged from coalition work, their absence can derail progress, especially if they fail to keep their own constituencies informed. Another source of distrust emanates from long-standing perceived inequalities among members, such as active membership of licensed practical nurses or certified nursing assistants in a nursing coalition. To overcome distrust, leaders and members must work diligently on including these potentially disenfranchised members. To achieve inclusion, leaders may meet individually with these individuals, seeking their advice and asking for their assistance in the mission of the coalition. In the end, people must feel valued or treasured for all their participation and contributions to the enterprise.

## CONTROL FREAKS AND PROTECTING TURF

The tendency to hold control and "turf" can happen at the individual member level and at the coalition level. At the individual level, there are those in whom coalition success breeds a new brand of person—one who knows "the truth" and is always willing to share it. These individuals need to be gathered back into the fold and made to feel that their ideas are worthy, but at the same time, they

must understand that they do not possess all the answers to the work at hand.

The same holds true at the coalition level, when coalitions become successful and an upstart coalition or other group appears to be invading the coalition's territory. This is a time for reflection among coalition members. Are the coalitions competing? Why is another group forming? What does this all mean? Are there opportunities for collaboration among the coalitions? Or joining of forces?

## POOR HANDLING OF DIFFERENT PERSPECTIVES

By their very nature, coalitions consist of individuals representing constituencies with differing perspectives on issues. For example, hospital associations are concerned with maintaining an adequate nursing workforce to preserve patient safety and quality of care, but at the same time, they must be pragmatic about the economic viability of their member hospitals. And nursing is only one component of their issues in the vast array of reimbursement concerns, financial viability, competition, certificates of public need, and so on. Nurses associations' primary advocacy concerns are on the practice of registered nurses. Consequently, hospital and nurses associations' perspectives frequently collide over practice issues such as mandatory overtime and staffing ratios. Both organizations are concerned with quality and safety of care, however. It is at these intersection points that coalitions can be effective.

If coalition goals are meaningful and relevant to these disparate members, then the members will have a vested interest in keeping the coalition together. Therefore all have a responsibility to see that they stay focused on the mission and goals while appreciating differences in their perspectives. Sometimes staying focused is easier when coalitions are grassroots phenomena, with local or regional interests. In these coalitions, many members may in fact be bona fide members of several constituent groups. For example, at a statewide level, the coalition member representing the hospital association may be a nurse executive who also belongs to the nurses association in addition to a specialty nursing organization such as the state chapter of the association of critical care nurses. That one individual could conceivably understand the potential conflicting nature of representation for specific coalition agenda items. For that person, maintaining a strict position representing one association becomes a difficult task. Although messy, this interplay is what makes statewide or regional coalitions more effective.

The task of appreciating differences while moving forward on meeting coalition goals is easier if members commit to attend meetings and join in the work of the coalition. That said, coalition leaders have a responsibility for seeking diversity of opinions at meetings and working toward achieving decisions with which members can live. It may be that some strategies have to be abandoned because the coalition cannot achieve consensus. There may be situations in which members will agree to disagree and conduct their disagreements in the open without rancor. The latter situation can happen when members respect one another, having worked together over time in the coalition (Bolton & Guion, 2002b).

## FAILURE TO ACT

Coalitions begin with fire in their bellies. Unfortunately, going from words to action is sometimes more difficult than members had originally thought. Some coalitions formulate and reformulate action plans ad infinitum without getting to the action piece. However, action is the coalition's currency. Without action, there will be no funds to support the work. The failure to move forward most probably resides with weak leadership, and resolution of the problem may require a coup d'état to replace that leadership. At some point members will have to determine that they are not moving forward. Then they leave, they arrange a takeover, or they assist the leaders to move toward action.

## LOSING BALANCE

Coalition leaders and members wear out. Managing, leading, and working in coalitions drain energy. All members are entitled to personal lives and must know that they do not have to keep their coalition jobs for life. Each person must assess his or her readiness to step aside and support the leadership and membership activities of new incumbents. Therefore coalitions should set in place a means for leadership succession planning at regular intervals.

# POLITICAL WORK OF COALITIONS

Should coalitions speak out on issues that matter to them? Should nursing coalitions speak out for nursing? Of course. But advocacy work has its up sides and down sides.

## REASONS TO ADVOCATE

Nursing coalitions that are established to advocate for particular legislative initiatives will be successful if the initiatives are enacted into law. At that point, the coalition will have met its goal, and it may disband. Alternatively, it may envision another goal and begin work toward accomplishing that.

## REASONS NOT TO ADVOCATE

When coalitions advocate for certain positions, they run into opposition from stakeholders who are opposed to those positions. The further coalitions go out on the limb, the more people line up to saw off the limb. In fact, coalitions stand to lose their financial support if they go too far. In addition, there are legal restrictions on advocacy by tax-exempt groups in lobbying, so coalitions may be forced to pull back if they become too forcefully active. Therefore, coalitions should choose their battles carefully, making certain that they are willing to accept the consequences of winning or losing.

## HOW TO ADVOCATE WITH GRACE

The solution, of course, is to proceed with care. Advocacy, by its very nature, involves risk. Coalition members should work out their differences and carefully select the words they will use when advocating for positions. Coalition members should agree in advance on the advocacy approaches they will take that will not jeopardize their legal status as well as disenfranchise funders and members. Here are some effective approaches, using the five *R*s (derived from Berkowitz & Wolff, 2000).

- *The right preparation.* Advocating spokespersons should know their facts by researching the issue and doing their homework. When presenting, members should know what they want to say and how to say it.
- *The right communicator.* The coalition should select the right persons to deliver the message.

These individuals should be media savvy, knowledgeable on the issues, and able to communicate with the intended audiences. Building relationships with the audiences in the community is very important.

- *The right message.* The coalition should agree on the message that will be given. The messengers should state clearly why decision-makers should adopt their point of view, show why those reasons are in the decision-makers' own best interests, back up their reasons with facts, and give successful examples of similar decisions made.

- *The right request.* The coalition should decide itself which requests will be made to whom and when. At the time of request delivery, the requests should be feasible for the decision-maker to act on. These requests may be for legislative initiatives, support for a community-based program, or any other aim of the coalition.

- *Repetition.* The coalition should start back at the beginning and repeat as necessary. This means that each coalition initiative will most likely need an iterative process for working on its goals.

Coalition work can be extremely exciting and fulfilling. By bringing together individuals who represent varying perspectives, coalitions can achieve their goals through active involvement of these diverse members and their constituencies. Leaders must emerge or be selected who are passionate about the cause and who can simultaneously attend to detail and create an organized structure for the coalition work. Coalitions must meet regularly and take action on their decisions. In the end, coalitions must advocate for their mission. Nursing coalitions must advocate for nursing, knowing that nursing is critical to the public's health care needs. Finally, nurses lead coalitions, and they are active members of coalitions created by other stakeholders committed to improving health.

## Key Points

- Coalitions can be an effective political strategy to influence health policy.

- The more diverse the constituencies represented for a common goal, the stronger the power of the coalition.

- Coalitions must continually reinvigorate and reinvent themselves if they are to sustain their work.

## Web Resources

**Building Coalitions: Structure**
*http://wch.uhs.wisc.edu/docs/PDF-Pubs/Structure-11.pdf*

**Building Coalitions: Turf Issues**
*http://wch.uhs.wisc.edu/docs/PDF-Pubs/TurfIssues-12.pdf*

**Coalition Building**
*http://wch.uhs.wisc.edu/01-Prevention/01-Prev-Coalition.html* or
*http://edis.ifas.ufl.edu/FY496*

**Coalition Building 1: Starting a Coalition**
*http://ctb.ku.edu/tools/en/sub_section_main_1057.htm*

**Planning for Change: A Coalition Building Technical Assistance System**
*www.c-pal.net/pdf/coalition_building.pdf*

## REFERENCES

Berkowitz, B., & Wolff, T. (2000). *The spirit of the coalition.* Washington, DC: American Public Health Association.

Bleich, M. (2003). Managing, leading, and following. In P. Yoder-Wise (Ed.), *Leading and managing in nursing* (3rd ed.). St. Louis: Mosby.

Bolton, E. B., & Guion, L. (2002a). Building coalitions: Structure. Retrieved May 17, 2005, from *http://wch.uhs.wisc.edu/docs/PDF-Pubs/Structure-11.pdf.*

Bolton, E. B., & Guion, L. (2002b). Building coalitions: Turf issues. Retrieved May 17, 2005, from *http://wch.uhs.wisc.edu/docs/PDF-Pubs/TurfIssues-12.pdf.*

Community Tool Box. (2005). Coalition building 1: Starting a coalition. Retrieved May 15, 2005, from *http://ctb.ku.edu/tools/en/sub_section_main_1057.htm.*

Hegge, M. (2005). Using data to influence nursing workforce policy. In B. Cleary & R. Rice (Eds.), *Nursing workforce development: Strategic state initiatives.* NY: Springer.

Jaworski, J., & Flowers, B. (1998). *Synchronicity: The inner path to leadership.* San Francisco: Berrett-Koehler.

Rice, R. (2005). The evolution of state nursing workforce initiatives. In B. Cleary & R. Rice (Eds.), *Nursing workforce development: Strategic state initiatives.* NY: Springer.

## Lessons from the Long-Term Care Coalition

*"Great discoveries and improvements invariably
involve the cooperation of many minds."*

ALEXANDER GRAHAM BELL

Coalition building—bringing together groups and individuals to achieve a common goal for their mutual self-interest—is often the secret of winning important policy issues. The process of forging a coalition, keeping it together, and developing the strategies that allow all partners to engage and participate according to their level of interest and capacity is an art. This vignette is the story of one coalition, the Long-Term Care Campaign (LTCC). As every nurse knows, providing resources, services, and insurance for the long-term care of people with chronic diseases or disabilities is a major health crisis today and one that will grow with the aging of the "baby boomers." This example, a coalition that was designed to bring long-term care to the top of the public agenda—and that existed only from 1987 to 1991—may seem a strange choice, because the goal still has not been met. Funding from the sponsors ended, and the health care debate moved on to President Clinton's health care reform initiative. But it is a good mini–case study and contains important lessons about building a broad coalition to bring a "hidden" issue to national attention so that solutions can be found.

### WHY BUILD COALITIONS?

Nurses and nursing need to focus more on coalition building to become leaders for system-wide changes to solve major health problems. Coalition building to create campaigns around important issues will extend organizational outreach, increase nurses' influence, and build confidence in our strength to affect policy and legislation. It can help ensure that at every "table" where the future of health care and the structure and financing of health care are discussed—whether for federal policy, the future of the health care industry, state health care decision-making, or the responsibilities of various health professions—the voice of nurses is heard and heeded. There is a corollary: nurses can't win major health changes just by themselves. Changing the health care debate to meet the goals of nurses will require the active grassroots support of new players with a shared interest in the outcomes.

As the health care professionals most trusted by the public, nurses have a potentially powerful voice. To be effective *leaders*—and really see concrete systems changes—nurses need to engage more broadly than in the traditional professional coalition partnerships with doctors, the pharmaceutical industry, and hospitals. All of these are, to some degree, discredited in the public view, have less public support, and are seen to be too self-interested. That is not true for nurses! These players need nurses just as much, if not more, than we need them.

### THE LONG-TERM CARE CAMPAIGN

The LTCC was created in 1987 by Families USA (a health advocacy group), the Alzheimer's Association, and AARP. These founding partners were faced with a difficult reality: long-term care was seen as a personal problem and was not discussed as a societal problem. Yet this was a personal problem faced by a vast number of American families who were at dual risk: they might be unable to afford the long-term care that they or their family members needed, or they might be able to provide the care, yet face financial devastation. How could the partners make this a public issue and forge meaningful solutions when there was no demand for changes in public policy?

**145**

The LTCC was organized to create that demand around a vision for the future with a clear statement of principles, not a piece of legislation. The principles, hammered out with the lead partners and ratified by all of the more than 150 organizations that joined the effort, supported a national long-term care social insurance program for citizens who required long-term care because of chronic illness, injury, or disability, regardless of age, that would be funded by a Medicare-like plan with shared financing from individuals, employers, and the federal government. The principles called for covering care in a variety of settings—the home, nursing homes, independent living facilities, and respite care situations. The watchwords of the principles were "Quality, Accessibility, and Affordability," and there were no legislative prescriptions.

The campaign structure was minimal, "lean and mean," and flexible. The national campaign provided the framework, the outreach to engage coalition partners from organizations large and small, and the tools to make the job an easy one for volunteers, but the work and the direction of the campaign were decided largely at the grassroots level. Volunteer state coordinators were connected through shared materials, conference calls, and meetings. Organizational representatives became the steering committee and met frequently in Washington. Champions were recruited in the Congress and Senator Jay Rockefeller of West Virginia became the very active public leader. He had special interest, passion, and knowledge about the issue because his mother had Alzheimer's disease.

In order to raise the level of the debate, we used the 1988 general election as a major organizing vehicle—wherever the election campaign was active, the LTCC was actively putting pressure on the candidates and their campaigns to take a stand on long-term care. We targeted states of particular interest to the national media. Other states came on board because of the interest and commitment of local leaders, who came from every walk of life and type of organization.

The LTCC created a variety of organizing activities for national, statewide, and local groups and made advocacy fun. Everyone from the novice to the committed activist was encouraged to participate and get satisfaction from participation. The LTCC felt like a movement. People wanted to give their time and energy because there was a sense of movement toward a goal that kept them active. That was done by creating a series of small but sustaining wins that built momentum.

There were lots of opportunities for creative local activities that were knitted together through a common communications strategy to build public understanding and support. All the activities were designed to engage the press and gain "free media." Activists interviewed public officials who were caregivers and recruited them to speak out on behalf of solving the long-term care crisis. Governors and mayors were asked for proclamations. Long-term care days were held in state legislatures and Congress. People requiring long-term care and their family caregivers became part of the campaign, and public officials and the media were invited to visit their homes. The "face" of the campaign was made up of real people with real stories to tell about love and caring, responsibility and lack of support, financial hardship and sacrifice. Long-term care gradually became seen as a problem for our society—a problem for all of us to solve, not just a private issue for individual families.

Most important was a sophisticated communications strategy to show the national importance of the grassroots organizing and the support of so many different groups. The national media focus was a roll-up of the state and local activities and the faces and voices of real caregivers. The LTCC developed a nationwide list of families who were facing critical long-term care issues—seniors, children, the disabled; families—who were willing to talk to the press and be examples in the press. These unusual spokespersons had a central clear message: "We are responsible families doing all we can to take care of our loved ones, but we need help with a serious problem that could face your family, too." It was extremely effective in making the demand for long-term care visible. Developing solutions to meet this demand became a central issue in the 1988 presidential campaign. There were candidate forums (including one in Florida with the two presidential candidates), TV specials, state resolutions to Congress, and mayoral and gubernatorial proclamations of Long-Term Care Days.

The coalition did not survive long after Inauguration Day for President George H. W. Bush and was dissolved in 1991. With no support from the Administration, new and pressing priorities for the lead organizations, diminished resources, and a loss of momentum in the field, the coalition folded. Long-term care is still a vision, not a reality. But we shifted the view of long-term care from a personal responsibility to one that must involve our entire society. As long-term care looms for the aging activist baby boomer generation, we believe that another coalition will emerge to move the issue to the next level.

## Lessons Learned

We learned many lessons about building successful coalitions—those that will stay together to address important issues of the times:

1. *Know where you are going.* Have a clear vision statement of values and goals in a simple statement of principles that organizations and individuals can relate with and sign on to. Take the time to bring leading groups on board. Target your activities to where they will have the most effect.

2. *Think about groups with political clout.* The LTCC was one of the first national issue campaigns to reach out for "unlikely allies," particularly seniors over 55, who were often caregivers themselves and were concerned about the enormous gap in Medicare coverage related to long-term care. Seniors are a politically powerful voting bloc with great concerns about health care. Seniors register and vote, and politicians listen.

3. *Bring a wide range of supporters together.* Although it is easy to form a coalition with the usual health care players, it is seldom effective. Washington, DC and state capitals are full of such groups, and most are ineffective. The really effective coalitions include grassroots supporters, not just national groups. The LTCC reached out beyond health professionals and seniors to those with chronic diseases and their families and organizations, disability groups, small business organizations, and the public at large. Now there are new opportunities to reach the public using Internet-based

organizing and outreach vehicles like Get Active, an online business for helping membership organizations use technology to recruit, retain, and engage their members *(www.getactive.com)*.

4. *Grow the funding base while you grow the coalition.* The primary takeaway from the LTCC was the need to grow the funding base at the same rate as the grassroots base grows. Because the coalition was dependent on organizational funding, when the lead organizations changed their priorities, the coalition had a diminished funding base. Now there are new strategies and approaches to grow a base of individual givers through Internet-based organizing. For example, *Moveon.org*, the first truly effective progressive Internet-based campaign, started life with a budget in the thousands and raises almost all of its millions directly from activists on the web.

5. *Keep the coalition simple and flexible to react quickly to changing situations.* Effective advocacy takes place when the design includes different types and levels of activity to suit different levels of commitment and time availability. The design is personal: If I only want to spend 2 minutes writing a letter or sending a decision-maker an e-mail, I should be able to do that. If I want to form a coalition in my hometown and commit to that level of activity, the coalition should develop the tools that will allow me to do that.

6. *Respect differences and provide the "glue" to bring everyone together.* Although it is organizations that sign up for coalitions, it is individuals who do the actual work and make time in their busy lives for coalition activities. Never expect everyone to be active; some organizations will never do a thing, but having their name on the letterhead is worthwhile. A range of activities or action steps will help organizations and individuals stay involved, and a virtual community through a Website and e-newsletters or action alerts helps everyone feel part of one effort.

7. *Plan for the long-term, and celebrate short-term incremental wins.* The game plan for winning major issues extends over a long time (for example, several sessions of Congress), and building momentum over time is tough. Continuous feedback allows individuals to be connected, to

feel that they are influencing the direction of the coalition, and to be fully active participants.

8. *Create a strong message and communications strategy.* An effective coalition uses a series of tools including the press, the Internet, articles, and reports. Internal communications with coalition partners build strength. At the core must be a clear, strong message that resonates with the public intellectually and viscerally.

9. *Keep advocacy activities interesting, and lift the voices that count.* Top-down advocacy is a thing of the past. It is not enough to rely on national organizations; there is a need to build support at the local and state levels. Internet-based advocacy is key, particularly to attract younger activists. Relatively inexpensive software is available to make it achievable for almost any coalition.

Coalition building led by nurses could make a powerful difference in the delivery of care by reaching out to other stakeholders; educating, engaging, and mobilizing a wider and wider circle of people to advocate; using effective communications; and finding champions among public officials. Nurses see health care "up close and personal" and have the patient's interests as well as their own at heart. Unlike almost everyone else in the complex health care industry, with major health care policy issues (other than licensing issues) nurses are seen as not having a vested interest in the results but rather as advocates for better care.

There is no doubt that major improvements are needed in health care. There are unmet needs, challenges, and opportunities to lead on issues that can be pivotal to change the way health care decisions are made, patients treated, disease prevented, and resources allocated. The long-term care problem certainly still needs to be solved! Nurses need to be effective coalition builders to be leaders for better health policies—not only for nursing—because they understand, better than anyone else, the needs of patients for a much better health care delivery system.

# Harnessing the Power of the Media to Influence Health Policy and Politics

Diana J. Mason, Catherine J. Dodd, & Barbara Glickstein

*"Congress shall make no law…abridging the freedom of speech, or of the press, or of the right of the people peaceably to assemble, and to petition the Government for redress of grievances."*

U.S. CONSTITUTION, FIRST AMENDMENT

*"Whoever controls the media—the images—controls the culture."*

ALLEN GINSBERG

Our government is of the people, by the people, and for the people. James Madison once said that "a people who mean to be their own governors must arm themselves with the power which knowledge gives"(Madison as cited in Harris, 2005, p. 90). Real democracy requires an informed citizenry and free and open debate on issues and alternatives. The first amendment of our Constitution protects the "freedom of the press" for the purpose of ensuring that all voices are heard. Policy decisions should consider the interests of all the people and protect the most vulnerable in society.

The first amendment gives the press constitutional protection not afforded any other enterprise in the country. Many would argue that this protection is essential because the press plays a crucial watchdog role in our system of government. Indeed,

a true free press, one not wholly owned by a handful of corporate interests as is becoming the case today, should serve to monitor and report on the unchecked power of the president and Congress (Kalb, 1997; Labaton, 2004). Many in and outside of journalism are passionate about protecting the press's rights and freedoms as essential for an open society and democracy. In 2005, *New York Times* journalist Judith Miller refused a grand jury's request to provide her sources for a story she had worked on but never published (although others did) that involved the revelation of the identity of an agent of the Central Intelligence Agency. The agent's husband, a former diplomat, had angered the Bush administration by publicly not substantiating its claim that Iraq's Saddam Hussein had purchased uranium for nuclear weapons. She went to jail instead, believing that that protection of sources is fundamental to a free press.

The last decade of the century was considered "the information age," and now we are in the "telecommunication age." Information is crowded into "sound bites" and visual images that communicate instant messages and shape public opinion. Although some argue that sound bites represent superficial communications, Jamieson (2000, p. i) counters that they can be significant: "Substantive soundbites are the stuff of which the best news stories are made."

Certainly, instant messaging is changing the role of the individual in our government. Today, political leaders and well-financed special interest groups use the wonders of modern technology—television, telephone, satellite, cable, and personal computers—to send scientifically tested and well-crafted messages in an instant and, almost as quickly, to receive feedback from members of the public who have access to these media. In fact, telecommunication systems have provided people with direct access to policymakers. It is transforming our nation from representational government to a direct democracy. Our constitution, the doctrine that protects freedom of the press, was designed to separate the rulers from the ruled. Every citizen can participate in electing representatives who conduct the business of government. The founders of our country created a representational republic (Grossman, 1997). But that is changing.

Representatives today are listening to the instant feedback from their constituents who have the means and motivation to communicate and are modifying their positions based on these public opinions. Lawrence Grossman (1997), former president of NBC News and Public Broadcasting Service, questions whether this new "electronic republic" will make government more responsive to the people or whether it will be manipulated by individuals pursuing their own ends at the expense of those without access to telecommunications or motivation to participate.

In addition, the media profoundly influence who gets elected to public office. An effective media strategy can shift voters' decisions late in the campaign. In fact, no candidate for national or state office can expect to capture voters' commitment on election day without a well-designed media campaign. Indeed, such media strategies have become the prime stimulus for escalating costs of running a campaign. Candidates either have to bring their personal wealth to their campaigns or have to be willing to spend the majority of their time in fund-raising. Will this distort who can run for public office and whether our public officials are representative of the constituency they serve?

Today the media imbue in us the message that success equals money and possessions. Over the past few decades "news reporting" has changed in terms of what is important because it is influenced by who invests in the media in terms of ownership and advertising. Solomon (2005) points out that "economic progress is more newsworthy than human needs or accomplishments." Headlines no longer reveal how many people saw a new movie release and what the story is about; the news reports how much the movie earned or "grossed." New innovations in education or success stories are not in the news; the cost per pupil is covered. Health care is not covered from the human interest perspective; it is covered in terms of how much money the industry earned, or cost. Nursing, the major labor cost in health care, is all but invisible.

In the 1990s, nurses became increasingly concerned about their invisibility in the media (Buresh, Gordon, & Bell, 1991; Sigma Theta Tau International, 1998). Although gains have been made, this invisibility limits nursing's ability to advocate for health policy (Chaffee, 2000). Nurses are viewed by the public and by policymakers as credible, moral, and trustworthy, and they must participate in the new "electronic republic." This chapter discusses the role of the media in policy and politics and provides nurses with strategies to access and use the media to promote healthy public policies.

## POWER OF THE MEDIA

A classic example of the power of media in shaping health policy arose during the first months of William Jefferson Clinton's presidency. When President Clinton took office in 1992, one of his primary domestic policy priorities was the guarantee of comprehensive health care coverage for every American. In September of 1993, he proposed the Health Security Act to Congress and the public with the hope and anticipation that this would become landmark legislation. The nursing community was particularly supportive of this legislation because it recognized advanced practice nurses as important providers of primary care. Clinton's proposal initially had substantial public support, because many believed the country had a moral imperative to extend health care coverage to all who live here.

However, according to an analysis by the Annenberg Public Policy Center of the University of Pennsylvania (1995), two curious characters, Harry and Louise, had a tremendous impact on shifting the public's sentiments, dashing the hopes of President Clinton and nurses, who saw the legislation as an important remedy for an ailing health care system.

Harry and Louise were characters in a series of television advertisements sponsored by the Health Insurance Association of America (HIAA), which adamantly opposed the president's plan. Actors portrayed this couple voicing grave concerns about the bill. They said, "Under the President's bill, we'll lose our right to choose our own physician," and "What happens if the plan runs out of money?" Although the advertisements were not the only reason for the demise of the Health Security Act, Harry and Louise effectively planted fear and negativity in the hearts and minds of many citizens within the span of 60 seconds. Suddenly, many of those Americans who had been concerned about the growing numbers of uninsured became more concerned about how the bill would affect their own health care options and withdrew their support from the Act.

What many do not realize about the Harry and Louise commercials is the fact that the target audience was not the public, directly. Rather, it was policymakers and those who could influence how the public perceived the issue: journalists. The ads originally aired in the country's major media centers: Washington, DC; Los Angeles; New York City; and Atlanta. They were seen and reported on by journalists. In fact, the ads got more air time by becoming part of the journalists' news stories. Many people who saw the ads did so through viewing them as part of the evening news, not as a paid advertisement (Annenberg Public Policy Center of the University of Pennsylvania, 1995).

The Harry and Louise commercials are an example of a deliberate media strategy to mobilize a public constituency around a public policy issue. It is one illustration of the power of the media in policy and politics. The media saturate this nation and much of the world with images that change people's opinions, shape their attitudes and beliefs, and transform their behavior (McAlister, 1991).

## INDIVIDUAL VERSUS AGGREGATE FOCUS

Schmid, Pratt, and Howze (1995) argue that individual-focused interventions for changing health behaviors are limited in long-term effectiveness; rather, these authors maintain that community- or aggregate-focused interventions hold the greatest promise for improving the health of communities. An example of aggregate-focused interventions is public policy such as U.S. sanitation laws, which had a dramatic effect on the health and quality of life for many people. The media provide a potentially powerful aggregate approach to influencing public policies that can promote health. Certainly, the media can be viewed as a political tool. Turow (1996, p. 1240) notes, "Journalists now recognize that public discussions of medicine are necessarily political— i.e., they are ultimately about the exercise of social power."

The media's power arises from their ability to get a message to large numbers of people or to key people instantly. Talk radio, which has proliferated in the past decade and has become more popular because of long commuting times and cellular phones, is a volatile medium. Talk radio charted a different course after 1987 when Ronald Reagan repealed the Fairness Doctrine, a Federal Communications Commission (FCC) rule established in 1947 under President Franklin D. Roosevelt and designed to minimize any possible restrictions on free speech caused by limited access to broadcasting outlets. Before the rule was repealed, in order to get or keep an FCC broadcast license, a station had to "devote reasonable attention to coverage of controversial issues of public importance" and provide "reasonable although not necessary equal" opportunities for opposing sides to express their views. Roosevelt felt that the airwaves belonged to everyone. He did not want commercial radio broadcasting to become another for-profit industry (Wallace, 2005).

Today, most talk radio has become a big business that is motivated by revenue. The loudest and most provocative radio voices often produce higher ratings and command higher prices for advertising. Information presented by talk show hosts and their callers is not screened by editors for accuracy and objectivity. Talk show hosts are often chosen for their provocative style rather than their broadcast skills (Rehm, 1997). Nurses can play an important role in providing fair and factual information on health issues and concerns when talk radio is misrepresenting issues. (*Getting Free Media Coverage for Nursing Issues,* following this chapter, provides more information on calling in to talk radio.)

The Internet is increasingly taking center stage as a vehicle for sharing information and shaping public opinion. It provides uncensored access, speed, and a snowballing effect in which the message can take on a life of its own. The first notable demonstration of the power of the Internet in political campaigns occurred in 1994. Former Speaker of the House of Representatives Tom Foley (D-WA) was defeated by an Internet campaign against him launched by Richard and Mary Hartman of Spokane, Washington. The year before his defeat, the headline for a story in the *High County News,* a biweekly newspaper serving 11 Western states, was "Tom Foley Thrives in a Very Republican District" (Koberstein, 1993). The Hartmans launched a "De-Foley-ate Congress" campaign over the Internet. "Politicos Blazing Cyberspace Trail" was the headline in the July 17, 1995 issue of *Computerworld* after Foley's defeat. The article noted, "Move over, talk radio. The Internet's World Wide Web is fast becoming a new weapon for politicos as well as a battleground for next year's elections" (Betts, 1995). The Hartmans had shown the power of the Internet for political campaigns, particularly for controlling messages to defeat a candidate. Ten years later, Howard Dean showed the Internet's power for building a grassroots constituency and fund-raising when he, a relatively unknown governor from Vermont, became John Kerry's leading opponent in the Democratic primary race for president.

In addition, bloggers have proved to be quite influential in shaping public policy debates and political campaigns. In the University of Southern California's *Online Journalism Review,* Glaser (2004) reported on a survey he conducted, asking key leaders in journalism what they considered to be the most important developments in the media realm related to the Internet and technology. At the top of the list was how bloggers gained credibility and shaped the way media reported on the 2004 elections.

Two Pew surveys conducted in early 2005 show that 16% of U.S. adults (32 million) are blog readers and that 6% of the entire U.S. population has created a blog. That's 11 million people, or 1 in 17 American citizens (Rainie, 2005a; 2005b).

Paid or commercial advertising, including pop-ups and banners on Websites, also influences the public's perceptions and knowledge about health issues. Each of us is now confronted with thousands of paid messages per day. Commercial advertising is found on cereal boxes, on milk cartons, in journals, in magazines, in newspapers, at bus stops, on billboards, even on the sides of buses. Television ads often include text on the screen because many people use a "mute" button during the commercials. Wireless phones offer another opportunity for advertisers because they are so popular, particularly with young adults who are harder to reach via TV and print. New technology, more widely available in Europe, uses transmitters installed in billboards to beam out text messages to the phones of people walking by. This is another high-tech method to deliver a message that may be available in the near future as wireless phones and short-range technology advance in the United States.

In 1997 the Food and Drug Administration (FDA) changed the rules and regulations governing pharmaceutical advertising to consumers. Direct-to-consumer advertising is now prevalent in news magazines, in train stations, on television, on the radio, and everywhere the public travels. Consumers in turn ask their providers for these advertised drugs, which are often more costly than generic forms. This commercial advertising has contributed to increases in health care spending that began during the late 1990s and has put prescription drug coverage on the agenda of state and federal policymakers (Learner, 2005).

Although FDA regulations require that the ads not misrepresent the product, pharmaceutical companies carefully select images that send messages beyond the stated or printed word. For example, the FDA sent letters to the manufacturers of drugs used to treat human immunodeficiency virus (HIV), cautioning them about their advertising. Many of these ads showed strong and healthy-looking individuals engaged in strenuous physical activity.

In San Francisco the director of sexually transmitted disease prevention and control services at the city's department of health said the ads were false portrayals of HIV-infected clients. He also suggested that the ads contributed to risky behavior because the impression from the ads is that HIV is easily manageable with medication.

## NURSING AND THE MEDIA

Two studies during the 1990s documented nursing's invisibility in the media (Buresh et al., 1991; Sigma Theta Tau International, 1998). Commissioned by Sigma Theta Tau International Nursing Honorary Society, the *Woodhull Study on Nursing and the Media* found that nurses were included in health stories in major print media (newspapers and news magazines published in September 1997) less than 4% of the time, even when they would have been germane to the story. An even more disturbing finding was the fact that nurses were represented in health care industry publications less than 1% of the time. Buresh and Gordon (2000) suggest that findings such as these could be systematic journalistic bias against nursing. But they also note that nurses are not proactive in accessing the media. (See Buresh and Gordon's book *From Silence to Voice: What Nurses Know and Must Communicate to the Public*, 2003.)

In the mid 1990s, organized nursing mounted a strategic campaign to shape public opinion about the importance of what nurses contribute to health care. During this decade the cost-focused reengineering, restructuring, and downsizing of health care organizations led many organizations to eliminate nursing positions and replace nurses with unlicensed assistive personnel. In response to the ANA campaign slogan "Every Patient Deserves a Nurse," the New York State Nurses Association invested several million dollars to launch a media campaign with the message "Every Patient Deserves an RN—a Real Nurse" (Sheridan-Gonzalez, & Wade, 1998). Television, radio, and print ads appeared in targeted areas throughout the state, including the capital city of Albany, where policymakers and their staff would see the ads. The campaign offered a "hospital evaluation kit" that people could use to evaluate the adequacy of nursing in their hospital, and the association distributed

75,000 kits. Policymakers talked about the campaign, as did nurses' neighbors, friends, and families. It put nursing on the public's agenda and created support for nursing's legislative agenda.

Beginning in 2004 with the recall election of Arnold Schwarzenegger to the governorship of California and his subsequent attempts to halt progress on mandated minimum nurse-patient ratios in that state, the California Nurses Association engaged in a sophisticated and aggressive media campaign designed to discredit the governor and his motives. (See *California Nurse Staffing Ratios* following Chapter 18.) Their efforts were described in a *TIME Magazine* story, "Nursing a Grudge: The Governor's decision to allow bigger hospital work loads has ignited a bitter battle in California":

…the nurses have produced a Hollywood caper of a showdown, putting unrelenting pressure on Schwarzenegger to back down…Nurses have buzzed his fundraisers with "Air Arnold" planes that drag banners reading DON'T BE BIG BUSINESS'S BULLY!…When the A&E channel ran a biopic called See Arnold Run, the California Nurses Association punctuated it with commercials of R.N.s denouncing him as "driven by greed and profits," part of a $100,000 TV campaign. Their full-page ads in Washington and California newspapers accused him of kowtowing to the hospital lobby to "put vital health policy up for sale"…According to a recent Gallup poll, nurses are more popular than he is. (Roosevelt, 2005)

And when all of the governor's ballot initiatives failed in the 2005 elections, the California Nurses Association's "indefatigable nurses" were credited with being a leading force in the defeat (Sharp, 2005).

Nurse researchers need to be more proactive in communicating their work to journalists. In many cases researchers can and should be turning to their institutional public relations department for expertise and support in developing press releases and pitching stories to journalists. But the public relations people will need the researcher's help in describing the relevance of the research to journalists. Most journalists are not interested in conceptual frameworks and details beyond descriptive and summary statistics. They want to know why the research would be of interest to the public, what the primary findings were, and how these findings can be used. Some doctoral programs now require that their students define both the policy and public relevance of their research. A more aggressive approach to public dissemination of nursing research would enhance the public's perception of nursing as a science while promoting research utilization, including by policymakers.

## GETTING ISSUES ON THE PUBLIC'S AGENDA

What the media do or do not cover is equally powerful in determining what issues are considered by policymakers. Here are a few examples:

- The epidemic of HIV and acquired immunodeficiency syndrome (AIDS) is recognized as having been exacerbated by a lack of coverage by the media and journalists who saw it as a problem limited to promiscuous gay men and drug abusers (Shilts, 1987).
- When the front page of an influential newspaper carries a headline and story about the use of nurse practitioners as primary care providers, the issue is "on the agenda" of policymakers and the public.
- In 2000, the front page of *USA Today* reported on a study of family presence during resuscitation and invasive procedures published in the *American Journal of Nursing*. This and other widespread television, radio, print, and Internet coverage prompted debates on the issue and pressure on health care institutions to examine and change their policies.
- Walt Bogdanich and his colleagues at *The Wall Street Journal* published a front-page article in February 1987 on the misreading of Pap smears by laboratory technicians that left some women with a misdiagnosis. One year later, Congress passed the Clinical Laboratory Improvement Amendments, requiring minimum standards for laboratory operations and technician training (Otten, 1992).
- In recent years, the media has increased their coverage on the obesity epidemic in this country. Extensive reviews of both Eric Schlosser's book *Fast Food Nation* and Morgan Spurlock's documentary *Super Size Me*, both exposé's of the fast food industry, placed major fast food companies on the defensive and caught a lot of

people's attention. The Physician's Committee for Responsible Medicine, a nonprofit organization that promotes preventative medicine, organized a screening of the film *Super Size Me* at the Library of Congress that drew more then 400 Hill staffers. Six weeks after the film opened, McDonald's introduced the "Adult Happy Meal"—which included a pedometer, water, and a salad—and they phased out the "super size" option from their menu. McDonald's denies that the film had any influence on their decision.

Milio (2000) points out that policymakers are increasingly relying on "information brokers" to be informed about policy matters. Public officials often first learn about an issue through the press. In fact, a bill can be wallowing in the mire of legislative bureaucracy with no hope of passage until media highlight the issue that the bill addresses. For instance, many states and local communities had considered policies to restrict teenagers' access to cigarettes, but it took a media exposé on the deliberate targeting of adolescents by a cigarette manufacturer through the "Joe Camel" ads to get some of the legislation passed.

Brodie, Hamel, Altman, Blendon, and Benson (2003) analyzed data from 39 surveys of the public about news stories that were conducted by the Henry J. Kaiser Family Foundation and the Harvard School of Public Health between August 1996 and December 2002. They found that the media are the primary source of health information for more than 50% of public, and 40% follow health policy stories.

Although the news media are instrumental in getting issues onto the agenda of policymakers, non-news entertainment television programs can mobilize public constituencies around an issue. Turow (1996) points out that non-news television entertainment is particularly loaded with rhetoric that often stereotypes power relationships and may be more successful than the news in shaping people's images of the world.

Highly viewed TV presentations of medicine hold political significance that should be assessed alongside news. The television show "ER" aired an episode in which seniors needed emergency care because the husband took the wife's medications when they could not afford to buy the drugs prescribed for each of them. Another episode showed the plight of a poor minority patient who did not receive the same treatment referral as a white, well-insured patient. The popular White House–inspired "West Wing" series covered ergonomic regulations for workplace injuries, abortion, the death penalty, homophobia and hate crimes, homelessness, clean air, Cuban refugees, and tax cuts. "Law and Order SVU" has produced episodes focusing on the illegal trade of human organs for transplantation and the international trafficking of girls and women. In the past few years we have witnessed an increase in ads for these programs during the nightly news on network television. This conflation of news and entertainment is designed to boost corporate ratings and revenue.

Like the rhetorical struggles in news about medicine, series such as "ER," "House," "Grey's Anatomy," "Scrubs," and "Chicago Hope" are ultimately about power. Every week they act out ideas about the medical system's authority to define, prevent, and treat illness. Such programming can shape people's expectations, beliefs, and opinions of medicine, nursing, and health care (Brodie et al., 2001). Unfortunately, these programs seldom portray nurses and nursing accurately. The Center for Nursing Advocacy was founded to address media's misrepresentations of nurses and nursing in such programs, advertising, film, and art. (See *Changing Poor Portrayals of Nurses in the Media: The Center for Nursing Advocacy*, following this chapter.)

## EVALUATING PUBLIC POLICY

Media can also highlight the outcomes of a public policy. In 1989, New York decided to try to reduce the mortality rate after cardiac bypass surgery by requiring all hospitals to report on the case mix, risk factors, and outcomes of this surgery. The state analyzed these data, developed a method for ranking hospitals on their mortality rates, and released these rankings to the public. The media responded with feature stories highlighting "the best" and "the worst," or which hospital outranked another in the same community. In addition, one newspaper won a court case requiring the state to release the ranked data by individual surgeon. Unfortunately, not all journalists knew statistics well enough to realize

that some of the differences in rankings that they were highlighting were not statistically significant or clinically meaningful. As a result of such misinterpretations of the data, the state decided to educate journalists about the outcome initiative, interpretations of the data, and the need to emphasize what hospitals and surgeons were doing to improve the quality of care. Subsequent media coverage has highlighted the high-quality improvements that were made. Although the state once feared that the media coverage could undermine the effort to push for public reporting of medical outcomes, the program is now considered a model that has been replicated in other states and for other conditions or procedures (Chassin, Hannan, & DeBuono, 1996).

Public reporting of outcome data is now expected of health plans and institutions (Marshall, Shekelle, Davies, & Smith, 2003). Yet, Werner and Asch (2005) point out that the impact of such reporting on quality of care is largely undocumented and could have detrimental effects—for example, by making facilities and physicians reluctant to care for patients with high-risk or complex conditions even though many reporting systems adjust for risk. Nevertheless, public reporting of nurse-patient ratios by hospitals and nursing homes is being promoted in federal and state legislative proposals put forth by nursing and other organizations concerned about inadequate staffing. Senator Daniel Inouye and Congresswoman Lois Capps have sponsored such legislation, known as the "RN Safe Staffing Act" in the Senate and the "Quality Nursing Care Act" in the House.

## CAMPAIGNING AND ELECTION OUTCOMES

Media can determine who gets elected to public office. When a candidate running for public office wakes up to a news report on his or her own questionable financial dealings, the candidate worries, even if the story is unfounded. The image of the candidate in the minds of many can be tarnished forever. Similarly, the candidate's campaign manager and staff will read the letters to the editor of the newspaper to see which issues and positions are of concern to a community. They will also stage *media events*. These are a type of on-site press conference at a place that provides the visual images (for television and press photos) representative of an attention-getting problem that the candidate commits to resolve through policy initiatives.

The presidential election in 2000 was controversial, not just because of chads and other balloting problems, but because the news media called the outcome of the Bush-Gore race before the votes were tallied sufficiently to accurately predict who would be the next president. When one television news anchor said that Bush had won, then later retracted the statement, both Republicans and Democrats cried foul, recognizing that a premature call on the outcome of a race can actually change what those who have not yet voted decide to do (including whether to even go to the polls and bother to vote in a race that has already been called). In fact, media coverage of elections has become quite controversial and a focal point for discussions of ethics in journalism.

In the 2004 presidential campaign, John Kerry attempted to play his strength as a Vietnam veteran against George W. Bush's unexplained absence from the National Guard in Texas. But this strategy backfired when a group calling itself Swift Boat Veterans for Truth organized to question his claims about his service in Vietnam. The group called into question Kerry's patriotism for speaking out against the war when he completed his second assignment in Vietnam, questioning whether his Medal of Honor was deserved and suggesting that his anti-war speech before Congress undermined the safety of his fellow soldiers who remained in Vietnam. The group prepared hard-hitting ads that aired relentlessly in key states such as Florida and Pennsylvania; created a Website and blogs devoted to discrediting Kerry; and produced a documentary, e-mail alerts, and press releases to deliver their message. Although the group included some of Kerry's fellow soldiers who served with him in Vietnam, questions arose about its alignment with the Republican party and the source of funding for an expensive multimedia campaign *(www.rubyan. com/politics/archives/ 002153.html)*.

During the primaries for the 2004 presidential elections, Howard Dean showed the power of the Internet for political campaigns by using it for grassroots fundraising and messaging. Using the Internet, he raised more money than any other Democratic candidate before the primary elections using *MeetUp.com,* a Web tool for forming social groups, and bloggers (Wolf, 2004). This electronic strategy is now being called a *distributed campaign* and is viewed as a bottom-up rather than a top-down approach to political campaigns. (See *Distributed Campaigns: Using the Internet to Empower Activism,* following this chapter.)

## WHO CONTROLS THE MEDIA?

The profession of nursing is to health care as the profession of journalism is to the media. Nurses do not control the health care industry. It is controlled by corporate interests and the investors in the health care industry: the pharmaceutical industry, the medical technology industry, and the insurance industry, to name only a few. The government subsidizes the industry through reimbursement for health care and medications, as well as funding of biomedical research. The economic success of the health care industry depends on the government—on who gets elected and who is in power. In 2002, Congress passed a reform to the Medicare program adding a limited prescription drug benefit that prevents bulk discounting of drugs because of the power of the pharmaceutical lobby and their support of political candidates.

Similarly, journalists do not control the media industry. The industry is owned and controlled by six major corporations that "control 90 percent of what Americans read, see and hear for news" (Harris, 2005, p. 83). In 2003 the FCC, made up of political appointees reflecting the dominant party's priorities, voted to ease the restrictions on cross-ownership between different news entities. Harris quotes a *Washington Post* op-ed by Ted Turner (founder of CNN) published just prior to the FCC vote, in which Turner suggests that easing the restrictions on cross ownership between newspapers, TV, and radio, "will extend the market dominance of the media corporations that control most of what Americans read, see, or hear" and "give them more power to cut important ideas out of the public debate" (Harris, 2005, p.83).

The corporations are concerned about their advertisers or their "commercial interests" and about the government officials that regulate the industry and control their commerce; so the media corporations apply filters to determine what to air and print.

The filters reflect the need to please their best-paying advertisers and key elected officials so their reporters will not be denied access to them and regulations won't restrict their commerce. In addition, sometimes profit motives of the for-profit media corporations can lead to "paid news." In 2005 one of us (D. Mason) was surprised to be given a proposal for the production of television footage to promote a study being published in the *American Journal of Nursing*. The production company provided the option of "guaranteed placement" of the story on Fox News and NewsWatch for over $10,000, raising questions about the legitimacy and ethics of such "news" outlets.

Many people rely on National Public Radio and Public Television for news and analysis. In 2000 the conservatives began to act on their belief that these publicly supported media outlets are too liberal. The Republican-dominated U.S. House of Representatives and Senate threatened to reduce funding for the Corporation for Public Broadcasting, causing the "public media waves" to become more reliant on corporate donations. The picture became more threatening when President Bush appointed Kenneth Tomlinson to be the corporation's chairman; Tomlinson promptly hired a researcher to secretly monitor "liberal bias" in public radio and television. Tomlinson was criticized for politicizing public broadcasting in an era when independent journalism is diminishing in the United States (Stolberg, 2005).

Another parallel between nursing and journalism is the issue of ethical conduct. Nurses are exposed to unethical and unsafe practices in health care, and in some cases they report unethical unsafe practices to regulatory agencies—sometimes risking their jobs to do so. The profession of nursing has a code of ethics that guides nurses. The Code of Ethics of the Society of Professional Journalists instructs journalists to "Seek Truth and Report It," elaborating, "Journalists should be honest, fair, and courageous in gathering, reporting and interpreting information…[And they should] be free of obligation to any interest other than the pubic's right to know" (Cohen, 2005, p. 145).

Unfortunately, there is no agency that regulates unethical coverage or publishing, so there is no whistle to blow. The mainstream media will not report on their own bias. Blogs and websites will report on it; however, Internet news readers read the sources that most closely align with their values. Subscribers to the Center for American Progress (a Democratic think tank) do not read the news and analysis from the Cato Institute (a Republican think tank) and vice versa. It is essential that nurses assess their sources of information and participate in setting the record straight when issues have been misreported or inadequately covered.

## FOCUS ON REPORTING

One can argue that individual journalists are equally responsible for their choice of issues to cover and how they cover them. Getting to know the nature and quality of a particular journalists' work can help you to decide how much trust to place in it.

- Do they frequently misrepresent issues?
- Are their stories sensationalized, overplayed, or exaggerated?
- Do they present all sides of an issue with accuracy, fairness, and depth?

Journalists rarely have the same depth of knowledge about a topic as insiders. *Atlantic Monthly* national correspondent James Fallows (1996) provides an informative critique of and challenge to the media in his book *Breaking the News*. He argues that the media have contributed to a public cynicism of politics and policymakers that has resulted in a largely uninvolved citizenry. This is due partially to journalists' having limited expertise on particular issues; as a result they often cover only the political dimensions of an issue rather than the details of the policy options.

In addition to the Harry and Louise commercials, the media influenced the demise of President Clinton's Health Security Act in other ways that demonstrate this point. Dorfman, Schauffler, Wilkerson, and Feinson (1996) reported that in-depth analysis and explanation of the issues and the legislation were scarce in local news coverage; the focus tended to be superficial coverage of the risks and costs of the legislation to specific stakeholders. In fact, Milio (2000) notes that full debate of approaches to remedying an ailing health care system was not available to most citizens, because the single-payer alternative was rarely covered by the press. In an analysis of media coverage of the issue, the Annenberg Public Policy Center (1995, p. iv) found that the press concentrated on only a few of the alternative proposals for health care reform, focused reporting on strategy rather than on the pros and cons of proposals, magnified the impact of negative fear-based advertisements by focusing on them, and "had a tendency to filter both elections and policy debates through a set of cynical assumptions, including the notion that politicians act out of self-interest rather than a commitment to the public good."

In reality, few journalists have the breadth of knowledge about science, time, and editorial support to provide thorough reporting on health issues that have policy implications. This results in less-than-adequate reporting on important issues, such as how communities should respond to the West Nile virus. Roche (2002) examined print media coverage of the risks and tradeoffs of approaches to reducing the mosquito population to reduce the incidence of and mortality from West Nile encephalitis. None of the newspapers or magazines examined gave any information about risk of mortality from pesticide exposure or the cost; larviciding was rarely discussed, and no report compared larviciding with targeting adult mosquitoes. Roche concluded that the public is "operating 'in the dark' in evaluating the question of whether pesticides should be deployed."

Journalists usually report on television, radio, and the Internet based on information "released" to "the press" by various groups and organizations. Some journalists investigate beyond what is "released." Unfortunately, many are often prevented by their editors or producers from presenting all the facts. Editors and producers answer to the corporations that own the media outlets that censor or dilute what can be aired or published. For example, in 2004 ABC's *Nightline* devoted an entire show to honoring the U.S. men and women who had died in the Iraq War by reading their names and showing their photographs at a time when the Bush administration wanted to avoid such images for fear that they would undermine support for the war in Iraq. Many ABC affiliates around the country, owned by the Sinclair

Broadcasting Group, were prevented (censored) from airing the special because it was "contrary to the public interest" (Harris, 2005, p. 87).

## ANALYZING THE MEDIA

Although this chapter advocates that nurses more frequently and effectively use the media as a political tool, the first obligation that all nurses have is to be knowledgeable consumers of media messages. Nurses must seek out factual unbiased information from many sources before taking positions on policy issues and be able to critically evaluate media messages, assess who controls the media, and identify whose vested interests are being protected or promoted. Nurses should add *Mediachannel.org* and *Mediareform.net* to their Internet favorites and evaluate their sources. When nurses assess patients and families, they get information from as many sources as possible; assessing the media is no different. Box 9-1 provides an exercise for analyzing newspaper reporting critically.

### WHAT IS THE MEDIUM?

The first step is to ask yourself where you get your information and news.

- What television and radio news-related programming do you regularly tune in to? Do you read a daily newspaper?
- What is the station's, program's, or paper's reputation? Is it known for balanced coverage of health-related issues? Is it partisan?
- Does it cover national as well as state and local issues?
- Is it a credible source of information about health issues and policies?

These questions provide a basis for you to judge whether the information and news that you are getting are credible and representative of a broad sector of public opinion. For any particular issue of concern you will want to sample various media presentations of the issue and evaluate their messages and effectiveness.

### WHO IS SENDING THE MESSAGE?

Who is sponsoring the message and why? Part of understanding what the real message is about

---

**BOX 9-1**   How to Analyze Newspaper Reporting

The following exercise on how to analyze a newspaper expands one that was developed by Douglas (1991) for Fairness and Accuracy in the Media (FAIR), a national media watch group that critically analyzes news reports to raise consciousness about, and to correct, bias and imbalance.

- Get a recent copy of two or more national newspapers. Find an issue of concern and compare the papers on their coverage of the issue.
- First, note where the article is placed. Is it on the front page? Is it buried amid advertisements in a small portion of one column in the last section of the paper? Why do you think it received front, or last, page coverage?
- Second, note who wrote the article. The reputation of journalists can give you a sense of what bias might appear in the reporting, whether the coverage is likely to be balanced, and whether this journalist is someone who is known for in-depth investigative reporting.
- Third, what are the sources of information that are reported in the article? Every time a government official (e.g., president, other administration official, congressional representative, or staff) says something, highlight the passage with a

yellow marker. This includes "anonymous high-placed public officials" whose names and formal titles are not included. Every time the source is nongovernmental, highlight the passage with a pink marker. With a blue marker, note every time a woman or a person of color is mentioned or quoted. Now compare these passages. The ratio of yellow to pink to blue suggests what and who are routinely considered most important.

- For health reporting, note how often journalists quote or refer to nurses as opposed to physicians. How might the article be different if nurses were a primary source of information on the topic?
- What is the focus of the article? Does it present all sides of an issue? Is the coverage confined to the politics of an issue, rather than the content of the issue itself? (Fallows, 1996)
- Do any photographs included in the article reflect the issue and the people involved in it? If it is a story on some aspect of patient care, for example, does the photograph include and name nurses who are providing the care? Or are only the physicians shown and named?
- Who sits on the board of directors of a newspaper, and what interests do they represent? What is or is not being said in the editorials that might be directly or indirectly critical of these interests?

---

comes from knowing who is behind the message. You could interpret the real message behind the Harry and Louise commercials against President Clinton's health care reform legislation once you knew they were sponsored by the HIAA. If the legislation had passed, the majority of insurance companies would have been locked out of the health care market. Instead, their media success left them in control of health care in the United States. Similarly, questions arose during the 2004 presidential campaigns about who was behind the Swiftboat ads that claimed John Kerry had not performed honorably as a Vietnam soldier despite being awarded two medals of honor for heroism for his service there.

For news media, ask the following questions: Who owns this medium? What are the owner's biases? In addition, more and more newspapers are using the Associated Press (AP), or other major national papers, as their source for stories. The AP does not

investigate; they attend events, accept news releases, and file reports. If newspapers are using abridged stories from other papers, the news slant or bias of the other paper reflects the bias or slant of the paper you are analyzing.

## WHAT IS THE MESSAGE AND WHAT RHETORIC IS USED?

What is the ostensible message that is being delivered, and what is the real message? What rhetoric is used to get the real message across? In the continuing debate on Social Security, the Bush administration attempted to create a "crisis" of solvency that needed immediate reform. Economists and organizations like the AARP were successful in pointing out that the government's own actuaries demonstrate that the Social Security Trust is solvent through 2042 and that the fund will begin to spend more than it is receiving only in 2018, so there is no immediate crisis. Bush's messages have also appealed to individual self-interest in talking about an "ownership society" and "private accounts," which are contrary to the purpose of the Social Security system, which was set up in 1935 to protect all of society—especially the elderly, the widowed, and the disabled. Bush's message avoids talking about the Trust's solvency because his proposals actually contribute to insolvency sooner than the current condition.

In 2005, pollster Frank Luntz of the Luntz Research Companies provided an analysis of the rhetoric used in the 2004 campaign and outlined rhetoric that Republicans should use to win legislative battles and political campaigns in 2006. Asking, "How does a president with a 50% approval rating...," the unpublished document provides language for the major issues that would confront the federal Republican policymakers. For example:

Sometimes it is not what you say that matters but what you don't say. Other times a single word or phrase can undermine or destroy the credibility of a paragraph or entire presentation...[E]ffectively communicating the New American Lexicon requires you to stop saying words and phrases that undermine your ability to educate the American people. So from today forward YOU are the language police. From today forward these are the words never to say again. (Luntz, 2005, Appendix, p. 1)

One of the words "never to say" is "privatization/private accounts." Rather, the document advocates the phrase "personalization/personal accounts." The report notes that "Many more Americans would *personalize* Social Security than *privatize* it... Personalizing Social Security suggests *ownership* and *control* over your retirement savings, while privatizing it suggests a profit motive and winners and losers. "BANISH PRIVATIZATION FROM YOUR LEXICON" (Appendix, p. 1). Democrats were well aware of this difference in language and consistently framed the issue as "privatization."

On health care, the document admonishes never to say "healthcare choice" but rather to say "the right to choose," noting:

This is an important nuance so often lost on political officials. Almost all Americans want "the right to choose the healthcare plan, hospital, doctor and prescription drug plan that is best for them," but far fewer American actually want to make that choice. In fact, the older you get, the less eager you are to have a wide range of choices. One reason why the [Medicare] prescription drug card earned only qualified public support was that it offered too many choices and therefore created too much confusion for too many senior citizens. (Appendix, p. 4)

Every issue has "spin doctors" who develop believable messages based on focus groups and polling. As messages get repeated in the media, they become normalized and believable. It is essential to be attentive to the language used in media messages—whether delivered directly by policymakers or pundits or advocates—and evaluate the credibility, bias, and intentions of information sources. What and whom should we believe?

Images also convey important messages. As the Luntz document notes, "Language is your base. Symbols knock it out of the park.... The American people cannot always be expected to directly grasp the connection between your policies and your principles. Symbols bridge this gap, so use them" (Section 2, p. 2). The document promotes the obvious symbols of the American flag and Statue of Liberty. But consider the symbols used by health insurance companies to advertise to employed individuals and families. These ads use pictures of healthy active adults and bright-eyed children. Health insurers have never used images of obese individuals or people disabled by arthritis to attract new members to their insurance products. These are examples of targeted media messages in which images are symbols to augment carefully crafted rhetoric to sway a target audience to believe or act in a particular way.

## IS THE MESSAGE EFFECTIVE?

Does the message attract your attention? Does it appeal to your logic and to your emotions? Does it undermine the opposition's position?

## IS THE MESSAGE ACCURATE?

Who is the reporter, and what reputation does the reporter have? Is the reporter credible, with a reputation for accuracy and balanced coverage of an issue? What viewpoints are missing? Whose voice is represented in the message or article?

## RESPONDING TO THE MEDIA

One of the most important ways to influence public opinion is to respond to what is read or seen or heard in the media. *Getting Free Media Coverage for Nursing Issues* (following this chapter) describes the power and use of letters to the editor and of listener call-ins to talk radio programs. There are several other ways to respond to the media: writing an opinion editorial, mobilizing grassroots efforts to boycott sponsors and call producers, being proactive, and saying thanks.

### WRITING AN OPINION EDITORIAL

Opinion editorials ("op eds") allow more in-depth response to current issues and provide a way to get an issue on the public's agenda. Although they are often solicited by a newspaper or magazine, particularly in large cities, local community papers are often eager to receive editorials that describe an important issue or problem, include a story that illustrates the impact of the problem, and suggest possible solutions.

Nurse Teri Mills (2005) took advantage of Nurses' Week in 2005 to submit an op ed on nursing to the *New York Times*; it was published on May 20. See Box 9-2 for a reprint of her piece, "America's Nurse." Not only did she include a hook to the recent event of Nurses' Week in the first paragraph, but she went on to suggest an idea that many would consider rather provocative: "dethrone the surgeon general and appoint a National Nurse" (p. A25). The *Times* receives many more submissions than it can print, so it clearly helped to have a timely topic, concisely and clearly written in a conversational style, and with an unexpected or provocative slant.

### MOBILIZING GRASSROOTS EFFORTS TO BOYCOTT SPONSORS AND CALL PRODUCERS

For commercial media, disturbing programs and stories can be suppressed by threatening to boycott the sponsors who bought advertising time or space attached to the program or by expressing concerns to the producers, editors, or station managers. A successful grassroots effort by nurses arose in response to the airing of *Nightingales*, a prime-time television

program that portrayed nurses as mindless sex objects. Nursing organizations contacted their members and asked them to write to the producers and sponsors of the program, noting that they would not buy the sponsor's products. When a sponsor knows that a group of more than 2 million people (with family, friends, and professional colleagues) doesn't like the program their ads are paying for, they'll think twice about continuing to sponsor such programs. *Nightingales* was canceled by the network before the first season was over.

As noted in the opening to this chapter, the Center for Nursing Advocacy has picked up this mission and is building a grassroots network of nurses to change media's misrepresentations of nurses. Nurses can and should support this work and can do so through its web site, *www.nursingadvocacy.org*. The Taking Action that follows this chapter describes some of its successes, often by contacting the ad or program's sponsors and mobilizing other nurses to do so.

Contacting producers can also be done proactively to ensure appropriate representation of nurses or an issue. A powerful example came in the 1960s with the airing of *Dr. Kildare* and *Ben Casey*, two television programs featuring smart, caring, "nice guy" physicians. The American Medical Association (AMA) actively encouraged the producers to present these images:

In return for showing their organization's seal of approval at the end of each program, AMA physicians demanded the right to read every script and make changes in the name of accuracy. To them, however, accuracy also meant a proper doctor's image. During the height of its power in the 1960s, the AMA Advisory Committee for Television and Motion Pictures tried to make sure that with few exceptions the physicians who moved through doctor shows were incarnations of intelligent, upright, all-caring experts. AMA physicians were even insistent about the cars their TV counterparts drove (not too expensive), the way they spoke to patients (a doctor could never sit on even the edge of a female patient's bed), and the mistakes they made (which had to be extremely rare).... [Later] Doctors' organizations expressed anger that the programs were holding nurses and psychologists to the same status as MDs. (Turow, 1996, p. 1241)

Although the AMA's influence over television programming waned in the 1970s, physicians are

**BOX 9-2**   Example of A Nurse's Op Ed: The *New York Times,* May 20, 2005

### AMERICA'S NURSE
### By Teri Mills

*Teri Mills teaches nursing at Portland Community College, Portland, Ore.*

SO, national Nurses' Week has come and gone and what happened? Nothing, despite estimates that by 2020 there will be 400,000 fewer nurses than are needed in this country. Drastic action is required. And here's the action I suggest: dethrone the surgeon general and appoint a National Nurse.

Here's why. Prevention is the best way to lower health care costs. If people take care of themselves and don't get sick, well, you know the rest. And who better to educate Americans on how to take better care of themselves than nurses?

After all, nurses are considered the most honest and ethical professionals, according to a recent Gallup poll. It's the nurse whom the patient trusts to explain the treatment ordered by a doctor. It is the nurse who teaches new parents how to care for their newborn. It is the nurse who explains to the family how to comfort a dying loved one.

Meanwhile, the surgeon general, the nation's head doctor, is all but invisible. If you went to a supermarket and asked 10 people the surgeon general's name or to describe his or her role, it's unlikely that you would find anyone who could. (It's Richard H. Carmona, by the way.)

Now, I'm not saying that a National Nurse will become a household name immediately. But given all

that's at stake—the health of a nation—and given the surgeon general's inability to connect with Americans, it seems to me that we should at least give nurses a try.

Here's what I'd have the National Nurse do. She or he would highlight health care education through 15-minute weekly broadcasts that would also be available on the Internet. The emphasis would be on prevention: how to have a healthy heart; how to raise your teenagers without going crazy; how to avoid being swept into the growing tide of obesity.

The Office of the National Nurse would yield benefits in a multitude of ways. The informational programs would decrease dependence on a health care system that is not only expensive but at times inaccessible, especially for those who lack insurance or live in rural areas. Through the office, nurses could sign up for a National Nurse Corps that would organize activities to enhance health in their communities.

A National Nurse would give public recognition to the valuable work that nurses perform each day; if we're lucky, the National Nurse would help stem the nursing shortage by attracting people to the profession. A National Nurse won't solve all of our country's health care problems, but one would definitely improve the situation. America has a history of honoring great nurses—from Clara Barton to Susie Walking Bear Yellowtail. Isn't it time we did so again?

Readers should note certain characteristics of this op ed piece:
- It's short—454 words.
- It hooks to a national event—Nurses' Week.
- It defines a problem—the shortage of nurses and its impact on the people.
- It's provocative—it suggests that we replace a widely accepted national physician position with a national nurse position.
- It includes details or examples—what the person in this role might do.
- It describes the potential impact of the idea—and in one paragraph!

frequently consulted on health-related entertainment programs. Nurses have also served as consultants, and sometimes they have volunteered their services to a producer.

### SAYING THANKS

One of the most important strategies that nurses can use to influence the media is to thank the journalist who did a fine job in covering an issue of importance on nursing and health care. This can be

done in person or in writing. It goes a long way toward developing a relationship with the journalist that can be of help later when you have a story or an issue you would like covered.

### GETTING THE MESSAGE ACROSS

Getting your message to the appropriate target audience requires careful analysis and planning.

For example, you might want to target a message to local homeowners, many of whom watch a particular TV station's evening news. To get television coverage, you must have a visual attraction. California nurses staged a media event on a senior health issue by staging a "rock around the clock" marathon, with seniors in rocking chairs outside an insurance company. They received press coverage of the event, which elicited some supportive letters to the editor as well as some negative press from seniors who said that they were stereotyping elderly persons. See Box 9-3 for guidelines for getting your message across and Box 9-4 for a sample press release.

## MEDIA ADVOCACY

Harnessing the media for your own purposes is an important strategy if you are seeking public support for health-promoting policies. Media advocacy is the strategic use of mass media to apply pressure to advance a social or public policy initiative (Dorfman, Wallack, & Woodruff, 2005; Jernigan & Wright, 1996; Wallack & Dorfman, 1996). It is a tool for policy change—a way of mobilizing constituencies and stakeholders to support or oppose specific policy changes. It is a means of political action (DeJong, 1996).

Often, well-financed lobbies will develop public marketing messages and air them in only the districts where there are "swing votes" in Congress. Those constituents see the ads and call their member of Congress. The ads usually portray only part of the information. One of President George W. Bush's earliest actions was to propose a $1.6 trillion tax cut. Television and radio ads were aired using the voice of former Democratic President John F. Kennedy explaining why a tax cut would be good for the economy. The ads were aired in states with Democratic U.S. senators who were considered "swing" votes, meaning that they might be persuaded to vote for the tax cut with the Republicans if they heard from their constituents.

Media advocacy differs from social marketing and public education approaches to public health. Table 9-1 delineates some of these differences. Media advocacy defines the primary problem as a power gap, as opposed to an information gap, and therefore mobilization of groups of stakeholders is

needed to be able to influence the process of developing public policies.

The example of tobacco control illustrates the focus of media advocacy. The dangers of smoking were well known, albeit not admitted by tobacco companies until 1997. During the past 30 years, public policies that attempted to limit smoking created "a shift in the acceptability of smoking" (Wallack & Dorfman, 1996, p. 298). Advocates have also focused on the tobacco producers instead of the users. As Wallack and Dorfman (1996, p. 298) summarized, "In tobacco control, as in other public health issues, the challenge we face is to change the environment, and media advocacy provides a tool to help us meet that challenge." Because the tobacco settlements enriched state budgets, some states have used the money to reframe the public's thinking about tobacco and gain public support for stricter anti-smoking policies. Fichtenberg and Glantz (2000) report that such a campaign launched by California was associated with a reduction in deaths from heart disease. More recently, nurse researcher and educator Ruth Malone started a grassroots group called Nightingales for nurses who want to participate in nurse-led anti-smoking campaigns. (See the vignette by Ruth Malone, "The Nightingales Take on Tobacco.")

The success of Mothers Against Drunk Driving (MADD) is another illustration of the power of media advocacy. Over the past two decades, MADD developed a policy agenda aimed at preventing drunk driving. They developed a "Rating the States" program to bring public attention to what state governments were and were not doing to fight alcohol-impaired driving. Then, after a national press conference just after Thanksgiving, the beginning of a period of high numbers of alcohol-related traffic accidents, MADD representatives held local press conferences with their state's officials and members of other advocacy groups to announce the state's rating. Local and national broadcast and print press coverage resulted in the exposure of an estimated 62.5 million people to the story. Subsequently, action was taken in at least eight states to begin to address the problem of drunk driving (Russell, Voas, DeJong, & Chaloupka, 1995). Its success has led to an even more radical organization

**BOX 9-3** Guidelines for Getting Your Message Across

The following guidelines will help you shape your message and get it delivered to the right media:

### THE ISSUE

- What is the nature of the issue?
- What is the context of the issue (e.g., timing, history, and current political environment)?
- Who is or could be interested in this issue?

### THE MESSAGE

- What's the angle or "so what"? Why should anyone care? What is news?
- Is there a sound bite that represents the issue in a catchy, memorable way?
- Can you craft rhetoric that will represent core values of the target audience?
- How can you frame nursing's interests as the public's interests (e.g., as consumers, mothers, fathers, women, taxpayers, health professionals)?

### THE TARGET AUDIENCE

- Who is the target audience? Is it the public, policymakers, or journalists?
- If the public is the target audience, which segments of the public?
- What medium is appropriate for the target audience? Does this audience watch television? If so, are the members of this audience likely to watch a talk show or a news magazine show? Or do they read newspapers, listen to radio, or surf the Internet? Or are they likely to do all of these?

### ACCESS TO THE MEDIA

- What relationships do you have with reporters and producers? Have you called or written letters or thank-you notes to particular journalists? Have you requested a meeting with the editorial board of the local community newspaper to discuss your issue and how the members of the board might think about reporting on it?
- How can you get the media's attention? Is there a "hot" issue you can connect your issue to? Is there a compelling human interest story? Do you have a press release that describes your issue in a succinct, compelling way? (Box 9-4 provides a sample press release.) Do you have other printed materials that will attract journalists' attention within the first 3 seconds of viewing it? Are there photographs you can take in advance and then send out with your press release? Can you digitalize the images and make them available on a website for downloading onto a newspaper?
- Whom should you contact in the medium or media of choice?

- Have you been getting prepared all along? Are you news conscious? Do you watch, listen, clip, and track who covers what and how they cover it? What is the format of the program, and who is the journalist? What is the style of the program or journalist?
- Who are your spokespersons? Do they have the requisite expertise on the issue? Do they have a visual or voice presence appropriate for the medium? What is their personal connection to the issue, and do they have stories to tell? Have they been trained or rehearsed for the interview?

### THE INTERVIEWS

- Prepare for the interview. Get information on your interviewer and the program by reviewing the interviewer's work or talking with public relations experts in your area. Select the one, two, or three major points that you want to get across in the interview. Identify potential controversies and how you would respond to them. And rehearse the interview with a colleague.
- During the interview, listen attentively to the interviewer. Recognize opportunities to control the interview and get your primary point across more than once. What is your sound bite? Even if the interviewer asks a question that does not address *your* agenda, return the focus of the interview to *your* agenda and to *your* sound bite with finesse and persistence.
- Try to be an interesting guest. Come ready with rich, illustrative stories. Avoid yes or no answers to questions.
- Know that you do not have to answer all questions and should avoid providing comments that would embarrass you if they were headlines. If you don't know the answer to a question, say so and offer to get back to the interviewer with the information.
- Avoid being disrespectful or arguing with the interviewer.
- Remember that being interviewed can be an anxiety-producing experience for many people. It's a normal reaction. Do some slow deep-breathing or relaxation exercises before the interview, but know that some nervousness can be energizing.

### FOLLOW-UP

- Write a letter of thanks to the producer or journalist afterward.
- Provide feedback to the producer or journalist on the response that you have received to the interview or the program or coverage.
- Continue to offer other ideas for stories on the same or related topics.

**Date press can release a story** *and* **whom to contact for more information, including phone number and e-mail address**

**Focused header to get journalist's attention**

**Place of release** *and* **primary focus of release**

**Quote**

**Explanation of release's focus, making it self-explanatory**

**Quote on impact**

**Background, with enough detail that a journalist can write story without additional information**

**Description of person or organization issuing release**

**Hash marks indicating end of release**

---

**BOX 9-4**   Sample Press Release

For Immediate Release:                          Contact: Stacie Paxton
April 5, 2001                                                272-226-7747
                                                        spaxton@netnet.com

### REP. CAPPS INTRODUCES BIPARTISAN BILL TO ADDRESS NATION'S NURSING SHORTAGE CRISIS

#### Former Nurse Fights to Ensure More RNs Enter and Remain in the Workforce

Washington, DC—Representatives Lois Capps (D-CA), Sue Kelly (R-NY), Rosa DeLauro (D-CT), and 25 other members yesterday introduced landmark, bipartisan legislation to address the nursing shortage crisis facing our nation's hospitals, nursing homes, and other health institutions. Similar legislation was introduced in the Senate today by Sens. John Kerry (D-MA) and James Jeffords (R-VT).

"As a registered nurse, I know that patient care will be compromised if we don't address this crisis immediately," said Rep. Capps. "My bill will encourage more people to enter the nursing profession by providing incentives that other service careers already provide."

The Nurse Reinvestment Act establishes a National Nurse Service Corps to provide educational scholarships to nurses who commit to serve in a health facility determined to have a critical shortage of nurses. Grants would also be available to help individuals at any level of the nursing profession—from a nursing aide to an individual pursuing a doctoral degree—obtain more education. The bill also provides funding for public service announcements and supports nursing recruitment grants for educational facilities. In addition, it would expand Medicare and Medicaid funding for clinical nursing education and reimburses some home health agencies, hospices, and nursing homes for nurse training.

"Nurses are a critical part of our health care system," said Capps. "Fewer people are entering the nursing profession, and the current RN workforce is aging. If Congress doesn't act now to attract more individuals
into this profession, this shortage will turn into a major crisis that will be felt by every American needing medical attention."

According to the National League of Nursing, the number of individuals graduating from nursing programs declined 13% between 1995 and 1999 and this decline is expected to continue. Today, the average registered nurse (RN) is 45 years old, and by 2010, 40% of the RN workforce will be over 50. Capps worked closely with the American Nurses Association, American Organization of Nurse Executives, American Association of Colleges of Nursing, and other groups to develop legislation to address the documented shortage of individuals entering the nursing profession.

Capps—an RN for 41 years—earned her nursing degree at the Pacific Lutheran University in Tacoma, Washington. She has worked as a nursing instructor in Oregon, as head nurse at Yale New Haven Hospital, and as a school nurse in Santa Barbara County for more than 20 years.

###

**TABLE 9-1** Media Advocacy Versus Social Marketing and Public Education Approaches to Public Health

| MEDIA ADVOCACY | SOCIAL MARKETING AND PUBLIC EDUCATION |
|---|---|
| Individual as advocate | Individual as audience |
| Advances healthy public policies | Develops health messages |
| Changes the environment | Changes the individual |
| Target is person with power to make change | Target is person with problem or at risk |
| Addresses the power gap | Addresses the information gap |

Adapted from Wallack, L., & Dorfman, L. (1996). Media advocacy: A strategy for advancing policy and promoting health. *Health Education Quarterly, 23*(3), 297. Copyright 1996 by Sage Publications. Reprinted by permission of Sage Publications.

with a more prohibitionist stance that caused its founder, Candy Lightner, to resign from the group (Hanson, 2005).

Getting on the news media agenda is one of the functions of media advocacy (Wallack, 1994). With numerous competing potential stories, media advocacy employs strategies to frame an issue in a way that will attract media coverage. But *how* the message is presented is as important as simply getting the attention of the news media. The demise of the Health Security Act demonstrates this point. It got on the media's agenda, but the important messages were lost in the discussion of managed competition and the strategic use of the Harry and Louise commercials.

## FRAMING

Getting on the agenda and then controlling the message require *framing* (Dorfman et al., 2005). Framing "defines the boundaries of public discussion about an issue" (Wallack & Dorfman, 1996, p. 299). *Framing for access* entails shaping the issue in a way that will attract media attention. It requires some element of controversy (albeit not over the accuracy of advocates' facts), conflict, injustice, or irony. The targeted medium or media will shape how the story is presented. For example, television requires compelling visual images. If a broad audience is to be reached, several media need to be targeted. It also

helps to attach the issue to a local concern or event, anniversaries, or celebrities or to "make news" by holding events that will attract the press, such as releasing research or in some other way being "newsworthy" (Jernigan & Wright, 1996).

*Framing for content* is more difficult than framing for access. Although a compelling individual story may gain access to the media, there is no guarantee that the reporter will focus on the public policy changes that are needed to address problems illustrated by the individual. Wallack and Dorfman (1996) note that this framing "involves the difficult process of 'reframing' away from the usual news formula" (p. 300). The authors suggest that this reframing can be accomplished by the following:

- Emphasizing the social dimensions of the problem and translating an individual's personal story into a public issue
- Shifting the responsibility for the problem from the individual to the corporate executive or public official whose decisions can address the problem
- Presenting solutions as policy alternatives
- Making a practical appeal to support the solution
- Using compelling images
- Using authentic voices—people who have experience with the problem
- Using symbols that "resonate with the basic values of the audience" (Wallack & Dorfman, 1996, p. 300)
- Anticipating the opposition and knowing all sides of the issue

Jernigan and Wright (1996, p. 314) argue that media advocacy is most effective when it is "linked to a strong organizing base and a long-term strategic vision." Training and designating spokespersons are important to controlling the message.

## *Key Points*

- The media in our society are tremendously powerful and may be the single most influential force shaping public policy and political campaigns.
- Understanding how you might be influenced by media requires thoughtful, critical analysis of news and advertising meant to promote specific

values and perspectives deemed essential for advancing a specific policy or political agenda.

- Strategic use of the media requires framing an issue to access media and to get your message across to the public or target audience.
- Nurses, both individuals and groups, can influence public policy by engaging in media advocacy and being proactive in shaping media portrayals of the profession and policy matters.

## *Web Resources*

> **Project for Excellence in Journalism and the Committee of Concerned Journalists**—site provides information on research, resources, and standards for improving journalism
> *www.journalism.org*
> **J-Lab: The Institute for Interactive Journalism**—a center of the University of Maryland's Philip Merrill College of Journalism that "helps news organizations and citizens use new information ideas and innovative computer technologies to develop new ways for people to engage in critical public policy issues"
> *www.j-lab.org*
> **Pew Center for Civic Journalism**—was created by the Pew Charitable Trust to stimulate innovations in reengaging the public in public life, including matters of public policy
> *www.pewcenter.org*
> **Henry J. Kaiser Family Foundation**—partners with the Harvard School of Public Health to survey the public about key health issues and publishes the Kaiser/Harvard News Index, a report of the leading health news issues followed by the public
> *www.kff.org/kaiserpolls*
> **John S. and James L. Knight Foundation**—provides philanthropic support to promote excellence in journalism and the education of journalists
> *www.knightfdn.org/default.asp*

> **Poynter Institute**—a school dedicated to teaching and inspiring journalists and media leaders; it provides an "Ethics On-Call" service for journalists to get advice on ethical issues in journalism.
> *www.poynter.org*
> **Mediachannel.org**—nonprofit site that focuses on global media issues, offering analysis of news and commentaries from an international network of media issues, organizations, and publications
> *www.mediachannel.org*
> **Free Press**—nonpartisan organization working to involve the public in media policymaking and to craft policies for more democratic media
> *www.freepress.net*

## REFERENCES

Annenberg Public Policy Center of the University of Pennsylvania. (1995). *Media in the middle: Fairness and accuracy in the 1994 health care reform debate.* Philadelphia: Annenberg Public Policy Center.

Arnold, K. (2003). Journals, the press, and press releases: A cozy relationship. *Science Editor, 26*(5), 169-170.

Betts, M. (1995). Politicos blazing cyberspace trail. *Computerworld.* Retrieved August 29, 2005, from *www.politicsonline.com/coverage/computerworld.*

Brock, D. (2004). *The Republican noise machine: Right-wing media and how it corrupts democracy.* New York: Three Rivers.

Brodie, M., Foehr, U., Rideout, V., Baer, N., Miller, C., Flournoy, R., & Altman, D. (2001). Communicating health information through the entertainment media. *Health Affairs, 20*(1), 192-199.

Brodie, M., Hamel, E. C., Altman, D., Blendon, R., & Benson, J. M. (2003). Health news and the American Public, 1996-2002. *Journal of Health Politics, Policy and Law, 28*(5),927-950.

Buresh, B., & Gordon, S. (2000). From silence to voice. *Journal of Nursing Scholarship, 32*(4), 330-331.

Buresh, B., & Gordon, S. (2003). *From silence to voice: What nurses know and must communicate to the public.* Ithaca, NY: Cornell University Press.

Buresh, B., Gordon, S., & Bell, N. (1991). Who counts in news coverage of health care? *Nursing Outlook, 39*(5), 204-208.

Chaffee, M. W. (2000). Health communications: Nursing education for increased visibility and effectiveness. *Journal of Professional Nursing, 16*(1), 31-38.

Chassin, M. R., Hannan, E. L., & DeBuono, B. A. (1996). Benefits and hazards of reporting medical outcomes publicly. *New England Journal of Medicine, 334*(6), 394-398.

Cohen, E. D. (2005). Corporate Media's Betrayal of America. In Cohen (Ed.), *News Incorporated.* Amherst: Prometheus Books.

DeJong, W. (1996). MADD Massachusetts versus Senator Burke: A media advocacy case study. *Health Education Quarterly, 23*(3), 318-329.

Dorfman, L., Schauffler, H. H., Wilkerson, J., & Feinson, J. (1996). Local television news coverage of President Clinton's introduction of the Health Security Act. *Journal of the American Medical Association, 275*(15), 1201-1205.

Dorfman, L., Wallack, L., & Woodruff, K. (2005). More than a message: Framing public health advocacy to change corporate practices. *Health Education and Behavior, 323,* 320-336.

Douglas, S. J. (1991). Reading the news in more than black and white. *EXTRA!, 4*(7), 1, 6.

Fallows, J. (1996). *Breaking the news: How the media undermine American society.* New York: Vintage Books.

Fichtenberg, C. M., & Glantz, S. A. (2000). Association of the California tobacco control program with declines in cigarette consumption and mortality from heart disease. *New England Journal of Medicine, 343*(24), 1772-1777.

Glaser, M. (2004). Bloggers, citizen media and Rather's fall—Little people rise up in 2004. Online Journalism Review. Retrieved August 28, 2005, from *www.ojr.org/ojr/stories/041221Glaser.*

Grossman, L. K. (1997). The electronic republic. In T. Walker & C. Sass (Eds.), *Perspectives: Readings on contemporary American government.* Alexandria, VA: Close Up Foundation.

Hanson, D. J. (2005). Mothers against drunk driving: A crash course in MADD. Retrieved January 29, 2005, from *www.alcoholfacts.org/CrashCourseOnMADD.html.*

Harris, J. (2005). To be our own governors. In Cohen (Ed.), *News incorporated.* Amherst, Prometheus Books.

Jamieson, K. H. (2000). *Everything you think you know about politics...and why you're wrong.* New York: Basic Books.

Jernigan, D. H., & Wright, P. A. (1996). Media advocacy: Lessons from community experiences. *Journal of Public Health Policy, 18,* 306-329.

Kalb, M. (1997). The value of a free press. In T. Walker & C. Sass (Eds.), *Perspectives: Readings on contemporary American government.* Alexandria, VA: Close Up Foundation.

Koberstein, P. (1993). Tom Foley thrives in a very Republican district. High County News. Retrieved August 28, 2005, *www.hcn.org/servlets/hcn.Article?article_id=29.*

Labaton, S. (2004, June 23). Senate votes to restore media limits. *New York Times,* C1.

Learner, N. (2005, August 8). Sen. Frist: DTC Advertising Drives Up Rx Drug Costs. *FDA News.* Retrieved January 29, 2006, from *http://www.fdanews.com/cgi-bin/udt/sc2.display.ppv?client_id=wbi_wdl&inv_id=20711&sid=44390&view=V.*

Luntz, F. (2005). *The new American lexicon.* Alexandria, VA: The Luntz Research Companies. Retrieved September 16, 2005, from *www.dailykos.com/story/2005/2/23/3244/72156.*

Marshall, M. N., Shekelle, P. G., Davies, H. T. & Smith, P. C. (2003). Public reporting on quality in the United States and the United Kingdom. *Health Affairs (Millwood), 22*(3), 134-148.

McAlister, A. L. (1991). Population behavior change: A theory-based approach. *Journal of Public Health Policy, 12,* 345-361.

Milio, N. (2000). *Public health in the market: Facing managed care, lean government and health disparities.* Ann Arbor, MI: University of Michigan Press.

Mills, T. (2005, May 20). America's Nurse. *New York Times,* A25.

Otten, A. L. (1992). The influence of the mass media on health policy. *Health Affairs, 11*(4), 111-118.

Rainie, L. (2005a). New data on blogs and blogging. Commentary, May 2, 2005. Retrieved September 11, 2005, from *www.pewinternet.org/ppf/p/1083/pipcomments.asp.*

Rainie, L. (2005b). The state of blogging: Pew Internet and American Life Project data memo, January 2, 2005. Retrieved September 11, 2005, from *www.pewinternet.org/ppf/r/144/report_display.asp.*

Rehm, D. (1997). Talk radio and the public dialogue. In T. Walker & C. Sass (Eds.), *Perspectives: Readings on contemporary American government.* Alexandria, VA: Close Up Foundation.

Roche, J. P. (2002). Print media coverage of risk-risk tradeoffs associated with West Nile encephalitis and pesticide spraying. *Journal of Urban Health, 79*(4), 482-490.

Roosevelt, M. (2005, March 7). Nursing a grudge. *Time Magazine.* Retrieved January 29, 2006 from: http://time-proxy.yaga.com/time/magazine/article/qpass/0,10987,1032330,00.html?ticket=T%3Av1%3A7316ecaf50fb8f3b246dea29458db9b0%3A113856 0284%3A%252Ftime%252Fmagazine%252Farticle%252Fqpas s%252F0%252C10987%252C1032330%252C00.html&q=2.50.

Russell, A., Voas, R. B., DeJong, W., & Chaloupka, M. (1995). MADD rates the states: Advocacy event to advance the agenda against alcohol-impaired driving. *Public Health Reports, 110*(3), 240-245.

Schmid, T. L., Pratt, M., & Howze, E. (1995). Policy as intervention: Environmental and policy approaches to the prevention of cardiovascular disease. *American Journal of Public Health, 85*(9), 1207-1211.

Sharp, K. (2005, November 11). The woman behind Arnold's defeat. *Berkeley Daily Planet.* Retrieved on January 29, 2006, from *www.mindfully.org/Reform/2005/Woman-Defeat-Arnold11nov05.htm.*

Sheridan-Gonzalez, J., & Wade, M. (1998). Every patient deserves a nurse. In D. J. Mason & J. K. Leavitt (Eds.), *Policy and politics in nursing and health care* (3rd ed.). Philadelphia: Saunders.

Shilts, R. (1987). *And the band played on.* New York: St. Martin's Press.

Sigma Theta Tau International. (1998). *The Woodhull study on nursing and the media: Health care's invisible partner.* Indianapolis: Sigma Theta Tau Center Nursing Press.

Solomon, N. (2005). Big money, self-censorship and corporate media. In Cohen (Ed.), *News Incorporated.* Amherst, Prometheus Books.

Stolberg, S. G. (2005, July 1). Researcher's appraisals of commentators are released. *New York Times,* A13.

Turow, J. (1996). Television entertainment and the U.S. health care debate. *Lancet, 347,* 1240-1243.

Wallace, D. (2005, April). Host. *Atlantic,* 67.

Wallack, L. (1994). Media advocacy: A strategy for empowering people and communities. *Journal of Public Health Policy, 15,* 420-436.

Wallack, L., & Dorfman, L. (1996). Media advocacy: A strategy for advancing policy and promoting health. *Health Education Quarterly, 23*(3), 293-317.

Werner, R., & Asch, D. (2005). The unintended consequences of publicly reporting quality information. *Journal of the American Medical Association, 293,* 1239-1244.

Wolf, G. (2004). How the Internet invented Howard Dean. Wired Magazine. Retrieved August 28, 2005 from *www.wired.com/wired/archive/12.01/dean.html.*

# Taking Action
Catherine J. Dodd

## Getting Free Media Coverage for Nursing Issues

*"The need for a powerful nursing voice has never been greater."*

SUZANNE GORDON

In 1987 after Congresswoman Nancy Pelosi was elected to the U.S. House of Representatives, I was asked to join her staff because of the effective role I played in coordinating a "Nurses for Pelosi" effort within her campaign. I quickly learned many lessons in working for a member of Congress. One of my first assignments was to rotate through the early morning "letter to the editor" clipping and faxing job in the office. This meant leaving the house by 5 AM to purchase the first issue of the morning paper at an all-night newsstand and arrive at the San Francisco Congressional Office by 5:30 AM to read, clip, and fax back to Washington, DC, the editorial page with the letters to the editor so that they would be on Congresswoman Pelosi's desk by 9 AM. Why? Because newspaper subscribers tend to be homeowners, and homeowners vote in every election.

Letters to the editor reflect what voters are thinking about local issues. The editor of the editorial page usually does not publish a letter until more than one letter on the same issue has been received, so published letters reflect the views of lots of voters. A catchy, well-written letter to the editor that is published has much more political weight than a personal lobbying letter on an issue. (So if you are going to write just one letter, write the letter to the editor; better, though, is to write your lobbying letter, as well!)

This in no way means that Congresswoman Pelosi concerned herself only with homeowners and newspaper subscribers. She represented a district that is overwhelmingly Democrat, so her reelection was certain. She is an advocate for voters and those unable to vote—children and the many noncitizens who live in San Francisco. She still listens to and is concerned about what the voters think.

### LETTERS TO THE EDITOR

Today, in campaigns for ballot initiatives as well as candidates, press staff are orchestrating letters-to-the-editor campaigns to show "voter support" of candidates and issues. For statewide issues and candidates, only six different letters are needed. Six basic letters are drafted and faxed to six volunteer letter submitters in the geographic area of every major daily in the state. The letter submitters put the text of the letter on their personal letterhead and fax the same letter to the same paper to which five other people are faxing their letters. The same plan works for local issues, as well. Major papers like to demonstrate the breadth of their circulation, so they frequently publish letters received from nearby cities and suburbs. Editors of the editorial page want to be viewed as fair, so they will attempt to balance the number of letters written by women and men. This gives women an excellent chance of being published, because women do not write as much or as often as men.

In a graduate class on health policy and politics at San Francisco State University, I offered nursing students extra credit for every letter to the editor they write. In 1994, California voters passed Proposition 187, a mean-spirited, antiimmigrant initiative that, among other things, denied prenatal and emergency care to undocumented persons. After the election and just before Thanksgiving, a student who had immigrated from Russia with her family wrote a letter to the editor about how our country's first immigrants would not be celebrating Thanksgiving. They would be hiding from immigration officials had Proposition 187 been the law of the land at that time. It was published with headlines on Thanksgiving day and was the subject of several days' worth of subsequent letters supporting the provision of prenatal care and education to undocumented people. Those extra credit points had a lasting effect. Other students report the therapeutic effect of writing a letter about something that makes them feel angry or passionate and knowing that, if published, it will reach tens of thousands of readers (Box 9-5).

---

**BOX 9-5**   Letter to the Editor

The following letter was published on March 14, 2004, leading off the letters section of the Sunday edition of the *Detroit Free Press*. It was written by nurse Antonia Villarruel, a professor of nursing at University of Michigan School of Nursing and a contributor to this book. The title is added by the newspaper.

**Word length:** This is 206 words; letters should adhere to the word limits provided in the letter guidelines. Letters that exceed the limit are much less likely to be published.

**Opening paragraph** lays out the problem or issue. An opening that challenges prevailing thought, provokes controversy, or provides an engaging anecdote or statistic will be more likely to draw in the reader—and the editor.

**Arguments** for your position are clearly stated.

**Opposing arguments** are acknowledged and countered.

**Concluding statement** provides a challenge or direction for different thinking or action.

**Signature** includes the letter writer's name, title, affiliation, city, and state. Some papers use a style that does not include RN and degrees. In such cases, a title or affiliation can identify the letter writer as likely to be a nurse, but this could also be worked into the letter—e.g., "As a nurse researcher, I have studied the interventions to reduce teen pregnancy...."

### COMPREHENSIVE INFORMATION IS THE BEST SEX ED

Adolescents shouldn't be having sex. Adolescents shouldn't get pregnant, get HIV or STDs. On those points, policymakers, parents and health professionals can agree. But regardless of what we think, the reality is that adolescents are having sex, they are getting pregnant, and they are at risk for HIV and STDs.

Clearly, the abstinence message needs to be delivered loud and clear at home, in schools and during encounters with health professionals. But we can't legislate abstinence. Our research and practice experience tells us that providing adolescents with the knowledge and skills about how to negotiate abstinence is important. So is similar content about negotiating and using contraceptives and condoms.

The major fear is that teaching youths about condoms and contraceptives will promote more sexual activity. This isn't true. Providing information doesn't promote sex. In fact, once given the information, many adolescents recognize that sex isn't like it is on television. Many decide they are simply not ready.

Health care providers, parents, schools and policymakers have similar concerns: How can we ensure the safety and health of our state's most valuable resources, our youths? We need to consider what adolescents tell us they need. Our message has to move beyond promoting what we think they should do.

—Antonia M. Villarruel
Associate Professor Director
Center for Health Promotion
The University of Michigan School of Nursing
Ann Arbor

Reprinted with permission of the *Detroit Free Press*.

## TALK RADIO

A similar strategy can be used for radio talk shows, which reach hundreds of thousands of people at one time. (General commercial radio audiences, as opposed to public radio listeners, cannot be categorized as perennial "always" voters.) Radio talk shows can be used to educate the public about new treatment modalities, changes in the quality of care, dangerous patient care situations, or any number of issues that concern nurses. Having a group or "radio response squad" of well-prepared registered nurses listening to a talk show and prepared to call in on an issue or during an "open" session can be an effective advertising tool. Callers should be cautioned to write down the three points they want to make and practice them on a friend. If they get to the producer and are asked what their position is, they should be neutral and have a question they want to pose. (If an on-air caller just expressed your position, the producer will not air another caller with the same position.) Once on the air, callers should make their point and say, "I will stay on the air for your response," being prepared to defend their statements. "Taking a response off the air" allows the host or talk show guest to have the last word.

Regardless of the medium, if you are advocating for the public (as opposed to advocating for nursing's professional interests), always identify yourself as a registered nurse. The public trusts and values nurses, and your message will carry more clout.

## *Lessons Learned*

- Letters to the editor can put issues onto policymakers' agendas.
- Letters need to be timely, short, and to the point.
- Prepare your key messages before calling into talk radio.

---

# *Taking Action*   Ryan W. Ozimek

## *Distributed Campaigns: Using the Internet to Empower Activism*

*"Any sufficiently advanced technology is indistinguishable from magic."*

ARTHUR C. CLARKE

A flurry of new techniques for political campaigning emerged during the 2004 presidential election, especially when it came to effectively using the Internet as a tool to reach new supporters and mobilize activists. With the lessons learned from the 2000 presidential election, and the heavy competition among Democratic presidential candidates, campaigns extended their outreach plans from door-to-door campaigning to viral Internet marketing.

One of the important online campaign methodologies created during this tumultuous campaign season was the concept of distributed campaigns. A distributed campaign is an Internet-based campaign that contains a viral aspect and whose success depends on the viability of three important online campaign components: Websites, networks, and message delivery methods.

As opposed to more traditional online campaign models, where content and messages are pushed from the top of a campaign (i.e., a campaign headquarters) down to the grassroots supporters, the distributed campaign model turns this concept on its head. Rather than campaign leadership providing the messaging, the grassroots effectively provides the messaging itself, virally spreading the content over various ad hoc communities.

## THE PURPOSE OF A DISTRIBUTED CAMPAIGN

The purpose of the distributed campaign model is to go beyond the core supporters, and reach out to those swing voters at the margins. The goal is to allow the grassroots communities to take greater ownership of the campaign, giving them more incentive to stay involved and provide content that will attract fellow citizens.

Viral campaigns are as old as advertising itself. People place a great amount of trust in messages exchanged between members of their community and place less trust in those provided by outside agents. For instance, if your friend provides you information about a candidate whose message resonates closely with your friend's beliefs, his message to you will likely be more effective than a 30-second television spot by the same candidate. Even if the message is identical, the trusted relationship between you and your friend will make the message more compelling, and in the end more effective.

## A BRIEF HISTORY OF DISTRIBUTED CAMPAIGNS

With the 2004 presidential election season providing the roots of distributed campaigning, its history can be summarized quite quickly. Facing battles against Washington, DC insiders, Democratic presidential candidate and Vermont Governor Howard Dean and his campaign staff knew that their differentiator against the eight other Democratic candidates would need to be a campaign relying heavily on grassroots support. Although most of the Democratic candidates turned to their established national bases, Dean grew a grassroots community following that quickly became the most vocal in the race for the presidency.

"Deaniacs," as they were called, provided Dean an incredibly powerful grassroots community. At the beginning of the campaign, Dean created a Website that was similar to that of his competition, full of messages and events driven by the campaign's headquarters. To allow for the growth of online Dean supporter communities, technologically savvy supporters began creating "Deanspaces," online communities that could quickly be created and easily managed not by the campaign headquarters, but rather by the niche communities themselves. For instance, nearly every state had a Deanspace, which allowed supporters in any state to self-identify themselves as Dean supporters and self-organize events, fundraising drives, and even mass e-mail campaigns.

The fascinating aspect of Deanspaces was that the campaign headquarters provided no catalyst and very little sustained support, but the communities thrived regardless. Suddenly, grassroots supporters had the tools they needed to reach out to the margins, reaching constituents that would have otherwise never been reached by the campaign headquarters. In just a few months hundreds of Deanspaces were created, raising tens of thousands of dollars for Dean and bringing together thousands of homegrown events, popularized by *www.meetup.com*. A distributed campaign was created, sustained, and grown without much effort required by the campaign headquarters.

## ONLINE TOOLS THAT FACILITATE SELF-ORGANIZATION

Distributed campaigns may require less hands-on support from a campaign headquarters than the traditional online campaign, but they need tools that are both easy to use and easily distributable to a variety of audiences. There are four core online tools that have proven most effective in the creation of a distributed campaign: Websites (including blogs and community forums), e-mail, petitions and surveys, and action centers (including write-your-representative forms, contact media forms, and other outbound individualized messaging efforts).

### Websites

One of the first places to start your distributed campaign is with a Website. When constituents first become interested in your campaign, they will want to learn more about it without having to commit heavy resources or time. A Website gives your campaign a virtual home where people can peruse your literature, learn more about your positions, and decide whether they are interested in becoming more involved, all without a single direct touch to anyone on your campaign. This autonomy empowers visitors to make decisions on their own, so it is important that your messaging and interactivity on the site aid in leading people down a path that makes decisions about your campaign easy.

So far, we have discussed only the broadcast mechanisms of a Website, in which messages are simply pushed from your campaign down to the visitors; however, this methodology fails to meet one of the most important pillars of distributed campaigns by not facilitating horizontal or upstream communication. To bridge this gap, distributed campaigns should include blogs and forums.

## Blogs and Forums

The order in which these two Internet tools are implemented is important to the distributed campaign's success. As we will discuss next, blogs are much easier to implement and maintain than forums. You should take into account the size of your campaign as well as the human resources you have to maintain the Website. If your team has only one or two people to manage the entire Website, it might be most effective to focus only on a blog. If you have more than two people who can provide support for your Web site, your campaign should be able to effectively support a forum in addition to a blog.

Blogs are, at their core, simply easy ways for your campaign to provide information to your supporters while simultaneously allowing feedback. In the context of this discussion, we will assume that your campaign does not have a content management system or a Website manager that easily allows a nontechnical person to maintain all the content on your Website. A blog fills this role nicely for smaller, grassroots campaigns by enabling you to easily and frequently post content on your Website. Blogs keep Websites fresh, and in any campaign, freshness is what keeps people hungry to stay involved.

Although a blog can simply be your tool to update content on your Web site, they have been most effective when written with a personal voice. For instance, your "issues" page or "about us" page holds detailed information about your campaign,

but information that is normally written from an organizational perspective. Your blog, on the other hand, should be updated on a regular basis.

The blog provides an excellent opportunity for a campaign to retrieve information from its supporters. Built into most blogs is the ability to easily collect comments for each posting made to the blog. Campaigns often have a top-down structure, in which information is handed out only after careful consideration and development from the top of the campaign. A blog turns this process on its head. Blogs require the campaign headquarters to be comfortable with allowing the community of supporters to create content that is then published on the campaign's Website. Of course, administrators of the blog will have ultimate control of the content that is placed on the site's comment section; however, editing or censoring of information on the blog and its comments should be avoided unless the content is extremely damaging or vulgar.

Creating blog entries and keeping track of comments can be a difficult task to keep up with during a campaign. For campaigns that have the capacity to take the next step of interactivity with their constituents, a distributed campaign would include a forum or community chat room, where discussions and communication can be started by members of the community.

Forums provide the first level of multi-channel communication in a distributed campaign. Essentially, in a distributed campaign this is the first opportunity for the campaign to allow its supporters to have content creation and management abilities. Many positive results can be derived from a forum. Forums, in their self-developing ways, allow certain members of the community to immediately rise to the top. For instance, once campaign supporters have an outlet to post their concerns or ideas, the rest of the community can then provide peer review of these ideas and respond accordingly. During the 2004 presidential election, the Dean campaign took ideas from supporters who had risen to the top in peer review, and then took action on them. When the campaign was preparing for a speech Dean was to give in New York, they looked to the forums and the online community for help. Supporters had posted an idea of having a red bat placed on the

Website; the bat would fill up as more money was raised for the campaign. Within hours, campaign manager Joe Trippi made sure that when Dean went on stage in front of the press and New York supporters, he had a red bat in his hands and told everyone that he was running a different campaign: he was listening directly to his supporters.

Although most campaigns will not have the Dean press coverage, the story highlights an important point. Forums that allow supporters to post their ideas, with the community weighing the benefit of these ideas for the campaign, essentially create a new layer of campaign management. By carefully monitoring what the community writes in the forums, a campaign can retrieve information from a great source of self-selected supporters. In addition to watching the forums for new ideas, it's also important for the campaign management to "prune" the forum. *Pruning* is a term used to describe the process of going through the postings on a forum and making sure they are being placed in the right place and that they are acceptable to be read by a wide variety of potential visitors.

## E-Mail

Creating a Web site that attracts visitors takes more than simply posting great content. You need to find ways to draw visitors to your site so that they can read all the content that you've placed there. One effective way to get the message out about your distributed campaign is e-mail. When e-mail is used in conjunction with the distributed campaign, information can be quickly passed along among friends and families faster than by simply posting information on the Website.

To be successful, and to improve the chances of drawing supporters back to your Website, it's important that every e-mail sent by the campaign include a few key elements:

1. The e-mail should have a prominent link to the Website, as well as contact information for the campaign.
2. The e-mail should be written with brevity and should be to the point. The point of these e-mails isn't to convey complex messages, but rather to attract readers to the Website to learn more,

become involved in the campaign, and spread the word about the campaign to others.
3. Each e-mail should make it easy to forward the e-mail to friends. For instance, you can include a small form in your HTML e-mail that has three blank fields in which the reader can enter the e-mail addresses of friends to have the e-mail forwarded.

Although the actual creation of content for an effective campaign e-mail is outside the scope of this section, the key to a distributed campaign is simply to make sure that the campaign includes an e-mail component. Sending e-mails to your constituents is an important way to get in touch with your supporters who are not visiting your Website (or Websites) regularly and to provide them reasons to visit the site and get involved. A distributed campaign should consider sending e-mails to its supporters at least once a week.

## Petitions and Surveys

Once e-mails have brought more potential supporters to a campaign's Website, the campaign now has an opportunity to learn more about the new supporters. Blogs and forums allow the campaign to take a generalized, qualitative approach to understanding its supporters; however, these online tools don't provide the degree of detail that managers need to clearly understand the opinion of supporters. In a distributed campaign, in which individuals become closely connected with the online community, supporters are more likely to answer honestly and candidly to surveys created by the campaign. Using surveys allows a campaign to quantify the opinions of its supporters as well as understand the effectiveness of campaign messages used by the campaign.

In addition to surveys, online petitions can be used to create collective action among a distributed campaign community. For instance, a community can create a petition to send to the campaign headquarters to say that the community does not believe that the campaign's messaging is in the best interest of the community. By allowing a community to self-generate a petition like this, the campaign can receive additional demographic information that it couldn't collect through a survey, simply because the campaign management likely wouldn't already know the right questions to ask. Though a community petition, the community leaders are able to send a strong message upstream, providing information that can be critical in maintaining support among communities.

## ACTION CENTERS

We have discussed ways in which a campaign can work to create interactivity among its supporters within the organization. The main goal of a campaign's efforts, however, is often outward facing. Once supporters have been brought together and have built a community, the campaign must then give them the tools necessary to take appropriate action on behalf of the campaign. These tools are commonly called *action tools* and can range from online form letters that can be sent to legislators to systems that let supporters write letters to their editors.

Currently the nonprofit and advocacy technology marketplace is still young in the development of these action centers. When building action centers, there are essentially two paths of development that an organization can take. One path is to work with other nonprofit organizations, such as Democracy In Action *(www.democracyinaction.org)*, that provide online action centers for campaigns and advocacy groups. Organizations such as these make it extremely easy for a campaign to use a suite of action tools that it can then hand off to its supporters.

For instance, in our earlier definition of a distributed campaign, we summarized that the most effective (and efficient) way to spread a message is through trusted bridges (e.g., between friends or family members). The Dean campaign started to do this through the use of Deanspaces. The next step is to allow each of these distributed campaign communities to have its own set of action tools. A campaign might have 10 distributed campaign communities, then have a contest between each of the communities to see which can send the most letters to their community's legislators on behalf of the campaign. By creating a contest like this, a campaign can invigorate leadership within communities and thereby distribute management down to

the communities, without stressing the campaign's top management.

## WHY DISTRIBUTED CAMPAIGNS MAKE GOOD SENSE

Distributed campaigns make extremely good sense strategically for several reasons:

1. *They create more engaging Websites.* In a traditional online campaign, the same group of individuals who are maintaining the entirety of the campaign, from phone calls to strategy, are also creating top-down messaging on the Website. This normally produces tunnel vision and messages that are strictly staying on the prescribed talking points. The output: Websites that lack interactivity or excitement.

   A distributed campaign passes some of the content creation and site management down to the grassroots, where information doesn't need to pass by campaign management to be posted. The content on distributed sites is normally more engaging, because it can be written with a personal "voice." In addition, because the purpose of a distributed site is to write for a particular niche audience, the content often is more attractive for particular groups than more generic messaging from the campaign headquarters.

2. *They enable efficient message distribution.* By building trusted bridges between constituents, a distributed campaign allows effective distribution of messages. Efficient distribution can be measured by both the pure numbers of e-mails sent or by the number of actions taken by supporters based on those e-mail messages. The number of messages sent is increased by creating a network of supporters at the margins who will then send the e-mails to friends and family members who would otherwise not have been reached by the campaign. Once the messages are received, the number of individuals who then turn to the campaign (or distributed community sites) and take action is often increased because the messages in the e-mails were more appropriately targeted to the niche audience.

3. *They allow evaluation of messages.* All of the tools that have been detailed here assist in the evaluation

of campaign messages. From blogs to surveys, all the tools we've listed allow a campaign to evaluate messages in ways that a simple campaign Website simply can't.

4. *They move people up the ladder of engagement.* In traditional online campaigns it can be very difficult to increasingly engage supporters without heavy campaign management. In a distributed campaign the giving of ownership to niche communities heavily engages supporters. As supporters become more involved in the campaign using the distributed network, the likelihood that they will move up the ladder of engagement and reach out to others, increases dramatically.

## DISTRIBUTED PROTECTION AGAINST ATTACKS

Although no one will likely confess to purposefully attempting to hack or harm another campaign's Website, in any online campaign protection of your Internet infrastructure is critical. Traditional campaigns require heavy oversight by a small group of high-level technologists. Because these individuals are often heavily depended on for other tasks, it's critical that their security risk evaluations be automated. A properly designed distributed campaign allows a campaign manager (not a technologist) the ability to easily suspend a site or simply take it offline. This might require a bit of extra preparation up front, but this can help alleviate problems that might arise in the future. Because the nature of a distributed campaign is to hand over administration rights to individuals not necessarily involved in the day-to-day operations of the campaign headquarters, it is essential that campaign management have an emergency cord to pull in case a site is attacked by the opposition. Finally, although it might be tempting to censor comments posted on distributed sites

that don't support your campaign's main messages, it's important not to do so. Removing nonsupportive posts shows that your distributed campaign is actually just another top-down campaign. Visitors want to see that there is balance in messaging, even if sometimes that includes skepticism of your campaign. If a Website has defamatory information posted on its forums or site, however, it's critical for the main campaign management to have the ability to easily and effectively take down either the inflammatory postings or the site in its entirety.

## *Lessons Learned*

- During the presidential elections of 2004, the Internet became a major influential force through blogs, online forums, and carefully designed use of e-mail.
- A distributed campaign moves the center of action of a political campaign from the headquarters to the grassroots.

## *Web Resources*

**Democracy In Action**
*www.democracyinaction.org*
**PICnet**
*www.picnet.net*
**Personal Democracy Forum**
*www.personaldemocracy.com*
**MeetUp.com**
*www.meetup.com*

## Talking the Right Talk about Nursing

*"Insanity: doing the same thing over and over again and expecting different results."*

ALBERT EINSTEIN

Several weeks ago, when I was visiting San Francisco, I had coffee with some newfound acquaintances. One of the women asked me why I'd come to town. I told the group that I was speaking at a nursing conference. "Oh, nurses, nurses are great," the woman, who was in her mid-sixties, exclaimed. "I was recently in the hospital having surgery and the nurses were so great. They were so nice. They stopped by to talk to me. One of them even gave me a back rub."

I agreed with her. But, I probed, did she know that her nurses did more than stop by to chat and give her back rubs? Had she had any postsurgical complications? I asked.

"Not a one," she said. Her doctors were the very best, she explained.

Was she aware that the nurses were also key in making sure she didn't get a postsurgical infection, develop a blood clot in her leg, pneumonia, or a urinary tract infection?

"Really?" she asked. "The nurses?"

"Yes, the nurses. Let me ask you a question," I continued. "Did you leave the hospital with any medications?"

She rolled her eyes. "Did I ever!"

"And who taught you about how to safely take the medications?"

She thought for a moment. "Well, the doctor mentioned something about it. But I guess it was the nurse who really went through it all with me," she said.

"I'm sure she did," I said, and for the next half hour we continued what was essentially a mini–teach-in on what nurses actually do.

This wasn't a forced march through the world of nursing. The women I was talking to were genuinely interested and asked multiple questions. What do nurses really do? How much do they get paid? (Not enough, I explained.) What about their working conditions? ("They need improvement," I said.) How many patients are they taking care of these days? (Too many—eight to ten, sometimes even more.) "Oh my goodness," the woman who'd recently been hospitalized exclaimed yet again. "That can't be good. Isn't that too many?"

Which led to a discussion about the kind of resources and working conditions nurses need to provide good nursing. I told my friends about the staffing ratio legislation that had been passed in California and suggested they should call their political representatives to support similar regulations nationwide. They all said they would.

I have no idea if my friends followed up on my suggestion, but I do know they left the table understanding more about nursing than they did when they sat down for coffee.

### EDUCATING THE PUBLIC WORKS

For the past 17 years I've been having conversations like this with friends and journalists and political representatives and policymakers. And I know that talking the talk works. Nurses can convince people that what they do is really important and help them understand why they, as non-nurses, should learn more about nursing. Such conversations can also help people understand that they need to do more to support nurses' attempts to obtain the social resources necessary for high-quality care.

I know many nurses don't only walk the walk in their daily practice; they talk the right talk when they get out of the hospital or other health care setting. The problem is that not enough nurses talk compellingly and convincingly about their work.

**177**

Instead of talking about their knowledge and their actual daily practice, too many nurses focus on their virtues—on how kind, holistic, and humanistic they are. Instead of amplifying their caring narrative by talking about their medical and technical knowledge, nurses talk mainly about how emotionally available they are. Instead of talking about the money and resources needed to finance their work, nurses often pretend that they aren't interested in money and that they can somehow produce good nursing care out of thin air.

I've become convinced that when nurses move beyond virtue and include medicine and money in their narrative of practice they can overcome the deeply rooted stereotypes that often prevent people from understanding the consequential nature of nursing work. In fact, explaining about nursing—talking the talk—is critical if nurses are going to be able to continue walking the walk—providing high-quality nursing care to sick and vulnerable human beings.

Why do nurses need to take action on the communication front?

Because in almost every country in the world, nursing is under threat. Administrators and policymakers are constantly threatening to replace registered nurses with poorly educated—and therefore cheaper—workers. Although hospitals and health systems obsess about nurse recruitment, they do little to assure nurse retention. Thus, nurses are given patient loads that are too heavy or are constantly told they can easily be replaced by less-skilled workers. They are expected to contribute unpaid labor to keep hospitals afloat, or they themselves are floated from units in which they have great expertise to units in which they have little. And when they ask for a raise or better working conditions, they risk being scolded for being too selfish and not sufficiently devoted to their patients.

This occurs because administrators—and the broader public—don't seem to grasp that nurses don't work for love but for money, and are not simply extra pairs of hands and feet but knowledge workers with specific skills. Imagine how a physician would respond if someone told him he was charging too much and should be more altruistic? (When it comes to physicians, the mantra is "if you

don't pay them enough, you won't attract the best and the brightest." When was the last time you heard someone saying that about nursing?) I have learned that after patients leave the operating room, their lives depend not just on the best neurosurgeon but also on the best neurosurgical nurse. Yet not enough members of the public understand this simple fact.

## QUESTIONS FOR NURSES

As you read this, ask yourselves this question: How many of you believe that the public trusts you as an RN, trusts nurses?

Then ask yourself whether you think most members of the public understand what nurses really do and the contributions they really make to the health care system?

In my experience, when I am giving a lecture and ask these two questions, hundreds of hands are raised when I ask question number one, but only a few flutter up when I ask question number two. So here's the paradox: If people trust nurses, but don't understand what nurses do, why do they trust nurses? Because nurses are nice? Sweet? Kind? Selfless? Or because nurses are knowledgeable and intelligent, save lives, prevent suffering, and save money?

Unfortunately, I think even grateful patients may value nurses because the patients think nurses are nice—not because they think nurses really know their stuff.

Why is this? It's not only because patients have been raised on traditional stereotypes about nursing. It's also because nurses do not educate the public in ways that reverse those stereotypes.

## NURSING: DIFFUSE, VAGUE, INDEFINABLE?

When I ask nurses to describe their work, very often they respond with, "Oh, it's too hard to talk about nursing. It's too diffuse, too vague, and too indefinable." But I have written thousands of pages about nursing, and I am not a writer of fiction. I have been able to write about nursing because nurses have described their work to me and because I have observed their work and asked them questions about it.

After much reflection and reading dozens of studies I have concluded that nurses are fundamentally rescue workers. Using their considerable knowledge—and their brains, not just their hearts—they rescue patients from the risks and consequences, not only of illness, disability, and infirmity, but also of the treatment of illness. And they protect patients from the risks that occur when illness and vulnerability make it difficult, impossible, or even lethal for patients to perform the activities of daily living—ordinary acts like breathing, turning, going to the toilet unassisted, coughing, or swallowing. Even the most caring and emotion-laden activities in which nurses engage are part of this rescue work. In forging nurse-patient relationships, nurses rescue patients from isolation, loneliness, fear, and anxiety—even terror.

## WHAT NURSES DO—IN A SOUND BYTE

Nurses save lives, prevent complications, prevent suffering, and save money. Why do nurses have such a hard time explaining something so clear and concrete? I think it's because they've been educated and socialized to focus on their virtues rather than their knowledge and their routine everyday practice. Indeed, I believe many of the problems of modern nursing stem from what nurse historian Sioban Nelson and I call the virtue script in nursing (Gordon, 2005; Gordon & Nelson, 2005).

When asked to describe their work, nurses all too often focus on their honesty, and trustworthiness, their holism and humanism, their compassion and their caring. While these attributes are a critical part of nursing, nurses often articulate caring work in a way that sentimentalizes and trivializes the complex caring skills nurses must acquire through education and experience. After all, knowing when to talk to a patient about a sensitive issue; when to provide sensitive or disturbing information; when to move in close to hold a hand or move away to a respectful distance—all of these are complex decisions a nurse makes that are based on equally complex skills and knowledge the nurse has mastered. But all too often the fact that caring is a skill is left out of the nursing story.

Nurses are still talking about themselves—or allowing themselves to be talked about—in the most highly gendered, almost religious terms and allowing themselves to be portrayed with the most highly gendered, almost religious images. Indeed, as Nelson and I argue, with the best intentions in the world, many modern nursing organizations and nurses reproduce and reinforce traditional images of nursing as self-sacrificing, devotional, altruistic, anonymous, silent work. These images reflect the religious origins of the profession, when nurses in religious orders were socialized to sacrifice every shred of their individual identity, to be obedient members of an anonymous mass. They hark back to an era when nurses were taught not to claim credit for their work and accomplishments but were instead supposed to view themselves as divine instruments who willingly assigned the credit for their accomplishments to God, the Bishop, the Abbess, or the Mother Superior. Most importantly, these images reflect a time when nurses were taught not to talk about a good deed because that suggested the sin of pride. What nurses could accept were compliments for their deferential behavior and angelic virtues.

## THE PROBLEM OF NURSES' VISIBILITY

The problem of nursing visibility did not disappear with the movement to professionalize nursing that grew in the nineteenth century. In the nineteenth century, reformers like Nightingale adapted a religious framework to help women who wanted and needed to work outside of the home to find purposeful paid work. Being paid to work with strange men's naked bodies would hardly have been considered respectable.

Nurse reformers helped women navigate the passage to this particular kind of paid work by borrowing religious templates. The nun's coronet was modified into the nurses' cap. In English-speaking countries, nurses were called *sisters*. Nurse reformers desexualized nurses by asking them to wear the ugliest uniform possible. Nursing students were not allowed to marry and were shut in cloisterlike dormitories near the hospital. Nurses were said to be self-sacrificing and morally superior beings who would create order out of the chaos of the nineteenth-century hospital.

Focusing on nurses' virtues also helped nurses in what was to become a long battle with medicine over the highly contested terrain of the hospital.

Before the nineteenth century very few doctors had ever set foot in a hospital. In the nineteenth century, doctors were moving into the hospital in greater numbers and wanted to control the institution. They were not pleased to see a group of women who wanted authority and education competing for public regard. Doctors were happy to have trained nurses but only if they were their servants. They wanted nurses to know what to do and how to do it but not why they were doing it. Because nursing at this time was feminized, women with no political, legal, economic, or social power had to make a deal with medicine. The deal was that nurses could have virtues but no knowledge. Again, the religious template allowed nurses to negotiate this passage to purposeful work by making them safe from medicine (Gordon & Nelson, 2005).

In the nineteenth century, nursing was thus constructed as self-sacrificing, anonymous, devotional, altruistic work. Although this formulation served women in that era, contemporary nurses—whose situation has dramatically changed—still use it to legitimate their work to the public. Look or listen to the images that nurses mobilize to talk about their work. In 2000 the International Council of Nurses chose a pure white heart as the symbol of contemporary nursing. For nurses week in 2002 the American Nurses Association used the slogan "Touching Lives, Lifting Spirits," with an angelic figure hovering in the background. In 2000 the Quebec Order of Nurses defined nursing as "an expertise straight from the heart." And in 2002 the Ohio Health System celebrated nursing with the following (Ohio Health Brochure, 2002):

*People believe there are beings*
*That come to you in your darkest hour*
*Guide you when your life hangs in the balance*
*Cradle you.*
*Calm you.*
*Protect you.*
*Some people call them guardian angels.*
*We call them nurses.*

Or consider what was on notepad paper to advertise St. Mary's Hospital in Madison, Wisconsin: "You're wrapped with love in our quilt of caring."

## THE VIRTUE SCRIPT

These messages are so pervasive that they create a social feedback loop that reinforces and then reproduces the nineteenth-century view that nurses are sentimental workers who may even act as agents of a higher power (God or the physician). Through a complex historical process nurses inherit these virtuous images. Nurses then stress these images when they discuss their work. Once this virtue script is relayed by nurses to other health care professionals, the public, patients, and the media, these groups broadcast the messages to an even wider audience. This audience then closes the social feedback when the idea is projected back onto its source—nurses who then have to "live" the ideal.

One of the most critical participants in the social feedback loop is the mass media. In stories or headlines about nurses in newspapers and magazines, nurses are often portrayed as self-sacrificing, self-effacing angels of mercy.

In 2001 the *Toronto Star* ran a story about a nurse who had founded a community health care center dedicated to serving children and adolescents. The nurse, Ruth Ewert, after identifying a glaring lack of adolescent health care services, raised money to found a center to provide the needed health care. The headline, instead of reflecting her knowledge, courage, and persistence, introduced her as an "angel in our midst" (Taylor, 2002).

In the spring of 2003 the *New York Times* ran an article, "Premature Births Rise Sharply, confounding Obstetricians," on the rising number of premature births (Brody, 2003). The article featured a photograph of a nurse reaching tenderly toward a premature infant in a neonatal intensive care unit in what could be considered a nurturing act reserved for mothers. The lengthy article, filled with quotes from numerous physicians, demonstrates their scientific knowledge on the subject; there is only one quote from a nurse, and nurses never comment on the science involved in caring for premature infants. The article further supports physicians' quest for knowledge by saying, "Doctors can save most premature babies, but they haven't found a way to stop premature births." Such depictions of nurses have serious impacts. Nurses are excluded from the process of scientific curiosity and discovery and from the act of rescuing babies from complications and saving their lives—which is precisely what nurses who work with such babies do. If health care administrators and policymakers are allocating scarce resources, to whom will they give the money—the "tenders" or the "savers"?

To effectively promote what they really do, nurses need to extricate themselves from this social feedback loop. The public knows that nurses are kind and caring and compassionate. They know nurses talk to patients more than doctors do. What the public doesn't know is that nurses' caring is a skilled activity and that nurses also participate in medical cures and have technologic and scientific know-how. How can nurses inform them that doctors don't do all the curing and that nurses make a difference in medical outcomes—thereby saving lives, preventing suffering, and saving money?

They can do this by talking about their work in the ways that Bernice Buresh and I outline in our communications guidebook, *From Silence to Voice: What Nurses Know and Must Communicate to the Public* (2003) and by broaching some taboo subjects—what I call the three Ms—medicine, money, and mortality.

## Medicine

One of the things nurses need to talk about is their knowledge of medicine and the fact that they participate in the processes of cure, of medical innovation, and of diagnosis, prescription, and treatment. As I have observed nurses over the years, I have watched them deny, not claim, their participation in these activities. Although I have written a great deal about caring in nursing work, I am often uncomfortable with the way discussions of caring skirt perilously close to traditional female-gender stereotypes. Rather than depicting caring as a skill—what Benner calls the "skill of involvement"—it almost seems as if nurses trivialize their caregiving skills by adopting the very sexist self-definitions that have been consistently used to denigrate and sentimentalize their work. When I first went into the hospital to observe nurses, for example, I noticed how often nurses would almost robotically repeat

the phrase, "Nurses care and doctors cure." Or they recited the other popular mantra, "Nurses are the patient's advocate." Or the equally popular, "Doctors take care of diseases, and nurses take care of the people who have them." Some academics and nurses' organizations translated these thoughts into more official-sounding statements used in the definition of nursing diagnosis, which puts nurses in charge of the "human response to illness," while doctors are in charge of what—the inhuman response?

When I was writing my book *Life Support: Three Nurses on the Front Lines* (Gordon, 1996), I followed nurses on an oncology unit for 2 years. I watched these nurses administer chemotherapy, make sure it was effective, manage patients' nausea and vomiting, patrol for infection, and make sure patients survived. Yet the nurses insisted that "nurses care and doctors cure." I was puzzled by this formulation because nurses actually did much of the curing. Why, I wondered, were nurses then giving this critical activity away to medicine? I wondered. Why were they allowing doctors to claim credit—as the nuns gave credit to God—for the work they did? Nurses always tell me that doctors get the adulation and admiration they get because they have power over life and death. Don't nurses have the same power?

When nurses tell their stories, they need to clearly explain that they are part of, not apart from, the medical system, medical knowledge, and medical innovation and cure. Indeed, they must explain that medical progress and high-quality patient outcomes cannot exist without nurses' participation.

Whenever I do a workshop I ask nurses to do the following exercise.

Describe a situation in which the concrete, routine daily activities of your work make a difference to patients. I ask nurses to recount their story in clear, ordinary language that a non-nurse or non–health care professional would understand. I ask them to explain what they are doing and why they are doing it, and I ask them, if possible, to integrate facts and statistics into their stories. Most importantly, I ask them to combine, not counterpose, their medical and technical skills and practice and their caring and educational roles.

Yet all too often, nurses will actually downplay their medical, technical skill, and knowledge or counterpose the emotional and physical. In a typical anecdote, an oncology nurse in a masters program wrote that, "People may think the most important part of being an oncology nurse is inserting an IV, accessing a port-a-catheter, administering anti-nausea medication, or infusing chemotherapy. This is not true. The part of my job that makes the greatest impact is educating a patient to take care of himself safely and efficiently at home."

But the cancer patient isn't going to make it home at all if his IV isn't inserted correctly, his port-a-catheter safely accessed, and his nausea managed. The patient may die if his chemotherapy is incorrectly infused. The nurse taking care of the patient—since she wasn't a social worker—had to know a lot more than family dynamics. Why not combine rather than counterpose, as in the following:

As an oncology nurse I do a number of critical things. I administer chemotherapy to cancer patients. As I do this I make sure their IVs are inserted correctly. If they are not, toxic chemotherapy drugs won't go into their veins and can leak under their skin, sometimes causing irritation or burns so severe that the patient may require a skin graft. I access devices that deliver chemotherapy directly into their subclavian veins carefully so that patients don't develop central venous catheter line infections, which can kill patients and cost millions. I make sure patients do not develop the kind of nausea and vomiting that could leave them dehydrated and malnourished, requiring additional hospitalization, and I make sure the chemotherapy is delivered into their veins so their cancer will go into remission. Once all this is accomplished the patient is able to go home, and I make sure to educate the patient so he or she can recognize any symptoms of infection that might result from the chemotherapy or deal with the many emotional problems cancer patients face.

## Money

I think it is also critical for nurses to talk to patients about money—about why they need it and deserve it. As I said before, when asked about money (i.e., salaries), nurses the world over often repeat the mantra, "It isn't about the money." Isn't it? In fact, the nursing crisis is all about money. It's about our social failure to pay nurses what they deserve and to

allocate sufficient health care resources to give nurses what they need to do their work. It's a product of the expectation that nurses will continue to contribute their free labor to making the health care system work by forfeiting their coffee and lunch breaks. It's about our refusal to hire enough staff to allow RNs to leave their units to get the additional clinical education needed to keep up with new developments in medicine and nursing.

Nursing is an organized institutional intervention. Nurses need financial resources to do their work. If we focus exclusively on the hospital, nurses need IV tubing, syringes, sheets, pillowcases, beds, and meds. No matter how kind, competent, and well intentioned they are, good nurses need social resources in order to produce good nursing. Nurses must learn to talk the money talk. Nurses must also learn to connect their rescue work to money—to explain to administrators, policymakers, and political representatives that not having enough nurses wastes money.

Before I sat down to write this essay I was in Iowa, where I met the Governor of Iowa, Tom Vilsack, in a restaurant. Governor Vilsack was actually considered as a running mate to John Kerry in the 2004 presidential race and is apparently considering a run for President as a Democratic candidate in 2008. I had about 5 minutes with him. I gave him my new book, *Nursing Against the Odds*, and began to talk to him about nursing. When he looked at the book, he said to me, "Ms. Gordon, you know the only thing hospitals and administrators care about when it comes to nursing is money. All they care about is how to save money."

"Governor," I replied, "I understand that, but you know the policies that hospitals and health systems are pursuing when it comes to nursing are in fact wasting money not saving it. For example, consider this. A hospital administrator feels under pressure to save money and lays off a nurse who earns $40,000 a year. So the unit is short staffed and the nurses can't turn patients enough or properly check patients for a little red spot on the hip, or ankle, or sacrum that can become a 2-inch craterlike bedsore that goes all the way down to the bone. So three patients develop bedsores that cost $40,000 to heal. Do the math: you haven't saved $40,000; you've just spent $80,000 unnecessarily. Or a unit is short staffed and nurses can't give patients pain medication after surgery, so patients are in so much pain that they won't cough or walk or move. As a result, two patients develop pneumonia and have to be sent to the ICU for a week—which costs more than $200,000. Or they develop blood clots in their legs that delay discharge, plus the medications they are on cost $12,000 for a 3-month supply."

The governor had never heard these statistics connected to nursing. Hopefully he gave them some thought.

So here's an idea. Do the following exercise. You have 5 minutes to explain why nurses are important to a political representative, health care administrator, or journalist. In clear, comprehensible language, explain to this person why the policies the state is pursuing are not cost effective and why proper nursing care is.

Or how about borrowing the slogan used by the Australian Nursing Federation—"Nurses: You can't live without them"—and adapting it to struggles for better pay and working conditions. "Value nurses. You can't live without them."

**Mortality**

Finally, I think nurses must talk about mortality. They must explain why the neoliberal market model of health care simply doesn't capture the reality of health care work. Taking care of sick people is simply more demanding than the work of most other professions or occupations. Nurses, like doctors and other clinicians, work with the sickest, most vulnerable people in our societies. Nurses are dealing with people who are ipso facto not at their best. They may be in pain, depressed, sullen, irritable, anxious, and sometimes angry, maybe even violent. Nursing is hard, emotional, and physical work, even under the best of circumstances: when there are plenty of RNs; when collegial relationships are the norm between doctors and nurses; when nurses have administrative support from hospital executives and managers; when clinicians know what's wrong with a patient and what to do about it; and when pay is good.

That's why sociologist Daniel Chambliss (1996), in his book *Beyond Caring*, reminds us of the pitfalls

of likening a hospital to any other business organization that processes goods and services.

In one crucial respect, the hospital remains dramatically different from other organizations: *in hospitals, as a normal part of the routine, people suffer and die.* This is unusual… Only combat military forces share this feature. To be complete, theories of hospital life need to acknowledge this crucial difference, since adapting themselves to pain and death is for hospital workers the most distinctive feature of their work. It is that which most separates them from the rest of us. In building theories of organizational life, sociologists must try to see how hospitals resemble other organizations…but we should not make a premature leap to the commonalities before appreciating the unique features of hospitals that make a nurse's task so different from that of a teacher or a businessman or a bureaucrat. (p. 16)

The combination of difficult patients, taxing schedules, and arduous physical work means that nurses need a set of complex rewards. They must feel that they make enough money and benefits; they have to feel that they can enjoy a sense collegiality on the job; they need to feel that they are respected and that they have good working conditions; and, perhaps most important, they need to feel that they make a difference to the patients for whom they sacrifice so much on a daily basis.

This is why I believe that the non-nursing public must begin to more actively support nurses and fight for nursing care. I believe those of us who are non-nurses—people whom you have educated about nursing—must understand the connection between high-quality nursing care and their survival. We must understand that unless we are hit by a truck and die instantly, or die in our sleep—which is a death most of us wish for and few of us actually get—most of us will depend on nursing care sooner or later. And if we need it later we will need it longer. We need to understand that it's way too late to worry about whether a nurse will answer your buzzer when you're flat on your back in a hospital. We potential patients and sometime patients need to fight for nursing when we're healthy if we are to be assured of high-quality nursing care when we're sick. But the public will never fight for nursing if nurses do not talk the talk that will help them support and sustain their practice.

## *Lessons Learned*

- Nurses must talk about their work in credible, compelling ways that highlight not only their care and compassion but also the scientific, medical, and technical work they do.
- Nurses must be alert to the images their hospitals, organizations, and associations use to depict nursing work. They need to move beyond images of nurses as virtue workers, angels, and saints to images of serious, knowledgeable professionals engaged in serious, consequential work.
- Nurses need to talk about some taboo subjects—their contributions to cure and medical treatment, their need to be adequately paid, and the fact that their work is unique because, on a daily basis, so many nurses deal with suffering and death.

### REFERENCES

Brody, J. E. (April 8, 2003). Premature births rise sharply, confounding obstetricians. *New York Times*, D5.

Buresh, B., & Gordon, S. (2003). From silence to voice: What nurses know and must communicate to the public. Ithaca, NY: Cornell University Press.

Chambliss, D. (1996). *Beyond caring: Hospitals, nurses, and the social organization of ethics*. Chicago: University of Chicago Press.

Gordon, S. (1996). *Life support: Three nurses on the front lines*. New York: Little, Brown.

Gordon, S. (2005). *Nursing against the odds: How health care cost-cutting, media stereotypes, and medical hubris undermine nurses and patient care*. Ithaca, NY: Cornell University Press.

Gordon, S., & Nelson, S. (2005). An end to angels. Moving away from the virtue script toward a knowledge-based identity for nurses. *American Journal of Nursing, 105*(5), 62-69.

Ohio Health Brochure. (2002). *Celebrate Nursing Excellence Week*. May 5-12. Columbus, OH: Ohio Health System.

Taylor, B. (February 9, 2002). Angel in our midst. *Toronto Star*, T1.

---

## *Taking Action*     Sandy Summers & Harry Jacob Summers

## Changing Poor Portrayals of Nurses in the Media: The Center for Nursing Advocacy

*"Our way is not soft grass; it's a mountain path with lots of rocks."*

DR. RUTH WESTHEIMER

In November 2004 "Dr. Phil" McGraw, the television psychologist, told his millions of viewers that in his career he had seen many "cute little nurses" out to "seduce and marry" physicians "because that's their ticket out of having to work as a nurse." A nurse e-mailed us the news at the Center for Nursing Advocacy. Within a couple of days, the Center had posted an analysis of Dr. Phil's comments on our Website, *www.nursingadvocacy.org*, along with a letter that supporters could e-mail to the

"Dr. Phil" show. Even though the timing was less than ideal—we launched our campaign the Wednesday before Thanksgiving—over 1400 nurses and supporters wrote letters to the show over the ensuing 5-day period. Many letters expressed controlled fury.

The following Monday, the show's public relations officer called the Center to negotiate a resolution. "Dr. Phil" immediately issued a message of support for nurses, made a lengthy on-air statement of support (stopping short of an admission of error or an apology), and promised to do a future show on nurses in the media, although as of mid-2005 he appeared only to have inserted a few comments on the subject in a show about his sister's recovery from a severe injury. Although "Dr. Phil" may not have responded in an ideal way, the show clearly heard nurses' voices, and at least some of its viewers saw his fairly positive follow-up statements.

Sad to say, many who broadcast or publish influential negative images of nurses continue to do so with impunity. Nurses' objections are often ignored—if they are even expressed. However, that is changing as the Center helps nurses to advocate for accurate portrayals of them and their work.

## FOUNDING THE CENTER FOR NURSING ADVOCACY

In 2001 a small group of us who were graduate students at Johns Hopkins University School of Nursing was discussing the nursing crisis, which was becoming a major threat to global health. It seemed to us that one of the most fundamental problems (if not the most fundamental problem) was the disconnect between what nursing is and what society thinks nursing is. We felt we had to do something about it (Figure 9-1).

As our first effort, we decided to tackle the most influential purveyor of inaccurate nursing images: the NBC television show "ER," which reaches perhaps hundreds of millions worldwide. Having watched many episodes of the show, we believed that its nursing portrayal, dramatic power, and global reach together likely contributed greatly to poor public understanding of the profession. Later we found research confirming this. A 2000 JWT Communications study of U.S. youth in grades 2 to 10 found that the students got their strongest impression of nursing from "ER," and that they knew more about the major nurse character's love life than they did her professional work—a finding that is quite consistent with the show's approach to its lone major nurse character. The school kids also said that they saw nursing as a technical field "like shop," and a "girl's job" that was not good enough for private school students. After crafting a letter and convincing many nursing leaders to join us in signing it, we sent it to the producers of "ER." We requested and got a conference call with a key producer and the show's "medical advisor." And while we wish the call had produced more tangible positive results onscreen, that was the beginning of our media advocacy. We came to believe that we had to change

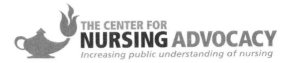

### THE CENTER FOR NURSING ADVOCACY
*Increasing public understanding of nursing*

> **The Mission of the Center for Nursing Advocacy**
>
> The Center for Nursing Advocacy seeks to increase public understanding of the central, front-line role nurses play in modern health care. The focus of the Center is to promote more accurate, balanced, and frequent media portrayals of nurses and increase the media's use of nurses as expert sources. The Center's ultimate goals are to foster growth in the size and diversity of the nursing profession at a time of critical shortage; strengthen nursing practice, teaching, and research; and improve the health care system.

the way the world sees nursing if we were to change the way it treats nursing.

Several of us decided to form a permanent group to tackle this key problem, to which no other U.S. nursing group was exclusively dedicated. Consulting with prominent figures who had worked on the nursing image problem, we formed an informal advisory committee and began some basic advocacy under the name The Nursing Vision. One friend, a nonprofit professional who would become our treasurer, advised us to contact the Maryland Association of Non-Profits (MANO), whose mission is to provide nonprofit organizations with critical technical assistance and support. MANO helped us get organized and determine how to get started.

After Sandy's graduation from Hopkins in 2002, we became a Maryland nonprofit corporation, The Center for Nursing Advocacy, and we also established a Website to facilitate our work. The Center began with a volunteer staff of three. We also had a board that included prominent nursing leaders interested in the nursing image. In the summer of 2004, after considerable effort, the Center obtained 501(c)(3) tax-exempt status from the IRS, a milestone in the start-up of a U.S. charitable organization.

### What Have We Accomplished with the Media?

The Center's Website acts as a clearinghouse of information and advocacy on public understanding of nursing; it offers detailed information on media campaigns, basic information about nursing and the nursing crisis, dozens of reviews and comments on media products such as television shows, films, and books, and many hundreds of analyses of news products relevant to nursing from around the world. We send regular e-news alerts to thousands of supporters. The Website is a basic resource for the media, health care professionals, and the public. As of early 2006, the site was getting about 150,000 page-views per month and contained over 900 pages, many of considerable length. The Center speaks with the press frequently about public understanding of nursing. We issue press releases and have generated extensive coverage for our activities in the mainstream and nursing press, including significant U.S. coverage in early 2006 for our annual Golden Lamp Awards, which recognize the best and worst media portrayals of nursing. We sparked major global coverage for two large campaigns: our "ER" campaign in 2003 and our campaign about a global ad campaign by the Skechers shoe company in 2004. Table 9-2 provides a list of some campaigns we've undertaken and the impact of these efforts.

The Skechers campaign is a good example of our work. The ad in question, one of three suggestive ones in a campaign oriented toward different jobs, offered a blatant "naughty nurse" image. Pop star Christina Aguilera appeared in a dominatrix scenario, wearing a short white dress revealing cleavage and little red hearts on her exposed bra, a garter belt, and white stockings. She mock-threateningly held an enormous silver syringe over her patient (also Aguilera). Skechers' planned campaign included extensive print and point-of-sale ads around the world. We contacted the company first and asked them to pull the ad. When they didn't respond, we posted an analysis of the ad, including a photo, and set up a form e-mail letter so nursing supporters needed only to enter their contact information and click on the send button. Many wrote original letters, strengthening the power of the campaign. In 2 weeks, over 3000 e-mails from nursing supporters flooded Skechers. A week after we began our campaign, a national Christian advocacy group launched an e-mail campaign about all three ads, including the two that showed Aguilera in teacher-student and

cop-arrestee scenarios. This group managed to generate over 15,000 letters, but only the nurse ad was pulled.

Other campaigns against harmful advertising images have required fewer letters, and in a number of cases phone calls from the Center have been enough. Pennzoil and Physicians Formula cosmetics company pulled "naughty nurse" print ads after about 100 letters to each company. Disney, which had retailed Jessica Rabbit naughty nurse pins to "celebrate" Nurses Week in 2003 and 2004, agreed to pull the products after about 300 letters. After Chicago radio shock jock Mancow posed in drag as a "naughty nurse" in imitation of a blink-182 CD cover, it took only a few phone calls from the Center to persuade the station owner to pull the ad. Another "naughty nurse" billboard, placed by a "massage parlor" owner in Texas, came down after one call from us. After calls from the Center, online quiz-master Tickle agreed to pull a stereotype-laden online nursing test designed to pull readers to the Monster job Website. And Wal-Mart, which had placed an ad in nursing journals suggesting that nurses did not have to be "brain surgeons" to know that the company offered a good deal on scrubs, quickly agreed to pull the ad after one phone call from the Center and one letter from a supporter. Wal-Mart also worked with us in developing a new ad without the negative implications for nurses.

The Center has also had success in influencing the federal government's conduct with regard to the nursing image. Beginning in late 2004, a Center campaign persuaded the U.S. Department of Health and Human Services to change the name of its prominent annual "Take a Loved One to the Doctor Day" campaign to "Take a Loved One for a Checkup Day," which does not exclude advanced practice nurses.

The news media and Hollywood, whose effects on public health views and actions have been well documented, have been far more difficult for nurses to influence. In addition to the basic stereotypes that color most of the public's views of nurses, this difficulty may be in part because many creators of those media products believe they already know about nursing, and perhaps because in such cases we are trying to change the actual product, rather

**TABLE 9-2** Campaigns Leading and Not Leading to Immediate Changes in Media

| MEDIA SOURCE | REASON FOR CAMPAIGN | NUMBER OF LETTERS OR OTHER CONTACTS | RESPONSE FROM MEDIA SOURCE |
|---|---|---|---|
| **CAMPAIGNS LEADING TO IMMEDIATE CHANGES IN MEDIA** | | | |
| U.S. Dept. of Health and Human Services | Annual "Take a Loved One to the Doctor Day" campaign name excluded APRNs 2002-2004 | 375+ | Changed campaign name to "Take a Loved One for a Checkup Day" in 2005; thanks offered to nurses, but no apology |
| Skechers | Worldwide "naughty nurse" print and point of sale ads, 2004 | 3000+ | Withdrew the ad, but no apology |
| Dr. Phil Show | "Wanna-be Mrs. Welby" statements by host, 2004 | 1400 | On-air statements of support for nurses, but no apology |
| "Today" Show | Journalists and American Medical Association president suggested patients put their safety at risk by visiting nurse practitioner-staffed quick clinics, 2005 | 3500+ | Show producer promised to work with the Center on future nursing story ideas, but no apology |
| Gillette | Commercial featuring "naughty nurse" lured into bed with patient by his TAG body spray, 2005 | 650 | Pulled the ad and made a telephone apology, but provided no written apology |
| Pennzoil | Naughty nurse print ad, 2004 | 100+ | Ads pulled from circulation, but no apology |
| Disney | Jessica Rabbit naughty nurse pins, 2003 and 2004 | 300+ | Pins removed from sale, but no apology |
| Clairol | Nurse abandoning patient to wash hair and have sexual fantasy in television commercial, 2003 | 30+ and one person with connection to Clairol management | Withdrew the commercial, plus an apology |
| Wal-Mart | Nurse too dumb to be a brain surgeon print ad, 2005 | The Center + 1 | Changed commercial to focus only on bargain hunting |
| "Jeopardy!" | Question suggesting nurse practitioners provide care only for minor ailments, 2004 | The Center + 2 | Featured a positive question on nursing on 2005 show; no apology |
| Good Housekeeping | Feature with 75 physician health ideas encouraged patients to lie to triage nurses and bribe nurses with treats to get better care, 2005 | 200+ | Letter to the editor printed, with editor's note stating that many nurses had objected; health editor agreed to work with nurses on future articles |

*Continued*

**TABLE 9-2** Campaigns Leading and Not Leading to Immediate Changes in Media—cont'd

| MEDIA SOURCE | REASON FOR CAMPAIGN | NUMBER OF LETTERS OR OTHER CONTACTS | RESPONSE FROM MEDIA SOURCE |
|---|---|---|---|
| **CAMPAIGNS LEADING TO IMMEDIATE CHANGES IN MEDIA—cont'd** | | | |
| Clamato | Naughty nurse television commercial, 2005 | The Center + 1 | Withdrew the commercial, no apology |
| Mancow "shock jock" radio station | Chicago billboard featured Mancow imitating naughty nurse image on blink-182 CD cover, 2004 | The Center + 1 | Billboards pulled down; station manager delivered a telephone apology |
| Physician's Formula Cosmetics | Naughty nurse print ad, 2004 | 100+ | Ads quickly pulled from circulation, plus an apology |
| Tickle online quiz master | Encouraged career seekers to take "Who's Your Inner Nurse" quiz, which featured nurses as caring but shallow physician-mate-seekers, 2005 | The Center + 3 | Grudgingly and slowly removed the quiz but refused to replace it with Center's revised quiz "because Tickle didn't write it"; no apology |
| **CAMPAIGNS NOT LEADING TO IMMEDIATE CHANGES BY MEDIA** | | | |
| "ER" | Handmaiden image in which physicians perform much nursing work and nurses perform menial tasks; campaign started 2001 | 1500+ and one show sponsor | One conference call; occasionally, more accurate plotlines, notably in late 2005; basic approach only marginally improved |
| "Grey's Anatomy" | Physicians perform nearly all nursing work and get credit for it; physician characters deliver vicious, unrebutted anti-nurse slurs | 1000+ | Unproductive telephone call with ABC executive; show producers refuse to communicate |
| "House" | Brilliant physicians provide virtually all care. Mute nurses push gurneys and clean up stool. | 300+ | Show producers refuse to communicate |
| "Scrubs" | Physicians perform all meaningful work; the sole nurse has only a love life, with little professional responsibility or drive | 165+ | Show producers refuse to communicate |

**TABLE 9-2** Campaigns Leading and Not Leading to Immediate Changes in Media—cont'd

| MEDIA SOURCE | REASON FOR CAMPAIGN | NUMBER OF LETTERS OR OTHER CONTACTS | RESPONSE FROM MEDIA SOURCE |
|---|---|---|---|
| **CAMPAIGNS NOT LEADING TO IMMEDIATE CHANGES BY MEDIA—cont'd** | | | |
| American Medical Association | Association president makes media statements questioning safety of nurse practitioner care, though research shows it is at least as good as physician care, 2005 | 3700+ | Refused to take calls from the Center or respond in any way |
| Virgin Mobile Canada | Naughty nurses in high-profile publicity stunt and point of sale ads, 2005 | 250+ | Refused to apologize for stunt and refused to remove ads |
| Jib Jab | Naughty nurse online video and various apparel, 2005 | 200+ | Adamantly refused to remove the products |
| 3 Wishes Lingerie | Full line of naughty nurse lingerie, 2004-present | 55+ | Designed new, even naughtier nurse lingerie |
| Bras n' Things Lingerie, Australia | At least one naughty nurse lingerie item, 2005 | 60+ | Removal of print ads and Internet catalog of the lingerie, but it remains for sale |
| Hamilton and Bradford collections | Nurse-angel and nurse–teddy bear figurines, 2004-present | The Center + 2 | No response and no removal of merchandise from sale |
| "The Nurse" cigar shop, Bangkok, Thailand | Sales clerks dress in naughty nurse outfits and sell cigars and wine, 2003-present | 50+ | No response and apparent continued use of name of shop and nursing outfits |

than merely a means of advertising it. In addition to the "Dr. Phil" campaign, we have ongoing campaigns regarding NBC's "ER" and "Scrubs," Fox's "House," and the ABC hit "Grey's Anatomy."

"Grey's Anatomy" focuses on nine or ten surgeons, but they seem to spend about half their time doing nursing work. When nurses do appear, they tend to be peripheral subordinates. Even one remarkable scene in which a veteran nurse guided an intern step by step through a rescue of a patient in cardiac tamponade gave all credit for saving the patient's life to the intern. The show's intern characters have repeatedly used the word "nurse" as a grave insult—for example, "You're the pig who called Meredith a nurse."

"House" is perhaps even more addicted to "physician nursing." The hit show's six physician characters constantly do key care tasks that nurses do in real life. The rare nurse characters tend to be silent, barely visible clerks, like wallpaper that assumes human form to move or hold objects. Although the show mostly pretends that nurses do not exist, some late 2005 episodes indicated that its physician heroes consider nurses to be unskilled clean-up staff who are good for handling stool and patients who have fallen down.

The sitcom "Scrubs" focuses mainly on four physician characters and one nurse. Once again, the physicians do most of the nursing, and although the show has occasionally touched on real nursing issues, for the most part it conforms to the prevailing view of nurses as physician assistants without significant scientific expertise. Indeed, the moral of one horrific 2003 episode was that it is the nurse's job to be quiet and do whatever physicians tell her. The major nurse character is a positive one, but plotlines involving her have focused almost exclusively on her personal life.

"ER" probably makes more of an effort with nursing than other major network shows, but it still perpetuates the classic handmaiden stereotype. The major characters consist of about seven to nine physicians and one nurse. Nurses are presented as skilled assistants to the physicians, who dominate and spend significant time doing nursing tasks, such as performing triage and defibrillation, educating patients, giving medications, and (at times) hiring, firing, and supervising nurses. Meanwhile, though nurses sometimes make substantive contributions to patient care, they also spend a lot of time answering phones, opening suture trays, and having or discussing romantic relations with the physicians. Senior physicians display contempt for nursing, an attitude the show presents as nasty but not necessarily unfounded. Furthermore, the physicians generally get all credit for patient outcomes. In the fall of 2005, "ER" introduced PhD-prepared nurse manager Eve Peyton, a character who displayed nursing clinical expertise heretofore unseen on prime time network television. Peyton was manipulative and could be harsh, but she also challenged physicians' care plans, displayed mastery of evidence-based practice, and was a vigorous nursing advocate. The character appeared in six episodes, but she left abruptly after the show effectively turned her into a street thug. She was summarily fired after she decked an uncooperative patient dressed as Santa Claus and poured urine on him, later swearing at her colleagues as she left the emergency department.

We had a campaign protesting the use of an orangutan playing a nurse on the campy NBC soap opera "Passions" from 2003 to early 2005, but the show refused to do anything in response to nurses' concerns. The portrayal ended only when the monkey's owner moved to Florida. Some people thought we were wrong to bother objecting to it, arguing that nobody would really think a monkey could do a nurse's work. However, one nursing union told us that during recent contract negotiations with a major hospital corporation, a management representative told them that nurses didn't deserve a raise because the hospital could train monkeys to do a nurse's job.

In general, network hospital programs present nurses as peripheral handmaidens or ignore them altogether, and they show physician characters doing much of the exciting, important work that nurses really do. Yet many nurses still watch and defend such programs. It appears that some do not understand the extent to which the media, including fictional media, affects the real world. Yet these effects are well established in the public health and other professional communities, and Hollywood itself has been eager to claim credit for having a positive impact on health and social issues when it can. (We have extensive FAQs on our website to help nurses, students, and the public learn more about this.) Part of the problem may be that many nurses, busy with hard science courses in an often compressed curriculum, do not receive extensive training in media awareness or textual analysis generally. It may also be that, as Suzanne Gordon has suggested (see her Taking Action), many nurses have been socialized to accept abuse and disrespect without complaint as part of the profession's enduring "virtue script." Moreover, what Gordon has aptly termed the "medical superstar narrative" remains a strong social force even among nurses. And of course television is a powerful, arguably addictive medium. People do not appreciate criticism of their favorite shows. Even so, we urge nurses to look closely at what these shows are really telling the world about nursing. We analyze many key episodes in great depth to help nurses think about the messages they are really sending. Then we encourage nurses to take action with our easy, quick form letters.

### HOW WE'VE DONE IT

We believe the progress we have been able to make is due mainly to our ability to motivate nurses to speak up about their work, and our ability to create and efficiently display significant analysis of relevant media products and nursing issues.

## Power of Technology

One key factor is the powerful information technology offered by the Internet, which allows a tiny organization to develop a very large Web presence and spearhead powerful advocacy campaigns. It is unlikely that we could have anything like the impact we have now without the Web as our main platform.

## Lessons About Advocacy

We have also learned several key things about this type of advocacy. One is that nurses respond with greater force to certain types of harmful images, notably "naughty nurse" images, which may call into question their status as serious professionals in an especially basic way. Motivating action based on "handmaiden" or "angel" imagery is more difficult. In addition, the easier it is for people to act, the more likely they are to do so. We therefore offer supporters model "instant letters" that take only seconds to send to the objects of campaigns, as well as providing detailed contact information. Different types of media products may require different approaches. Advertisers appear to be far more sensitive than the entertainment media. Therefore in 2004 we started a campaign asking the companies who advertise on "ER" to pressure the show to do better, and we plan to employ this tactic more in the future. In doing our work, we have often used humor and other creative elements in ways that are not typical of charitable and advocacy organizations, pursuing an approach that we have called "entertainment advocacy." This approach elicits various reactions from supporters, the objects of our campaigns, and the public. We believe it is often effective at making the sometimes dry and repetitive work of an advocacy organization more engaging, and in letting media creators know that we understand what they do. However, there are obvious trade-offs involved. Not everyone appreciates advocacy that includes satirical elements, and some have found certain of our analyses to be flippant or unworthy of a serious advocacy organization. Many others do appreciate them, and we feel that the work of history's great satirists (such as Jonathan Swift) demonstrates that our approach is fully consistent with the pursuit of serious policy aims.

## Volunteer Help

Another fundamental factor in our influence so far has been our ability to put together willing and capable people to offer significant skilled volunteer assistance. As a practical matter, the Center operates with less than two full-time equivalents. Sandy has two decades of diverse experience in a variety of clinical nursing, nonprofit, and for-profit management settings, but she has been able to work full time with little or no salary because of support from her spouse. Our senior advisor (Harry, her husband) is a veteran attorney with experience in nonprofit work and media analysis; he has worked for the Center without pay. The Webmaster (Sandy's brother) recently retired after a career spent founding and leading a major computer-aided manufacturing software firm; he has worked without pay. Taken together, we have contributed extraordinary amounts of unpaid time to the Center. Recently the Center hired a talented high school student as a part-time project associate—the only Center staffer ever to be paid market rate. In this respect the Center's model to date—have skilled, committed relatives willing and able to devote time to the cause—may have limited general applicability. Trying to effect social change solely with a few volunteers does present potential costs that not everyone may choose to bear. These include considerable lost income, perpetual underdog status, and significant personal stress, including difficult family choices, particularly when core personnel have young children. But we hope our work does show what can be done with limited personnel if they are committed.

## Resources

Staff resources have been a key early challenge, and the limited funding for paid workers is an obvious limitation on our work. Another chronic issue for us has been fund-raising. Up until this point, we have primarily sought individual supporting members, although we have received two modest institutional grants. We have focused primarily on programming, rather than fund-raising, in part because we subscribed to an "if we build it, they will come" theory. We believed we needed to show potential funders that we had the capacity to do this important work. In addition, because we have been able to operate at a very basic level without significant funding, we have also felt compelled to do what we could on the programming side. No doubt every nonprofit feels that its work is desperately needed, and we have often felt overwhelmed by everything that requires our attention. We constantly have difficulty choosing not to work on issues that we lack the resources to pursue effectively. For now, programming continues to absorb the vast majority of our time, although now that our Website has grown significantly, we do hope to focus more on fund-raising.

## WHY NURSES SHOULD GET INVOLVED

Sometimes people wonder why we care so much about nursing's media image or what difference it makes in terms of fixing the nursing crisis. Public understanding of the profession matters because what people see affects what they think, and what they think affects what they do. The media's effect on health-related views and actions is well documented, and public health and medical professionals have worked hard for decades to affect how the media portrays health care. Nurses—whose profession is in the midst of global crisis—must do the same. Most non-nurses still do not know that nurses are skilled clinicians who save lives and improve outcomes every day. We need a sustained effort not just to counter bad images but also to foster positive ones. Research suggests that nursing's image has been a problem for many decades.

Nurses themselves bear some responsibility for the public's low understanding. We have often failed to explain ourselves, yielding the media spotlight to physicians and hospital executives, who may send messages to nurses that the media spotlight is not their rightful place. But our patients need a stronger nursing profession so that they can get the care that they need from us. Article 9.4 of the U.S. Code of Ethics for Nurses encourages "nurses [to] work individually as citizens or collectively...to bring about social change."

More public understanding of nursing will lead to more financial and political support. That will lead in turn to increased funding for nursing research, education, and clinical practice, including better staffing, a key factor in the shortage. Indeed, decisions on nurse staffing levels and the allocation of resources for nursing are often made by people who are not nurses and who know little about what we do—even if they work in the same hospital. And when society undervalues nurses, it does not listen to the health information nurses have been trained to impart.

In summary, we believe that resolving the nursing crisis and improving public health depend on a better understanding of nursing.

## HOW NURSES CAN GET INVOLVED

Nurses can and should work to improve public understanding of their work in many ways. These range from the most local to the most global, from personal contacts to the influential mass media, from distributing male nurse "action figures" to all the kids you know, to using the Internet, which is now a critical global vehicle for social progress (Figure 9-1).

The Center for Nursing Advocacy's Website (*www.nursingadvocacy.org*) is a hub of action. It works to help nurses work as a cohesive force to increase what society knows about their profession. It encourages nurses, the media, and society as a whole to think more deeply about the way nursing is presented (Box 9-6).

The action page on the Center's Website lists myriad ways to increase public understanding. For instance, our free e-mail news alerts help supporters stay on top of the latest relevant media products and encourage supporters to contact those who create the products, to send thanks or encourage improvement. For some truly egregious media depictions, we create "instant letters" for those who don't have the time or inclination to compose an original letter. It takes just a minute to fill in your contact information and hit "send." Of course, original letters are even more effective, and the Website makes those easy to create and send as well. Other ideas discussed on the site include acting as expert resources for journalists and creating nurse-centered works in a variety of media. Faculty can easily find material for class project ideas to assign their students. And we have an in-depth resources section that students can use in building scholarly projects.

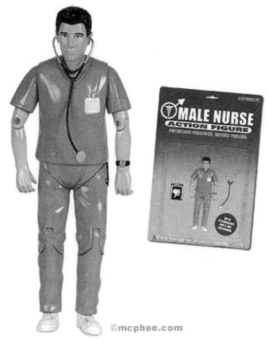

©mcphee.com

**Figure 9-1** Male Nurse Action Hero. This figure made the Top Ten selections of Best Media Portrayals of Nurses in the Second Golden Lamp Awards from the Center for Nursing Advocacy. This is one of the very few professional nurse action figures of which we've heard. Some of the packaging is questionable, such as the use of the term "male nurse," the medical symbol (the caduceus) instead of the nursing symbol (the lamp), and the phrase "Physicians prescribe, nurses provide," which seems to undervalue the contributions of bedside and advanced practice nurses. Despite these problems, when we tried out the action figure on our children, there was an immediate halt to comments such as "Men can't be nurses." That alone is worth a fortune to nursing, which remains no more than 10% male in most nations. The company that distributes the figure describes it as follows: "Armed with a stethoscope and a clipboard holding an x-ray, this 5¼" tall, hard plastic Male Nurse Action Figure is ready to treat your symptoms and fix what ails you. Male nurses make up 6% of the nurses in the United States and only slightly more in Australia and the United Kingdom, but this number is growing. These men are blazing the trail as role models and mentors for generations to come. Thank a male nurse today!"

---

**BOX 9-6** Supporting the Center's Work

Go to *www.nursingadvocacy.org* to make a donation, become a member, or sign up to be a Center Representative!

We encourage nurses and nursing students to become Representatives of the Center at their schools and workplaces and within their nursing organizations. Representatives circulate our news alerts to their discussion boards, listservs, or blogs; promote dialog about nursing media issues; and encourage others to become members of the Center. (To increase the strength of the Center, we really need more member support so that we can hire more staff.) Some Representatives give presentations at their hospitals, schools, or union meetings to help spread the word about our work. We have a presentation on DVD already prepared that we can send out, which makes it very easy for anyone to deliver the message in his or her own setting.

---

Other parts of the Website function as an informational and analytic resource for nurses, the media, and the public. Our FAQ and positions page answers some of the more basic or provocative questions we have heard. Many nursing faculty use these to help teach their professional development classes and build professional self-esteem among future nurses. We also offer in-depth reviews of films, books, television programs, and other media products to show how they affect nursing's image, as well as to stimulate discussion. We encourage nurses to create art featuring accurate nursing images—including television shows, books, Websites, comic books, and paintings—to help educate the public about nursing.

Considering the constraints, we believe the Center has made real strides in building the capacity to help nurses analyze and respond to media images, and to encourage them to be more proactive in promoting public understanding of their life-saving work. We hope to teach the world what nurses do, to empower nurses individually and as a profession, and to improve the health of our patients. We hope all nurses and friends will join us at *www.nursingadvocacy.org* to help build a profession that's second to none.

## *Lessons Learned*

- Many of the problems confronting nurses are connected to misrepresentation of nurses and nursing in the media.
- The Center for Nursing Advocacy focuses on improving portrayals of nurses in the media and can be accessed at *www.nursingadvocacy.org*.

- The Center needs and welcomes nurses' support through their donations, participation in Center campaigns to challenge poor media portrayals of nursing, and volunteering to represent the Center in their places of work and organizations.

# Research as a Political and Policy Tool

Donna Diers & Lynn Price

*"We are drowning in information but starved for knowledge."*

JOHN NAISBITT

Research by itself does not make policy. Politics intervene. The research doesn't get to the right people. Policy agendas shift. The quality of the research may count for little in the face of the power of special interests or election politics. On the other hand, clever, targeted research may sneak in to influence policy without a great deal of traditional political advocacy.

Research may be a tool to help carve policy, if it is in the right hands and is carefully sharpened and skillfully applied. But because research design is never perfect and probabilistic reasoning does not satisfy legislators who want a quick and simple "Does it work?" answer, the role of research in policymaking is more complicated than it looks.

Policy decision-making is frustrating to people in action-oriented disciplines such as nursing and tiresome to those who believe the action that should follow from the data is obvious. The making of *public* policy is even more involved because by definition it includes the acts of government or governmental agencies shaped by the will of the people, whether by formal vote, lobbying, or contributions to political campaigns. Finally, public policymaking, at least in the United States, is *public* to some degree, inviting the participation of all who want a piece of the action,

no matter how ignorant or biased those participants may be.

In an analysis of "morality policy," Mooney (2001) identifies some public and private policy issues that profit less from research than from interest group influence and polling. Morality policy issues include abortion, clinician-assisted suicide, needle exchange included in human immunodeficiency virus (HIV) care, and anything having to do with sex or "sins" such as gambling, smoking, or drug use.

*Public* policy is just one policy venue. *Private* policy generated by nongovernmental agencies (the Joint Commission on the Accreditation of Healthcare Organizations [JCAHO], for instance) or even by institutions may also be fed by research or may ignore research in favor of administrative or political pressure as a way to make decisions.

In this chapter we try to tease apart the relationships between research and policy to suggest the rich and varied ways in which nursing research can become part of the policy process. We begin with a point of view on what research is, then move to discussing how research fits with the agenda-setting part of the policy process—shaping the agenda then getting on it. A mini case study on the use of data to shape the "nursing shortage" agenda shows how intricate this work is. Because regulation has become such a formidable way of implementing policy in the new millennium, we move to considering the relationship between research and regulation. Before we turn the conceptual corner toward "so what does this all mean for research?" we stop off briefly to deal with the role of special interests at the research-policy interface.

## WHERE POLICY HAPPENS

We use "happens" to suggest that there is less rigor to policymaking or implementation on the basis of research than might be fervently wished. Policy decision-making happens in many ways, on a continuum from nearly accidental to carefully orchestrated, and in many places and not always where or how you might think.

The most obvious places for policy decision-making are the legislative branch public policy forums—state and national legislatures. But policymaking also happens in neighborhood associations, in town meetings, at aldermanic hearings, and in the offices of the executive branch agencies who craft regulation. Tip O'Neill, who long served as Speaker of the U.S. House of Representatives, said "all politics is local" (O'Neill & Hymel, 1994, p. xii). It's true. And in nursing, it is at the hospital nursing unit and service level—in the community clinic and Visiting Nurse Association, the primary care office practice, the birthing center, and the school health service. "Private" policy is as real as the more familiar territory of public policymaking and has the same need for evidence. The rules for use of data ought to be the same, but as policy and political actors change, so do considerations about research.

## WHAT IS RESEARCH?

Even legislatures have been run over by the evidence-based bandwagon.

A morning spent listening to public testimony before the Connecticut General Assembly's Committee on Public Health brought uncounted examples of legislators demanding, "What's the evidence?" For example, a committee member was heard to worry that although it might be all right for advanced practice nurses (APRNs) to prescribe in hospitals and nursing homes, it is not all right in the outpatient setting because there is no physician close at hand. The clever nurse lobbyist might take

the occasion to query on what evidence base the committee member relies.

For our purposes, research is systematic collection and/or analysis of existing data. We also include systematic reviews and meta-analyses in this definition. These are approaches to aggregating data over a number of studies. The powerful Institute of Medicine (IOM) reports on health care quality are systematic reviews, for example and we will advert to them later (IOM, 2000, 2001, 2004).

Research includes case studies, sample surveys or polls, epidemiologic investigations of incidence and prevalence, various forms of correlational design, and the alleged gold standard of study design, the randomized controlled clinical trial or RCCT. We include data mining—drilling into existing administrative data, letting the data lead rather than hypothesizing in advance—as a type of research because of the power of this method in institutional policymaking and program support. Cheung, Moody, and Cockram [2002] have made a strong case for data mining in nursing's interests.

One way to think about how research can be used is to "demonstrate the difference nurses make" (Jennings, 2003). This approach attempts to get nursing into discussions of health care policy writ large. The overarching category for such research is health services research, and it deals with how care or service is practiced and how that is related to outcomes. Nursing health services research is still in its infancy, which means there are wide-open opportunities for developing this part of the discipline. Thinking of nursing as part of health services delivery opens up audiences for nursing's contribution to quality of care and outcomes, the major policy agendas for the millennium. Health care administrators, epidemiologists, planners, and economists are slowly coming to understand that they ignore nursing as part of service delivery at their peril.

Car seat regulation, children in foster care, access to mental health services, genetic testing and discrimination, nutritional supplements—these are all things that come to nurses in practice. Nurses are already designing research to inform policy debates over such issues (Drenkard & Ferguson, 2002; Gottesman, 2001; Shelton, 2002; Williams & Martin, 2003; Xue &

Cohen, 2004). Our evidence—supplied by research and evaluation—informs policy, and because we are nurses the evidence comes with unquestioned clinical credibility. Although research alone will not save us, it is a powerful tool to get us to the horse-trading negotiations that do produce policy.

As a tool for politics and policy, research joins narrative storytelling or anecdote, to be pulled carefully out of the drawer when the opportunity or necessity surfaces (McDonough, 2001). "Give us the stories," cry the legislators. "We've got to have the stories." Narratives and anecdotes help laypersons connect the impact of the policy on our patients and our practice. Legislators are generally laypersons.

## SHAPING THE AGENDA

The first step in policymaking is shaping the agenda. John Kingdon (1995) is the master agenda-setting analyst. He asks the question, "Why do some problems come to occupy the attention of governmental officials and other policymakers more than other problems?" And the answer, he says, lies in how policymakers learn about issues and how the issues come to be defined as problems.

Policymakers have children and aged parents, and anyone's heart strings are tugged by stories of sick children or elders who need resources that aren't there. Legislatures hold public "concept hearings," inviting interested parties to present their ideas for new policy. Generally, the way to get early attention to a policy vacuum is through a clever anecdote or personal story and if possible, by bringing the sweet little child with cancer and letting her run around the room, charming the Committee.

Sometimes policy is made strategically by interested parties. The strategy is to make visible the research about the problem. "Patient safety" is the contemporary shining example. Surely patients should be safe while in the hands of health care professionals. Who could argue? The boldface headlines were all the same across the world when the IOM's first report, *To Err is Human: Building a Safer Health System* (2000), came out. The report stated that "98,000 patients died unnecessarily in U.S. hospitals." It is interesting to note that the effect of this publicity went directly to regulation rather than to legislation. How does anyone write a law to improve patient safety when the research itself suggests the problems were not "bad apples" (providers) but systems of care? We will return to this point later.

Aiken, Smith, and Lake (1994) pushed nursing to the forefront of the policy agenda with their study of Medicare mortality in hospitals. Surely undue mortality is the ultimate measure of patient safety, and this study, published as it was in *Medical Care* (which despite its name is a journal of the American Public Health Association, which specializes in health services research) got the kind of headlines we have longed for. Suddenly nurses were visible as contributors to quality of care. Suddenly the big consulting firms that market themselves to hospital nursing leadership for leadership training started to focus on hospital culture change to support professional nursing practice that doesn't kill patients (a new revenue target for them).

What made this research so powerful was a combination of things: a large sample of national administrative data; a policy hook to the Medicare program; a well known, respected author with considerable personal authority; publication in a highly regarded interdisciplinary professional journal; and a title for the article that put it right in your face: "lower Medicare mortality among a set of hospitals known for good nursing care." Timely publication, just at the beginning of what has become a three-report IOM commitment to patient safety, was also a factor. The agenda was already being set—patient safety—but nursing wasn't in on it until Aiken brought it forward.

The timing was not coincidental. Aiken's long trail of policy-related research has often shaped agendas, especially in the area of the relationship of nursing practice to patient outcome and the environments for practice. She and others have done ground-breaking work on various aspects of the nursing shortages, introducing important changes in the way nursing shortages had been perceived before as either the result of an unsatisfying profession or simply "refrigerator nurse" cycles: nurses who work only long enough to buy an appliance for the family. Her early work on environments for practice seized the moment for what was then the high-profile patient population: those with AIDS. Her studies showed that specialized AIDS units produced better outcomes. Of course "specialization" is nursing.

Nursing specialization at the unit level has not been studied often, but where it has the implications are clear. Where nursing units can concentrate patients with similar conditions, nurses can get good at the work (Czaplinski & Diers, 1998; Diers & Potter, 1997). This has large institutional policy implications when hospitals try to decide how to configure bed allocations. (All politics are local…)

When trying to affect the local policy environment, it is sometimes possible to build on research done elsewhere, by offering a metaanalysis of all research on the policy topic to date. This aggregate approach can result in findings that are more persuasive to policymakers, because the findings are consistently replicated across studies. A good example of this approach can be found in the review of nurse practitioner (NP) research published in the *British Medical Journal* (Horrocks, Anderson, & Salisbury, 2002). Horrocks and colleagues reviewed 23 observational studies and 11 randomized controlled trials conducted in the United States and Britain since 1973. Each of the 34 studies reviewed compared the care of NPs and physicians, looking at various aspects of practice, such as prescriptive habits, patient satisfaction, and how often referrals were made by the clinician. Horrocks and co-workers (2002) nicely summarized which variables were used by each study and how many studies used any particular variable.

The results? This metaanalysis confirms what has been known since the earliest studies on advanced practice nursing in primary care: that patients derive more satisfaction from encounters with NPs than with physicians, that there are virtually no significant differences between NPs and physicians in referral or prescriptive practices, and that patient outcomes for NPs are as good as, and sometimes better than, those for physicians. But as important for policy debate is the fact that all of that information, collected over 30 years, is now handy and summarized (Horrocks et al., 2002).

Horrocks and colleagues conducted this study in the current policy climate of the British National Health Service, which is struggling like most health systems to provide good care with limited resources. The "systematic review" was done to answer for policymakers "whether nurse practitioners can provide care at first point of contact equivalent to doctors in a primary care setting" (Horrocks et al., 2002, p. 819). The researchers identify further questions that need be answered, including economic analysis, but the answers are, one hopes, definitive with regard to basic safety and competence of NP care, even for the policymakers unfamiliar with the role.

In China, government is the only policymaker. "Administrators play an important role…by influencing government with relevant data" (Lui, 2004, p. 150). Huaping Lui, a nurse administrator, recognized that the contemporary staffing standards and workload ratios were based on 1978 standards of number of hospital beds. Her study looked at length of stay and patient diagnosis in two large urban hospitals in China to begin to develop a new methodology for allocation of nursing resources. This may be the first step in adjusting workload ratios for contemporary practice, which would be a huge policy change nationally and locally for Chinese hospitals.

## GETTING ON THE AGENDA

A classic paper by Cobb, Ross, and Ross (1976) distinguishes among three models of agenda building: the outside initiative, the mobilization model, and the inside initiative model. "Out" and "in" mean outside and inside the policymaking machinery. The inside model proposes that there are some issues that never go "outside" the internal governmental sphere because they are too arcane, controversial, or complex. Many of these issues deal with regulatory change or highly technical legislation detailing the mechanics of particular federal or state programs. Here, research and other forms of lobbying information go straight to the legislators or federal agencies without necessarily playing to the public media.

The recent success of organized nursing to change the way in which Medicare will pay for services of NPs is an example of the inside model. There is no huge public interest in the rules Medicare uses for paying practitioners; this is not an intriguing problem to the American Association of Retired Persons

(AARP), for example, which ordinarily cares a lot about Medicare. But reimbursement rules and rates are of enormous interest to the nursing profession, which undertook to change Medicare law.

Under Medicare the services of NPs could be billed only as "incident to" the provision of medical care by a physician, and NPs could not receive direct reimbursement for their work. Nursing organizations banded together to convince the Medicare program that it would be in its financial interest to let NPs bill in their own names, albeit at a lower rate (85% of allowable physician charge) (Price & Minarik, 1998, 1999). Nursing's issues were identity and autonomy as well as recognition for services rendered. If NPs cannot bill in their own names, with their own Medicare provider numbers, there will never be any national data about their safety or effectiveness. The data analyzed in an internal government study indicated that NPs would be "worth" 97% of physician fees based on actual work and costs of practice, including overhead and malpractice insurance (Sharp, 1996). The eventual compromise rate of 85% was all the traffic could bear.

Organized medicine saw this and other recent changes in regulation for nurse-midwives and nurse anesthetists as a challenge to its hegemony. Some 49 physician organizations petitioned the Health Care Financing Administration (now CMS—Centers for Medicare and Medicaid), but as a "Citizens Petition," to restrict billing to physicians (American Medical Association [AMA] "Citizens Petition" sent to HCFA, 2000). Some 250 nursing organizations responded (Nursing's response to AMA "Citizen's Petition" sent to HCFA, 2000). None of this activity hit the major public media. The issue is simply too technical. Even the usual attention the AMA gets in the public media did not happen this time. New actors, including consumers and, one would argue, nursing are blunting the so-called "iron triangle" of power elites: physicians, hospitals, and legislators or regulators.

The "outside" model is "hit 'em on the head to get their attention." The 98,000 unnecessary deaths revealed by the first IOM collection of patient safety studies is an example. Many a piece of legislation is passed in response to a crisis. Witness the Patriot Act after 9/11, and the emergency Sunday afternoon passage of legislation to change the legal oversight of the Terri Schiavo case.

The involvement of celebrities is one way to catalyze attention. Recent examples abound: The late Christopher Reeves, Michael J. Fox, Mary Tyler Moore, and Nancy Reagan made pleas for support of stem cell research to work on diabetes, Parkinson's disease, Alzheimer's disease, and spinal cord injury. Nursing was fortunate to attract the interest of Dana Delaney, the television actress who played a Vietnam era nurse in "China Beach," to assist in the effort to get veterans benefits for women veterans of the Vietnam era (Rasmussen, 1991).

Where advanced practice nursing has made progress on issues that have to do with our parochial interests, such as licensure, scope of practice, third-party reimbursement, and prescriptive authority, the progress has generally been made by sophisticated political minuet rather than data-based argument. On these issues we have not had sufficient data and still do not. For example, there is very little literature on the effect of granting APRNs prescriptive authority. If nurses can prescribe, do we do it? Do we do it right? How often do we consult a physician, even with full-scope prescribing authority? Yet prescribing authority in one form or another exists in most states (Phillips, 2005) over the opposition of physicians and pharmacists and essentially without data.

Contemporary nursing's political strategy involves hooking APRN concerns to expand scope of practice and prescribing authority to the "managed care" agenda, which is about money, not practice. Although the research on the cost-effectiveness of advanced practice nursing is still slim, it has been cleverly analyzed and combined with regulatory options by Barbara Safriet, an attorney and former Associate Dean of the Yale Law School, in a monograph that is often made part of public testimony (Safriet, 1992). Having this information compiled by an attorney who is not a nurse has the effect of making the data even more powerful, because the information does not seem self-serving. Her recent update in 2002 uses her experience in a Pew Foundation–funded task force to produce a "primer" for policymakers, because her experience taught her how ignorant policymakers are about nursing and advanced practice (Safriet, 2002).

# GETTING OUR ACT TOGETHER: A MINI CASE STUDY ON USE OF DATA

The American Nurses Association (ANA) took the very unpopular stance of supporting Medicare in the mid 1960s because Medicare would bring access to care, which meant more nursing jobs. But two decades later, organized nursing resisted the implementation of the Diagnosis Related Groups (DRG)–based Prospective Payment System under Medicare, which would pay hospitals a calculated fixed rate per discharged patient. In 1983 the ANA provided public testimony against this legislation on the basis of predictions of nursing jobs lost. By the mid 1980s the effect of the payment system was being felt in hospitals that had cut registered nurse (RN) positions because a decreased length of stay (LOS) was anticipated. LOS dropped like a rock, but intensive care unit (ICU) days rose, and the demand for nursing went through the ceiling. Shorter lengths of stay mean that the "easy" days of nursing at the beginning and end of the stay are gone, and all of the "sick" days are concentrated in the shorter stay.

The American Hospital Association (AHA), stimulated by the American Organization of Nurse Executives (AONE), did several quick and dirty surveys. The average community hospital RN vacancy rate rose from 4.4% in 1983 to 11.3% in December 1987.

The National League for Nursing (NLN) concluded that the supply of associate degree graduates would exceed demand in 2000 and that the supply of baccalaureate- and master's-prepared nurses would be under demand by about 0.5 million each.

At the same time, the Division of Nursing of the Bureau of Health Manpower of the Health Services and Resources Administration in the U.S. Department of Health and Human Services (1984), which collects data on nursing numbers and employment rates, was reporting that there was no shortage of nurses.

So already there are four different sets of numbers. The ANA's agenda is jobs: more nurses. AONE's agenda is recruitment and manpower: more nurses. NLN's agenda is education and the health of schools of nursing in the supply pipeline: more nurses.

The agenda of the Division of Nursing, as part of the executive branch of government, is to decrease federal expenses: Less funding is needed because there are enough nurses.

The nursing shortage data, flawed as they were, pushed hospitals even in rate-regulated states to raise salaries so that nursing staff could be hired and retained. But within 5 years, something happened, and now conventional wisdom held that highly paid nurses were part of the cause of escalating health care costs and should be reengineered and downsized out in favor of lower-paid, unlicensed personnel. California was savaged by managed care.

Buresh and Gordon (2000) report the fight for "safe hospital staffing" legislation in California. It is a remarkable story of political sophistication and coalition building between unions and nursing to eventually pass the first state law that mandates nurse/patient staffing ratios. The effort involved changing the political landscape to help elect a Democrat as governor and a sophisticated media campaign. About 5 years passed between the first, unsuccessful bill and the one signed by Governor Gray Davis in 1999. The story illustrates many of the facets of politics and policy reflected throughout this book, including using the media to advantage, framing the issues correctly, and building coalitions.

The California Nurses Association commissioned a study that analyzed 18.2 million patient discharges and other hospital and government data that linked nurse staffing to patients. The study documented increased nursing workloads and the second lowest ratio of nurses to patients in the nation. Then, in a brilliant move, they commissioned a public poll to measure how frightened Californians were about their access to nursing. Spetz (2001) points out that the California Department of Public Health put itself in a difficult position because there were no data to determine what a "safe" staffing ratio might be. That California had been the first state to embrace managed care made this effort all the more important as a signal to the industry, "Enough already!"

The agenda that is now being shaped is not about nursing resources being a number of warm bodies. It is about the working conditions for nursing (Aiken et al., 2001; Demir, Ulusoy, & Ulusoy, 2003; Hertting, Nilsson, Theorell, & Larsson, 2004;

Nursing Workforce, 2001; Reeves, West, & Barron, 2005). In the long run, that will be a more effective strategy for the profession, although how that translates into public policy or regulation is a much more subtle question. It is not at all clear that the proper fix for nursing working conditions could or should be a matter of public policy. It might be a matter for accreditation, for example. Hospitals must retain their accreditation status to be able to collect reimbursement from Medicare, even though accreditation is a private function in the United States. It might also be driven by patients and market demand; if the public becomes more aware of the relationship between safe care and nursing presence, consumer demand could alter current hospital practice in a highly competitive business.

The research that will inform the next round of policy discussions about nursing shortages should move away from the warm-body-count methodology to concentrate on what the nature of nursing's work is in the new millennium, how the working environment conditions affect work, and what the outcomes are. There may be more fat to be cut out of the American health care delivery system, but it won't be in nursing. The future demands that we all understand more about the relationship of practice to outcome.

That work will require different education for nurse researchers—more emphasis on health services research—and more to the point, a recognition of the essentiality of nursing in managing health care operations: how the work of patient care and service delivery gets done. Linda Aiken has given us a huge gift with her conceptual work on the relationship of nursing to outcomes (Aiken, Sochalski, & Lake, 1997). Now, research needs to be designed to look at nursing where the work happens—the hospital nursing unit, the clinic, the home care visit, and so on. Then we need to add those studies up in metaanalyses and systematic reviews—after, of course, making them locally available for policy decision-making.

There will always be a place for clinical research on patients and their care. From a policy perspective, however, the research that will carry the discipline farther faster will be health services research. The policy and political climate is very ripe now, on the heels of the IOM safety reports, and also in reaction

to the slash-and-burn restructure, merge, or die action that characterized the 1990s. Suzanne Gordon, a journalist who specializes in nursing, had collected masses of evidence about what studies show about the effects of the madness of the recent past, and she is using that body to bring the consequences on nursing to larger public attention (Gordon, 2005).

## RESEARCH AND REGULATION

Values set the policy. Policy codifies the values. Legislation translates them. Regulation implements them. This is the process in the best of all possible worlds.

But regulation is coming to be more important in health care than even legislation, through accreditation, standard setting, and other efforts that become absorbed into public standards.

The CMS administer the Medicare and Medicaid programs. From the beginning of the Medicare legislation, the administrative agency had a mandated quality agenda. In their first attempt to meet that requirement, the agency published mortality rates from every hospital in the United States. One, in California, had an 89% mortality rate, which shocked newspaper readers. It was not a hospital; it was a hospice, and one might wonder why it didn't have a 100% mortality rate.

This embarrassing faux pas caused the agency to realize that measuring quality by mortality required data on processes of care that were not available in the administrative data reported to them (Jencks & Wilensky, 1992). They needed another way to deliver on their quality mandate.

Among other things, they put together a Cooperative Cardiology Project in four pilot states. The states tested whether clinical guidelines developed by the American College of Cardiology regarding early treatment for acute myocardial infarction (MI) could be assessed through a sampling of discharge patient records. The guidelines were just lying around, waiting for someone to find them. The MI guidelines became CMS's first set of quality indicators and were immediately swept up by the JCAHO, then the Leapfrog Group, playing "me too." The Leapfrog Group *(www.leapfroggroup.org)* is a group of Fortune 500 companies that have simply declared themselves in the game of health care quality.

The Internet provides the platform to make available quality data in the form of standard metrics (measurements), even if they aren't the most interesting metrics. In early 2005 the CMS put on the Internet a hospital comparison program *(www.cms. gov)* in which it is possible to compare any hospital with the whole country at least for the metrics that have been agreed on—none of which, at the moment, translates easily into nursing.

All of this, and other quality efforts, have forced the creation of a National Quality Forum, a membership organization *(http://qualityforum.org)* to try to coordinate all these quality measurements that otherwise will drive health care organizations into the poorhouse.

The Magnet Hospital recognition program of the American Nurses' Credentialing Center *(www. nursingworld.org/ancc)* makes a part of its anointing of hospitals a requirement that they submit data on a selected set of "nurse sensitive" patient outcome metrics (e.g., fall rates, pain assessment) to the ANA's database *(www.nursingquality.org)*. This will create a database for research, although there will be no comparison statistics from non-Magnet hospitals.

The adoption of private standards by public programs is a uniquely American phenomenon. There is no public testimony or access to the decisions of private organizations as there is in federal or state legislation and regulation. That may mean that the information for decision-making in private organizations might itself be an occasion for public policymaking, as has begun by the extension of federal oversight for human informed consent provisions from federally funded research to *any* research in which human subjects are enrolled. Toward the end of the Clinton administration, the federal regulatory agency (Office of Inspector General [OIG]) had considerably expanded its investigations and used the power to halt research and issue fines (Kalb & Koehler, 2002) for violations.

## SPECIAL INTERESTS AND RESEARCH

Support (funding) for health care research comes from many sources including public funds from

government (National Institutes of Health); some state health departments; charitable foundations (e.g., the Robert Wood Johnson Foundation, W.K. Kellogg Foundation, Commonwealth Fund, Pew Charitable Trust); advocacy groups; and for-profit entities such as pharmaceutical and medical device companies. In fact, government is no longer the largest funder of biomedical research; the pharmaceutical industry is (Field, Baranowski, Healy, & Longacre, 2003). It takes no great degree of cynicism to suspect that research that does not serve industry interests may well never appear in public.

Recent entrants into the research funding arena are variously open or disguised special interest groups. Organizations with "family" in their titles tend to have a pro-life agenda. Organizations with "economy" in their titles may have an organized labor agenda. One interesting example is the Connecticut Center for the New Economy *(www.ctneweconomy. org),* whose website never mentions where its funds come from: unions. Many advocacy groups have funds to either do their own research or make grants or negotiate contracts to do it for them. The research tends, not surprisingly, to support the policy agenda of the advocacy organization.

The Agency for Health Care Policy and Research (AHCPR) (now the Agency for Healthcare Research and Quality [AHRQ]) is funded by a 1% "tax" on National Institutes of Health (NIH) research, originally to support evaluation of the use of public monies for medical scientific research (Gray, 1992). In the 1990s the agency convened multidisciplinary committees, nearly always including nurses, some chaired by nurses, to review literature in particular areas—pain, urinary incontinence, depression in primary care—and develop publicly available guidelines in two forms: one for consumers and one for health professionals. The process is fairly straightforward, essentially nonpolitical, grinding hard academic work—which then went public.

One of the topics picked was low back pain. The expert panel reviewed the science and generated its report and guidelines, which said that 8 of 10 patients with acute back pain will recover in a month or so without therapy; surgery benefits only 1 in 100 patients; and much diagnostic imaging is unnecessary. Were the practice guidelines implemented, there would be billions of dollars of savings and patients would be protected from unnecessary surgery. The American Academy of Orthopedic Surgeons endorsed the guidelines. But the North American Spine Society, a group of surgeons, was outraged and got the attention of two Republican Texas representatives, who agitated to cut off the Agency's funding. To make a very long story short, the Agency came close to losing all of its funding. There was, of course, no requirement that anybody ever use the guidelines, but the transfer to regulation wasn't far away (AHCPR drops guideline development, 1996).

Research isn't completed until it is peer reviewed and published. The extent to which special interests have influenced this process is not something easily determined. Deyo and colleagues (1997) collected their own and others' experiences. They showed that the ox gored by the spine studies was the manufacturer of a pedicle screw sometimes used in spinal fusion. The manufacturer was being sued by patients alleging poor results. Attorneys for the defendant tied up researchers for a long time with subpoenas for detailed records. Another pedicle screw manufacturer unsuccessfully sought a court injunction to prevent the Agency from publishing its guidelines.

Simon, one of the coauthors of the Deyo paper mentioned in the preceding paragraph, was caught in another controversy when research by his team questioned the value of immunodiagnostic tests often used to support disability and liability claims for chemical sensitivity. He went crosswise of plaintiff's attorneys, laboratories, and advocacy organizations for people with disabilities. Allegations of scientific misconduct were made to the federal Office of Research Integrity and the Medical Board in Washington where Dr. Simon worked for group health. Individual patients were contacted and encouraged to attack his credibility.

Psaty, another coauthor of the Deyo paper, and his colleagues had studied calcium channel blockers, diuretics, and beta-blockers and found that the short-acting calcium channel blockers were associated with an increased risk of MI. The media's handling of the story played up the risk and downplayed the science, and the manufacturers of calcium channel blockers were annoyed. The pharmaceutical companies funded mass mailings to physicians from an "opinion leader" in hypertension management without identifying the source of funding for the mailing.

An article entitled "Thyroid Storm" (Rennie, 1997) describes the story of an investigation that took 9 years to reach print because it called into question the superior efficacy of Synthroid, a synthetic thyroid preparation (Dong et al., 1997). The study had been funded by the manufacturer of Synthroid, and several other preparations were tested. The investigators had submitted the manuscript to *JAMA* with a cover letter saying that the sponsor of the research disagreed with the conclusions. The results showed that all the synthetic thyroid preparations were bioequivalent. The manufacturer of Synthroid checked the files and found an agreement to the original funding that gave them the right to approve any potential publication.

The manuscript was peer reviewed and eventually approved for publication, but it was abruptly withdrawn when the manufacturer brought legal action. The company was being considered for acquisition by another pharmaceutical firm, and the comparative efficacy of its most important product was at issue. The company did a reanalysis of data, reaching conclusions opposite to those of the original study, and published its findings in a new journal for which the company's investigator was an associate editor. The situation reached the notice of the *Wall Street Journal*.

The issue became a matter of public policy when the U.S. Food and Drug Administration entered and alleged that the company had mislabeled its product's efficacy, a violation of federal law, using the results of its own reanalysis. That apparently brought all parties to the table, and eventually the company agreed not to challenge publication of the original manuscript.

Those of us who like to read the very fine print of the annual publication of the CMS rules in the *Federal Register* were intrigued when in 2002 the CMS allowed the evidence from one and only one research study, funded by the Johnson and Johnson company and published in the *NEJM,* to create *in advance of FDA approval* a payment mechanism for drug-eluting stents (Hensley, 2002; *Federal Register,* 2002). (The *Wall Street Journal* headline writer got the agency wrong: it was the CMS, not the FDA. See, this stuff is tough!) In the same regulatory announcement, the CMS denied the request of a different manufacturer, Guidant, for a similar exception, on the grounds that the only research available was the company's own, a distinction that escaped many readers. Guidant's stock plummeted (Guidant plunges, 2002). And the CMS is probably very sorry to have done this, because now they must deal annually with every device and drug manufacturer who wants the same privilege. For example, in the rules for fiscal 2005 there were 10 new proposals for essentially the same deal, all of which the CMS turned down (*Federal Register*, 2004). And one wonders why the administrative costs of health care in the United States exceed those of any other country in the world?

Vioxx, a painkiller made by Merck, was voluntarily removed from the market when data suggested that long-term use increased cardiac risk. A report in the *New York Times* (Berenson, 2005) details the pressure the researchers were under by Merck to redefine causes of death associated with the drug's use as "unknown" to deflate the statistics.

It is getting increasingly difficult to tell the difference between honest scientific agreement and profit-driven market initiatives in the public press. And, of course, patients bear the brunt of this.

## RESEARCH DESIGN FOR POLICY

It should be obvious by now that the quality of research may have little to do with its impact on policy. There are, however, some ways in which research can be made more useful and usable in policy decision-making.

In the first place, research can be used to help *define a problem*, particularly to determine how big it is. The new research about nursing staffing and working conditions may be an example. Aiken and colleagues (2001) have an international study that suggests that the working condition issues in the United States are similar to those in Canada and Scotland, and to a lesser extent in Germany. They suggest that working conditions predict nurses' intentions to stay or leave their present positions and that work is bringing the environment for care into the political and health policy environment in totally new ways. For example, if it were realized that the working environment for nursing makes a difference in nursing recruitment and retention, then perhaps

local decision-makers might make the working environment a priority. (All politics are local…)

*Aggregating studies* in the form of systematic literature reviews or metaanalyses are becoming an important research strategy. Metaanalyses and similar reviews are now embedded in Internet-based resources, especially the Cochrane Library in the United Kingdom (*www.cochranelibrary.com*).

Health care data systems in the United States are fed from a merger of data from the billing system and data from patient records, made computer readable in international disease coding systems. These data are the source for most health services research because they are publicly reportable to Medicare and to most state data depositories. Nurses have generally not known about these incredibly rich data sources, which, because they originate in hospitals, nursing homes, and home care agencies, are also available at the local level. Nursing homes are mandated to use a standard minimum data set (MDS), which is much more than minimum. Home care agencies use a different standard data system (OASIS), prescribed by government. Although nurses may complain about having to fill out these tedious forms, the data they produce are very nurse-friendly. Hospital data can also be used for nursing when nurses understand what the data are and how to read them (Diers, Weaver, Bozzo, Allegretto, & Pollack, 1998). *Data mining* in existing administrative data is an increasingly important policy-related strategy. The advantage of using administrative data is that they are always there, produce very large samples, are inexpensive to access and, if they also include economic measures such as costs, appeal to policymakers.

*Policy evaluation* is another way to use research to shape or change policy. Sikma and Young (2003) report an exquisite example of a study designed to evaluate the effect of allowing nurses in Washington State to delegate certain functions to assistive personnel in nursing homes. The study design used case study methods to address the concerns of multiple stakeholders.

Pickiness about research design is not always relevant when the goal is to boil down a collection of disparate studies or other data to make a policy point. This is not at all the same as fudging the numbers. Politicians and policymakers are generally not entranced by arcane academic standards for methodologic technicalities. The gathering of NP literature by the Office of Technology Assessment (OTA, 1988), as well as Safriet's (1992, 2002) use of OTA and other studies, read, to the academic eye, as insufficiently critical of the studies cited. The study commissioned by the California Nurses Association to buttress their policy agenda for setting nursing staffing ratios had holes in it large enough to drive Gov. Schwarzenegger through. But to do an academic critique on this work is surely beside the point of having this information gathered by an unbiased critic, on the one hand, and an adroit use of administrative data and policy survey techniques on the other.

## IN THE END

The *American Journal of Nursing* (AJN) is increasingly becoming a forum for linking research and practice to policy. *AJN's* ANA and paid subscription circulation is larger than *NEJM's* and *JAMA's*. The largest circulation scholarly journal in nursing, *Journal of Nursing Scholarship*, for Sigma Theta Tau, does not take policy positions. The two new (since 2000) policy journals in nursing, *Policy, Politics, & Nursing Practice* and *Nursing and Health Policy Review* are becoming important venues for nursing policy thinking.

Research is not something to be plugged in when a policy or political crisis rears up. Timing is everything. Nurses, as politicians, policymakers, and researchers, need to keep (or have access to those who keep) such close touch with what is happening in the policy and political environment that we can anticipate trends and design studies to address them. We need to have networks of information, which is simpler now with the Internet and Google, MEDLINE, Lexis-Nexis, and all the other computer tools.

These, then, are the multiple and simultaneous strategies:

- Keep or find nursing data. Find and use the computerized information systems in the practice or the institution. Find the decision support people who know how to get data out. Policymakers want to know how big a problem is. How many patients, victims, families are affected? Policymakers also want to know how small a problem is: Connecticut

NPs argued successfully for their ability to sign for handicapped parking privileges because they were already doing it and the inconvenience of having to get a physician's cosignature would not prevent the issuance of more stickers, something the policymakers as parkers were already annoyed about.

- Think about your research in a policy context: What needs policy attention? Car seats? The ability of NPs to prescribe home care? The contents of vending machines in schools? What?
- Think about local replication as a policy strategy. If it works "there," maybe it will work here, too.
- Some specialty nursing journals have a regular "column" or "department" for brief policy-related research—*Pediatric Nursing, Nurse Practitioner, Advance for Nurse Practitioners, Clinical Nurse Specialist*. Use them for your own data presentation. Published research is generally more powerful than unpublished research, and research is generally more powerful than anecdote.
- When possible, collect the research and produce a research synthesis or metaanalysis.
- Use the public relations department in your hospital, university, or workplace. They know how to do the "dirty" work of publicity, from which we shy away.

## *Key Points*

- Research can inform public policy; at other times it will have no impact on so-called "morality" policy issues.
- Data from research can be used to get an issue on the agenda of policymakers, including at the local institutional level.
- Special interest groups sometimes manipulate research or attack researchers when they don't agree with the findings of studies.
- Nurses must think carefully and strategically about the research that is needed to further their policy agendas.
- There is a wealth of administrative and clinical data for nurses to mine; we must not miss the opportunity to think about the policy implications of such data.

*Web Resources*

> **Health Affairs**—a policy journal published by Project Hope
> *www.healthaffairs.org*
> **Henry J. Kaiser Family Foundation**—for state health issues
> *www.kff.org*
> **Rand Corporation**—for evidence-based clinical research
> *www.rand.org/health*
> **Agency for Healthcare Research and Quality**
> *www.ahrq.gov*

## REFERENCES

AHCPR drops guideline development. (1996, June). *HSR Reports*, p. 4. Association for Health Services Research, 1130 Connecticut Ave. NW, Washington, DC 20036.

Aiken, L. H., Clarke, S. P., Sloan, D. M., Sochalski, J. A., Busse, R., et al. (2001). Nurses' reports of hospital quality of care and working conditions in five countries. *Health Affairs, 20*(3), 43-53.

Aiken, L. H., Smith, H. L., & Lake, E. T. (1994). Lower Medicare mortality among a set of hospitals known for good nursing care. *Medical Care, 32*(8), 771-778.

Aiken, L. H., Sochalski, J., & Lake, E. T. (1997). Studying outcomes of organizational change in health services. *Medical Care, 35*(11), NS6-NS17.

AMA *"Citizens' petition" sent to HCFA.* (2000, June 27). Nursing World/Legislative Branch. Retrieved July 24, 2000, from *www.nursingworld.org/gova/federal/agencies/hcfa/hcfaama.htm.*

Berenson, A. (2005, April 24). Evidence in Vioxx suits shows intervention by Merck officials. *New York Times*, CLIV (53), p 1 et seq.

Buresh, B., & Gordon, S. (2000). *From silence to voice: What nurses know and must communicate to the public.* Ottawa: Canadian Nurses Association.

Cheung, R. B., Moody, L. E., & Cockram, C. (2002). Data mining strategies for shaping nursing and health policy agendas. *Policy, Politics, & Nursing Practice, 3*(3), 248-260.

Cobb, R., Ross, J. K., & Ross, J. H. (1976). Agenda building as a comparative political process. *The American Political Science Review, 70,* 125-138.

Czaplinski, C., & Diers, D. (1998). The effect of staff nurse specialization on length of stay and mortality. *Medical Care, 36*(12), 1626-1638.

Demir, A., Ulusoy, M., & Ulusoy, M. F. (2003). Investigation of factors influencing burnout levels in the professional and private lives of nurses. *International Journal of Nursing Studies, 40*(8), 807-827.

Deyo, R. A., Psaty, B. M., Simon, G., Wagner, E. H., & Omenn, G.S. (1997). The messenger under attack: Intimidation of researchers by special interest groups. *New England Journal of Medicine, 336*(16), 1176-1179.

Diers, D., & Potter, J. (1997). Understanding the unmanageable nursing unit with case-mix data. *Journal of Nursing Administration, 27*(11), 27-32.

Diers, D., Weaver, D., Bozzo, J., Allegretto, S., & Pollack, C. (1998). Building a nursing management analysis capacity in a teaching hospital. *Seminars for Nurse Managers, 6*(3), 108-112.

Division of Nursing, Bureau of Health Manpower, Health Research Services Administration, U.S. Department of Health and Human Services. (1984). *The registered nurse population: Findings from the national sample survey of registered nurses, November 1984.* Washington, DC: Division of Nursing.

Dong, B. J., Hauch, W. W., Gabertoglio, J. G., Gee, L., White, J. R., Bubp, J. L., & Greenspan, F. S. (1997). Bioequivalence of generic and brand-name levothyroxine products in the treatment of hypothyroidism. *Journal of the American Medical Association, 277*(15), 1205-1213.

Drenkard, K., & Ferguson, S. (2002). Genetic testing and discrimination: Case example—Virginia. *Pediatric Nursing, 28*(1), 71-73.

*Federal Register.* (2002). Drug-eluting stents. *Federal Register, 67*(148), 50003-50007.

*Federal Register.* (2004). Add-on payments. *Federal Register, 69*(154), 49000-49206.

Field, R. I., Baranowski, B. J., Healy, R. A., & Longacre, M. L. (2003). Toward a policy agenda on medical research funding: Results of a symposium. *Health Affairs, 22*(3), 224-230.

Gordon, S. (2005). *Nursing against the odds.* Ithaca, NY: Cornell University Press.

Gottesman, M. M. (2001). Children in foster care: A nursing perspective on research, policy, and child health issues. *Journal of the Society of Pediatric Nurses, 6*(2), 55-64.

Gray, B. H. (1992). The legislative battle over health services research. *Health Affairs, 11*(4) 38-66.

Guidant plunges on court ruling. (2002, October 2). Retrieved October 2, 2002, from *http://money.cnn.com.*

Hensley, S. (2002, August 1). FDA agrees to pay 17% premium for drug-coated stents. *Wall Street Journal*, D4

Hertting, A., Nilsson, K., Theorell, T., & Larsson, U. S. (2004). Downsizing and reorganization: Demands, challenges, and ambiguity for registered nurses. *Journal of Advanced Nursing, 45*(2), 145-154.

Horrocks, S., Anderson, E., & Salisbury, C. (2002). Systematic review of whether nurse practitioners working in primary care can provide equivalent care to doctors. *British Medical Journal, 324*(7341), 819-824.

Institute of Medicine (IOM). (2000). *To err is human: Building a safer health system.* Washington, DC: National Academies Press.

Institute of Medicine (IOM). (2001). *Crossing the Quality Chasm: A new health system for the 21st century.* Washington, DC: National Academies Press.

Institute of Medicine (IOM). (2004). *Keeping Patients Safe: Transforming the work environment of nurses.* Washington, DC: National Academies Press.

Jencks, S. F., & Wilensky, G. R. (1992). The health care quality improvement initiative. *Journal of the American Medical Association, 268*(7), 900-903.

Jennings, B. M. (2003). Research about nursing: An agenda whose time has come. *Policy, Politics, & Nursing Practice, 4*(4), 246-249.

Kalb, P. E., & Koehler, K. G. (2002). Legal issues in scientific research. *Journal of the American Medical Association, 287*(1), 85-91.

Kingdon, J. W. (1995). *Agendas, alternatives, and public policies* (2nd ed.). New York: HarperCollins.

Lui, H. (2004). Pursuing an evidence base to change nurse staffing policy in China. *Nursing Administration Quarterly, 28*(2), 150-152.

McDonough, J. E. (2001). Using and misusing anecdote in policy making. *Health Affairs, 20*(1), 207-212.

Mooney, C. Z. (2001). *The public clash of private values: The politics of morality policy.* New York: Chatham House.

Nursing's response to AMA "Citizens' Petition" sent to HCFA. (2000, August 17). Nursing World/Legislative Branch. Retrieved December 4, 2000, from *www.nursingworld.org/gova/federal/agencies/hcfa/ama.htm.*

Nursing workforce: Emerging nurse shortages due to multiple factors. Report to the Chairman, Subcommittee on Health, Committee on Ways and Means, U.S. House of Representatives. U.S. General Accounting Office GAO-010944, July 2001. Retrieved February 23, 2002, from *www.gao.gov.*

Office of Technology Assessment (OTA). (1988). *Nurse practitioners, physician assistants and certified nurse-midwives: A policy analysis.* Washington, DC: U.S. Government Printing Office.

O'Neill, T., & Hymel, G. (1994). *All politics is local.* New York: Bob Adams/Random House.

Phillips, S. J. (2005). A comprehensive look at the legislative issues affecting advanced nursing practice. *The Nurse Practitioner, 30*(1), 14-47.

Price, L., & Minarik, P. (1998). More on Medicare reimbursement: Clarification of direct billing and "incident to" billing. *Clinical Nurse Specialist, 12,* 246-249.

Price, L., & Minarik, P. (1999). Update on federal Medicare rules affecting advanced practice nurses. *Clinical Nurse Specialist, 13,* 90-91.

Rasmussen, E. China Beach memoirs. October 24, 1991. *Nurseweek.* Retrieved March 14, 2005, from *www.nurseweek.com/news/features/01-10/chinabeach.html.*

Reeves, R., West, E., & Barron, D. (2005). The impact of barriers to providing high-quality care on nurses intentions to leave London hospitals. *Journal of Health Services Research and Policy, 10*(1), 5-10.

Rennie, D. (1997). Thyroid storm. *Journal of the American Medical Association, 277*(15), 1238-1243.

Safriet, B. (1992). Health care dollars and regulatory sense. *Yale Journal on Regulation, 9*(2), 417-488.

Safriet, B. (2002). Closing the gap between *can* and *may* in health-care providers' scopes of practice: A primer for policymakers. *Yale Journal on Regulation, 19*(2), 301-334.

Sharp, N. (1996). Nurse practitioner reimbursement: History and politics. *Nurse Practitioner, 21*(3), 100, 103-104.

Shelton, D. (2002). Failure of mental-health policy—incarcerated children and adolescents. *Pediatric Nursing, 28*(3), 278-281.

Sikma, S. K., & Young, H. M. (2003). Nurse delegation in Washington State: A case study of concurrent policy implementation and evaluation. *Policy, Politics, & Nursing Practice, 4*(1), 53-61.

Spetz, J. (2001). What should we expect from California's minimum nurse staffing legislation? *JONA, 31*(3), 132-140.

Williams, L. E., & Martin, J. E. (2003). Car seat challenges: Where are we in implementation of these programs? *Journal of Perinatal & Neonatal Nursing, 17*(2), 158-164.

Xue, Y., & Cohen, S. S. (2004). Dietary supplements: Policy and research implications for nurses. *Policy, Politics, & Nursing Practice, 5*(3), 149-159.

# POLICYSPOTLIGHT

# From Practice to Policy: Improving Wound Care Outcomes

Elizabeth A. Ayello, Sharon Baranoski, & Courtney H. Lyder

*"In the middle of difficulty, lies opportunity."*
ALBERT EINSTEIN

Wounds, particularly ones that are chronic or nonhealing, pose a special challenge in the United States. Not only are they seen in every health setting, but they are a significant health policy issue in the United States because they are costly, both financially and emotionally. Venous ulcers (formerly called *venous stasis ulcers*) are the most commonly occurring peripheral vascular ulcer. The incidence and prevalence of pressure ulcers has attracted the attention of regulatory agencies and prompted efforts to reduce their rates. As the number of Americans with diabetes mellitus continues to escalate, neuropathic ulcers of the foot remain the leading cause of nontraumatic amputations.

## CREATING CLINICAL PRACTICE GUIDELINES

With a goal of enhancing quality, appropriateness, and effectiveness of health care services, early initiatives to contain costs resulted in the development of clinical practice guidelines. In the 1990s the Agency for Healthcare Research and Quality (AHRQ), formerly the Agency for Health Care Policy and Research (AHCPR), developed and released professional clinical practice guidelines along with consumer versions of pressure ulcer prevention (guideline no. 3) and pressure ulcer treatment (guideline no. 15) (Panel for the Prediction and Prevention of Pressure Ulcers In Adults, 1992; Bergstrom et al., 1994). The multidisciplinary panels that developed these guidelines followed a rigorous process that included an extensive literature review, public testimony at open forums, information from consultants, and peer and pilot reviews of guideline draft documents.

Health professionals have used nursing research to provide updates to the original recommendations of the AHRQ Clinical Guidelines. The Wound, Ostomy, and Continence Nurses Society (WOCN) has recently revised the pressure ulcer guidelines and developed guidelines for arterial, venous, and neuropathic ulcers (Ratliff, 2005).

Numerous guidelines for foot ulcers in persons with diabetes mellitus exist. The first guideline is from the American Diabetes Association (ADA). It is based on the 1999 Consensus Development Conference on Diabetic Foot Wound Care. Other guidelines for the prevention and treatment of diabetic foot ulcers by the following organizations exist or are nearing completion:

- International Working Group on the Diabetic Foot (IWGDF)—International Consensus on the Diabetic Foot
- American Pharmacology Association
- American College of Foot and Ankle Surgeons
- Infectious Diseases Society of America
- Wound Healing Society

A summary of the commonalities among these numerous guidelines provides clinicians with a "cohesive framework for assessing and managing patients with diabetic foot wounds" (Frykberg, 2005, p. 210).

Regardless of the source, the guidelines provide a basis for care protocols developed by leading experts in wound care. Despite these guidelines, achievement of reduction in the numbers of these wounds, use of the practice guidelines for treatment, or consistent dissemination has yet to be realized. What follows is a discussion of some of the exemplars of wound care policies that nurses working collaboratively have made a reality.

## WOUND CARE POLICIES FOR LONG-TERM CARE

Pressure ulcers are a serious problem in the long-term care setting (LTC). The number of residents with pressure ulcers in LTC has been reported as ranging from 2.3% to 23.9% (Cuddigan, Ayello, & Sussman, 2001) to a federal mean of about 9% (Centers for Medicare and Medicaid Services [CMS], 2005). LTC has a long history of regulation for pressure ulcers. For LTC, Tag F-314 is the federal regulation on pressure ulcers. It states that "based on the comprehensive assessment of a resident, the facility must ensure that a resident who enters the facility without pressure sores does not develop pressure sores unless the individual's clinical condition demonstrates that they were unavoidable. (Although the regulatory language of Tag F-314 uses the term *pressure sores*, CMS acknowledges that the widely used nomenclature in practice is *pressure ulcers* and uses pressure ulcers throughout the document.) The intent of this regulation is that a resident in an LTC facility will not develop a pressure ulcer unless the clinical condition is such that the ulcer is unavoidable." The revision of Tag F-314 has corrected the problem with lack of clarity about what constitutes "unavoidable," as it now states what defines an avoidable or an unavoidable pressure ulcer.

### The Process for Revision of Tag F-314

On November 12, 2004, CMS not only released but made immediately effective its *Guidance to Surveyors for Long Term Care Facilities*, which is available at *http://new.cms.hhs.gov/manuals/downloads/ som107ap_pp_guidelines_ltcf.pdf.* The federal Tag F-314 on pressure ulcers did not change, but the way that the guidance is interpreted over the 40-page document did change significantly. The document consists of two sections. The interpretation section (pp. 130-155, including references) provides a common language and overview of evidence-based care for both surveyors and clinicians on pressure ulcer prevention and treatment. The investigative protocol (pp. 156-167) is an important part of the survey process, as it determines whether the pressure ulcer was avoidable or unavoidable, as well as the adequacy of the facility's interventions and efforts to prevent and treat pressure ulcers.

The revised guidance was the outcome of a 3-year project by CMS to reinterpret Tag F-314. In January 2001 a panel was convened. It was chaired by an outstanding CMS nurse leader, Beverly Cullen. Members of the panel included CMS employees, surveyors, stakeholders, and wound care experts. Two of the authors, Ayello and Lyder, served as the wound care nurses on the panel. The panel used the best available evidence on pressure ulcers. After several meetings an initial draft went out for public comment in 2002. All public comments were read and discussed by the panel. A second round of public comment occurred in 2003. This was again followed by a thorough review of all comments by the panel members. After the committee reached consensus and revision of the document, it was sent to CMS for circulation and approval. Before release of the revised guidance, Dan Berlowitz, MD, the National Pressure Ulcer Advisory Panel (NPUAP) president at that time, along with the nurse consultants and a state surveyor, developed the educational program, which explained the major points of the revised guidance. This educational program was mandatory for surveyors and was Web-broadcast for satellite training.

## Policy Options

The revised Tag F-314 has several new sections. It includes a definition not just of pressure ulcers, but of other ulcers, such as arterial, venous, and neuropathic ulcers, so they can be readily differentiated from pressure ulcers. Other definitions help

to determine if a pressure ulcer is avoidable or unavoidable. Other information provides new clarity in pressure ulcer risk assessment parameters, staging, healing measurement, and current treatment modalities including infection management, dressings, support surfaces and pressure relief, debridement, and nutrition.

The implications for revised Tag F-314, including the anticipated impact on the quality of pressure ulcer care and facility compliance, have been discussed in the literature (Fleck, 2005; Lyder, 2005). The educational bar for surveyors and clinicians has been raised. It is helpful, though, that facilities have a single resource to guide them in their preparation for surveys as well as prevention and treatment of pressure ulcers (Fleck, 2005). Not only must facilities examine and revise their pressure ulcer policies and procedures for concurrence with the guidelines, but they must be aware of the new categories of deficiencies that could lead to facility citations and to their associated monetary penalties. The possibility of increased citations as well as the severity of citations have raised some concern among facilities. No longer does the lowest level, a level 1 citation (no actual harm, with potential for minimal harm) exist for pressure ulcers. This is because CMS views the failure of a facility to provide appropriate care to prevent or heal pressure ulcers as more than minimal harm. Instead, pressure ulcer citations can involve only the higher levels of 2 to 4, as follows:

- Level 4—Immediate jeopardy (e.g., a resident admitted with a stage IV pressure ulcer fails to show signs of healing)
- Level 3—Actual harm (e.g., a resident developed multiple avoidable stage II pressure ulcers)
- Level 2—No actual harm with potential for more than minimal harm (e.g., a resident developed an avoidable stage I pressure ulcer)

It is hoped that the clinical examples of possible negative resident scenarios included in the revised guidance will provide an objective and consistent way of measuring noncompliance in LTC.

## WOUND CARE POLICIES IN HOME CARE

The Outcome and Assessment Information Set (OASIS) assessment and document tool was mandated on October 1, 2000 for use by all

Medicare-certified home care agencies. OASIS is a group of data elements that represent core items of a comprehensive assessment. It provides the basis for measuring patient outcomes for the purpose of outcome-based quality improvement in the home care arena (Abraham, 2005). CMS has finalized two rules relating to home health agencies (HHAs). One rule revises the existing conditions of participation (CoPs) by requiring home care to collect data. The other expands the new CoPs by requiring HHAs to report OASIS data to their state survey agency. This collection and reporting of OASIS data allows CMS and agencies to have continual objective standardized information on patients and their responses to home health interventions (Stephens, 2004).

Skilled nursing and rehabilitative services for wound care provided in the home are covered under Medicare and by other payers. Wound care services generally fall into the categories of observation and assessment, teaching or training, and direct hands-on care (Motta, 2001).

The Medicare Regional Home Health Intermediary Manual (HIM-11) fully explains the types of wounds that usually qualify as reasonable and necessary for home health care. The complexity of wound types, treatment plans, and wound dressings and supplies presents a unique challenge for HHAs. One of those challenges is balancing care needs with cost-effective treatment modalities. Medicare pays HHAs under a prospective payment system (PPS) based on a 60-day episode of care. Wound care dressings, and supplies (gauze, saline, wound cleansers, tape, and so on) are bundled under this 60-day payment episode. Wound care dressings and supplies, exclusive of durable medical equipment, are considered part of the care provided and cannot be billed separately. This has created a financial burden for many agencies.

CMS data on wound care patients shows that the home health case mix report indicates that 37% of patients have a pressure ulcer, a stasis ulcer, or a surgical wound. Surgical wounds constitute the largest patient population at 27%, followed by pressure ulcers (7%) and stasis ulcers (3%) (Johnston, 2005). Arterial and diabetic wounds are not tracked by the OASIS data system and are not included in the numbers just cited.

### Partnering with Nurses

CMS partnered with WOCN to develop the OASIS Guidance Document for classification of wounds. The wound OASIS items were developed by consensus among the WOCN's panel of experts. The specific items related to wound care are items listed as MO 440 through 488, pressure ulcers, stasis ulcers, and surgical wounds. The system for wound classification uses terms such as *not healing, partially granulating, fully granulating,* and *no observable pressure ulcer, stasis ulcer, or surgical wound.* Definitions of these terms were provided by the WOCN's expert panel. This guidance document was developed to provide continuity to definitions and collection of the data elements.

OASIS data will provide agencies with the opportunity to measure clinical outcomes and the financial impact of wound care treatments. Agencies can analyze the data and benchmark their performance with other, similar agencies. Important quality improvement changes can then be implemented to improve patient care, as well as agency efficiency and effectiveness. Agencies can gather data that will support a better understanding of their patient population, facilitate patient and staff education, and help increase the overall outcomes of their wound interventions.

As the population continues to age, and baby boomers become home health patients, an effective wound program will be at the forefront of successful outcomes for home care agencies across the country. It is expected that CMS will be updating and changing several of the OASIS items in the future.

The Medicare Payment Advisory Commission (MedPAC), an independent federal body that advises the U.S. Congress, has recommended exploring a Pay for Performance (P4P) system for home health. Speculation is that this system will be implemented within the next 2 years. P4P is a practice that attaches reimbursement to performance indicators such as outcomes, utilization, or process tracking measures (Twiss, Lang, & Rooney, 2005). Many believe that the OASIS assessment and documentation tool will form the foundation of a P4P model in home care, as it most closely meets MedPAC's measurement criteria. It is critical that

HHAs prepare by analyzing their outcome data on wound care and institute improvements in pressure ulcer, stasis ulcer, and surgical wound treatment.

## WOUND CARE POLICY IN ACUTE CARE

The emergence of patient safety as a priority for hospitals has been fueled by a 1999 Institute of Medicine Report, *To Err is Human*. In this report it was determined that up to 98,000 patients die annually because of medical errors, making them the eighth leading cause of death in the United States (Institute of Medicine, 1999). Furthermore, countless patients may be injured during a hospital stay. Although hospitals are not directly regulated by CMS, this federal agency has much influence on the care practices of U.S. hospitals.

In 2002, CMS and Qualidigm (Connecticut Quality Improvement Organization) began a 3-year project to investigate medical errors among Medicare beneficiaries in U.S. hospitals. The Medicare Patient Safety Monitoring System (MPSMS) is a collaboration among CMS and the U.S. Food and Drug Administration, Centers for Disease Control and Prevention, Agency for Health Care Research and Quality, and leading health care associations (Hunt, Verzier, Abend, & Lyder, 2005). This federal project aims not only to identify adverse medical events in hospitals, but to ensure that hospitals provide safe environments for patients. To ascertain hospital adverse medical rates, over 40,000 medical records of hospitalized Medicare beneficiaries were obtained. Through validated algorithms, each medical record is painstakingly reviewed for the identification of medical adverse events.

In 2004, pressure ulcer was added as a clinical condition to be tracked by CMS through the MPSMS. This was predicated on the fact that the cumulative prevalence of pressure ulcers among hospitalized patients aged 55 years and older has been reported to be as high as 30% (Cuddigan et al., 2001). Hospital-acquired pressure ulcers have been associated with a greater risk of death within 1 year of hospitalization (Barczak, Barnett, Childs, & Bosley, 1997). Not only do hospital-acquired pressure ulcers result in death and other adverse outcomes for patients, they can also increase hospital liability (Bennett, O'Sullivan, DeVito, & Remsburg, 2000). The development of pressure ulcers in hospitalized patients can result from a breakdown in the institutional system of care delivery, because the prevention of pressure ulcers requires the cooperation and skill of the entire medical team (Lyder, Grady, Mathur, Patrello, & Meehan, 2004). Moreover, it was determined that the development of pressure ulcers can be significantly influenced by the actions of health care providers. To that end, the development of a pressure ulcer can be considered a medical error.

The identification of pressure ulcers as a patient safety issue has huge implications for hospitals. Hence, their development may imply that a medical error has occurred. Given the increasing litigation related to hospital-acquired pressure ulcers, hospitals will need to take a more proactive stance to reduce their pressure ulcer incidence rates. Proper education of clinical staff and implementation of national pressure ulcer guidelines will ideally position hospitals to reduce their incidence rates.

## *Lessons Learned*

- Partnering nurse clinicians with members of regulatory agencies has resulted in the establishment of national benchmarks for wound care.
- The power of specialty organizations to work collaboratively with policymakers to create practice guidelines is critical to improving wound care nationally.
- With a shifting emphasis on prevention and future policies by CMS on wound care, nurses must be ready to provide testimony on best practices to influence policy decisions.

## *Web Resources*

**Centers for Medicare and Medicaid Services—Action Plan (for Further Improvement of) Nursing Home Quality**
*www.cms.hhs.gov/quality/nhqi/NHActionPlan.pdf*

*Continued*

*Web Resources — cont'd*

**Guidance to Surveyors for Long Term Care Facilities**
*http://new.cms.hhs.gov/manuals/downloads/ som107ap_pp_guidelines_ltcf.pdf*
**National Guidelines Clearinghouse (NCG)**
*www.guideline.gov*
**National Quality Measures Clearinghouse**
*www.qualitymeasures.ahrq.gov*
**Wound, Ostomy, and Continence Nurses Society**
*www.wocn.org*

## REFERENCES

Abraham, P. R. (2005, March/April). Case mix coding: Data reveals reimbursement and diagnosis snafus. *Remington Report, 13*(2), 50-54.

American Diabetes Association (ADA). (1999). Consensus development conference on diabetic foot wound care. *Diabetes Care. 22,* 1354-1360.

Barczak, C. A., Barnett, R. I., Childs, E. J. & Bosley, L. M. (1997). Fourth national pressure ulcer prevalence survey. *Advances in Wound Care, 10*(4), 18-26.

Bennett, R. G., O'Sullivan, J., DeVito, E. M., & Remsburg, R. (2000). The increasing medical malpractice risk related to pressure ulcers in the United States. *Journal of the American Geriatric Society, 48,* 73-81.

Bergstrom, N., Bennett, M. A., Carlson, C. E., et al. (1994). *Treatment of pressure ulcers. Clinical practice guidelines, no. 15.* AHCPR Publication No. 95-0652. Rockville, MD: U.S. Department of Health and Human Services. Public Health Service, Agency for Health Care Policy and Research.

Centers for Medicare and Medicaid Services (CMS). Action Plan (For Further Improvement of) Nursing Home Quality. Retrieved January 5, 2005, from *www.cms.hhs.gov/quality/nhqi/ NHActionPlan.pdf.*

Cuddigan, J., Ayello, E. A., & Sussman, C. (Eds.). (2001). *Pressure ulcers in America: Prevalence, incidence, and implications for the future.* Reston, VA: National Pressure Ulcers Advisory Panel.

Fleck, C. A. (2005). New CMS pressure ulcer guidelines. *Extended Care Product News, 97,* 37-42.

Frykberg, R. G. (2005). A summary of guidelines for managing the diabetic foot. *Advances in Skin and Wound Care, 18,* 209-214.

Hunt, D., Verzier, N., Abend, S., & Lyder, C. (2005). *Fundamentals of Medicare patients' safety surveillance: Intent, relevance, and transparency.* U. S. Agency for Health Research and Quality for the Patient Safety Advances Compendium. Rockville, MD: Agency for Healthcare Research and Quality.

Institute of Medicine. (1999). *To err is human: Building a safer health system.* Washington, DC: National Academy Press.

Johnston, P. (2005, May/June). Quality wound management: Linking staff education and wound care competency. *Remington Report, 13*(3), 28-30.

Lyder, C. H. (2005). Pressure ulcers in long-term care: CMS initiative. *Extended Care Product News, 97,* 19-20.

Lyder, C., Grady, J., Mathur, D., Patrello, M., & Meehan, T. (2004). Preventing pressure ulcers in Connecticut hospitals using the plan-do-study-act model for quality improvement. *Joint Commission Journal of Quality and Safety, 30,* 205-214.

Motta, G. J. (2001). Regulatory issues and reimbursement. In D. L. Krasner, G. T. Rodeheaver, & R. G. Sibbald (Eds.), *Chronic wound care: A clinical source book for healthcare professionals* (3rd ed). Wayne, PA: HMP Communications.

Panel for the Prediction and Prevention of Pressure Ulcers in Adults. (1992). Pressure ulcers in adults: Prediction and prevention. Clinical practice guidelines, no. 3. AHCPR Publication No. 92-0047. Rockville, MD: U.S. Department of Health and Human Services. Public Health Service, Agency for Health Care Policy and Research.

Ratliff, C. R. (2005). WOCN's evidence-based pressure ulcer guideline. *Advances in Skin & Wound Care, 18,* 204-208.

Stephens, E. D. (2004, November/December). The financial and clinical benefits of outcome based quality improvement: Better care at less cost. *Remington Report, 12*(6), 30-31.

Twiss, A., Lang, C., & Rooney, H. (2005, March/April). Pay for performance preparedness. *Remington Report, 13*(2),18-22.

# FALLS AND PUBLIC POLICY: CREATING A BLUEPRINT FOR CHANGE

Deanna Gray-Miceli

*"Change your thoughts and you change your world."*
                                        NORMAN VINCENT PEALE

As I traveled home from a conference hosted by the John A. Hartford Foundation in Washington, a conversation unfolded with an older couple waiting for the same train. The gentleman asked me, "What do you do?" I replied, "I'm a nurse and have a special interest in older people who fall." I quickly discovered that I was speaking to a trustee of the Robert Wood Johnson Foundation whose elderly mother recently had been institutionalized after a fall. As an advocate, I offered help. We exchanged business cards at the end of the conversation. I felt as though I had offered some much-needed information about her fall that appeared to be a surprise. Why did they not know the seemingly obvious cause of their mother's fall? Had no explanations been given by her care providers? Had the providers attributed the fall to old age? How could the fall have been prevented? How would the institution improve its ability to prevent falls in the future?

## FALLS AS A PUBLIC HEALTH PROBLEM

### Scope and Magnitude of Falls

Falls are a major public health problem, with no geographic boundaries or age predilections, as evidenced by the following statistics:

- Falls rank as the sixth leading cause of fatal unintentional injuries among infants under 1 year of age and adults 55 to 64 years of age in the United States (National Center for Injury Prevention and Control, 2003).

- Falls account for 49% of deaths among adults aged 60 to 69 and 66% of deaths among adults aged 70 or older (Runyan et al., 2005).

- In 1999, among people of all ages, nearly 4 million emergency department visits and 4.2 million office-based physician visits were because of falls (Runyan et al., 2005).

Table 10-1 illustrates the pervasiveness of home injuries resulting from fall events across all age groups. Health care facilities also experience a similarly high rate of falls that are injurious.

- In nursing homes, nearly 75% of residents experience a fall each year (Rubenstein, Josephson, & Robbins, 1994).

- In 2000, over 7 million persons of all ages were treated in hospital emergency departments in the

**TABLE 10-1** National Estimates and Rates for Nonfatal, Unintentional Home Injuries Caused by Falls, by Age Group (United States, 1998)

| AGE GROUP (IN YEARS) | NUMBER (PERCENT) | RATE PER 100,000 (95% C1) |
|---|---|---|
| 0-14 | 1,520,728 (27.2%) | 2541 (2060-3021) |
| 15-24 | — | — |
| 25-44 | 1,237,064 (22.1%) | 1491 (1127-1856) |
| 45-64 | 908,480 (16.2%) | 1603 (1245-1960) |
| 65-74 | 522,156 (9.3%) | 2902 (1991-3812) |
| >75 | 1,090,768 (19.5%) | 7669 (5986-9351) |
| Total | 5,596,700 (100%) | 2081 (1864-2297) |

From Runyan, C. W., Perkis, D., Marshall, S. W., Johnson, R.M., Coyne-Beasley, T., et al. (2005). Unintentional injuries in the home environment in the United States. Part II: Morbidity. *American Journal of Preventive Medicine, 28,* 80-87.

**213**

United States for nonfatal injuries due to falls (National Center for Injury Prevention and Control, 2003).

- Serious injuries from falls include hip fracture, (Williams-Johnsons, Wilks, & McDonald, 2004).
- For those 75 years of age and older, falls are the leading cause of the 50,000 deaths that arise from traumatic brain injury (Adekoya, Thurman, White, & Webb, 2002).
- Estimated economic costs of fall-related injuries sustained in the home totaled over $90 billion in 1998 (Zaloshnja, Miller, Lawrence, & Romano, 2005).

Besides the physical injury, costs, and loss of work, falls—especially serious ones—often change lives forever (Gray-Miceli, 2001).

### The Need for a Public Policy Response

Given the impact of falls on individuals, families, and society, a policy response is essential if falls are to be uniformly reduced across all sectors of society. We must ask: Are we doing enough to prevent falls from occurring? What can society do to better understand and prevent falls at home, in the community, and in health care facilities?

This policy spotlight will lay a foundation for developing a public policy response to falls, illustrating the myriad policy options aimed at the primary and secondary prevention of falls. These options include increasing public and provider awareness of the multifactorial nature of fall prevention and management, developing public health initiatives that will provide technical assistance to local health departments and health care organizations, and suggesting changes in the current use of the public health surveillance system. These policy responses will be illustrated through the example of New Jersey's decision to introduce fall-related goals into their health agenda for the new millennium (New Jersey Department of Health and Senior Services [NJDHSS], 2001), with the outcome of the hiring of a clinical scholar to develop statewide fall-prevention initiatives. I am that clinical scholar. As a geriatric nurse practitioner, I was able to play a role in lessening the burden of statewide morbidity and mortality from falls in New Jersey.

### FACTORS INFLUENCING THE PRIMARY PREVENTION OF FALLS

Early in my employment in state government, I realized that one of the most daunting challenges I faced was how to implement an unfunded initiative. In addition, I had to consider how to implement a fall-prevention initiative within a large, complex public health system. Indeed, I learned that other states share this challenge. Infrastructure issues complicate the prevention of falls by any public health system. Such issues include the following:

- A lack of coordinated services across programs and services that have clients who experience falls
- A lack of funding to support initiatives developed
- An underutilized public health surveillance system

One positive factor serving as a catalyst for change, however, is that all service providers, stakeholders, and public health officials are committed to promoting the health, safety, and general welfare to the public they serve. Therefore there was a vested interest in the aims of the initiative among administrative officials of three divisions within the public health department—Aging and Community Services, Long-Term Care Systems, and Health Care Quality Oversight. The idea that the health of New Jersey residents could be improved through a fall-prevention initiative engendered their interest and support.

### DEVELOPING A POLICY RESPONSE

A national policy for fall prevention does not currently exist. Rather, action plans exist such as those based on national objectives identified in *Healthy People 2010*, as well as those adopted within individual state plans on aging in New Jersey, Washington, California, and Florida, for example. Although embryonic, there is a movement toward a national public policy for fall prevention. California is leading the way in the development of a prototype model, funded by the Archstone Foundation. It is uniting academic schools of public health and medicine and the state department of health. But those involved in this initiative acknowledge the constraints imposed by limited resources.

In the absence of a national public policy for fall prevention, local and state health departments have adopted elements of a well-developed injury prevention paradigm recommended by the State and Territorial Injury Prevention Director's Association (STIPDA). The blueprint for injury prevention overall can also guide fall prevention by focusing efforts on:

- Statewide and local data collection and analysis
- Program design, implementation, and evaluation
- Coordination and collaboration
- Technical support and training
- Policy development

Although many factors contribute to the absence of a national public policy for fall prevention, none is more salient than the societal context of how falls are perceived by the public and health care providers. If fall prevention is to occur at an aggregate level, societal views of falling, data collection about falls, and databases must be revamped.

### Societal Views of Falls

When we think about falls we tend to think about injuries. It's almost expected that after a fall, an injury will follow, particularly in the elderly. Although this is sometimes the case, it is not always so. A long-standing misconception is that falls are largely a result of environmental accidents. Indeed, falls are still recognized and often managed as isolated events rather than as possible syndromes or outcomes related to other multiple factors and causes. Changing this misconception is paramount if we are to fully embrace the concept that falls should be prevented among all age groups.

Falls can be attributed to the following:

- Medications (Kelly et al., 2004; Leipzig, Cumming & Tinetti, 1999; Neutel, Perry, & Maxwell, 2002)
- Chronic diseases (Shaw, 2002; Stolze et al., 2004)
- Acute diseases (Ooi, Hossain, & Lipsitz, 2000; Mukai & Lipsitz, 2002)
- Environmental conditions (Gill, Williams, Robinson, & Tinetti, 1999; Connell, 1996).)
- Age (Davies, Steen, & Kenny, 2001)
- Idiopathic phenomena

Two other major factors shape the misconception of falls as accidents: how fall data are coded and an underdeveloped public health surveillance system for fall prevention.

### Data Obtained about Falls: The E Code Nomenclature

The International Classification of Diseases (ICD, 2001) provides health providers with a tool for coding disease entities and events for diagnosis and reimbursement. This international reference classifies falls as events associated with external causes of injury—"E" codes. E codes refer to environmental events and circumstances that are the mechanism responsible for the injury. Table 10-2 identifies examples of E codes available for fall coding. This listing of available E codes is limited, because it does not include falls that occur for other reasons, such as adverse effects of medications, acute illnesses, or chronic diseases.

Should a serious disease-related event occur within a person and result in a fall (e.g., severe anemia causing generalized weakness and a fall, or cardiac syncope causing a sudden blackout and a fall), use of the current E code classification will not capture these antecedents. Expansion of this current E code nomenclature must occur if we are to understand and prevent falls within a population such as the elderly, who experience falls as a result of disease-related causes (e.g., "fall related to syncope" or "fall related to orthostatic hypotension"). Note that in order for these changes to be applied to practice, a more comprehensive and uniform post-fall assessment is needed that can identify such causes.

In the long run, the use of the current listing of E codes without further expansion to other causes

**TABLE 10-2**   Examples of Accidental Falls: E800-E999 Codes

| FALLS OCCURRING (IN OR FROM) | ASSIGNED E CODE |
| --- | --- |
| Burning building | E890.8 |
| Fall on or from sidewalk curb | E880.1 |
| Fall from chair | E884.2 |
| Fall from bed | E884.4 |
| Unspecified fall | E888.9 |

From *International classification of diseases* (ICD)-9-CM (9th revision). (2001). Los Angeles, CA: Practice Management Information Management.

creates two problems: (1) it perpetuates a notion that falls are all extrinsically caused by environmental conditions, and (2) it limits linkages to other variables that together can help build the science of all fall-related occurrences. Any public policy that includes monitoring data by use of E codes must first consider the multifactorial nature of falls and represent this information in an expanded classification of falls. State departments of health have the authority to introduce new codes of diseases or conditions into existing databases and to trend data accordingly.

## Underutilization of Public Health Surveillance Systems

In almost all state databases, fall and injury data are collected. Fall-related data exist in both administrative and surveillance databases. Typically data are extrapolated from these sources to trend the incidence of falls related to demographic characteristics such as age or gender, time of the fall or injury, geographic distribution of fall and injury rates, associated fatalities, and emergency department visits or hospitalization rates. Linkages of fall-related variables to data concerning specific medications or specific diseases are less common.

Clearly a policy is needed for establishing a comprehensive data registry that would include the various factors that can contribute to the occurrence of falls and subsequent injuries. This registry could tabulate and trend incidences and prevalence of falls across all age groups as they occur in relation to other comorbid conditions, disease states, and medications. Furthermore, this registry could form the foundation for *data-based* clinical programs and services. In clinical practice settings, this sort of information is vital in order to allocate resources and plan care appropriately. A registry such as this could also help to develop the much-needed classification scheme for coding of fall-related events, other than the current E codes.

***Lack of a uniform reporting mechanism from health care facilities.*** In health care facilities such as nursing homes, in which the rate of falls is the highest, there exists no uniform reporting mechanism. The best estimates of fall rates are not necessarily derived from the Minimum Data Set

(MDS), the largest repository of national data from nursing homes, but rather on quarterly summaries and aggregate incident reports. The entry of a fall into the MDS is conditional, entered under certain circumstances, and not universal. The MDS captures Medicare beneficiaries' annual admissions and readmissions for patients having a significant change in their function, such as that resulting from injury. It does not represent the majority of residents, many of whom are long-stay residents covered by Medicaid.

When data from the MDS are used for surveillance (not its intended purpose), problems arise for the clinician and the older resident. Consider the following example. A resident falls; the RN performs an assessment then enters the information about the fall into the MDS. When asked to identify the time frame of the fall occurrence, such as within 30 days or between 31 and 180 days, the RN enters "within 30 days." This fall occurrence is identified in the MDS system as "yes" or "no," but the fall frequency is not. You may wonder whether this really matters. From a clinical standpoint, it matters a great deal. If a fall occurrence is once per patient per 30 days, one check is entered, signaling a trigger for reassessment. But if the older adult falls eight times in 30 days, still only one check is entered. The clinical implications of one fall versus several falls are enormous. Greater medical attention is clinically warranted for the resident who falls frequently, as a standard of appropriate medical and nursing care. In addition, plans of care and level of supervision might need to change accordingly. Changing this fall-related variable from a "check" to a number can significantly influence patient care and clinical practice.

Table 10-3 outlines a blueprint for addressing a lack of uniform data reporting for falls.

## FALL POLICY IN NEW JERSEY
### Extent of the Problem

For the first time since 1998, *unintentional injuries* has taken the position as the fifth leading cause of death in New Jersey (NJDHSS, 2002). In addition:

- In addition to motor vehicle deaths, falls were the leading cause of injury deaths for those 65 years and over (NJDHSS, 2002).

**TABLE 10-3** Selected Components of a Blueprint for Fall Reform

| Issue: Lack of uniform documentation and fall reporting |
|---|

| POSSIBLE SOLUTION | POSSIBLE OUTCOME(S) |
|---|---|
| Uniform documentation of fall events | Consistent information Determine Fall Patterns |
| Standardized Post-Fall Assessment (age-appropriate) | Develop programs and services |
| Uniform case definitions of fall types | Expand current fall taxonomy |
| Uniform reporting of fall incidences to state Departments of Health | Estimate fall incidence/ prevalence so that targeted programs can be identified |
| Addendums to E codes reflective of all possible fall etiologies | Linkages of falls to all associated events |
| Public Health Fall Surveillance Registry integrated across multiple departments | Aggregate fall incidence and prevalence Develop interventions based on demography and geography |

- The rate of traumatic brain injury from falls is highest in the oldest age groups (65 years and over), although falls are also the leading cause of traumatic brain injury for those under 15 years of age (NJDHSS, 2004).
- In the labor force, falls occur more often among workers age 55 years and older, accounting for 18% of fatal work-related injuries (NJDHSS, 2003).

Given the populations affected and the extent of the impact of falls, New Jersey had to address how to develop a comprehensive, effective policy that could be implemented without an infusion of substantial new funds. For each policy initiative developed, consideration was given to the ease of implementation and to the potential for high impact in terms of service provision and/or data acquisition.

In the early 1990s a committee within the Bureau of Health Statistics at NJDHSS focused on injury prevention across the lifespan. Shortly thereafter the governor-appointed Osteoporosis Council was established, mainly to monitor the high rate of hip

fractures in the state. The epidemiology of injury, its incidence, and its magnitude documented the need for focused attention in this area, including the recognition that falls needed to be included as an integral part of an injury prevention program.

Two objectives related to seniors were included in *Healthy New Jersey 2010.* Objective 4 calls for reducing the death rate per 100,000 population from falls of persons aged 65 and over to 12 for persons aged 65-84 years and to 105 for persons aged 85+ years. Objective 8 calls for reducing annual hospitalization rates for hip fractures among seniors 65 years of age and older. Although the objectives and deliverables for 2010 are clear, less clear are what initiatives should be introduced that can be successfully adopted, when should they be introduced, and by whom. Delays occurred because we needed a formalized strategic plan, which might include a governor-appointed task force or proposed legislation.

Several initiatives were considered. Selection of the initiatives and finalization occurred through ongoing dialogue with representative stakeholders. Ease of implementation through existing programs without incurring high costs was a major consideration, along with the option's fit within the context of a public health model. Therefore the options proposed had to address either the primary or the secondary prevention of falls and related injuries. Supporting evidence for the likelihood of success of any one option was also obtained through a review of the literature on effective, evidenced-based interventions.

Primary prevention concerns health promotion and health protection, with a focus on preventing the fall from occurring at all. Targeted high-risk populations and high-risk behaviors for falls occurring among seniors in the community fit into this category. The secondary prevention of falls concerns the early diagnosis and treatment, with a goal of preventing prolonged disability or complications from falls. Options that targeted high-risk populations within health care facilities or patients who have already fallen fit into this category.

### Primary Prevention

*Fall prevention tool kit initiative.* Within the scope of primary prevention, development of a Fall Prevention Tool Kit was selected as one of the first initiatives. This Tool Kit is a series of educational brochures that focused on falls across all age groups, their multifactorial causes, associated high-risk situations, and their prevention and management. Content in the brochures provide the foundation for viewing falls as not simply the result of environmental accidents but as having common causes among people of all ages that are preventable. The Fall Prevention Tool Kit contains three brochures geared toward a general public with low literacy; the brochures focus on (1) general knowledge about falls, (2) medications and fall-related events, and (3) environmental and high-risk hazards. Costs for the brochure were drawn from existing budget lines. The major disadvantage associated with the Fall Prevention Tool Kit is the inability to formally monitor its impact in terms of fall incidence reduction.

Brochures were printed and made available for distribution to the many community-based programs serving older adults in the Aging and Community Services Division. Public Health employees, many of whom are caregivers to children and older adults, were also targeted recipients of the Tool Kit. In terms of dissemination, aside from the existing programs targeting older adults and falls, this brochure will be used in New Jersey Health Fairs, throughout the Department of Personnel (for employee caregivers), and through the Division of Occupational Safety. Information contained within the brochures will be posted online on the state's health promotion Website. It is anticipated that the Fall Prevention Tool Kit will be used in other, related projects.

***The first health initiative.*** At the request of the administrative officials, we partnered with First Health, New Jersey's major vendor for pharmaceutical assistance to over 400,000 seniors. This initiative involved the development of a pharmaceutical intervention for older adults at risk of falling because the geriatric literature has documented that prescribed medications have been associated with falls. This initiative, involving consumers, pharmacists, and prescribers, carries a low price tag; it includes a single mailing to the beneficiaries, the Fall Prevention Tool Kit, and a follow-up survey of the intervention's effectiveness.

As of 2005, more than 1500 individuals had been identified as potential recipients of information about high-risk medications linked to falling. Plans are underway for identified persons, and their prescribers to receive the informational Fall Prevention Tool Kit and to respond to a survey about its usefulness.

### Educational Videotape for Fall Prevention for Seniors

Consistent with a primary prevention initiative for increasing public awareness is the idea of compelling videotapes marketed for seniors that incorporate state-of-the-science information about the multifactorial nature of falls, injuries and their prevention. The main consideration of this initiative was funding for the development of a product, not necessarily dissemination. One of my major roles has been to apply for the grant funding that would allow for the production of the video. This video will become an important adjunct to the Fall Prevention Tool Kit for fall prevention. Funding is pending.

### Secondary Prevention

***Technical assistance initiative.*** Additional initiatives were requested for inclusion in the plan for Public Health Priority Funding. Areas previously targeted in this plan included Senior Health Initiatives related to osteoporosis, injury prevention, and arthritis. The opportunity to add a public health initiative related to fall prevention was seized. If supported, this initiative will provide access for technical support to any of New Jersey's 21 community-based Area Agencies on Aging. In a recent needs survey conducted on these 21 county offices on aging, data were collected related to existing fall prevention services and potential interest in collaboration on the development of fall-prevention activities. Of the 21 counties, 13 responded, all identifying this as a priority need for stakeholders.

The major disadvantage of implementing this objective relates to a lack of consolidated manpower in fall prevention. However, including this initiative sets the stage for many other important projects such as training opportunities for RNs serving high-risk age groups in the community. It is expected that linkages to public health schools will help in implementing this initiative.

Inquiries about this provision have been received from county offices on aging and health care organizations. The state is working on developing memoranda of agreement to provide technical assistance to interested health care organizations that are academically based. In-house program development regarding fall prevention and injury reduction is targeted for RNs serving the thousands of older residents in New Jersey who are at high risk of falling or who have fallen.

***Reducing falls in hospitalized older adults.*** The New Jersey legislature sanctioned the development of a training initiative directed at providers in acute care hospitals. In February of 2005, New Jersey joined several other states in the nation to make adverse event reporting mandatory. Public Safety Law requires that acute care institutions report adverse events, including falls, to the New Jersey Department of Health. A group of administrative officials supervises the enactment of this legislation and its outcomes. As part of a quality improvement initiative, the DHSS has partnered with the Health Care Quality and Oversight Division to offer a training workshop on fall prevention to all general hospitals.

This training program directed at increasing knowledge about falls and their causes was constructed and discussed with the administrative officials overseeing the Health Care Quality and Oversight Division for hospitals. We have planned a 2-day workshop over three cycles, free of charge, for designated hospital personnel involved in patient care and patient safety. The targeted audience is 50 general hospitals, each appointing three representatives. The content of the program will help these facilities to develop their own quality improvement initiative or best practice approach, including policy and procedures related to evidence-based assessment and intervention for fall prevention and management. The major advantage of this initiative will be the ability to evaluate its effectiveness in the primary and secondary prevention of falls.

The first cycle of workshops was delivered in October and January of 2006, with training provided to 14 hospitals and 42 employees. All participants developed and implemented a fall prevention initiative on one or more hospital units. Important outcomes realized were team collaboration and best practice approaches to reduce falls. Participants received continuing education credits. Long-term outcomes being measured are reductions in fall incidence and associated injuries.

## Lessons Learned

These fall-prevention initiatives are in progress or have been implemented successfully thus far and can serve as a model for other policy initiatives aimed at reducing the incidence of falls and their consequent injuries. Those replicating this work should consider the following points:

- Design initiatives with ease of implementation in mind and without a large monetary outlay unless funding is not an issue.
- We still need long-term data on important outcome measures such as fall incidence and prevalence to demonstrate the cost benefit of these initiatives. The aggregate costs of falls and injuries to the victims, their families, and the state will need to be considered.
- There are many interrelated factors for consideration when developing a public policy for reducing falls. All factors are equally important, ranging from increasing knowledge or changing myths and preconceived ideas about falls to analyzing how fall-related data are coded, collected, and analyzed.
- Changing the current perception of falling and developing the data systems for fall surveillance is not easy and will require the understanding and support of key stakeholders and administrative public officials.
- The issue of a lack of resource allocations and budget appropriations is of national importance if there is to be a public policy approach to reducing falls and their associated injuries in the United States.

## Web Resources

**National Center for Injury Prevention and Control, Centers for Disease Control and Prevention (CDC)—A Tool Kit to Prevent Senior Falls.**
*www.cdc.gov/ncipc/pub-res/toolkit/toolkit.htm*
**New Jersey Department of Health and Senior Services (NJDHSS)—Healthy New Jersey 2010. Volume I: A Health Agenda for the First Decade of the New Millennium.**
*www.state.nj.us/health/chs*

## REFERENCES

Adekoya, N., Thurman, D. J., White, D. D., & Webb, K. W. (2002). Surveillance for traumatic brain injury deaths—United States, 1989-1998. *MMWR Surveillance Summaries, 51*(10), 1-14.

Connell, B. R. (1996). Role of the environment in falls prevention. *Clinics in Geriatric Medicine, 12*(4), 859-880.

Davies, A. J., Steen, N., & Kenny, R. A. (2001). Carotid sinus hypersensitivity is common in older patients presenting to an accident and emergency department with unexplained falls. *Age and Ageing, 30*(4), 273-274.

Gill, T. M., Williams, C. S., Robinson, J. T., & Tinetti, M. E. (1999). A population based study of environmental hazards in the homes of older persons. *American Journal of Public Health, 89*(4), 553-556.

Gray-Miceli, D. L. (2001). Changed life: A phenomenological study of the meaning of serious falls to older adults (doctoral dissertation, Widener University, 2001). *UMI Dissertation Abstracts* (UMI No. 30005877).

*International classification of diseases* (ICD)-9-CM (9th revision). (2001). Los Angeles: Practice Management Information Management.

Kelly, K. D., Pickett, W., Yiannakoulias, N., Rowe, B. H., Schopflocher, D. P., et al. (2004). Medication use and falls in community-dwelling older persons. *Age and Ageing, 32*(5), 503-509.

Leipzig, R. M., Cumming, R. G., & Tinetti, M. E. (1999). Drugs and falls in older people: A systematic review and meta-analysis: Cardiac and analgesic drugs. *Journal of the American Geriatrics Society, 47*(1), 40-50.

Mukai, S., & Lipsitz, L. A. (2002). Orthostatic hypotension. *Clinics in Geriatric Medicine, 18*(2), 253-268.

National Center for Injury Prevention and Control, Centers for Disease Control and Prevention (CDC). (2003). Injury research agenda. Retrieved February 19, 2006, from *www.cdc.gov/ncipc/pub-res/research_agenda/02_introduction.htm.*

National Center for Injury Prevention and Control, Centers for Disease Control and Prevention (CDC). (2005). A tool kit to prevent senior falls. Retrieved February 20, 2006, from *www.cdc.gov/ncipc/pub-res/toolkit/toolkit.htm.*

Neutel, C. I., Perry, S., & Maxwell, C. (2002). Medication use and risk of falls. *Pharmacoepidemiological Drug Safety, 11*(2), 97-104.

New Jersey Department of Health and Senior Services (NJDHSS). (2001). Healthy New Jersey 2010. Volume I: A health agenda for the first decade of the new millennium. Trenton, NJ. Retrieved February 19, 2006, from *www.state.nj.us/health/chs.*

New Jersey Department of Health and Senior Services (NJDHSS). (2002). New Jersey health statistics 2002. Trenton, NJ. Retrieved February 19, 2006, from *www.state.nj.us/health/chs.*

New Jersey Department of Health and Senior Services (NJDHSS). (2003). NJ census of fatal occupational injuries 2003, Trenton, NJ. Retrieved August 10, 2005, from *www.nj.gov/health/eoh/survweb/odispubs.htm.*

New Jersey Department of Health and Senior Services (NJDHSS). (2004). Central nervous system injury, 2000. Trenton, NJ. Retrieved December 20, 2005, from *www.state.nj.us/health/chs/tbi00/index.html.*

Ooi, W. L., Hossain, M., & Lipsitz, L. A. (2000). The association between orthostatic hypotension and recurrent falls in nursing home residents. *American Journal of Medicine, 108*(2), 106-111.

Rubenstein, L. Z., Josephson, K. R., & Robbins, A. S. (1994). Falls in the nursing home. *Annals of Internal Medicine, 121*, 442-451.

Runyan, C. W., Casteel, C., Pekis, D., Black, C., Marshall, S. W., et al. (2005). Unintentional injuries in the homes in the United States. Part I: Mortality. *American Journal of Preventive Medicine, 28*(1), 73-79.

Runyan, C. W., Perkis, D., Marshall, S. W., et al. (2005). Unintentional injuries in the home environment in the United States. Part II: Morbidity. *American Journal of Preventive Medicine, 28*, 80-87.

Shaw, F. E. (2002). Falls in cognitive impairment and dementia. *Clinical Geriatric Medicine, 18*(2), 159-173.

Stolze, H., Klebe, S., Zechlin, C., Baecker, C., Friege, L., & Deuschl, G. (2004). Falls in frequent neurological diseases—prevalence, risk factors and etiology. *Journal of Neurology, 251*(1), 79-84.

Williams-Johnson, J. A., Wilks, R. J., & McDonald, A. H. (2004). Falls: A modifiable risk factor for the occurrence of hip fractures in the elderly. *West Indian Medical Journal, 53*(4), 238-241.

Zaloshnja, E., Miller, T. R., Lawrence, B., & Romano, E. (2005). The costs of unintentional home injuries. *American Journal of Preventive Medicine, 28*(1), 88-94.

# chapter 11

# Conflict Management: A Critical Part of Politics

Alma Yearwood Dixon

*"Conflict builds character. Crisis defines it."*

STEVEN V. THULON

It had been a long and difficult shift. As too often happens, nurses called in sick. The census was high, and the patients required several different treatments and procedures. Sitting in the conference room, the nurse was determined to finish the endless paperwork so that she could leave on time. In fact, if she hurried she might be able to leave a little early—perhaps get to the post office before it closed, to mail the package she had been carrying all week. She might even make it to the cleaners. A smile crossed her face as she relished the thought of some time to complete errands that all needed to be accomplished but that too often had to wait because she simply ran out of time. Not enough time was starting to feel like her lifestyle, but maybe today would be different. Then she heard her name called to answer a page from the Emergency Department. Her heart sank, and for good reason. True to form, the ED nurse on the phone said he was sending up a patient. She knew the patient probably had been in the ED all shift and could have been sent up earlier. Her anger started to rise as she struggled with how to respond to the ED nurse's call.

Whenever two people interact, the potential for conflict exists because of the unique way that each person perceives the situation, processes information, and forms an opinion. Conflict within the work setting is a natural occurrence as people define and

work toward common goals. The need to work for a "common good" facilitates conflict resolution. However, the current environment in health care has resulted in increased discord among staff, who are being engulfed by changes dictated by socioeconomic forces outside the profession. These changes are driving nursing education and practice in profoundly different ways. Consensus building and teamwork are more difficult because the players and the playing field are unfamiliar. Therefore nurses need to acquire new skills in conflict resolution and the art of negotiation.

## TYPES OF CONFLICT

Conflict can be defined as the internal discord that occurs as a result of incongruity or incompatibility in ideas, values, or beliefs of two or more people. As opposed to a misunderstanding, conflict is more than a failure in interpretation; it usually represents some combination of a perceived threat to power or social position, scarcity of resources, and differing value systems. Conflict induces incompatible or antagonistic actions between two people or among groups (Ury, 2000).

Conflict can take many forms. It can occur in a concentric fashion, beginning with incompatible personal thoughts, values, perceptions, or actions (intrapersonal conflict). It can then radiate to differences in relationships between individuals (interpersonal conflict) or groups of people (intergroup conflict) and to incompatibility with organizational demands, policies, or procedures (organizational conflict).

## INTRAPERSONAL CONFLICT

Intrapersonal conflict occurs within the individual nurse and represents an internal struggle to clarify values, perceptions, or needs. Nurses hold many responsibilities, including responsibility to the organization, to superiors, to peers, and ultimately to patients as well as to their individual families. These responsibilities may conflict, and that conflict may be internalized. It is imperative that the nurse practice self-awareness and gain the skill in taking a personal inventory to resolve intrapersonal conflict as soon as it is felt in order to avoid impairments in physical or emotional health. This type of conflict can occur when a nurse is challenged to behave in ways that are not consistent with beliefs about professional ethics and practice, although the action may achieve organizational goals. For example, no matter where they practice, nurses are constantly challenged to question what they personally believe about health care and the practice of nursing with questions such as the following:

■ Is high-quality care sacrificed with shortened hospital stays?

■ Am I sacrificing high-quality care when I am forced to work overtime?

■ If I say no, will I have a job?

■ What is my response to a patient who is either racist or sexist when interacting with me?

■ What do I do when I cannot compromise what I believe in?

Intrapersonal conflict can serve as the impetus for personal growth and change. According to Kritek (1994), conflicts are teaching experiences that call forth a commitment to courage, self-honesty, and learning. Recognizing that conflict resolution requires an exploration of alternatives, "one is divested of the illusion of a belief in 'the one right way,' [and] the doors open to a myriad of ways, each with some truth and some distortion" (Kritek, 1994, p. 21). And, as Lappe and Perkins (2005) suggest, our troubled world, with its global-wide warring factions will only improve when as individuals we accept responsibility to face the conflict and view it as an opportunity for mutual engagement and learning, rather than trying to keep the lid on conflict or using conflict as a means of dominating a situation.

## INTERPERSONAL CONFLICT

Conflict between individuals can be manifested by angry, hostile, or passive behaviors. These behaviors may be verbal, nonverbal, or physical. According to Brinkman and Kirschner (1994), interpersonal conflict occurs when the emphasis is placed on differences between people, and as a result, "united we stand, divided we can't stand each other" (p. 38).

Interpersonal conflict can impair working relationships, hinder productivity, and damage morale. Brinkman and Kirschner (1994) suggest strategies of blending and redirecting to resolve conflict in a timely and efficient manner. Blending involves reducing differences by finding common ground and mutual understanding, and redirecting is a process of using the rapport to change the trajectory of the communication toward a positive outcome.

To accomplish these strategies, one must be able to communicate and to listen until the issue is understood. The following steps are suggested:

1. Demonstrate listening and understanding by posture, voice volume, and action.
2. Backtrack or repeat some of the words used.
3. Assess nonverbal communication.
4. Clarify meaning and intent.
5. Summarize what was heard.
6. Confirm to find out whether understanding was reached.

These steps to careful listening and understanding facilitate conflict resolution by enabling the participants to define the problem clearly and by setting a climate for cooperation. Grover (2005) suggests that when assessing nonverbal communication, one should include all nonverbal cues such as facial expressions, eye movements, hand movements, posture, and use of personal space. Taken together, verbal and nonverbal communication are important indicators of messages sent and received in interpersonal relationships.

## INTERGROUP CONFLICT

*After 20 years as a nurse manager, it seemed to her that after you beat a dead horse a zillion times, it should be dead! She was so tired of the conflict between the nurses and the doctors. What amazed her most was that over the years no matter who the players were, the dialogue never changed. Well, perhaps she had to admit that the new nurses were more direct in their responses. However, the theme of lack of appreciation, lack of respect, and so on, really hadn't change over time. It was difficult to get the physicians and nurses to remove the blanket statements that implied that all nurses don't follow orders or are unavailable or all doctors are rude and act like gods.*

*No matter how many times she needed to repeat the exercise, she insisted on separating the person from the problem in order to address the problem without attacking the person involved, knowing that personal attacks hamper communication and conflict resolution. Marveling at how some staff members held onto grudges, she spent considerable time focusing on the present and not on past injustices and hurt feelings. She was firm with rules that prohibited personal attacks on others, backstabbing, and sarcasm. This enabled her to stay in the present and focus only on the problem at hand. Or, as she would often say, "Let's beat that old horse one more time!"*

Intergroup conflict occurs between two or more groups of people, departments, or organizations. When intergroup conflict occurs, the participants form cohesive teams that "circle the wagons" against the other teams, who are perceived as the enemy with opposing views. Each team tends to recognize only the positives within its membership and only the negatives within the other teams. Typical behaviors include "we/they" language, gossip and blaming, backstabbing, and sabotage.

The resolution of intergroup conflict involves a process of identifying shared goals, focusing on the benefits of differences and diversity, valuing the input of all team members, and clarifying misperceptions.

## ORGANIZATIONAL CONFLICT

Organizational conflict can reflect intrapersonal, interpersonal, and intergroup conflict. This form of conflict may occur between superiors and their subordinates or between staff and management. It usually concerns policy, power, and status. In contrast, horizontal conflict involves individuals with similar power and status in the organization.

It usually occurs over discord related to authority, expertise, or practice issues.

Organizations are large, complex social systems with interacting forces that exert influence on nursing in all practice and education settings. These influences include the constant pressures of shrinking resources and financial constraints, the expanding needs and expectations of clients, the increasing militancy of nurses and students, and the persistent problems of interprofessional competition. These influences add to the prevalence of organizational conflict.

Nurses are required to function with political astuteness and prudent skill in identifying the subtle forces that have an impact on practice. They are required to make a realistic assessment of the circumstances, discern the obvious, and grasp and comprehend the obscure. Effective nurses have a grasp of the situation, with a logical shrewdness. However, when faced with conflict, too many nurses resort to a spontaneous emotional response without thinking of circumstances or consequences.

Effective organizations are composed of competent individuals who are able to practice in environments where differences are both valued and used as the impetus for constructive change. Organizational conflict that is not resolved can result in warring factions, reduced productivity, and disruption of teamwork.

## CONFLICT RESOLUTION

Conflict resolution involves a process of negotiation toward a mutually acceptable agreement. Methods for resolving conflict may result in win-lose solutions or, ideally, in win-win solutions.

### WIN-LOSE SOLUTIONS

According to Roe (1995), win-lose solutions can be categorized in the following manner:

1. *Denial*, or *withdrawal*, involves attempts to get rid of the conflict by denying that it exists or by refusing to acknowledge it. If an issue is not important, or if it is raised at an inopportune time, denial may be an appropriate strategy. However, if the issue is important, it will not go away and may grow to a point at which it becomes unmanageable and builds to a greater complexity.

2. *Suppression,* or *smoothing over,* plays down the differences in the conflict, and the focus is placed on areas of agreement rather than on differences. Smoothing over may be appropriate for minor disagreements or to preserve a relationship. It is especially inappropriate when the involved parties are ready and willing to deal with the issue. It is important to note that the source of the conflict rarely goes away, and the conflict may surface later in a more virulent form.

3. *Power* or *dominance* methods to resolve conflict allow authority, position, majority rule, or a vocal minority to settle the conflict. Power strategies result in winners and losers, and the losers do not support the final decision in the same way that the winners do. Although this strategy may be appropriate when the group has agreed on this method of resolution, future meetings may be marred by renewal of the struggle.

4. *Compromise* is considered a mutual win-lose method of conflict resolution that involves each party's giving up something (losing) to gain and meet in the middle (winning). In our culture, compromise is viewed as a virtue. However, bargaining has serious drawbacks. For example, both sides often assume an inflated position because they are aware that they are going to have to "give a little," and they want to buffer the loss. The compromise solution may be watered down to the point of being ineffective, and there is often little real commitment to the solution. Furthermore, compromise may result in antagonistic cooperation because either or both parties perceive that they have given up more than the other. Despite these drawbacks, compromise can be useful when resources are limited, when both sides have enough leeway to give, and when this solution is necessary to forestall a total win-lose stance.

## WIN-WIN SOLUTIONS

The goal of win-win solutions is to manage discord so that the conflict is a constructive impetus for growth, innovation, and productivity. Two win-win strategies are collaboration and principled negotiation.

**Collaboration.** The goal of collaboration is for everyone to win: No one has to give up anything.

According to Marquis and Hurston (1994), "In collaboration, both parties set aside their original goals and work together to establish a supraordinate goal or common goal. Because both parties have identified the joint goal, each believes they have achieved their goal and an acceptable solution. The focus throughout collaboration remains on problem solving, and not on defeating the other party" (p. 290).

This approach to conflict resolution requires that all parties to the conflict recognize the expertise of the others. Each individual's position is valid, but the group emphasis is on solving the problem rather than on defending a particular position. All involved expect to modify original perceptions as the work of the group unfolds. The belief is that ultimately the best of the group's collective thinking will emerge because the problem is viewed from varied vantage points rather than one limited view.

Gardner (2005) identifies 10 lessons in collaboration that are useful in conflict resolution. The lessons include:

- Having an awareness of self including preconceived notions, values, and goals
- Valuing diversity in thought and feelings
- Focusing on a model of conflict that views it as a natural occurrence that provides the opportunity for deeper understanding
- Recognizing that, like clinical excellence, collaboration and conflict resolution are life-long learning skills

**Principled Negotiation.** Principled negotiation is a method of conflict resolution that is used as an alternative to positional bargaining. It was developed by the Harvard Negotiation Project and can be summarized in four basic steps, as identified by Fisher, Ury, and Patton (1992):

1. *Separate the people from the problem.* This step recognizes that all players in the negotiation are human beings with emotions, felt needs, deeply held values, and different backgrounds, experiences, and perceptions. Therefore each person views the world from a selective vantage point, and perceptions are frequently confused with reality.

Because conflict is a dynamic process that begins on an intrapersonal level and expands to include relationships among people, it is easy to understand that negotiations are often clouded by the problem and the relationships. Therefore conflict resolution that results in a battle over wills and positions fosters identification of the positions with personal egos. Those positions are defended against attack and become nonnegotiable. Saving face becomes necessary to reconcile future decisions with past positions. Moreover, arguing over positions endangers ongoing relationships and entangles the relationship with the problem.

In separating the people from the problem, one must pay careful attention to perception, emotion, and communication. Attempts are made to see the situation from the other person's viewpoint and to have an empathetic understanding of the other point of view. This includes suspending judgment and actively listening. The parties each work to avoid blaming the other for the problem or putting the worst interpretation on each action and instead discuss each perception. Emotions are valued, and creative ways are sought for their expression.

2. *Focus on interests, not on positions.* Interests define the problem, and the conflict in positions is usually a conflict among needs, desires, concerns, and fears. Interests are the motivators behind positions, and identifying them allows for alternative positions that satisfy mutual interests. Dirschel (1993, p. 164) explains:

Identify the facts and feelings behind each side's desires and concerns. Behind opposing positions often lie shared and compatible interests. If the focus is on positions rather than interests, the parties will have difficulty brainstorming other options, because they will be intent on keeping their bottom-line positions.

3. *Invent options for mutual gain.* Having only one answer to a dispute is counterproductive and leads to negotiations along a single dimension. Wiser decision-making involves a process of selection from a large number of possible solutions. The more options identified, the more chances there are for creative, productive solutions for all parties concerned.

Successful negotiations that result in several options are often impeded by seeking the single answer because it is believed that resolution to discord requires narrowing the gap between positions rather than broadening the options available. Negotiations that are bound by a "fixed-pie" approach also dictate win-lose battles because there are only a few good options to go around. (The fixed-pie approach is based on the assumption that options for resolution of a conflict are limited, as opposed to the belief that creative thinking can lead to more and better options.)

The process of brainstorming is one method to invent options without judging them. Participants in the exercise are encouraged to identify as many ideas as possible without judgment or criticism. Attempts should be made to invent ideas that meet shared interests. Shared interests can serve as common denominators in the resolution process. These interests need to be explicit and stated as goals.

4. *Insist on using objective criteria.* To ensure a wise agreement between opposing wills involves negotiation on some basis of objective criteria. These criteria need to be based on a fair standard and, ideally, be prepared in advance of the agreement. Discussion of the criteria, rather than of positions to be gained or lost, allows for deferment to a fair solution instead of bruised egos and hurt relationships.

Fisher and colleagues (1992, p. 14) conclude that, "In contrast to positional bargaining, the principled negotiation method of focusing on basic interests, mutually satisfying options, and fair standards typically results in a wise agreement. The method permits you to reach a gradual consensus on a joint decision efficiently without all the transactional costs of digging into positions only to have to dig yourself out of them."

The settings in which nurses practice and teach will continue to require expertise in conflict resolution as the challenges of transforming health care continue. According to Kritek (1994), negotiating often occurs at an "uneven table," at which some participants are at a disadvantage that others do not acknowledge. Uneven tables represent situations in which the assurance of justice, equity, or fairness is uncertain or unlikely. The nurse is challenged to recognize conflict as an impetus to change that requires personal growth, while choosing a method of conflict resolution depends on personal style and the situation. The recommendations outlined in the Web Resources are useful no matter what method you use to resolve the conflict.

## Key Points

- There is more than one method of conflict resolution; varied strategies can assist nurses in coping with intrapersonal, interpersonal, intergroup, and organizational conflict.
- Positional negotiating limits the development of creative options that can lead to win-win solutions.
- Principles negotiating requires that parties separate the people from the problem, focus on interests rather than position, and be creative in brainstorming options for a win-win solution.
- Competence in managing interpersonal and organizational discord will be essential as work groups become more diverse and the chance for differing viewpoints increases.
- Nurses can play a pivotal role in facilitating an environment in which conflict is used to enhance the exploration of new approaches and alternatives to problems.

## Web Resources

**Center for International Development and Conflict Management**
*www.cidcm.umd.edu*
**Harvard Negotiation Project**
*www.pon.harvard.edu/research/projects/hnp.php3*

**Harvard Negotiation Project's Clearinghouse**—resources on negotiation
*www.pon.org/catalog/index.php*
**International Association for Conflict Management**
*www.iacm-conflict.org*

## REFERENCES

Brinkman, R., & Kirschner, R. (1994). *Dealing with people you can't stand*. New York: McGraw-Hill.

Dirschel, K. (1993). Dynamics of conflict, and conflict management. In D. J. Mason, S. W. Talbott, & J. K. Leavitt (Eds.), *Policy and politics for nurses* (2nd ed.). Philadelphia: Saunders.

Fisher, R., Ury, W., & Patton, B. (1992). *Getting to yes: Negotiating agreement without giving in* (2nd ed.). New York: Penguin.

Gardner, D. (2005). Ten lessons in collaboration. *Online Journal of Issues in Nursing, 10*(1), 2.

Grover, S. (2005). Shaping effective communication skills and therapeutic relationships at work: The foundation of collaboration. *AAOHN Journal, 53*(4), 177-182.

Kritek, P. B. (1994). *Negotiating at an uneven table*. San Francisco: Jossey-Bass.

Lappe, F., & Perkins, J. (2005). *You have the power: Choosing courage in a culture of fear*. New York: Jeremy P. Tarcher/Penguin.

Marquis, B. & Hurston, C. (1994). *Management decision-making for nurses* (2nd ed). New York: Lippincott.

Roe, S. (1995). Managing your work setting: Positive work relationships, conflict management, and negotiations. In K. W. Vestal (Ed.), *Nursing management: Concepts and issues* (2nd ed.). Philadelphia: Lippincott.

Ury, W. (2000). The third side: Why we fight and how we can stop. New York: Penguin.

# POLICYSPOTLIGHT

## ALTERNATIVE DISPUTE RESOLUTION: A TOOL FOR MANAGING CONFLICT

Phyllis Beck Kritek

*"If the only tool you have is a hammer, you tend to see every problem as a nail."*

ABRAHAM MASLOW

Policy emerges through a political process shaped by context—shifting forces that may appear to be chosen, yet are often capricious or alternately serendipitous. I think health care policy in the United States is no exception. Examples illuminate this point:

- Instant messaging and instantaneous news coverage create information exchanges that can amplify both caprice and serendipity.
- Following U.S. Census Bureau data, we can keep tabs on the expanding number of citizens without health care coverage, which rose to 45 million by 2003, or 15.6% of the population, 11.4% of children. Young adults (aged 18 to 24 years) were the least likely to have coverage, with nearly a third (30.2%) without coverage (National Coalition on Health Care, 2005).
- End-of-life decisions, often a painful and private human dilemma, become national news, best exemplified by the tragedies associated with the end of Terri Schiavo's prolonged existence in a persistent vegetative state. This public drama, which now includes a readily accessible Internet copy of her autopsy, split the nation and created a frenzy of policy discussions and conflicts. Enhanced longevity has increased the number of age cohorts interacting about this and other human dilemmas concerning health and health care.

- The disproportionately large groups of "baby boomers" are aging with reluctance, with Botox and Cialis as indicators of the struggle. The baby boomers control the health care enterprise and are uncertain about the traits and behaviors of those who will take their jobs, leading to tensions across generations. It is estimated that 80% of the boomers will not retire when they reach retirement age; it is unclear what they will be doing (American Association of Retired Persons [AARP], 2004).
- Malpractice insurance for physicians and claims against them have expanded exponentially, health care costs continue to increase, and technology daily creates new options for interventions without concurrent deliberations about their ethical and fiscal consequences. Physicians play a leadership role in both dominant political parties—Bill Frist for the Republicans and Howard Dean for the Democrats—and their status as physicians is persistently noted as germane. The global nursing shortage has reached crisis proportions, and although work environment problems continue to explain much of the shortage, there is little evidence, outside of nursing, of the political will to significantly alter these conditions.

These examples merely scratch the surface of the contextual factors shaping health care policy and politics today, yet they serve as markers for the sense of malaise and frustration that can shape responses to the services that many people believe are most central to their continued well-being: their health care. We are a nation struggling with health care policy and politics.

It is within this context, I believe, that conflict management in health care arenas becomes urgent, and the delineation of principled conflict management becomes a moral choice with implications. Because we humans use language to understand and communicate our ideas, our first task in understanding this urgency, and its moral undergirding, is to define terms.

## DEFINING OUR TERMS

Conflict tends to be one of the most emotionally charged terms shaping any dialog on policy issues in health care, a response easily understood after studying a formal dictionary definition of the word. *Conflict* is defined as "fight, battle, war; competitive or opposing action of incompatibles; antagonistic state or action; mental struggle; the opposition of forces or persons" (Merriam Webster, 1996). It is not difficult to grasp the discomfort associated with the term. Even those who like conflict tend to like it only as an arena in which they can seek to dominate or win a fight.

This is a patently "western worldview" definition, standing in sharp contrast to alternative views of complementarity exemplified by the "eastern" symbolism of yin and yang or Barry Johnson's (1996) (consistent with reference list) description of polarity management, in which the tension of opposites is the path to expanded understanding and transformative insights. Although the latter may be a worldview embraced in theory, it is not the coin of the realm, perhaps best demonstrated by the repeated description of our culture as one that is "litigious." We anticipate battle, largely in the hope of winning. Hence, understanding conflict involves both the actual formal definition that shapes cultural discourse—and therefore politics and policy—and also the connotation, which does not posit conflict management as a goal. In the main, when engaged in conflict, we aim to prevail.

*Management* is another useful term. Among the many definitions available, the ones that serve as focus here include "to handle or direct with a degree of skill; to succeed in accomplishing, to achieve one's purpose" (Merriam Webster, 1996). Returning to the prior definition of conflict, however, one finds also that managing can mean "to make and keep compliant," a clue to the dilemma of the meaning of management in our culture, where the manager can either direct one with skill or try to keep one compliant. It is for this reason that the inclusion of the idea of "principle" emerges.

*Principled* in this discussion refers to behaviors "exhibiting, based on, or characterized by principle." *Principle* in turn refers to "a comprehensive or fundamental law, doctrine, or assumption; a rule or code of conduct. In health care, that is shaped by the age-old adage of "do no harm" (Merriam Webster, 1996). The American Nurses Association (ANA) Professional Code of Ethics (ANA, 2001) translates this dictum for nurses, and indeed addresses the issue of conflict in health care with some degree of specificity. What is posited in an emphasis on the guidance of principle is that managing conflict is shaped by a code of conduct that encourages and discourages selected behaviors.

All of this, of course, is done within a practice, where we as individuals do not succeed so much as we "carry out, apply; do or perform; work at repeatedly in order to become proficient." Although we aver that we wish to become skillful in the arena of politics and policy, it is indeed largely a practice. We hope to practice politics, which can involve "the total complex of relations between people living in society" and "the relations or conduct in a particular area of experience," in this case health care (Merriam Webster, 1996). As becomes increasingly apparent, the juxtaposition of these concepts provides a beginning sketch of a conceptual map of the inherent complexity of conflict management in health care within a political agenda—an insight that helps explain the extraordinary immobility that often shapes efforts at health care reform and the extraordinary frustration of persons seeking health care today.

There is one other term lurking here: *policy.* It exacerbates the situation. References to policy often assume dictionary definitions such as "prudence or wisdom in the management of affairs" and "a high level overall plan embracing the general goals and acceptable procedures" (Merriam Webster, 1996). These serve as my referents in this discussion. Policy, however, can also mean "management or procedure based primarily on material interest," a definition that begins to unveil the dilemmas faced not only by principled policymakers, but more immediately by health care providers, including nurses, who often feel imprisoned in "health care cost containment" as the primary and sometimes only concern in policy discussions. This also may explain why the United States is the only "developed" country that has not defined health as a human right, why we struggle in the debate over universal coverage of health care, and why we elect to call health care an "industry." Material interest is important to us. And it writes our history in important ways.

## A BRIEF HISTORY OF ALTERNATIVE DISPUTE RESOLUTION

*Conflict management* is a phrase, among others, used to refer to a burgeoning field most often labeled *Alternative Dispute Resolution* (ADR). Although there previously were varied antecedent delegalization movements in the United States (Harrington, 1982), ADR mushroomed in the 1960s and came of age in the 1990s (Dukes, 1996), the former in part a response to heightened societal conflict and an attendant litigation explosion. This led a variety of groups and individuals to search and test out mediation and its corollaries as an "alternative" to litigation, hence ADR. The backdrop used was the historical and practical experiences of labor and industrial dispute resolution and international diplomacy practices. The theoretic focus that has emerged emphasizes the replacement of decisions based on power (such as authoritarianism and competition) or based on rights or entitlement (such as litigation and adjudication) with a preference for decisions based on relationships and the interests of the disputants.

Scholars, centers, organizations, and legislation followed, applying ADR to a variety of conflict arenas including labor and industrial disputes but also consumer, community, family, environmental, organizational, governmental, and international disputes. The primary focus of these initiatives was to create mediation options for disputants by which they could reduce their obstacles to communication, explore alternatives, transcend adversarial behaviors, and address the needs of all parties with the assistance of a "third party," who was described as "neutral," a mediator (Folberg & Taylor, 1984).

Health care, it should be noted, has been slow to join this shift toward noncoercive dispute resolution.

Currently, the dominant ADR professional organization, a product of the merger of three prior major organizations, is the Association for Conflict Resolution (ACR). It has 18 professional interest groups at this time. These sections provide a useful snapshot of current areas of practice and specialization, and so I list them here to that end: Commercial, Community, Consumer, Court, Crisis Intervention, Education, Environment and Public Policy, Family, Health Care, International, Ombuds/Ombudsman, Online Dispute Resolution, Organizational Conflict Management, Research, Restorative and Criminal Justice, Spirituality, Training, and Workplace. Although the scope of practice arenas is extensive at this point in the history of ADR, and although health care is one of those arenas, it is not the most developed or integrated.

## HEALTH CARE: THE LAST FRONTIER IN ALTERNATIVE DISPUTE RESOLUTION

Robson and Morrison (2003) posit that ADR in health care is the last big ADR frontier, and they list four health care characteristics that explain why it may be less likely to use conflict management approaches in solving its problems. These include the fact that health care is a complex adaptive system, which makes it harder to understand; the widespread inequalities and imbalances of power, knowledge, and control; the widely divergent "cultures" and value systems of the various professional and nonprofessional groups working within the system; and the difficulty inherent in identifying the parties who should sit at the table. I would add that the reliance on litigation as a problem-solving device is a difficult behavior to overcome.

Harvard School of Public Health provided pioneering work in bringing ADR education to the health care community through its certificate program, directed by Dr. Leonard Marcus, where I served as an instructor for several of the early training programs. There have been no analogous health-focused certificate programs offered to date, however, and this program is currently not being offered. Debra Gerardi (an RN/JD) and her partner, Ginny Morrison, principals in Health Care

Mediations, Inc. *(www.healthcaremediations.com)*, have developed a core curriculum of programs titled "Curing Conflict" that has been offered to various health care communities numerous times, and I have been providing comparable training to nursing communities for 19 years. These efforts exemplify an investment in health care mediation training and practices. Their paucity, however, presents a sharp contrast to the overall development of programs in ADR. This stands in sharp contrast to the growing number of formal training programs available, described briefly in Box 11-1.

This is an admittedly truncated history of ADR and tends to provide highlights rather than exhaustive analysis. I have included it to provide an additional snapshot of the context of conflict management in health care. Simply stated, the resources, training programs, and personnel are available for implementing conflict management in health care. The field of health care itself, however,

---

**BOX 11-1    Expansion of Alternative Dispute Resolution: Graduate Programs**

First master's program (1982) and subsequent doctoral program in alternative dispute resolution (ADR) offered at George Mason University, Fairfax, Virginia.

By 1998, 13 universities offered graduate degrees in dispute resolution (Kroll, 1997).

■ Today, Peterson's reports 38 graduate programs, largely linked to other disciplines such as law, industrial relations, public policy, sociology, political science, and environmental science (Peterson's, 2005).

　■ Nine of the programs are at Syracuse University
　■ Seven of the programs are at George Washington University
　■ Two are at Pepperdine

　This indicates that some universities are creating cultures focused on conflict management

■ Only George Washington reports a program with a health focus, housed in the School of Public Health, with an emphasis in several degree offerings.

■ Some more recent options probably do not yet appear in Peterson's because of the rapid development of these programs.

---

has proven itself a reluctant, sometimes anxious, participant. Equally troubling are the findings often debated in the health care ADR community but recently documented by Anderson and D'Antonio (2004). ADR professionals have serious misconceptions about health care that "impede their ability to provide effective conflict-resolution services" (p. 15). More specifically, the assumptions ADR professionals make about the health care community and its various subcultures are often at odds with the self-perceptions of the participants in the health care community. For example, Anderson and D'Antonio discovered that whereas ADR professionals expected physicians to report that their primary sources of conflict were insurers and patients, physicians themselves reported that their greatest sources of conflict were other physicians and administrators (p. 16). In addition, the historic tensions between physicians and lawyers enter into these relationships, as many ADR practitioners are lawyers. The reluctance among health care providers to embrace ADR can be exacerbated by these preconceptions and historic disconnections. Hence, the bridge between these two communities is often fragile at best, sustained by a limited number of interested parties.

In lieu of investing in ADR, the health care community has invested in other related or contrasting services and programs. Certainly, the existence of ombudspersons has addressed some of the concerns of patients and their families about care or experiences that they view as troublesome. The human resources division of many health care systems and hospitals has integrated some cursory training on conflict management into their educational programs, a practice that can frustrate providers who recognize the implicit oversimplification in short courses that fail to grapple with the inherent complexity in health care conflicts. Ethics committees attempt to address the moral dilemmas that confront health care providers today and provide reasoned reflection on options and opportunities. And finally, the legal representatives of health care communities often view disputes as their terrain, where the use of the justice system is accessed using traditional approaches and models. All of these factors shed some light on the current reluctance of health care communities to become active participants in ADR.

## GOVERNMENTAL ALTERNATIVE DISPUTE RESOLUTION POLICIES

### International Alternative Dispute Resolution

The study of ADR's integration into existing governmental policy in the United States is an instructive exercise in shifting norms and values. The early implementation of ADR involved its use in international diplomacy, most apparent in the creation of the United States Institute of Peace (USIP). The USIP Website aptly describes its history and purpose as follows:

The USIP is an independent, nonpartisan federal institution created by Congress to promote the prevention, management, and peaceful resolution of international conflicts. Established in 1984, the Institute meets its congressional mandate through an array of programs, including research grants, fellowships, professional training, education programs from high school through graduate school, conferences and workshops, library services, and publications. The Institute's Board of Directors is appointed by the President of the United States and confirmed by the Senate (USIP, no date).

USIP is a low-profile agency, rarely referenced in the popular media, despite its extensive publication and public policy background work. It is perhaps a sign of the times that its most recent public media visibility was linked to the August 2003 President Bush recess appointment (hence, without congressional review or approval) of a controversial new board member, Daniel Pipes. Pipes, a Middle East scholar who founded and directs the Middle East Forum, is a prolific author with strongly stated opinions, often arguing that there is no use for negotiation or diplomacy in the Israeli-Palestinian conflict, one best solved by a total Israeli military victory.

Because his anti-Muslim views were well documented in his writings and perceived by many as racist, his appointment was highly controversial, evoking a spate of national editorials, perhaps best exemplified by the comment from the *Chicago Tribune* (April 30, 2003): "The institute is a quasi-governmental think tank dedicated to international peace and conflict-resolution. Pipes, who seems to invite conflict, is far from the ideal candidate." This anecdote exemplifies the complexity of using ADR approaches in international diplomacy and may help explain the resistance to ADR that characterizes many individual responses to its potential.

### Federal Agency and State Level Alternative Dispute Resolution Initiatives

The coming of age of ADR in the 1990s was in part manifested in emergent federal policy. This is best exemplified by a series of Public Laws: 101-552 in 1990, 102-354 in 1991, 104-320 in 1996, and 105-315 in 1998. The first two introduced and amended what became in 1996 the Administrative Dispute Resolution Act authorizing and encouraging federal agencies to use arbitration, mediation, negotiated rule making, and other consensual methods of dispute resolution, further expanded by the 1998 law to include all 94 federal court districts.

This legislation essentially normalized and eased the process of using ADR within all federal agencies. It encouraged agencies to design ADR systems that fit the unique needs of a given agency, supporting a range of ADR processes as options. These included binding arbitration, conciliation, cooperative problem solving, dispute panels, early neutral evaluation, facilitation, fact finding, mediated arbitration, minitrials, settlement conferences, nonbinding arbitration, ombudsmen (later changed to gender neutral *ombuds*), partnering, and peer review panels.

During the ensuing years, various federal agencies have implemented this legislation, with initial emphasis on employee disputes. This implementation can be traced by visiting the Websites of the various agencies (see the general information Website *www.eeoc.gov/federal/adr/clearinghouse*). Subsequent to the 1996 legislation, in 1998 President Clinton issued a memorandum to the heads of executive departments and agencies creating a "Working Group" to facilitate and encourage agency use of ADR methods. Colsky (2002) provides a brief but informative discussion of the various groups enabling this implementation process.

Because these federal initiatives were largely motivated by an interest in decreasing the costs associated with litigation, not surprisingly, ADR is gradually filtering down to grassroots communities. An example of interest to health care providers is a mediation program initiated by the Centers for Medicare and Medicaid Services, those agencies that fund and regulate the country's largest health insurance program. Under the aegis of quality control, a "Beneficiary Complaint Response Program" was initiated in September 2003 and offers beneficiaries mediation for complaints associated with "perceptions of clinical quality of care issues and communication," noting that this is only the initial focus of the mediation program, with an implicit expectation of expansion to other kinds of patient complaints (Centers for Medicare and Medicaid Services, 2004).

State level interest in the use of ADR has also grown, in part through the efforts of the ADR community and in part as a result of the filtering-down process from federal initiatives. Executive orders are most often the tool of choice for encouraging the use of ADR practices for state government disputes. At this time at least nine states have such executive orders aimed at the implementation of dispute resolution processes: Alabama, Florida, Massachusetts, Minnesota, Montana, New Mexico, Oregon, Pennsylvania, and Utah.

Federal and state initiatives have created a climate in which ADR is gradually becoming normalized. Incursion into health care disputes places this potential for normative policy within the health care community's purview and demonstrates the importance of informed awareness of local, state, and national ADR developments that may change current health care practices and policies. It is in the interest of all health care providers to become aware of these developments.

## PRINCIPLED CONFLICT MANAGEMENT

As is apparent from the federal initiatives outlined above, there is a range of practices that fall within the general description of ADR. All assume a dispute in which parties are pursuing their own interests. All posit that a nonadversarial process can create the conditions for a resolution of the dispute. Whereas some processes are formal, structured, supervised, and recorded, others are more informal. Selection of an appropriate process is theoretically unique to the dispute and the disputants. In practice, this may be determined more by programs, resources, and policies available or even imposed.

Knowing that a range of options exists is important in crafting ADR policy. Maintaining a wide scope of options is an inherent assumption of ADR; in practice, this range may be dramatically reduced. As choice diminishes, the freedoms associated with moral agency incrementally decline, because conflicts often have embedded in them competition between two valued principles (e.g., justice and compassion). When options are narrowed to a limited number of solutions to such a competition, the range of solutions to a moral dilemma go unexplored. Hence, under such circumstances, principle-based ADR may become a more elusive goal.

ADR, like all fields of human endeavor, has a variety of worldviews embedded in its practices. Because all involve some type of negotiation, the worldview about the nature of negotiation is a critical prior assumption. Some practitioners embrace *distributive negotiation*, emphasizing each disputant's goal as "getting what I want" in the process, tolerating "dividing the pie" with little regard for the outcomes for others (Mayer, 2000, p. 148). This approach is familiar to readers of some business literature in which negotiation is described as successfully prevailing, often without principled guidelines shaping the process.

An approach more congruent with the "do no harm" ethical commitment of health care providers is one that is integrative in nature, in which negotiations aim to create outcomes that meet all parties' essential needs and maximize benefits for everyone (Mayer, 2000, p. 151). Although *integrative negotiation* focuses on interests, it views the parties as partners and emphasizes relationship, communication, education, and the use of a principled process. As is apparent, this approach better approximates my description of and commitment to "principled" conflict management.

Although the differences between distributive and integrative approaches to ADR are substantive, they are often not noted by proponents of one or another ADR initiative. In addition, few educational or training programs clearly report their worldview as part of their marketing. It has been my experience that many of the "canned" training programs available are dissatisfying to health care providers because they emphasize distributive processes and hence abrade the moral sensibilities of many health care providers.

Bush and Folger (Bush & Folger, 1994; Folger & Bush, 2001) are ADR theorists and practitioners who have added a further dimension to worldview options, introducing *transformative mediation*, which explores the transformative potential of conflict resolution for all parties, including the mediator, and focuses on strengths instead of weaknesses and compassion instead of selfishness. Their work has created a practitioner community and a sizable body of literature and is noteworthy for its congruence with the worldview of health care providers, particularly nurses.

A further factor to consider in exploring principled conflict management is the personal style of the individual serving as guide in the journey, variously a mediator, facilitator, or third-party neutral of some type. The latter designation is the most noteworthy, because neutrality is more an ideal than a reality. In addition, the degree of commitment to self-reflection and self-evaluation of such persons varies widely within the field of ADR. While the field continues to refine a code of ethics, there is no assurance that any given practitioner will manifest adherence to such a code.

These observations highlight the potential dangers lurking in the effort to create and implement ADR policy in health care and may in part explain some of the resistance reported to its implementation in health care communities. The deterrents to implementation in health care reported by Robson and Morrison (2003) referenced previously are germane in this context. If selected parties are not present at a negotiation, or organizational complexity and diversity of values are ignored or minimized, outcomes will be altered. The power, knowledge, and control inequalities and imbalances are of particular interest to nurses.

My personal investment in ADR nearly 20 years ago was significantly altered by the latter issue. I was repeatedly advised to "set an even table," that is, to ensure that there were no power, knowledge, or control inequalities. I reported to my teachers that indeed I personally had never sat at an even table. Although they noted that my observation was

insightful, they did not provide solutions to my dilemma. This quandary became the motivating force for writing the book that describes alternatives: *Negotiating at an Uneven Table: Developing Moral Courage in Resolving Our Conflicts* (Kritek, 2002). It essentially tackles the tough question of knowing you are at an uneven table. This is a critical factor in dealing with health care ADR, in which these imbalances shift and change regularly.

The observations of Anderson and D'Antonio (2004) about the significant differences between perceptions of the health care providers and ADR professionals concerning health care conflict adds a further dimension to the need to engage in a critical appraisal of the worldviews of ADR professionals in the health care environment. Resistance to ADR may in part express health care practioners' frustration with ADR professionals' inability to understand health care environments where they practice, or most disturbingly, that ADR providers may exacerbate conflict by furthering troublesome conditions, not the least of which is an assumption about sustaining power imbalances. Nurses are well advised to evaluate the options available to them when asked to embrace ADR. In principle, it is a rich and promising resource that can greatly improve work conditions for nurses; in practice, applied carelessly, it can further the very problems most onerous for nurses. An informed nursing community can ensure that optimal conflict management systems are put in place. As becomes apparent, one may want to embrace principled ADR and may find that the rules of the game further conflict, ignore critical variables, exclude important participants, or neglect central values of the health care community. Resistance under such conditions is understandable, perhaps even laudable. The journey toward effective ADR in health care is daunting, and oversimplification will serve no one well. In addition, health care communities may find it in their self-interest to create their own conflict management systems before they are imposed, either legislatively or in some other fashion.

## DE FACTO POLICY AND DELIBERATE CONSCIOUS POLICY

Although discussions of policy tend to focus on formal conscious efforts to create statements of "prudence or wisdom in the management of affairs," often policy is far less overt, public, deliberate, wise, or scrutinized. A recent initiative of the USIP is a useful case in point. In an effort to better understand the negotiating styles of various nations, invitational workshops were convened to explore the topic with subsequent written reports made available (see *www.usip.org/pub*). Reports are available on Russian (1998), French (2001), and German (2003) styles, and a book on Korean (2003) styles is also marketed. In July 2000 a workshop on United States style was convened, with a report made available in October 2002.

Three statements from the workshop summary are germane here:

1. U.S. negotiators have a distinctive style: forceful, explicit, legalistic, urgent, and results-oriented. Although these traits inevitably vary according to personalities and circumstances, a recognizably pragmatic American style is always evident, shaped by powerful and enduring structural and cultural factors.
2. While American diplomats tend to see themselves as tough but fair bargainers, most foreign practitioners regard the United States as a hegemonic power that is less concerned to negotiate than it is to persuade, sermonize, or browbeat negotiating counterparts into acceding to American positions.
3. Culture significantly influences how U.S. negotiators use language and time. They tend to be blunt and legalistic while employing a conceptual vocabulary drawn from such diverse fields as labor relations, Christian theology, and sport. They are uncomfortable with silence and ignore body language. They enter a negotiation with their own timeframe and usually press for an early agreement, especially if the issue at stake has political significance at home. (USIP, 2002)

One has to admire USIP for its candor. The images presented clearly point toward distributive negotiation, and the exercise of power, rather than the exploration of interests, to achieve goals. If indeed this is the norm in the United States, then policy and politics are infused with this "style" assumption. The point of departure appears to be more competitive than cooperative or collaborative, and the exercise of power, with unstated entitlement signals built in, is assumed.

Not surprisingly, power expressed in this sense refers not to agency or the ability to act, the primary definition of power available in the dictionary, but rather the opportunity to exercise power "over" others, the intent to control another or others, in this case even communicating that one has the "right" to do so. Entitlement assumes the implicit marginalization of those without power. Marginalized individuals and groups are defined in part by that lack of power and the limitations on their degrees of freedom. This may all be well intentioned, and indeed argued from a moralistic perspective, yet is nonetheless a process of hegemonic power.

Exploring policy and politics about conflict management is germane in light of this snapshot about the national style of negotiating. If policies are crafted from this point of view, marginalization is implicitly structured into the emergent policy. This possibility adds further impetus to the health care community in noting that it is in its self-interest to craft ADR policy before others craft it on its behalf. "Do no harm," as Dworkin (2002) notes, is the most difficult ethic.

As a group that has historically been frustrated with its efforts at the exercise of influence and power in health care environments, nurses interested in ADR policy development are wise to reflect on these issues. Policies could readily emerge that may exacerbate this situation. Certainly, assumptions of entitlement by various groups within the health care community have often left nurses feeling marginalized. In addition, nurses often harbor unresolved anger at the abuses they have experienced in their work world, making them vulnerable to aggressive modes of negotiation.

Debra Gerardi, the previously referenced nurse lawyer providing "Curing Conflict" training programs, serves as the health care sector editor for Mediate.com, a primary information resource in ADR. Her thoughtful editorials can provide a useful and readily accessible roadmap for health care communities willing to take on the challenge of crafting their own investments in ADR (see, for example, Gerardi, 2002, 2003). Only through becoming better informed will nurses make the "wise" policy choices about ADR and its implementation in their work environments. Nurses, however, have been tentative in their responses to the opportunities afforded them by ADR policy crafting.

## CONFLICT MANAGEMENT STYLES IN NURSING

Nursing's reluctance to embrace ADR is noteworthy in the context of the mushrooming evidence about the impact of conflict in nursing work environments. One of the finest examples of such documentation was the report of a VHA survey on the negative impact of physician disruptive behavior on nurse satisfaction and retention (Rosenstein, 2002), followed by a subsequent study reporting that nurses were as disruptive as physicians and that both groups' behaviors altered clinical outcomes in seriously deleterious ways (Rosenstein and O'Daniel, 2005). Box 11-2 illustrates how principled conflict management might be used to address physician abusive behavior.

Another useful example is the documentation sponsored by the American Association of Critical-Care Nurses (AACN) of the seven topics of crucial conversations especially difficult for health care professionals (Box 11-3); the documentation points to sites of discomfort and eventual conflict (AACN, 2005). The evidence that conflict exists and is troublesome is overwhelming.

Yet, while there is a great deal of literature available acknowledging the conflicts experienced by nurses, there is limited research available exploring nursing's preferred styles of managing this conflict. Valentine (2001), however, has provided a salient report about nurses' responses to conflict—essentially providing a metaanalysis of research conducted on nurses' preferred conflict management styles in which the Thomas-Kilmann Conflict Mode Index (Thomas & Kilmann, 2002) provided measures. The TKI is the most accepted tool for such appraisals and hence provides data that can be compared with that in other populations. Valentine's outcomes are informative.

While only 10 studies were available for Valentine's scrutiny, a pattern did emerge. Of the five management styles measured by the TKI (Table 11-1), nurses' strongest preference was for conflict avoidance, followed by compromise and accommodation, the latter often confused with collaboration. The least-used modes were competition, and strikingly, collaboration, the mode most often recommended in

---

> **BOX 11-2** Alternative Dispute Resolution and Physician Abusive Behavior: An Example
>
> One of the most familiar dilemmas nurses face is verbal abuse from physicians. Historically this has been dealt with through accommodation, avoidance, compromise, and often deep-seated but silent anger and resentment. The effective use of alternative dispute resolution (ADR) skills could alter this pattern.
>
> Dr. Schwartz is the offending physician, let's say a surgeon. Nurse Laudent is the supervisor of the operating room in which the verbal abuse occurs. Nurse Laudent would first not engage in any response during the verbal abuse, not trying to deal with the conflict while it was hot. After the event, a careful conflict analysis would reveal whether this was a system-wide problem or a single-person event. If a single-person event, which is increasingly true, then a policy dealing with verbal abuse may be an option. If Dr. Schwartz is resistive to intervention, the responsible party for enforcing a policy about the behavior in question is the chief of the service. Rather than lodging a complaint, Nurse Laudent would make a formal appointment with the chief of surgery to discuss a proposal for a policy on verbal abuse. The meeting would not aim at accusations but at optimizing the OR work environment for everyone.
>
> Policy would identify consequences if verbal abuse were to occur. Nurse Laudent would negotiate with the chief of surgery to evoke a commitment to application of consequences. Because this involves potential disciplinary action of a colleague, it would be critical for Nurse Laudent to be clear that medicine would discipline medicine, and in cases in which nurses engaged in verbal abuse, Nurse Laudent would discipline nurses. Included in this series of negotiations would be meetings with nurses and surgeons to elicit their support of the policy and explain the rationale of improved work environment. Included in these meetings would be Dr. Schwartz. This would all be quite open and public and, if possible, would include electronic communication, posting of the policy in public view, etc.
>
> Although this is somewhat oversimplified, it does map out the possibilities.

---

**BOX 11-3** Silence Kills: The Seven Crucial Conversations for Health Care

Seven categories of conversations that are especially difficult, yet essential:
1. Broken Rules
2. Mistakes
3. Lack of Support
4. Incompetence
5. Poor Teamwork
6. Disrespect
7. Micromanagement

---

**TABLE 11-1** The Thomas-Kilmann Conflict Mode Index Measures Described

| CONFLICT MODE STRATEGIES | OUTCOMES |
| --- | --- |
| **AVOIDING** | |
| Does not pursue own concerns or that of the other; does not address the conflict; withdrawal and suppression | Unassertive Uncooperative Short-term resolution |
| **COMPROMISING** | |
| Find expedient, mutually acceptable solution that partially satisfies both parties; give up something to satisfy other | Moderately assertive Moderately cooperative Short-term resolution |
| **ACCOMMODATING** | |
| Neglects own concerns to satisfy concerns of the other; minimizes differences; emphasizes similarities; self-sacrificing | Unassertive Cooperative Short-term resolution |
| **COMPETING** | |
| Pursues own concerns at expense of other; focuses on winning; power-oriented; shows low concern for other; uses whatever it takes to win | Assertive Uncooperative Short-term resolution |
| **COLLABORATING** | |
| Works with other party to find solution that fully satisfies both parties; confronts issues; explores underlying concerns | Assertive Cooperative Long-term resolution |

From TKI individual instrument booklet (Thomas, K. W., & Kilmann, R. H. [2002]. *Thomas-Kilmann conflict mode index.* Palo Alto, CA: CPP).

current literature on work environment enhancement and patient safety (see, for example, IOM, 2004).

These three preferred modes of conflict all generate outcomes that fail to resolve the conflict, leave all parties somewhat dissatisfied with the compromise, or put us at disadvantage as we forego our interests to accommodate others. They are also short-term solutions, so they actually simply smooth over the conflict so it can return another day—and it does. These preferences may be helpful in understanding nurses' conflict-aversive behaviors. We nurses have learned over time, albeit in part because of our own styles of conflict management, which outcomes are likely to prove unsuccessful and unattractive to us.

What the TKI outcomes demonstrate is that a reframed worldview about conflict and its resolution is both timely and important to nurses. A readiness to integrate ADR into our practices and policies is clearly in our self-interest. The alternatives we are currently using not only are ineffective but may actually be deleterious to our patients' well-being. They are clearly deleterious to our well-being.

## THE NURSE AS HEALTH CARE DIPLOMAT

The good news is that nurses actually have substantive ADR values, responsibilities, and skills in place. Nurses essentially function as health care diplomats, negotiating the myriad of difficult conversations and disconnections that shape today's health care environment. This has only recently begun to be formally recognized and discussed, in part because of the salient discussions in the IOM report focused on transforming nurses' work environments (IOM, 2004).

Within this report, the IOM exploration of nurses' roles notes, "RNs spend a large amount of time integrating patient care" (IOM, 2004, p. 98). Shortell, they note, calls this "clinical integration" (Shortell, Gillies, & Anderson, 2000a), and McCloskey, Bulechek, Moorhead and Daley (1996) call this "indirect care", estimating that 25% to 40% of nurses' work time is dedicated to such indirect care activities. Using either description, or a third one I am calling "health care diplomat," what the IOM report documents is that the current health care environment "requires that nursing staff communicate and coordinate with a wide variety of health care workers who participate in a patient's health care" (IOM, 2004, p. 100). Referencing Shortell, they posit, "The increased complexity of health care often requires that patients be cared for by multiple providers with specialized expertise in diverse roles for a single or across multiple episodes of care" (Shortell et al., 2000b). Health care diplomats, nurses, handle the complex cross-communication implicit in this complexity of care. Happily, they come well equipped for the challenge. Table 11-2 summarizes the values, responsibilities, and skills inherent in both nursing's traditions and in the educational and practice expectations of nurses and nurse managers.

This list of existing ADR competencies (see Table 11-2) warrants scrutiny, because any other health care occupation community desirous of becoming ADR competent would need to master these in order to serve as the system's diplomat. Nurses are uniquely advantaged in terms of readiness to master ADR because they already possess these needed competencies. They therefore serve as a critical ability base for nurses wishing to add ADR competencies to their repertoire.

## LESSONS FROM THE FIELD

This advantage can be easily squandered, however, in light of needed additional competencies. Nearly 20 years of teaching hundreds of nurses about ADR has taught me a good deal about what is still needed. Nurses still struggle with selected necessary values, work responsibilities to be integrated, and negotiation and mediation skills to be added or enhanced. These are summarized in Tables 11-3, 11-4, and 11-5 and are essentially self-explanatory. As is obvious, the fact that they are readily understood does not imply that they are readily or easily acquired. Individual nurses will need to reflect on these needed competencies and make informed decisions. The tables do provide checklists of learning opportunities for nurses interested in improving their

**TABLE 11-2** Existing Alternative Dispute Resolution Nurse Competencies

| CHECKLIST | NURSE COMPETENCIES |
|---|---|
| | **VALUES** |
| _____ | Belief in the worth and value of each human person |
| _____ | Commitment to quality of services provided |
| _____ | Advocacy for patients and families |
| _____ | Sensitivity to patients and families and their needs |
| _____ | Fairness in treatment of patients and families |
| _____ | Compassion |
| _____ | Care and concern for others |
| _____ | Commitment to constructive work environments |
| | **RESPONSIBILITIES** |
| _____ | Surveillance |
| _____ | Physiologic therapies |
| _____ | Helping patients compensate for loss |
| _____ | Providing emotional support |
| _____ | Educating patients and families |
| _____ | Integrating care |
| _____ | Documentation of activities and outcomes |
| _____ | Seeking information needed |
| _____ | Supervision |
| | **SKILLS** |
| _____ | Communication with diverse individuals |
| _____ | Relationship competencies |
| _____ | Knowledge of system and its processes |
| _____ | Listening ability |
| _____ | Monitoring and anticipation of adversity |
| _____ | Systems-based conceptual thinking |
| _____ | Connectivity with entire organization |
| _____ | Intuition |
| _____ | Critical thinking |
| _____ | Differential diagnosing |
| _____ | Awareness of importance of timing |
| _____ | Sense of humor |

Copyright by Phyllis Beck Kritek, RN, PhD, FAAN, 2005.

diplomacy capabilities and are presented in a format that encourages a commitment to learning.

Some precautions may be useful. It is important that nurses not leave mastery of ADR to "outsiders" with a limited understanding of the health care

**TABLE 11-3**   Alternative Dispute Resolution Value Cultivation Checklist for Nurses

| COMMITMENTS | PROFESSIONAL VALUES TO BE CULTIVATED |
|---|---|
| _____ | Courage to face and transform conflict |
| _____ | Compassion with those with whom I differ |
| _____ | Embracing diversity as an opportunity and an advantage |
| _____ | Forgiveness |
| _____ | Pursuit of mission congruence as a challenge |
| _____ | Inclusiveness in my relationships |
| _____ | Justice as a complex but worthy goal |
| _____ | Manifesting "do no harm" as a lifestyle |
| _____ | Peacebuilding |

Copyright by Phyllis Beck Kritek, RN, PhD, FAAN, 2005.

**TABLE 11-4**   Alternative Dispute Resolution Responsibilities Checklist for Nurses

| COMMITMENTS | PROFESSIONAL RESPONSIBILITIES TO BE INTEGRATED INTO WORK ROLE |
|---|---|
| _____ | Differentiating between critical thinking and judging others |
| _____ | Differentiating between humor and ridicule |
| _____ | Differentiating between problems and essential polarities |
| _____ | Differentiating between accommodation and collaboration |
| _____ | Becoming willing to overtly own my own power |
| _____ | Publicly committing to my professional code of ethics |
| _____ | Acknowledging and owning my role in conflicts on the job |
| _____ | Anticipating that the "other side" can teach me something |
| _____ | Understanding the manifestations of oppression |
| _____ | Confronting and mastering my fear of retribution |
| _____ | Detaching from the need for the "right answer" |
| _____ | Detaching from mindsets of powerlessness |
| _____ | Detaching from "victim-think" |
| _____ | Detaching from deprivation expectation |
| _____ | Imagining that conflict can even be fun |
| _____ | Learning from conflicts I experiences |

Copyright by Phyllis Beck Kritek, RN, PhD, FAAN, 2005.

environment or with an unintended tendency to perpetuate the problems most onerous to nurses, such as power imbalances. Although administrative personnel and human resource managers may provide some introductory information about ADR, it is noteworthy that the competencies are complex and challenging, and giving them a cursory nod serves no one well. The effort to oversimplify the work of conflict resolution will invariably lead to frustration and dissatisfaction with outcomes. It is hard work.

Hence, nurses are wise to beware of the "quick fix" for enhancing their ADR competencies, becoming vigilant about assurances that these can be achieved with one class, or using only one process, or embracing only one person's views as informative. ADR will not support the illusion of the "one best way," and if it is presented as such, it is wise to be skeptical at best.

Nurses, like most health care providers, are educated to focus on the most problematic dimension of a patient's health status. As a result, we go for the worst situation first and may be prone to do so with conflict resolution. It is therefore useful to note that mastering conflict resolution will require a counterintuitive decision to handle the easiest conflicts first, gaining mastery and confidence in the process.

Identifying those factors that make health care environments unique will become increasingly important in ensuring that the ADR practices introduced show congruence with the environment. Nurses are uniquely well equipped to make these determinations and would be wise to position themselves as the vanguard in clarifying the issues and identifying preferred practices.

Having made a commitment to enhancing ADR competencies, nurses may find it useful to place their learning squarely in the center of our traditions as health care diplomats and peacemakers. We are good at this; we can become much better. We also have demonstrated an increased readiness to move beyond the silence of accommodation; ADR becomes an arena where speaking out becomes imperative. We have a history of comfort

**TABLE 11-5**  Alternative Dispute Resolution Skills Checklist for Nurses

| COMMITMENTS | NEGOTIATION AND MEDIATION SKILLS TO BE ADDED OR ENHANCED |
|---|---|
| _____ | Picking my tables deliberately |
| _____ | Conducting a careful and complete conflict analysis |
| _____ | Identifying when the conflict is actually a system problem, not a person problem |
| _____ | Discovering the interests of everyone participating in the conflict |
| _____ | Asking questions often and well |
| _____ | Asking others how I might help in the conflict |
| _____ | Acknowledging the strengths of others in a conflict |
| _____ | Doing my homework before trying to deal with the conflict |
| _____ | Learning to observe myself objectively during a negotiation |
| _____ | Reframing all aspects of a conflict before trying to deal with it |
| _____ | Generating numerous options before selecting one |
| _____ | Creating the unimagined option |
| _____ | Clarifying all possible choices and their consequences |
| _____ | Knowing my boundaries and maintaining them |
| _____ | Using integrative and constructive humor |
| _____ | Following up on a process to see it through to its conclusion |
| _____ | Creating closure |
| _____ | Affirming my outcomes |

Copyright by Phyllis Beck Kritek, RN, PhD, FAAN, 2005.

with innovation and discovery. Treating our learning about ADR as such a process will serve us well.

What we are about, of course, is creating a culture of conflict competence and principled conflict management. It is my conviction that no group within health care is better equipped to do so. In addition, as the Gallup Poll on citizens' rating of honest and ethical professions demonstrated (Carroll, 2003; Moore, 2004), we can be trusted to pursue these efforts in a manner that evokes trust from our patients and their families. This too is a salient advantage.

## GETTING STARTED

As is obvious, the first challenge is a commitment to the steady expansion of ADR competencies. Although it would be encouraging if nurse leaders were in the vanguard of this commitment, individual nurses can take action without this advantage. All that is required is the political and personal will to do so. We do not need to blindly replicate the adversarial patterns of others; we can introduce and demonstrate a more effective model, and in the process display our ability to "take the high road." Courses, books, and tapes on ADR abound; any nurse can decide to become a more competent health care diplomat. A concrete example of how this might lead to altered behavior is described in Box 11-2.

Applying ADR in health care can then become both informative and gratifying. Arenas abound. Workplace relationships are an obvious starting point. Nurses can enhance their ability to become effective diplomats in organizational conflict. They can improve their ability to create change, alter cultures, and introduce conflict management systems into their workplace. ADR can substantively alter the tone, focus, and intent of nurses' legislative initiatives, and indeed, the way they are pursued.

Using Table 11-5 as an action guide, nurses can take more time to identify the optimal site for legislative initiatives, picking ones where they can make a difference, have influence, and further the public health of citizens. Current Medicaid drug coverage is a useful example. A careful and complete conflict analysis demonstrates that this is a system problem. Who are the parties we can build coalitions with, and what will they ask of us? What are the interests of the legislators who must take action? Since most are concerned about constituent satisfaction, emphasizing this issue is probably more effective than simply stating it is a good and noble thing to address. Options for solving the problem are important, and starting a negotiation without multiple options simply leads to a discussion that becomes a complaint. Asking legislators to explain their position and their solution to this dilemma can quickly highlight deficiencies in an existing position. Letting the legislator reveal this is far more effective than making an accusation. These are a few ways that negotiating skills alter how we might pursue public policy initiatives. In all such cases, group action is best, so engaging larger groups becomes a goal.

"Selling" ADR is something of a challenge, yet it readily fits pressing health care system dilemmas. Obvious motivations would include improving patient safety through better communication and cost containment through improved problem solving processes. The latter issue of cost containment is significant, because conflict is very costly. Table 11-6 provides a checklist of the cost factors associated with unresolved conflict in organizations and can be adopted to demonstrate this fact.

Some situations in which ADR can be integrated and "practiced" include governmental and health care organization negotiations, workplace negotiations, communication in our professional organizations, public discourse where we present nursing's viewpoint, and community activism. These are a few examples that demonstrate the multiple uses of the competencies, once enhanced. Practicing where it is most likely to be successful is important in building competency.

## CREATING A CULTURE OF PRINCIPLED CONFLICT MANAGEMENT

A culture of principled conflict management would address myriad "problems" that have daunted nurses for decades. Although not all conflicts can be resolved, and many are complex and resistant to change, many are quite amenable to ADR approaches, with solutions that can be both successful and gratifying. If the majority of amenable conflicts were addressed in this fashion, the cultures of health care could be altered substantively, making each of these various cultures amenable to principled conflict management.

There is an obvious need for education and continued professional development, and nurses need to request assistance. Integrating diplomat roles into formal evaluation protocols, rewards, and recognition would make a powerful statement supporting such efforts. Integrating the role into the work of educators, researchers, administrators, and practitioners would effectively expand our understanding of the promise of ADR for health care communities, for nurses, and for our patients and their families.

**TABLE 11-6** Health Care Organization Conflict Cost Factors Estimate Form

| FACTORS ASSOCIATED WITH CONFLICT THAT CONSUME A HEALTH CARE ORGANIZATION'S RESOURCES | ESTIMATED ANNUAL COST |
|---|---|
| Wasted time for employees | _____ |
| Bad decisions made during conflicts | _____ |
| Lost or resigned employees | _____ |
| Unnecessary restructuring | _____ |
| Sabotage | _____ |
| Theft | _____ |
| Strained cross-professional communication | _____ |
| Disruptive behavior of personnel | _____ |
| Damage to property | _____ |
| Lowered job motivation | _____ |
| Lowered job morale | _____ |
| Lost work time | _____ |
| Verbal abuse and its sequelae | _____ |
| Employee replacement | _____ |
| New employee orientation | _____ |
| Health costs associated with job stress | _____ |
| Staffing disruptions | _____ |
| Scheduling dilemmas | _____ |
| Absenteeism | _____ |
| Tardiness | _____ |
| Work not completed before shift ends | _____ |
| Errors | _____ |
| Failure to rescue | _____ |
| Falls and injuries | _____ |
| Patient safety neglect | _____ |
| Endless pointless meetings | _____ |
| Meetings focused on power distribution | _____ |
| Repetitious policy manifestos | _____ |
| Provider career changes | _____ |

Copyright by Phyllis Beck Kritek, RN, PhD, FAAN, 2005.

I would like to give Mohandas Gandhi, a model of nonviolent conflict management, the last word: "We must be the change we hope to see in the world."

## Lessons Learned

- ADR has come of age and is now increasingly embedded in national and state policy and practices; it is gradually "showing up" as an expectation in health care environments.
- Worldview shapes our approaches to ADR; nurses are advised to create their own ADR

initiatives congruent with nursing's ethics and traditions rather than having them imposed externally.

■ Nurses possess substantive ADR competencies already, and could be a powerful ADR resource in health care once they strengthen and expand these baseline abilities, particularly in their role as health care diplomats.

■ Creating a culture of principled conflict management competence would have a powerful impact on addressing many of the most troublesome challenges facing health care today and substantively alter both political practices and emergent policy.

## *Web Resources*

**Association for Conflict Resolution**—the major professional organization for ADR scholars and practitioners in the United States; provides information on membership, specialization groups, emerging certification programs, educational offerings, ethical codes, and related information
*www.acrnet.org*

**CDR Associates**—one of the most well-established and respected ADR companies, with 35 years of experience in both the training and practice of ADR; course offerings are a particularly useful resource
*www.mediate.org*

**Conflict Resolution Information Source**—information resource managed by the Conflict Resolution Consortium at the University of Colorado; a free online clearinghouse indexing over 25,000 webpages, books, articles, audiovisual materials, events, and news articles
*www.crinfo.org*

**Conflict Resolution Network Canada**—showcases some of the rich work being done in Canada in the field of ADR, including educational and training programs, reading resources, and news in the field
*www.crnetwork.ca*

**Health Care Mediations, Inc.**—a successful conflict management company headed by a nurse, Debra Gerardi; demonstrates the impact a nurse can have in changing work environments
*www.healthcaremediations.com*

**Institute for the Study of Conflict Transformation**—an organization whose purpose is to study and promote the understanding of conflict and intervention processes from a transformative perspective; provides options for persons interested in the work of Bush and Folger on transformative mediation, including educational and organizational resources
*www.transformativemediation.org*

**Peacemakers Trust**—Canadian charitable organization dedicated to research and education on conflict transformation and peace building; provides extensive bibliographies, case studies, and related resources
*www.peacemakers.ca*

**U.S. Institute of Peace**—an independent, nonpartisan federal institution created by Congress to promote the prevention, management, and peaceful resolution of international conflicts
*www.usip.org*

**U.S. Office of Personnel Management**—part of the official site of the federal government's human resource agency; provides a resource guide for ADR techniques and practices in federal agencies, along with bibliographies, Websites, and information from the ADR Act of 1996, which mandated the use of ADR processes for all agencies
*www.opm.gov/er/adrguide*

## REFERENCES

American Association of Critical-Care Nurses (AACN). (2005). Silence kills: The seven crucial conversations for healthcare. Final report cosponsored by Vitalsmarts. Retrieved June 10, 2005, from *www.rxforbettercare.org/SilenceKills.pdf.*

American Association of Retired Persons (AARP) (Prepared for AARP by Roper ASW). (2004). *Baby boomers envision retirement II—Key findings: Survey of baby boomers' expectations for retirement.* Washington, DC: AARP.

American Nurses Association (ANA). (2001). *Code of ethics for nurses with interpretive statements.* Washington, DC: American Nurses Association.

Anderson, C., & D'Antonio, L. (2004, Fall). Empirical insights: Understanding the unique culture of health care conflicts. *Dispute Resolution Magazine,* 15-18.

Bush, R. A. B., & Folger, J. P. (1994). *The promise of mediation: Responding to conflict through empowerment and recognition.* San Francisco: Jossey-Bass.

Carroll, J. (2003). Public rates nursing as most honest and ethical profession. Retrieved February 13, 2004, from *www.gallup.com/poll.*

Centers for Medicare and Medicaid Services. (2004). *Mediation: A new option for medicare beneficiaries to resolve complaints filed through a QIO.* Retrieved January 24, 2005, from *http://new.cms.hhs.gov/BeneComplaintRespProg/Downloads/3a.pdf.*

Colsky, A. (2002). The federal government and ADR: How things get done. Retrieved June 30, 2005, from *http://mediate.com/articles/colsky1.cfm#.*

Dukes, E. F. (1996). *Resolving public conflict: Transforming community and governance.* Manchester, UK: Manchester University Press.

Dworkin, A. (2002). Heartbreak: The political memoir of a feminist militant. New York: Basic Books.

Folberg, J., & Taylor, A. (1984). *Mediation: A comprehensive guide to resolving conflicts without litigation.* San Francisco: Jossey-Bass.

Folger, J. P., & Bush, R. A. B. (Eds.). (2001). *Designing mediation: Approaches to training and practice within a transformative framework.* New York: Institute for the Study of Conflict Transformation.

Gerardi, D. (2002). Hope for healthcare—Returning civility and cooperation to health care. Retrieved July 7, 2005, from *http://mediate.com/pfriendly.cfm?id=1043.*

Gerardi, D. (2003). The tipping point: Managing conflict to create culture change in health care. Retrieved July 7, 2005, from *http://mediate.com/pfriendly.cfm?id=1449.*

Harrington, C. (1982). Delegalization reform movements: A historical analysis. In R. Abel (Ed.), *The Politics of Informal Justice* (Vol. 1). New York: Academic Press.

Institute of Medicine. ( 2004). *Keeping patients safe: Transforming the work environment of nurses.* Washington, DC: National Academies Press.

Johnson, B. (1996). *Polarity management: Identifying and managing unsolvable problems.* Amherst, MA: HRD Press.

Kritek, P. B. (2002). *Negotiating at an uneven table: Developing moral courage in resolving our conflicts* (2nd ed). San Francisco: Jossey-Bass.

Kroll, C. (1997). Graduate programs in dispute resolution keep growing. Retrieved June 30, 2005, from *http://mediate.com/articles/krollc.cfm.*

Mayer, B. (2000). *The dynamics of conflict resolution: A practitioner's guide.* San Francisco: Jossey-Bass.

McCloskey, J., Bulechek, G., Moorhead, S., & Daley, J. (1996). Nurses' use and delegation of indirect care interventions. *Nursing Economic$, 14*(1), 22-33.

Merriam-Webster. (1996). *Merriam Webster Collegiate Dictionary.* (10th ed.). Springfield, MA: Merriam-Webster.

Moore, D. W. (2004). Nurses top list in honesty and ethics poll. Retrieved January 14, 2005, from *www.gallup.com/poll.*

National Coalition on Health Care. (2005). Health insurance coverage. Retrieved June 30, 2005, from *www.nchc.org/facts/coverage.shtml.*

Peterson's. (2005). Graduate programs in dispute resolution and alternative dispute resolution. Retrieved June 30, 2005, from *http://www.petersons.com/fts/code/smplrslt.asp?cpage=2&anyQuery=dispute+resolution&volume=GR&sponsor=1.*

Robson, R., & Morrison, G. (2003). ADR in healthcare: The last big frontier. *ACResolution,* Spring, 1-6. Retrieved June 27, 2005, from *http://mediate.com/articles/robmorr1.cfm.*

Rosenstein, A. H. (2002). Original research. Nurse-physician relationships: Impact on nurse satisfaction and retention. *American Journal of Nursing, 102*(6), 2634.

Rosenstein, A. H., & O'Daniel, M. (2005). Disruptive behavior and clinical outcomes: Perceptions of nurses and physicians. *American Journal of Nursing, 105*(1), 54-64.

Shortell, S., Gillies, R., & Anderson, D. (2000a). *Remaking health care in America* (2nd ed.). San Francisco: Jossey-Bass.

Shortell, S., Jones, R., Rademaker, A., Gillies, R., Dranove, D., et al. (2000b). Assessing the impact of total quality management and organizational culture on multiple outcomes of care for coronary artery bypass graft surgery patients. *Medical Care, 38*(7), 207-217.

Thomas, K. W., & Kilmann, R. H. (2002). *Thomas-Kilmann conflict mode index.* Palo Alto, CA: CPP.

United States Institute of Peace (USIP). (2002). U.S. Negotiating Behavior. Special Report 94. Retrieved December 12, 2002, from *www.usip.org/pubs/specialreports/sr94.html.*

United States Institute of Peace (USIP). (no date). USIP home page self-description. Retrieved April 14, 2005, from *www.usip.org.*

Valentine, P. E. B. (2001). Gender perspective on conflict management strategies of nurses. *Journal of Nursing Scholarship, 30*(2), 69-74.

# chapter 12

# Health Policy, Politics, and Professional Ethics

Leah L. Curtin

"To see what is right and not do it is want of courage."

CONFUCIUS

In order to frame our discussion of policy, politics and ethics, I will present some actual situations: a "no-admit" list, dying with dignity, and Health Insurance Portability and Accountability Act (HIPAA) horror stories.

## CASE STUDY I: A NO-ADMIT LIST

A graduate student asked about the use of a no-admit list and described the following situation.

*A 29-year-old male with diagnoses of bipolar disorder, substance use disorder, and antisocial personality disorder comes to the emergency department (ED) one midnight shift under a law enforcement Baker Act. This law permits a 72-hour involuntary placement for psychiatric assessment. The law says the patient is to be admitted to the nearest Baker Act receiving facility. The ED staff provided me with the following unsolicited information: "Get rid of this guy fast, he's trouble"; the patient is an "abuser of the system," they say, and he has assaulted several health care workers. He is a drain on overextended resources because his behavior requires constant intervention to maintain safety.*

*I find in our assessment office that the patient is on a "do not admit" list. The unit nursing staff on duty*

*that night provides me with the information that this patient assaulted a nurse on one of the adult psychiatric units and was jailed and charged for this offense. The nurse sustained permanent damage to her knee and currently has a restraining order against this patient.*

*At this time the patient is calm and cooperative during my assessment—other than making continuous, aggressive requests to smoke and several attempts to leave the ED without an escort to do so. The psychiatrist on call was new to this facility, as was I at the time, so we were unaware of the patient's history and past treatment record. In addition, the psychiatrist and I had a previous positive professional relationship at another facility and I knew that he respected my recommendations. Before calling him, I make inquiries at area psychiatric units and find out that earlier in the day this patient left treatment at a facility 70 miles away and is not welcome back because of his aggressive behavior. The local community mental health facility also is not amenable to a referral because this patient assaulted personnel there in the past. My colleague at the community center says that this patient has "burned all his bridges in a hundred mile radius."*

*I now have a great deal of information from various sources about this patient. To pose this question realistically and succinctly, do I say, "Doc, this guy is bad news and the unit will have your head and mine if we admit him" or "Doc, this patient is suicidal with a plan and we have the closest bed"? What about the* law*? How legal is a "do not admit" list, and what are my ethical obligations particularly when administration is aware of this patient's situation and has opted to not address options that might break the cycle of continued abuse of acute services and the abuse of resources this facilitates?

## CASE STUDY II: DEATH WITH DIGNITY

The Oregon Health Department published an accounting of Oregon's experience with the first Death with Dignity Act in the nation, excerpts from which follow:

*Physician-assisted suicide (PAS) has been legal in Oregon since November1997, when Oregon voters approved the Death with Dignity Act (DWDA) for the second time… In response to a lawsuit filed by the State of Oregon on November 20, 2001, a U.S. district court issued a temporary restraining order against Attorney General Ashcroft's ruling pending a new hearing. On April 17, 2002, U.S. District Court Judge Robert Jones upheld the Death with Dignity Act. On September 23, 2002, Attorney General Ashcroft filed an appeal, asking the Ninth U.S. Circuit Court of Appeals to overturn the District Court's ruling, which was subsequently denied on May 26, 2004 by a three-judge panel. On July 13, 2004, Ashcroft filed an appeal requesting that the Court rehear his previous motion with an 11-judge panel; on August 13, 2004, the request was denied. On November 9, 2004, Ashcroft asked the U.S. Supreme Court to review the Ninth Circuit Court's decision and on February 22, 2005, the court agreed to hear the appeal. Arguments were held during the Supreme Court's term beginning in October of 2005, and in a stunning blow to the Bush Administration, the Supreme Court upheld the Oregon*

law in January of 2006; thus Oregon's law remains in effect.

*The Death with Dignity Act allows terminally ill Oregon residents to obtain and use prescriptions from their physicians for self-administered, lethal medications. Under the Act, ending one's life in accordance with the law does not constitute suicide. However, we use the term "physician-assisted suicide" because it is used in the medical literature to describe ending life through the voluntary self-administration of lethal medications prescribed by a physician for that purpose. The Death with Dignity Act legalizes PAS, but specifically prohibits euthanasia, whereby a physician or other person directly administers a medication to end another's life. To request a prescription for lethal medications, the Death with Dignity Act requires that a patient must be:*

- *An adult (18 years of age or older)*
- *A resident of Oregon*
- *Capable (defined as able to make and communicate health care decisions)*
- *Diagnosed with a terminal illness that will lead to death within 6 months*

*Patients meeting these requirements are eligible to request a prescription for lethal medication from a licensed Oregon physician.† To comply with the law, physicians must report to the Department of Human Services (DHS) all prescriptions for lethal medications within 7 working days of prescribing the medication. Reporting is not required if patients begin the request process but never receive a prescription. In the summer of 1999 the Oregon legislature added a requirement that pharmacists must be informed of the prescribed*

---

*Section 1867 of the Social Security Act imposes specific obligations on Medicare-participating hospitals that offer emergency services to provide a medical screening examination (MSE) when a request is made for examination or treatment for an emergency medical condition (EMC), including active labor, regardless of an individual's ability to pay. Hospitals are then required to provide stabilizing treatment for patients with EMCs. If a hospital is unable to stabilize a patient within its capability, or if the patient requests, an appropriate transfer should be implemented.

---

†To receive a prescription for lethal medication, a patient must fulfill the following steps: (1) The patient must make two oral requests to his or her physician, separated by at least 15 days. (2) The patient must provide a written request to his or her physician, signed in the presence of two witnesses. (3) The prescribing physician and a consulting physician must confirm the diagnosis and prognosis. (4) The prescribing physician and a consulting physician must determine whether the patient is capable. (5) If either physician believes the patient's judgment is impaired by a psychiatric or psychologic disorder, the patient must be referred for a psychologic examination. (6) The prescribing physician must inform the patient of feasible alternatives to assisted suicide including comfort care, hospice care, and pain control. (7) The prescribing physician must request, but may not require, the patient to notify his or her next of kin of the prescription request.

*medication's ultimate use. Physicians and patients who adhere to the requirements of the Act are protected from criminal prosecution, and the choice of legal physician-assisted suicide cannot affect the status of a patient's health or life insurance policies. Physicians, pharmacists, and health care systems are under no obligation to participate in the Death with Dignity Act... The Department of Human Services (DHS) is legally required to collect information regarding compliance with the Act and make the information available on a yearly basis... Although five fewer patients ingested lethal medication in 2004 compared with 2003, the trend has been upward since legalization. In 1998, 16 Oregonians used PAS, followed by 27 in 1999, 27 in 2000, 21 in 2001, 38 in 2002, 42 in 2003, and 37 in 2004. Paralleling the upward trend in the number of deaths are the ratios of PAS deaths to total deaths: in 1998 there were 5.5 PAS deaths per every 10,000 total deaths, followed by 9.2 in 1999, 9.1 in 2000, 7.0 in 2001, 12.2 in 2002, 13.6 in 2003, and an estimated 12/10,000 in 2004...Compared with all Oregon decedents, PAS participants in 2004 were more likely to have malignant neoplasms (78%), to be younger (median age 64 years), and to have more formal education (51% had at least a baccalaureate degree). During the past 7 years, the 208 patients who took lethal medications differed in several ways from the 64,706 Oregonians dying from the same underlying diseases. Rates of participation in PAS decreased with age, but were higher among those who were divorced or never married, those with more years of formal education, and those with amyotrophic lateral sclerosis, HIV/AIDS, or malignant melanoma...* (http://oregon.gov/DHS/ph/pas/docs/year7.pdf).

## CASE STUDY III: HIPAA HORROR STORIES

In the wake of HIPAA, many a strange situation has arisen. Consider the following: According to surveys, an average of 150 people from nursing staff to x-ray technicians to billing clerks have access to a patient's medical records during a typical hospital stay. In the office of an individual health care practitioner or small group practice, virtually everyone has access to a patient's protected health information. Although many of these individuals have a legitimate need to

see all or part of the patient's record, until HIPAA no laws governed who those people are or what information they are allowed to see. Now, failure to provide adequate protection can result in serious breaches of privacy with grave consequences. You may have seen news stories in which a camera pans over a dumpster overflowing with unshredded medical charts. News anchors follow up with and interview patients, bringing them the very file discovered amid the trash. Hearing such horror stories is grounds for worry about the safety of your own health information, even if an annual checkup is the extent of your physician visits.

This very issue of privacy is at the heart of HIPPA, which went into effect on April 14, 2003. Thanks to HIPAA, it's easier for terminally ill patients to obtain health insurance. Federal standards now exist for the availability of health insurance and the electronic transmission of patient medical information. Regulations of fraud and abuse have been strengthened. Also, charts in doorway pockets now face inward so people walking down the hallway can't read them. One effect of HIPAA is that individuals now have to sign a Notice of Privacy Practices from health care providers. This notice outlines the provider's privacy policies. The most important provision of HIPAA is the privacy rule. This rule covers an individual's "protected health information." This type of information includes bills, claims, prescriptions, data, lab results, medical opinions, and even appointment histories. All health care providers, health maintenance organizations (HMOs), and health insurers must comply with this privacy rule if they electronically store health information (www.cms.hhs.gov/hipaa).

However well intentioned and even necessary the legislation, it has unintended consequences. Consider the following actual situation:

*Mrs. B., an 83-year-old widow, suffers from Parkinson's disease. She resides in an assisted-care facility, where she receives full assistance. She has only one child, a daughter who also has serious health problems and lives approximately 75 miles away. Recently, Mrs. B. suffered a serious urinary tract infection, high fever, and some mild disorientation. Subsequently she was transported by ambulance to the hospital, her parting words being, "I don't want you to tell anyone where I am or what's wrong with me, especially not my daughter!" instructions that she also gave to hospital staff. Although Mrs. B.'s daughter was frantic with worry, no one would tell her where her mother was or what was wrong with her not even when she was able to arrange a ride to visit her mother, only to find her "missing." All information was withheld according to the provisions of HIPAA, even though Mrs. B., once she recovered, could not remember giving anyone instructions to withhold information from her daughter.*

## THE ENDS AND THE MEANS

Why bring these particular situations to your attention? Principally this: Each involves a variation of the same question—that is, what means can be legitimately used to achieve an end that someone (or a political party, or even the electorate) believes to be good? We have laws that require screening, stabilizing, and treating all people who come to an ED (a good) even though it may enable abuse of the system (an evil), as in Case Study I. In Case Study III the law (HIPAA) seeks to protect the privacy of patients (a good) even though it may cause anxiety for family members and even patients themselves (an evil) on occasion. In Case Study II the situation is far more ambiguous and controversial because it is a generally accepted principle of both law and ethics that killing a person is wrong—and therefore encouraging suicide is wrong. Others believe that enabling medically assisted suicide is a good because it promotes personal autonomy and therefore respects the dignity of individuals facing inevitable and painful deaths. The difference is this: In Cases I and III the law provides for a good (equity of access in Case I and privacy in Case III) which may occasionally produce an evil (abuse of the system in Case I and psychologic suffering in Case III); in Case II the law enables what is generally considered an evil (killing, or suicide) in order to produce a good (autonomy and relief of suffering). This inevitably leads to a discussion of whether or not the ends can ever justify the means.

The ends-and-means argument often is explained as follows. We can cut a man open (an evil means) to save his life (a good end). We can remove a perfectly healthy kidney from one person (an evil means) to transplant it to save the life and health of another (a good end). And we admire the person who sacrifices his life (an evil means) to save the life of his friend (a good end). If our intention (to produce good) can justify the means (doing an evil), then can we not torture one man (an evil means) to gain information that might save another person's life or even the lives of many people (a good end)? Is it acceptable to risk some people's well-being in order to help many people? (For example, in developing the hepatitis B vaccine, mentally retarded children at a home in Buffalo, NY were given various strains and strengths of the vaccine and then exposed to the virus—an evil means used to determine what type and strength of vaccine should be used on the general public, a good end.) Can we assure the election of a person whom we believe to be of superior quality (a good end) by corrupting the political process (an evil means)? All of which provide an introduction to some of the murkier aspects of the theory that "the ends justify the means."

## A FEW THINGS THAT MUST BE SAID

Before we get into more ticklish problems, it is important to note that cutting a person open, even to save his life, is not a good thing unless the person consents to it. Similarly one cannot "steal" one person's kidney even to save another; rather, the consent of both donor and recipient is required. The prisoner does not choose to be tortured, although it is very tempting to justify "beating the facts out" to protect innocent lives. But hard as it is to say, if a man can be tortured on the suspicion that he may know something subversive, who is safe from governmental oppression? For we, just as they, are members of society. The price we pay for freedom and human rights is to grant them to all people, not just a favored few. And yes, it is risky, and yes, it may reduce our "efficiency" and in some cases even lead to loss of life. But the alternative is that *no one* has rights (i.e., just claims), rights become the privilege of a favored group while all other individuals are utterly helpless before the power of the state.

Certainly the electorate does not consent to the corruption of the electoral process—and even if a majority did approve of breaking the rules of fair engagement to ensure that a particular candidate was elected, would that make it right? Would it not end up threatening the very foundations of a free society (because the foundation of a republic lies in the honesty of its electoral process)? Without honest elections, those in power have all the power to ensure that they stay there!

As for the children used in medical research, the consequence of these and other cases that came to light in the 1970s was the establishment of institutional review boards and stringent guidelines that were put in place to curtail medical research. Why? Because our laws require us to protect the well-being of the vulnerable, even though sacrificing the vulnerable may end up benefiting large numbers of the general population. Put another way, if the human rights of patients, organ donors, and children can be sacrificed to expediency, so can your rights and mine. Therefore it is in the public's best interest to protect children (and prisoners and other vulnerable people), even at the cost of slower development of medical treatments.

Gandhi, one of the twentieth century's most principled political leaders, taught and demonstrated through his life and political actions that there is no difference between ends and means—that, in fact, what we choose to do (the means) is what actually is manifest in the world, regardless of what we intend to produce (the ends) (Gandhi, 1958). In short, the means *are* the ends, because the means are what we have chosen to bring into existence. Another author puts it this way: "One man in the twentieth century led us back into morality as a practical thing... and that was Mohandas Gandhi. His greatest contribution to the discussion of politics and morality was his insistence that 'the distinction that the Cartesians and the Marxists had made between ends and means was a false distinction'. Gandhi demonstrated that the means were the end; that how you did things determined the end, that violence as a means to solving a problem was in fact the nature of the solution. He was able to destroy the mightiest empire in history without the use of a single gun. So the proof he gave was that morality was not impractical, and what is practical and worth practicing is only morality" (Kidder, 1994, p. 222).

# ETHICS: RIGHT AND WRONG

Ethics has to do with right and wrong in this world, and politics has everything to do with what happens to people in this world! Moreover, both ethics and politics have to do with making life better for oneself and others. Surely both deal with power and powerlessness, with human rights and balancing their claims, with justice and fairness—and, yes, with good and evil. And good and evil are *not* the same as right and wrong. Right and wrong have to do with adherence to principles; good and evil have to do with the intent of the doer and the impact the deed has on other people. Surely politics involves justice in the distribution of social goods; fairness and equity in relationships among and between people of different races, genders, and creeds; and access to education and assistance when one is in need. And, yes, it has to do with intent and social impact (good and evil).

According to a contemporary philosopher, the discipline of ethics proposes to identify, organize, examine, and justify human acts by applying certain principles to determine the right thing to do in specific situations (Wellman, 1975). Although the goodness of an action lies in the intent and integrity of the human being who performs it, the rightness or wrongness of an action is judged by the difference it makes in the world. Therefore the principles applied in ethical analysis generally derive from a consideration of the duties one person owes another by virtue of commitments made and roles assumed, and/or a consideration of the effects that a choice of action could have on one's own life and the lives of others.

## PROFESSIONAL ETHICS

A professional ethic is built around three essential components:

1. *Its purpose.* All professions develop in response to a social need—one that the members of the profession promise to meet. Put in legalistic terms, this need (along with the power and privileges society grants to the profession to help the professionals meet the need) and the profession's promised response to it constitute the profession's contract with society.

2. *The conduct expected of the professional.* The ethical code developed and promulgated by the profession—its code of ethics—describes the conduct society has a right to expect from professionals as they go about the business of the profession. However, it is not a list of prescribed do's and don'ts but rather an articulation of those values that, in fact, outline the scope of the profession's practice and the relationships that ought to pertain between its members and the lay public, among the practitioners of this profession, between the practitioner and the profession itself, and between the professional and the community within which he or she practices.

3. *The skills and outcomes expected in professional practice.* Nursing's standards of practice state with some precision the obligations of nurses in specific areas of practice. Clearly, each of these components is dynamic—that is, subject to change and reevaluation as the profession grows, as knowledge increases, and as social mores and expectations develop. This is not to claim that there are no constants (e.g., a general imperative to respect persons), but rather to say that the meaning and application of the imperatives change.

Professional ethics is the study of how personal moral norms apply or conflict with the promises and duties of one's profession. Society demands that professionals be held to a separate moral standard of conduct because the choices professionals make affect other people's lives more than their own. Generally speaking, the kinds of choices that fall within this context encompass: (1) the human rights of the patient and the degree to which he or she is capable of exercising them; (2) choices about the technical options available and their appropriate application to the human being as well as the "value options" open to patients—whether or not and to what extent they want or reject the technical options; (3) choices about research and learning on human beings; (4) choices about resource allocation in situations of scarcity; (5) choices about futile care and patient autonomy; (6) choices about the preeminence of one's own self-interest—ranging from exposure to biologic and other workplace hazards, to recompense for services rendered, to weighing an institution's interests into the equations; and

(7) questions of law and regulation—what laws are needed to assure the public's well-being, and to assure some equity in the distribution of resources. It is unbelievably easy to justify—for the sake of financial security, for the sake of research, for the sake of the "greater good," even for the sake of our own intellectual curiosity—sacrificing the comfort, well-being, or even the very lives of other people—even, or most particularly, *because* they are in our power. Therefore to an increasing extent there is public oversight of health care practice and health care research.

As members of the profession face specific ethical quandaries, they are obliged morally and sometimes even legally to keep in mind the promises their professions both infer and imply. Once the profession as a whole adopts a code of ethics, the professional views the occupation and all of its requirements as an enduring set of normative and behavioral expectations. Thus, the ethics of a profession not only delimit the role and scope of its activities and prescribe the nature of the relationship that should exist between its members and the public but also establish duties that professionals owe to one another and to the profession itself. Codes of professional ethics also usually include a pledge to exert one's best efforts to maintain the honor of the profession and to uphold its public standing. The reason for this is that a profession's members *cannot* practice effectively without the public's trust—and although this is true for all professions, it is especially so for the politician, whose reputation is undercut as intense media scrutiny lays every infraction of every politician before the entire public. Thus it is that the U.S. House Ethics Manual prescribes as a member's first duty: "to conduct himself at all times in a manner which shall reflect creditably on the House of Representatives" *(www.house.gov/ethics)*.

Unfortunately, professions develop unevenly because the professionals who comprise them are in diverse states of awareness, intellectual attainment, and commitment. Member's perceptions of their roles and their character traits affect the problems they see, the personal presence they bring to them, the manner in which they address them, and the reservoir of personal resources they can call on to serve another day. At the same time, their moral commitments (or lack of them), as repeated in hundreds of their colleagues, create or destroy the credibility of the profession. In no profession is this truer than in politics because the stakes are so high, the power so great, and the temptations so insistent.

Just as the license to practice nursing does not include a permission to practice it poorly but rather presupposes an obligation to practice it well, election to office carries with it a compelling obligation to serve all of the people well all of the time *(www.house.gov/ethics)*. If election to office entails an obligation to work for the good of all, then the power to govern entails an obligation to judge and to monitor well one's own conduct and the conduct of one's colleagues. Therefore each member of a profession shares the obligation of assuring that every member follows established standards and codes.

Now, given that our motives are pure, what about nurses' political activities? One of the most tempting endeavors in the world is either to make an exception of oneself before the fact, because, of course, we mean well, or to excuse one's conduct for very much the same reasons. So we must honestly ask ourselves if our own Political Action Committees should act primarily to advocate for nurses' interests (e.g., seeking money for nursing education and research, addressing workplace issues such as mandatory overtime or registered nurse (RN) ratios, supporting opportunities for professional growth such as advanced licensure). Although a good case can be made that what is good for nurses and nursing is good for patients, one must ask, "Is it always good for the nation?" This is most particularly the case in light of the fact that the vast majority of nurses work in institutions for the care of the sick and elderly and that the vast majority of nurses' specialties are disease focused. That is, nurses, despite a perfunctory nod to wellness, are primarily engaged in caring for the sick and in augmenting the practice of medicine.

Although the practice of medicine has existed since ancient times, it is important to realize that the practice of curative or clinical medicine had virtually zero impact on human survival until about 1950, when antibiotics became available to the general population (McKeown, 1976). This observation, although thoroughly documented, runs counter to the common impression that improvements in our health and life expectancy are a result of medical progress. This is not true. The dramatic improvement in health and life expectancy from 1900 to 1950 (from 49 years in 1900 to 74 by 1950) is due almost entirely to an improved standard of living, a sufficient and clean food supply, social justice, public sanitation, vaccination, personal hygiene, and other such public health measures (Canadian Institute for Advanced Research, 1994). Moreover, the practice of professional medicine was not available to most people until the mid twentieth century, so even if there had been effective treatments, only a few people would have had access to them (Evans, Barer, & Marmor, 1994). But more fundamentally, until the mid 1900s the medical procedures that were available were as likely to hasten as to retard death (Black, Morris, Smith, & Townsend, 1982).

The obvious result of these largely social and environmental improvements is that most people began living long enough to age—and with age comes an increased risk for chronic illnesses and their acute manifestations. However, modern medicine as practiced in the United States of America has little to do with treating anything other than the acute manifestations of chronic illness. Although in the 50 years between 1950 and 2000, life expectancy increased to 80 years (about 30 additional years for the average person born in America), only 5 of those years are attributable to clinical medicine, and most of clinical medicine's contributions come from improved perinatal and early childhood care (Peterson, 1996).

Put another way, 100 years ago in 1900 when there was not any effective medicine, a person who survived to age 65 was expected to live an additional 11 years (to age 76). Today, with massive amounts of medical technology, a person who survives to age 65 has an average life expectancy of 80 years—an additional 15 years of life (U.S. Bureau of the Census, 2001). This means that there has been a gain of only 4 years of life over the last 100 years for those who survive to the age of 65. Moreover, of that additional 4 years, 3 can be attributed to public health measures, and only 1 year to clinical medicine *(www.fis.org/public/slide 6)*.

Society may be better served by determining what keeps populations healthy—and medical and nursing care have little to do with it! At least since the ancients wrote the book of *Leviticus*, people have known that the conditions surrounding where you live and work affect your health. We have always known that poverty isn't good for anyone and that whether people are well nurtured or well housed or have unhealthy lifestyle habits (e.g., drinking, smoking) affects their health. Moreover, we have learned that the *effectiveness of treatment* is heavily influenced by where people live and their relationships with those with whom they live. All of these are markers of social and environmental conditions, not of quality or access to medical care! So, even though the determinants of health (not illness) are found where, and with whom, people are in the world, we lobby for "health" legislation and funding and research that focus on diagnosis, treatment, and even prevention of disease as isolated events in isolated individuals.

When one explores the field of public health research, one begins to realize that the nature of the factors that cause disease can be better understood *in light of what produces healthy people*, and that *social* rather than *medical* interventions make a far greater contribution to the health of any community. Thus, a good case could be made that to advance the health of the population, nurses should be advocating for social and environmental change, not funding for more research and treatment for the ill...that far from advocating for their own advantage, or even the best interests of the ill, nurses and physicians should be lobbying for better environmental conditions, nutrition, education, and social supports for young families.

However, the principles of distributive justice, indeed the personal security of every member of society, are affected by whether or not someone will care for them if they are injured or ill or when they become elderly. Therefore what is in the profession's best interests and the patients' (those who are ill) best interests does indeed promote society's best interests—as long as this concern does not undermine the economic viability of that society. So, it is possible to reconcile competing interests; in fact, that's what politics is all about, on every level.

To frame this discussion, a review of the principles of distributive justice is in order.

## PRINCIPLES OF DISTRIBUTIVE JUSTICE

Health care professionals, who are ideally situated to make micro-distributive decisions and whose social role enables them to speak with authority to the general population about the impact of resource allocation decisions on the health and welfare of various segments of the population, must not allow social decisions to influence their clinical decisions. For one thing, their ethical codes require—and for good reason—that health care professionals act in the best interests of the person on whom they are laying hands (Frankl, 1959). For another thing, the will of the citizenry, as expressed through the votes of their elected representatives, should determine the distribution of the resources they have so diligently (if unwillingly) supplied to their governments. In general, the principles of distributive justice ought to be used to guide decision-making at the sociopolitical levels. They are:

1. *To each the same thing.* One of the simplest principles of distributive justice is that of strict or radical equality. The principle says that every person should have the same level of material goods and services. Even with this ostensibly simple principle, some of the difficult specification problems of distributive principles can be seen; specifically, construction of appropriate indexes for measurement, and the specification of time frames. Because there are numerous proposed solutions to these problems, the "principle of strict equality" is not a single principle but a name for a group of closely related principles.

2. *To each according to his need.* The most widely discussed theory of distributive justice in the past three decades has been that proposed by John Rawls in *A Theory of Justice* (Rawls, 1971) and *Political Liberalism* (Rawls, 1993). Rawls proposes the following two principles of justice: (1) Each person has an equal claim to a fully adequate scheme of equal basic rights and liberties, and (2) social and economic inequalities are "to be to the greatest benefit of the least advantaged members of society" (Rawls, 1993, pp. 5-6). These principles give fairly clear guidance on

what type of arguments will count as justifications for inequality.

3. *To each according to his ability to compete in the open market place.* Aristotle argued that virtue should be a basis for distributing rewards, but most contemporary principles owe a larger debt to John Locke. Locke argued people deserve to have those items produced by their toil and industry, the products (or the value thereof) being a fitting reward for their effort. His underlying idea was to guarantee to individuals the fruits of their own labor and abstinence. According to some contemporary theorists (Feinberg, 1970), people freely apply their abilities and talents, in varying degrees, to socially productive work. People come to deserve varying levels of income by providing goods and services desired by others (Feinberg, 1970). Distributive systems are just insofar as they distribute incomes according to the different levels earned or deserved by the individuals in the society for their productive labors, efforts, or contributions.

4. *To each according to his merits (desserts).* Merit-based principles of distribution differ primarily according to what they identify as the basis for deserving. Most contemporary proposals regarding merit fit into one of three broad categories (Miller, 1976, 1989):
   - Contribution: People should be rewarded for their work activity according to the value of their contribution to the social product.
   - Effort: People should be rewarded according to the effort they expend in their work activity.
   - Compensation: People should be rewarded according to the costs they incur in their work activity.

## NOW TO THE NITTY-GRITTY

Ethical theory is relatively unambiguous and rational. Unfortunately the real world—whether it be the world of organizational politics or the world of national health policy development—is, generally speaking, murky at best. It operates on opinion, emotion, and, as often as not, relationships. Therefore to a great extent one could say that what is wrong in relationships is also wrong in politics—so that, for

example, lying to further a political aim is as wrong as lying to a friend, a loved one, an employer, or a patient.

When people ask whether it is right to lie about something (e.g., the number of people affected by a particular disease) to get funding for research and/or treatment of patients with a particular disease, in a word the answer is yes. It is wrong. Why is lying wrong? It's wrong because it undermines the foundation of any relationship: trust. In like manner, lying to further a political agenda is wrong—not only because it undermines trust, but also because it fosters further dishonesty. Judging by the amount of political dishonesty reported in the media, one is led to the conclusion that there is a lot of lying going on! Adding to it—telling more lies to further our own agenda—will only make matters worse. Already I can hear people say, "But the worst of the worst will win if we don't lie!" Perhaps, but if you choose to join the worst of the worst in their lies, then the worst of the worst has already won.

Is it right for nurses to endorse a powerful candidate even though they oppose his positions on a number of social issues? Perhaps that might be a good move. The answer is yes, it may indeed be the right thing to do. Remember, politics is about relationships, and relationships cannot prosper when one party insists that the other party must agree with them on every (or even any) issue. "In the end, to thrive—even to exist—invariably means to tolerate in oneself a certain degree of inconsistency, but that is a far cry from deserting one's sense of right and wrong. It means, rather, that this is a world chock-full of small mindedness and inequity, a world in which greed and vanity are encouraged—*promoted*—at every turn. Each of us should know which lines she will not cross—would not even consider crossing—both in one's professional life and in the world at large, and those principles must remain inviolate" (Stein, 1982, p. 149). It is not wrong to compromise; compromise is part of the give and take of relationships, and it is part of the give and take of politics.

Well, one might ask, if it's acceptable to compromise, can it be acceptable to distort an issue to manipulate public opinion or to win the support of a particular congressman? Here one must be very careful, because deliberate distortion is lying by intent if not by actual fact. One can frame a discussion in a manner that is more acceptable to a certain constituency without lying. For example, in the health care arena, one can use words that appeal to known values; words like *tradition, legitimate authority*, and the like tend to appeal to conservatives, whereas other words like *autonomous* and *experimental* tend to appeal to liberals. Knowing the target audience and framing the issue in words that will help them listen (or at least not harden their opposition) is smart, not unethical.

Now, back to the issue of nurses' (and others') lobbying activities: Here compromise is in order. It is not wrong for a clearly defined group to support legislation and policies that push forward the best interests of the members of that group, provided that it is done honestly and openly and within the legitimate boundaries set by law. However, any professional group has a duty, imposed on it by both its social role and its code of ethics, to push forward laws and policies that protect or advance the best interests of those whom they serve. And finally, any citizen, particularly a knowledgeable one, has a civic duty to speak out for the common good.

The issues are not easy, nor are their proposed solutions. But ignoring them not only may lead to social disaster, it will also place the onus of decision-making on nurses and physicians. The real irony of the situation is that *health policy questions are resolved everyday on our clinical units*. Why? The health care system as it is currently structured and financed leaves access and decision-making up to insurers and to individuals who work at the "point of care." Resources to provide care are shrinking, as government and third party purchasers (employers who represent small and large businesses, alike) pressure the system to control, if not shrink, spending.

How much is too much to spend on medical care? This question is not easily answered at either the micro-level or the macro-level. On the micro-level it is handled a bit more easily, as individuals decide whether to spend their money on food or drugs or to see a physician because they or their children are suffering a certain symptom. As we move incrementally from the individual to the social level, matters become more complex.

For example, on March 11, 2004, the *Boston Globe* ran an article about a 79-year-old woman who is now completely paralyzed from Lou Gehrig's disease (Kowalczyk, 2004).

When Barbara Howe was diagnosed with Lou Gehrig's disease, she knew that it would cripple her before killing her. Therefore she repeatedly told her daughters and doctors and nurses to do whatever it took to keep her alive as long as she could appreciate her family. Howe also discussed end-of-life care with her family and physicians. Nonetheless, she ended up in a situation that neither she nor her family foresaw: long before her death, she was unable to make the slightest gesture while her doctors and her family argued in court about whether she still wanted everything done to keep her alive, given the advanced stage of her disease and the fact that she had been unable to communicate anything for more than 3 years.

Mrs. Howe did not leave the hospital from the time of her admission on November 15, 1999 until the time of her death in 2004. Blue Cross and Blue Shield of Massachusetts stopped covering her hospital stay in 2002. Her physicians and nurses believed that she was in pain and that keeping her alive was tantamount to torture. However, the patient's oldest daughter, who was her mother's health care proxy, disagreed, stating that it was her belief that her mother still recognized family members when they entered the room and would not have wanted to die at that point. The daughter also said that when she sensed that her mother no longer appreciated her family, she would have the ventilator turned off.

Howe's case epitomizes a shift in American medicine, one outcome of patients and families who are more educated and opinionated about health care—and more suspicious that physicians may deny care because of soaring costs.

As late as August of 2000, Mrs. Howe told her physicians that being alert was more important to her than being pain free—even though she suffered from constant headaches and facial pain. She also indicated that she wanted to continue receiving aggressive care, even though her ability to interact was fading fast. At the beginning of 2001, she could follow people with her eyes and move one finger.

By the end of the year, even these tiny gestures had disappeared.

In July 2001 the hospital's end-of-life committee reviewed the case. During this meeting, the patient's daughter insisted that her mother wanted aggressive treatment as long as she was able to enjoy and respond to her family. The ethics committee agreed to honor the request. However, shortly thereafter, Howe lost the ability to blink and to lubricate her eyes. Subsequently the dry tissue of her right cornea tore, and the end-of-life committee met immediately to reconsider her situation. As quoted by the journalist, the chairman of the ethics committee, Dr. Edwin Cassem (a psychiatrist and Jesuit priest), wrote in the minutes of the ethics committee, "There is now 100 percent unanimous agreement that this inhumane travesty has gone far enough. This is the Massachusetts General Hospital, not Auschwitz" (Kowalczyk, 2004, p. 7F).

The next day, surgeons removed Howe's right eye. Later that month, the hospital's lawyers asked the Probate and Family Court to intervene, but they ruled that there was not sufficient cause to remove the patient's daughter as her health care proxy. However, the judge did urge the daughter to refocus her assessment from the patient's wishes to the patient's best interests.

On January 13, 2004 physicians and nurses again asked Massachusetts General's end-of-life committee to order withdrawal of life support, saying the patient was now in danger of losing her left eye, which was taped shut except when her daughters visited. The daughter returned to court, saying her mother's left eye had improved; she said that when the patient was in danger of losing it, she would allow the hospital to turn off the ventilator. On February 22, 2004 the parties met with the probate judge for 2½ hours but failed to agree on a course of action (Kowalczyk, 2004). Barbara Howe died at the age of 80, 26 days before a court settlement would have allowed the hospital to turn off her ventilator (Kowalczyk, 2005).

The Howe case, so far at least, has not progressed beyond the local level—and that is difficult enough. The next case, though, went to state supreme courts and to federal courts, as well as to local, state, and national legislatures. What follows is a summary of

testimony given in the Terri Schiavo case in the Pinellas County Circuit Court.

Terri Schiavo, 25, was found unconscious by her husband in the early morning of February 25, 1990. She had suffered a full cardiac arrest. Defibrillation was performed seven times during initial resuscitative efforts, with eventual restoration of a normal cardiac rhythm. The initial serum potassium level was 2.0, undoubtedly the cause of her cardiac arrest. Terri had a history of erratic eating habits, including probable bulimia, with a major weight loss several years before this event. In November of 1992, Michael Schiavo won a malpractice suit against Terri's physicians for failing to diagnose her health problems leading up to the cardiac arrest resulting directly from her eating disorder (George W. Greer, Circuit Court, Pinellas County, Florida, File No. 90-2908-GD-003).

Terri was in a coma for approximately 1 month, and then her condition evolved into a persistent vegetative state (PVS). Four board-certified neurologists in Florida consulting on her care—James H. Barnhill, Garcia J. Desousa, Thomas H. Harrison, and Jeffrey M. Karp—diagnosed her PVS. The initial computed tomography (CT) scan on the day of admission, February 25, 1990, had normal findings, but further CT scans documented a progression of widespread cerebral hemisphere atrophy, eventually resulting in CT scans in 1996 and 2002 that showed extreme atrophy, specifically, "diffuse encephalomalacia and infarction consistent with anoxia, hydrocephalus ex vacuo, neural stimulator present." Clinical examinations over the years were entirely consistent with the diagnosis of permanent vegetative state secondary to hypoxic-ischemic encephalopathy (George W. Greer, Circuit Court, Pinellas County, Florida, File No. 90-2908-GD-003).

For purposes of rational discussion, it helps to make some important distinctions, such as the distinction between a coma and a PVS. "A coma is a profound or deep state of unconsciousness. An individual in a state of coma is alive but unable to move or respond to his or her environment. Coma may occur as a complication of an underlying illness, or as a result of injuries, such as head trauma. A persistent vegetative state (commonly, but incorrectly, referred to as "brain-death") sometimes follows a coma. Individuals in such a state have lost their thinking abilities and awareness of their surroundings, but retain non-cognitive function and normal sleep patterns. Even though those in a persistent vegetative state lose their higher brain functions, other key functions such as breathing and circulation remain relatively intact. Spontaneous movements may occur, and the eyes may open in response to external stimuli. They may even occasionally grimace, cry, or laugh. Although individuals in a persistent vegetative state may appear somewhat normal, they do not speak and they are unable to respond to commands" *(www.ninds.nih.gov/disorders/coma/coma.htm).*

Another problem that needs to be addressed is whether or not feeding is a medical intervention, especially whether or not a permanent feeding tube could be considered a "futile medical intervention," and therefore could be legitimately withdrawn. Although feeding per se is not a medical intervention, tube feedings may indeed be considered one. At any rate, the courts in the Schiavo case held this to be so (George W. Greer, Circuit Court, Pinellas County, Florida, File No. 90-2908-GD-003). If Schiavo could have been fed by mouth and swallow her food, the courts may have taken a different position. However, whether Terri was fed via a PEG tube or fed orally, she was still in a permanent vegetative state, and feeding her would not have not resulted in any change in her clinical condition, except she would probably die much sooner were attempts made to feed her orally—that is, the feeding tube could not improve her medical condition. If feeding is not a medical treatment, can medical personnel refuse to provide it, or remove a feeding tube if it already is in place? The answer is unclear and may depend on the patient's wishes and values, or those of a legal guardian. In the Schiavo case, despite her parents' monumental efforts, Schiavo's husband repeatedly was recognized by the courts as her legal guardian.

Although numerous court cases have irrefutably established a patient's right to refuse medical treatment, few have dealt with a patient's right (if there is one) *to undergo* medical treatment when all medical authorities agree that the treatment is useless. Although a case can be made that a right to refuse treatment isn't worth much if there is no right to treatment, one must ask if there is a right "to treatment that can in no way benefit one." Surely not even the most zealous advocates for universal access to health care would insist that patients have a right to medical treatments that do not benefit them and that may, indeed, harm them.

How much can any one citizen, or family, demand from society? This is, indeed, a political question that, according to the best information available to us, should not be answered in a manner that undermines support for policies that improve living and working conditions, provide support for young families, reduce domestic and social violence, and assure fair wages, educational benefits, and a clean environment, for these are the elements of a health-producing society (Black, Morris, Smith, & Townsend, 1982). And the questions do not stop at difficult cases, or even with a determination of futility. In fact, these questions must be asked about such well-established programs as Medicare. Is it right to assure medical care for the elderly (surely a good thing) by taxing the incomes of all workers (if not an evil thing, at least it is not a fair thing, because they must support a program to which they themselves have no access, especially when many of these workers lack insurance for themselves and their families)? Some may say the answers to such questions of domestic policy are a matter of political philosophy—and, indeed, they are. But they also are matters of ethics: of what is right and wrong. And they are matters that health professionals cannot escape.

## Key Points

- The end can never justify the means, because the means one chooses to use are precisely what is brought into this world.
- Political means must be used to set policy, not to determine events in individual cases.
- If advocating for policies that cover all the costs of the care of the sick undermines support for policies that improve living and working conditions, provide support for young families, reduce domestic and social violence, and assure fair wages, educational benefits, and a clean environment for

the population at large, it actually will increase the amount of illness in a population.

- A professional ethic is built around three essential components: (1) the purpose of the profession; (2) the conduct expected of the profession articulated in ethical codes; and (3) the results or skills expected as articulated in standards of practice.

- Ethics and politics have much in common. Each has to do with right and wrong in this world. Each has to do with making life better for oneself and others. Each deals with power and powerlessness, with human rights and balancing their claims, and with justice and fairness.

## Web Resources

---
**Baylor College Center for Medical Ethics and Health Policy**
*www.bcm.edu/ethics*
**Curtin Calls**—site of Leah Curtin, with focused area on ethics
*www.curtincalls.com/Frame/Ethics*
**Hastings Center**—an independent, nonpartisan, and nonprofit bioethics research institute founded in 1969 to explore fundamental and emerging questions in health care, biotechnology, and the environment
*www.thehastingscenter.org*
**Nursing Ethics**—an international journal on ethics for health care professionals
*www.nursing-ethics.com*
**NursingEthics.ca**—a Canadian-based site for resources on nursing ethics
*www.nursingethics.ca*
---

## REFERENCES

Black, D., Morris, J. N., Smith, C., & Townsend, P. (1982). *Inequalities in health: The Black report.* Harmondsworth, Middlesex, England; New York: Penguin Books.

Canadian Institute for Advanced Research. (1994). *The determinants of health.* CIAR publication #5. Toronto: CIAR.

*Ethics manual for members, officers, and employees of the U. S. House of Representatives.* Retrieved August 23, 2003, from *www.house.gov/ethics/Ethicforward.html.*

Evans, R. G., Barer, M. L., & Marmor, T. R. (Eds.). (1994). *Why are some people healthy and others not? The Determinants of Health of Populations.* New York: Aldine DeGruyter.

Feinberg, J. (1970). *Justice and personal desert, doing and deserving.* Princeton, NJ: Princeton University Press.

Frankl, V. (1959). *Man's search for meaning.* Boston: Beacon Press.

Gandhi, M. (1958). *The collected works of Mahatma Gandhi.* Publications Division, Ministry of Information and Broadcasting, Government of India, New Delhi.

George W. Greer, Circuit Court, Pinellas County, Florida, File No. 90-2908-GD-003.

Kidder, R. M. (1994). *Shared values for a troubled world: Conversations with men and women of conscience.* San Francisco: Jossey-Bass.

Kowalczyk, L. (2004, March 11). Hospital, family spar over end-of-life care. *Boston Globe,* 2F-8F.

Kowalczyk, L. (2005, June 8). Woman dies after battle over care. *Boston Globe,* 2F.

McKeown, T. (1976). *The role of medicine: Dream, mirage or nemesis?* Oxford: Basil Blackford.

Miller, D. (1976). *Social justice.* Oxford: Clarendon Press.

Miller, D. (1989). *Market, state, and community.* Oxford: Clarendon Press.

Peterson, P. G. (1996). Will Americans grow up before they grow old? *Atlantic Monthly, 9.* Retrieved September 14, 1996, from *http://pqasb.pqarchiver.com/theatlantic/doc/9765211.html?MAC=5a3ab40de384a55bc545988.*

Rawls, J. (1971). *A theory of justice.* Harvard, MA: Harvard University Press.

Rawls, J. (1993). *Political liberalism.* New York: Columbia University Press.

Stein, H. (1982). *Ethics and other liabilities.* London: St Martins Press.

U.S. Bureau of the Census. (2001). *Statistical abstract of the United States 2000.* Washington, DC: U.S. Government Printing Office. Retrieved July 6, 2001, from *www.census.gov/prod/2001pubs/c2kbr01-2.pdf.*

Wellman, C. (1975). *Morals and ethics.* Glenview, IL: Scott, Foresman.

# The U.S. Health Care System

Sue Thomas Hegyvary

*"We are not just one good Health Affairs article away from solving the problems of the U.S. health care system."*

IAN MORRISON

The U.S. health care system is a highly complex, pluralistic entity, praised by some, denounced by others. Its biomedical progress has led the world for decades, but its costs are the highest in the world. It enables unprecedented and often unimaginable treatment for some people, but its doors remain closed to millions of others. Clear descriptions and wider understanding of this gargantuan system are needed, and the goal for this chapter is to provide them.

Both informed analyses and everyday opinions indicate that the U.S. system has some serious problems and that reform is needed. Discussions about reform too often lack a base of systematic evidence, like declaring a diagnosis and treatment plan without first taking a careful history and performing a physical examination. This chapter does not provide a recommended plan for health care reform. Instead it provides a wide base of evidence, in international context, about characteristics of the U.S. system. This information and discussion should enable readers to reach their own conclusions about the strengths and deficits of the U.S. health care system and to consider viable alternatives for change. In this chapter the term "U.S. health care system" pertains to the composite of health care services in the country, including both public and private sectors, and encompassing structures, processes, and outcomes of the system.

## EVOLUTION OF AN OPEN SYSTEM IN U.S. HEALTH CARE

Systems can be described in various ways, and no one approach is a standard for assessing health care systems. An important foundation for assessing and planning health care systems is clarity of the organizational concepts of "open" and "closed" systems. Although "open" might sound positive and "closed" negative, the terms indicate differences in definition and function; they are not value statements. Furthermore, they are not separate elements of a dichotomy; they are points on a continuum.

## OPEN VERSUS CLOSED SYSTEMS

The major distinguishing feature of an open versus a closed system is the relationship of people and functions within the system to those outside it (Thompson, 1977). A closed system is internally structured and controlled, its membership is clearly defined, and its processes are buffered from external influence. The nearest approximations of a closed system historically in U.S. health care are the Group Health Cooperative and Kaiser Permanente systems, which were prototype managed care systems and have been in existence since the mid-twentieth century. They are internally self-governing and self-regulating, including structures, finances, and member enrollment. They are simultaneously the insurer, the regulator, the employer of health personnel, and the provider of services for designated enrollees. Yet they still must be concerned with their external environments, such as regulatory and accrediting agencies, as well as competition from other providers, so they cannot be completely closed systems.

In concept, if the structure and functions of one of these systems were expanded to national level, covering all Americans and including services now contracted to other providers, it would be a national health service (NHS). However, note that neither Group Health Cooperative nor Kaiser Permanente has ever been a governmental system; they are in the private sector. This point is important in the following discussion of international assumptions and comparisons of health care systems, because a common assumption about systems that provide universal coverage is that they are necessarily public. The Veterans Administration and other federal agencies that fund or provide health care also have many characteristics of closed systems in both funding and people served, but they too are subject to external regulation and influence.

At the other end of this continuum are open systems. Open-system entities are characterized by continuous reciprocity in major components of the system. People inside the system constantly interact and negotiate with people outside the system (e.g., patients, payers, contractors, physician groups, and others). Open systems might look more chaotic than closed systems, but their openness can be by design. The U.S. health care environment is an open system, both by design and by default; some call it a "patchwork" of systems (Heinrich & Thompson, 2002). Americans historically have distrusted centralized government, so decentralization and pluralism have long been defining characteristics of American life, including health care services. The U.S. health care system has evolved as an increasingly open system, composed of many diverse components. It is an open system, yet extensive types of regulation prevent it from being a true "open-market" system.

Organizational and systems theories indicate that effectiveness and survival of systems require continuous adaptation in response to both internal and external changes. If systems become too complex to function efficiently and effectively, adaptations falter, resulting in less-than-desirable outcomes for the system and the population it is supposed to serve. Many citizens and analysts believe the U.S. system has reached or exceeded this extreme type of open system.

Although these concepts and definitions are based on many decades of observations and studies of organizations, not of whole countries or entities as complex as national health care systems, they are useful in analyzing and understanding the evolution and function of health care systems.

## SENTINEL EVENTS IN U.S. HEALTH CARE

Health care historically has been perceived as separate from general societal institutions, protected from the world of commerce and competition, and held apart as bordering on the sacred. Health care facilities (i.e., hospitals) were exempt until recently from most of the rules governing business organizations, in part because of their dominant history as religious and military institutions. They could and did function as relatively closed systems. Some important events in U.S. health care history illustrate defining moments in the evolution of the system.

**Opposition to Centralized Government.** Since the founding of the country, Americans have opposed strong centralized government. In the early twentieth century many reformers advocated "sickness insurance" like that for workers in Germany, but national health insurance never received much political support. The Shepherd-Towner Act of 1921 set the stage for national funding for decentralized programs by providing matching funds to states for prenatal and child health centers. Public health nurses in these centers reduced maternal and infant mortality by teaching women basic hygiene and how to care for themselves and their families. This program was considered highly successful. However, it was discontinued in 1927 after the American Medical Association (AMA) convinced legislators that it was excessive federal interference with local health care services (Heinrich & Thompson, 2002; Starr, 1982). Perhaps more an issue of professional dominance and medical economics than of political ideology, it established the power of the AMA over health care legislation. It also set the stage for the focus of health services more on the desires of providers than on the needs of the public.

**The Rallying Cry against "Socialized Medicine."** Concerns about both cost and availability of medical care in the economically difficult 1930s led to formation of the Committee on the Costs of Medical Care. In its final report the committee opposed compulsory health insurance but endorsed group practice for provision and payment of medical care. Denouncing the proposals as socialized medicine, the AMA succeeded in preventing enactment of even voluntary health insurance. In 1943 a bill before the U.S. Senate to create comprehensive and universal health insurance was defeated because of strong opposition led by the AMA. A few years later, national health insurance was part of Truman's successful campaign for the presidency, but again accusations of socialism, including by the AMA, led to its defeat. However, the AMA supported one of Truman's proposals, the Hill-Burton Act for hospital construction, and the bill passed (Heinrich & Thompson, 2002; Starr, 1982). The American Nurses Association (ANA), with a much larger membership than the AMA, repeatedly supported proposals for national health insurance (Woods, 1996). However, the influence of the ANA and other professional organizations was never equal to that of the AMA. Thus, although the emotionally charged term *socialized medicine* is ill defined and based on many misperceptions of European systems, its use remains a successful tactic against expansion of national programs of health care financing.

**Passage of Medicare and Medicaid.** Despite the opposition of the AMA, but with the support of the AFL-CIO labor unions and professional organizations such as ANA, Medicare and Medicaid programs were enacted in 1965 as an amendment to the Social Security Act of 1935. Medicare was established as a federal insurance program for payment of acute medical services for people who are age 65 and older, are permanently disabled, or have end-stage renal disease. Medicaid was set up as federal funding to states, with matching state funds, to provide health care for poor people and to cover some long-term care services. These programs provide a partial "safety net," but they do not fund comprehensive services, and their restrictions on eligibility exclude coverage for many people without health insurance (Bodenheimer & Grumbach, 2002).

**Rise of Hospitals and Biomedical Enterprise.** Rapid expansion of hospitals as the center for provision of medical care, growth of medical group practices, increased availability of payment through Medicare and Medicaid as well as from private insurers, and burgeoning advances in biomedical sciences led to a heyday for growth of the American health care industry. Calling health care an industry spurred the impassioned resistance of health professionals because of the religious and humanitarian origins of health care. Paradoxically, those beliefs were not expressed as support for universal coverage for health care, even during the social upheavals of the 1960s. Dominant behaviors have indicated and reinforced the cultural emphasis on individuality, not on social welfare, and the desire to retain health care as a partitioned sector with great emphasis on rights and prerogatives of providers.

The dramatically expanding medical sciences and services were focused quite successfully on treatment of acute conditions, leading to increasing specialization and fragmentation of health care services and relegation of public health to lesser status and importance. The "technologic imperative" reigned, with acute care treatment at any cost for those who could pay. Those trends continued well into the 1970s, as hospitals became high-tech tertiary care centers with insurance reimbursement for expenses of providing services. Hospital networks expanded to create vertically integrated systems, combining primary, secondary, and tertiary care as single corporate entities. The number of for-profit conglomerates increased. This era further solidified the emphasis on medical treatment of acute illness in hospitals, without systematic attention to health promotion, community and population health, or needs of people unable to pay. Agencies such as community health centers, home care services, nursing homes, and public health agencies functioned on very limited funding, outside the mainstream of hospital-based biomedical enterprise (Bodenheimer & Grumbach, 2002; Garrett, 2000).

**From Reimbursement to Payment.** After failure of voluntary cost controls, the beginning of prospective payment in 1983 opened a new era in U.S. health care. That change was a true paradigm shift; it was not just evolutionary, it was revolutionary. No longer would providers be reimbursed for expenditures; they would receive lump-sum payment per patient on the basis of diagnosis, according to the national schedule with some regional variations. If they spent less per patient, they kept the difference. If they spent more, they had to absorb the deficit. Thus, hospitals were required to operate as businesses, with accountability for services and budgets. Payments from Medicare and Medicaid were reduced. Vertically integrated systems had already been created after President Nixon signed the Health Maintenance Organization Act in 1973 (Millenson, 1998). After prospective payment began in 1983, these integrated systems expanded in far greater numbers to balance costs and coordinate services by combining levels of care, from primary care to the most advanced and acute specialty care, forming relatively closed systems. This movement began in the 1970s and increased as mergers and acquisitions became common approaches to managing costs and positioning for survival in a competitive market. Shock waves swept through the health care industry for the next two decades as hospitals unable to compete were forced to close. Lengths of stay decreased, putting great pressure on home care agencies, nursing homes, and of course patients and families (Bodenheimer & Grumbach, 2002; Williams & Torrens, 2002). Seemingly, medical practice would have been highly affected by these changes. However, physician's selection of practice location, their productivity, and their satisfaction have been linked not as much to the changes in the marketplace as to their compensation (Conrad et al., 1998; Zierler, et al., 1998).

**Failed Reform.** National reform of health care was a high priority of the Clinton administration in the 1990s. Fraught with political controversy from the beginning, proposed reforms failed. Despite widespread dissatisfaction with various aspects of the health care system, no coherent plan for national policy or system-wide reforms has been on the public agenda since then. Emphasis on primary care increased, but more recently the proportion of U.S. physicians in primary care has decreased (Biola et al., 2003; Pinnacle Health Group, 1999), and the success of managed care is widely questioned (Dudley & Luft, 2003). The focus on prescription drug costs and inclusion of prescription drug benefits in Medicare have consumed both political and public attention, to the extent that some people appear to believe that treating this problem would cure the ills of the health care system. Further, powerful stakeholders including the AMA, insurance companies, and employer groups remain effective in blocking more comprehensive national programs (Quadagno, 2004).

Efforts for effective change continue, locally and nationally, publicly and privately, but they have not come close to resolving some long-standing problems and the still-increasing costs. Whether all those problems can ever be resolved to the satisfaction of whole populations is doubtful, given that every health care system in the world is undergoing change because of costs, dissatisfaction of some stakeholders, and less than desired outcomes. Assessing the U.S. health care system in international context enhances understanding of the complexity of the health care system in the United States, reasons for its variance from those of other advanced countries, and insights into possible directions for change (Fried & Gaydos, 2002; Powell & Wessen, 1999).

## THE U.S. HEALTH CARE SYSTEM IN INTERNATIONAL CONTEXT

Efforts in recent decades to identify a "best" health care system have generally been focused mostly on structure and financing. Other analysts have looked primarily at outcome measures such as life expectancy and infant mortality. More recently, the amount of health care expenditures has garnered much attention as a predictor of overall outcomes. No one approach is complete, and every approach contains problems that limit comparisons. This analysis is presented not to suggest that identifying a "best" system is possible or even desirable but to portray the U.S. system along several dimensions.

This information does not include the historical or cultural context of sentinel events in other countries, and that information would be useful in more detailed analyses.

## HEALTH SYSTEMS PERFORMANCE

An important attempt to assess national health care systems around the world was the initiative of the World Health Organization (WHO) to measure health systems performance (HSP). The WHO definition of a health system is one that "includes all actors, institutions and resources that undertake health actions—where a health action is one [with] the primary intent to improve health.... Four key functions determine the way inputs are transformed into outcomes that people value: resource generation, financing, service provision and stewardship." An assumption basic to WHO analyses is that the ultimate and permanent responsibility for performance of a country's health system lies with government (WHO, 2001a, 2001b).

WHO analysts used their HSP measure to assess national health systems in all countries of the world. The HSP includes five indicators: overall level of population health; health inequalities or disparities within the population; overall level of health system responsiveness (a combination of patient satisfaction and how well the system performs); distribution responsiveness within the population (how well people of varying economic status are served by the system); and the distribution of the health system's financial burden within the population (WHO, 2001b). This measure has been controversial because it is based on opinion surveys of WHO experts throughout the world, and the databases for making determinations are unclear and possibly inconsistent (Blendon, Kim, & Benson, 2001). However, it warrants mention, regarding both the indicators and the results for different countries. The HSP measure yields scores on each aspect of a country's system and also allows ranking of countries according to their overall scores. On a scale from 0 to 100 it indicates the extent to which a country achieves the goals in each of the five indicators in relation to its resources (WHO, 2001a).

In the latest survey the overall HSP score for the United States was 84. The United States scored highest in the world in level of responsiveness (i.e., quality). However, the overall score of 84 placed the United States thirty-seventh of 191 countries because of unequal access to services within the population and lack of fairness of financing. Countries in Western Europe, plus Japan and Singapore, scored highest overall (Table 13-1). Despite questions about the validity and reliability of the HSP, the results for the United States appear consistent with widescale perceptions of U.S. health care, both inside and outside the country.

Such comprehensive efforts to assess and compare health care systems are difficult. More common are national comparisons of certain aspects of systems, including structure and financing, health care expenditure, and outcomes in population health. Exploring these characteristics enhances clarity about the U.S. system as well as possible areas for change.

## STRUCTURE AND FINANCING OF HEALTH CARE SYSTEMS

Although details of implementation vary within and among countries, national health care systems of the world can be categorized in three types: NHS, mandated insurance model, and entrepreneurial model (Fried & Gaydos, 2002; Roemer, 1993). Because structures and financing are so closely linked, they are considered together. A major dimension in this categorization is the degree of central authority of the government: highest in an NHS, lowest in an entrepreneurial model. Financing and performance of selected countries to illustrate types of systems are shown in Table 13-1.

**National Health Service.** The most easily understood type of system is that of an NHS. It is clearest because it denotes one comprehensive national system for structure, coordination, financing, control, and delivery of services. Among currently functioning systems it most approximates an all-inclusive, closed type of system. The prime example is the health care system of the United Kingdom (UK), established in 1948. All components of the NHS are centralized, including funding mostly from taxation, governmental determination of health policy, governmental payment of health

**TABLE 13-1** Health System Expenditures, Sources of Funding, and Performance Score, by Type of System in Selected Countries, 2001

| TYPE OF SYSTEM AND COUNTRY | PERCENT OF GDP USED FOR HEALTH CARE | EXPENDITURES PER CAPITA (INTERNATIONAL DOLLARS) | PERCENT OF GOVERNMENT FUNDS | PERCENT OF PRIVATE FUNDS | PERCENT OF PRIVATE FUNDS: OUT-OF-POCKET EXPENSE | HEALTH SYSTEM PERFORMANCE SCORE (RANK)* |
|---|---|---|---|---|---|---|
| **NATIONAL HEALTH SERVICE** | | | | | | |
| United Kingdom | 7.6 | 1989 | 82.2 | 17.8 | 55.3 | 92 (18) |
| **MANDATED INSURANCE** | | | | | | |
| Australia | 9.5 | 2699 | 67.9 | 32.1 | 61.4 | 88 (32) |
| Canada | 9.5 | 2792 | 70.8 | 29.2 | 52.3 | 88 (30) |
| Germany | 10.8 | 2820 | 74.9 | 25.1 | 42.4 | 90 (25) |
| Japan | 8.0 | 2131 | 77.9 | 22.1 | 74.9 | 96 (10) |
| Singapore | 3.9 | 993 | 33.5 | 66.5 | 97.0 | 97 (6) |
| Sweden | 8.7 | 2270 | 85.2 | 14.8 | 100.0 | 91 (23) |
| **ENTREPRENEURIAL** | | | | | | |
| USA | 13.9 | 4887 | 44.4 | 55.6 | 26.5 | 84 (37) |

From World Health Organization (WHO). (2001). World health report 2000: World Health Organization assesses the world's health systems. Retrieved March 27, 2004, from *www.int/whr2001/2001/archives/2000/en/press_release.htm* and *www.who.int/whr/2000/en/annex10_en.pdf;* and World Health Organization (WHO). (2001). About health systems performance. Retrieved April 5, 2005, from *www.who.int/health-systems performance/about.htm.*
*GDP,* ross domestic product.
*Range of 0 to 100.

care personnel, and governmental ownership of facilities. The NHS provides a full range of services, but some very expensive types of treatment might not be provided. A critical feature of this type of system is the designation of "global budgets." Overall expenditures are capped, and various methods are used to stay within spending limits, including restrictions on the types of services that can be provided in the NHS (Bodenheimer & Grumbach, 2002; Thai, Wimberley, & McManus, 2002).

The broad foundation of the NHS is a pervasive network of general practitioners and primary care services, with local, regional, and national coordination. Every person using the NHS must have a general practitioner as the "gatekeeper," and people choose their general practitioners. Frontline primary care also includes NHS-Direct, an organized arrangement for access to district nurses-on-call, via telephone or the Internet, for every resident of the United Kingdom (Clark, 2000; Schoen et al., 2004). Thus, the basic element of the NHS is primary care, with referrals to hospitals and

specialists as necessary. Over 60% of physicians in the United Kingdom are primary care practitioners. Governmental cost controls pertain to all parts of the NHS, including physician payment, hospital costs, and pharmaceutical expenditures (Bodenheimer & Grumbach, 2002).

About 13% of NHS funding comes from employer-employee contributions, but the United Kingdom separates health insurance from employment (Bodenheimer & Grumbach, 2002). Everyone has coverage, regardless of employment status. Although comprehensive health care services are provided through public funding for everyone in the United Kingdom, excluding specifically restricted types of treatment, the United Kingdom allows a parallel private system for both health care services and private health insurance. About 11% of the population uses private services. People choosing to use the private system still must pay the taxes that support the NHS, and they pay for the private care in addition. Reasons for choosing private-sector services include perceptions of waiting time and quality of services in NHS facilities, as well as desire for preferential treatment. Practitioners who are salaried employees of NHS are permitted to engage in fee-for-service private practice in addition to their work in NHS. Many general practitioners maintain private practice and are paid from NHS funds for services rendered to patients who are covered under NHS (Bloor & Maynard, 2002; Bodenheimer & Grumbach, 2002).

The NHS in the United Kingdom continues to undergo various reforms (Stevens, 2004), but the basic premises and principles of the system remain intact. It is the prototypic comprehensive single-payer national system, with universal access to governmentally provided health care. The NHS has adequate levels of acceptance and success to have remained intact for over a half-century. The Canadian system is sometimes compared with that of the United Kingdom. However, Canada has varied systems in different provinces, and it does not have the single unified structure of an NHS. Canada also has a large private sector, and private providers by law may not duplicate the services provided and paid for by the government. Physicians are paid on a fee-for-service basis. Canada's national health insurance, as in the United Kingdom, is separate from employment (Bodenheimer & Grumbach, 2002; Conference Board of Canada, 2005).

Additional countries have or are establishing centralized, public, comprehensive health care systems. Affluent countries with many elements of this model are Norway and Sweden. Sweden is regarded in this discussion as predominately in the mandated insurance model, though its system is mixed, with many characteristics of an NHS implemented regionally. Other variations of this model, still with the intent of a centrally controlled comprehensive system, exist in middle-income Costa Rica and in lower-income Sri Lanka (Dow & Saenz, 2002; Roemer, 1993).

**Mandated Insurance Model.** A national health service and mandated universal coverage are not synonymous, and systems with mandated insurance coverage have a seemingly endless range in form. The defining principle in the mandated insurance model is that the national government

sets policy that all people are covered for health care services. Setting policy for universal coverage might be all the government does. Or the government might also fund or provide basic services to people without other coverage. People do not have to be covered in the same way, and coverage is not necessarily through public funds. When it is provided through public funds, again the methods might vary, including global budgets, tiered services, or the requirement of cost-effectiveness analysis before new drugs or treatments are approved, as in Australia. Analogous to the requirement for universal basic education, either public or private, the baseline in this model is health care coverage for the entire population. How that policy is implemented at the provider-patient level has many different versions of quasi-open systems, with varying degrees of governmental regulation. Often called the "social insurance" model, it began in Germany in the late nineteenth century.

This type of system has deep historical roots in the hundreds of types of "sickness insurance" within guilds or occupational groups in Europe in the nineteenth century. It was adopted in Germany in 1883 for lower-paid workers, not as a matter of social philosophy, but as a result of governmental negotiations with labor unions. Workers and employers were required to share the cost of sickness insurance. More-affluent people remained in the private market. The rapidly emerging model, although not without controversy, had the critical support of physician groups. Mandatory coverage for workers soon became a political concept far beyond the origins of sickness insurance, resulting in a firmly established employment base for insurance, a model that spread rapidly to many other European countries (Basch, 1999; Roemer, 1993).

Germany in the 1880s had more than 20,000 small local sickness funds, and in the 1990s more than 1000 of them were still in operation (Basch, 1999). With mandated coverage, everyone must be part of some fund. The German government does not fund or deliver the services; it regulates and monitors the system. The concept of mandated coverage has been adopted in many countries, including France, Japan, Austria, Belgium, Switzerland, Australia, New Zealand, and the Netherlands (Basch, 1999;

Fried & Gaydos, 2002), with more recent extensions in Mexico, India, and other countries (Fried & Gaydos, 2002; Roemer, 1993). Although the overall principle in this model is mandated universal coverage, some countries such as Japan, with physician ownership of many hospitals, support considerable levels of entrepreneurship (Ikegami & Campbell, 2004).

The mandated insurance model now is the most common type of health care system throughout the developed world and also in many developing countries, but structures, financing, and delivery of care vary widely. A government might provide insurance from tax revenues, or funding is sometimes a combination of employment-based insurance with a "safety net" public assistance program for unemployed people. Levels and quality of services are not uniform within countries; tiers of service exist in many countries by design, in others by default. So the principle of universal coverage does not assure equal access to all types of health care services, and every country has some forms of de facto rationing of services (Reinhardt, Hussey, & Anderson, 2004; Twaddle, 2002).

A major variation of the mandated insurance model that approaches the entrepreneurial model is the health care system in Singapore (Basch, 1999). Until a major reorganization in 1984, Singapore had an NHS like that of the United Kingdom, with publicly provided health care services financed by general taxation. The new system had four founding principles: free choice for consumers; self-accountability and self-reliance; free market competition; and the government as provider of last resort, with at least minimal services for people unable to pay. The resulting system is based on compulsory medical savings accounts (MSAs), funded through required percentages of income that increase with age, up to a specified amount in the account. Employers match the individual savings. The MSA is personally owned, analogous to a pension fund; it is not part of a pooled public fund. It remains part of a person's assets, even as part of one's estate at death. Basch (1999) described it not as health insurance, but as a forced savings plan. The MSA pays for a person's medical expenses as much as possible, although catastrophic illness is covered through a general tax-based fund, as are basic health care services for people unable to pay. The Singapore government maintains control over the system, including facilities and health care personnel. Because some types of very expensive treatment are excluded, people may choose to pay for such services privately. This mandated yet somewhat open system exists in a unique societal context, and it appears to have been very successful there. Although the cultural and political contexts differ greatly, the guiding principles and provisions in Singapore are echoed in many discussions of reforms in the United States.

**Entrepreneurial Systems.** The major example of a predominately entrepreneurial system is that of the United States (Fried & Gaydos, 2002; Roemer, 1993). The word *entrepreneurial* denotes private enterprise, so the term is somewhat misleading. Nearly half of the health care services in the United States are publicly funded through Medicare, Medicaid, the Veterans Administration, and other public programs (Bodenheimer & Grumbach, 2002), yet services to people enrolled in these programs are provided largely in the private sector. This type of system is an extreme type of open system, with limited central control, no national policy for universal coverage, and a wide and changing mix of providers and linkages among providers. It also contains a vast web of regulations, so its function as an open and entrepreneurial system is limited and sometimes contradictory. A few other countries (e.g., Thailand and Pakistan) have many elements of an entrepreneurial system (Roemer, 1993; Twaddle, 2002), and some other countries such as the Netherlands and Mexico (Johnson, Carillo, & Garcia, 2002) have made changes toward the pluralistic and entrepreneurial system of the United States (Thai, Wimberley, & McManus, 2002; Twaddle, 2002). Discussion of the U.S. system follows, after consideration of other dimensions of the international context.

## HEALTH CARE EXPENDITURES

Recent findings in a study of global health showed that the factor with greatest explanatory power in groups of transitional and developed countries (but not in developing countries) was health care expenditures (Hegyvary, Berry, & Murua, 2006). This finding pertained to groups of countries, not necessarily to individual countries. In the group of 79 transitional countries and the group of 27 advanced countries (including the United States), spending more on health care contributed to longer life expectancy and lower death rates of infants and children under age 5 years. However, the United States differed from others in the group of advanced countries. Americans spent the most by far, but their longevity and child survival were marginal to the rest of the peer group.

In 2001 the United States reported the world's highest per capita expenditure on health care, $4887 per person, international dollars (World Bank, 2002, 2003) and the highest percentage of gross national product consumed for health care (see Table 13-1). These figures far exceeded those of any other country. At the same time the United States was the major exception among peer countries in that it alone did not provide some form of universal or "safety net" coverage for people unable to pay, and 47 million Americans lack health insurance (Krisberg, 2005). Expenditures have continued to rise; Smith, Cowan, Sensenig, Catlin, and Health Accounts Team (2005) reported a per capita expenditure of $5670 in the United States in 2003, with continued increases in spending. The percent of the U.S. gross domestic product (GDP) spent for health care rose from 13.3% in 1993, to 14.1% in 1999, to 15.3% in 2003 (Smith et al., 2005), compared with an average of about 8% in peer countries (World Bank, 2003).

These findings and similar results in other reports lead to many questions. One pertains to the actual accounting for health care costs and the comparability of data from different countries. Analysis of validity and reliability is lacking, and greater standardization of databases is needed for valid comparisons. Still, the U.S. expenditure is so much higher than that of comparable countries that even with some margin of error in the data the overall results warrant attention.

The reasons for the high expenditures in the United States are the subject of much debate and acrimony. Proposed reforms contain implicit assumptions about the parts of the system at fault for the high expenditures. Advocates for a single-payer system assume that multiple payers cause increased costs and decreased efficiency. Proponents of governmental control of the pharmaceutical industry assume that the costs of prescription drugs and profits of pharmaceutical companies are the culprits. Others point to limiting physicians' incomes, providing more out-of-hospital services, or other measures based on the assumed locus of excessive costs. Table 13-2 shows that *all* parts of the U.S. health care system have had increased expenditures from 1993 to 1999 to 2003 (not adjusted for inflation). However, the proportional share of expenditures has changed substantially in only two areas: the proportion spent on hospital care has decreased, and the proportion for prescription drugs has greatly increased (Smith et al., 2005).

The categories of national health expenditures (NHE) listed in Table 13-2 account for 95% of NHE in the sample years. About one third of NHE was for hospital care, and hospital costs continued to rise in actual expenditures during this time. However, the proportion of NHE spent for hospital care decreased from 36.1% in 1993, to 32.2% in 1999, to 30.7% in 2003. Similarly, both home health services and nursing home care also had increased expenditures during that time, but their proportion of the NHE also decreased.

The second most-expensive category, physicians and clinical services, accounted for a steady 22% of NHE. "Other professional services" also were steady at about 3%, as were dental services at about 4.4%. Although the percentages of NHE were stable in these categories, their actual expenditures nearly doubled. Expenditures for nursing services are not visible in these categories. Nursing costs are usually included by location of care: hospitals, the home, and nursing homes. Numbers of health personnel are shown in Table 13-3, indicating that, compared with the selected peer countries, the United States had a much larger number of physicians, a mid-range number of nurses, pharmacists, and dentists, but a negligible number of midwives (WHO, 2005).

A current major focus of national ire about health care expenditures is the pharmaceutical industry. Indeed, expenditures for prescription

**TABLE 13-2** National Health Expenditures (NHE) in the United States, by Category, Amount, and Percent of Total, 1993-2003 (in Millions of Dollars)

| | 1993 | | 1999 | | 2003 | |
|---|---|---|---|---|---|---|
| NHE total | $888.1 | | $1222.2 | | $1678.9 | |
| NHE % of GDP | 13.3 | | 14.1 | | 15.3 | |
| | US$ | % | US$ | % | US$ | % |
| Hospital care | 320.0 | 36.1 | 393.4 | 32.2 | 515.9 | 30.7 |
| Physician or clinical services | 201.2 | 22.6 | 270.9 | 22.2 | 369.7 | 22.0 |
| Other professional services | 24.5 | 2.7 | 36.7 | 3.0 | 48.5 | 2.9 |
| Dental services | 38.9 | 4.4 | 56.4 | 4.5 | 74.3 | 4.4 |
| Home health care | 21.9 | 2.5 | 32.3 | 2.6 | 40.0 | 2.4 |
| Nursing home care | 65.7 | 7.4 | 90.7 | 7.4 | 118.8 | 6.6 |
| Prescription drugs | 51.3 | 5.8 | 104.4 | 8.5 | 179.2 | 10.7 |
| Durable medical equipment | 12.8 | 1.4 | 17.2 | 1.4 | 20.4 | 1.2 |
| Program administration and net cost of private insurance | 53.3 | 6.0 | 73.3 | 6.0 | 119.7 | 7.1 |
| Governmental public health | 27.2 | 3.1 | 41.2 | 3.4 | 53.8 | 3.2 |
| Research | 15.6 | 1.7 | 23.7 | 1.9 | 40.2 | 2.4 |
| Construction | 16.2 | 1.8 | 18.3 | 1.5 | 24.5 | 1.4 |

From Smith, C., Cowan, C., Sensenig, A., Catlin, A., & Health Accounts Team. (2005). Health spending growth slows in 2003. *Health Affairs,* *24*(1), 185-194.

**TABLE 13-3** Health Personnel per 100,000 Population in Selected Countries, 2001

| | AUSTRALIA | CANADA | GERMANY | JAPAN | SINGAPORE | SWEDEN | UNITED KINGDOM | UNITED STATES |
|---|---|---|---|---|---|---|---|---|
| MDs | 249 | 209 | 362 | 201 | 140 | 305 | 166 | 549 |
| RNs | 774 | 1009 | 950 | 821 | 424 | 977 | 496 | 772 |
| Midwives | 60 | 1 | 12 | 19 | 11 | 67 | 43 | 1 |
| Pharmacists | 72 | 80 | 58 | 171 | 28 | 60 | 59 | 68 |
| Dentists | 42 | 56 | 78 | 72 | 26 | 94 | 40 | 59 |

From World Health Organization (WHO). (2005). Human resources for health. Retrieved April 7, 2005, from *http://globalatlas.who.int/GlobalAtlas/ DataQuery/home.asp.*

drugs, a category that includes the costs of research and development in pharmaceutical companies, more than tripled during the target decade. The proportion of NHE consumed for prescription drugs was 5.8% in 1993, 8.5% in 1999, and 10.7% in 2003. This category is the only one that showed such a dramatic rise in proportional expenditure during the decade, with the exception of research, which was a much smaller expenditure. Analyzing this

sector is difficult. Without question, prices and profits have increased. However, the short- and long-term cost savings through use of highly effective pharmaceutical agents must be part of the analysis.

Administrative activities are a hidden source of great expense, in part because of the complex web of regulations. The database for Table 13-2 did not include overall administrative costs. Woolhandler, Campbell, and Himmelstein (2003) compared costs of health care administration in the United States and Canada in 1999. They found that administrative costs in the United States accounted for 31% of health care expenditures, or US$1069 per capita. Administrative costs in Canada accounted for 16.7% of expenditures, or US$307 per capita. Further, the national health insurance program in Canada had an overhead of 1.3%, but the overhead of private insurers was higher in Canada (13.2%) than in the United States (11.7%).

Similarly, Reinhardt, Hussey, and Anderson (2004) examined health care spending in 30 highly advanced countries. They reported that the U.S. expenditure per capita in 2000 was $4631, compared with the peer-group median of $1983. They and others suggested that the increased expenditure in the United States does not buy more care; instead, it is a matter of the capacity for pricing (Anderson, Reinhardt, Hussey, & Petrosyan, 2005). Anell and Willis (2000) showed in their resource profiles that the types of expenditures, not simply the amounts, are important in international comparisons.

Widescale implementation of managed care, in the form of health maintenance organizations (HMOs) or preferred provider organizations (PPOs), occurred in the United States to control costs, to establish a strong primary care base, and to create more closed, seemingly more controllable systems. In 2004, 39% of Americans were enrolled in managed care organizations, about one third of them in HMOs and two thirds in PPOs. However, managed care penetration varied greatly by state, as shown in Table 13-4. Penetration was greatest among commercial insurers (91.2%), followed by Medicaid (60.3%), and only 12.5% of Medicare enrollees (Managed Care Fact Sheets, 2004a, 2004b). Managed care has not been popular or successful in the Medicare population because elderly people tend to have multiple chronic illnesses and the costs of their care are high.

One of the goals of managed care is to decrease costly services and to control physicians' practices by using capitation and incentives to limit expenditures. At the same time, however, recent reports have indicated that chief executives of managed care organizations had the largest earnings in history (Kazel, 2003). Satisfaction with managed

**TABLE 13-4** Highest and Lowest Managed Care Penetration in U.S. States, 2004, by Percent of State Population

| HIGHEST | | LOWEST | |
|---|---|---|---|
| California | 48.0 | North Dakota | 0.3 |
| Connecticut | 39.1 | Mississippi | 0.4 |
| Massachusetts | 37.4 | Wyoming | 2.2 |
| Rhode Island | 31.6 | Alabama | 2.8 |
| Maryland | 30.8 | Idaho | 2.9 |
| New Mexico | 30.8 | Arkansas | 5.3 |
| Hawaii | 29.7 | South Carolina | 6.1 |
| Wisconsin | 28.4 | Kansas | 6.4 |
| Kentucky | 28.3 | Nebraska | 7.5 |
| Colorado | 27.3 | Oklahoma | 7.9 |

From Managed Care Fact Sheets. (2004). HMO penetration, by state and region, 2004. Retrieved April 3, 2005, from *www.mcareol.com/factshts/factstat.htm*.

care varies among both providers and consumers (Schur, Berk, & Yegian, 2004), and overall reduction in national expenditures is not evident.

## HEALTH CARE OUTCOMES

Two commonly cited indicators of population health at the national level are life expectancy and infant-child mortality. Hegyvary, Berry, and Murua (2006) studied the distribution and determinants of these outcomes in 161 countries at the turn of the twenty-first century. Life expectancy and infant-child mortality rates in selected advanced countries are shown in Table 13-5. The United States ranked lowest among these peer countries. However, caution is necessary in interpreting international differences in infant and child mortality. The data reported by WHO and the World Bank pertain to deaths per 1000 live births. At issue is the definition of a "live birth." In some countries infants under a minimum gestational age or of extremely low birth weight are not considered viable and therefore might be reported as fetal deaths instead of infant deaths. A further complication is efficiency of the system of registration of births (Joseph & Kramer, 1997; Kramer et al., 2002), so that a delay of a day or two in registering births results in lack of reporting of infant mortality during that time. These differences have been reported among advanced countries, including

**TABLE 13-5** Life Expectancy and Infant-Child Mortality in Selected Countries, 2002

| | AUSTRALIA | CANADA | GERMANY | JAPAN | SINGAPORE | SWEDEN | UNITED KINGDOM | UNITED STATES |
|---|---|---|---|---|---|---|---|---|
| **LIFE EXPECTANCY AT BIRTH*** | | | | | | | | |
| Male | 78.0 | 77.2 | 75.6 | **78.4** | 77.4 | 78.0 | 75.8 | **74.6** |
| Female | 83.0 | 82.3 | 81.6 | **85.3** | 81.7 | 82.6 | 80.5 | **79.8** |
| **HEALTHY LIFE EXPECTANCY*** | | | | | | | | |
| Male: at birth | 70.9 | 70.1 | 69.6 | **72.3** | 68.8 | 71.9 | 69.1 | **67.2** |
| Female: at birth | 74.3 | 74.0 | 74.0 | **77.7** | 71.3 | 74.8 | 72.1 | **71.3** |
| Male: at 60 | 16.9 | 16.1 | 15.9 | **17.5** | **14.5** | 17.1 | 15.7 | 15.3 |
| Female: at 60 | 19.5 | 19.3 | 19.0 | **21.7** | **16.3** | 19.6 | 18.1 | 17.9 |
| Infant mortality[†] | 4.8 | 5.2 | 4.5 | 3.8 | **2.9** | 3.4 | 5.6 | 7.1 |
| Under-5 child mortality[†] | 6.4 | 7.2 | 6.0 | 5.3 | 5.7 | **3.9** | 7.0 | 8.6 |

*From World Health Organization (WHO). (2005). Statistics by country or region. Retrieved April 7, 2005, from *www3who.int/whosis/country/indicators.cfm*.

[†]From World Bank. (2003). World Bank Group: Data and statistics. Retrieved March 20, 2003, from *www.worldbank.org/data*.

Japan, Canada, and France (Office of Technology Assessment, 1993; Sepkowitz, 1995). Some of the higher infant mortality in the United States might be the result of greater use of heroic measures to deliver and sustain unviable, extremely low-birth-weight infants of very low gestational age, and the norm of reporting deaths of all newborns as "infant mortality." The extent of this reported lack of reliability of data across countries is not known. Still, even if some differences in the data exist, the higher levels of child mortality and the shorter life expectancy both at birth and at age 60 in the United States, compared with peer countries, are not consistent with the much greater expenditures for health care.

Another indicator of health care outcomes is major causes of death. Table 13-6 shows differences among selected peer countries for the two leading causes of death in all these countries in 2002: cancer and cardiovascular diseases. The United States had the lowest reported rate of cancer deaths and mid-range deaths from cardiovascular diseases for both

men and women. Table 13-7 shows U.S. deaths from cancer, cardiovascular diseases, diabetes, mental disorders, and suicides from 1979 to 2000, for men and women. The greatest change was the reduction in deaths from cardiovascular disease, a probable indication of success in health promotion and health care services. The percentage of deaths from cancer in the United States increased somewhat for men but not for women. Keeping this cause of death relatively low in relation to peer countries is a positive outcome of the health care system. In contrast, and undoubtedly important in the coming years, is the doubling of diabetes among American men and its tripling among women, most likely related to obesity and lifestyles. Deaths from mental disorders doubled for men and quadrupled for women. However, deaths from suicide remained nearly stable for men and they decreased for women, likely an indicator of successful treatment of depression, the major cause of disability in the United States and in most regions of the world (National Alliance on Mental Illness, 2003).

**TABLE 13-6**   Percent of Deaths from Cancers and Cardiovascular Diseases, by Sex, in Selected Countries, 2002

| | PERCENT FROM MALIGNANT NEOPLASMS* | | PERCENT FROM DISEASES OF CARDIOVASCULAR SYSTEM† | |
|---|---|---|---|---|
| | MALE | FEMALE | MALE | FEMALE |
| Australia | 30.2 | 25.2 | 35.4 | 42.2 |
| Canada | 29.9 | 27.6 *H*‡ | 34.1 | 36.1 |
| Germany | 28.2 | 22.3 | 41.8 | 52.0 *H* |
| Japan | 34.4 *H* | 27.0 | 27.5 *L* | 34.8 *L* |
| Singapore | 29.5 | 27.6 | 36.5 | 37.6 |
| Sweden | 24.5 | 21.7 *L* | 45.0 *H* | 46.0 |
| United Kingdom | 28.0 | 23.5 | 39.2 | 39.2 |
| United States | 24.3 *L* | 21.8 | 37.2 | 41.1 |

From World Health Organization (WHO). (2005). Table 1. Numbers and rates of registered deaths. Retrieved May 7, 2005, from *www3.who.int/whosis/mort/table1_process.cfm.*

*ICD-10: C00-C97

†ICD-10: I00-I99

‡H = Highest in this column; L = Lowest in this column.

Notes: Cancer death rate higher in men than in women, all countries. Cardiovascular death rate higher in women than in men, all countries. Cardiovascular deaths, both men and women, higher than cancer deaths, except Japanese men.

**TABLE 13-7**   Percent of All-Cause Mortality in the United States, by Selected Causes

| | MALIGNANT NEOPLASMS | | CARDIOVASCULAR DISEASES | | DIABETES MELLITUS | | MENTAL DISORDERS | | SUICIDE | |
|---|---|---|---|---|---|---|---|---|---|---|
| | MALE | FEMALE | MALE | FEMALE | MALE | FEMALE | MALE | FEMALE | MALE | FEMALE |
| 2000 | 24.3 | 21.8 | 37.2 | 41.1 | 2.7 | 3.1 | 1.5 | 2.3 | 2.0 | 0.5 |
| 1995 | 24.0 | 22.5 | 38.6 | 44.2 | 2.2 | 2.9 | 1.4 | 2.2 | 2.0 | 0.5 |
| 1990 | 24.1 | 22.9 | 39.9 | 45.9 | 2.0 | 2.6 | 1.0 | 1.3 | 2.2 | 0.6 |
| 1985 | 22.5 | 21.7 | 44.4 | 50.1 | 1.4 | 2.2 | 0.9 | 0.9 | 2.1 | 0.6 |
| 1979 | 21.1 | 21.1 | 47.5 | 53.7 | 1.3 | 1.1 | 0.7 | 0.6 | 1.9 | 0.8 |

From World Health Organization (WHO). (2005). Table 1. Numbers and rates of registered deaths. Retrieved May 7, 2005, from *www3.who.int/whosis/mort/table1_process.cfm.*

Despite the relatively low numbers of primary care providers and emphasis on specialty medical care in the United States, the United States ranked very high among peer countries on some aspects of preventive care. Those results indicated that some aspects of primary care are provided in specialty practices (Schoen et al., 2004).

## DISCUSSION

What accounts for this mixed profile of the health care system in a country as rich and powerful as the United States? Several interpretations are possible, particularly:

- Lack of national health care policy for the entire population
- Lack of primary health care
- Problems in areas identified as determinants of health outcomes
- Social and political ideology

## NATIONAL HEALTH CARE POLICY

De facto historical and current health care policy has indicated support of an entrepreneurial model, with mostly employment-based insurance, other than governmental funding for special populations such as from Medicare, Medicaid, and the Veterans Administration. Lacking is an articulated national policy, as exists in all peer countries and in most transitional countries, that health care services are available in some form to the entire population. Without a coherent and highly visible national policy, an open-system, entrepreneurial approach can be taken to extreme, leaving full coverage of the population to the discretion of providers who must compete in the marketplace to survive. Without incentives to provide full coverage, such services require voluntary efforts that often cannot be sustained over time. An example is the "faith-based initiatives" advocated by the Bush administration for provision of many such services. These initiatives might work for some people for a while, but they remain marginal to mainstream services provided in health care networks, and they further complicate and fragment a "patchwork" system.

Having a national policy does not preclude having a largely private-sector system for delivery of services, as illustrated in countries such as Germany and to a considerable extent even in Canada. The clearest example of a definitive national policy for an otherwise mostly entrepreneurial system is Singapore. Historical precedents consistently have indicated that enacting any national policy requires support of major stakeholders.

## LACK OF PRIMARY HEALTH CARE

Studies have shown that the strength of a country's primary care system is associated with reduced mortality, lower costs, higher patient satisfaction, and comparable quality of patient outcomes (Health Evidence Network, 2004). The shift toward managed care in the 1980s and 1990s included emphasis on provision of "primary care" as the point of entry to a system. In theory it is intended to be both the clinical foundation and the organizational gatekeeper for access to a vertically integrated system, with focus on comprehensive and integrated care (Starfield, 2001). In practice, however, services are often more sequential than integrated. Primary care practitioners assess and treat conditions that do not require more expensive specialty

care, often on a capitated basis and often with salaried personnel. When necessary, they refer patients to specialty practitioners, and in most managed care systems patients may not go to specialists without referral from the primary care practitioner. Physicians in several areas of practice (internal medicine, family practice, pediatrics, obstetrics-gynecology, and some say also psychiatry) provide primary care, as do many nurse practitioners. Dissatisfaction with many aspects of managed care and HMOs has undermined the provision of primary care services (Schur et al., 2004).

A related concept, often erroneously considered synonymous with primary care, is primary "health" care. This community-wide focus on health, espoused in repeated statements from WHO (2003), includes the "application of the relevant results of social, biomedical and health services research and public health experience" (p. 9). Thus, medically oriented primary care is part of but not synonymous with primary health care. Primary care is often focused on diseases: their detection, treatment, and prevention. In primary health care the emphasis is on health promotion for both person and community, including promoting healthy lifestyles, providing health education and counseling, helping people to manage and cope with chronic illness while also assessing for signs and symptoms that require further medical treatment, and linking health services with the many other determinants of individual and community health. Primary health care is especially important for infants and children. Major improvements in child survival have been reported in many countries as a result of community-based primary health care (Basch, 1999). This concept is reminiscent of the Shepherd-Towner Act of 1921, which had clinical success but political failure.

Although primary health care pertains to everyone, it might have the greatest effect on people with least access to a full range of health care services. Lack of primary health care services often is evident when people have advanced health problems before they seek treatment, resulting in the need for more expensive treatment than otherwise may have been needed (Health Evidence Network, 2004; Kunitz & Pesis-Katz, 2005).

## ATTENTION TO DETERMINANTS OF HEALTH OUTCOMES

Increasing attention has been given in recent years to societal determinants of health. The most comprehensive study of country-level health to date indicated three dimensions that explained global life expectancy and child mortality in 2000: resources, empowerment, and demography. In the group of 55 least-developed countries, the strongest determinant of better health outcomes was demography, specifically low birth rates, followed by greater equality of incomes and higher enrollments in secondary and tertiary education. High birth rates continued to have negative effects in the group of 79 transitional countries, but more important as birth rates declined was the adequacy of health care resources (i.e., health care expenditures and numbers of health personnel). In all groups of countries, empowerment via secondary and tertiary education was an important explanatory factor, and higher levels of democracy and civil rights characterized the healthiest populations (Hegyvary, Berry, & Murua, 2006).

Those findings cannot be applied to individual countries except for purposes of assessment and identifying hypotheses. However, the overall findings are consistent with conditions in the United States, which was marginal to peer countries on several important factors. The birth rate in the United States was second highest among its peer countries. Enrollment in secondary education, particularly of girls, was lower than that of most peer countries. Rates of poverty, child malnutrition, illiteracy, and income inequality were higher than those of peer countries. At the same time, U.S. spending for health care far exceeded that of any country in the world, illustrating a possible point of diminishing returns on health care spending unless underlying societal determinants of health, as well as the nature of expenditures, are addressed. Better health at all ages in the United States is most likely among White, better-educated, and higher-income people, indicating significant variations in subpopulations by social factors as well as race and ethnicity (Macintyre & Ellaway, 2000; World Bank, 2002, 2003).

## SOCIAL AND POLITICAL IDEOLOGY

Ideological beliefs and assumptions underlie national health care systems and provision of services. A prime example is the statement that both health and health care services are human rights, widely accepted at the Alma Ata Conference sponsored by WHO in 1978 (Hall & Taylor, 2003). Participants set goals to be achieved globally by the end of the twentieth century, specifically the "Health for All" initiative. Some indicators were defined, importantly regarding health systems and primary health care, and notable efforts were undertaken in many countries. However, the meaning and reality of "health for all" was not clear, including the question of whether everybody in the world ever would or could be healthy. In some sectors the slogan was changed to "Health care for all," which appeared clearer but still lacked definition of what constitutes the health care services for everyone. Is it the provision of a designated set of basic or primary health care services? Or is it everything that might be done to maximize health for every person? Or is it simply a right of access to specified health care services as prescribed in countries with mandated health insurance? The question of rights is further complicated by the fact that no other type of goods and services, except compulsory education, is publicly provided as a right—not food, shelter, or other basic human needs. These questions are undercurrents in debates about health care in every country, especially as costs of health services increase around the world.

Another assumption articulated in WHO documents is that the ultimate responsibility for performance of the country's health system lies with government. This assumption follows from the statements about health care for all. However, it is not universally accepted in its entirety, and it might be categorically rejected, especially in the private sector, where the large majority of health care services in the United States are provided. This debate is deeply rooted in differences in societal values that characterize countries and define the context in which health systems evolve.

In their decades of study of social values in many countries, Inglehart (1999) and Inglehart and

Baker (2000) found that the United States consistently differed in social values from peer countries in Western Europe, Japan, Australia, and New Zealand. Two scales were particularly important in their studies: survival versus self-expression, and traditional versus secular-rational values. Among industrialized countries, the United States had one of the highest scores on individual self-expression, indicating great value placed on individuality, quality of life, happiness, and trust. At the same time, the United States showed a more traditional orientation than did any peer country except Ireland. Traditional values were largely related to religion and religious doctrine. The converse orientation toward secular-rational values, found in all other peer countries, was less focused on religion and more on social and interpersonal freedoms. On the basis of religious (in this case, Christian) doctrine, as well as the statement in the U.S. Constitution to "promote the general welfare," one might expect that the United States would place higher priority on health care for all than do populations with secular-rational values. However, data consistently show the contrary.

Countries highest in self-expression and secular-rational values (e.g., Western European countries, Japan, Australia, and New Zealand) had the longest life expectancy and lowest child mortality (Hegyvary, Berry, & Murua, 2006). Inglehart and Baker (2000) concluded that development is shaped by cultural heritage, such that modernization need not follow one distinct path. They also said, "Industrializing societies in general are not becoming like the United States. In fact, the United States seems to be the deviant case" (Inglehart & Baker, 2000, p. 49). How much Americans are willing to pay for that marginality, with higher health care costs for less desirable outcomes, is the fundamental question.

## SUMMARY

The U.S. health care system is unique in the world in its level of decentralization, entrepreneurship, level of expenditure, and high quality of some services, combined with less than optimal health outcomes in the American population. Evidence indicates particular points of problems, specifically

lack of a coherent national health care policy, lack of universal coverage for health care, low levels of primary care and primary health care in comparison with peer countries, high costs of administrative activities, and limited attention to societal determinants of health.

The Conference Board of Canada (2005) concluded that: "There is no single equation that gives the optimal balance between low-cost and high-quality health care" (p. 1). The varied approaches to the provision of health care in peer countries indicate that no one type of system has superior outcomes or uniform public acceptance. Systems evolve in unique social and cultural contexts, as products of their history, politics, and social values. Thus, improvement of structures, processes, and outcomes of the U.S. health care system could result from various approaches. Evidence indicates that simply putting more money into the system has not resulted in desired improvements.

Historical and cultural characteristics of the United States, short of paradigmatic change in values and political ideology, are inconsistent with enactment of a centralized, closed type of health care system. Piecemeal changes in components of both open and closed systems can have unanticipated consequences, like squeezing a balloon. Given the societal context of the United States, major improvements require governmental leadership, with cooperation of both public and private sectors. If that is not achieved, trends indicate that the United States will remain marginal to peer countries in costs, health system performance, and health of the population.

Comparisons of international health care systems do not provide evidence of a "best" system, nor do human systems of any type, open or closed, health care or other, portray ultimate "truth" of social values. Health care systems are the ever-changing products of a people's dominant perceptions, historical and contemporary, about life's truths for them. Thus, systems can be expected to vary widely, for both beneficence and utilitarian purposes. The more effective and tangible the results of human systems, the more they will endure while others struggle to adapt and survive. No population is the lesser because its systems require change. It is only the lesser if it steadfastly refuses to change in the face of consistent evidence of the need for change, as well as evidence of inconsistency between its espoused values and its deeds.

## Key Points

- The U.S. health system is an entrepreneurial type of open-but-regulated system, one of only a few in the world.
- Public funds account for nearly half of U.S. health care expenditures, but the provision of services is largely in the private sector.
- Health care expenditures in the United States are the largest in the world, as indicated by both expenditures per capita and the percent of the GDP.
- Categories with largest proportional expenditures are hospital care, administration, physician and clinical services, and prescription drugs.
- Major outcomes, such as life expectancy and infant-child mortality, are marginal to those in peer countries.
- Death rates from cancer are low in comparison with peer countries and have remained relatively stable over two decades as a percentage of all-cause mortality; deaths from cardiovascular diseases have significantly decreased, indicating successful treatment and prevention in at least these important specialty areas.
- Quality of U.S. health services provided has been ranked highest in the world, but overall health system performance has been ranked thirty-seventh in the world, the latter largely attributed to lack of universal access to services and lack of fairness of financing. However, preventive care in the form of screening for major diseases ranks very high among peers.
- Access to services is not universal, and over 47 million people do not have insurance coverage for health care services. The extent to which this population accounts for the marginality of the United States in relation to peer countries is unclear.

- The large majority of physicians are in specialty or subspecialty practice, and the proportion in primary care practice has decreased.
- Compared with peer countries, the United States has more physicians, average numbers of nurses, dentists, and pharmacists, but extremely few midwives.
- Attempts at major national reforms have failed because of powerful stakeholders and longstanding social and political values.

## Web Resources

**Agency for Healthcare Research and Quality**
*www.ahrq.gov*
**The Commonwealth Fund (Working to Improve Health Care Quality and Coverage)**
*www.cmwf.org*
**National Center for Health Statistics**
*www.cdc.gov/nchs*
**The National Coalition on Health Care**
*www.nchc.org*
**U.S. Health Resources and Services Administration**
*www.hrsa.gov*

## REFERENCES

Anderson, G. F., Reinhardt, U. E., Hussey, P. S., & Petrosyan, V. (2005). It's the price, stupid: Why the United States is so different from other countries. Retrieved May 4, 2005, from *www.chiff.com/a/HLFH703cost.htm*.

Anell, A., & Willis, M. (2000). International comparison of health care systems using resource profiles. *Bulletin of the World Health Organization, 78*(6), 770-776.

Basch, P. F. (1999). *Textbook of international health* (2nd ed.). New York: Oxford University Press.

Biola, H., Green, L. A., Phillips, R. L., Guirguis-Blake, J., Fryer, G. E. (2003). The U.S. primary care physician workforce: Minimal growth 1980-1999. *American Family Physician, 68*, 1483.

Blendon, R. J., Kim, M., & Benson, J. M. (2001). The public versus WHO on health system performance. *Health Affairs, 20*(3), 10-20.

Bloor, K., & Maynard, A. (2002). In K. V. Thai, E. T. Wimberley, & S. M. McManus (Eds.), *Handbook of international health care systems*. New York: Marcel Dekker.

Bodenheimer, T. S., & Grumbach, K. (2002). *Understanding health policy: A clinical approach*. New York: Lange Medical Books/McGraw-Hill.

Clark, J. (2000). Old wine in new bottles: Delivering nursing in the 21st century. *Journal of Nursing Scholarship, 32*(1), 11-15.

Conference Board of Canada. (2005). Key findings. Retrieved April 10, 2005, from *www.health.gov.ab.ca/resources/publications/pdf/Conference_Board2.pdf*.

Conrad, D. A., Marcus-Smith, M. S., Cheadle, A., Maynard, C., Kirz, H. L., et al. (1998). Primary care physician compensation method in medical groups: Does it influence the use and cost of health services for enrollees in managed care organizations? *JAMA, 279,* 853-858.

Dow, W. H., & Saenz, L. B. (2002). Costa Rica. In B. J. Fried & L. M. Gaydos (Eds.), *World health systems: Challenges and perspectives.* Chicago: Health Administration Press.

Dudley, R. A., & Luft, H. S. (2003). Managed care in transition. In P. R. Lee & C. L. Estes (Eds.), *The nation's health* (7th ed.). Sudbury, MA: Jones and Bartlett.

Fried, B. J., & Gaydos, L. M. (Eds.). (2002). *World health systems: Challenges and perspectives.* Chicago: Health Administration Press.

Garrett, L. (2000). *Betrayal of trust: The collapse of global public health.* New York: Hyperion.

Hall, J. J., & Taylor, R. (2003). Health for all beyond 2000: The demise of the Alma-Ata declaration and primary care in developing countries. *Medical Journal of Australia, 178*(1), 17-20.

Health Evidence Network. (2004). *What are the advantages and disadvantages of restructuring a health care system to be more focused on primary care services?* Copenhagen: World Health Organization. Available at *publicationrequests@euro.who.int.*

Hegyvary, S. T., Berry, D. M., & Murua, A. (2006). *Global distribution and determinants of life expectancy and child mortality* (manuscript submitted for publication).

Heinrich, J., & Thompson, T. M. (2002). Organization and delivery of health care in the United States: A patchwork system. In D. J. Mason, M. W. Chaffee, & J. K. Leavitt (Eds.), *Policy and politics in nursing and health care* (4th ed.). Philadelphia: Saunders.

Ikegami, N., & Campbell, J. C. (2004). Japan's health care system: Containing costs and attempting reform. *Health Affairs, 23*(3), 26-36.

Inglehart, R. (1999). Globalization and postmodern values. *Washington Quarterly, 23*(1):215-228.

Inglehart, R., & W. E. Baker. (2000). Modernization, cultural change, and the persistence of traditional values. *American Sociological Review, 65,* 19-51.

Johnson, A., Carrillo, A. M., & Garcia, J. J. (2002). Mexico. In B. J. Fried & L. M. Gaydos (Eds.), *World health systems.* Chicago: Health Administration Press.

Joseph, K. S., & Kramer, M. S. (1997). Recent trends in Canadian infant mortality rates: Effect of changes in registration of live newborns weighing less than 500 g. *Canadian Medical Association Journal, 156*(2), 161-163.

Kazel, R. (2003). CEO compensation: Accomplishments translate into healthy paychecks. Retrieved May 12, 2005, from *www.hmocrisis.com/forum_052203.html#33.*

Kramer, M. S, Platt, R. W., Yang, H., Haglund, B., Cnattingius, S., & Bergsjo, P. (2002). Registration artifacts in international comparisons of infant mortality. *Paediatric and Perinatal Epidemiology, 16*(1), 16-22.

Krisberg, K. (2005). 45 million Americans now lack health insurance. The Nation's Health. Retrieved May 7, 2005, from *www.apha.org/tnh/index.cfm?fa=Adetail&id=97.*

Kunitz, S. J., & Pesis-Katz, I. (2005). Mortality of white Americans, African Americans, and Canadians: The causes and consequences for health of welfare state institutions and policies. *Milbank Quarterly, 83*(1). Retrieved June 15, 2006, from *www.milbank.org/quarterly/8301feat.html.*

Macintyre, S., & Ellaway, A. (2000). Ecological approaches: Rediscovering the role of the physical and social environment. In L. F. Berkman & I. Kawachi. *Social epidemiology.* Oxford: Oxford University.

Managed Care Fact Sheets. (2004a). HMO penetration, by state and region, 2004. Retrieved April 3, 2005, from *www.mcareol.com/factshts/factstat.htm.*

Managed Care Fact Sheets. (2004b). National HMO Enrollment. Retrieved April 3, 2005, from *www.mcareol.com/factnati.htm.*

Millenson, M. L. (1998). Managed care makes a name for itself in the years following the federal 1973 HMO act. *Healthplan, 39*(4), 62-68.

National Alliance on Mental Illness. (2003). Nation's voice on mental illness. Retrieved May 12, 2005, from *www.nami.org/Content/ContentGroups/Helpline1/Major_Depression.htm.*

Office of Technology Assessment. (1993). *International health statistics: What the numbers mean for the United States.* Washington, DC: Office of Technology Assessment.

Pinnacle Health Group. (1999). Physician statistics summary. Retrieved May 5, 2005, from *www.phg.com/aritclepf_p005.htm.*

Powell, F. D., & Wessen, A. F. (1999). *Health care systems in transition: An international perspective.* Thousand Oaks, CA: Sage.

Quadagno, J. (2004). Why the United States has no national health insurance: Stakeholder mobilization against the welfare state, 1946-1996. *Journal of Health and Social Behavior, 45*(Extra issue): 25-44.

Reinhardt, U. E., Hussey, P. S., & Anderson, G. F. (2004). U.S. health care spending in an international context, *Health Affairs, 23*(3), 10-25.

Roemer, M. I. (1993). *National health systems of the world. Volume 2: The issues.* New York: Oxford University Press.

Schoen, C., Osborn, R., Huynh, P. T., Doty, M., Davis, K., et al. (2004). Primary care and health system performance: Adults' experiences in five countries. *Health Affairs, 23*(Suppl 2), W4-487-503.

Schur, C. L., Berk, M. L., & Yegian, J. M. (2004). Public perceptions of cost containment strategies: Mixed signals for managed care. *Health Affairs, 23*(Suppl 2), W4-516-525.

Sepkowitz, S. (1995). International rankings of infant mortality and the United States' vital statistic natality data collecting system—failure and success. *International Journal of Epidemiology, 24*(3), 583-588.

Smith, C., Cowan, C., Sensenig, A., Catlin, A., & Health Accounts Team. (2005). Health spending growth slows in 2003. *Health Affairs, 24*(1), 185-194.

Starfield, B. (2001). Basic concepts in population health and health care. *Journal of Epidemiological Community Health, 55,* 452-454.

Starr, P. (1982). *Social transformation of American medicine.* New York: Basic Books.

Stevens, S. (2004). Reform strategies for the English NHS. *Health Affairs, 23*(3), 37-44.

Thai, K. V., Wimberley, E. T., & McManus, S. M. (2002). *Handbook of international health care systems.* New York: Marcel Dekker.

Thompson, J. A. (1977). *Organizations in action.* New York: McGraw-Hill.

Twaddle, A. C. (2002). *Health care reform around the world.* Westport, CT: Auburn House.

Williams, S. J., & Torrens, P. R. (2002). *Introduction to health services* (6th ed.). Albany, NY: Delmar.

Woods, C. Q. (1996). Evolution of the American Nurses Association's position on health insurance for the aged: 1933-1965. *Nursing Research, 45*(5), 304-310.

Woolhandler, S., Campbell, T., & Himmelstein, D. U. (2003). Costs of health care administration in the United States and Canada. *New England Journal of Medicine, 349*(8), 768-775.

World Bank. (2002). *World Development Indicators* (CD-ROM). Washington, DC: World Bank.

World Bank. (2003). World Bank Group: Data and statistics. Retrieved March 20, 2003, from *www.worldbank.org/data*.

World Health Organization (WHO). (2001a). World Health Report 2000: World Health Organization assesses the world's health systems. Retrieved March 27, 2004, from *www.int/ whr2001/2001/archives/2000/en/press_release.htm* and from *www.who.int/whr/2000/en/annex10_en.pdf*.

World Health Organization (WHO). (2001b). About health systems performance. Retrieved April 5, 2005, from *www.who.int/health-systems performance/about.htm*.

World Health Organization (WHO). (2003). Primary health care: A framework for future strategic directions. Geneva: WHO. Retrieved August 29, 2005, from *www.who.int/chronic_ conditions/primary_health_care/en/phc_report_oct03.pdf*.

World Health Organization (WHO). (2005). Human resources for health. Retrieved April 7, 2005, from *http://globalatlas. who.int/GlobalAtlas/DataQuery/home.asp*.

Zierler, B. K., Marcus-Smith, M. S., Cheadle, A., Conrad, D. A., Kirz, H. L., et al. (1998). Effect of compensation method on the behavior of primary care physicians in managed care organizations. *American Journal of Managed Care, 4*(2), 209-220.

# **POLICY**SPOTLIGHT

## THE NATIONAL HEALTH SERVICE IN THE UNITED KINGDOM

Tony Leiba

*"Unless we change our ways and our direction, our greatness as a nation will soon be a footnote in the history books, a distant memory of an offshore island, lost in the mists of time like Camelot, remembered kindly for its noble past."*

MARGARET THATCHER

Evolution and not revolution is the underlying precept of the National Health Service in the United Kingdom, a system started in 1948 that continues to be supported by the public. This discussion presents a brief history of the National Health Service and examines the recent reforms to the system. Particular focus is directed to recent governmental reform to enable the development of the private sector through a finance initiative and foundation hospital trusts. The foundation hospital trusts, although they are fully part of the National Health Service, are locally controlled and have greater freedom to manage their own affairs. Finally, the relevance of these health care policies on nursing is addressed.

### BIRTH OF THE NATIONAL HEALTH SERVICE

Before 1948, health services were obtained from three sources: charity and voluntary provisions; private health care in hospitals (with mainly insurance-based payment); and Poor Law hospitals. The charity and voluntary hospital provisions were financed from endowments, unpaid medical specialists and consultants, trade unions, and payments from wealthier patients. These were the teaching hospitals, and many were exclusively for paying patients. The Poor Law hospitals or infirmaries took in the destitute sick. These hospitals were financed by local governments and were later referred to as *munici-pal hospitals.* All these institutions became part of the National Health Service Act in 1948.

The National Health Service Act of 1946 formed part of a wider process of social change and reform as an element of the developing welfare state. The legislation passed during the 1940s laid the foundation for the welfare state. The surveys of Booth (1903) in London and Rowntree (1901) in York had decisively shown that the greatest causes of poverty were low wages and interruption of earnings because of sickness, unemployment, and old age. These pressures led the 1906 Liberal government to produce a program of welfare legislation. World War II accelerated the need, but it was the Labour government in the early postwar years that finally implemented the program.

Some of the provisions of the welfare state included:

- 1944 Education Act to combat ignorance and provide free universal education for children according to their age, aptitude, and ability. This was to be financed through general taxation.
- 1945 Family Allowance Act to alleviate child poverty to provide a universal system of payments for each child through school and financed by general taxation.
- 1946 National Industries Insurance Act to attack want and to alleviate poverty. All working people would contribute. Entitlements provided cradle-to-grave coverage for maternity, sickness, unemployment, widowhood, and retirement.
- 1946 National Health Service Act to combat disease by providing universal comprehensive service, free at the point of use and financed by taxation and national insurance.
- 1948 National Assistance Act to provide a financial safety net for those either inadequately or not covered by insurance. Local authorities were to provide care, assistance, and rehabilitation for elderly, mentally ill, and disabled people and provide housing for homeless people.
- 1949 Housing Act to combat squalor. Local authorities were empowered to make grants for property improvement or conversion.

The population responded favorably to the National Health Service. The services were to be comprehensive, universal in coverage, and free of charge at the point of use. The intention was to plan, integrate, and distribute services more effectively and to enable equality of health care access. Freedom of choice was upheld by doctors, who could refuse patients, and by patients, who could change doctors.

When the National Health Service started, physicians won many concessions, including an independent contractor system for general practitioners (GPs); the option of private practice and access to pay beds for their private patients in National Health Service hospitals; a system of distinction awards for hospital consultants; and a major role in the administration of the service. The hospital consultant is the highest grade for medical staff. Such individuals lead a group of doctors and are in control of a certain number of beds. They are given monetary rewards known as *distinction awards* for long service. To secure the cooperation of the medical profession, Aneurin Bevan said that he had "stuffed their mouths with gold" (Able-Smith, 1964, p. 480).

Between the years 1946 and 1948, local authorities and voluntary bodies lost control of the hospitals, along with their properties. The intention was to extend all necessary services to those who wished to use them, regardless of financial means. A tripartite structure of hospital services, family GP services, and local health authority services was created.

The services were "to secure improvement in the physical and mental health of the people and the prevention, diagnosis and treatment of illness" (Merrison Report, 1979, p. 8). The service was designed to meet health needs wherever and whenever they arose. However, there was no occupational health or comprehensive family planning service. Industrial medical services and the armed services were also not part of the system.

Alongside a free-at-the-point-of-delivery health service was a fee-paying service—in reality forming a two-tier system of health care. Some GPs had separate waiting rooms for so-called panel (non–fee-paying) patients, away from private fee-paying patients, and hospitals had separate units or rooms assigned for private fee-paying patients. This was a concession made to the doctors for their cooperation with the development of the National Health Service. It enabled them to work in the National Health Service in a salaried position while retaining their private practice. There were also private hospitals and private residential homes.

## THE NATIONAL HEALTH SERVICE REFORMS AND MODERNIZATION

Major reforms of the National Health Service began in the 1980s. These reforms sought to introduce market principles into a centrally planned and publicly financed health service. At the time there was major growth in the private sector, particularly in certain types of care, such as non-urgent hospital care. The cost of private care was financed by personal medical insurance or as an employment benefit to white-collar and some blue-collar workers and their families. There was increasing competition for patients between the public and private systems, mainly through glossy pictorial advertisement of facilities and services. Although health care continued to be financed centrally, the reforms sought to ensure that resources were used efficiently and that the services provided were responsive to patients and providers. In essence the government argued that the reforms were intended to modernize the structure of the National Health Service and not retreat from the principles on which it was established in 1948 (Ham, 1998).

## PRIVATE HEALTH CARE

The private sector of the health services has always consisted of more than pay beds. It includes the commercial sale of medicines, drugs, and appliances by pharmacists and supermarkets; private care by GPs and hospital-based consultants who also work for the National Health Service; private hospitals, nursing homes, and clinics; and private practices outside the National Health Service of dentists, doctors, nurses, chiropodists, physiotherapists, osteopaths, and chiropractors. It incorporates a list of drugs (and requires patients to pay the full cost of any drug not on the list); dental and prescription charges from which some groups are exempt; and optical services with exemptions for children and the poor.

Throughout the 1980s, privatization was encouraged because it created an increase in the number of total health facilities, thus relieving pressure on the National Health Service. It prevented the National Health Service from becoming a monopoly supplier and employer and enabled consumers to have more choices by providing an alternative to the National Health Service (Le Grand & Robinson, 1984).

## SOCIAL, ECONOMIC, AND POLITICAL ASPECTS OF PUBLIC AND PRIVATE HEALTH CARE

The government since 1979 has favored the growth of free-market health initiatives. Since coming to power in 1997, the Labour government has continued to support the private-public mix of services. There have been a variety of incentives to support the expansion of private health care, which have included:

- Revised consultants' contracts, enabling all consultants to undertake private practice
- Phasing out of pay beds from National Health Service hospitals and encouraging the development of private hospitals
- Support for people paying into private health insurance through tax relief for the low paid and the elderly
- Incentives such as tax concessions for small businesses and relaxed planning rules to encourage private hospital building (Rayner, 1986)

The government was keen to promote collaborative arrangements between the National Health Service and the private sector, in particular the contractual use of private facilities by the National Health Service, to ease the pressure for beds and reduce waiting lists.

Developments in private health care have raised a number of important policy questions. First, will a two-tier system result from the existence of public-private health care? Laing (1995) argues that the private sector has become increasingly heterogeneous with a diverse structure, clientele, and services. For example, private nursing homes and abortion clinics do not cater only to wealthy clients. Second, is private health care of a superior quality to public health care? Higgins (1988) stated that concerns about safety were voiced because of the geographic location and isolation of private hospitals and the use of part-time staff with limited experience. He argues that there is little evidence to suggest that private health care is of superior quality to public health care.

Second, experiences from other countries suggest that fee-for-service health care may disadvantage patients by encouraging unnecessary tests and treatments. Although the emergence of a two-tiered system has threatened the notion of equal access to health care regardless of ability to pay, the most privileged groups, who gain most from the private sector, also benefit from the public sector. Therefore private-sector growth does not necessarily exacerbate inequalities in health care provision.

Third, an argument for private health care is that it extends choice and convenience for patients. Challis and Bartlett (1987) found that a small minority of patients using nursing homes were able to exercise choice about when to enter care, which home to choose, or even when to change homes. However, in reality, the geographic variation in the distribution of such homes limits the choices available to elderly people.

According to Baggott (2004), it is difficult to estimate the size of the private sector. It consists of private for-profit organizations as well as individual practitioners working partly or wholly in a private capacity. It includes health services from acute hospitals, nursing homes, dentistry, and alternative medicine. Therefore any estimate of its size depends on how private health care is defined. Laing and Buisson (2001) state that the private sector provided 19% of hospital and nursing home services in the United Kingdom in 2000. In addition, the private sector provided 1% of maternity care, 13% of elective surgery, over 50% of abortions, and over 80% of long-term nursing and residential care for the elderly. Its share of the GP service is small—about 3%—and its contribution to dental services is 38%.

The private sector, boosted by the government's intention to expand partnerships with the public sector, engages in joint working initiatives. Such partnerships are demonstrated in treating patients on a contract-out basis, sharing equipment, cooperating in training, and enabling medical companies to buy surplus National Health Service property. The government also insisted that the National Health

Service catering, laundry, and cleaning services should be offered to private contractors to provide the most economic use of limited resources. Usually value for money is defined in terms of economy, efficiency, and effectiveness. Essentially it requires that limited resources be used to deliver a health service that is first and foremost effective (Department of Health and Social Security [DHSS], 1983). However, private contractors employed by the public hospitals were accused of poor standards that may also have contributed to poor standards of hygiene and cleanliness and thereby to hospital-acquired infections (Office of Health Economics, 1987).

The private sector, although still controversial, is a growing enterprise. Supporters contend the following:

- National Health Service waiting lists are reduced when patients use private-sector services
- The competition improves standards of care
- Delays in receiving health care are reduced, and private care provides special amenities such as a single room, a telephone, and access to a particular provider
- More choice is offered to the public, and greater freedom is afforded to doctors who might otherwise emigrate
- Better financial discipline curbs abuse, reduces waste, and decreases time spent on trivial complaints
- Most important, privatization has provided much needed revenue for the health system

In contrast, those who argue passionately about the disadvantages of the private sector claim that it does the following:

- Encourages health care professionals to leave the National Health Service
- Moves private practices to affluent areas
- Enables the jumping of the queue
- Deters treatment of patients who cannot afford the charges
- Could never provide comprehensive coverage for all health care situations such as mental illness, learning disability, long-term rehabilitation care, and long-term geriatric and dementia care
- Creates a two-tiered system of health care—those who can afford private treatment and those who cannot

Critics argue that the private sector draws resources away from the National Health Service. They argue that this creates incentives to build up private caseloads, resulting in poorer service for National Health Service patients (Keen, Light, & Mays, 2001). The other main criticism is that the private sector makes an insufficient contribution to research and development and staff training yet benefits from having the National Health Service as a backup service.

Since the early 1980s an increasing number of people have been covered by private medical insurance. Private medical subscriptions were paid for by large businesses as fringe benefits for their employees (Laing & Buisson, 1994). The General Household Survey (1987) investigated the occupation of those who had private medical insurance and obtained the following figures:

- Professional, 27%
- Employers and managers, 23%
- Intermediate (nonmanual), 9%
- Skilled manual, 3%
- Semi-skilled, 2%
- Unskilled, 1%

There clearly is a relationship among social or occupational class, private medical insurance, and the use of private health care.

The private sector involvement is about redefining the National Health Service. It is being changed from a centrally run health provider to a system in which different health care providers—public, private, and voluntary—have common standards. The expansion of the private sector is being achieved in the following ways:

- Through the private finance initiative sometimes referred to as the *public private partnership*
- By using the concordat, an agreement of cooperation between the Department of Health (DoH) and the private sector to bring private hospitals and nursing homes into the mainstream of National Health Service service provisions
- By developing foundation hospital trusts
- By establishing a new regulatory board to oversee these provisions

These public and private developments will enable public and patient involvement through patient forums. These will provide input into how

> ### Glossary
>
> *Concordat:* An agreement of cooperation between the Department of Health and the private sector to bring private hospitals and nursing homes into the mainstream of National Health Service service provisions.
>
> *Consultant:* The hospital consultant is the highest grade of medical staff and is a specialist, leading a firm of doctors and controlling a quota of beds.
>
> *Foundation hospital trust:* Initiative committed to increasing the scope and range of private sector activity within National Health Service services.
>
> *General practitioner:* Family physician.
>
> *National Health Service executive:* A member of the Department of Health who develops health policy and provides strategic leadership to the National Health Service.
>
> *Panel patients:* Non–fee-paying patients.
>
> *Private finance initiative:* One of a range of government policies to increase private sector involvement in the provision of public services.
>
> *Strategic health authorities:* They act as a bridge between the Department of Health and local National Health Service services to provide strategic leadership for improvements in health and well-being and adequate local health services.

local services are run and will be represented on the boards of all National Health Service organizations.

## THE PRIVATE FINANCE INITIATIVE

The private finance initiative is a partnership in which private capital is used to finance public sector projects such as new hospital buildings. This is particularly helpful to overcome decades of underinvestment in buildings and equipments. However, Gaffney and Pollock (1997) argue that reliance on private investment inflates the scale of capital schemes to levels that far exceed more-prudent public proposals, as bidders try to improve their rates of return. This cost escalation puts new demands on public revenue, which in turn leads to the search for new funding streams. This can result in a decreased bed capacity, untested changes in health care provisions, and use of more public funds than the private system was meant to replace. Therefore, profit and returns on capital become more of a priority, and the National Health Service ends up paying more for less.

## FOUNDATION HOSPITAL TRUSTS

Foundation hospital trusts are a part of the government's 10-year program of reform known as the *National Health Service Plan for England* (DoH, 2000), under which market-oriented and pro-business policies continue to be implemented. Health is a devolved function, and so foundation hospital trusts do not apply in Scotland, Wales, and Northern Ireland. The Scottish, Welsh, and Northern Ireland parliaments have not decided to go along with the development of foundation hospital trusts.

This initiative is a commitment by the government to increase the scope and range of private sector activity within National Health Service services by creating independent foundation trusts. These foundation trusts and hospitals will have National Health Service assets transferred to their ownership and control. They will be granted a license to operate by an independent regulator. They will be freed from National Health Service controls and will be accountable not to the Secretary of State for Health but to a board composed of employers, staff, and local residents, some of who will be locally elected. They will have greater freedom to set their own terms and conditions of service, giving them the ability to vary the pay and conditions package for staff and to contract out clinical and nonclinical services. They will be able to borrow for capital investment, generate income, and have greater control over the retention of the proceeds of land assets (DoH, 2003).

Before the foundation hospital trusts became a reality in April 2004, National Health Service trusts remained heavily regulated from the center, constrained in their ability to retain any surpluses they generated, in their ability to borrow from the private sector, in their access to capital, and in their ability to set their own conditions of service. The foundation hospital trusts will be able to address these issues and so change the National Health Service from a monolithic centrally run monopoly provider to a system in which different health providers, public and private, work with a common ethos and standards.

## REGULATION OF THE FOUNDATION HOSPITAL TRUSTS

The legislation for foundation hospital trusts provides for an independent regulator to state what services will be provided by a licensed foundation hospital trust. Foundation hospital trusts are therefore required to meet reasonably the demand for regulated health services (Mohan, 2003). This, however, leaves room for interpretation of what is "reasonable," thus allowing foundation hospital trusts to be selective in their choice of patients. This could result in patients being treated not in the hospital of their choice nor in the hospital nearest to them. Mohan (2003) wondered how the independent regulator would protect the rights, if any, of patients who want to be treated in a hospital of their choice near to their home?

Supporters of foundation hospitals and trusts claim that it will modernize the National Health Service and empower staff, democratize the service, and stimulate innovation. Opponents are concerned that the effect will be to drive a stake through the fundamental principle of the National Health Service, resulting in competition among hospitals and trusts rather than cooperation. Furthermore, the reforms signal a move away from the pursuit of equality to an agenda of consumer choice and preference, with citizenship entitlements becoming defined in terms of the opportunities available to individuals in markets. Opponents also argue that as the delivery system becomes more dependent on profits and returns to shareholders, new inefficiencies and transaction costs will make universal health care unsustainable, as there will be a gradual reduction in National Health Service services paid out of taxation and free at the point of use. High-quality care could be sacrificed. Health care will become a lottery decided at the local level (Mohan, 2003).

In August 2004 the Secretary of State for Health, the Right Honourable John Reid, asked the Healthcare Commission to offer advice on the difficulties, challenges, and experiences of the first 20 National Health Service foundation trusts. The commission prepared its report after analyzing performance data and interviewing more than 700 people. These included governors, trust directors, and health staff, as well as people in the local health community. The report concludes that foundation trusts have made hospitals more responsive to local communities and accelerated investment in patient care. However, in the period looked at there is no evidence to show that foundation trusts have improved the quality of care provided to patients. The commission has asked for a further review when the trusts will have been on operation for a longer period and when there will be data on their impact on service quality (Healthcare Commission, 2005).

### RELEVANCE TO NURSING

There is a strong argument that the public-private initiatives in the National Health Service could lead to labor market distortions, greater privatization of the nursing workforce, and greater disparities in pay among nurses working in different hospitals. Foundation hospitals and trusts have greater autonomy than other National Health Service hospitals and trusts to vary the terms and conditions for staff.

The Royal College of Nursing (RCN) has taken steps to study the reality of nursing practice and patients' experiences in the private sector (RCN, 2001). With the expectation that the private sector is set to expand, concern has been growing about the long-term effect on the principles of the National Health Service and how these changes will affect the quality of nursing care and patient outcomes.

The RCN (2001) reported increases in nursing workloads, higher patient dependency, and increases in early patient discharges, which created added pressure on community staff. Often there were inappropriate early discharges, increased readmission rates, and long waits in accident and emergency units. Patients were placed on inappropriate wards with staff not properly trained for their conditions. The RCN report demonstrated increases in nonregistered staff such as health care assistants and agency nurses. Registered nurses reported having less contact with patients, and patients expressed concern that the nurses always seemed to be busy. Patients believe the clinical environment has improved and are happy with new facilities that enable them to have nicer private rooms, gyms, shops, and gardens. Nursing staff comment that the new hospital designs enabled improved observation of patients. Both nurses and patients are positive about

the appearance of the buildings, but they complain of the loss of parking spaces with increased charges. On the other hand, staff facilities were reported to have deteriorated, staff meals were more expensive, and staff accommodations were reduced (and when present were considerably more expensive).

### NURSING INVOLVEMENT IN POLICY

The RCN (2004) stated that nurses were not involved in the development of the new initiatives. However, the RCN has been a part of the consultation and negotiation processes when hospitals apply to become foundation hospital trusts. On receiving the application, the Secretary of State requires the applying hospital to demonstrate that they have the support of the RCN. Whether or not the RCN supports an application depends on whether trusts show commitment to the RCN's standards for quality. The quality criteria are used to assess the trust's performance. They cover four main areas: governance, human resource management, service delivery, and National Health Service principles. The RCN monitors all foundation hospital trusts; should a foundation hospital trust fail to meet the quality criteria, the RCN will notify the governors of the foundation hospital trust, the government through the local Member of Parliament, and the regulator of all foundation hospital trusts.

### NURSING EDUCATION

Since the mid 1990s, nurse education in the United Kingdom has been wholly located within the higher education sector. Although all preregistration nurses are now university educated, few nurses receive degrees. The vast majority of nurses receive diplomas, and only 10% receive degrees. In fact these are the same 10% who received degrees before the wholesale incorporation of nurse education into universities. Nursing courses are either diploma courses, in which most nurses are enrolled, or degree courses, in which only a minority of students are enrolled. Nurses have pointed out that there is limited research differentiating the performance of a diplomat versus that of a graduate. It is difficult to recruit individuals with the appropriate level of education and academic ability because of the innumerable opportunities that women now have for entering other professions. Women still make up the majority of entrants into nursing (Burke & Harris, 2000).

Should nursing be an all-graduate profession? The RCN has made its views clear, asserting that nurses need degree-level education in order to move forward in the twenty-first century and have equal status with other health care professionals (Hancock, 1997). The National Health Service administrator has indicated that the National Health Service does not want an all-graduate profession because of the financial implications (Newton, 1997). Burke and Harris (2000) argued that the rapidly changing policy agenda is one of the reasons why graduate nurses would be of value to the National Health Service. Such nurses would be able to interpret, implement, and evaluate policy, critically analyze policy, and bring to clinical practice leadership, assertive, reflective, and critical skills.

## Key Points

- The British health system is now a public-private system, attempting to provide more-efficient and cost-effective services with common standards for the public.
- Both supporters and detractors agree that the newer private system has enabled services that could not be provided only in the public sector.
- The changes in the National Health Service have increased opportunities for profit, a reduction in entitlements to free care, and greater inequity.
- Nursing is only beginning to become involved in influencing policy decisions, primarily through the RCN in the private sector.

## Web Resources

> **Department of Health**
> *www.dh.gov.uk*
> **Royal College of Nursing (RCN)**
> *www.rcn.org.uk*

## REFERENCES

Able-Smith, B. (1964). *The hospitals, 1800-1948*. London: Heinemann.

Baggott, R. (2004) *Health and health care in Britain*. Basingstoke: Palgrave.

Booth, C. (1903). *Life and labour of the People in London*. London: Macmillan.

Burke, L., & Harris, D. (2000). Education purchaser's views of nursing as an all graduate profession. *Nurse Education Today, 20*, 620-628.

Challis, L., & Bartlett, H. (1987). *Old and ill. Private nursing homes for elderly people*. Mitcham: Age Concern.

Department of Health (DoH). (2000). *The NHS plan*. London: HMSO.

Department of Health (DoH). (2003). *Health and social care (Community Health and Standards Bill)*. London: DoH.

Department of Health and Social Security (DHSS). (1983). Competitive tendering in the provision of domestic catering and laundry services. *Health Circular, 83*, 18.

Gaffney, D., & Pollock, A. M. (1997). *Can the NHS afford PFI?* London: British Medical Journal.

General Household Survey. (1987). London: HMSO.

Ham, C. (1998). Population centred and patient focused purchasing: The UK experience. In P. Spurgeon (Ed.), *The new face of the NHS*. London: Royal Society of Medicine Press.

Hancock, C. (1997). The graduate nursing debate. RCN view. England Graduate Nursing Conference, Harrogate Management Centre, November 18, London.

Healthcare Commission. (2005). *The Healthcare Commission's review of the NHS foundation trusts*. London: Healthcare Commission. Retrieved July 25, 2005 from *www.health-carecommission.org.uk*.

Higgins, J. (1988). *The business of medicine*. Basingstoke: Macmillan.

Keen, J., Light, D., & Mays, N. (2001). *Public-private relations in healthcare*. London: Kings Fund.

Laing, W. (1995). *Laing's review of private health care*. London: Laing & Buisson.

Laing, W., & Buisson, R. (1994). *Private medical insurance update*. London: Laing & Buisson.

Laing, W., & Buisson, R. (2001). *Laing's healthcare market review 2001/2002*. London: Laing & Buisson.

Le Grand, J., & Robinson, R. (Eds.). (1984). *Privatisation and the welfare state*, London: Allen & Unwin.

Merrison Report. (1979). *Report of the Royal Commission on the National Health Service*. Cmnd 7615, London: HMSO.

Mohan, J. (2003). *Reconciling equity and choice? Foundation hospitals and the future of the NHS*. London: Catalyst.

Newton, G. (1997). The graduate nursing debate. An NHS executive perspective. England Graduate Nursing Conference, Harrogate Management Centre, November 18, London.

Office of Health Economics (OHE). (1987). *Hospital acquired infection*. London: OHE.

Rayner, G. (1986). Health care as a business: The emergence of a commercial hospital sector in Britain. *International Journal of Health Services, 17*, 197-216.

Royal College of Nursing (RCN). (2001). *Response to the commons Health Select Committee inquiry into the role of the private sector in the NHS*. London: RCN.

Royal College of Nursing (RCN). (2004). *The right foundation*. London: RCN.

Rowntree, S. (1901). *Poverty: A study in town life*. London: Macmillan.

## COULD A NATIONAL HEALTH SYSTEM WORK IN THE UNITED STATES?

Kristine M. Gebbie

*"There are always alternatives."*

MR. SPOCK, *STAR TREK*

The United States is often singled out as the only economically developed country on the globe that does not assure universal access to health services for its population, although it spends more than any other nation. For example, 2005 comparisons show that the median percentage of gross domestic product invested in health services by economically developed countries is 8.5%, whereas in the United States it is over 14%. The median expenditure is just over $2000 (USD) per capita, but the United States spends over $5000. Yet the United States has fewer hospital beds (2.9 per 1000 people compared with the United Kingdom, which has 3.9 per 1000 people) and fewer professionals (e.g., 7.9 nurses per 1000 compared with a median of 8.9 per 1000 or with the United Kingdom, which has 9.2 per 1000). Furthermore, the United States has nearly 50 million people with no health insurance, many more with limited access to care, and the insured with widely varying degrees of access based on geography, type of insurance, and barriers such as language or cultural gaps (Anderson, Hussey, Frogner, & Waters, 2005).

Near universality of access is achieved in other countries through a variety of arrangements, including government-operated care systems, government-managed finance systems, and government-mandated financing. In the United States, moves toward a universal system have been made at several points during the twentieth century, most recently in the 1993-1994 proposal by President Clinton that died without ever coming to a vote in Congress. The issue is one for serious concern, because this country, which spends so much more on health, is far from leading the planet on measures of health such as length of healthy life lived or proportion of infants living to their first birthday. Exploring the potential for a national health system can reveal strengths and weaknesses and begin to answer whether it is possible in the United States.

### POSSIBLE APPROACHES TO A NATIONAL SYSTEM

The two major approaches to a national system that have been successfully used elsewhere are through some form of financing that is universal or through a service system of some kind that is universally available. For each of these there are at least two structural options, and each will be briefly discussed in turn.

### Universal Payment

Universal payment as a route to a national health system assumes that the lack of access to services is primarily associated with lack of ability to pay and therefore that if funds were available, the services would follow. This discussion of payment will not take up the problematic reality of such an assumption. It is notable, however, that even some people who have financing for care are unable to get access because practitioners are not available for reasons such as geographic maldistribution, professional workforce shortages, or some form of social discrimination (e.g., denial of Medicaid to some immigrants, or provider prejudice regarding sexual orientation).

***National tax.*** The simplest form of universal payment would be a national program in which tax funds are used to pay providers for care rendered as needed. The tax could be a special one (such as that currently used to support Medicare for those over 65) or some portion of general revenues. The payment from this single national payer could go directly to those providing care (as in the province-based single-payer system of Canada) or could be managed through contracts with fiscal intermediaries (as is now the case for Medicare). If truly universal, there would be little or no administrative burden for enrollment, as everyone would automatically be eligible. There would be a need to negotiate with providers of care for fee levels and methods of reimbursement; a single payer controlling all health dollars would be a formidable bargaining agent for hospitals and clinicians to confront. The fear of such a single agent clearly affects policy decisions, such as the prohibitions on national contracts for lower-cost drugs under the Medicare drug benefit legislated in 2003. This program is to be managed through the usual range of nongovernmental providers, each of which may negotiate with manufacturers for lower prices. However, the most powerful negotiator, the nation-wide Medicare program as a whole, is prohibited from negotiating for a single lowest price for all seniors across the country.

***Multiple payers.*** Alternately, a universal payment system could be constructed with multiple payers. For example, all employers, no matter how small or large, could be required to provide a certain level of health insurance for all employees and their families, with Medicare continuing for those over 65 or disabled and a form of Medicaid used for the unemployed and their families. This less-monolithic system is the heart of the rejected Clinton plan and shares features with that in place, for example, in Germany. It allows for a range of payment mechanisms, with more room for bargaining and less sense of the government as the overwhelming controller of the purse strings. For a system such as this to work successfully, there would have to be rules governing the components of coverage and dual coverage in families with more than one worker. The employment-based coverage would be financed as it is now, with funds that would otherwise be available for wages or other benefits; coverage for those not in working families would require tax support, as it does now to the extent that they are available. Although this might be more palatable to practitioners or institutions, many employers, especially those with few employees, would find the mandate objectionable.

## Universal Care

A more radical approach to a national health system would be to make the actual provision of care universal.

***National health system.*** This is the approach begun after World War II in Great Britain, with the National Health Service. National tax dollars (general or special taxes) are used to pay primary care providers throughout the country for basic health services and to pay specialists and hospitals for their share of needed services. This essentially makes the provision of care a government service, whether the caregivers and hospital staff are put directly on a government payroll or are employed by contract. The managers of the system are obligated to find sources of care for everyone throughout the country; to do so, they might need to make differential fees available to recruit providers—for example, to serve remote areas. This approach also lends itself to careful investment in only as many hospital beds and specialized services as population size and health statistics suggest are needed, with a clear disincentive for continuing the expensive practice of having large numbers of excess beds or competing diagnostic services. It is for this reason that Britain, as most other countries, invests far less in multiple, identical pieces of diagnostic equipment. For example, the United Kingdom has only 5.5 magnetic resonance imaging (MRI) units for each million in the population, compared with the United States at 8.2 per million (Anderson et al., 2005). There are many fears, however, that such a system has too many incentives to control cost and not enough incentives to be user friendly or of high quality.

***State-based system.*** Universality could be achieved with similar results but greater flexibility by placing the requirement for access on the states through some combination of funding incentives and penalties. Expecting each state to use its tax authority and funds provided through national tax resources to assure access for everyone would allow each state to employ and deploy its own preferred mix of generalists and specialists, community-based and hospital-based services. Within a national minimum expectation, states with more income could choose a richer mix of services, but no one would be without access to care. This approach to national minimums and state options on organization and final mix of services is the overall structure for our present Medicaid system. There are risks here, as even states with a relatively high income level could adopt a more miserly approach to access for health and illness services.

For providers of care, either form of a universal care system presents a far more radical change from current realities than a move to assure payment for care for everyone. Such centralized control of purse strings makes it far less likely that individual entrepreneurs or entrepreneurial systems would survive. And it is not clear that the current infusion of private capital into development of pharmaceuticals or equipment would continue, or whether a leveling of incomes across types of providers might prove discouraging to those considering entering a health profession.

## THE PARTICIPANTS

Understanding the debate about universal coverage in the United States is almost impossible without at least some awareness of the groups that have participated in the arguments that have kept the system as it is now. These include myriad groups that maintain political and economic power through the present nonstructure:

- *For-profit insurance companies*, which might not be allowed to sell competing products at whatever price they can command
- *Pharmaceutical and technology manufacturers*, which might experience limits in the volume of what can be sold or have to face monopsonistic buying power

- *Medium-sized and small businesses* that believe that they would be forced to pay either taxes or premiums beyond what is affordable
- *Health professionals*, particularly those in small group, fee-for-service practices, who perceive that their degree of freedom may become limited

From other perspectives there are also groups whose focus is more on what is currently missing and therefore that speak out on behalf of change:

- *Labor unions*, aware of the vulnerability of their members to arbitrary changes in work-related and retiree coverage
- *Advocates for population groups* with decreased access in the current system
- *Health professionals in salaried positions*, particularly those in system-oriented organizations such as public health agencies and community-based health centers
- *Businesses* that have grasped the potential economic benefit of leveling the cost playing field by bringing everyone to the table

Although neither of these perspectives is absolutely the purview of one political party or the other, the Republican party and those identified as farther to the right on the political spectrum are more identified with opposition to any form of mandated universality. The Democratic party and those identified as farther to the left on the political spectrum have been traditionally more identified with the campaigns for comprehensive approaches.

## BARRIERS TO RESOLVING THE LACK OF UNIVERSALITY

Describing ways that universality could be achieved does not deal with the reality that universality of access to care or funding for care has not been popular in the United States. The history of care and payment has been a blend of entrepreneurship, private charity, and public charity.

### American Enterprise

Entrepreneurs have been free to develop care or care products and sell them freely, subject for just over 100 years to the strictures of federal and state safety regulation and professional licensing laws. Private groups, particularly religious ones, have offered hospitals, clinics, and home care and other services to those unable to purchase such services for themselves, although this charity role has diminished in the face of rising costs and a greater number of reimbursement programs. Governments have offered public hospitals, various clinics, and a few finance systems, to assure that the neediest citizens have had access to at least the rudiments of care. There is a personal cost to these "free" services, paid in such currency as extended waiting time for care or loss of personal dignity.

## Incrementalism

Over the latter half of the twentieth century the United States edged closer toward universality with the convergence of specialized programs such as Medicare, community and migrant health centers, expanded Medicaid, state insurance purchasing initiatives, and the Child Health Insurance Program. However, these positive moves on the part of governments have been offset by the growing number of jobs that do not offer a health insurance benefit either for workers or for worker families or do so at a cost that is not affordable. Furthermore, these incremental moves are open to the fluctuations in year-to-year budgets and changing political philosophies. There is no indication that this trend will be reversed any time soon.

## Political History

It is also important to remember that the political history of the United States is one of suspicion about government and a reluctance to use government as the solution to a problem. The election of 2004 returned to office a party that has consistently run against government, proposes tax cuts in part so that the funds will not be there to tempt Congress to spend, and that touts private solutions to social concerns. The 2005 proposals to make major changes in the Social Security Administration suggest that even this most basic of social contracts among citizens and their government is in danger of being negated.

Recollecting multiple panel discussions and academic presentations during the 1993-1994 health reform debate, the overall impression was that, while people were willing to agree that lack of access to care is a problem, they were divided about whether this improvement should be publicly financed and reluctant to support either spending more money or giving up some of their own current services in order to make it possible. If this is accurate, it means that decision-makers were receiving sufficiently mixed messages that any action they took would please only a few. There is a history of abrupt reversal of public policy on catastrophic coverage for seniors in the 1980s (Congress enacted in one session and repealed in the next a system of higher Medicare taxes that assured a limit on personal expenditures for extremely high medical expenses, in large part because of anger by seniors claiming they were misled regarding the increased premiums they would have to pay for this protection) and the disastrous 1993-1994 health reform debate (when President Clinton attempted to keep his campaign promise of health care for all by sending to Congress a complex proposal developed largely behind closed doors by a panel headed by his spouse; the idea died an agonizing death through attacks by every established interest that stood to lose control or funding). Those events, coupled with the conflicting views of the public, make it seem highly unlikely that any major effort to achieve universality will be attempted in the near future. Even the most popular of changes, creating a Medicare prescription drug benefit, was accomplished by crafting a benefit that is incomplete, complex, and extremely confusing to many participants. For example, the period of full implementation in January of 2006 led to many individuals being denied access to medication essential to the management of chronic mental illness, with an echo effect of increased hospitalization costs.

## POTENTIAL POSITIVE FORCES

Despite the negatives, there are some forces that might push the country in the direction of universality.

## A Balancing Act

The major force is the conundrum of balancing cost and quality without leaving an even larger number of individuals without care. A number of states attempting health reform and universal coverage in the 1980s and 1990s dealt with this problem extensively. The problem can be described as similar to trying to get complete control of a large, slightly underfilled balloon: when you grab on one place, it simply bulges out in another. The expectation that the care system will achieve a higher quality of error-free care may require additional staff, different staff, or new information systems, all of which entail cost. Under the existing system, adding any staff or capital equipment without jeopardizing quality or raising cost can be accomplished by reducing the number of individuals cared for. If, however, it is very clear that no one can be moved outside—that is, left without care—we will be forced to have the dialogue needed to make a collective agreement on all three points: how much care, of what quality, and at what cost. However, no state has the legal authority to require participation in any state-specific universal plan on the part of Medicare or companies choosing to self-insure and thereby be exempted from state regulation by ERISA*, so state efforts have at best had only partial success and for limited periods of time.

### Economics Matter

The sense that there is a problem has dissipated since the wave of support for health reform in 1992 and 1993, when President Bill Clinton tried to live up to his campaign promise of providing universal access to care. Because those who are uninsured are disproportionately from often-disenfranchised groups, their concerns have not been heard. Emergence of a larger group more representative of the economic and ethnic mix of the nation would make the problem real. Many hope that awareness of the problem would be rekindled if the economy

were to take a serious downturn, bringing home to many more individuals the reality that under the present nonsystem they are only one paycheck or one layoff away from being unable to finance needed health care for themselves and their families. There is a resurgence of reports from large employers that they are experiencing crippling increases in costs for health insurance for employees (even if they ignore families and retirees). The most well known of these complaints is from General Motors: When the cost of materials and labor is broken out per vehicle manufactured, the attributable cost of health insurance exceeds the cost of raw metals used. Public awareness of such stories can stimulate the political will to make the needed changes.

### The Public's Role

Public awareness and concern may be, in the end, what makes the change possible. A policy change such as that needed in the United States to develop a comprehensive and inclusive national health policy can happen only when there is a confluence of a perceived problem, a potential solution, and the political will to act. The potential solutions are many and have been in circulation for many years. The exact combination of funding and organization that would achieve universality in the United States may not be known, but its component parts are most likely already within the policy menu. What is missing is a widespread awareness that there really is a problem, coupled with the political will to solve it.

However, the use of an awakened public to make as major a change as national health a reality in the United States is unlikely because it would take a sustained lobbying effort that lasts longer than one election cycle and is loud enough to be heard over the voices of the currently enfranchised nonsystem. The fears of clinicians, hospitals, suppliers, employers, and insurance companies that they will lose autonomy and face tough regulation and even tougher price negotiations means that they will argue loud and long against any single national voice about health. And there is no way to achieve true universality, or a truly national system, without that single national voice.

---

*The Employee Retirement Income Security Act (ERISA) exempts self-insured health benefits plans from regulation by the states, meaning that self-insured companies may limit benefits, arbitrarily change coverage, or exempt certain conditions in ways that would otherwise be limited by state law if coverage were offered through ordinary insurance companies. When the law was enacted in 1974 the focus was primarily on eliminating duplicate oversight of pension plans for companies operating in many states. Hawaii had a mandate for universal employment-based insurance that predated ERISA and is the only exemption to the law.

## *Key Points*

- A national system can work only if we make a national decision that access to care is a basic human right.
- The debate about a national system is confused because of confusing terminology and lack of understanding of what is done elsewhere.
- The debate about a national system is rooted in our political history and should be entered with a full appreciation of our past efforts.

## *Web Resources*

Information about current debates about improved coverage and movements toward universal coverage can be followed through the Websites of major professional associations such as the following:
**American Hospital Association**
*www.aha.org*

**American Medical Association**
*www.americanmedicalassociation.org*
**American Nurses Association**
*www.ana.org*
**American Public Health Association**
*www.apha.org*
These foundations have a particular interest in health reform:
**Commonwealth Fund**
*www.commonwealthfund.org*
**Henry J. Kaiser Family Foundation**
*www.kff.org*
**Milbank Memorial Fund**
*www.milbank.org*
**Robert Wood Johnson Foundation**
*www.rwjf.org*

### REFERENCES

Anderson, G. S., Hussey, P. S., Frogner, B. K., & Waters, H. R. (2005). Health care spending in the US and other industrialized countries. *Health Affairs, 24*(4), 903-914.

# *Taking Action*   Alice Sardell

## *Community Health Centers: A Successful Strategy for Improving Health Care Access*

*"We really want people who cannot afford health care—the poor and the indigent—to be able to get good primary care at one of these community health centers, and not in the emergency room of hospitals across the United States of America."*
PRESIDENT GEORGE W. BUSH, JANUARY 27, 2005

There are currently more than 1000 community health centers (CHCs) serving 15 million people at 5000 sites all over the United States. These programs provide medical, dental, mental health and substance abuse services, nutrition counseling, outreach, transportation, and other social services to uninsured patients as well as those with Medicaid, Medicare, SCHIP, and even private health insurance. Community health centers include programs serving migrant workers and the homeless.

CHCs are located in areas designated by the federal government as medically underserved and serve all residents of a geographic catchment area, without regard to insurance status or ability to pay. About half of all health centers are in urban areas, and half are in rural areas. They are primarily funded by a mix of public insurance (Medicaid and Medicare) and federal grants. Patients served by CHCs are poorer, sicker, and more likely to be persons of color than the general U.S. population (National Association of Community Health Centers [NACHC], 2005).

CHCs are unique health service institutions in several important ways. First, they are a community-oriented, culturally sensitive model of health care services integrated with social and educational services. Second, they are governed by consumer boards that by federal law must have a majority of members who receive care at the health center. Third, they are "safety net providers," caring for people who do not have health insurance.

These health care institutions were first funded as "neighborhood health centers" as part of the War on Poverty in 1965, one aspect of President Lyndon B. Johnson's Great Society program. They were created by activist physicians and federal government officials—"policy entrepreneurs"—who believed that disparities in health status were intimately linked to social, economic, and political inequalities. Health centers were to treat whole communities, not just individuals, and to provide jobs as well as health services. Although these programs were products of the "political stream" or policy environment of the 1960s, they survived the end of the War on Poverty and subsequent political challenges during the more conservative Nixon and Reagan Administrations. Not only did they overcome these challenges, but they became institutionalized as part of the federally funded heath care system. In fact, health centers were the only domestic social program that was expanded during President George W. Bush's first term in office (2001 to 2004) and then targeted for further expansion during his second term.

The policy history of the CHC program explains how a program providing care to communities with very few political resources and therefore little political influence was able to survive and to grow in an era in which less and less attention was paid to problems such as poverty and inequality. This history illustrates how supporters within federal executive agencies and Congress nurtured the program during its first decade until an effective national advocacy organization for health centers was built. This national organization, its state partners, and local health centers then successfully created broad support for health centers that is bipartisan and exists across ideological boundaries. The story of the survival of the CHC program is a story about the creation of a "policy network" supportive of CHCs. The story of its expansion is a tale of skilled policy advocates who have been able to frame the argument for health center funding in a way that fits within a political environment vastly different from the one in which it was born.

## CREATION OF NEIGHBORHOOD HEALTH CENTERS

The first neighborhood health centers were funded in 1965 as demonstration programs by the Community Action Program established by the Economic Opportunity Act (EOA) of 1964. The goal of this legislation was to eliminate the causes of poverty in the United States. Health was not initially one of the areas in which programs were to be established, but early on it became clear that participants in the educational and training programs that were established, such as Head Start and the Jobs Corps, suffered from lack of access to health care. The very first health demonstration programs were created by two medical educators, Dr. H. Jack Geiger and Dr. Count Gibson, of Tufts University Medical School. The model of the two centers that they established, one in a Boston housing project and one in a poor rural area of Mississippi, combined comprehensive health services based on a public health–social medicine perspective, community development, and the training and employment of community residents. Health center staff in Mississippi found that children in the community had recurring episodes of malnutrition and dysentery. In response they organized residents who decided to construct wells and establish a farm cooperative to feed themselves and their children. Other health centers funded under this program, which was authorized by an amendment to the

EOA by Senator Edward Kennedy (D-MA), also provided community development and employment opportunities as well as health care services. For example, a neighborhood health center in Brooklyn, NY gave preference in hiring to local residents, and health center staff facilitated the creation of a community organization to rehabilitate housing in the area. By the end of 1971 there were 100 neighborhood health centers funded under Kennedy's 1966 amendment.

The original neighborhood health center model contained four elements: social medicine, decentralized community-based care, community economic development, and community participation. From the social medicine perspective, health status is shaped by the physical and social environment, and treatment includes intervention in that environment. Health care was to be community based by offering services to all of the residents of a specific geographic catchment area (rather than to those who fit within certain disease or health insurance categories) and by employing community residents to serve as a bridge between patients and professional staff. These workers, often called *family health workers,* made home visits and provided health education and advocacy services along with health care. The recruitment, training, and employment of these workers was also an example of the way in which neighborhood health centers were venues for community economic development. Finally, "maximum feasible participation" of the poor was required of all programs funded under the EOA. The operationalization of this concept involved conflict between project administrators (many of whom were employed by hospitals, medical schools, and health departments in the early years) and health center consumers during the program's early years. When health centers received a separate federal program authorization in 1975, community governance became a central component that defined the program (Sardell, 1988).

Policy innovation in the United States most often requires that one or more individuals "invest their resources—time, energy, reputation, and sometimes money" in advocating for a new policy idea. John Kingdon calls these advocates "policy entrepreneurs" (Kingdon, 1995, p. 122). Policy advocacy is most successful when entrepreneurs in and outside of government work together to support a new policy or program. This is what happened in the case of the creation of the neighborhood health center program. Activist physicians and federal Office of Economic Opportunity (OEO) officials worked together to create a policy that would provide greater access to health care services to low-income populations and to provide services that were different from those offered by "mainstream" medical institutions. In addition, Senator Kennedy became convinced that health centers should be the major program for serving underserved communities. He acted as an advocate for the program within Congress, deflecting opposition to both anti-poverty programs and to "socialized medicine." When President Nixon took office the political environment changed. President Nixon was not supportive of the social programs initiated by the Johnson Administration. Yet during the Nixon Administration, sympathetic federal officials' policy protected the program until its advocates outside of government grew stronger (Sardell, 1988).

## THE SURVIVAL AND INSTITUTIONALIZATION OF THE HEALTH CENTER PROGRAM

Beginning in 1968 the Public Health Service (PHS) within the Department of Health, Education and Welfare (DHEW) also provided funding for the establishment of about 50 comprehensive health centers in low-income areas. The involvement of the PHS in primary health services had been historically limited to the funding of categorical disease programs. However, the 1960s was a period in which socially concerned health professionals, administrators, and social scientists joined the agency as an alternative to serving in the military during the Vietnam War. Some of these individuals became policy entrepreneurs within the PHS on the issue of comprehensive health service programs in low-income areas. They were supported in their efforts to fund these programs by top DHEW officials appointed by President Johnson.

Although the Nixon Administration did not support the neighborhood health center program, there were civil servants in the PHS, as well as the

OEO, who acted from inside the government to protect it. As the OEO was phased out, decisions as to the timing of the transfers of individual programs from the OEO to DHEW were made in ways that would protect more politically vulnerable programs (for example, programs in the South, where local elected officials were not supportive). In addition, agency officials awarded technical assistance grants to newly formed state health center associations and (in 1973) to the National Association of Neighborhood Health Centers, an organization created in 1970.

Key congressional leaders such as Senator Kennedy and Congressman Paul Rogers (D-FL) (chairmen of the committees with jurisdiction over public health programs) also supported the health center program during the presidencies of Richard Nixon and Gerald Ford. When health centers were first funded by the OEO, it was expected that as the program grew, it would be primarily financed by Medicare and Medicaid payments. But this had not happened, both because many patients treated at health centers were not enrolled in the Medicaid program and because the Medicaid program in many states did not reimburse for the many non-medical services that health centers provided. In 1972 DHEW announced that it planned to phase out federal grants to health centers. However, in opposition to the wishes of the Nixon and Ford administrations, Congress in 1974 and 1975 passed legislation specifically describing "community health centers" and authorizing grant funding for them. The legislation was vetoed by both Presidents, but in 1975 Congress overrode President Ford's veto. The creation of the program took place within the wider context of intense conflict between presidents who aimed to reduce the role of the federal government in social policy and a liberal Democratic Congress that wanted to preserve the social programs of the Great Society. This congressional action was a critical point in the history of the program because it now had its own legislative authority that defined the characteristics of "community health centers."

A CHC has to have a consumer-dominated governing board. This board establishes general policies for the center, has fiduciary responsibility,

and appoints its executive director. A majority of board members have to be consumers who use its services. When enacted, this was the most rigorous community participation provision in any health service program up to that time. This legislative provision, reaffirmed many times, has meant that community-based primary care programs that don't have such a governing board structure, such as those run by hospitals, cannot receive federal grants as CHCs (Sardell, 1988). This provision has also enabled advocates to frame CHCs as embodying "local control" in public policymaking, an aspect of the program that has appealed to Republicans as well as Democrats.

The Ford administration (1974 to 1977) attempted to reduce CHC program funding and to end categorical grant programs in health. Within that political environment, federal program officials initiated changes that helped to expand congressional support. New program monitoring systems were established that provided measurable performance criteria for the health centers so that congressional concern with efficiency was addressed. In addition, "rural health initiatives," smaller-scale, basic medical programs were funded. More centers could be funded because they required fewer resources than the large urban centers. And rural, white congressional districts could potentially become a part of the health center constituency. These changes were part of the "institutionalization" of the health center program (Sardell, 1988). Over time, the cost-effectiveness of CHCs has been one of the major arguments made for increasing support for this model of care. Further, since the 1980s, members of Congress from rural districts and states have been important champions of CHCs.

In the same period that federal agency officials were making decisions that would ultimately strengthen congressional support for CHCs, an organization representing the health centers themselves was created. Today this organization is one of the most effective advocacy organizations in Washington. Beginning in 1975 the NACHC (*www.nachc.org*) began to focus on educating members of Congress and their staffs about the value of CHCs. A policy analyst was hired, a weekly newsletter on policy events was published, and the

Association initiated an annual "Policy and Issues Forum" in Washington, DC, which brought together health center consumers and staff to learn about policy issues and speak to members of Congress about them. The following year a Department of Policy Analysis was created. Beginning in 1978 the NACHC functioned as part of the policy network supportive of the CHC program. During the following decades, membership in NACHC grew, as did the organizational infrastructure.

## COMMUNITY HEALTH CENTERS AND THE POLICY ENVIRONMENT: ADMINISTRATION SUPPORT AND ADMINISTRATION CHALLENGE

President Jimmy Carter (1977 to 1981) appointed federal officials who were very supportive of the CHC program. In fact, some had been policy entrepreneurs in various areas of health and social policy during the Johnson administration. There were funding increases for CHCs during the Carter administration. In addition, the rural health initiative concept of smaller centers was extended to urban areas, and the focus on management efficiency continued (Sardell, 1988). A reimbursement system that provided support for health centers was begun with the enactment of the Rural Health Clinic Services Act. This legislation, supported by the Carter administration, increased the Medicare and Medicaid rate paid to rural health clinics and allowed reimbursement for the services of nurse practitioners and physicians assistants.

In contrast to the Carter administration's support, health center appropriations were reduced during the early years of the Reagan administration (Lefkowitz, 2005). President Reagan also proposed that health centers, along with 10 other programs, be combined into a health services block grant to the states. Congress rejected this and instead enacted a primary care services block grant only for CHCs and only if states volunteered to administer the program—a block grant in name only. The block grant was later repealed and the federal CHC program reauthorized. During the Reagan era (1981-1989) NACHC worked to prepare health centers to respond both programmatically and politically to a policy environment of increased

state involvement in health policy decisions and to increased market competition resulting from the growth of managed care. Primary care associations were to be developed at state and regional levels, and the NACHC provided technical assistance to enable health centers to successfully become part of the world of managed care (Sardell, 1988).

## BROAD POLITICAL SUPPORT FOR COMMUNITY HEALTH CENTERS IN THE CURRENT ERA: AN EXPLANATION

During the Presidency of George H.W. Bush (1989 to 1993) Congress again increased funding for the health center program through the appropriations process. In addition, the staff of Senator John Chafee (R-RI) and the NACHC initiated legislation that dealt with the problem of low Medicaid and Medicare reimbursement rates for services delivered at CHCs. Under the Federally Qualified Health Center (FQHC) program, which became part of Medicaid in 1989 and Medicare in 1990, CHCs and "look-alikes" (clinics that did not get federal grant monies under the CHC program but had the characteristics of CHCs) would have special Medicaid and Medicare reimbursement rates that were closer to actual costs than regular per-visit rates paid by Medicaid in many states. As a result, health centers were able to collect higher reimbursements for Medicaid and Medicare patients. Medicaid became the major source of revenue for health centers, rather than federal grant funds. From 1990 to 1998, the proportion of health center revenues *from federal grants substantially decreased* from 41% to 26%.

Although Bill Clinton, a Democrat, was elected president in 1992, it was bipartisan support from both Houses of Congress and advocacy from within the public health bureaucracy that protected the health center program during the Clinton years. The Clinton administration's focus was on a national health reform plan that would restructure care for everyone; there seemed to be less interest within the administration on health care institutions designed exclusively to serve the traditionally underserved. Yet congressional and bureaucratic champions successfully fought to continue such separate programs within the Clinton Health Security Act, and Congress continued to increase funding for health centers in the budgets enacted during the Clinton Presidency. There was almost a 65% increase in federal appropriations for the health center program between 1995 and 2001 (Lefkowitz, 2005).

Republican George W. Bush was elected president in 2000 as a conservative who would look outside government for the solutions to social problems. Yet he has embraced CHCs, a program created by liberal Democratic President Lyndon Johnson in the 1960s. In 2001, in his first year of his first term in office, Bush proposed a 5-year initiative to expand health center sites to serve 6.1 million new patients. Congress supported funding for this initiative, and as of 2005 there were three million new patients being treated at CHCs (NACHC & George Washington University, 2005). In January of 2005, President Bush talked about the need for access to health care and called himself "a big backer of expanding CHCs to every poor county in America" (quoted in NACHC & George Washington University 2005). In his budget for fiscal year 2006, the President included an additional $304 million to reach the original 5-year capacity goal (Stevenson, 2005). This expansion would be part of a budget that slashed spending for a wide variety of domestic programs including food stamps, home energy assistance, training grants for health professions, veterans' benefits, and Medicaid (Pear, 2005a). Expanding CHCs in low-income areas was to be a budget priority.

What explains the support that CHCs, programs serving ethnic minorities and the poor, have from President George W. Bush, a Republican conservative? First, are policy arguments based on data that show that health centers provide access to high-quality health care for underserved populations in a cost-effective way. For example, studies comparing uninsured patients who receive care at CHCs with uninsured patients who do not find that CHC patients are less likely to wait to seek care and are more likely to report having a usual source of care and to receive preventive health counseling. Low-income minority women who are uninsured or have Medicaid are more likely to have had cancer screening tests if they are patients at health centers than similar women who are not health center patients (Proser, 2005).

Health centers are also central in efforts to reduce ethnic and racial disparities in health status. One way in which this occurs is by offering enabling services such as health and nutrition education, outreach, language translation, and transportation. Health centers have, since 1999, participated in Health Disparities Collaboratives established by the U.S. Department of Health and Human Services. These Collaboratives seek to eliminate racial and ethnic disparities in chronic disease through a patient empowerment model of chronic disease management (NACHC, 2003).

It is important to note here that nurse practitioners and other advanced practice nurses are central to these efforts (Hawkins, 2005). In fact, the number of nurses employed in CHCs has been increasing as the numbers of patients served has increased. In 2004, 10,625 nurses worked at health centers, including 2199 nurse practitioners, 350 nurse midwives, and 8076 other nurses. In the same year health centers employed 6680 physicians (Health Resources and Health Services Administration, 2004). Since 2000 the number of nurses employed at health centers has increased by almost 30%, with the largest increase, 41%, in the number of nurse practitioners and nurse midwives (personal communication, Dan Hawkins, November 13, 2005).

Second is the expansion of the policy network to include conservative members of Congress, so that network now includes an ideologically diverse set of policymakers.

Beginning as early as the 1980s, policy staff at NACHC worked with moderate and conservative Republicans as well as Democrats on issues of concern to health centers (Hawkins, 2005). This process of building relationships on a bipartisan basis became critical when the Republicans gained control of Congress in 1994 and then in 2000 when Bush was elected President. In addition to the liberal Democrats and moderate Republicans who were program supporters in its formative years, health center champions in Congress in the current period include powerful Republican conservatives such as Senators Orin Hatch of Utah and Christopher "Kit" Bond of Missouri and Representative Henry Bonilla of Texas. In fact, Senator Bond and Congressman

Bonilla brought the idea of expanding health centers to the attention of George W. Bush during his first campaign for the presidency (Hawkins, 2005). The policy arguments discussed above and the fact that these lawmakers have health center users among their constituents suggest reasons for their support.

Third, it is the relatively long experience and high levels of skill of the officials and staff of the CHC advocacy community that has successfully wedded policy arguments with grassroots political activity. As of 2005 the Department of Policy Analysis of the NACHC has 13 full-time and three part-time staff members, including three whose focus is on state-level issues. Primary care associations at the state and regional levels, together with the NACHC, have successfully met a series of policy challenges to the program's continued existence and growth and have helped to create the very broad support enjoyed by the CHC program 40 years after its creation.

## THE FUTURE OF COMMUNITY HEALTH CENTERS

Between 1999 and 2004, the population using CHCs increased by almost 50%. This was the largest growth in patients served since the beginning of the program in the 1960s. This increased demand for health center services reflects an increase in the number of uninsured and poor Americans. In the current period* 91% of health center patients have incomes at or below 200% of the federal poverty level (FPL) as compared with 31% of the U.S. population, and 40% are uninsured, in contrast to 15.6% of the overall population. Patients who have Medicaid as their health insurance constitute 35.7% of the health center population and 12.4% of the U.S. population. In terms of ethnicity, a little less than two thirds of the health center population and one third of the U.S. population are people of color. The proportion of low-income and uninsured patients seen at health centers increased more rapidly than did the

proportion of these groups in the general population, whereas the proportion of Medicaid patients at many health centers decreased. In addition, the proportion of health center visits for chronic illness has increased in recent years. Therefore health centers are treating more individuals with greater medical needs than ever before.

Health centers continue to provide an array of services that decrease the experience of fragmented service delivery. For example, both the proportion of health centers providing dental care and mental health services and the number of patient visits for these services has increased during the last few years. In 2004, more than 70% of health centers nationwide provided these services (NACHC, 2005).

Although some supporters may view CHCs as primarily cost-effective alternatives to emergency rooms, others value their provision of a comprehensive, culturally competent, broad array of health services and their structure of community governance. Even in nations with universal health insurance, institutions similar to CHCs provide health care to isolated and vulnerable populations (Wilensky & Roby, 2005). The future of CHCs, is, of course, linked to policy developments in the larger health care system. These include the training of a diverse workforce in the delivery of health services based on the CHC model, the availability of capital funds to CHCs, and the future of Medicaid.

As discussed earlier, Medicaid provides more than a third of the revenues of health centers. This revenue not only provides care for patients who are insured by Medicaid, but also supports the health center infrastructure that cares for patients without any health insurance (Hawkins & Rosenbaum, 2005). Health centers generally operate with no excess revenue and thus are financially fragile. Medicaid is the most "reliable payer," paying the highest percentage (87%) of charges of any revenue source in 2004 (NACHC, 2005). President Bush's initiative to expand the number of health center sites does not address the issue of ongoing operational funding. Clearly, the financial future of CHCs is linked to the future of Medicaid and to health insurance generally.

---

*Data on the health center population are from 2004; data on the overall U.S. population are from 2003 (NACHC, 2005).

During the last decade Governors have argued that their states need a larger role in decision-making about eligibility and benefits within the Medicaid program. Congress has been discussing ways to cut Medicaid spending, including giving more authority to the states (Pear, 2005b). The NACHC has taken a leading role in the debate over the future of Medicaid, organizing a coalition of providers to argue for Medicaid policies that reimburse preventive and primary care and preserve benefits while reducing costs (Hawkins, 2005). Medicaid is a very complicated and controversial policy issue, but its importance to the future of CHCs is an example of the intimate interrelationship between models of health care delivery and systems for health care financing.

## Lessons Learned

The policy history of CHCs illustrates several aspects of the process of advocating for health care innovation.

1. First is the crucial importance of understanding the political stream or general political environment and framing policy solutions in ways that fit that environment. Socially concerned health professionals and others created neighborhood health centers as part of the War on Poverty, and health center advocates today frame their policy arguments in terms of current health policy concerns.

2. Second is that program survival and institutionalization during the 1970s was the result of the actions of federal officials who were ideologically and personally committed to health center programs and helped to create a nongovernmental advocacy organization to represent them. The resulting health center policy community consisted of federal agency officials, members of Congress, and the NACHC.

3. Third, the current expansion of health centers as a central plank of Bush administration health policy is the result of the development of long-term relationships with members of Congress from across the political and ideological spectrum and policy arguments made in terms of access, the reduction of health disparities, and the cost-effectiveness of the program.

## Web Resources

**Association of Health Center Affiliated Health Plans**
*www.ahcahp.org*
**Health Disparities Collaboratives**
*www.healthdisparities.net*
**National Association of Community Health Centers**
*www.nachc.org*
**National Center for Farmworker Health**
*www.ncfh.org*
**National Health Care for the Homeless Council**
*www.nhchc.org*
**National Rural Health Association**
*www.nrharural.org*
**Primary Care Associations**
*www.nachc.com/primcare/srpcalist.asp*

## REFERENCES

Hawkins, D. R. Jr. (2005, October 31). Phone interview with Daniel R. Hawkins, Jr., Vice President for Federal, State, and Public Affairs, NACHC.

Hawkins, D., & Rosenbaum, S. (2005). Health centers at 40: Implications for future public policy. *Journal of Ambulatory Care Management, 28,* 357-365.

Health Resources and Health Services Administration. (2004). Bureau of Primary Health Care, Uniform Data System (UDS) Reports for Section 330 Grantees. Retrieved February 12, 2006, from *www.bphc.hrsa.gov/uds/data.htm.*

Kingdon, J. (1995). *Agendas, alternatives, and public policies* (2nd ed.). New York, HarperCollins.

Lefkowitz, B. (2005). The health center story: Forty years of commitment. *Journal of Ambulatory Care Management, 28,* 295-303.

National Association of Community Health Centers (NACHC). (2003). *Special Topics Brief #2, The role of health centers in reducing health disparities.* Prepared by Michelle Proser. Washington, DC: NACHC.

National Association of Community Health Centers (NACHC). (2005). *The safety net on the edge.* Washington, DC: NACHC.

National Association of Community Health Centers (NACHC) & George Washington University. (2005). *A nation's health at risk III.* Washington, DC. Prepared by Michelle Proser, Peter Shin, and Dan Hawkins.

Pear, R. (2005a, February 8). Domestic programs subject to Bush's knife: Aid for food and heating. *New York Times,* A22.

Pear, R. (2005b, October 30). Congress weighs big cuts to Medicaid and Medicare. *New York Times,* A1.

Proser, M. (2005). Deserving the spotlight: Health centers provide high-quality and cost-effective care. *Journal of Ambulatory Care Management, 28,* 321-330.

Sardell, A. (1988). *The U.S. experiment in social medicine: The Community Health Center Program, 1965-1986*. Pittsburgh: The University of Pittsburgh Press.

Stevenson, R. W. (2005, February 8). President offers budget proposal with broad cuts. *New York Times*, A1.

Wilensky, S., & Roby, D. (2005). Health centers and health insurance: Complements, not alternatives. *Journal of Ambulatory Care Management, 28*, 348-356.

# POLICYSPOTLIGHT

## THE POLITICS OF LONG-TERM CARE

Charlene Harrington

*"He who wants to warm himself in old age must build a fireplace in his youth."*

GERMAN PROVERB

Long-term care (LTC) is one of the fastest growing areas of health care, as the U.S. population is growing older and has a greater number of chronic illnesses and disabilities. In 2004 there were an estimated 36.3 million individuals aged 65 and over living in the United States (12% of the U.S. population), including 4.9 million individuals aged 85 and over (U.S. Census Bureau, 2005). The former number is expected to have increased to 18% of the population by 2025 (Congressional Budget Office [CBO], 2002). With the aging of the population, the demand for LTC and the need for nurses and other personnel to provide services is growing rapidly. Box 13-1 includes statistics on who is working in this field, demonstrating that about 300,000 registered nurses (RNs) and over 2 million other workers provide LTC services in the United States.

With total LTC expenditures of $150.8 billion in 2004 (Smith, Cowan, Sensenig, Catlin, and the Health Accounts Team, 2005), LTC is a critical sector, but one that receives little attention from the nursing profession. Why have nursing associations historically focused on acute care rather than LTC?

First, the majority (59%) of RNs work in acute care, but the proportion of nurses employed in acute care has declined (from 68% in 1984) as LTC and other employment settings increase (Health Resources and Services Administration [HRSA], 2001). Second, many RNs join the American Nurses Association through collective bargaining units associated with hospital employment. RNs who work in LTC are the poor cousins of acute care RNs, making 12% less per year than nurses working in acute care (HRSA, 2001). Because there are so few RNs in each individual nursing home, home health agency, and hospice program, most are not a part of collective bargaining units. RNs in LTC are more likely to be supervisors or managers than RNs in hospitals (HRSA, 2001). The unions in LTC (such as the Service Employees International Union) usually bargain for nonlicensed nursing personnel and/or for service employees rather than for RNs. Moreover, many RNs in LTC, working for low wages and benefits, may find the dues for joining a nursing organization unaffordable, and/or they may not understand the benefits of membership. Others belong to industry trade association groups through their employers (such as the American Health Care Association).

Nursing associations need to be more active in advocating for LTC, even though the RN membership

---

**BOX 13-1** Facts about Long-Term Care

- About 17,000 U.S. nursing homes take care of 1.6 million nursing home residents at any given point in time (over 2.5 million patients with short stays are discharged annually) (National Center for Health Statistics [NCHS], 2003).
- Of the total 1 million nursing home employees, 143,000 (only 13.5%) are RNs; the other employees are nursing aides and orderlies, licensed practical nurses, administrators, housekeeping and dietary staff, and other employees (NCHS, 2003).
- About 55,141 residential care facilities with 1.77 million beds provide services to individuals in the United States (these include so-called board and care, assisted living, group homes, and other types of facilities) (Harrington, Chapman, Miller, Miller, & Newcomer, 2005).
- Residential care facilities do not provide skilled nursing care, although a growing number of facilities have recognized the value of registered nurses (8,140 RNs work in such facilities) (HRSA, 2001).
- Home health and hospices programs (11,400 programs) served over 7.8 million patients in 2000, with 1.46 million patients at any given time (NCHS, 2003).
- An estimated 129,000 RNs work in home health, and 19,000 RNs work in hospice programs in the United States (HRSA, 2001).
- An estimated 1.2 million home and personal care workers, including those who are self-employed or unpaid family workers, provided assistance to individuals living at home in 2003 (Chapman, Kaye, and Newcomer, 2005).

---

from LTC is not large. LTC is an important growing area that not only employs many RNs but also employs nursing personnel and personal assistants. Many families, including those of nurses, need formal and informal LTC for older people as well as a growing number of children and middle-aged individuals (LaPlante, Harrington, & Kang, 2002). Nurses need to be concerned about ensuring access to high-quality LTC at a reasonable cost.

This policy spotlight focuses on some of the policy and political issues facing nursing in LTC. First, it reviews the problems with the quality of nursing home care and the poor enforcement of federal quality regulations. Second, it examines nursing

home staffing and reimbursement policies. Third, it discusses the need for more home and community-based services (HCBS). Finally, nurses are urged to become advocates for older and disabled people who need LTC services.

## POOR QUALITY OF CARE AND WEAK REGULATORY ENFORCEMENT

Poor nursing home quality has been documented since the early 1970s and culminated in passage of the Omnibus Budget Reconciliation Act (OBRA) of 1987 to reform nursing home regulation (Wunderlich & Kohler, 2001). Although it was expected that OBRA 1987 would improve the survey and enforcement system and ultimately improve quality, these expectations have yet to be realized. A number of studies and reports have described the poor quality of some nursing homes (Page, 2003; Wunderlich & Kohler, 2001; Wunderlich, Sloan, & Davis, 1996). In 2003, 90% of nursing homes received a total of about 105,000 deficiencies for failure to meet federal regulations, for a wide range of violations of quality standards that result in unnecessary resident weight loss, pressure ulcers, accidents, infections, decline in physical functioning, and many other problems (Harrington, Carrillo, and Crawford, 2004a). Studies have also documented the serious quality problems related to the ongoing problems with the federal and state survey and enforcement system including the complaint investigation process (General Accounting Office [GAO], 1998, 1999a, 1999b, 2000, 2002a, 2002b).

State surveyors are often unable to detect serious problems with quality of care and allow most facilities to correct deficiencies without penalties (GAO, 2002b). When violations are detected, few facilities have follow-up enforcement actions or sanctions taken against them (Harrington, Mullan, & Carrillo, 2004b). The continued widespread variation in the number and type of deficiencies issued by states shows that states are not using the regulatory process consistently (GAO, 2003). Many state officials admit they are unable or are unwilling to comply with federal survey and enforcement requirements (Harrington et al., 2004b).

U.S. Senate committees held a series of hearings between 1998 and 2003 regarding the nursing home studies by the GAO (now called the *Government Accountability Office*) and have repeatedly urged the Centers for Medicare and Medicaid (CMS) to improve the survey and enforcement process (GAO, 2003). Between 1998 and 2002 the average number of deficiencies per facility increased, but the percent of facilities given deficiencies for causing harm or jeopardy to residents declined from 24% in 2000 to 17% in 2003 (Harrington et al., 2004a). The GAO (2003) found that 39% of the facilities reported by state surveyors as having *no* deficiencies *did* in fact have actual harm deficiencies. Some state survey agencies are downgrading the scope and severity of deficiencies, and many states still are not referring cases for immediate sanctions (GAO, 2003).

In 2003 the GAO found that state surveys were problematic for reasons including the continued predictability of standard surveys, the inadequacy of state consumer complaint investigation policies and procedures, the fact that 15 states still did not have toll-free hotlines for complaint reporting, and the fact that some states did not investigate complaints in a timely fashion (GAO, 2003). Problems with poor state investigation and documentation of deficiencies and large numbers of inexperienced state surveyors in some states were found, and the federal oversight of state activities was still found to be inadequate.

State officials report that problems in their ability to enforce the federal regulations are related in part to inadequate federal and state resources for their regulatory activities. States received less than half of 1% of the total expenditures on nursing facilities in the United States in 1999 for regulatory activities, and state regulatory budgets have been declining (Walshe & Harrington, 2002). The federal-state nursing survey process gives the appearance that government is doing something about the quality of care problems, but in reality the enforcement system does little to change or improve the system and generally does not remove the most serious violators from the system. To ensure the safety of residents, greater standardization and stringency are needed in the survey and enforcement process, and poor performing facilities should have their certification revoked.

## INADEQUATE NURSING HOME STAFFING LEVELS

Low nurse staffing levels are the single most important contributor to poor quality of nursing home care in the United States. Over the past 25 years numerous research studies have documented the important relationship between nurse staffing levels, particular RN staffing, and the outcomes of care (Page, 2003; Harrington, Zimmerman, Karon, Robinson, & Beutel, 2000b; Wunderlich et al., 1996; Wunderlich & Kohler, 2001). The benefits of higher staffing levels, especially RN staffing, can include lower mortality rates; improved physical functioning; less antibiotic use; fewer pressure ulcers, catheterized residents, and urinary tract infections; lower hospitalization rates; and less weight loss and dehydration (Page, 2003; Wunderlich et al., 1996; Wunderlich & Kohler, 2001). Three separate IOM reports have recommended increased nurse staffing in nursing homes, particularly RN staffing.

Since 1997 the average U.S. nursing home has provided a total of 3.6 hours per resident day (hprd) of RN, licensed vocational nurse (LVN) and licensed practical nurse (LPN), nursing assistant (NA), and Director of Nursing time (Harrington et al., 2004a). Of the total time, most (60% or 2.2 hours) is provided by NAs, who have an average of 11 residents for whom to provide care. RNs and LVNs each must care for about 34 residents, although nurses usually have many more residents on nights, weekends, and holidays (Harrington et al., 2004a). The most disturbing finding is that average RN staffing hours in nursing homes has declined by 25% since 2000, with RNs having been replaced by NAs (Harrington et al., 2004a). This has reduced the quality of care at a time when nurse staffing levels are already inadequate to protect the health and safety of residents (CMS, 2001).

Staffing is the best predictor of good processes of nursing home care (for example, preventing weight loss). Schnelle and colleagues conducted a study to determine if there were differences in the quality of care processes among selected California nursing homes with different staffing levels (Schnelle et al., 2004). They found that nursing homes in the top 10th percentile on staffing (4.1 hprd or higher) performed significantly better on 13 of 16 care processes implemented by NAs, compared with homes with lower staffing. Residents in the highest-staffed homes were significantly more likely to be out of bed and engaged in activities during the day and receive more feeding assistance and incontinence care. The study concluded that there is a relationship between facility reports of total staffing and the quality of care processes (e.g., assisting with eating) (Schnelle et al., 2004).

Widespread quality problems were found in most nursing homes: inadequate assistance with eating (only 4 to 7 minutes of assistance); verbal interactions during mealtime only 28% of the time; false charting (inaccurate documentation of feeding assistance, toileting, and repositioning); toileting assistance only 1.8 times on average in 12 hours; residents not turned every 2 to 3 hours; over half of residents left in bed most of the day; walking assistance only one time a day on average; and widespread untreated pain and untreated depression (Schnelle et al., 2004). Comparing the results of the staffing study findings with studies of eight separate quality indicators (weight loss, bedfast condition, physical restraints, pressure ulcers, incontinence, loss of physical activity, pain, and depression), Schnelle and colleagues concluded that staffing levels were a better predictor of high-quality care processes than the eight quality indicators that were examined (Schnelle et al., 2004). These findings suggest that discharge planners and consumers should rely on indicators of the amount of nursing staff rather than on clinical indicators when selecting nursing homes.

A CMS (2001) report found that staffing levels for long-stay residents that are below 4.1 hours per resident day (hprd) result in negative consequences for residents (if below 1.3 hprd for licensed nurses and 2.8 hprd of NA time). NA time should range from 2.8 to 3.2 hprd, depending on the care residents need, just to carry out basic care activities (CMS, 2001). This amounts to 1 NA per seven or eight residents on the day and evening shifts and 1 NA per 12 residents at night. When actual staffing levels were compared with the target goals recommended by the CMS report (2001), 97% of all facilities were found to be operating below the desired level in 2001. The recommended nurse staffing

level in the CMS (2001) report was similar to the 4.5 hprd level recommended by experts (Harrington et al., 2000a). Consumers should be informed about each facility's nurse staffing levels compared with the target goals identified in the CMS (2001) report.

Unfortunately, CMS has not agreed to establish minimum federal staffing standards that would ensure that nursing facilities meet the 4.1 hprd, mostly because the potential costs were estimated to be at least $7 billion in 2000 (CMS, 2001). Most nursing homes are for-profit entities and are unlikely to voluntarily meet a reasonable level of staffing with regulatory requirements. If staffing levels are to improve, minimum federal staffing standards are needed, along with additional government funding to pay for the staffing.

Many states have begun to raise their minimum staffing levels since 1999, although two states eliminated their ratios (Harrington, 2005). California (3.2 hprd) and Delaware (3.29 hprd) have established high standards for direct care, and Florida established a 3.6 hprd total licensed and licensed minimum standard. These new standards are improvements but are still well below the 4.1 hprd level recommended by the CMS 2001 report. Efforts to increase the minimum staffing standards that are case mix adjusted should continue to have the highest priority at the state and federal levels.

## NURSING FACILITY REIMBURSEMENT REFORM

Medicaid nursing home reimbursement methods and per diem reimbursement rates are of great importance because they influence the costs of providing care. In 2003, Medicaid paid for 48% of the nation's total $110.8 billion nursing home expenditures, Medicare paid for 12%, consumers paid for 28%, and private insurance and other payers paid for 8% (Smith et al., 2005). Overall, the federal and state government paid for 60% of nursing home expenses.

Medicaid reimbursement policies have primarily focused on cost containment rather than other important goals including equitable payment to providers, access for those eligible for Medicaid, and quality of care. The majority of states have adopted Medicaid prospective payment systems

(PPSs) for nursing homes that set rates in advance of payments, based on past allowable costs rather than paying facilities based on actual past costs (Swan, Harrington, Studer, Pickard, & deWit, 2000). PPS methodologies are successful in controlling reimbursement growth rates, but facilities tend to respond by cutting the staffing and quality levels.

Medicaid nursing home payments were an average of $115 per day across the nation, whereas Medicare rates for freestanding facilities were $269 in 2000 (Scully, 2003). In 2000, Medicaid rates fell short of costs by $9.78 per day in nursing homes, for an estimated shortfall of about $3.5 billion for the United States (Scully, 2003). Low Medicaid reimbursement rates are a direct contributor to low nursing home staffing levels. Grabowski (2001) found that an increase in Medicaid reimbursement rates improved quality as measured by an increase in the use of RN staff and a reduction in deficiencies in the tightest regional markets. Another study found that low wages are a direct contributor to inadequate staffing levels in nursing facilities (Harrington & Swan, 2003). Facilities are not likely to increase staffing without adequate Medicaid reimbursement rates.

To make matters worse, Congress passed Medicare PPS reimbursement for implementation starting in 1998 to reduce overall payment rates to skilled nursing homes (Medicare Payment Advisory Commission [MedPac], 2002). Under PPS, Medicare rates are based in part on the resident case mix (acuity) in each facility to take into account the amount of staffing and therapy services that residents require. Skilled nursing homes, however, do not need to demonstrate that the amount of staff and therapy time provided is related to the payments allocated under the PPS rates.

As a result of Medicare PPSs, nursing home professional staffing decreased and regulatory deficiencies increased, showing the negative effect of Medicare PPSs (Konetzka, Yi, Norton, & Kilpatrick, 2004). As noted previously, the level of RN staffing in U.S. nursing homes has declined by 25% since 2000 (Harrington et al., 2004a). The average hours for licensed practical or vocational nurses held steady during the period, whereas the hours for NAs increased to replace the lost RN hours.

One policy option is to revise the Medicare PPS formula to specify the minimum proportion of Medicare payments that must be used for nurse staffing (RNs, LPNs, and NAs) and therapy services. If the minimum amount of payments for nursing and therapy services were regulated, nursing homes would be prevented from cutting nurse staffing.

Despite the Medicare PPS rate cuts, excess profits have grown because Medicare does not limit the profit margins of nursing homes. A GAO (2003) study of Medicare profit margins found that the median margins for freestanding skilled nursing facilities were 8.4% in 1999 and increased to 18.9% in 2000. The median total margins for all payers were less (primarily because of low Medicaid payment rates). Facilities with very high profits appear to be taking profits at the expense of quality. California nursing homes with net income profit margins greater than 9% were found to have higher deficiencies and poorer quality of care (O'Neil, Harrington, Kitchener, & Saliba, 2003). Strict limits on administrative costs and profit margins under Medicare and Medicaid PPS could be instituted to reduce the excess profit taking by nursing homes.

Poor quality of care in nursing homes has been associated with low wages and benefits and high employee turnover rates (Harrington & Swan, 2003). In 2002 the average median hourly wage for NAs was only $8.57 (CMS, 2001). State Medicaid rates generally reinforce the current low wage and benefit levels. Nursing home wages and benefits are substantially lower than those of comparable hospital workers (National Center for Health Statistics [NCHS], 2003) and lower than those in many jobs in the fast food industry and other unskilled jobs and generally well below the level of a living wage. A recent CMS study (2001) found that NA wages and benefits need to be raised by 17% to 22% in order to retain employees in long-stay facilities (or an average of $1.45 to $1.89 per hour on an average hourly wage rate of $8.57 nationally). They also estimated that rate increases are needed for RNs (4.5% to 7%) and for LVNs (3.3% to 4.5%) nationally in order to stabilize the workforce. Congress and CMS should ensure that state Medicaid rates include adequate amounts for nursing wages and benefits.

## HOME AND COMMUNITY-BASED SERVICES

LTC services that are needed for long periods (more than 90 days) are focused on providing assistance with limitations in activities of daily living and supporting those with cognitive limitations and mental illness. Over 13.2 million adults (over half under age 65) living in communities in the United States received an average of 31.4 hours of personal assistance per week in 1995 (LaPlante et al., 2002). Only 16% of the total hours were paid care (about $32 billion), leaving 84% of hours to be provided by informal caregivers. Only 33% of the $84 billion Medicaid LTC expenditures were for home and community care, whereas 67% was spent on institutional care in 2003 (Burwell, Sredl, & Eiken, 2004).

One reason for the high institutional spending is the oversupply of institutional LTC beds and the undersupply of HCBS (Harrington, Chapman, Miller, Miller, & Newcomer, 2005). Although the number of nursing home beds grew and the aged population increased over the past decade, it is surprising to note that the average certified nursing facility occupancy rates in states declined from 90% in 1995 to only 85.5% in 2003 (Harrington et al., 2004a). Therefore an excess supply of nursing home beds exists in many states. Low nursing home occupancy rates can lead to financial problems for facilities, higher charges, and higher public reimbursement rates to cover the cost of unused beds. The reductions in nursing home facility occupancy rates are probably related to the growth in residential care and assisted living facilities as substitutes and to the rapid growth of HCBS (Harrington et al., 2005).

There are increased pressures to expand HCBS, especially in the Medicaid program. The public increasingly reports a preference for LTC provided at home over services in institutions, and this is encouraged by reports of serious nursing home quality problems (Kitchener et al., 2005). In addition, the 1990 Americans with Disability Act (ADA) and the subsequent legal judgment in the 1999 Olmstead Supreme Court decision require that states must not discriminate against persons with disabilities by refusing to provide community services when these are available and appropriate (Rosenbaum, 2000).

In response to the increased demand, participation in the Medicaid HCBS waiver program (which provides alternatives to institutional care) rose by 258% and expenditures increased by 553% from 1992 to 2001 (Kitchener, Ng, Miller, and Harrington, 2005). Combined Medicaid home health, personal care services, home and community based waiver service served 2.1 million participants and expenditures were $21.99 billion in 2001 (Kitchener et al., 2005). Total HCBS services increased by 630% compared with a growth of 224% for institutional care between 1990 and 2002 (Burwell, Sredl, & Eiken, 2004).

In spite of the growth in HCBS, there is strong evidence that the current supply of HCBS is inadequate. State Medicaid program directors report that many disabled groups are not served by existing HCBS programs and that state programs lack adequate funding and have waiting lists (Kitchener, Ng, & Harrington, 2004). In 2001, only 29 states had Medicaid personal care attendant programs, and many states have limited services under their HCBS waiver programs. In 2002, over 158,000 individuals were on waiting lists for HCBS across the country (Kitchener et al., 2004). Some states have rapidly expanded their HCBS programs, whereas others still lag behind, relying heavily on institutional services (Kitchener et al., 2004). Medicaid HCBS programs urgently need more funding to expand access to care at home and to prevent institutionalization.

One way to ensure choice in LTC services is to support a policy advocated by many disabilities groups: the proposed Medicaid Community-Based Attendant Services and Supports Act (MiCASSA) of 2005 (Harkin, 2005). MiCASSA would mandate that all states develop a plan for the coverage of community-based attendant services, using a uniform federal definition of services that assist individuals in accomplishing activities of daily living and related support services to standardize services across states. States would be given additional federal Medicaid funding to allow them to establish personal attendant services (while assuring that states maintain the existing services), and states would be required to set up quality control and monitoring systems for HCBS.

The main opposition to MiCASSA is the potential costs if additional Medicaid participants request new LTC services. One recent study estimated the costs to address the unmet needs (LaPlante, Kaye, Kang, & Harrington, 2004). Although the plan is costly, the nation could afford to pay for this additional care, to prevent the wide number of negative consequences of unmet needs, such as weight loss, falls, loss of functioning, and pain and suffering.

## PUBLIC FINANCING OF LONG-TERM CARE

The only segment of the U.S. population whose cost of LTC is fully covered consists of individuals who live below the poverty threshold and are enrolled in Medicaid. Except for short-term postacute care, the rest of the population must either pay for care out of pocket or resort to privately purchased LTC insurance. The financially crippling cost of LTC (as much as $50,000 to $60,000 per year) is one of the great fears confronting persons who are otherwise self-supporting. Yet, relatively few individuals have either the means or motivation to insure themselves privately. Only about 10% to 20% of the elderly can afford to purchase LTC insurance (GAO, 1991; Wiener, Illston, & Hanley, 1994).

If individuals "spend down" to the poverty threshold, they can become Medicaid eligible as a last resort, making LTC a means-tested program. The spend-down requirements not only constitute a hardship to the patient and a social stigma but create dependence on public assistance that would be unnecessary if the entire population were insured. Means-tested programs create financial incentives that encourage individuals to divest their income and assets to qualify for services (Harrington, Heller, & Geraedts, 2002).

A mandatory social insurance program offers distinct advantages. If everyone paid into the system, individuals would have access to coverage when they are chronically ill or disabled without the humiliation of having to become poor to receive services (Harrington et al., 2002). By expanding the Medicare program to include LTC, the payment of LTC contributions early in a worker's life could "prefund" at relatively affordable Medicare rates LTC services that generally are required late in life. Thus, the financial risk could be spread across the entire population so that individual premium costs or taxes would be relatively manageable, in comparison with the costs of insurance purchased when individuals are older and at high risk of needing LTC.

Other countries such as Germany and Japan have adopted public long-term insurance systems that can serve as models for the United States. For example, the goal of the 1995 German LTC insurance system is to provide protection and coverage for persons requiring LTC (Geraedts, Heller, & Harrington, 2000). The German LTC program consists of a mandatory system in which employees and their employers make equal contributions into the LTC insurance program and the unemployed are paid for by the government (Geraedts et al., 2000; Cuellar & Wiener, 2000).

In Germany, three levels of care needs (high, medium, and low) were established, based on need for assistance with two or more activities of daily living (e.g., bathing, dressing, and toileting) (Geraedts, et al., 2000). Three choices of types of care are provided in Germany: (1) informal caregivers, who receive cash payments; (2) formal care services at home (payments are made directly to providers); and (3) institutional care services (payments are made directly to the facilities) (Geraedts et al., 2000). Germany also pays the pension benefits for those who assume a large burden of informal caregiving. The program's goal is to prevent unnecessary institutionalization by focusing on disease prevention and rehabilitation and services at home. Germany provides care to 72% of recipients at home and allocates 44% of LTC expenditures to full-time institutional care, an admirable goal worthy of replication in the United States (Geraedts et al., 2000).

The area of greatest concern for any type of new entitlement program is cost. The German system has built in a number of features to control costs, including establishing maximum payment rates, copayments and cost sharing, and per-beneficiary limits on institutional expenditures (Harrington et al., 2002). The major contribution of the German LTC insurance program has been to dispel the myth that public LTC insurance is not affordable. Because LTC is a predictable need for a relatively large segment of the population, it can be covered by insurance for a reasonable cost if the plan is mandatory so that the risk is spread across the population. The nation should focus on the public financing of LTC insurance that would ensure that all citizens have adequate, high-quality LTC when they need such services.

## SUMMARY

We need a vision for advocacy in LTC that is multi-dimensional and long range. Political efforts are needed at the local, state, and national levels. Community mobilization, public education, legislative reform, and legal actions are all needed to bring about policy changes to ensure access to high-quality LTC services. Consumer advocates and ombudsmen have taken a lead in reform efforts, but they need help to make progress.

Organized nursing needs to place its considerable political influence into LTC reform, including improving the quality of nursing home care and expanding home and community-based services. These efforts could improve the lives of residents in nursing homes as well as those who need LTC services in the home and community. Nursing should act not only because of its concern for all those individuals who need LTC but also to ensure that nurses themselves and their families and friends will have access to high-quality, appropriate LTC in the future.

## Key Points

- Many nursing homes in the United States have a poor quality of care because they have inadequate nurse staffing levels (RNs, LVNs, and NAs).
- Consumers prefer home and community-based services, but there is an inadequate supply of such services.
- Medicare does not cover LTC (only short-term nursing home, home health, and hospice care), so most individuals must pay for their care out of pocket or become poor before Medicaid will pay for their LTC.
- Nurses need to advocate for a higher quality of care, greater access to LTC services, and adequate public funds to pay for LTC.

## REFERENCES

Burwell, B., Sredl, K., & Eiken, S. (2004). *Medicaid long term care expenditures in FY 2003.* Boston, MA: Medstat.

Centers for Medicare & Medicaid Services (CMS). (2001). *Appropriateness of minimum nurse staffing ratios in nursing homes. Report to Congress: Phase II Final.* Volumes I to III. Baltimore: CMS (prepared by Abt Associates).

Chapman, S., Kaye, S., & Newcomer, R. (2005). *Home and personal care workers by state. Tabulations from the 2003 American community survey for U.S. Census Bureau.* Center for Personal Assistance Services. Retrieved December 10, 2005, from *http://pascenter.org/state_based_stats/acs_workforce_state.php.*

Congressional Budget Office (CBO). (2002). The looming budgetary impact of society's aging. Washington, DC: CBO. Retrieved December 11, 2005, from *www.cbo.gov/showdoc.cfm?index=3581&sequence=0.*

Cuellar, A. E., & Wiener, J. M. (2000). Can social insurance for long-term care work? The experience of Germany. *Health Affairs, 19,* 8-25.

General Accounting Office (GAO). (1991). *Long-term care insurance: Risks to consumers should be reduced.* Report to the Chairman, Subcommittee on Health, Committee on Ways and Means, House of Representatives. GAO/HRD-92-14. Washington, DC: GAO.

General Accounting Office (GAO). (1998). *California nursing homes: Care problems persist despite federal and state oversight.* Report to the Special Committee on Aging, U.S. Senate. GAO/HEHS-98-202. Washington, DC: GAO.

General Accounting Office (GAO). (1999a). *Nursing homes: Additional steps needed to strengthen enforcement of federal quality standards.* Report to the Special Committee on Aging, U.S. Senate. GAO/HEHS-99-46. Washington, DC: GAO.

General Accounting Office (GAO). (1999b). *Nursing homes: Complaint investigation processes often inadequate to protect residents.* Report to Congressional Committees. GAO/HEHS-99-80. Washington, DC: GAO.

General Accounting Office (GAO). (2000). *Nursing homes: Aggregate Medicare payments are adequate despite bankruptcies.* Testimony before the Special Committee on Aging, U.S. Senate. GAO/T-HEHS-00-192. Washington, DC: GAO.

General Accounting Office (GAO). (2002a). *Nursing homes: More can be done to protect residents from abuse.* Report to Congressional Requestors. GAO/HEHS-02-312. Washington, DC: GAO.

General Accounting Office (GAO). (2002b). *Nursing homes: Quality of care more related to staffing than spending.* Report to Congressional Requestors. GAO/HEHS-02-431R. Washington, DC: GAO.

General Accounting Office (GAO). (2003). *Nursing home quality: Prevalence of serious problems, while declining, reinforces importance of enhanced oversight.* Report to Congressional Requesters. GAO-03-561. Washington, DC: GAO.

Geraedts, M., Heller, G. V., & Harrington, C. (2000). Germany's long-term-care insurance: Putting a social insurance model into practice, *Milbank Quarterly, 78,* 375-401.

Grabowski, D. C. (2001). Does an increase in the Medicaid reimbursement rate improve nursing home quality? *Journal of Gerontology: Social Sciences, 56B*(2), S84-S93.

Harkin, T. (2005). S. 401 and H.R. 910: The Medicaid Community-Based Attendant Services and Supports Act (MiCASSA) of 2005.

Retrieved December 11, 2005, from *http://thomas.loc.gov/cgi-bin/query/D?c109:1:./temp/~c109Z50Q0B::*.

Harrington, C. (2005). Nurse staffing in nursing homes in the United States. Part I. *Journal of Gerontological Nursing, 31*(2), 18-23.

Harrington, C., Carrillo, H., & Crawford, C. (2004a). *Nursing facilities, staffing, residents, and facility deficiencies, 1997-03.* San Francisco: University of California. Retrieved December 11, 2005 from, *www.nursinghomeaction.org/public/245_1267_9316.cfm.*

Harrington, C., Chapman, S., Miller, E., Miller, N., & Newcomer, R. (2005). Trends in the supply of long term care facilities and beds in the U.S. *Journal of Applied Gerontology, 24*(4), 265-282.

Harrington, C., Heller, G. V., & Geraedts, M. (2002). Commentary on Germany's long term care insurance model: Lessons for the United States. *Journal of Public Health Policy, 23*(1), 44-65.

Harrington, C., Kovner, C., Mezey, M., Kayser-Jones, J., Burger, S., Mohler, M., Burke, R., & Zimmerman, D. (2000a). Experts recommend minimum nurse staffing standards for nursing facilities in the United States. *Gerontologist, 40*(1), 5-16.

Harrington, C., Mullan, J., & Carrillo, H. (2004b). State nursing home enforcement systems. *Journal of Health Politics, Policy and Law, 29*(1), 43-73.

Harrington, C., & Swan, J. H. (2003). Nurse home staffing, turnover, and casemix. *Medical Care Research and Review, 60*(2), 366-392.

Harrington, C., Zimmerman, D., Karon, S.L., Robinson, J. and Beutel, P. (2000b). Nursing home staffing and its relationship to deficiencies. *Journal of Gerontology: Social Sciences, 55B*(5), S278-S287.

Health Resources and Services Administration (HRSA), Department of Health and Human Services, Bureau of Health Professions, Division of Nursing. (2001). The *registered nurse population, March 2000: Findings from the national sample survey of registered nurses.* Washington, DC: HRSA.

Kitchener, M., Ng, T., & Harrington, C. (2004). Medicaid 1915 home and community-based services waivers: A national survey of eligibility criteria, caps, and waiting lists. *Home Health Care Services Quarterly, 23*(2):55-69.

Kitchener, M., Ng, T., Miller, N., & Harrington, C. (2005). Medicaid home and community-based services: National program trends. *Health Affairs, 24*(1), 206-212.

Konetzka, R. T., Yi, D., Norton, E. C., & Kilpatrick, K. E. (2004). Effects of Medicare payment changes on nursing home staffing and deficiencies. *Health Services Research, 39*(3), 463-487.

LaPlante, M., Harrington, C., and Kang, T. (2002). Estimating paid and unpaid hours of personal assistance services in activities of daily living provided to adults living at home. *Health Services Research, 37*(2), 387-415.

LaPlante, M. P., Kaye, H. S., Kang, T., & Harrington, C. (2004). Unmet need for personal assistance services: Estimating the shortfall in hours of help and adverse consequences. *Journal of Gerontology: Social Sciences, 59B*(2), S98-S108.

Medicare Payment Advisory Commission (MedPac). (2002). *Report to Congress: Medicare payment policy.* Washington, DC: MedPac.

National Center for Health Statistics (NCHS), Centers for Disease Control and Prevention, Department of Health and Human Services. (2003). *Nursing homes: What has changed, what has not? The National Nursing Home Survey.* Retrieved February 10, 2006, from *www.cdc.gov/nchs/data/nnhsd/NursingHomes1977-99.pdf.*

O'Neill, C., Harrington, C., Kitchener, M., & Saliba, D. (2003). Quality of care in nursing homes: An analysis of the relationships among profit, quality, and ownership. *Medical Care, 41*(12), 1318-1330.

Page, A. (Committee on the Work Environment for Nurses and Patient Safety, Institute of Medicine [IOM]). (Ed.). (2003). *Keeping patients safe.* Washington, DC: National Academies Press.

Rosenbaum, S. (2000). *Olmstead V L. C.: Implications for older persons with mental and physical disabilities.* Washington, DC: American Association of Retired Persons [AARP].

Schnelle, J. F., Simmons, S. F., Harrington, C., Cadogan, M., Garcia, E., and Bates-Jensen, B. (2004). Relationship of nursing home staffing to quality of care? *Health Services Research, 39*(2), 225-250.

Scully, T. (2003). *CMS Health Care Industry Market Update. Nursing Facilities.* Washington, DC: Centers for Medicare and Medicaid Services (CMS).

Smith, C., Cowan, C., Sensenig, A., Catlin, A., and the Health Accounts Team. (2005). Health spending growth slows in 2003. *Health Affairs, 24*(1), 185-194.

Swan, J. H., Harrington, C., Studer, L., Pickard, R. B., & deWit, S. K. (2000). Medicaid nursing facility methods: 1979-1997. *Medical Care Research and Review, 57*(3), 361-378.

U.S. Census Bureau, American Community Survey Office. (2005). Estimates of the resident population by selected age groups for the US and states and for Puerto Rico: July 1, 2004. Washington, DC: U.S. Census Bureau, July 1, 2004. Retrieved March 27, 2005, from *www.census.gov/popest/states/asrh/SC-est2004-01.html.*

Walshe, K., & Harrington, C. (2002). The regulation of nursing facilities in the US: An analysis of the resources and performance of state survey agencies. *Gerontologist, 42*(4), 475-486.

Wiener, J. M., Illston, L. H., & Hanley, R. J. (1994). *Sharing the burden: Strategies for public and private long-term care insurance.* Washington, DC: The Brookings Institution.

Wunderlich, G. S., & Kohler, P. (Committee on Improving Quality in Long-Term Care, Division of Health Care Services, Institute of Medicine [IOM]). (Eds.). (2001). *Improving the quality of long-term care.* Washington, DC: National Academies Press.

Wunderlich, G. S., Sloan, F. A., & Davis, C. K. (Committee on the Adequacy of Nurse Staffing in Hospitals and Nursing Homes, Institute of Medicine [IOM]). (Eds.). (1996). *Nursing staff in hospitals and nursing homes: Is it adequate?* Washington, DC: National Academies Press.

# EVOLVING POLICY IN HOME HEALTH CARE

Karen B. Utterback

*"One doesn't discover new lands without consenting to lose sight of the shore for a very long time."*

ANDRE GIDE

Health care services delivered in the home have been an important part of the health care delivery system in the United States for well over a hundred years. During the early years, care was primarily delivered by Visiting Nurse Associations and the funding came mostly from philanthropic and benevolent funds. In 1965, health care services in the home became a more-prevalent part of the health care delivery system when Congress enacted the Medicare and Medicaid programs. This legislation included home health services as a benefit of both programs and provided a predictable reimbursement mechanism for care delivery in the home (National Association for Home Care [NAHC], 2004).

In 1981, President Ronald Reagan signed the Omnibus Budget Reconciliation Act; this legislation gave states the option to set up Home and Community-Based Services (HCBSs) Waiver programs. The design of these programs provides enhanced community support services in an effort to avoid unnecessary institutional care. The program encourages the development and delivery of new kinds of services such as home modification, transportation, respite, personal care, and homemaker services (Centers for Medicare and Medicaid [CMS], 2005c).

In 1982, Congress passed and President Reagan signed into law legislation establishing hospice care as a Medicare-covered benefit and as an optional benefit for states under their Medicaid programs. This provided yet another increased opportunity for care delivery in the home.

In recent years, care delivered in the home setting has grown significantly. In 2001, over 2.42 million patients received home health services and over 594,000 patients received hospice care (CMS, 2005d). In 2004, there were over 275 HCBS waiver programs operating in 49 states and the District of Columbia and serving over 700,000 people annually (Smith & Jackson, 2004).

Currently "self-directed" care models are developing within the HCBS waivers. Called "cash and counseling demonstrations," they are designed to allow flexibility in care delivery; such as allowing the beneficiary to arrange, manage, and pay for services on his or her own. The program is designed to give beneficiaries more choices among types and sources of services, including incentives to seek out lower-cost services to maximize available cash. Early analysis of these programs has shown high levels of patient satisfaction and fewer unmet needs for services relative to traditional Medicaid programs (Frieden, 2004). Critics of these models argue that quality controls and requirements designed to protect the beneficiary when a licensed and/or certified provider is used to deliver the care are bypassed, and as a result outcomes and patients themselves may suffer (Halamandaris, 2005).

The incentive for states to explore new and innovative models such as the "cash and counseling" model is largely a result of rising costs of state Medicaid budgets and the lack of resources to fund them. These financial difficulties, and the reality that the care needs will increase as the population ages and the prevalence of chronic illness rises, have forced leaders and policymakers at local, state, and federal levels to be more innovative and creative in their approach to meeting these care needs (Congressional Budget Office, 2004).

## ISSUES AND TRENDS IN HOME-BASED CARE SERVICES

### The Need

According to the U.S. Census Bureau, the population over age 65 will increase by nearly 42 million people by the year 2050, an 8.3% growth in this segment of the population (U.S. Census Bureau, 2004). This aging demographic, combined with an increasing prevalence of chronic illness, is forcing the United States to rethink its health care delivery model. The Rand Corporation estimates that half of the U.S. population—or 157 million Americans—will have a chronic condition by 2020. It is estimated that 81 million of these individuals will suffer from two or more chronic illnesses and will account for over 80% of the health care spending in the United States (Information Technology Association of America [ITAA], 2004). Given that 90% of older individuals have a chronic condition and 70% have more than one chronic illness (Wu & Green, 2000), it may be assumed that many of these older Americans will need effective and coordinated management of heart disease, cancer, and other chronic illnesses. This will include multiple provider types and a heightened level of care coordination at a time when the number of available health care workers, including nurses, is decreasing (Anderson, 2002).

Much of the care needed to manage chronic illness can and will be delivered in the home setting. Currently home-based services provide a foundation for care to many of the elderly and chronically ill. The projected population increases and incidence in illness will, however, bring new stressors to the home-based care system.

### Transformational Change

In early 2005 the CMS held meetings with various stakeholders to discuss the need for "transformational change in the health care system." The word *transformational* was used intentionally to suggest a more aggressive approach in bringing about change than typically would be taken on a national scale (NAHC, 2005b). CMS intends to use its Quality Improvement Organizations (QIOs) to drive this change. It will be based on the six aims for quality improvement in health care that are a result of the Institute of Medicine study, "Crossing the Quality Chasm: A New Health System for the 21st Century." These are safety, effectiveness, patient-centeredness, timeliness, efficiency, and equity. CMS identified four strategies to achieve the aims: measuring and reporting performance; using health information technology more effectively; redesigning the process of care delivery; and changing organizational culture (NAHC, 2005b).

An estimated 10 million children and adults in the United States currently need access to long-term care services. These services are necessary for assistance with activities of daily living, meal preparation, medication management, and managing a home. In 2001, Medicaid spent $75.3 billion for long-term care services; the majority of that expenditure was for nursing home care, with only 29% spent for home-based services. The funds spent on home-based services included care provided through the home health benefit, optional state plan services, and waiver programs (Crowley, 2003).

According to a survey by MetLife published in 2004, there are approximately 1.6 million nursing home residents, who experience an average nursing home stay of 2.4 years and costs of nearly $112 billion annually. The average cost of a nursing home stay is $192.00 per day, or $70,080 annually. In contrast, the average hourly wage of a home health aide is $18 per hour; using an assumption that aide services are provided for 8 hours per day, 365 days per year, the cost would be less than $53,000 annually. Assuming even 30% of this care was provided in the home setting the savings would be nearly $10 billion annually (MetLife, 2004). Home-based services are and will be at the center of the transformational change needed in our health care delivery system for primarily two reasons: HCBSs are substantially less costly than institutional care, and patients prefer to remain in their homes as long as possible.

It is unclear what the exact form and time line for this transformational change will be. President George W. Bush and U.S. Department of Health and Human Services (HHS) Secretary Mike Leavitt have designed a roadmap to meet their goals for the next 10 to 15 years. The roadmap includes a move to electronic health records, an increasing focus on wellness and prevention, and recognition of the value of individual responsibility in health decisions. The growing aged population, the prevalence of chronic illness, and increasing health care costs as a percent of the gross domestic product (GDP) are drivers that could increase the pace of instituting processes to meet the policy goals (HHS, 2005).

### Use of Technology

Technology to date has been slow to be adopted by health care providers, despite consumer interaction with sophisticated forms of technology to streamline and manage virtually all other aspects of their lives. The adoption of an electronic health record will present significant benefits and challenges over the coming years. Concerns exist among providers and individuals about the cost of adoption, as well as privacy and security issues. However, for consumers, the increasing use of the Internet by those over 65 years of age is a good example of the developing appreciation of the use of technology in health care. A survey for the Pew Internet & American Life Project found that 66% of adult internet users seek health-related information on the Internet. This is up from 63% just 2 years ago (Kaiser Family Foundation, 2005).

In April 2004, Executive Order 13335 was signed by President George W. Bush to establish the office of National Health Information Technology. The purpose of this new office is to examine and encourage information technology adoption by health care providers in order to improve the management of patients, maintain wellness, and prevent medical error and injury, including the use of electronic health records. Widespread adoption of technologies such as these is believed to be crucial to decreasing medical errors and to improving efforts to manage chronic illness through a disease management (DM) approach to care (Institute of Medicine, 2001).

### Disease Management

Increasing the health care delivery system's focus on prevention, wellness, and patient accountability is strongly supported through adoption of a DM approach to care by the direct care providers, including home-based service providers. The DM approach has demonstrated effectiveness and cost savings but to date has largely been used by the payers and has not yet significantly influenced the practice patterns of direct care providers.

The components of DM include population identification; evidence-based practice guidelines; collaborative practice models; patient self-management education; process and outcome measurement; and routine reporting and feedback loops (Disease Management Association of America [DMAA], 2005). These components and capabilities will be needed by providers at all levels to effectively and efficiently manage the growing population with and prevalence of chronic illness in the home setting. Changes to the current culture, new incentives, and new tools to support the use of evidence-based, collaborative care are essential to supporting this change.

A challenge to widespread adoption of a DM model for care is related to the current lack of interoperability among health care providers. Increased interoperability will be necessary between health care providers and individuals in order improve provider collaboration and to involve the patient directly in their care. These are essential components of the DM model and contribute to the prevention of costly hospital stays and the use of emergency rooms and to the improvement of the quality of life for the chronically ill individual.

### Centers for Medicare and Medicaid Demonstration Projects

CMS is taking the lead to create changes in health care provider culture and provide new incentives to improve the care of the chronically ill. The Medicare Modernization Act of 2003 (MMA) included mandates from Congress to CMS to initiate a number of demonstration projects designed to improve collaboration, reward cost savings, and improve quality of life for chronically ill beneficiaries. Examples of demonstration projects currently underway include the Chronic Care Improvement Program (CCIP) and the Care Management of the High Risk Beneficiary (CMHRB). Each of these programs focuses on care delivery outside of institutions—that is, primarily in the home—and is designed to facilitate provider and patient collaboration. The programs include reimbursement methodologies that are risk based and focused on the overall wellness of the beneficiary (CMS, 2005b).

## PUBLIC AND PRIVATE POLICY INITIATIVES

### Public Initiatives

There are a number of public and private initiatives that point to the importance of the home as a strategic care site for health care delivery. Public projects include: The World Health Organization's Healthy Cities Initiatives, the Bush administration's New Freedom Initiative, and the Pay for Performance models. Private efforts include Bill Gates' Grand Challenges in Global Health and Newt Gingrich's Center for Health Transformation.

In 1988 the World Health Organization (WHO) launched its Healthy Cities Project. The project was based on the premise that the health of people living in cities and towns is strongly determined by their living and working conditions. This initiative provides policy and planning solutions for urban health problems and focuses on changing the way individuals and communities think about health. Currently the initiative has active projects in 44 states and 475 cities in the United States and in over 1000 European cities in 30 countries (CityNet Healthy Cities, 2005). These programs strive to ensure healthy lifestyles for all people and to focus on quality of life issues. Examples include health education programs, Internet-based newsletters, and printed materials focusing on health prevention and healthy lifestyles. A good example of a robust collection of services and education targeted toward establishing and supporting health life styles is Minneapolis's Health Cities/Thriving Families Project.

Quality of life is a strong theme in health care today—nearly as strong as the issues surrounding cost. In 1999 the U.S. Supreme Court ruled that "unjustified institutional isolation of persons with disabilities is a form of discrimination" and that states must provide community-based services and reasonable accommodations to these individuals in order to afford them the opportunity to avoid

institutionalization if possible. This ruling, known as the Olmstead Decision, has and will continue to influence the way states choose to provide long-term care services to their residents (CMS, 2005a). It can no longer be assumed that as long as nursing home beds are available, placing individuals in need of assistance into those beds is the right or prudent thing to do. Institutionalization should be an option of last resort. Many states have struggled to make the appropriate resources available for individuals with disabilities. Executive Order 13217 called on the federal government to assist states and localities to swiftly implement the resources necessary to support the Olmstead Decision. CMS, under the umbrella of HHS, has instituted a number of initiatives to support the efforts of the states. Examples include programs such as, "Ticket to Work and Work Incentives Improvement Act," the "Real Choice Systems Change Grants," and the "New Freedom Initiative." Each of these programs provides grant opportunities for states to experiment with new delivery models and combinations of services that encourage and enable the individual to remain in the home. Examples of innovation that can be achieved with programs like these are evident in the work being done in Arkansas with the Real Choice Systems Change Grant, through which the state has created a number of Internet-based directories for assistance in accessing available resources and educational offerings and have run public awareness campaigns to recruit direct support professionals to provide assistance in the homes of the disabled.

### Private Initiatives

The increasing level of concern about the future viability of our health delivery system is further evidenced by a look to the private sector. Bill Gates, founder of Microsoft, formed and funded a project called "Grand Challenges in Global Health." The project was kicked off in May 2003 with a solicitation for scientific and technologic innovation aimed at removing a critical barrier to solving an important health problem in the developing world with a high likelihood of global impact and feasibility (Varmus et al., 2003). Examples of health issues that meet the grand challenge definition include

HIV/AIDS, malnutrition, and the lack of access to medical care. The scope of the initiative is broad and may include breakthroughs in the areas of surveillance, prevention, detection, diagnosis, and treatment of disease. Technologic breakthroughs are included in the list of the grand challenges. These technologies are focused on population identification and tools to improve care management at the point of care. Technologies such as these will be essential in the management of chronic illness in the aging population in future years.

Political leaders from differing viewpoints are developing policy options. Newt Gingrich, former U.S. Congressmen and Speaker of the U.S. House of Representatives, formed the "Center for Health Transformation." This foundation is dedicated to "envisioning" the health care system of the future and moving its political agenda forward. In May 2005, the center published an "Open Letter" to Congress supporting a bipartisan bill introduced into the U.S. House by Representatives Tim Murphy (R-VA) and Patrick Kennedy (D-RI) entitled "21st Century Health Information Act of 2005." The bill is expected to play an important role in modernizing health care and moving our systems into the information age. Senator Hillary Clinton (D-NY) is working with the Republican leadership of the Senate to develop a companion bill. Specifically, the bill supports the Regional Health Information Organizations (RHIOs) being tested and studied by Dr. David Brailer, National Coordinator for Health Information Technology's group and provides some exceptions to the Stark and Anti-Kickback laws in order to allow hospitals to equip community providers with the technology infrastructure to support health care information technology adoption. These exceptions to the Stark and Anti-Kickback laws are necessary in order to allow the hospital system or health network to provide the information technology tools needed by the physicians to support the development of the RHIO and enable patient information to be shared seamlessly among providers. Currently the Stark and Anti-Kickback laws prohibit physicians from referring patients for "designated health services" (including inpatient, outpatient, and home health services, among others) that would be paid for by Medicare or Medicaid to entities in or with which the physician has financial arrangements, whether through compensation, ownership, or investment (Gingrich, 2005a).

Another project of the Center for Health Transformation is the "Long Term Living Project." The purpose of this project is to identify and support efforts to assure independent living for seniors for as long as possible and encourage and support active healthy aging. The project is focused on solutions that will allow individualized care to be delivered in the home through the use of technology and services (Gingrich, 2005b).

## THE FUTURE

The future of health care will depend strongly on home-based services, if for no other reason than the home is the only care setting with enough beds to house the rapidly aging population. To ensure that care delivery is efficient and effective, changes are critical. The current delivery model claims to have the patient at the center; however the various providers interacting with the patient have little formal interaction, and much of the information needed is left up to the patient to communicate among providers. In a changing delivery model the relationship between providers and the patient will be much more dependent on collaboration and seamless access to needed information to support clear concise communication and continuity of care delivered largely within the home.

Innovations such as telemonitoring and sensor technology hold great promise to support the changes necessary to provide increased communication and collaboration, enabling patients to remain comfortably and safely in their homes despite their chronic illness and care needs. Examples of this enabling technology include monitoring devices designed to collect objective and subjective information that are simple for the individual to use and can effectively detect subtle changes in condition. The information collected can alert health care providers to intervene in the individual's care early in the period of exacerbation, potentially avoiding injury, emergent care, or hospitalization.

Sensor technology can track an individual's movements and alert care givers or health care providers of actions that may pose a risk to the individual's well-being, all without hindering the individual's movement or activity. These technologies range from simple devices, such as the "I've fallen and can't get up" alert systems, to sophisticated sensors that unobtrusively collect data about a patient's weight, bodily functions, dietary consumption, and location; such sensors are currently in various stages of design. The cost of these technologies can range from less than $35 per month for simple technologies such as personal emergency response systems (PERS) to several hundred dollars per month, depending on the sophistication and frequency of the monitoring sessions. Costs may well be within reach, to allow the "baby boomer" generation the opportunity to remain in their own homes and to allow the shrinking health care workforce to be able to manage their care needs both safely and effectively.

A study released in late 2004 by the New England Healthcare Institute revealed that congestive heart failure patients receiving remote physiologic monitoring had 32% reduction in rehospitalizations, a 25% reduction in health care costs, and a 2% increase in quality-adjusted life years. Results similar to these comparing the use of remote patient monitoring are becoming common in the literature (New England Healthcare Institute, 2004).

## IMPORTANCE OF NURSING INVOLVEMENT

Nurses play a vital role in monitoring and understanding these data and in appropriately managing ongoing patient needs. This new role and its responsibilities bring both opportunity and challenge. Work is underway to help define many of the issues related to scope of practice, ethics, and legalities. Nurses leading the way in this new practice setting include Carolyn M. Hutcherson, MS, RN, who has been instrumental in recognizing and communicating legal issues that are unique to telenursing, and Loretta M. Schlachta-Fairchild, RN, PhD, C, who has been instrumental in defining standards of practice related to telenursing (Hutcherson, 2001).

Changes are well underway to the structure and culture of our health care delivery system, to strengthen the home as the center of care delivery,

and technology advances will further enable and support the vision for aging in place. These factors working together will insure the home's presence at the center of our delivery model for years to come.

## Key Points

- The home has long been an important setting for health care delivery, and as the population ages and the prevalence of chronic illness increases, the importance of the home will undoubtedly increase.
- CMS has a critical role in monitoring, in providing incentives for innovative care, and in paying for the largest group of recipients of home care—those receiving Medicare and Medicaid.
- Some of the most significant innovations that will influence future care delivery are the use of Internet technology to monitor care and educate people in their homes.

## Web Resources

**American Telehealth Association**—telenursing special interest group
*www.atmeda.org/about/aboutata.htm*
**Arkansas Real Choice Initiative**
*www.arkansas.gov/dhhs/aging/realchoice.html*
**Center for Health Transformation**
*www.healthtransformation.net/home*
**Center for Health Transformation—Long Term Living Project**
*www.gingrichgroup.com/projects/ Long_Term_Living*
**Centers for Medicare and Medicaid Services Demonstration Projects**
*www.cms.hhs.gov/researchers/demos*
**Centers for Medicare and Medicaid Services—Home Health Providers**
*www.cms.hhs.gov/providers/hha*
**CityNet—Healthy Cities Initiative**
*www.iupui.edu/~citynet/cnet.html*
**Grand Challenges in Global Health**
*www.grandchallengesgh.org*

*Continued*

## Web Resources — cont'd

**MedPac**
*www.medpac.gov*
**Minneapolis's Healthy Cities/Thriving Families**
*www.ci.minneapolis.mn.us/dhfs/docs/ JulySept2005.pdf*
**National Association for Home Care**
*www.nahc.org*
**New Freedom Initiative**
*www.hhs.gov/newfreedom*
**Office of the National Coordinator for Health Information Technology**
*www.hhs.gov/healthit*
**Quality Improvement Organization**
*www.cms.hhs.gov/qio*
**Real Choice Systems Change Grants**
*www.cms.hhs.gov/systemschange*
**Social Security Administration—Ticket to Work**
*www.ssa.gov/work/Ticket/ticket_info.html*
**Stark Law**
*www.ebglaw.com/article_350.html*

## REFERENCES

Anderson, G. (2002). Testimony to Subcommittee on Health of the Committee on Ways and Means, U.S. House of Representatives. Retrieved August 1, 2005, from *http:// waysandmeans.house.gov/legacy/health/107cong/4-16-02/ 107-80final.htm*.

Centers for Medicare and Medicaid Services (CMS). (2005a). Americans with Disabilities Act/Olmstead Decision. Retrieved April 1, 2005, from *www.cms.hhs.gov/pf/printpage. asp?ref=http://63.241.27.78/olmstead/defualt.asp?*.

Centers for Medicare and Medicaid Services (CMS). (2005b). Demonstration projects. Retrieved August 1, 2005, from *www.cms.hhs.gov/researchers/demos*.

Centers for Medicare and Medicaid Services (CMS). (2005c). Home and Community-Based Services Waiver Program: Program history. Retrieved August 1, 2005, from *www.cms. hhs.gov/medicaid/1915c/history.asp*.

Centers for Medicare and Medicaid Services (CMS). (2005d). Statistics. Retrieved April 1, 2005 from *www.cms.hhs.gov/ researchers/pubs/datacompendium/2003/03pg8687.pdf* and *www.cms.hhs.gov/researchers/pubs/datacompendium/2003/ 03pg8485.pdf*.

CityNet Healthy Cities. (2005). Overview of healthy cities. Retrieved April 1, 2005, from *www.iupui.edu/~citynet/booklet.htm*.

Congressional Budget Office. (2004). *Financing long-term care for the elderly*. Washington, DC: U.S. Government Printing Office.

Crowley, J. (2003). *Medicaid and the uninsured: An overview of the Independence Plus initiative to promote consumer-direction of services in Medicaid*. Washington, DC: Kaiser Commission.

Disease Management Association of America (DMAA). (2005). Definition of disease management. Retrieved August 1, 2005, from *www.dmaa.org/definition.html*.

Frieden, L. (2004). Consumer directed health care: How well does it work? Retrieved April 1, 2005, from, *www.ncd.gov/ newsroom/publications/2004/consumerdirected.htm*.

Gingrich, N. (2005a). Bipartisan bill is progress toward a 21st century intelligent health system. Retrieved May 1, 2005, from *www.healthtransformation.net/project/health_information_ technology/984.cfm*.

Gingrich, N. (2005b). Long term living project. Retrieved August 1, 2005, from *www.healthtransformation.net/projects/ Long_Term_Living*.

Halamandaris, V. (2005). Halamandaris works with National Governors Association on "Rebalancing" Medicaid expenditures: Six states spotlighted as models for providing home-/ community-based services in future. *National Association for Home Care Report*, E-issue 281, 1. Retrieved May 1, 2005, from *www.nahc.org/NAHC/CaringComm/eNAHCReport- mbrs/05/050513.html*.

Health and Human Services (HHS). (2005). Secretary Mike Leavitt's 500-day plan. Retrieved May 1, 2005, from *www.hhs.gov/500DayPlan/500dayplan.html#HealthCare*.

Hutcherson, C. (2001). Legal considerations for nurses practicing in a telehealth setting. Online *Journal of Issues in Nursing*, 6, 3. Retrieved August 1, 2005, from *www.nursingworld.org/ ojin/topic16/tpc16_3.htm*.

Information Technology Association of America (ITAA). (2004). Chronic care improvement: How Medicare transformation can lives save money, and stimulate an immerging technology industry. E-Health White Paper. Retrieved August 1, 2005, from *www.itaa.org/isec/docs/chioniccare.pdf*.

Institute of Medicine. (2001). Crossing the quality chasm. Retrieved May 2005, from *http://books.nap.edu/html/ quality_chasm/reportbrief.pdf*.

Kaiser Family Foundation. (2005). U.S. consumers increasingly using Web sites to find health information. Retrieved May 1, 2005, from *www.kaisernetwork.org/daily_reports/print_report. cfm?DR_ID=30147&dr_cat=3*.

MetLife. (2004). Analysis from federal long term care insurance program and MetLife Mature market Institute. Retrieved August 1, 2005, from *www.metlife.com/Applications/Corporate/ WPS/CDA/PageGenerator/0,,P250~S692~AP,00.html*.

National Association for Home Care (NAHC). (2004). Basic statistics about home care, updated 2004. Retrieved August 1, 2005, from *www.nahc.org/NAHC/Research/04HC_Stats.pdf*.

National Association for Home Care (NAHC). (2005b). CMS discusses auspicious "transformational change" for home health, broader health care system. *National Association for Home Care Report*, E-issue 271, 2. Retrieved April 1, 2005, from *www.nahc.org/NAHC/CaringComm/eNAHCReport- mbrs/05/050428.html*.

New England Healthcare Institute. (2004). Remote physiologic monitoring: Innovation in the management of health failure. NEHI Innovation Series. Retrieved April 1, 2005, from *www. nehi.net/CMS/admin/cms/_uploads/docs/HF%20Report.pdf*.

Smith, G., & Jackson, B. (2004). Summary of results: National Quality Inventory Survey of HCBS Waiver Programs. Prepared for U.S. Department of Health and Human

Services and Centers for Medicare & Medicaid Services. Retrieved April 1, 2005, from *www.consumerdirection.org/pdf/InventoryReport.pdf*.

U.S. Census Bureau. (2004). Projected population of the United States by age and sex: 2000 to 2050. Retrieved April 1, 2005, from *www.census.gov/ipc/www.usinterimproj*.

Varmus, H., Klausner, R., Zerhouni, E., Acharya, T., Daar, A., & Singer, A. (2003). Grand challenges in global health.

Retrieved April 1, 2005 from *www.sciencemag.org/cgi/reprint/302/5644/398.pdf*.

Wu, S. Y., & Green, A. (2000, October). *Projection of chronic illness prevalence and cost inflation*. RAND Corporation.

# **POLICY**SPOTLIGHT

## MENTAL HEALTH PARITY: WILL IT EVER HAPPEN?

Judith B. Krauss & Cynthia Kline O'Sullivan

*"A sound mind in a sound body is a short but full description of a happy state in this world."*

JOHN LOCKE

Despite recent federal and state legislative efforts to correct inequities, mental health care is subject to less insurance coverage and more access restrictions than medical or surgical care. This spotlight highlights key forces behind these inequities, which have prompted advocates and legislators to push for policies to achieve parity of coverage for mental and physical illnesses. We discuss the concept of mental health parity and address specific opportunities for improving mental health care through changes in public policy.

### THE REALITY, COSTS, AND CONSEQUENCES OF MENTAL ILLNESS

Mental illness affects individuals regardless of race, ethnicity, socioeconomic status, age, or geographic area. In 2000, mental illnesses ranked first, above all other conditions including cardiovascular and musculoskeletal disorders, for causing disability among citizens of all ages in the United States, Canada, and Western Europe. Including alcohol

and drug use disorders, the causes of disability due to mental disorders were attributed to 36% of the cases among these countries. The mental disorders most associated with disability consisted of depression, bipolar disorder, and schizophrenia, and constituted 24% of the causes of disability overall that year (World Health Organization, 2001). Nationally, between 1 and 5 children and youth are estimated to have some type of mental health problem (Department of Health and Human Services [DHHS], 1999). Of Americans over 55, almost 20% experience mental disorders that are not a function of the typical aging process, such as anxiety, depression, posttraumatic stress disorder (PTSD), schizophrenia, and substance abuse disorders (DHHS, 1999).

A major government-sponsored survey of more than 9000 Americans, known as the National Comorbidity Survey Replication, indicates that during their lifetimes, almost half of the American population will meet the criteria for four broad categories of mental illness: anxiety disorders (such as panic disorder and PTSD), mood disorders (such as major depression and bipolar illness), impulse-control disorders (such as attention deficit and attention deficit hyperactivity disorder), and substance abuse. Mental illness frequently manifests in an individual's life by the teenage or early adult years. In fact, by the age of 14 half of those who will ever be diagnosed with a mental disorder show signs of the disease, and by age 24 three quarters will show signs; yet many will go undiagnosed or receive improper treatment (Kessler et al., 2005).

Every year, approximately 6% of adults in the United States are so affected by mental illness that they are unable to perform routine activities of daily living. This disability lasts an average of 3 months and results in lost wages and productivity. It is estimated that untreated mental illness costs U.S. businesses about $79 billion a year as a result of absenteeism and lost productivity (Kessler et al., 2005).

One of the most distressing outcomes of mental illness, which may be preventable with adequate diagnosis and treatment, is suicide, estimated to cause more deaths each year than homicide or war (WHO, 2001). Suicide among 15- to 19-year-olds numbers 9.5 per 100,000, with girls twice as likely as boys to attempt suicide, but boys four times more likely than girls to die by suicide. The rate for boys has increased threefold since the early 1960s, and continues to rise among African-American and Native American male adolescents. Annual state expenditures for medical costs associated with completed or attempted suicides by youths aged 20 or younger is nearly $1 billion (DHHS, 1999).

Suicide among adults aged 65 and older is the highest of any other age group, with white males over age 85 making up the largest subgroup (DHHS, 1999). Studies have reported that the majority of older adults who commit suicide do so within 1 month of seeing their primary care providers (PCPs). This sobering statistic suggests that primary care practitioners may have inadequate knowledge about the diagnosis of mental health problems, especially depression, in the elderly. Furthermore, even when diagnosis has been made through accurate symptom recognition, psychiatric treatment of elderly patients by primary care practitioners is frequently inadequate (Lyness et al., 2002).

Only slightly over half of those who need mental health treatment actually receive it, and do so after delaying for 10 years or more. Factors that contribute to an individual's postponement of treatment include inattention to early warning signs,

inadequate health insurance, and unwillingness to seek treatment because of the stigma associated with mental illness (Kessler et al., 2005).

## MENTAL HEALTH CARE AND STIGMA

Although a detailed history of mental health care in the United States is well beyond the scope of this spotlight, it is important to understand the role of stigma and its influence on historical patterns of care as the context for current inequities in coverage of mental health services.

Treatment of mental illness in the United States has its roots in early sixteenth-century Europe and seventeenth-century colonial America. What we now recognize as symptoms of psychiatric disorders were not viewed as an illness, but were seen as a form of demoniac possession and witchcraft to be destroyed. Early treatment theories grew out of this highly stigmatized view.

The first major pattern of care was institutional, and it took three centuries for institutional care to move from treatment consisting of torture and punishment, to a form of humane but benign neglect, to state and county asylum care and the first signs of real treatment. Still, the major goal during the seventeenth, eighteenth, and nineteenth centuries was to "protect" society from the "insane," and the unintended consequence was to preserve the stigma associated with mental illness (Krauss & Slavinsky, 1982).

The second major pattern of care in the latter half of the twentieth century was deinstitutionalization and the community mental health center movement. Prompted by early successes with psychoactive drugs and psychosocial treatment, pressure from social liberals who deplored the dehumanizing effects of institutionalization, and fiscal conservatives who wanted to shift the burden of care from the states to the federal government, this movement was the first public recognition that the stigma of mental illness and resultant isolation were worse than the illness itself. Of course it took nearly the remainder of the twentieth century to discover that deinstitutionalization alone was not enough and to develop the treatment armamentarium we now accept as commonplace. In the meantime, large numbers of people with serious mental disorders who had also suffered the ravages of years of institutionalization were "on the streets" with very little intervention, symptomatic, socially dysfunctional, and frightening to the general public. Stigma was alive and well (Krauss & Slavinsky, 1982).

The third pattern of note emerged at the end of the twentieth century—the "Decade of the Brain"—and involved the recent advances in understanding the neurobiology of psychiatric disorders. With increased knowledge about the neurobiologic determinants of mental illness came the medicalization of mental health treatment. The growing evidence of the biologic basis of mental illness and the development of more effective medications with fewer side effects led to the hope of normalization and more equitable treatment of those with mental illness. However, there is a long way to go before the centuries of stigma associated with mental illness will be overcome.

Mental illness is still difficult to diagnose, in part because of a lack of clear biologic markers and definitive laboratory or radiologic tests that can confirm diagnosis and in part because of the fact that many people with mental illness are treated by PCPs unfamiliar with the diagnostic process and taxonomy. The personality and behavioral changes that occur as a result of some mental illnesses are difficult for many nonpsychiatric practitioners to understand, and this misunderstanding further fuels the stigma.

Unfortunately, stigma extends to inequity in insurance coverage for mental health care and the behavioral and cognitive services of mental health professionals. When people with mental illness experience discrimination in treatment or health care reimbursement, the illness itself often hampers their ability to navigate the political and administrative labyrinths necessary to counter the effects. For all of these reasons, the mental health parity movement was born.

## MENTAL HEALTH PARITY DEFINED

Private, public, and group health insurance plans often provide lower levels of coverage for the treatment of mental illness compared with the treatment of other illnesses. Coverage might be limited through the use of annual or lifetime dollar limits; higher copayments or cost sharing by the insured; or limits on the number of covered inpatient or outpatient days. The simplest definition of mental health parity evolved from efforts to correct such insurance inequities and refers to *mental health benefit parity*—meaning that insurance coverage would be comparable for mental illness treatment and medical or surgical treatment with the same out-of-pocket expenses resulting from copayments, deductibles, or limits on visits. However, there is also what is known as *supply-side inequity*, which has to do with managed care strategies to keep costs down—such as discounted fees for service and capitation—that might discourage practitioners from treating such patients; gate-keeping and utilization review, which can restrict access to mental health services; and more-stringent definitions of medical necessity, which can also limit access to care (Burnam & Escarce, 1999, Thomas & Leavitt, 2002). An expanded definition of mental health parity also addresses these inequities, although they are harder to measure and to legislate.

Two scenarios provide a practical illustration:

■ Your spouse develops diabetes. Before the diagnosis being made, a PCP performs an initial evaluation, orders diagnostic tests, and initiates insulin injections or oral medications. At some point the PCP refers your spouse to a specialist for additional evaluation and treatment consultation. Every few weeks until his metabolic needs are adequately regulated, your spouse sees his PCP for follow-up. In addition, you and your spouse see a diabetes educator for lifestyle management, including helpful information on diet, exercise, and weight management. A visiting nurse comes to your home to evaluate any environmental concerns that might need to be corrected to reduce the risk of injury resulting from comorbid conditions, such as poor vision and peripheral neuropathy. If your spouse's condition becomes difficult to manage as an outpatient, he may require a brief hospitalization for more intensive monitoring and treatment. Your health care insurance covers 85% of your expenses, and the insurance company places no dollar or day limits on necessary medical visits or hospitalizations.

■ Your son is diagnosed with pediatric depression. It took almost a year to navigate the system and get a proper evaluation and diagnosis. You noticed that over a period of 6 months your son became increasingly withdrawn, engaged less with his kindergarten peer group, and spent more time daydreaming and acting out imaginary scenarios. Your pediatrician dismissed your concerns and assured you that this behavior was developmentally normal. Only after your son fell seriously behind in the classroom did the school offer vision and hearing testing, which proved normal. The school recommended that your son repeat kindergarten. Seeking explanations for the behavior change, you again consulted your pediatrician, who suggested neuropsychologic testing to rule out cognitive disabilities and an electroencephalogram (EEG) to rule out petit mal seizures. The EEG was easy to schedule, and 90% of the cost was covered by your insurance plan. It took 5 months to schedule the neuropsychologic testing, which was not covered by insurance and cost $1200. In the meantime, it was recommended that your son be evaluated by the school social worker. It took a month to receive the evaluation because she is the only social worker for three elementary schools (1500 students). She recommended further evaluation by a child psychiatrist, but none of the five psychiatrists recommended were taking new patients, so it took another 2 weeks to get a referral from your health insurance company. The treatment plan is for weekly counseling sessions with the psychiatrist for 12 to 24 months, and after several months, possibly antidepressant medications. The fee is $275 for the initial evaluation and $175 per week thereafter. Your health insurance limits outpatient mental health coverage to the first $500 annually. Over a 2-year period your out-of-pocket expenses could be well over $17,000 before even factoring in the cost of medication.

The scenarios illustrate the inequities in mental health insurance coverage contrasted with typical coverage for most medical or surgical illnesses and highlight the differences in benefit coverage as well as access to needed care. Despite legislative efforts, societal, political, and economic factors have prevented equality in diagnosis, treatment, and insurance for mental illness care. Many myths about mental health care persist and need to be dispelled before equity will be achieved.

## MYTHS OF MENTAL HEALTH CARE

### Myth #1

*Most people with mental illness are at fault for their situations and need to take personal responsibility to turn their lives around.*

### Fact

The stigma that still plagues mental illness fuels doubts about the validity of psychiatric diagnosis and treatment. Regier (2003) suggests that employers, insurers, legislators, and policymakers unrealistically fear that covering all psychiatric and emotional disorders in the fourth edition of the *Diagnostic and Statistical Manual* (DSM-IV) of the American Psychiatric Association (APA) will dramatically increase cost because of the overinclusiveness of the diagnoses contained in the DSM-IV and because some treatments might be sought for self-improvement rather than medical necessity. As a result, we hold mental health treatment to a higher standard than medical treatment. Regier (2003) points out that valid diagnostic theories follow major treatment advances in medicine as well as in psychiatry, noting that "syndrome-based diagnoses with no known causal mechanisms or disease theory enabled the control of cholera, pellagra, and dropsy (congestive heart failure) long before the cholera vibrio, niacin deficiency, or action of digitalis were understood" (p. 22). The DSM-IV is the accepted scientific standard for diagnosis in mental health and is based on a combination of known organic causes of psychiatric disorders as well as symptom patterns and observable signs such as mental status changes, organic impairment, functional disability, and psychomotor retardation. It is used by state Medicaid programs to determine eligibility for mental health services; is incorporated into more than 650 state and federal laws as the standard for defining mental disorders; and is one component of medical necessity for all managed behavioral health organizations, along with the published APA (2000b) evidenced-based practice guidelines

(Regier, 2003). Mental illness is no more a matter of poor self-control, laziness, or lack of will power than diabetes, and people with bona fide psychiatric diagnoses should not be held to a higher standard in order to gain access to covered treatment.

## Myth #2

*Mental illness is impossible to cure, and treatment is not very effective.*

## Fact

Effective treatments for quality care and recovery are now available for most serious mental disorders. The final report of the New Freedom Commission on Mental Health (2003) describes a number of treatments and services that have been developed in the mental health field whose effectiveness is well documented in the research literature, known as *evidence-based practices*, and also details a number of promising but less-well-studied "emerging best practices" (Boxes 13-2 and 13-3). In addition, the APA has published 11 evidence-based guidelines as a result of clinical trials of treatment efficacy and effectiveness for both psychosocial and psychopharmacologic treatments (APA, 2000b). The real problem is the delay in getting these treatments to the people who need them because of the lack of effective dissemination methods to promote broad use of the most effective practices, restrictive reimbursement policies, and the shortage of qualified health professionals in the mental health field.

## Myth #3

*Most of our states have mental health parity laws that require equal insurance coverage for both physical and mental illness. These laws have leveled the playing field.*

## Fact

Although 36 states as of 2005 had state mental health parity laws that were more comprehensive than the federal law (NAMI, 2005), a recent report by the General Accounting Office (GAO, 2000) demonstrated that access to needed mental health services as a result of such laws remains limited. Because each state's parity laws differ from the

---

**BOX 13-2  Examples of Evidence-Based Practices**

Evidence-based practice is defined by the Institute of Medicine (2001) as the integration of best-researched evidence and clinical expertise with patient values.

- Specific medications for specific conditions
- Cognitive and interpersonal therapies for depression
- Preventive interventions for children at risk for serious emotional disturbances
- Treatment foster care
- Multisystemic therapy
- Parent-child interaction therapy
- Medication algorithms
- Family psychoeducation
- Assertive community treatment
- Collaborative treatment in primary care

Adapted from New Freedom Commission on Mental Health. (2003). *Achieving the promise: Transforming mental health care in America. Final report.* DHHS Pub. No. SMA-03-3832. Rockville, MD: U.S. Department of Health and Human Services, Substance Abuse and Mental Health Services Administration.

---

**BOX 13-3  Examples of Emerging Best Practices**

Emerging best practices are treatments and services that are promising but less-thoroughly documented than evidence-based practices.

- Consumer-operated services
- Jail diversion and community reentry programs
- School mental health services
- Trauma-specific interventions
- Wraparound services
- Multifamily group therapies
- Systems of care for children with serious emotional disturbances and their families

Adapted from New Freedom Commission on Mental Health. (2003). *Achieving the promise: Transforming mental health care in America. Final report.* DHHS Pub. No. SMA-03-3832. Rockville, MD: U.S. Department of Health and Human Services, Substance Abuse and Mental Health Services Administration.

---

others', people are subject to problems in coverage if they move from one state to another, a situation that does not occur with other medical coverage, except if the change is associated with employment. Furthermore, because the states have their own mental illness parity laws, they are required to ensure compliance with these laws independent of federal support. Many states rely on state insurance commissions to enforce compliance by employers and private health insurance companies with respect to state parity laws; however, oversight for this role is often insufficiently funded and relies on complaints, allowing employers and insurance companies to slip out of compliance without penalty. In addition, parity laws tend to address only demand-side benefits such as copayments, deductibles, or limits on visits. Because most mental health coverage is provided through group plans, insurers and employers can use a variety of supply-side managed care techniques to control access, thereby reducing use (Burnam & Escarce, 1999).

## Myth #4

*Equal coverage for mental illness will cause insurance rates to skyrocket.*

## Fact

Studies by states regarding the effect of mental illness parity on health insurance rates to employers and patients have shown that comprehensive parity laws do not support this notion. For instance, Vermont, which has one of the most comprehensive laws, exceeding the federal law on every provision, found that since the state's enactment of its mental health parity law in 1998, insurance costs have not significantly increased, and 70% of employers surveyed were satisfied with the law in relation to its impact on employer health care expenses (Mathematica Policy Research, 1998).

## Myth #5

*If private health insurance doesn't pay for mental illness care, people with mental illness can get free treatment from state mental health systems.*

## Fact

Those who cannot continue to pay out of pocket for services without receiving reimbursement often stop their treatment. This situation illustrates a disparity in access to services based on ability to pay. Medicaid is the largest single financing source for mental health coverage, providing over half of

the funds for state and local community health services, as well as up to 52% of the funding for services received in the private mental health sector (Coffee et al., 2001). Those who qualify may obtain care through Medicare- and Medicaid-sponsored public health clinics and services. However, because of an increasing demand for care, the waiting lists for these clinics are long, and care generally goes to those who are the most acutely ill. Public mental health systems that treat the uninsured and those on public insurance have limited resources and must prioritize services to those with severe impairments because of mental or emotional problems. Those with mild or moderate mental health problems often cannot access the public system. Although Medicaid may pay for such patients to receive services from private providers, it does so at a lower rate than is typically charged. Patients must pay the difference out of pocket, and many low- or moderate-income families cannot manage such payments. Without treatment, individuals may become unnecessarily disabled or unemployed, resort to substance abuse, become homeless, be jailed, or attempt suicide. Untreated and undertreated mental illness is estimated to cost more than $100 billion each year in the United States (New Freedom Commission on Mental Health, 2003). This limitation in service may be described as a problem of parity in access to needed mental health services.

## LEGISLATIVE AND REGULATORY HISTORY OF MENTAL HEALTH PARITY

### Federal Initiatives

Treatment of mental illness has been a topic of some debate over the past several decades, and this debate continues to the present. A major constraint in mental illness treatment has been the limited funding available through public and private insurance programs. Recent developments to address the need for better funding include President Clinton's signing of the Mental Health Parity Act (MHPA) into law in 1996. Senators Pete Domenici (R-NM) and Paul Wellstone (D-MN) were bipartisan cosponsors of the bill, which was promulgated by DHHS, the Department of Labor, and the Treasury (Thomas & Leavitt, 2002). Under this law, mental health benefit caps were required to equal the lifetime limits for medical and surgical benefits. The law became effective on January 1, 1998. It has proved to be the first step before subsequent enactment of individual state parity laws, which are required to be at least as comprehensive as the federal law. Specific points regarding The Federal MHPA are summarized in Box 13-4.

The original Federal MHPA was scheduled to expire (legally referred to as *sunsetting*) on September 30, 2001, but President Bush signed legislation to extend the deadline until December 31, 2002. As of July 2005, subsequent reauthorization bills in Congress have granted 1-year extensions to the original MHPA every year since the first enactment (Mental Health Parity Reauthorization Act, 2003), but the federal law is at risk of sunsetting on December 31 of each year if not reauthorized. It is important to note that because the MHPA is a federal law, the more comprehensive state laws in many cases supersede it. However, the uncertain nature of federal reauthorization legislation has implications for employees of certain types of organizations who are not covered by state parity laws. Employers who are categorized as self-insured are protected through two federal acts: the Employee Retirement Income Security Act (ERISA) and the Public Health Service Acts, which provide employer exemptions from the state parity laws. Although these acts were never intended to cover issues regarding health insurance, they have essentially protected these employers from being required to comply with the more comprehensive state-mandated health insurance laws. For employees who work for such organizations, the Federal MHPA is essential; if it were allowed to sunset, they would not be protected by any mental health parity laws.

Other federal bills have been proposed by legislators to enhance the parity bills. Check the congressional Website (*http://thomas.local.gov*) for current legislation. Some of the legislation initiatives that try to equalizing coverage by eliminating outpatient visits and hospital day limits and equalizing required copayments and deductibles are opposed by insurance lobbyists. In addition, small business owners oppose them based on the anticipated cost increases resulting from lowering the small business exemption from 51 to 25 employees. Despite the merits of a bill such as the Positive Aging Act, implementing such a program is cited as too costly to warrant funding during budget deficit periods.

### State Initiatives

Many states have passed mental health parity laws that exceed the provisions of the federal law, and some have expanded original legislation to be even more inclusive. The Web Resources at the end of the chapter provide a list of locations where one can find updates on state parity laws. It is important to review the provisions of each law in order to evaluate how expansive or restrictive it is. Box 13-5 provides an illustrative comparison of three states: Vermont, which is considered to have a model parity law with broad inclusions; Louisiana, which exceeds federal standards by requiring equal coverage of medical and mental illnesses but only of specifically named disorders, making other coverage optional at the expense of the insured, and allowing a minimum limit on days in treatment; and Georgia, which on first blush appears to exceed the federal law, except that the provision includes the phrase "employers that choose to provide mental health benefits," thereby providing an

---

**BOX 13-4** Major Elements of the Federal Mental Health Parity Act of 1996

- A group health plan that does *not* impose an annual or dollar limit on medical or surgical benefits *may not* impose such a limit on mental health benefits.
- The provisions do not apply to *substance abuse* or chemical *dependency*.
- The group health plan *is not required* to include mental health benefits. Parity laws apply only to those plans that already offer mental health benefits.
- Exceptions are small businesses with fewer than 51 employees, group health plans whose costs increase at least 1% as a result of the Federal Mental Health Parity Act based on 6 months of actual claims data, and health plans included in the Employee Retirement Income Security Act.
- It does not mandate minimum or maximum outpatient visits or inpatient hospital days.

---

**BOX 13-5** Comparison of Three State Mental Health Parity Laws

- **Vermont, 1997 (Enacted January, 1998):** The law provides that health plans shall not establish any lifetime or annual payment limits, deductibles, copayments, coinsurance, or any other cost-sharing requirements, out-of-pocket limits, visit limits and any other financial component of coverage that places a greater financial burden on an insured than for physical health conditions. The law requires a single limit for mental health and physical health deductibles and out-of-pocket limits. The law requires parity coverage for mental illnesses and addictive disorders.

- **Louisiana, 1999 (Enacted January, 2000):** Mandates equitable coverage for severe mental illness including schizophrenia, schizoaffective disorder, bipolar disorder, pervasive developmental disorder (autism), panic disorder, obsessive-compulsive disorder, major depressive disorder, anorexia or bulimia, Asperger's disorder, intermittent explosive disorder, posttraumatic stress disorder, psychosis (not otherwise specified) when diagnosed in a child under 17 years of age, Rett's disorder, and Tourette's disorder. Policies must offer optional coverage for other mental disorders not covered in the list (at the expense of the policyholder). Minimum benefits are to include 45 inpatient days per year (an exchange of two partial hospitalization days or two residential treatment days per one hospital day may be provided) and 52 outpatient visits, including intensive outpatient programs. No small-business exemption.

- **Georgia, 1998 (Enacted April, 1998):** Requires larger employers (51 or more employees) that choose to provide mental health benefits to provide equal lifetime and annual caps for mental health benefits as are provided for other physical illnesses and provide the same dollar limits, deductibles, and coinsurance factors. Employers cannot impose separate outpatient and visit limits on the treatment of mental illnesses. Requires smaller employers (2 to 50 employees) that choose to provide mental health benefits to provide equal lifetime and annual caps for mental health benefits as are offered for other physical illnesses and provide the same dollar limits, deductibles, and coinsurance factors. "Mental illnesses" cover all brain disorders listed in the DSM-IV, including addictive disorders.

---

escape clause for those who do not wish to provide such coverage.

**Impact of State and Federal Initiatives**

Several government-sponsored studies of the effects of both state and federal parity laws have been completed. In May of 2000, the GAO published its report entitled *Mental Parity Act: Despite New Federal Standards, Mental Health Benefits Remain Limited.* The majority of employers were complying with the mental health parity law (86%). However, because of the federal law's limited scope, employers were able to reduce some benefits in order to offset improvements in others, resulting in the law having little impact on access to mental health services for most employees. For example, although most health plans have parity in lifetime expenditures allowed for both physical and mental illnesses, 65% of the plans restrict the number of outpatient visits and hospital days for mental health treatment more stringently than for other medical and surgical benefits. Furthermore, the GAO found that since the enactment of the federal MHPA, insurance claims costs increased negligibly, generally no more than 1% to 4%. However, because very few employers had submitted comprehensive reports to the GAO examining costs relative to parity legislation, there were incomplete data on cost increases, a problem that continues to hinder further forward legislation.

Oversight authority for addressing compliance and enforcement of the Federal MHPA is divided among state and federal agencies. The Agency for Health Care Research and Quality (AHRQ) is primarily responsible for addressing states not in compliance with the federal law. However, because most state parity laws are more comprehensive than the federal laws, state laws take precedence over the federal laws, and oversight authority is the responsibility of the individual states' insurance regulators. Other external groups such as labor unions may provide additional oversight for complaint-driven issues and in some instances have begun random audits on selected employers to evaluate compliance (GAO, 2000).

In an effort to examine the alleged private insurance company violations of parity laws some states

---

**BOX 13-6** Goals from the President's New Freedom Commission on Mental Health

**Goal #1: *Americans understand that mental health is essential to overall health*.** This goal requires more public education regarding the availability of services as well as education geared at reducing the stigma of mental illness. The best place to begin this education is through our primary care system; but in order to educate the public, primary care practitioners need to be educated first. Funding is needed to train primary care practitioners in the recognition and treatment of psychiatric disorders. In addition, because of the critical shortage of mental health practitioners, especially for children, incentive programs are needed to encourage new practitioners to enter the mental health field. Educational loan forgiveness programs would assist in this endeavor.

**Goal #2: *Mental health care is consumer and family driven*.** This goal requires that consumers and families be fully involved in working with all members of the health care team toward recovery. However, all too often, health care is driven by cost-containment goals of insurance companies rather than health care practitioners. The power of the managed care gate-keepers must be kept in check and not be allowed to dictate type and payment of service or limit the type of practitioner delivering the service.

**Goal #3: *Disparities in mental health services are eliminated*.** There are several disparities in the system that affect the poor, children, and the elderly. Other considerations include access to culturally competent health care and access to mental health care in rural and geographically remote areas. Realizing this goal will likely require incentive programs for all practitioners interested in working in underserved areas and underserved populations.

**Goal #4: *Early mental health screening, assessment, and referral to services are common practice*.** Education for those who work in our schools, community centers, and primary care areas is critical for this goal to be realized. This requires funding for research translation and dissemination.

**Goal #5: *Excellent mental health care is delivered, and research is accelerated*.** Disparities in care have been identified, and research is needed to understand the extent of the problems.

**Goals #6: *Technology is used to access mental health care information*.** Mental health care providers need access to information through the coordination of technology systems so that care is seamless and well informed. Consumers also need access to technology for education. Specific goals for this technology need to be defined so that it is useful and cost-effective. Users (physicians, nurses, mental health worker, social worker, and others) need to be involved with developing these systems to accomplish this goal.

Adapted from New Freedom Commission on Mental Health. (2003). *Achieving the promise: Transforming mental health care in America. Final report.* DHHS Pub. No. SMA-03-3832. Rockville, MD: U.S. Department of Health and Human Services, Substance Abuse and Mental Health Services Administration.

---

have formed partnerships in order to better track and focus efforts to relieve the problem. For example, the Connecticut chapter of NAMI has partnered with Connecticut's Attorney General to conduct a survey of citizens who feel their insurance company has improperly denied their mental health claims. It is also examining cost shifting from private insurers to public insurers for mental health services.

Finally, in response to the stigma that surrounds mental illness, unfair treatment limitations and financial requirements placed on mental health benefits, and the fragmented mental health service delivery system, President Bush launched the President's New Freedom Commission on Mental Health, which outlined six goals for the transformation of mental health care, identified in Box 13-6.

## HOW TO INFLUENCE MENTAL HEALTH PARITY POLICY

**Join Coalitions for Mental Health Reform.** Soon after the New Freedom Commission Report was released, five organizations with a history of sometimes conflicting mental health priorities came together to form a coalition called the *Campaign for Mental Health Reform*. This coalition has grown to include 16 partner members (see Box 13-7 for a list of coalition members). Together they work toward supporting the implementation of the commission's recommendations and other initiatives,

---

**BOX 13-7** Coalitions for Mental
Health Reform

**CAMPAIGN FOR MENTAL HEALTH REFORM**

*Founding members:* National Alliance on Mental
Illness, National Association of State Mental Health
Program Directors, American Psychiatric
Association, National Mental Health Association,
and Bazelton Center for Mental Health Law

*Partners:* American Academy of Child and
Adolescent Psychiatry, American Psychological
Association, Children and Adults with
Attention-Deficit/Hyperactivity Disorder, Depression
and Bipolar Support Alliance, Federation of
Families for Children's Mental Health, National
Association of County Behavioral Health Directors,
National Council for Community Behavioral
Healthcare, National Empowerment Center,
National Mental Health Consumers' Self-Help
Clearinghouse, Suicide Prevention Action
Network USA, United States Psychiatric
Rehabilitation Association

**COALITION FOR FAIRNESS IN MENTAL
ILLNESS COVERAGE**

National Alliance on Mental Illness, National
Mental Health Association, American Hospital
Association, American Managed Behavioral
Healthcare Association, American Medical
Association, American Psychiatric Association,
American Psychological Association, Federation of
Hospitals, National Association of Psychiatric
Health Systems

---

**BOX 13-8** Nursing Organizations
That Champion Mental
Health Parity

- American Nurses Association
- American Psychiatric Nurses Association
- American Academy of Nurse Practitioners

---

**BOX 13-9** Disease-Specific Advocacy
Organizations

- Manic Depressive Association
- Obsessive Compulsive Disorders Foundation
- Anxiety Disorders Association of America
- Trichotillomania Learning Center
- Juvenile Bipolar Research Organization
- Depression and Bipolar Support Alliance
- Children and Adults with Attention-Deficit/
  Hyperactivity Disorder

---

including evaluation of federal mental health block grants to states, addressing housing issues and the lack of inpatient psychiatric beds, and developing system interfaces with agencies such as Departments of Corrections.

Other coalitions have been formed to address specific aspects of mental illness care, including mental health parity. The Coalition for Fairness in Mental Illness Coverage represents consumers, families, health professionals, health care systems, and administrators who are interested in improving mental illness coverage (see Box 13-7 for a list of coalition members).

It is notable that neither of the two coalitions list nursing organizations as members, although there are some nursing organizations that have gone on record in favor of mental health parity (Box 13-8). It is essential that nurses join their professional organizations and urge those organizations to become active in coalitions like these. Nurses bring valuable expertise in patient education, patient advocacy, and family intervention. In addition, these coalition groups can be influential in advocating for coverage of services typically delivered by nurses; but they are unlikely to do so if nurses are not engaged in the organization.

In addition, there are many advocacy organizations that address specific disorders (Box 13-9), all of which try to leverage unified advocacy by focusing on individuals with specific diagnoses. All of these organizations have affiliated Scientific Advisory Boards to advise, educate, and promote professional leadership in these areas. Nurse researchers and expert nurse clinicians can participate on these boards. Public education is a core component of the mission statements of these patient groups through dissemination and translation of new scientific advances into the public arena. Nurses are particularly skilled in these areas and can make valuable contributions to such groups, at the same time promoting nursing as a profession.

Virtually all of these organizations and coalitions interact with state and national government agencies and legislators to promote mental health care reform and create more accurate perceptions about mental health and mental illness. Involvement with these groups is a good way for nurses to gain experience in the political process while advocating for vulnerable populations.

## Media Watch

Because of the stigma still associated with mental illness, many patients do not readily seek treatment and try to hide their illness. Consequently the general public gains most of its information about mental illness from the stereotypes portrayed in the media. Professional nursing organizations have long monitored the media for unrealistic and inaccurate portrayals of the nursing role. They should be encouraged to do the same on behalf of stigmatized patient populations, such as those with serious mental illness. Nurses can encourage their organizations to monitor print and film portrayals of mental illness, using letter-writing campaigns and pressure on advertisers to correct stereotypes. Nurses can also serve as professional advisors on projects in order to promote more accurate portrayals of mental illness.

## Lobby for Improved Primary Health Care Training

The New Freedom Commission (2003) highlighted the need for improved training of primary care clinicians in the recognition and treatment of psychiatric disorders. Nursing accreditation and education organizations should examine basic and advanced practice curricula to ensure inclusion of mental health and mental illness content in primary and acute care curricula. Nurses who work in high volume emergency departments or community health centers should lobby for the provision of collaborative psychiatric services as well as targeted in-service education to help improve both the medical and psychiatric care of people with mental illness. Specific mental illnesses are associated with particularly high levels of medical comorbidity, such as diabetes and poor oral health in patients with schizophrenia, and targeted interventions need

to be developed with a focus on these common medical problems.

A key example of the impact of a single event on the training practices of physicians stemmed largely from the death of one patient, Libby Zion. While an inpatient at a New York teaching hospital, Zion died as a consequence of an adverse drug interaction between meperidine, a narcotic analgesic, and an antidepressant medication in the monoamine oxidase inhibitor (MAOI) family. The medications had been ordered by an inexperienced, undersupervised, and fatigued surgical intern who was unfamiliar with the dangers of such drug interactions. As a consequence of this death, efforts to provide better supervision and to limit the number of hours that residents work have been developed, improving the training of many clinicians.

## Tracking State Parity Laws

Finally, successes in some states in providing progressive legislation regarding health benefits for the mentally ill have served as models for other states in demonstrating that the laws can be changed, with resulting improvements in care and long-term cost savings. As a useful first step, nurses may track their own state mental health parity laws, compare them with those of other states, and become active in proposing necessary revisions to state legislators. In addition, most mental health organizations also have advocacy Websites, which provide very helpful information related to pending legislation and other initiatives.

## Key Points

- There are ample opportunities for nurses to influence mental health parity policies, be it as citizen, clinician, researcher, or educator.
- People with mental illness are everywhere—patients in hospitals, members of our families, students in the school system, and colleagues at work.
- Regardless of specialty, nurses should be concerned about parity in mental health care and should stay informed about current public policy issues.

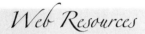

The Campaign for Mental Health Reform
*www.mhreform.org*
The Louis de la Parte Florida Mental Health
   Institute
*www.fmhi.usf.edu/parity*
National Alliance on Mental Illlness
*www.nami.org* (see Policy Updates)
U.S. Department of Labor
*www.dol.gov/dol/topic/health-plans/mental*

## REFERENCES

American Psychiatric Association (APA). (2000a). *Diagnostic and statistical manual of mental disorders* (4th ed.). Washington, DC: APA.

American Psychiatric Association (APA). (2000b). *Practice guidelines for the treatment of psychiatric disorders.* Washington, DC: APA.

Burnam, M. A., & Escarce, J. J. (1999). Equity in managed care for mental disorders. *Health Affairs, 18*(5), 22-31.

Coffee R. M., Graver, L., Schroeder, D., Busch, J. D., Dilonardo, J., Chalk, M., & Buck, J. A. (2001). *Mental health and substance abuse treatment: Results from a study integrating data from state mental health, substance abuse, and Medicaid agencies.* Rockville, MD: Substance Abuse and Mental Health Services Administration, Center for Substance Abuse Treatment & Center for Mental Health Services, U.S. Department of Health and Human Services.

Department of Health and Human Services (DHHS). (1999). *Mental health: A report of the Surgeon General.* Rockville, MD: U.S. Public Health Service.

General Accounting Office (GAO). (2000). *Implementation of the Mental Health Parity Act of 1996.* GAO/HEHS-00-95. Washington, DC: GAO.

Institute of Medicine Committee on Quality of Health Care in America. (2001). *Crossing the quality chasm: A new health system for the 21st century.* Washington, DC: National Academies Press.

Kessler, R. C., Berglund, P., Demler, O., Jin, R., Merikangas, K. R., & Walters, E. E. (2005). Lifetime prevalence and age-of-onset distributions of DSM-IV disorders in the National Comorbidity Survey Replication. *Archives of General Psychiatry, 62*(6), 593-602.

Krauss, J., & Slavinsky, A. (1982). *The chronically ill psychiatric patient and the community.* Boston: Blackwell Scientific.

Lyness, J. M., Caine, E. D., King, D. A., Conwell, Y., Duberstein, P. R., & Cox, C. (2002). Depressive disorders and symptoms in older primary care patients: One-year outcomes. *American Journal of Geriatric Psychiatry, 10*(3), 275-282.

Mathematica Policy Research. (1998). *The costs and effects of parity for mental health and substance abuse insurance benefits.* Washington, DC: Substance Abuse and Mental Health Services Administration, U.S. Department of Health and Human Services.

Mental Health Parity Reauthorization Act. (2003, December). Bill summary, 108th Congress. Retrieved February, 14, 2006, from *http://web.lexis-nexis.com/congcomp.*

National Alliance on Mental Illness (NAMI). (2005). State mental illness parity laws. Chart of state laws. Retrieved June 24, 2005, from *www.nami.org/printertemplate.cfm?template=/contentmenagement/html.display.*

New Freedom Commission on Mental Health. (2003). *Achieving the promise: Transforming mental health care in America. Final report.* DHHS Pub. No. SMA-03-3832. Rockville, MD: U.S. Department of Health and Human Services, Substance Abuse and Mental Health Services Administration.

Regier, D. (2003). Mental disorder diagnostic theory and practical reality: An evolutionary perspective. *Health Affairs, 22*(5), 21-27.

Thomas, N. S., & Leavitt, J. K. (2002). Mental illness parity: A call for nursing action. *Policy, Politics & Nursing Practice, 3*(1), 43-56.

World Health Organization (WHO). (2001). The *World Health Report 2001—Mental health: New understanding, new hope.* Geneva: WHO.

# The Department of Defense TRICARE Program: Health Care for the U.S. Military

Bonnie Mowinski Jennings

*"Let us endeavor to preserve the health of those who bravely enter the field of battle or expose themselves on the boisterous ocean in defense of their country."*
Surgeon Edward Cutbush

The U.S. health care system is in turmoil. This upheaval derives largely from the tension created between infinite health care needs and finite health care resources. The tension manifests in difficult tradeoffs among cost, quality, and access.

The U.S. Defense Health Program (DHP) is not immune to the turmoil, tension and tradeoffs occurring in civilian health care. In fact, increasing health care costs within the U.S. Department of Defense (DoD) prompted a dramatic change to military health care. A managed care program, TRICARE, was implemented in 1995 to control costs. This change left military beneficiaries—individuals eligible for care in the DHP—grappling with a new and far more complicated health program as well as one that continues to evolve. It left policymakers grappling with pressures from beneficiary groups, senior military leaders, and members of Congress.

Current DoD health policy issues relate largely to unabated increases in the cost of providing care to DoD beneficiaries despite the conversion to TRICARE. The DoD health policy issues can best be understood by placing them in the context of the government health programs as well as delineating key aspects of DoD health care.

## GOVERNMENT-SPONSORED HEALTH CARE PROGRAMS

The U.S. government sponsors six major health care programs that collectively provide coverage to about one third of the U.S. population and cost about $500 billion annually (Institute of Medicine [IOM], 2002). Of these, three are programs designed for individuals with high health care needs and low socioeconomic resources: Medicare, Medicaid, and the State Children's Health Insurance Program (SCHIP). The other three programs are designed for populations with which the federal government has a special relationship: the Indian Health Service (IHS), which cares for Native Americans; the Veterans Health Administration (VHA), which provides care to veterans with service-connected disabilities; and the DoD, which cares for eligible military beneficiaries.

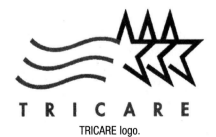

TRICARE logo.

323

## A DoD HEALTH CARE PRIMER

### Beneficiaries

The DHP provides health services for eligible beneficiaries from the uniformed services. These eligible beneficiaries include active-duty and retired personnel and their family members as well as survivors of deceased military. The U.S. uniformed services include the armed forces—Army, Navy, Air Force, Marine Corps—as well as the Coast Guard, the Public Health Service and the National Oceanic and Atmospheric Administration (Gidwani et al., 2005).

### Mission

The DHP enhances the security of the United States by providing health support for military operations as well as sustaining the health of the full complement of military beneficiaries. The mission is accomplished through the Military Health System (MHS) (Gidwani et al., 2005).

### Goals

The primary goals of the MHS are to improve force health protection and medical readiness. In other words, the MHS must sustain a healthy fighting force and ensure health care personnel are ready to deploy in support of the fighting force (Gidwani et al., 2005). In addition, health care is a known factor that enhances quality of life for service members and contributes to recruiting and retaining personnel (Jennings, Swanson, Heiner, Loan, & Hemman, in review; Military Officers Association of America [MOAA], 2005c; Shelton, 2001).

### Legislative Authority

Title 10 of the U.S. Code defines the DHP. It specifies the type of health care authorized (e.g., inpatient, outpatient, ambulance services, medications, prosthetic devices, hearing aids) by beneficiary type. Benefits vary for active-duty personnel, family members of active-duty personnel, military retirees, family members of military retirees, and survivors of deceased military members. Title 10 clearly states that medical and dental care for family members and retirees is subject to the availability of space, facilities, and staff. Therefore personnel losses and base closures may limit the "space available" to care for retirees.

### Forces Shaping Military Health Policy

*Interest groups.* Numerous groups work to give voice to issues that have the potential to affect all beneficiaries of the uniformed services—active-duty personnel, military reservists, military retirees, family members, veterans, and survivors of deceased active-duty personnel. To increase their political clout, 31 special interest groups united in 1985 as The Military Coalition. This powerful advocacy group has effectively argued to sustain or improve a variety of quality-of-life issues for military beneficiaries (Schwartz & Chaffee, 2002).

*Congressional influence.* The DHP is a part of the DoD budget. Therefore Congress passes the laws that define and fund the DHP. Particularly influential in decisions that affect the DHP are the Senate and House Armed Services Committees (the SASC and HASC respectively). For example, key provisions in the SASC mark-up of the Fiscal Year (FY) 2006 National Defense Authorization Act (NDAA) included an extension of TRICARE enrollment eligibility for children of members killed while on active duty as long as the children meet the conditions for a military identification card (MOAA, 2005b). The Senate and House Appropriations Committees are also extremely important in shaping the DHP.

Somewhat less obvious are the second-order effects of Congressional decisions on health care. For example, Congress determines the size of the military force. When force reductions occur, military health care staff across all three services—Army, Navy, and Air Force—are also downsized. Through other legislative acts, Congress can expand or contract the beneficiaries served by the MHS. For example, because medical benefits were extended to the family members of mobilized Guard and Reserve personnel, an additional 500,000 beneficiaries became eligible for DoD health care by the end of FY 2004 (Gidwani et al., 2005).

*Base realignment and closure.* In the 1960s, during the Kennedy administration, the DoD developed the base realignment and closure (BRAC) process to reduce the military base structure that was created during World War II. This process was initially conducted independent of Congressional involvement. Ultimately, economic and political pressures contributed to the signing of Public Law 95-82 in August 1977. As a consequence, DoD has to notify Congress when bases become candidates for closure or reduction. Since 1988 there have been four bipartisan BRAC commissions that collectively recommended closing 125 major military facilities and 225 minor military installations, as well as realigning operations and functions of 145 others (GlobalSecurity.org, 2005).

When a military base closes, health care facilities residing on those bases also close. For example, in May 2005 the Secretary of Defense announced recommendations from the fifth BRAC commission affecting a total of 180 military installations (MOAA, 2005b). After considerable deliberation and debate, these recommendations were approved by Congress in August 2005. Among their effects will be a major realignment of health care delivery in the Washington, DC area. For example, Walter Reed Army Medical Center (WRAMC) in Washington, DC will close, the Army hospital at Fort Belvoir in northern Virginia will be enlarged, and services at the National Naval Medical Center (NNMC) in Bethesda, Maryland will be expanded. In addition, the NNMC will change its name to Walter Reed National Military Medical Center. The announced closure of WRAMC was particularly disquieting because of its reputation as the "Harvard of military medicine" (Dao, 2005).

## THE MILITARY HEALTH SYSTEM BEFORE TRICARE: THE GOOD OLD DAYS

Before the implementation of TRICARE, eligible military beneficiaries believed they were entitled to "cradle-to-grave" health care. The health benefit was a part of the compensation package earned while serving on active duty. In addition, for those who retired from the military with at least 20 years of service, full health benefits continued as a part of the retirement package. Thus, military retirees envisioned life-long health care for themselves and their families. This care came from two sources: Military Treatment Facilities (MTFs)—military hospitals and clinics located worldwide—and the Civilian Health and Medical Program for the Uniformed Services (CHAMPUS), a fee-for-service (FFS) program available to retirees and family members

of both active-duty personnel and retirees. Although retirees age 65 and older were entitled to Medicare, the more common and expected avenue for care was through the military facilities. Beneficiaries were very comfortable with the long-standing traditions that defined the delivery of their health care.

In the 1990s the seeds of change were planted, however, as several events converged. The cost of care was rising in combination with bases closing, health care facilities disappearing, and military manpower being downsized. An initial response to these situations was a DoD initiative known as the *Coordinated Care Program* (CCP). Enacted in January 1992, CCP was intended to improve military health care business practices (Jennings, 1993). The effects of CCP were modest. However, they led to a more dramatic change in military health care. This program change was called TRICARE and it created considerable turbulence in the DoD health program. TRICARE was phased in worldwide over 3 years. Implementation began in the Pacific Northwest in March 1995; it was completed in June 1998, when the Northeastern region converted to TRICARE (Stoloff, Lurie, Goldberg, & Almendarez, 2000).

## THE BIRTH OF TRICARE

Like civilian managed care programs, TRICARE was implemented to reduce cost, preserve quality, and improve access to care. To achieve these goals, military health care resources from the Army, Navy, and Air Force were better integrated to create a more robust "direct care" system in military hospitals and clinics. Concurrently, direct care capabilities were supplemented by contracting with civilian providers to create "purchased care" networks (Gidwani et al., 2005).

Unlike civilian health care systems, TRICARE has a fourth mandate related to military operations or readiness. Active-duty military personnel must be in good health to ensure they can rapidly deploy anywhere in the world. Deployments could be for humanitarian reasons, as exemplified by the military assistance with the aftermath of hurricane Katrina that crippled the Gulf coast in August 2005. Deployments could also be for reasons of national security such as the war in Iraq. The readiness mandate typically has a profound effect on active-duty health care personnel. They must juggle meeting patient care needs while remaining proficient in their deployment roles. In addition, as health care personnel are deployed, there are fewer staff available to care for beneficiaries in the United States.

### TRICARE Program Options

TRICARE offers eligible military beneficiaries three insurance options. The centerpiece of the program, *TRICARE Prime*, is modeled after health maintenance organizations (HMOs). Active-duty personnel are automatically enrolled in TRICARE Prime at an MTF. Family members and retirees who choose TRICARE Prime may get their care through the civilian provider network or at the MTF, depending on capacity and provider availability. The other two TRICARE choices are an FFS option known as *TRICARE Standard* and a preferred provider organization (PPO) option known as *TRICARE Extra*. Each of the three TRICARE options differs with regard to enrollment requirements, out-of-pocket expenses, and the amount of government subsidy (Gidwani et al., 2005; IOM, 2002).

### Broken Health Care Promises

Concurrent with implementing TRICARE, the entire U.S. military was being downsized. As a consequence, the care limitations specified in Title 10 related to "space available" were put into play for the first time. This made it increasingly difficult for military retirees—a vocal and politically active group—to obtain health care in military facilities. Although beneficiaries typically hold TRICARE responsible for triggering the space-available clause, it was really the confluence of three factors—TRICARE implementation, manpower reductions, and BRAC decisions—that contributed to the change.

Regardless of the genesis, beneficiaries considered the activation of the space-available clause as breaching promises made to them when they entered active duty. Military service members believed they were entitled to "free" health care for life if they completed at least 20 years of service. It is not only older military retirees who are quick to address these broken promises. Present-day active-duty personnel comment that they expect to

have "full medical benefits" when they retire. As active-duty service members watch promised benefits change, however, they also acknowledge that "Congress can change that contract whenever they want to" (Jennings et al., in review).

### TRICARE TODAY

TRICARE currently provides health care to just over 9.1 million beneficiaries (Table 13-8). The direct care system involves numerous military facilities. These include 70 hospitals and medical centers, 18 of which are outside the United States, and 411 outpatient medical clinics, 102 of which are outside the United States. In addition, there are 417 dental clinics that provide care to active-duty personnel and 259 veterinary facilities. A total of 90,000 military personnel and 40,800 civilians staff these various TRICARE facilities (Gidwani et al., 2005).

Since its inception in 1995, TRICARE has evolved in substantial ways, four of which are highlighted here. Each of these illustrates the complexity of a health program governed by legislative action. Each also reflects important health policy implications.

1. *Improving access to care for active-duty personnel who live away from military facilities.*

   First, the FY 1998 NDAA directed DoD to provide a TRICARE Prime–like benefit to active-duty

**TABLE 13-8** Beneficiaries Available for Military Health Care in FY 2004 by Beneficiary Category

| BENEFICIARY CATEGORY | ELIGIBLE BENEFICIARIES* |
|---|---|
| Active duty | 1.81 |
| Active-duty family members | 2.41 |
| Retirees and family members <65 | 3.22 |
| Retirees and family members >65 | 1.72 |
| TOTAL | 9.16 |

Based on information in Gidwani, P. G., Bannick, R. R., Lurie, P., Goldberg, L., Kimko, D. D., et al. (2005). *Evaluation of the TRICARE Program. FY 2005 report to Congress.* Compiled by Altarum Institute, the Institute for Defense Analyses, and Mathematic Policy Research Institute on behalf of the Health Program Analysis and Evaluation Directorate, TRICARE Management Activity (TMA/HPA&E) in the Office of the Assistant Secretary of Defense (Health Affairs).

*In millions.

military personnel nationwide who were located more than a 1-hour's drive or 50 miles from an MTF. This program, known as TRICARE Prime Remote (TPR), went into effect October 1, 1999 (Stoloff et al., 2000).

Typical users of TPR are individuals assigned to recruiting and the Reserve Officers Training Corps (ROTC) programs. For example, because of BRAC decisions in years past, recruiters in Mobile, Alabama no longer have a military facility nearby. Likewise, many college campuses sponsoring ROTC programs are a distance from MTFs. Without TPR these individuals did not have reasonable access to care. The 2001 NDAA expanded TPR to all Uniformed Services. Family members of active-duty personnel were not included in the original 1998 legislation. NDAA-01 therefore also expanded the TPR benefit to families who accompany active-duty service members to the remote site (Stoloff et al., 2000).

2. *Keeping the promise of lifelong health care to retirees and their family members.*

Secondly, major TRICARE changes pertaining to Medicare-eligible military beneficiaries resulted from the 2001 NDAA. These changes were viewed as "the single greatest legislative victory for military retirees in 50 years" (Schwartz & Chaffee, 2002, p. 132). The bill enacted by this legislation was intended to rectify the broken promises to retirees in response to the lack of space-available care. Signed into law in October 2000, the bill mandated two programs to substantially expand benefits.

Through TRICARE for Life (TFL), which went into effect October 1, 2001, TRICARE became the second payer to Medicare for benefits covered by both Medicare and TRICARE. DoD beneficiaries eligible for Medicare can use TFL if they purchase Part B coverage. They are not eligible for TRICARE Prime, but they may use MTFs on a space-available basis, as well as Medicare, network, and nonnetwork providers. Of the 1.83 million DoD beneficiaries age 65 or over eligible for care in FY 2004, 1.65 million qualified for TFL because they had Part B coverage under Medicare (Gidwani et al., 2005; The Retired Officers' Association [TROA], 2001).

TRICARE senior pharmacy (TSRx), the second program, began in April 2001. It provides access to a full pharmacy benefit through either direct care

MTFs or purchased care in civilian facilities including contracted network pharmacies and a national mail order program (Gidwani et al., 2005; TROA, 2001). The cost of prescription drugs is rising faster than any other service offered by TRICARE, increasing by 40% from fiscal year 2002 to fiscal year 2004. It is noteworthy that only 9% of this increase is attributable to TSRx (Gidwani et al., 2005).

3. *Better administrative support to improve quality care and customer service.*

The third substantial change since the inception of TRICARE occurred in 2004. It pertained to the overall structure of TRICARE, principally the next generation of contracts. Known as TRICARE Next Generation (TNEX), the goals of these competitively awarded contracts concern sustaining high-quality care and improving customer service (Gidwani et al., 2005).

The most visible change from TNEX was the reduction of TRICARE regions from 12 to 3. The Western region is headquartered in San Diego, California, and TriWest Healthcare Alliance Corporation is the contractor partnered to supplement MTF care. The Southern region is headquartered in San Antonio, Texas, where Humana Military Healthcare Services was awarded the contract. Washington, DC is the headquarters for the Northern region, in partnership with Health Net Federal Services as the contractor. The effects of this transition remain to be determined.

4. *Expanding the beneficiary population.*

Finally, the number of TRICARE beneficiaries is growing. In 1998, when TRICARE implementation was completed worldwide, the eligible beneficiary population was about 8.3 million (Stoloff et al., 2000). By 2004 the beneficiary population had increased to 9.2 million, largely because of the activation of Guard and Reserve personnel in support of deployments related to national security (e.g., the global war on terrorism) as well as for humanitarian purposes (e.g., Indonesian tsunami relief). Military health benefits are now also available to the families of mobilized Guard and Reserve personnel (Gidwani et al., 2005). The number of health care personnel has not expanded, however.

This growing demand for care is occurring amid a diminishing supply of military hospitals, clinics, and health care personnel. Although DoD benefici-aries can get care in civilian health care facilities, not all health care providers will accept TRICARE patients because of the reimbursement rates. Language in the NDAA-04 mandated a market area survey to assess why providers were not accepting TRICARE patients. About 28% of the physicians who responded from the first markets surveyed indicated the problem was largely related to reim-bursement (Gidwani et al., 2005; MOAA, 2005a). TRICARE Standard reimbursement rates are tied to Medicare rates by law, a law believed to be based on a flawed formula (Medicare and TRICARE rates on block, 2005).

## BUDGET BATTLES: THE FUTURE OF TRICARE

Concerns about the cost of care were a strong cata-lyst leading to the creation of the TRICARE program. These same concerns will most likely shape the future of DoD health care because the cost of care continues to rise. In 2001 the DoD health budget was about $16 billion (Shelton, 2001). Expenditures in the Unified Medical Program (UMP), unadjusted for inflation, increased from $26.7 billion in 2003 (6.7% of the defense budget) to $30.4 billion in 2004 (a UMP growth of 13.4%). Estimates project UMP expenditures of $31 billion for 2005 (estimated at 7.6% of the defense budget), or a doubling of TRICARE costs since 2001. These increases are largely attributable to costs associated with TFL (Gidwani et al., 2005).

### Resource Wars

Budget battles pit DoD health care programs, weapons systems, and military manpower against one another. These battles were illustrated in an April 14, 2005 *New York Times* article. Despite TRICARE's goal of reducing or stabilizing the cost of care, the *Times'* projections are that TRICARE will soon claim more than 10% of the Defense budget, with 75% of the benefits going to retirees and veterans (Weiner, 2005). The Assistant Secretary of Defense for Health Affairs, Dr. William Winkenwerder Jr., concurred with this assessment, noting that if current trends are not abated, 75% to 80% of DoD health care funds will be spent on

caring for retirees and their family members (Gilmore, 2005).

### Victory or Defeat?

It appears that "the single greatest legislative victory for military retirees in 50 years" (Schwartz & Chaffee, 2002, p. 132) is now threatened. Interest groups such as the MOAA are speaking out to guard and protect health care benefits. Members of Congress are also taking a stand. For example, SASC Chairman Senator John Warner (R-VA) supports meeting obligations for the three competing needs—health care, weapons, and personnel. Other individuals argue that retiree health care does not reap a readiness benefit. MOAA mounts a counter-ing view by reminding Congress that, in the recent past, senior military officials such as the Joint Chiefs of Staff supported TFL and urged Congress to remedy military retiree health care problems because the perceived broken promises were exacting a toll on active-duty retention (TFL under fire, 2005). According to a former Chairman of the Joint Chiefs of Staff, "it is imperative to establish a method for funding health care benefits for retirees and their families in such a manner that this funding no longer competes with funding for operations, force struc-ture, and readiness. This will ensure that we always honor the national commitment we made long ago to our military retirees" (Shelton, 2001, pp. 57-58.)

A number of policy questions are embedded in these arguments. They range from issues specific to DoD structure to general issues about health care in the United States. They point out that managed care is not a panacea for controlling costs. They illustrate the increased consumption of health care resources by an aging population. They underscore that turmoil, tension, and tradeoffs are growing in all health care sectors.

### Sacrifice and Service to the Nation

Like civilian retirees who are expressing outrage as they watch promised health benefits dwindle (Barry, 2005), DoD beneficiaries are also infuriated about the possibility of losing an earned benefit. The anger is fueled by the lives of sacrifice and service expected of military personnel and their families. "We give our soldiers, sailors, airmen, and

Marines tremendous responsibility, and we put them in stressful and often dangerous environments thousands of miles away from home" (Shelton, 2001, p. 56). Often absent from civilian jobs is the life of "service and sacrifice defending the United States through multiple hot and cold wars" (TFL under fire, 2005, p. 26).

Emotional? Perhaps. But military personnel do what few Americans do—they support and defend the Constitution of the United States. In doing so, they may risk their lives and their health. As a consequence, they expect health care for themselves and their families when they retire (Jennings et al., in review; Jennings, Loan, Heiner, Hemman, & Swanson, 2004). In the words of military beneficiaries:

*I [expect military health care] to live up to what they told me when I entered boot camp. If you stay in the [military], you're going to have health care for life.* (60-year-old retired male officer)

*If I give the [military] 20 years of my life…I could be deployed anywhere, I could be fighting in a couple different wars. I'll give my life to this country and…I expect to be taken care of once I'm through. …I'm expecting full medical benefits when I retire.* (29-year-old male officer)

*My husband [who served 2 years in Viet Nam] and I…served 24 years in a field where he was gone most of the time, and our whole family sacrificed for this. That was a promise made in 1967, when he joined, that we were going to have health care for the rest of our lives.* (54-year-old female spouse of a retired officer)

## SUMMARY

Competing priorities—health care, weapon systems, or military manpower? What is the best way to balance these expensive programs? What modifications could be made to military health care to make it more cost effective? How much health care do military beneficiaries deserve? Who should be entitled to health care—active-duty personnel, retirees, families? These are the policy issues that are being debated now. These policy issues highlight the collision of finite resources and complex health care needs.

## Key Points

- The U.S. DoD operates one of the largest federal health systems—the MHS.
- Concerns about the cost of care were a strong catalyst leading to the creation of the TRICARE program—a managed care system in the MHS.
- The U.S. MHS has a dual mission—to provide high-quality health care to all eligible patients and to provide high-quality combat care for active-duty service members.

## Web Resources

> **TRICARE**
> *http://tricare.osd.mil*

## REFERENCES

Barry, P. (2005). Anxiety zone. Will the new Medicare law encourage employers to drop or keep their retiree drug plans? *AARP Bulletin, 26*(2), 14-17.

Dao, J. (2005, August 26). Taps plays for a hospital that tended all ranks. *New York Times*, A16.

Gidwani, P. G., Bannick, R. R., Lurie, P., Goldberg, L., Kimko, D. D., et al. (2005). *Evaluation of the TRICARE Program. FY 2005 report to Congress.* Compiled by Altarum Institute, the Institute for Defense Analyses, and Mathematic Policy Research Institute on behalf of the Health Program Analysis and Evaluation Directorate, TRICARE Management Activity (TMA/HPA&E) in the Office of the Assistant Secretary of Defense (Health Affairs).

Gilmore, G. J. (2005, February 4). DoD health care spending doubled in past four years. *MedNews*, article MN05406.

GlobalSecurity.org. (2005). Base Realignment and Closure (BRAC). Retrieved September 1, 2005, from *www.globalsecurity.org/military/facility/brac.htm*.

Institute of Medicine (IOM). (2002). *Leadership by example. Coordinating government roles in improving health care quality.* Washington, DC: National Academies Press.

Jennings, B. M. (1993). Nursing implications of the Department of Defense Coordinated Care Program. *Military Medicine, 158,* 823-827.

Jennings, B. M., Loan, L. A., Heiner, S., Hemman, E. A., & Swanson, K. M. (2004). *Expectations of military health care: An inductive analysis.* (Final report for Proposal N00-023). Bethesda, MD: TriService Nursing Research Program.

Jennings, B. M., Swanson, K. M., Heiner, S., Loan, L. A., & Hemman, E. A. (In review). *Health care experiences and expectations of military beneficiaries.* Manuscript submitted for publication.

Medicare and TRICARE rates on block. (2005, August). *Military Officer,* 30.

Military Officers Association of American (MOAA). (2005a, February 4). Legislative update. Retrieved April 28, 2005, from *legis@moaa.org*.

Military Officers Association of American (MOAA). (2005b, May 13). Legislative update. Retrieved May 16, 2005, from *legis@moaa.org*.

Military Officers Association of American (MOAA). (2005c, June 17). Legislative update. Retrieved June 17, 2005, from *legis@moaa.org* and *www.moaa.org*.

Schwartz, S. M., & Chaffee, M. W. (2002). Policy spotlight. Success through unity: A coalition's efforts to expand the U. S. Military Health Program. In D. J. Mason, J. K. Leavitt, & M. W. Chaffee (Eds.), *Policy and politics in nursing and health care* (ed 4). St. Louis: Saunders.

Shelton, H. (2001). Defense health care. The way ahead. *Retired Officer Magazine*, 53-58. Retrieved September 1, 2005, from *www.troa.org*.

Stoloff, P. H., Lurie, P. H., Goldberg, L., & Almendarez, M. (2000). *Evaluation of the TRICARE Program. FY 2000 Report to Congress.*

TFL under fire. (2005, June). *Military Officer*, 26.

The Retired Officer's Association (TROA). (2001). TRICARE for Life. The road to honoring health care commitments. *The Retired Officers Magazine*. Retrieved September 1, 2005, from *www.troa.org*.

Weiner, T. (2005, April 14). A new call to arms: Military health care. *New York Times*, C1.

# POLICYSPOTLIGHT

# THE U.S. VETERANS ADMINISTRATION: POLICY CHANGE FOR THE GREATER GOOD IN AN INTEGRATED HEALTH SYSTEM

Cathy Rick & Susan Pendergrass

*"If we keep on doin' what we always done, we'll keep on gettin' what we always got."*

BARBARA LYONS

Although every staff nurse is responsible for the quality and safety of care he or she provides to individual patients, it is equally important for all staff to understand and uphold organizational goals and initiatives. This organizational stewardship requires an understanding of the context of care and related internal and external forces that influence executive-level dilemmas and decisions. Putting things in context helps us all understand the "greater good"—how our individual work contributes to the profession and the health care industry as a whole.

## OVERVIEW OF THE VETERANS HEALTH ADMINISTRATION

The Veterans Health Administration (VHA) is a component of the highly complex governmental system that serves multiple stakeholders. Influenced by the dynamic complexities of the health care industry, the VHA operates within a highly political environment. The Department of Veterans Affairs (VA) is a part of the Executive Branch, governed by statute and regulations with oversight from Congressional committees, the General Accountability Office (GAO), and Executive Branch offices such as the Office of Personnel Management (OPM) and Office of Management and Budget (OMB). The Secretary of the VA is the highest-ranking official, and the Under Secretary for Health (USH) heads the VHA. Veterans Service Organizations are national representatives of the Veterans we serve, and each of the various organizations has a vested interest in the programs, services, and locations of the VA health care delivery system. In addition, professional organizations and labor organizations play a role in the "poly politics" of our health care system (Box 13-10).

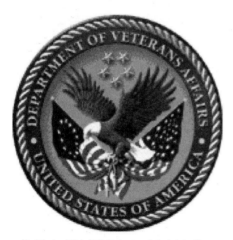

Emblem of the U.S. Veterans Administration.

## A Call for Comprehensive Change

Significant changes in health care delivery over the past decade have created the need to revitalize and reorganize the VA health care infrastructure to better serve our nation's veterans. As the largest integrated health care delivery systems in the world, the VA faces complex institutional and cultural challenges to keep pace with the demands associated with delivering care to over seven million enrolled veterans. These challenges drive the Capital Assets and Realignment for Enhanced Services (CARES) process, which is the most comprehensive review of the VA health care infrastructure ever conducted. The VA's mission to provide high-quality health care for America's veterans will never change. But how that care is provided—at what kind of facilities, where these facilities are located, and which medical procedures are used—must change over time.

---

**BOX 13-10**    Key External Oversight Bodies of the U.S. Veterans Health Administration

### GOVERNMENT ACCOUNTABILITY OFFICE

The Government Accountability Office (GAO) is an agency that works for Congress and the American people. Congress asks the GAO to study the programs and expenditures of the federal government. The GAO, commonly called the "investigative arm of Congress" or the "congressional watchdog," is independent and nonpartisan. It studies how the federal government spends taxpayer dollars. The GAO advises Congress and the heads of executive agencies (such as the Environmental Protection Agency [EPA], Department of Defense [DoD], and Department of Health and Human Services [HHS]) about ways to make government more effective and responsive. The GAO evaluates federal programs, audits federal expenditures, and issues legal opinions. When the GAO reports its findings to Congress, it recommends actions. *(www.gao.gov)*

### OFFICE OF MANAGEMENT AND BUDGET

The Office of Management and Budget (OMB) assists the president in the development and execution of his policies and programs. The OMB has a hand in the development and resolution of all budget, policy, legislative, regulatory, procurement, e-government, and management issues on behalf of the president. The OMB is composed of divisions organized either by agency and program area or by functional responsibilities. However, the work of the OMB often requires a broad exposure to issues and programs outside of the direct area of assigned responsibility. *(www.whitehouse.gov/omb)*

### OFFICE OF PERSONNEL MANAGEMENT

It is the job of the Office of Personnel Management (OPM) to build a high-quality and diverse federal workforce, based on merit system principles. The OPM works with the president, Congress, departments and agencies, and other stakeholders to implement human capital policies. OPM provides these federal departments and agencies with policies and guidance on managing human capital. *(www.opm.gov)*

### VETERANS SERVICE ORGANIZATIONS

Veteran Service Organizations (VSOs) consist of varied community-service organizations. The purpose of these organizations is to help foster, encourage, and promote programs serving veterans. There are multiple VSOs, each having a focused mission supporting diverse needs of disabled and war veterans and their dependents, including the widows and orphans of deceased veterans. *(www.va.gov/vso)*

The National CARES plan responds to this changing need. CARES enhances the VA's ability to offer greater access to high-quality health care closer to where most veterans live. To accomplish this in the environment of limited resources, it is critical to eliminate duplicate clinical and administrative services at VA facilities, increase efficiencies, and allow reinvestment of financial savings.

The CARES review process resulted in recommendations to consolidate services at 40 facilities—18 with small workload volume and 22 within close geographic proximity to other facilities or with multiple campuses. These changes have been referred to as "facility mission changes." Proposals projected a 42% reduction in vacant space, with demolition and divestiture as the primary methods to reduce vacant space. It was found that maintaining excess buildings and land required the VA to use medical care appropriations that could otherwise be used to provide direct medical care (Report to the Secretary of Veterans Affairs, 2004).

## HISTORY OF THE VETERANS AFFAIRS HEALTH SYSTEM

Until the mid 1990s the VHA operated largely as a hospital system, providing general medical and surgical services, specialized care in mental health and spinal cord injury, and long-term care (Perlin, Kolodner, & Roswell, 2004). VHA infrastructure and support facilities, many built in the aftermath of World War II, are not all configured for contemporary health care delivery, and some are no longer appropriately located. Moreover, with an average age exceeding 50 years, these buildings are becoming more costly to maintain. The CARES process is intended to address these issues, strategically realigning capital assets to enhance the health care infrastructure to better meet veterans' needs over the next 20 years (Perlin et al., 2004).

With a realignment of its more than 170 medical centers into Veteran Integrated Service Networks (VISNs), the VA sought to reinvent itself as a model system characterized by patient-centered, high-quality, high-value health care. VHA senior officials began this process by using many of the Baldrige principles of organizational improvement. A clear vision for the organization was developed, with an urgent desire to move away from traditional ways of doing business. A performance-based measurement system was introduced that both charged VISN leadership with clear expectations as well as reinforced key organizational priorities. This reinvention mandated structural and organizational changes, prioritization of resource allocation, and systems that would increasingly support the needs of patients, clinicians, and administrators. From 1995 to 2003, system-wide hospital admissions dropped from over 900,000 to 600,000 and outpatient visits rose from approximately 25 million to over 50 million annually.

## BALANCING POLICY AND POLITICS FOR SYSTEM-WIDE PLANNING

It is important to note that capital asset realignment does not occur in isolation; rather, many preparatory actions must occur before the organization initiates actions of this magnitude. The VA's strategic and capital planning must respond to governmental and budgetary timelines that have been a challenge to align internally. In the budget and capital planning process, the VHA must first complete internal assessments and develop local, regional, and national proposals. Proposals are analyzed and priorities identified, then a comprehensive plan is submitted as part of our annual congressional budget submission. The VA's capital and operations budget is obtained through congressional and presidential authorization. The OMB, within the presidential executive branch, requires budget submissions to clearly describe links to measurable outcomes (Performance and Accountability Report). These requirements demand extensive review and oversight in order to assure compliance with Congressional expectations for budget submissions.

Congress had become reluctant to provide capital funds without an established departmental strategic capital plan. Likewise in 1999 the GAO published a report critical of overhead cost for vacant VA space. These two factors and the organizational realignment of health care delivery provided the organizational readiness to begin a comprehensive capital asset assessment. Further urgency was felt as the agency determined that the life cycle replacement of its capital assets if completed at the current rate of congressional budget investment would take over 155 years.

In order to meet the demands of increasing and shifting (inpatient to outpatient) demand, the VA began to identify what types of facilities in what locations and which medical services were necessary in this evolving environment. The VHA priority was to provide expanded services in an outpatient environment and access to this care. Veterans and their service organizations and congressional representatives began to provide feedback concerning dissatisfaction with the need to travel long distances for primary care, the inability to obtain convenient appointments, and the lack of coordination of varied appointments, which necessitated numerous visits. The VHA refined its organizational priority to improve access to care by setting target goals and began an investment in establishing community-based outpatient clinics.

## CHARTING THE COURSE THROUGH THE CARES PLAN

The national CARES plan responds to the organizational priority of reorganization of care. CARES enhances the VA's ability to offer improved access to high-quality health care closer to where most veterans live and supports continuity of care for veterans served through a complete assessment of capital resources and alignment of these resources with enrollment and service use projections.

With an aging infrastructure of facilities (many were built in the 1940s) and the need to expand ambulatory and outreach programs, each of the more than 170 VA medical centers was charged with developing future-oriented proposals and plans to execute a transformation of assets and services. The system of 22 regional networks of integrated medical centers was used to develop a local approach to designing efficient and effective approaches for these plans. Before this, each medical center operated in a fairly isolated fashion without requirements to reduce duplication of services or coordinate programs with other VA medical centers in their general locale.

## CHALLENGES IN THE CARES PLANNING PROCESS

Although most stakeholders, VA leadership, and VISN personnel agreed on the need for some changes in the system, the challenges began with determining the necessary changes and weighing the impact of those changes at the local level. VA has some "built-in barriers" to change rooted in its decentralized operating model and the organizational boundaries that constitute the VISN structure. The organization of the VISNs, each having independent budgets and goals, does not always promote inter-VISN referral processes, communication, or cooperation. An additional barrier to change at the VISN level is the natural inclination toward preserving the status quo and the absence of real incentives for VISN leadership to change. Maintaining the status quo responds to stakeholder and community pressure to maintain a system, specific facilities, and methods of providing services that are familiar to veterans, staff, and others. This resistance to change is also based on fear of the unknown and of possibly losing services at local VA facilities. In addition, change can mean a loss of VA and community jobs or a shift in the configuration or location of VA staff (Report to the Secretary of Veterans Affairs, 2004).

### A Pilot Test of the CARES Process

The first step in the CARES process was a pilot project within one of the VISNs. A VISN in the Midwest region was chosen, as it had four large facilities in very close proximity, it had great need to modernize these facilities if they were to remain open, it served an area in which the veteran population was projected to decline, and the current budgets could not continue to meet infrastructure maintenance and service demand. Therefore this called into question the need for the current capital investment. As the agency began this pilot there was great concern from all stakeholders that this realignment would withdraw services from the local area. Both congressional representatives and advocacy groups began campaigns to influence the outcome of the pilot.

## PLANNING FOR NATIONWIDE IMPLEMENTATION AND EXTERNAL REVIEW

The pilot was conducted twice—first using an outside consultant, then again with an internal workgroup. The first consultant report was not seen by stakeholder groups as credible because of the consultant's perceived lack of understanding of the uniqueness of the organization and the healthcare needs of veterans, and the robustness of their financial analyses was questioned. Although the capital plan of the internal workgroup validated the basic conclusions of the first report, it refined and tailored the implementation steps and was finally accepted. What we learned from this pilot was that stakeholder communication was critical. We also needed a more standardized costing process and a more comprehensive forecasting model.

The next step in the process was to launch into a full assessment of all capital investments in the remaining VISNs. This was no small task for the agency. The VA, while relying on the health care administration to drive the planning initiative, also brought into the planning process its other divisions, Veterans Benefits and National Cemetery Administrations. Planning coordinators also used the opportunity to include potential partners such as the Department of Defense (DoD) into the process to ensure that all local capital asset sharing opportunities were identified and considered. The initial phase of the CARES process included an assessment of over 118 million square feet in 5044 buildings, with properties having an average age of 50.4 years. Although the VA is a national system and some standardization across the system is required, health care delivery and capital structure for this care is influenced by regional practice and referral patterns among the facilities within a geographic area. To be responsive to this the VA first looked at veteran population enrollment projections. The VISNs were then required to establish service market areas from which they could begin their assessment and planning actions. The markets were locally determined, taking into consideration geography, current assets within the area, and the levels of veteran population within the area that could sustain the need for services.

When conducting capital asset assessments, it is important to take into consideration that alterations in these investments involve many steps that require significant lead time. The VA obtains its capital budget from a separate congressional appropriation, and in the recent past this has not been sufficient to fund high-priority projects (only a half dozen major construction projects were started within a given year). In addition, projects take multiple years to be completed; therefore any capital planning activity must factor in this lead time as well as the scope of the project to meet future service needs. The VA used a 20-year planning cycle in CARES. Because the agency would need to assess staging of projects and the trend of service demand, it used 10- and 20-year projection planning horizons. This enabled the agency to assess how near term enrollment, use, and capital inventory would need to be addressed. Learning from the pilot, the agency invested in improving the demand forecast model. The model was refined to address reliance on VHA care, as many veterans have other health care options such as Medicare. It also adjusted for age, gender, mortality, morbidity, and migration patterns within its population and modeled against private and managed care practice patterns to name just a few factors within the actuarial model. As the VA used this model, both congressional and stakeholder groups questioned the validity of the model. This was more pronounced in areas in which the model showed a decline in the veteran population, and utilization projections therefore forced consideration in the plans for fewer or realignment of services. The model was presented at numerous congressional oversight hearings, and independent reviews of the model were conducted by these groups. Both found that it was a reasonable model from which to conduct capital planning, even as they recommended areas for improvement. These improvement recommendations were then incorporated into the next year's model projections.

## COMPLEX INTERNAL STEPS FOR IMPLEMENTATION

Steps in the CARES process included that the VISNs assess the existing capital investment through a comprehensive on-site visual examination, assign space to specific functions, and complete a standardized space assessment, from which gaps in service and capital were identified. Although stakeholders were not actively included in this assessment process, they were kept informed of the process through national and regional status reports. Once the specific planning initiatives were finalized by the VISNs, they were presented to the Under Secretary for Health for review and, when endorsed, sent to the Secretary, Department of Veterans Affairs for approval. It was during this process that it became apparent to the VA national leaders that in some VISNs capital initiatives that would require significant realignment were not always fully considered and brought forward. VISNs were required to rework their local plan. This led to stakeholder concerns, and once the plans were announced many stakeholders objected to the fact that they had not been actively involved or been given the ability to comment on specific plans.

## MORE FEEDBACK FROM EXTERNAL STAKEHOLDERS

With the increased stakeholder concern, advocacy groups began to petition their congressional representatives, and the capital planning process was in jeopardy. In response to significant stakeholder concern, the Secretary of the VA chartered a CARES Commission under the Federal Advisory Act. This Act formally establishes a process by which a federal leader can obtain stakeholder recommendations and mandates a process by which open public input is obtained. The CARES Commission examined the CARES planning process and the initiatives from this planning process and conducted regional and market public hearings in which local stakeholders were able to provide testimony. The following six factors were applied in the Commission's deliberations:

1. Impact on veterans' access to care
2. Impact on health care quality
3. Veteran and stakeholder views
4. Impact on the community
5. Impact on VA missions and goals
6. Cost to government

The Commission's year of intensive review of the VA plans to realign its infrastructure included 81 site visits to VA and DoD medical facilities and State Veterans Homes, 38 public hearings, 10 public meetings, and analysis of more than 212,000 comments received from veterans and stakeholders nationwide. The 16 commissioners unanimously agreed that the CARES process advances the VA's efforts to provide high-quality health care for the veterans it serves (Report to the Secretary of Veterans Affairs, 2004).

## NEXT STEPS

The Commission formally presented its findings to the VA Secretary through its recommendations on each of the VISN market plans. The Secretary was not bound by the Commission's decisions. He reviewed all decisions, visited many of the sites in which major conflict existed with regard to the plans, then published his final decisions. The CARES plan then became the blueprint from which the agency developed the congressionally required 5-year capital plan. Congress endorsed the CARES plan by requiring capital appropriation to fund the recommendations in the proposed CARES plan. Several facility plans remained in question, and Congress has ensured its ability to intervene in certain sites by requiring notification of any change in mission, realignment, or administrative changes. Thus the political interface continues even as the overall plan has been accepted.

## SUMMARY

The CARES planning initiative occurred over a 3-year period. What it accomplished was a full assessment of the current status of the agency's capital investments, identification of partnership opportunities with community and other federal agencies, and identification of gaps in service alignment and capital needs. Despite a good foundation in the dynamic environment of health care, this assessment will soon be either obsolete or not implemented unless further actions occur. The assessment needs to be incorporated into normal planning and business processes. The VHA has made the commitment to an annual update of the actuarial model and has taken the recommendations from the various stakeholder groups to improve the mental health service forecast model to better reflect the unique mental health services the VA provides. The long-term care model is also to be improved. The agency is currently in the process of realigning its planning process such that its capital planning can be more closely integrated into its budget and strategic planning process.

"The methodology developed for the CARES process will serve as a strategic resource for years to come on managing and realigning capital assts nationwide. In particular, this blueprint, with the refinements brought by the Commission's review, provides the underpinnings for an approach for medical care appropriations to more appropriately be used for providing direct medical care to our nation's veterans, rather than for maintaining outdated or underused infrastructure. Moreover, VA, by establishing a sound approach to realigning assets, has moved into a leadership role among other government agencies confronting similar issues" (Principi, 2004).

## Key Points

- The Department of Veterans Affairs Capital Asset Realignment for Enhanced Services (CARES) program is the VA's effort to produce a logical national plan for modernizing health care facilities.

- The influence of external stakeholders is significant in moving an organization forward, and they should be incorporated throughout major change processes.

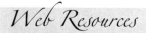

## Web Resources

**Department of Veterans Affairs CARES Business Plan Studies**
*www.va.gov/cares*
**U.S. Veterans Administration**
*www.va.gov*
**U.S. Veterans Health Administration**
*www.vha.gov*

### REFERENCES

Perlin, J., Kolodner, R., & Roswell, R. (2004). The Veterans Health Administration: Quality, value, accountability, and information as transforming strategies for patient-centered care. *American Journal of Managed Care, 10*(11), 828-836.

Principi, A. J. (2004, February). *CARES Commission Capitol asset realignment for enhanced services: Report to the Secretary of Veterans Affairs.* Washington, DC.

# POLICYSPOTLIGHT

## SUCCESSES AND STRUGGLES IN COMPLEMENTARY HEALTH CARE

Mary Jo Kreitzer

*"Society, community, family are all conserving institutions. They try to maintain stability, and to prevent, or at least to slow down, change."*
PETER F. DRUCKER

Consumer demand for complementary therapies has increased dramatically over the past 10 years. According to data released in 2004 by the Centers for Disease Control and Prevention, 62% of adults in the United States used some form of complementary or alternative medicine (CAM) therapy during the 12 months preceding the survey (Barnes, Powell-Griner, McFann, & Nahin, 2004). The most commonly used therapies were prayer, natural products such as herbs and nutritional supplements, deep-breathing exercises, meditation, chiropractic care, yoga, massage, and diet-based therapies. Consistent with other studies (Astin, 1998; Eisenberg et al., 1998), this study found that the majority of people use CAM as a complement to conventional biomedicine, not as an alternative. Reasons commonly cited for using complementary therapies include compatibility with personal values, desire to be actively involved with decision-making regarding care, dissatisfaction with conventional care or a perception that conventional care cannot adequately address symptoms or health conditions, and a preference for care that is more attentive to the whole person—body, mind, and spirit.

With the growth in the use of complementary therapies, many policy issues have surfaced that affect nurses, consumers, and health care organizations. Major issues include access to care and reimbursement for services, education and credentialing of providers, regulation of practice, funding of research, consumer education, and the creation of integrated care delivery systems.

The field commonly referred to as CAM is large, complex, and diverse. It is estimated to include over 1800 different therapies such as guided imagery, healing touch, and herbal medicine as well as culturally based systems of healing including traditional Chinese medicine, Ayurveda, homeopathy, and naturopathy. Even the title used to describe this continuum of healing approaches is laden with controversy and political considerations.

For many years the term *alternative medicine* was used to describe these healing approaches. They were viewed as part of the "counterculture" and often used in lieu of conventional care. The term itself implies an either-or mentality. As it became more apparent that these healing approaches were used in conjunction with conventional care, the phrase *complementary medicine* began to emerge. Although accurate for some consumers, others would argue that complementary approaches for conditions such as pain and stress management are primary and that the term *complementary* inaccurately and inappropriately deemphasizes their contribution and importance.

Within the discipline of medicine the preferred term is *integrative medicine*. The Consortium of Academic Health Centers for Integrative Medicine (CAHCIM), an organization of 29 medical schools, defines integrative medicine as "the practice of medicine that reaffirms the importance of the relationship between practitioner and patient, focuses on the whole person, is informed by evidence, and makes use of all appropriate therapeutic approaches, health care professionals and disciplines to achieve optimal health and healing" (CAHCIM, 2005). This definition is broad in that it could refer to any type of practitioner and patient and it highlights the importance of relationship-centered and whole-person care. Within the nursing literature, *complementary* or *integrative* therapies and healing practices are the terms more commonly used. For many in nursing, the term *medicine* is associated with the discipline and practice of medicine and therefore is not an acceptable term for a broad range of healing approaches practiced by many different types of health care professionals. In this chapter the terms *complementary therapies* and *CAM* are used interchangeably, given that CAM is the acronym or phrase most commonly used in national policy documents as well as the National Institutes of Health (NIH).

## USE OF COMPLEMENTARY THERAPIES WITHIN NURSING

The use of holistic approaches in nursing is not new. In fact, much of what is called "complementary therapy" has been within the domain of nursing for centuries. In her *Notes on Nursing*, published in 1860, Florence Nightingale described nursing as a holistic and integrated pursuit. Nightingale advocated that the role of the nurse was to help the patient attain the best possible condition so that nature could act and self-healing could occur. In addition to emphasizing good hygiene and sanitation, she also wrote about the importance of fresh air, light, touch, diet, and spirituality (Dossey, 2000).

Although nursing has a long tradition of focusing on caring, healing, and wholeness, concerns have been raised about the visibility of nursing in the contemporary complementary therapies or integrative medicine movement. The noted absence of nursing leadership within many national initiatives, underrepresentation of nurses among investigators successfully obtaining funding from NIH, inadequate focus on complementary therapies in undergraduate and graduate curricula, reimbursement issues for nurses providing complementary therapies, and significant differences in how boards of nursing are addressing the inclusion of complementary therapies in nurse practice acts led a group of nurse leaders to convene the Gillette Nursing Summit in 2002 (Kreitzer & Disch, 2003). The proceedings described a set of strategies that focused on ways to better align and position nursing relative to the integrative health care movement, thus assuring a more visible presence in decision-making forums that are shaping the future of health care in the United States.

## NATIONAL INSTITUTES OF HEALTH

In response to growing public interest in and use of complementary therapies, the U.S. Congress passed in 1991 Public Law 102-170, which provided $2 million to NIH to establish an office and an advisory panel to recommend a research program that would focus on promising unconventional medical practices. In 1993, as part of the NIH Revitalization Act, the Office of Alternative Medicine (OAM) was established within the Office of the Director of NIH. The purpose of the Office was to facilitate the evaluation of alternative medical treatment modalities and to disseminate information to the public via an information clearinghouse. In 1998, Public Law 105-277, the Omnibus Consolidated and Emergency Supplemental Appropriations Act, elevated the status and expanded the mandate of the OAM by authorizing the establishment of the National Center for Complementary and Alternative Medicine (NCCAM). NCCAM is one of 27 institutes and centers that comprise NIH. The mission of NCCAM is to explore CAM in the context of rigorous science, train CAM researchers, and disseminate authoritative information to the public and health professionals. Funding for NCCAM has increased significantly since its inception, as reflected in the fiscal year (FY) 2005 budget of $123 million.

## THE WHITE HOUSE COMMISSION ON COMPLEMENTARY AND ALTERNATIVE MEDICINE POLICY

Within the past 5 years there have been two national policy initiatives, the White House Commission on Complementary and Alternative Medicine Policy (2002) and the Institute of Medicine (IOM) CAM study committee (2005). Nurses were appointed to serve as members of both of these groups, and nurses provided testimony in open hearings that were part of the deliberations of both of these groups. President William J. Clinton issued an executive order (Executive Order No. 13147) in March 2000 that established the White House Commission on Complementary and Alternative Medicine Policy (WHCCAMP). The primary task of the commission was to provide the Secretary of Health and Human Services (HHS) with legislative and administrative recommendations for "ensuring that public policy maximizes the potential benefits of CAM therapies to consumers" *(www.whccamp.hhs.gov/finalreport.html)*. The 20-member commission focused on four areas:

- Education and training of health care practitioners
- Coordination of research to increase knowledge about CAM products
- Provision of reliable and useful information on CAM to health professionals
- Provision of guidance on the appropriate access to and delivery of CAM

The 29 recommendations addressed CAM information development and dissemination, access and delivery of safe and effective CAM services, coverage and reimbursement, use of CAM to promote wellness and health, the importance of incorporating CAM information in the education of health professionals, and the need for coordinated federal efforts. The final recommendation was that the president, Secretary of HHS, or Congress create an office to coordinate federal CAM activities and to facilitate the integration into the nation's health care system of those complementary and alternative health care practices and products determined to be safe and effective. With a change in administration at the executive level and within Congress, there has not been a clear mandate for implementing the White House

Commission recommendations, although a number of them are being reviewed and acted on incrementally within various public and private organizations and bodies at federal and state levels. As various policy issues regarding complementary therapies are addressed in this chapter, relevant WHCCAMP recommendations will also be highlighted.

## INSTITUTE OF MEDICINE REPORT ON COMPLEMENTARY AND ALTERNATIVE MEDICINE

In 2002, 16 NIH institutes, centers, and offices and the Agency for Healthcare Research and Quality (AHRQ) asked the IOM to convene a study committee to explore scientific, policy, and practice questions that arise from the significant and increasing use of CAM therapies by the American public. The report (National Academy of Sciences, 2005) emphasized that decisions about the use of specific CAM therapies should primarily depend on whether they have been shown to be safe and effective. The committee concluded that the goal should be the provision of comprehensive health care that:

- Is based on the best scientific evidence available regarding benefits and harm
- Encourages patients to share in decision-making about therapeutic options
- Promotes choices in care that include CAM therapies when appropriate

The committee also cited the need for tools such as guidelines that would aid conventional practitioners' decision-making about offering or recommending CAM, where patients might be referred, and what organizational structures are most appropriate for the delivery of integrated care. In recommending the development of such tools the Committee noted that the goal is to provide comprehensive care that is safe, effective, interdisciplinary, and collaborative. Recommendations were identified that would strengthen the Dietary Supplement Health and Education Act of 1994, expand research funding, promote teaching CAM content in health profession schools, and expand the number of providers able to work in integrated care.

## EDUCATION OF HEALTH PROFESSIONALS

In both the IOM and WHCCAMP reports, recommendations on educating health professionals were linked to improving care. The IOM report specifically mentions nursing in advising that health profession schools incorporate sufficient information about CAM into the standard curriculum at the undergraduate, graduate, and postgraduate levels to enable licensed health professionals to competently advise patients about CAM. Similarly, the WHCCAMP report recommends that conventional as well as CAM practitioners receive education and training to ensure public safety, improve health, and increase the availability and collaboration among qualified practitioners.

The extent to which nursing programs have incorporated content on complementary therapies is unclear. As documented in the Gillette Nursing Summit (Kreitzer & Disch, 2003), the perception among nurse leaders was that this area has received limited explicit curricular emphasis. It was also noted that within some nursing programs there is resistance to teaching what is perceived to be a fad or movement lacking in evidence that is being largely shaped and dominated by medicine. There are several nursing programs, however, that have been early leaders in integrating complementary therapies into nursing curricula. Three schools of nursing were recipients of NIH NCCAM R-25 CAM education grants: the University of Minnesota, the University of Washington, and Rush University College of Nursing. Each of these programs has extensive information on complementary therapies on its Website. (See the Web Resources at the end of the chapter.) In addition, there are several graduate nursing programs with an emphasis on complementary therapies:

- New York University holistic nurse practitioner program
- University of California at San Francisco adult nurse practitioner program
- College of New Rochelle Clinical Specialist master's degree in holistic nursing

Content on integrative therapies has been more readily integrated into nursing continuing education programs.

Within medicine a stronger and more-organized movement to integrate content on CAM is apparent. Eleven of 15 recently awarded NIH NCCAM R-25 CAM education grants were awarded to schools of medicine. An additional grant was awarded to the American Medical Student Association to support the development of curricula that will be integrated into medical schools across the country. Five years ago CAHCIM was formed to advance medical schools' integrative efforts in education, research, and clinical care. Twenty-nine medical schools participate in the consortium.

It is likely that an increased focus on complementary therapies in nursing education will occur. A document prepared by the American Association of Colleges of Nursing (AACN) titled *The Essentials of Baccalaureate Education for Professional Nursing Practice* (1998) is recognized as a nationally accepted standard that can be used in the accreditation process of the Commission on Collegiate Nursing Education. The Essentials document clearly recognizes the importance of complementary and holistic therapies. As described in Box 13-11, core competencies of baccalaureate-prepared nurses include the ability to perform a holistic assessment, demonstrate awareness of complementary therapies, administer pharmacologic and nonpharmacologic therapies, provide holistic care, and evaluate the usefulness of integrating traditional and complementary health practices.

For this policy initiative to be advanced, there is a need for faculty development and curriculum resources that include content on complementary therapies. In a recent survey of nursing faculty in a large university setting, over 90% indicate that clinical care should integrate the best of conventional and CAM practices, that health professionals should be able to advise patients about commonly used methods, and that CAM practices should be included in the nursing curriculum (Kreitzer, Mitten, & Shandeling, 2002). However, the majority of faculty does not feel prepared to teach content on complementary therapies. This suggests that from a faculty development perspective, opportunities need to be created for faculty to be exposed to information on complementary therapies and CAM practitioners.

---

**BOX 13-11    American Association of Colleges of Nursing: Examples of Baccalaureate Core Competencies**

- Perform a holistic assessment of the individual across the lifespan that includes spiritual, social, cultural, and psychologic assessment as well as a comprehensive physical examination.
- Use assessment findings to diagnose, plan, deliver, and evaluate high-quality care.
- Provide comfort and pain reduction measures including positioning and therapeutic touch.
- Develop an awareness of complementary therapies and their usefulness in promoting health.
- Administer pharmacologic and nonpharmacologic therapies.
- Provide holistic care that addresses the needs of diverse populations across the lifespan.
- Evaluate and assess the usefulness of integrating traditional and complementary health practices

From American Association of Colleges of Nursing (AACN). (1995). *The essentials of baccalaureate education for professional nursing practice.* Washington, DC: American Association of Colleges of Nursing.

## INTEGRATED CARE DELIVERY SYSTEMS

The IOM report (National Academy of Sciences, 2005) notes that in the United States there is a "distinct trend" toward the integration of complementary and alternative therapies within the conventional health care system. Evidence cited includes the increasing number of hospitals and health maintenance organizations (HMOs) offering CAM therapies, the increase in insurance coverage, and the growth in integrative medicine centers and clinics, many with close ties to medical schools and teaching hospitals.

According to American Hospital Association (AHA) surveys (Ananth, 2002), in 1998 only 7.9% of hospitals reported that they offered CAM services. By 2002 the number of hospitals offering CAM therapies had more than doubled to 16.6%. Seventy-five percent of hospitals offer community CAM education programs, and 49% offer CAM information on their hospital Websites. Of those hospitals not currently offering CAM services, 24% indicated that there were plans to do so.

## THIRD-PARTY REIMBURSEMENT

Although consumers are demanding access to CAM services and hospitals are increasingly offering CAM, reimbursement is a major policy issue. At present, access to CAM is largely limited to those who can afford to pay out of pocket. Reimbursement varies considerably region to region and is different based on the type of CAM services received. For example, Cleary-Guida, Okvat, Oz, & Ting (2001), in regional survey of insurance coverage, found that virtually all insurance carriers cover chiropractic care, and close to 40% cover acupuncture and 37% cover massage therapy. This pattern of reimbursement differs somewhat from that reported by Ananth (2002) who found in the AHA survey that CAM services most likely to be reimbursed included nutritional counseling (56%), chiropractic services (49%), and biofeedback (54%). Rather than provide across-the-board coverage for any type of CAM service, third-party payers seem more inclined to provide coverage for certain therapies for select conditions. For example, acupuncture may be reimbursed for people with chronic pain but not for a person wanting to use acupuncture to treat asthma.

In general, reimbursement is related to research evidence. As there is increased documentation of the safety, efficacy, and cost of a CAM therapy, there is an increased likelihood that it will be reimbursed.

There are two other trends in reimbursement that are important to note. Increasingly, third-party payers manage a portfolio of health plans that vary depending on the employer group. What a health plan covers and what it does not cover may depend more on the employer, who determines benefit coverage, than on the third-party payer who is managing the health plan. This has important implications for consumers who are advocating for increased reimbursement of CAM. Rather than lobby the health plan for changes, it may be more important to have input into decisions that the employer makes regarding selection of the health plan and what constitutes covered benefits.

Finally, over the past 5 years there has been an increase in the growth of health savings accounts (HSAs) and health care spending accounts. Individuals may establish HSAs that work much like independent retirement accounts (IRAs) but are directed toward medical expenses. Employers are also offering employees the option of establishing a health or medical savings account as part of their benefit package. The employee or employer makes contributions to the account, and it may be used to pay for unreimbursed health care expenses. Funds are controlled and owned by the account holder, and savings are rolled over every year and are portable. In some cases these accounts can be used to reimburse expenses associated with accessing complementary therapies. Health care spending accounts work in a similar manner. Employees can set aside pretax money to use for paying health-related bills, but generally all of the money must be spent within the fiscal year.

From a nursing perspective, when complementary therapies are provided in hospitals as part of nursing care, third-party reimbursement is not an issue, as the cost is folded into the overall cost of the hospitalization or these services are financially supported through philanthropy. Although this may enrich the role responsibilities of nurses and be beneficial to patients, adding this care component likely increases time demands for nurses and may not be associated with a commensurate increase or adjustment in staffing. Advanced practice nurses such as nurse practitioners who are providing complementary therapies as part of their primary care practice in outpatient settings face the same challenges and constraints as physician colleagues— that is, the services may or may not be reimbursed depending on the health plan, the patient's condition, and the type of service provided.

Both the White House Commission and the IOM reports addressed the policy issue of CAM coverage and reimbursement. The White House Commission recommended that insurers and managed care organizations offer purchasers (usually employers) the option of health benefit plans that incorporate coverage of safe and effective CAM interventions provided by qualified practitioners. The IOM recommendations were less prescriptive and focused on the importance of generating research that addresses the outcomes and costs of combinations of CAM and conventional medical treatments and models that deliver such care.

## REGULATION OF PRACTICE

As nurses work within interdisciplinary teams that include CAM practitioners, it is important to understand how CAM practitioners are regulated as well as how state boards of nursing regulate the practice of nurses who incorporate the use of complementary therapies into their practice. States vary considerably in the regulatory frameworks established to govern the practice of complementary therapies. From a policy perspective, what is often weighed is protection of public safety versus assuring the public access to complementary approaches to healing. As detailed in the White House Commission report, some states such as Minnesota provide almost unlimited freedom to practice, thus assuring consumers broad access to services. Unlicensed CAM practitioners in Minnesota must inform clients of their education, experience, and intended treatments, as well as possible side effects or known risks of treatments. Clients must sign an informed consent statement and are informed that complaints may be filed with the state department of health. In contrast, the state of Washington has adopted a much more tightly regulated environment. Washington provides licensure, registration, or exemption for various categories of CAM professionals. Regulations delineate the standards of practice; scope of practice; education and training requirements for licensure, registration, or exemption; and required professional oversight. In Washington, naturopathic physicians, acupuncturists, massage therapists, and chiropractors are licensed and regulated.

State boards of nursing have also varied in how they have approached the practice of complementary therapies by nurses. In a survey of boards of nursing, Sparber (2001) found that 47% of the boards permitted nurses to practice a range of CAM therapies and an additional 13% were in the process of discussing whether to allow nurses to practice such therapies. Minnesota (Minnesota Board of Nursing, 2003) is an example of a state that has adopted a formal statement on the use of integrative therapies in nursing practice. Rather than specify what therapies nurses can and cannot provide, the document states that nurses who employ integrative therapies in their nursing practice are held to the same accountability for reasonable skill and safety as they are with the implementation of conventional treatment modalities.

## RESEARCH

To advance the integration of complementary therapies, it is clear from a policy perspective that it is most critical to further develop the evidence base. Access to services is clearly tied to reimbursement, and reimbursement, in turn, is related to evidence. As noted in the IOM report (National Academy of Sciences, 2005), decisions about the use of complementary therapies should primarily depend on whether such therapies have been shown to be safe and effective.

The federal government through NIH established NCCAM. The mission of NCCAM (www.nccam.nih.gov) is to explore complementary and alternative healing practices in the context of rigorous science, to train CAM researchers, and to disseminate authoritative information on CAM to the public and professional communities. According to NCCAM's strategic plan for 2005 to 2009, the agency will concentrate on efforts that will yield the greatest impact on the health and well-being of people at every stage of life, and in particular will focus on research that will:

- Enhance physical and mental health and wellness
- Manage pain and other symptoms, disabilities, and functional impairment
- Have a significant impact on a specific disease or disorder
- Prevent disease or empower individuals to take responsibility for their own health
- Reduce selected health problems of specific populations

In addition to clinical research, basic science and health services research is necessary to help elucidate the mechanism of action underlying various complementary therapies and the cost effectiveness and outcomes associated with various models of care delivery that integrate CAM with conventional care.

In addition to NCCAM, other NIH centers and institutes fund research in complementary therapies including the National Institute for Nursing Research (NINR). Although funding for NCCAM, NINR, and CAM overall has increased over the past

5 years, in 2004 total NIH funding for CAM research was estimated to be $305 million, which constitutes less than 1% of the overall NIH budget in 2004 of $27.8 billion (NCCAM, 2005).

## Key Points

- As the field of complementary therapies continues to grow, nursing is well positioned to provide leadership in clinical care, research, and education; nurses have an understanding of patient care and health system needs that makes it imperative that they have input into policy formation and implementation within organizations and at state and national levels.

- Schools of nursing must prepare graduates who have knowledge and skills in complementary therapies.

- Care delivery systems must be designed to incorporate conventional and complementary health care services.

- An increase in funding for research is needed to determine the safety and efficacy of complementary and alternative interventions.

- Nurses should work with state boards of nursing on policies that accommodate the increased use of complementary therapies in nursing practice and maintain nurses' autonomy.

## Web Resources

**National Center for Complementary and Alternative Medicine**—information on research and funding opportunities
*www.nccam.nih.gov*

**Rush University College of Nursing**—information on complementary and alternative care
*www.rushu.rush.edu/nursing/CAM/index.html*

**University of Minnesota**—information on CAM at the University of Minnesota and access to free online CAM health professional education modules
*www.csh.umn.edu*

**University of Washington School of Nursing**—information on complementary and alternative care
*www.son.washington.edu/cam/*

**White House Report on Complementary and Alternative Medicine Policy**—the complete report
*www.whccamp.hhs.gov/finalreport.html*

### REFERENCES

American Association of Colleges of Nursing (AACN). (1998). *The essentials of baccalaureate education for professional nursing practice.* Washington DC: American Association of Colleges of Nursing.

Ananth, S. (2002). *Health Forum/AHA 2000-2001 Complementary and Alternative Medicine Survey.* Chicago: Health Forum.

Astin, J. A. (1998). Why patients use alternative medicine: Results of a national study. *Journal of the American Medical Association, 279*(19), 1548-1553.

Barnes, R., Powell-Griner, E., McFann, K., & Nahin, R. (2004, May 27). *Complementary and alternative medicine use among adults: United States, 2002. Advance data from vital and health statistics* (no. 343). Washington, DC: U.S. Department of Health and Human Services, Centers for Disease Control and Prevention, National Center for Health Statistics.

Cleary-Guida, M. B., Okvat, H. A., Oz, M. C., & Ting, W. (2001). A regional survey of health insurance coverage for complementary and alternative medicine: Current status and future ramifications. *Journal of Alternative and Complementary Medicine, 7*(3), 269-273.

Consortium of Academic Health Centers for Integrative Medicine (CAHCIM). (2005). Definition of integration medicine. Retrieved March 24, 2005, from *www.imconsortium.org/html/about.php.*

Dossey, B. M. (2000). *Florence Nightingale: Mystic, visionary, healer.* Springhouse, PA: Springhouse.

Eisenberg, D. M., Davis R. B., Ettner, S. L., Appel, S., Wilkey, S., Van Rompay, M., & Kessler, R. C. (1998). Trends in alternative medicine use in the United States, 1990-1997: Results of a national follow-up survey. *Journal of the American Medical Association, 280*(18), 1569-1575.

Institute of Medicine. (2005). *Complementary and alternative medicine in the United States.* Washington, DC: National Academies Press.

Kreitzer, M. J., & Disch, J. (2003). Leading the way: The Gillette Nursing Summit on Integrated Health and Healing. *Alternative Therapies in Health and Medicine Special Supplement, 9*(1), S2-S9.

Kreitzer, M. J., Mitten, D., & Shandeling, J. (2002). Attitudes toward CAM among medical, nursing and pharmacy faculty and students: A comparative analysis. *Alternative Therapies in Health and Medicine, 8*(6), 44-53.

Minnesota Board of Nursing. (2003). *Statement of accountability for utilization of integrative therapies in nursing practice.* Minnesota Board of Nursing. Retrieved May 22, 2005, from *www.nursingboard.state.mn.us.*

National Academy of Sciences. (2005). Complementary and alternative medicine in the United States. Retrieved March 28, 2005, from *www.nap.edu.*

National Center for Complementary and Alternative Medicine (NCCAM). (2004). *Expanding horizons in medical care: Strategic plan 2005-2009.* NIH Publication No. 04-5568. Washington, DC: U.S. Department of Health and Human Services, National Institutes of Health.

Sparber, A. (2001). State boards of nursing and scope of practice of registered nurses performing complementary therapies. *Online Journal of Issues in Nursing, 6*(3), 10.

White House Commission on Complementary and Alternative Medicine Policy. (2002). Final Report. Retrieved February 8, 2006, from *www.whccamp.hhs.gov/finalreport.html.*

# *Taking Action*    Susan Hassmiller & John Lumpkin

## The Role of Foundations in Improving Health Care

*"Philanthropy is commendable, but it must not cause the philanthropist to overlook the circumstances of economic injustice which make philanthropy necessary."*

MARTIN LUTHER KING, JR.

A patient was asked about her experience as part of the discharge process during a recent hospital visit. She responded, "Do you mean did I notice that the same nurse took care of me every day? Yes, I noticed, and it was wonderful. The last time I was here, I had a different nurse every day."

The impetus to develop a consistent working relationship between individual nurses and patients came from the regular quality-improvement meetings of the staff on the hospital unit participating in a Robert Wood Johnson Foundation (RWJF)–funded program called "Transforming Care at the Bedside" (TCAB). In this innovative program, frontline nurses are empowered to develop and present ideas to improve the quality of patient care and their own satisfaction with the work that they do. In several of the TCAB units the time that floor nurses spent doing nursing tasks on the experimental unit went from 35% to almost 70%, and turnover dropped to near zero. Many of the TCAB units in the 13 participating hospitals have waiting lists to work there. For many of the nurses in the

program, it was the first time that they felt as though their needs, concerns, and ideas were valued by management at the hospital. (For more on TCAB, see Box 13-12.) This is just one example of the role that foundations can play in providing the financial, technical, and knowledge-related resources to help nurses change their environment and improve the quality of care.

The mission of RWJF is to improve the health and health care for all Americans. Following in the footsteps of Robert Wood Johnson II, the RWJF has been engaged in programs to support the field of nursing, from support for nurse education to the development of interdisciplinary training vehicles in quality improvement at academic health centers. Recognizing the critical nature of the nurse staffing shortage and the central role that nurses play in the delivery of health and health care services, RWJF made nursing one of eight focus areas in 2002. The goal was to reduce the shortage in nurse staffing and to improve the quality of nursing-related care by transforming the way care is delivered at the bedside. The TCAB program has become the centerpiece of a nursing effort that has included work to improve hospital work environments in an effort to improve nurse satisfaction and ultimately the quality of patient care. Supporting the development of measures that link patient outcomes with nursing care is a project under current development that

## BOX 13-12   Transforming Care at the Bedside

Quality improvement in some hospitals involves a complicated bureaucracy in which innovation is stifled by layers of committees and approvals, and nurses on the units have little input into changes. "Transforming Care at the Bedside" (TCAB) is a partnership between the Robert Wood Johnson Foundation and the Institute for Healthcare Improvement with the goal of empowering frontline nurses to seek solutions to improve their work environments. Nurses use the "plan, do, study, act" (PDSA) mechanism of change to quickly identify and try innovations, sometimes on a daily or weekly basis. Changes are made around four themes:

- Patient-centeredness
- Lean (eliminating waste and inefficiencies)
- Staff vitality
- Reliability and safety
  Some examples of nurse innovations include:
- Smartly using technology, including cell phones and personal digital assistants (PDAs)
- Writing patient-stated goals on whiteboards in the patient's room
- Creating peace and quiet time
- Creating rapid-response teams to reduce cases of failure to rescue outside of critical care units
- Ensuring nursing control over workload through approaches such as a red-yellow-green workflow system (see *Transforming Care at the Bedside: Shadyside Hospital's Code Red* following Chapter 17)
- Decreasing documentation
- Instituting multidisciplinary rounds
- Conducting hourly safety rounds
- Creating "lift teams" for patient handling

will be important to provide nurses with recognition for the work they do.

## FOUNDATIONS: WHAT THEY ARE AND WHAT THEY FUND

A foundation is an organization that is established as a nonprofit corporation or a charitable trust under state law, with a principal purpose of making grants to unrelated institutions or entities or to individuals for scientific, educational, cultural, religious, health-related, or other charitable purposes (Schlandweiler, 2004). Foundations are regulated by the Internal Revenue Code (refer to 501(c)3 status),

and most can give grants only to nonprofit, charitable organizations and sometimes to individuals in the form of scholarships. By federal law most foundations must spend at least 5% of their year-end assets each year. Although foundations can use their funds to inform or educate on any issue, they are prohibited from lobbying or engaging in political activities.

In general, foundations have great freedom to fund what they want, consistent with their mission. A foundation's mission is generally established by the wishes of the individual or individuals who donated resources to the foundation, the direction of the foundation's board of directors, or a combination of the two. Some foundations are sharply limited in the categories they can fund or the geography they can serve by the enabling donation or at the direction of their board. Foundations are instrumental in funding ideas that are new, innovative, and otherwise untested. If it were not for foundations, many of our country's most pressing social problems, such as improving the quality of care for those at the end of life, would never get the attention they deserve. Most of the philanthropic dollars in this country go to causes that support education (25%), but health care gets the second largest number of dollars at 20% (Foundation Center, 2005).

There are approximately 73,000 grant-making foundations in the United States (Schlandweiler, 2004) that generally fall into one of the following four categories (Indiana Grantmakers Alliance, n.d.): *Private foundations.* This category includes family foundations created by individuals and families as vehicles for carrying out their charitable vision. The Packard Foundation and the Bill and Melinda Gates foundations are examples. Other private foundations are independent foundations that often were originally organized as family foundations, but over a period of time family involvement in the leadership declined. RWJF is an example. Some foundations maintain very close relationships with the industry that was built by their founder. For example, the Annie E. Casey Foundation has a board of directors largely composed of former UPS corporate leaders. Corporate foundations are another type of private foundation whose assets are derived primarily from contributions of a for-profit or not-for-profit company. The contributions may be from an initial endowment, periodic contributions, or both. Many maintain their ties to the parent corporation despite their existence as an independent entity. Hospital-related foundations that provide funding for community projects are an example.

*Public foundations.* These foundations receive at least one third of their income from the general public or other sources outside of the main funder. The Pew Charitable Trust (n.d.) is a public charity and the sole beneficiary of seven individual charitable funds established between 1948 and 1979 by two sons and two daughters of Sun Oil Company founder Joseph N. Pew and his wife, Mary Anderson Pew. Another type of public foundation is the community foundation, which is organized to serve specific geographic regions and receives its support from a variety of donors. The New York Community Trust is an example. Some public foundations are set up to collect funds from donors for a specific issue such as health or the arts. The National Endowment for the Arts is an example.

*Operating foundations.* These foundations are generally not grant-making organizations but primarily provide information about and analysis of health care issues to policymakers, the media, and the general public. The Kaiser Family Foundation is one example of an operating foundation, and their recent Chartbook on Medicare is an example of one of their many contributions.

*Corporate giving programs.* Corporate giving programs are grant-making programs established and administered within a for-profit corporation and are often administered by marketing or public relations staff. Grants made by these entities are often closely related to the parent company's profitability and business cycles. Gifts from corporate giving programs go directly to the receiving organization and are generally free from the reporting and other requirements of foundations.

Most foundations that have started in the last two decades have been as a result of the conversion of a not-for-profit health care provider or insurer into a for-profit organization or less commonly, through sales, mergers, joint ventures, or corporate restructuring. Because nonprofit organizations' assets are considered to be held in the public trust, state attorneys general have overseen many of these conversions. Conversion foundations are charged with funding health-related activities in their communities. The intent is that the converted assets be used in a manner consistent with the original nonprofit organization's mission. For example, the Colorado Trust funds accessible and affordable health care and programs that strengthen families with assets of over $191 million from the proceeds of the sale of PSL Healthcare Corporation (The Colorado Trust, n.d.).

## HOW FUNDERS MAKE DECISIONS

As the adage goes, if you have met one foundation, you have met one foundation. Each foundation is different, and each has its own unique process for making funding decisions. Some generalizations can be made, however.

### What Is Funded

Foundations will generally state up front on their Website what they will and will not fund. National foundations will screen proposal "fitness" before looking to see if the proposal is worthy of funding. For example, at RWJF we state clearly on our Website that we do not fund bricks-and-mortar types of projects. A proposal for building a building to house a new nursing school will be rejected without further review. Some foundations will accept unsolicited grants only at certain times during the year, and those dates will be on the Website. Some foundations solicit proposals as part of a developed program or in a specific content area. Proposals sent in outside that content area will be rejected. Finally, many foundations restrict the size of the initial inquiry to a set number of pages. Proposals beyond that size may be rejected without a review of the content.

### Evaluating the Proposal

Once a proposal has been received and it passes the "does it fit with what we do" screen, it will be reviewed by foundation staff related to the substance of the proposal. If it is a small foundation without significant staff, the proposal may go right to the board of trustees for a decision. A proposal will be reviewed based on some preliminary and basic questions:

- Do the applicants seem to have expertise in the area, and do they have the ability to do what they want to do?
- Is the project going to make a difference that lasts beyond the funding period (a concept that is called *sustainability*)?
- Does the applicant's organization have the organizational capacity and leadership structure to do what is proposed?
- Is the budget appropriate to what is being proposed (not too big and not too small)?

Foundations look on potential grantees as partners in effecting social change or, at the very least, partners to create action to solve a community problem. It is necessary that the applicant know the subject matter and can explain how the proposal fits with what is known in the field. Larger foundations have content matter experts for their areas of interest available for consultation. Often foundations look for applicant teams that include individuals who are known in their field. Other times foundations look for people with new approaches or want to broaden the numbers of partners they work with. Regardless, the proposal needs to demonstrate that the applicants know the territory.

## What's the Impact?

National foundations want to have an impact on a field. Frequently we look for programs that are innovative by addressing a new aspect of a problem, by addressing a problem a different way, or by applying a new or tested approach to newly affected or difficult-to-serve populations. Proposals that address an old problem in a way that has been proven to work tend to be less attractive. Many national foundations are willing to make a multiple-year commitment to a project but tend to see projects as having a beginning and an end. The project should have clearly stated goals, reasonable approaches to achieving those goals, and a clear plan to disseminate the findings or sustain the changes implemented without foundation funding.

Most foundations are no longer interested in funding a good program that will fade away when the funding ends. Our goal is to make a lasting difference for society.

## What's the Applicant's Capacity?

Foundations want to fund programs where they can get the most for their money, and they have a vested interest in the recipient organizations. As part of the fiscal due diligence process, each foundation will want to make sure that the applicant's organization has the capacity to complete the tasks proposed. We do realize that in some programmatic areas and in some communities organizational capacity is a problem and may include building organizational capacity as part of the grant. It is important for applicants to be direct about what they can and cannot do and where they need help.

## A Budget That Works

Finally, foundations review the budget for a project. This can be a show stopper. At one extreme the amount requested may be more than the foundation is willing to invest in the type of project. At the other extreme, the foundation may feel that the applicant underestimates what it will take to accomplish what is proposed. Either case will lead to a rejection of the project. Between the two extremes, the foundation's staff will be looking to see if the funds requested seem reasonable and consistent with what is being proposed. Generally, after looking at hundreds of budgets for grants, we get pretty good at identifying core costs versus extravagant costs.

After a review of the four areas, each proposal is assigned to a program staff person and goes through an internal review process and sometimes external reviews. But if we like the project and it stands up to the tests and we have the funds, we will fund it.

## DEVELOPING A FUNDING STRATEGY: HOW TO WORK WITH FOUNDATIONS

Let's assume that you are very interested in trying to find funding to start a mentorship program for new nurses. Foundations get many more proposals than they can possibly fund, so creating a funding strategy is very important. The two components that you have to know well from the onset are your own programmatic needs and a list of all the foundations that may be interested in funding your project. A list of health care foundations both nationally and in your region can be found at the Grantmakers in Health website *(www.gih.org)*. For grants of any kind, including health care grants, go to the Foundation Center Website at *http://fdncenter.org*.

Once you determine which foundations match your topic area, you will then need to go to the Websites of those foundations to make further determinations as to the specificity of their funding. For example, you might find a number of foundations interested in the topic of "nursing" but only a very small percentage that might actually be interested in a mentorship program for new nurses. However, a foundation might be interested in nurse retention, and you could frame your proposal for a mentorship project in terms of that priority. Foundations do tend to adopt specific areas within a topic, and these can change from year to year. If a Website is unclear as to whether your topic might be of interest to the organization, then either e-mailing them or calling might be helpful. Many foundations also have helpful ways for you to get answers to your questions, such as a letter-of-intent process. The most important thing to remember is that you should never develop a large multipage proposal and send it to a number of foundations on a random basis without first determining a foundation's specific needs and your actual chances of getting funded. You should always keep a record of where you sent a letter of intent and with whom you have had a conversation.

Foundations always seek to create the greatest leverage for turning project or demonstration work into actionable results. In this regard, you must have an idea ahead of time of how you will help foundations with this goal, including the identification of key stakeholders or people who will help turn results into action and policy. Knowing who your key stakeholders are and engaging them early, including the identification of an advisory committee, will be important. Throughout the lifespan of a project, especially those that are more long term and key to foundation strategy, foundations will use a host of mechanisms themselves to engage key stakeholders and inform policymakers, such as

newsletters, listserves, invitations to presentations, inclusion of stakeholders in opinion polls (both formal and informal), and use of video, Internet presentations and postings on the Foundation's Web site, and blast e-mails. Engaging the media will also be important and will include press releases and press briefings.

Foundations know that the more people and groups that are engaged in an area and the more money invested, the greater the likelihood that action will be taken and policies will be changed. Therefore foundations will most likely give preference to those projects that have important partnerships built in and extra sources of funding—either matching funds or in-kind resources. Funders know that with each additional key partner comes a potential layer of added influence that can only broaden and deepen the sustainability of the work. For example, as RWJF seeks to bring recognition to nurses and their role in improving the quality of patient care, we apply a variety of approaches from building the capacity of nurse leaders through leadership and media development activities, conducting and disseminating research that links nursing outcomes to quality of care and convening activities that bring nurses in contact with other key influencers of health care.

RWJF and other foundations also engage in demonstration projects in an effort to test and learn from potential good ideas. Examples of demonstration projects that went on to inform health care policy include the computerization of childhood vaccine records, simplifying the paperwork to enroll Medicaid-eligible children, the 911 emergency call system, and support for the development of the nurse practitioner role, including prescriptive authority. The W.K. Kellogg Foundation has been instrumental in efforts to build leadership capacity among diverse groups such as African-Americans and Native Americans, and the Gates Foundation is spearheading worldwide efforts to stop the spread of acquired immunodeficiency syndrome (AIDS) through prevention education and the development of an AIDS/HIV vaccine.

Once you get into the process, it will be the relationship you develop with a foundation officer that will help you most. Never make the mistake of believing that a foundation is an entity from which you might receive just money. Foundations are also important organizations with regard to intellectual capital. They are extremely thoughtful about the areas that they fund and many times are experts in your topic, so consider them partners in achieving your goals. Even if they are not experts themselves, they generally know who all the experts are in your area. Your program is always your program, but an experienced program officer can help you improve and/or finetune your approach. A list of the most important things to remember when working with a foundation follows:

- Know your own program and funding needs. Does the entire program need funding? Are there any partners that can be brought on to help fund segments?
- Do not chase money for money's sake. Know what you want to accomplish, and do not let a foundation or other funder dictate your mission. Foundations can have constructive ideas about shaping a program, but it should be your program.
- Be familiar with the foundation's Website and the possibility of a programmatic match before making any contacts. Understand the funders' needs and expectations.
- Know who you want to talk to and what their funding priorities and areas of expertise are.
- Prepare a sound byte version, a paragraph version, and a one-page version of what you hope to accomplish with foundation support, so that you're able to give the dose of information that is desired. The foundation will ask for a full proposal if they want it.
- Know the following about your proposal off the top of your head: intent, outcomes anticipated, measures of success, approximate funding required, duration, deliverables, potential for matching or in-kind funds, sustainability plans.
- If you are asked to submit a proposal, have someone who knows nothing about the topic read it and then describe in three sentences what you are asking the foundation to do. If they cannot, you have probably written it in "nurse" jargon instead of English.
- Never turn in any piece of work without first having a trusted editor review.

- Nurture foundation relationships. Be of service to the foundation; let them see your talents and skills by serving on advisory panels or reviewing papers if you are asked. Foundations are always "trying out" experts to see who might be useful for meeting their objectives. Foundations want to be successful, and just like any other organization they prefer to work with someone with a track record of success.
- Think about what else local funders offer besides money—for example, access to political or business leaders, technical assistance workshops for prospective grantees, convening capacity, and so on. Talk with the people you identify.
- Always look locally for funding first. If you can pilot something with local funding, you are in a better position to get national funding to bring your model to scale. Think about and work with others in the community on the same issue, as evidence of collaboration is always considered a plus by funders.
- Be visibly successful—"toot your own horn" about your agency and its good work. It is much better to have the funder hear about what you have been doing before they get the proposal.
- Don't give up. You may not get funded the first time around, but following the above recommendations will definitely get you closer to your goal.

## *Lessons Learned*

- Foundations are an important part of the nonprofit world and can be partners with nurses who are looking to develop innovative approaches to common problems.
- Foundations seek to fulfill their mission through investing in grantees whose programs and projects are consistent with that vision.
- Although the missions of foundations may vary and their approaches to funding differ, there are some basic approaches to applying for support.
- Understanding the mission of the foundation to which you are applying, in combination with a well-thought-out proposal with a sound budget, will increase the likelihood of funding.

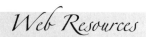

## Web Resources

> **Grantmakers in Health**
> *www.gih.org*
> **The Pew Charitable Trusts**
> *www.pewtrusts.com*
> **Robert Wood Johnson Foundation**
> *www.rwjf.org*

### REFERENCES

Foundation Center. (2005). Foundation Center Trends 2005 report: Foundations Today series 2005. Retrieved July 5, 2005, from *www.fdncenter.org/research/trendsanalysis/top100assets.htm.*

The Colorado Trust. (n.d.). About the Trust. Retrieved February 18, 2006, from *http://coloradotrust.org/index.cfm? fuseAction=AboutTheTrust.WhoWeAre.*

Indiana Grantmakers Alliance. (n.d.). Retrieved July 5, 2005, from *www.indianagrantmakers.org/resources/faqs/ about.cfm.*

Pew Charitable Trusts. (n.d.). History. Retrieved July 5, 2005, from *www.pewtrusts.com/about/about_subpage.cfm? page=a4.*

Schlandweiler, K. (Ed.). (2004). *Foundations fundamentals: A guide for grantseekers* (7th ed.). New York: Foundation Center.

# *Vignette*   Anita J. Catlin

## Neonatal Palliative Care: Moving a Vision Forward

*"There is one thing stronger than all the armies in the world: an idea whose time has come."*

VICTOR HUGO

### THE VISION

The vision was a loving death experience for a dying baby. The dream: to see a family hold and love their dying baby. The grandparents and clergy are present, there is singing, and the child is dressed in lovely baby clothes. There are no machines or lines other than a pain port. The lights in the room are dimmed, there is soft music playing in the background. The family is very satisfied that their child received the optimum of compassionate care.

### THE REALITY

The reality was often a nightmare, well described in an excerpt from a poem by neonatologist Lynne Willett (1998):

*Better that the last touch you feel is someone holding you,*

*Not crushing your chest with CPR, needles and the slime of K-Y jelly.*
*Better that you are warm and clothed*
*Not splayed out naked in the open with lights and blindfolds.*
*Better that you die now than go through days, weeks, months of that.*

In the early 1990s, babies were dying after multiple resuscitation attempts. Marginally viable babies were placed on ventilators and living only because of technologic support. Some babies were going home very impaired. Mothers were writing accounts of their despair over their infants' slow dying after technologic support (Alecson, 1995; Rogoff, 1995; Stinson & Stinson, 1983).

### SUPPORTING THE VISION WITH DATA

In 1995, I studied mothers whose children had survived from the NICU with severe impairments (Catlin, 1995). Disabled children were now growing up in the care of their mothers. And these mothers felt that they had not been given the right to request nontreatment of their very ill or very premature infants. These mothers told me that they felt that the neonatal physicians had made all the decisions, decisions that later shaped the trajectories of these mothers' lives. Putting on a good face, the mothers agonized in private—as Helen Harrison (2001), author and maternal advocate, would later say, "making lemonade." These parents began a listserve and talked about runaway technology and life with their growing and deaf, blind, autistic, or technologically supported children.

I decided that for my dissertation I would study how physicians made resuscitation decisions and which types of newborns they decided to keep alive with technology. The American Academy of Pediatrics Neonatal Resuscitation Program and my local Sigma Theta Tau chapter provided funding for a year of travel to interview physicians throughout the United States about resuscitation decisions.

## CARE WITHOUT CURE

What the physician participants in my 1998 study told me was troubling (Catlin, 1999). They resuscitated all newborns and supported all infants with technology. They reported no weight, gestational age, or medical condition criteria that they used for guidance. They had not heard about palliative care for newborns in internships or fellowships nor seen it in practice. None of the 54 physicians interviewed had ever planned the support for an infant in dying. They did, however, acknowledge the morbidity created when very, very small or very, very ill newborns were kept alive with no improvement. And they spoke of the sadness and burden they felt when seeing the outcomes of trading mortality for morbidity. Many physicians stated that they would be willing to embrace a palliative care model if it were presented by clinical leaders in the field.

Another study conducted in 1999 convinced me of the need for a palliative care model for newborns. With two colleagues I conducted a retrospective chart study of end of life care for infants and families in the NICU when ventilator support was withdrawn (Abe, Catlin, & Mihara, 2001). At that time the neonatal resuscitation protocol (Kattwinkel, 1998) never mentioned when resuscitation (or technologic life support) could be withheld or withdrawn.

No neonatal training book for either nurses or physicians described or even acknowledged that technologic interventions could be withheld or withdrawn. Although every book had a chapter on bereavement, the process of infant death was not mentioned. No article in the literature reported a process for ventilator withdrawal. What my colleagues and I found was little consistency in how end of life for newborns was handled, rare use of pain or symptom management, and little reported support of families while their infant was dying.

## SPREADING THE WORD

During the late 1990s and the early years of the twenty-first century, I began to speak publicly about better decision-making for marginally viable newborns and those who were born dying. In the beginning it was very hard. Some physician colleagues reacted quite negatively to my questioning of the technologic imperative in public forum. It was initially difficult for neonatal physicians to accept any goal other than "cure" for the extremely premature or very ill newborn. I traveled continuously, speaking wherever I was invited about ethical care delivery for newborns. Although I was chastised publicly and privately by important people in the field of neonatal medicine, I also garnered my supporters. As time passed, physician and nurse colleagues throughout the world seemed ready to support an addition to the "cure-only" model of care. My publications were picked up in the news, and e-mails began to arrive from Europe, the Middle East, Australia, and North and South America. Nurse and physician colleagues worldwide wrote to tell me, "Yes, we have gone too far with technology in neonatology, we need to hold back." A group of American nurses and physicians began ongoing communication. We met most often at the American Society of Bioethics and Humanities. A dedicated group of physicians (Brian Carter, Steven Leuthner, Marcia Levetown, Suzanne Toce, Deborah Campbell, and Byron Calhoun) and nurses (Winnifred Pinch, Joy Penticuff, Karen Kavanaugh, LizBeth Sumner, Irene Hurst, Lucia Wocial, and I) were all speaking publicly about compassionate comfort care for the marginally viable newborn. People began to listen, and we were championed by parents such as the

Millers, whose daughter Sydney was resuscitated against their will (Miller v. HCA, 2002), social worker Brenda Sumrall Smith, and Dr. William Silverman (Silverman, 2004), father of American neonatology.

Neonatologist Brian Carter and I began to work together on a study to create an actual protocol to assist practitioners with care of the dying baby. After submitting a proposal for this research, I was selected by the American Nurses Foundation to be an ANF Scholar; and they, along with my local Sigma Theta Tau chapter, gave us funding to conduct an 18-month-long Delphi study on compassionate neonatal dying. With 101 members on the Delphi panel, including physicians, nurses, parents, philosophers, administrators, psychologists, hospice experts, respiratory therapists, child life specialists, pharmacists, and a funeral director, we launched into a consensus-building project on end of life issues for newborns by addressing the following questions:

- What were the most ideal circumstances to support a family whose newborn child was dying?
- Who should be involved?
- What should be done, and how should it be done?
- What types of marginally viable newborns could be supported in a pain-free, dignified, and loving dying rather than be placed on a ventilator?
- If infants are removed from ventilatory support, what is the most compassionate way to do so?

We worked on the Internet, sending 13 questions and answers up and back, laboring over themes, sentences, and even words. Data collected were continually analyzed and sent back out for consensus. We sent the final document out for review. By 2001 we were disseminating this publicly, then we published the protocol in both the medical and the nursing literature (Catlin & Carter, 2002). In 2001 the National Perinatal Association awarded us the Model of Care Award in recognition of our contribution to the field of perinatal medicine.

Invitations followed from the American Academy of Pediatrics; Association for Women's Health, Obstetric and Neonatal Nursing; Academy of Neonatal Nursing; National Association for Neonatal Nursing; and state perinatal chapters. In 2003, I began working with hospitals and health care

systems on implementation of neonatal palliative care. For example, I met with physicians and nurses at Sutter Alta Bates Hospital in Berkeley, California and at the St. Boniface Hospital in Winnipeg, Canada to support newly developing palliative care programs for newborns. I arranged the meeting with local children's hospices, whom the neonatal staffs had never met, and helped develop a working plan for anticipated or sudden lethal illnesses in newborns. This national and international neonatal palliative care work was recognized with a nomination to the American Academy of Nursing.

In 2004, I was invited to speak about neonatal palliative care to the lead neonatal and obstetric researchers at a meeting convened by the National Institute of Health (NIH). Although the notion of palliative care was not immediately accepted, participants acknowledged that the technology had advanced beyond the ethics and that supportive community services for surviving children were lacking. When these leaders in the field at the NIH did not seem willing to endorse palliative care, I decided that the education must go to the public. Women who were pregnant were being screened for rare fetal anomalies but not being educated about previable births, which statistically were much more likely to occur. In an article called "Thinking Outside the Box: Prenatal Care and A Call for the Prenatal Advance Directive (Catlin, 2005)" I argued for education of all women about the number of weeks necessary for viable fetal development and the morbidity and mortality related to premature birth. Thus educated early, if preterm labor should occur, women could make an informed choice. This thinking was supported by Dr. Winnifred Pinch's longitudinal study of NICU parents (Pinch, 2002). "Mothers told me," she wrote, "'Next time I won't just blindly hand over my child.'"

The year 2004 brought chairing a national conference on neonatal ethics and palliative care, obtaining ELNEC certification, and writing guest editorials. A highlight of 2004 was a week of consultation with the Institute of Bioethics and the National Bioethics Committee of Portugal to teach about neonatal ethics. Countries outside of the United States were embracing the advanced technology, then suffering from similar problems of what to do when care does not cure.

## CONTINUED RESEARCH AND VISIONS

In 2005, I decided to study newborn children who are too sick to leave the hospital. These newborns have been supported with technology, but no one has ever recorded how many such children there are or what conditions they have. I know that wherever I go there are children on the neonatal intensive care unit celebrating their first birthdays. There are newborns with organ transplants who have never been out of doors. There are separated conjoined twins who live in a hospital or long-term care. When the alternative to palliative care for marginally viable newborns is supporting children with technology, we must explore what conditions cause children to be too sick to ever go home.

## THE PRESENT

As of 2006, neonatal palliative care continues to blossom. Nurses Dr. Roni Feeg, Dr. Cynda Rushton, and Lizbeth Sumner have been outspoken advocates for improved care for dying children. The City of Hope and Robert Wood Johnson Foundation ELNEC project is changing the face of pediatric palliative care by training hundreds of faculty, clinicians, and staff nurses in the principles of a compassionate, dignified, and pain-free death. Still, in all the pediatric training materials used by the ELNEC program and in most of the neonatal nursing or physician training books published, dying newborns are rarely mentioned. Colleagues Brian Carter and Marcia Levetown published the first text ever to discuss dying newborns in 2004 (Carter & Levetown 2004). Dr. Carol Kenner has included the end of life protocol in neonatal books she edits.

On July 26, 2005, I opened the *Wall Street Journal*. On the front page of the health section was an article titled "A New Approach for the Sickest Babies (Peterson, 2005)." My research partner Brian Carter was interviewed about the work in neonatal palliative care. The article showcased neonatal units around the nation that have created palliative care programs according to our protocol. Could this be the beginning of acceptance for the vision? And as a nurse, have I (and my many colleagues) had the

ability to help influence national health care policy? If so, this is extraordinarily fulfilling.

## *Lessons Learned*

- If you don't have data to show why your vision and change are needed, get the data through designing and conducting research of your own.
- Don't think that you have to be at a major university with national funding to create change. There are small sources of funding for all levels of researchers and local hospitals that are willing to host institutional review board approval.
- Share your data with media to put the issue on the public's and policymakers' agendas. Volunteer to speak frequently at any forum that will invite you.
- Read Eleanor Sullivan's book, *Becoming Influential* (2003), to guide your transition to policy maker.
- Work with an interdisciplinary team to move your vision forward whenever possible. Find colleagues that can support and encourage your ideas.
- Timing is important. If ideas are not at first accepted, be prepared to continue to create a context for change. And be tough skinned when chastised about trying to make changes.
- Involve the people who are affected by the health care policy. They, as were the parents here described, will be your champions.
- Participate in all national meetings that are about your topic. Make your work known.
- Advanced practice nurses have the ability and knowledge to influence the direction of health care. Use your colleagues as supporters, and you, too, will be able to keep a vision moving forward.

### REFERENCES

Abe, N., Catlin, A. J., & Mihara, D. (2001). End of life in the NICU: A study of ventilator withdrawal. *MCN: The American Journal of Maternal/Child Nursing, 28*(3), 141-146.

Alecson, D. G. (1995). *Lost lullaby*. Berkeley, CA: University of California Press.

Carter, B. S., & Levetown, M. (2004). *Palliative care for infants, children, and adolescents*. Baltimore: Johns Hopkins University Press.

Catlin, A. J. (1995). *Listening to the voices of women*. Unpublished manuscript (coursework). Chicago: Rush University College of Nursing.

Catlin, A. J. (1999). Physicians' neonatal resuscitation of extremely low birth weight preterm infants. *Image: Journal of Nursing Scholarship, 31,* 269-275.

Catlin, A. J. (2005). Thinking outside the box: Prenatal care and the call for a prenatal advance directive. *Journal of Perinatal and Neonatal Nursing, 19*(2), 169-176.

Catlin, A. J., & Carter, B. S. (2002). Creation of a neonatal end of life palliative care protocol. *Journal of Perinatology, 22*(3), 184-195; reprinted in *Neonatal Network, Journal of Neonatal Nursing, 21*(4), 37-44.

Harrison, H. (2001). Making lemonade: A parent's view of "quality of life" studies. *Journal of Clinical Ethics, 12*(3), 239-250.

Kattwinkel, J. (1998). *Textbook of neonatal resuscitation.* Elk Grove Village, IL: American Academy of Pediatrics.

Miller v. HCA. (2002). No. 01-0079, Texas Supreme Court. Retrieved February 11, 2006, from *www.supreme.courts.state. tx.us/historical/2003/sept/010079.htm.*

Peterson, A. (2005, July 26). A new approach for the sickest babies. *Wall Street Journal,* D1, D4.

Pinch, W. J. E. (2002). *When the bough breaks: Parental perceptions of ethical decision-making in NICU—Parental perceptions of ethical decision-making in NICU.* Lanham, MD: University Press of America.

Rogoff, M. (1995). *Silvie's life.* Berkeley, CA: Zenobia Press.

Silverman, W. (2004). Compassion or opportunism? *Pediatrics 113*(2), 402-403.

Stinson, R., & Stinson, P. (1983). *The long dying of baby Andrew.* Boston, MA: Atlantic Monthly Press.

Sullivan, E. (2003). *Becoming influential.* New Orleans: Prentice Hall.

Willett, L. (1998). Untitled poem. In Catlin, A. J. (Ed.), *Physicians opinions of resuscitation for extremely low birth weight neonates.* Dissertation. Chicago: Rush University.

# **POLICY**SPOTLIGHT

## THE POLITICS OF THE PHARMACEUTICAL INDUSTRY

Pamela J. Maraldo

*"There's a better way to do it...find it."*

THOMAS EDISON

The pharmaceutical industry has been under a barrage of relentless public fire for the last several years. Public perception of the industry trade group Pharmaceutical Research and Manufacturers of America (PhRMA) as an "evil empire" interested exclusively in profits has been fueled by a constant barrage of negative news coverage aimed at the entire industry. Following a scathing broadcast of the industry's lackluster performance by Peter Jennings, the June 13, 2002 issue of the *Wall Street Journal* published the results of a joint poll with NBC News showing that distrust of pharmaceutical companies was at an all-time high. Since then, the situation has grown worse (Maraldo & Lister, 2002).

Drug stocks began tumbling in the wake of a Texas jury's decision that Merck & Company's

Vioxx, its cyclooxygenase (COX)-2 inhibitor drug, was responsible for the death of Robert C. Ernest on all counts of negligence, wrongful death, and failure to take proper steps to alert physicians of possible dangers of Vioxx. Creating further erosion in the public trust of PhRMA, the industry is now even more suspect of putting profits ahead of patients' welfare.

Some consumer groups have launched a near-full-scale revolt over what they see as skyrocketing costs of prescription drugs in this country. The American Association of Retired Persons (AARP) led the charge, attacking PhRMA for what it perceived were exorbitant price increases. According to a report recently released by AARP, average prices of dozens of brand name prescription drugs widely used by elderly Americans have risen more than twice as fast as general inflation (Maraldo & Lister, 2002). Although annual change in overall prescription drug prices decreased from a high of 5.7% in

1999 to the 2004 increase of 3.3%, these increases include discount prices and continue to outpace the Consumer Price Index (Strunk, Ginsburg, & Cookson, 2005).

More government regulation seems to be on the horizon. Consumer groups, led by AARP, have been trying to persuade Congress and the Bush administration to use Medicare's vast clout to bargain directly with drug makers on prices. Under the new Medicare Modernization Act, which established the new drug benefit, Medicare is barred from such negotiating. By law, Medicare must accept prices negotiated by insurers, drug store chains, and pharmacy benefit managers, which lack Medicare's leverage. But the pressure is on.

Several states have already enacted laws requiring the use of generics whenever possible. The difference in inflation between name brand and generic drugs can be illustrated by statins—the drugs used to lower cholesterol. Early this year Pfizer raised the wholesale price of Lipitor, the best selling statin, to $2.17 each for the 10-mg pills and $3.15 each for the 20-mg pills. But there was no increase in the $1.18 wholesale price for Mevacor, an older statin (Strunk, Gingsburg, & Cookson, 2005).

Pharmaceutical companies have also recently experienced a spate of lawsuits initiated by state prosecutors. Filed on behalf of Medicaid, these suits allege that some drug companies have denied patients and state governments access to lower-priced versions of their medicines. Thirty-five states are working together in hopes of repeating the success of the nationwide campaigns that led to the $208 billion tobacco industry settlement. There are a number of class action suits from consumer groups; and, of course, the growing strength of generics as a result of increasing political support is part of the growing assault on the pharmaceutical industry.

Provider organizations have pushed back at PhRMA as well. According to the Health Care Advisory Board, Boston's Massachusetts General Hospital has instituted a new policy designed to restrict pharmaceutical company sales representatives' access to the hospital. In fact, only a few miles away from Pfizer's prized research facility in Groton, NY a sign on the door of the nearby Medical

Center says, "No drug reps allowed" (Maraldo & Lister, 2002).

Yet, a strong case could be made that where improvements in longevity and quality of life are concerned, we have PhRMA to thank. In the last century, drugs revolutionized medicine. Anyone who is old enough to remember life before World War II remembers the ravages of syphilis, pneumonia, and other infectious diseases in a world without the antibiotics we now take for granted. Women who lived before the discovery of oral contraceptives remember the damaging effects of pregnancy after pregnancy on their bodies and psyches. Selective serotonin reuptake inhibitors (SSRIs) have given many who have known the depths of despair a new lease on life.

Life-saving breakthroughs have long been the pharmaceutical industry's stock in trade. In some ways the pharmaceutical industry has done more for the advancement of people's health and the quality of life than any other sector of health care. A recent survey of 225 leading internists asked them to consider 30 medical and health care innovations and identify those whose loss would have the most adverse effect on their patients; 11 of the top 20 were drug therapies (Hunt, 2002).

## THE BLAME GAME

The path of blame in the health care system is a well worn one, with various sectors taking their turns on the hot seat. Public anger zeroing in on the pharmaceutical industry was once directed toward managed care companies, and before that, hospitals, and before that, physicians. Rising health care costs have been the bane of our economic existence for some three decades.

Furthermore, where drug spending is concerned, there is plenty of blame to spread around. Physicians often do not take the time to guide patients to less-expensive drugs that are as effective, and employers and insurers do not assume the responsibility for looking more deeply into the range of appropriate treatment therapies that they pay for.

Negative public perception is a major problem for the pharmaceutical industry. However, other players in the drug discovery process are not without blame. The U.S. Food and Drug Administration

(FDA) may head the list. Many policy observers believe that drug industry clout has led to influencing the research and testing agenda and having influential people in place inside the regulatory agencies.

Charged with ensuring the safety and quality of drugs on behalf of the public, investigations have demonstrated some truth to that charge. Business interests have appeared to supersede public health at the agency. During hearings on the risks and benefits of a controversial class of painkillers known as COX-2 inhibitors, Dr. David Graham, the FDA's associate safety director, accused the agency of suppressing a recent study that he conducted with Dr. Gurkirpal Singh of Stanford University demonstrating thousands of Vioxx-related deaths in the United States (Goldstein, 2005). "They don't want safety information [to go] out to the public," Graham charged in an interview, "because it will only highlight how inadequate their assessment of safety has been before the drugs have gotten onto the market." Graham said he was "told in very clear, emphatic and very terse, unfriendly tone of voice and terms, we were not to present these data. These data could not be presented."

The COX-2 inhibitor debacle created an avalanche of concern surrounding the release of studies that include critical clinical information. Adding more fuel to the need to release trial data, New York State Attorney General Eliot Spitzer sued GlaxoSmithKline for concealing negative information about the antidepressant medication paroxetine (Paxil). In August of 2004 as part of the settlement of that lawsuit, GlaxoSmithKline agreed to post on its corporate Website a summary of clinical-study reports for every company-sponsored trial of its medications completed after December 27, 2000 (Steinbrook, 2004).

In September of 2004, an organization of 11 general medical journals, including the *New England Journal of Medicine*, announced that "member journals will require, as condition of consideration for publication, registration in a public trials registry. Trials must register at or before the onset of patient enrollment" (Steinbrook, 2004). The policy was to be implemented in the summer of 2005.

To be sure, the pharmaceutical industry bears its share of responsibility for behaviors that are contrary to the public good. However, if the overall health care landscape is taken into account, culpability for the problems in health care can be a shared affair:

- Hospital costs are rising at a rate of 7% to 8% (inpatient, with outpatient costs rising at more than double that rate—16% to 17%) per year, but they constitute by far a larger percentage of (40%) of health care costs.
- Often the appropriate medication at the right time will be cost saving, as it may keep people out of hospitals and emergency rooms—cases in point are medications for asthma and diabetes.
- Premium costs of managed care companies are rising rapidly at the rate of 15% to 20% annually.

Therefore there are myriad other factors to consider in assigning the blame for rising health care costs. Indeed, studies cited by Klienke in the September/October 2001 issue of *Health Affairs* of the impact of pharmaceuticals on total health care costs demonstrated that they frequently cause overwhelming reductions in hospital costs (Klienke, 2001).

Attacking PhRMA alone is too simplistic—even though it may provide relief for our fears and frustrations with the system. The danger is emasculating an industry that has been very productive. If price controls become a reality, industry executives assert that the world can forget about new and better drugs. Consider protease inhibitor drugs, which have dramatically decreased deaths and hospitals costs for those with human immunodeficiency virus (HIV). If Congress had put price controls in place in the 1990s when the world was upset about prices, "there would be no protease inhibitors now" (Klienke, 2001).

Marketing curbs would also likely depress demand for new drugs and result in an increase in government outlays for research and development (R&D). Currently, the pharmaceutical industry actually spends more on medical research than National Institutes of Health (NIH). In 2002 the NIH annual budget was $24 billion. That same year, the drug industry's R&D budget was $32 billion (Klienke, 2005).

The complexity of the issue extends to concerns over price. On the surface, price increases are the major cause for concern. The real problem for PhRMA seems to lie in the question of value, not just price. Large increases in spending have been attributed to "me too" drugs with no significant clinical improvement over older medications. Expectations of an American public used to blockbusters—breakthroughs and cures—have been dashed after over a decade of "me too" drugs. During the 1990s, most of PhRMA's efforts were spent on "me too" drugs or drugs that used active ingredients already on the market (Hunt, 2002).

## SHAREHOLDER'S LAMENT

Constant pressure to grow sales and profit to achieve at least 10% revenue growth won't bring much sympathy from detractors of the industry, but the pressures are very real. Achieving 10% revenue growth would mean coming out with three to five blockbusters a year (Maraldo & Lister, 2002). Few manufacturers can meet such a target.

PhRMA must live and prosper in an investment sector ecology that is populated by a host of *other* players interested in maximizing their margins of profit for shareholders. Funders invest when they expect their investment will exceed what they can get from safer investments. Many are not certain that this will be the case in the future for PhRMA.

For many years, pharmaceuticals was the top-ranked industry in the annual Fortune 500 industry profitability rankings. Not any more: in 2004 pharmaceuticals were ranked only number three in return on sales, number 12 in return on assets, and number 13 in return on equity. And loyal shareholders are in pain: the average total annual return to shareholders between 1999 and 2004 was −1.4%! It is true that the performance of other economic sectors during that period was lackluster; however, investors have always considered pharmaceuticals to be somewhat resistant to the cyclic vagaries of other, less-essential commodities (Bary, 2004).

The industry's business model, which used to produce superior profits and happy shareholders year after year, consisted of the following key components:

- High fixed costs for discovering, developing, and launching blockbuster products
- A regular flow of innovative new products

- Payers willing to pay high prices relative to the low incremental unit product costs
- Patent protection that kept competition out sufficiently long to make the R&D and launch investments profitable (Angelmar, 2005).

Now this model is seriously called into question by investors and some in the industry itself. The drug sector is no longer a predictable producer of 10% or higher annual gains. Developing new versions of established drugs has been a saving grace strategy for the industry—less risky, less time consuming, and less expensive than starting from scratch in the drug discovery process. In addition, FDA policies favor improving on existing drugs that can be brought to market much more quickly and less expensively (Hunt, 2002).

The pressure to meet investor expectations will continue to rise, and more and more drugs are slated to come "off patent," making their less-expensive generic equivalents available to the public. Then there is the looming problem of imports, which threaten to take a chunk of the pharmaceutical industry's margins.

## THE IMPORTATION DILEMMA

Right in the FDA's own back yard, the City Council of Montgomery County, Maryland, recently added its name to a long list of cities and states that have defied federal law and passed legislation permitting citizens to buy medications in Canada. Moreover, 18 state attorneys general have written the Bush administration to urge passage of legislation allowing prescription drugs to be imported.

"Stopping good importation bills has a high, high cost not just in money, but in American lives," Dr. Peter Rost, a dissident Pfizer executive, declared at a rally on Capitol Hill in support of legislation that would allow imports. "Every day we delay, Americans die because they cannot afford life-saving drugs" (Rost, 2004).

During the presidential campaigns, John Edwards blasted the Bush administration for blocking the importation of drugs from Canada and told Americans, "We're not going to allow it." Senator John Kerry talked about prescription drug prices as well. Since the campaign the importation issue has been quietly pushed aside. Consumer advocates of all ages, however, continue to organize bus trips to Canada, where U.S. citizens can purchase cheaper drugs. (Savings run as high as 50%; some popular antidepressants cost twice as much here.)

In St. Paul, Minnesota, senior citizens journey for hours by bus to Winnipeg. Often the trips are funded in part by Senator Mark Dayton, a millionaire who donates his entire Congressional salary to fund the bus trips. This rebellion is being joined by a bipartisan coalition of governors, citizens, and state officials who are creating Web sites linking consumers to Canadian pharmacies. New Hampshire, for instance, includes a link to Canadadrugs.com on its official state Website. Even the Republican Governor Craig Benson recommends Canadadrugs.com, which is regulated by the Canadian government. So far, the FDA, faced with pressure from supporters of importation, has not acted to shut the sites down.

This movement is rapidly spreading throughout the nation. Recently Illinois and Wisconsin launched the nation's first state-sponsored program to help residents buy cheaper prescription drugs from both Europe and Canada. Some 24 states are considering legislation that would permit importation of drugs from Canada or elsewhere, and Connecticut, West Virginia, and Vermont are among several states that have already enacted proimportation laws.

Currently, one to two million Americans are defying federal law by using the Internet to purchase drugs from Canadian pharmacies. In the current conservative political climate, we are likely to see legislative attempts to open the floodgates to importation at the federal level thwarted. Yet, the issue of concerns over pricing is not likely to die easily, and consumer pressure to take action may become a political reality for Congress.

### ANTI-PhRMA OR ANTI-PROFIT?

Even though many cogent arguments continue to circulate as to why health care should not exist for profit and the fact that markets cannot be relied on to produce services that are essentially public in nature, like nursing and health care, the profit motive is alive and well in health care. The front page of *Barron's Weekly* recently touted the millions of dollars that can be realized because of new treatment discoveries in the works for diabetes. Perhaps the motives behind searching for cures should be more altruistic, but the health care system hasn't worked that way for a very long time.

Physician leaders like Arnold Relman, former editor of the *New England Journal of Medicine,* may express a desire to return to the good old fee-for-service days when health care was primarily not for profit, but even then there was plenty of profit hiding behind the 501(c)(3) nonprofit tax status. Perhaps things are now just more out in the open, and those who are profiting are a new cast of characters.

Many in nursing and medicine believe in the view espoused by Relman that our system is "expensive, inefficient inequitable and unpopular"; and that most of our ills derive from the fact that our system is market driven and so heavily commercialized (Relman, 2002). The other side of the argument is best articulated by Regina Herzlinger (2004), who writes *in support* of market-driven health care. Herzlinger and market-driven advocates hail the new discoveries of the genome that created the promise of phenomenal therapeutic advances. Many believe that we are truly on the verge of curing diseases such as Alzheimer disease, Parkinson's, diabetes, and heart disease as a result of the profit motive to make hay out of the new genetic knowledge.

The promise of personalized medicines or genome-derived drugs or genetic indicators for the therapy that best suits our individual responses and metabolic rates could be realized in the foreseeable future. Indeed, Millennium Pharmaceuticals has made strides with melastatin, a gene that produces a marker for skin cancer (Herzlinger, 2004).

Few would take issue with having the ability to use the right drug for the right person to improve health and reduce the costs of inappropriate treatments and side effects. It has been demonstrated in at least one study that 59% of the drugs frequently cited for adverse drug events were linked to genetic variations in patients' ability to metabolize the drugs (Herzlinger, 2004). Yet, most health policy experts dismiss the industry's promise of creating new drug therapies along these lines, because they focus on the "unsustainable strains" new discoveries will place on our ability to pay (Herzlinger, 2004).

Herzlinger believes that people should have access to the drugs they need, but not at the expense of new drug discovery.

Pharmaceutical companies have actually initiated a number of programs to provide drugs to those who can't afford them. In addition, many pharmaceutical companies donate generously to charitable activities ranging from providing acquired immunodeficiency virus (AIDS) drugs free of charge or cheaply to African nations, to relief funds and services during the 9/11 crisis, to efforts directed toward alleviating the burden of illness in third world countries.

Sometimes shareholders are not thrilled with the goodwill of the pharmaceutical industry. At Merck, Roy Vagelos, former Chairman and CEO of Merck, and his executive team decided in the 1980s to give away a drug that could cure river blindness in Africa—a move that to this day helps tens of millions of people in that part of the world. The decision, however, was controversial. Merck, a profit-making drug company, was clearly expected to earn profits from drugs coming out of its laboratories—not give them away free. Nonetheless, the goodwill resulting from the decision was invaluable. It seemed to energize the employees at Merck labs and instilled a deeper sense of purpose in the company.

## DIRECT-TO-CONSUMER ADVERTISING: A STEP IN THE RIGHT DIRECTION?

The pharmaceutical industry moved to align itself more with the consumer with direct-to-consumer (DTC) advertising. A highly controversial move, it began to be allowed when the FDA lifted its restrictions on drug companies' advertising in 1998. The results of the regulatory change have gotten mixed reviews. Used by pharmaceutical companies as a tool to raise awareness of disease areas and treatments, it has also been yet another target for criticism of the industry. Many consumer groups think DTC is a ruse to foist drugs on a gullible public and that the expenditure of billions of dollars on promoting drugs through expensive advertising serves only to create increases in the price of drugs sold to the public. Others believe that DTC has been revolutionary and a pioneer for consumer involvement—that the exposure to new drugs has been an educational

boon to consumers, helping them become more informed for conversations with doctors and nurses and others in health care delivery.

The role of public accountability in American society across a wide range of issues is increasing. Consumers are rapidly seizing control of their health care. Confronted with stark differences among providers and prices, and with out-of-pocket costs rising rapidly, Americans are learning to apply all they know about how to be a smart consumer of health care. Likewise, the system is learning to accommodate these savvy consumers, when it once took patients' loyalties for granted. The years of passive consumption under the fee-for service insurance model that protected consumers from the costs associated with more expensive choices are over. Bolstered by information technology, the consumer is playing a more and more active role. Increasingly, consumers are becoming more and more comfortable in their empowered roles.

The trend toward consumer empowerment has ignited a number of massive public education efforts. Ironically, the pharmaceutical industry has been something of a trailblazer in this consumer-driven era, bypassing the physician and moving directly to the consumer for advertising and promotion. Recognizing that health care is, at its heart, an information-based undertaking, DTC advertising was a bold move in many respects. But it hasn't gone far enough.

DTC behaviors in other industries often serve as models for the examination of our own practices. In this case the computer industry may offer a useful analogy. When Microsoft was blazing new trails with their first PC, Apple took keen notice of the fact that the lion's share of the Microsoft market was composed of "techies." All the rest of mainstream America, folks who did not yet have the technical expertise to venture into the high-tech product experience but liked the idea of using a PC, needed a more user-friendly machine. To address this need, Apple created the Macintosh, and with an ingenious marketing strategy dubbed the Mac the PC "for the rest of us."

"The rest of us" need legible package inserts, knowledgeable pharmacists who can answer questions, home delivery of prescription drugs (pizzas can be there in 15 minutes, why not a prescription?), and a better understanding of the differences between various drugs and treatment options. In spite of DTC's overly slick Madison Avenue style, the net result is more awareness on the part of consumers. That's not all bad.

## NURSING'S OPPORTUNITY WITH THE PHARMACEUTICAL INDUSTRY: TAKE THE ADHERENCE ISSUE PUBLIC

The pharmaceutical industry has a lot of work to do to restore the public trust. Many of the criticisms of the industry are well founded. Still, it seems misguided to move too far toward—overregulating an industry that has produced tremendous benefits in the past.

One thing is certain: We will always need drugs. PhRMA's dilemma demands a visible demonstration of sensitivity—and empathy, in particular—on the part of leaders to soothe the public's negative emotions, calm fears, and assuage anger. In this context, strategic partnerships with the nursing community would indeed be very furthering for PhRMA.

As pharmaceutical companies begin to look at ways to reestablish the public trust and increase goodwill with the public, the issue of nonadherence offers a key leverage point in communicating with the public—and nurses are the public's health educators of choice. According to the National Pharmaceutical Council, 10% of all hospital admissions are the result of pharmaceutical nonadherence, and 23% of all nursing home admissions are a result of people's inability to take their medications as prescribed (Levy, 1992).

Nonadherence results in lost productivity and premature deaths in addition to more hospital admissions, emergency-room care, physician visits, and occasionally surgeries. It is estimated that only about half of prescribed medicines are taken correctly (Maraldo & Lister, 2002). This problem drains an estimated $100 billion from our national economy every year and is blamed for the deaths of over 125,000 Americans annually (342 people every day) (Maraldo & Lister, 2002). There is also the personal side of the equation—the suffering and damage that occur when, for example, failure to

take contraceptives leads to unwanted pregnancies, failure to take estrogen-replacement medication causes osteoporosis, or failure to take hypertension medicine results in heart attack or stroke. Unless patients learn to take their medicines according to health care providers' instructions, and systems are in place to guard against adverse drug interactions, prescription drugs may not be used cost-effectively.

It is well established that nonadherence is a costly problem for employers, insurers, the health care system, and, last but not least, consumers. The nursing community should join with PhRMA to take the lead in addressing the problem with the public and should do so in a way that emphasizes the goal of health, rather than the goal of sales. Both sides have much to gain. Tackling the adherence issue represents a strategic opportunity to show the public that pharmaceutical companies are on their side. The overarching concept here is to create closer linkages with consumers that demonstrate value. Nurses have economic rewards to gain. The pharmaceutical industry is in a position to help finance initiatives that could assist nurses in developing new models of caring for patients with chronic disease and prevention—areas in which nursing care is what is needed and in which the greatest demand lies for the future.

A major education and awareness initiative by nurses on behalf of the industry would do a lot more than educate; it would communicate friendliness and respect. Over and over again it has been demonstrated that consumers willingly foot the bill when they perceive that something is worth it. And over and over again it has been demonstrated that the public trusts nurses.

If the goal of the pharmaceutical industry is to deliver the right drug to the right patient the first time, routinely integrating education into every patient encounter through nurses is a major opportunity. Innovative educational approaches could actually reframe the experience in the patient's mind to create a more positive relationship between pharmaceutical companies and consumers (Maraldo & Lister, 2002).

At a time when concerns about health care are escalating, it is striking to examine the trend toward alternative therapies. For example, in 1997,

Americans spent approximately $27 billion on providers of alternative health care including herbal preparations such as black cohosh, St. Johns wort, echinacea, and others. This is more than they spent in the same year on all conventional physician visits (Eisenberg, et al., 1998). In addition, the majority of this multi–billion-dollar spending represented out-of-pocket, nonreimbursable expenditures. Furthermore, this amount was more than double what consumers spent in 1990 (Maraldo & Lister, 2002). Americans are voting with their wallets to use more and more alternative practitioners. Alternative treatments are embraced with trust and acceptance, even when proof of efficacy is entirely absent. The pharmaceutical industry has been displaced as the "friend" of the public. It must regain this ground.

Members of the public are willing to trust their own instincts when it comes to their health care. Broad systemic solutions are needed for systemic complaints and concerns. In this age of technology, many revolutionary strategies, with nurses as the quintessential patient educators at the helm, are possible—such as the inclusion of easily and inexpensively reproduced CD-ROMs or videocassettes with each prescription filled. Such activities would likely have a beneficial effect on adherence, especially when dealing with topics some physicians are uncomfortable discussing, such as sexual problems.

At a time when health care delivery continues to be volume driven, physicians no longer have the time to educate their patients about serious aspects of pharmacologic therapies. Yet patient education must ultimately be a collaborative function. Pharmaceutical companies could take a major step in improving public perception by forming new strategic alliances with nurses, and nurses could take a step forward to suggest nurse-led innovations on the patient care side, in return.

## Key Points

- The pharmaceutical industry is experiencing a barrage of public anger. Some of it is legitimate; some of it is endemic to the way the heath care system operates—that is, the profit motive, and

FDA incentives encouraging the prevalence of "me-too" drugs in the past decade.
- The industry has contributed tremendous advances in the health of the nation, perhaps more so than other sectors. Advances have been made in genetics, and many more are on the horizon; it would be a mistake to slow the process of scientific discovery.
- Blame isn't useful in trying to fix our health care problems. The problem is a systemic one, with the wrong incentives and motivations in place. The pharmaceutical industry bears responsibility for its problems, to be sure, but others are part of the problem of rising costs.
- Using the right drug at the right time has been shown to be cost saving, keeping patients out of the hospital.
- Nursing has an opportunity to develop strategic partnerships with pharmaceutical companies to create new strategies and new models of care.

## Web Resources

**Better Management.com**—discussions of issues regarding the pharmaceutical industry business
*www.bettermanagement.com*
**Henry J. Kaiser Family Foundation**—information and analysis related to pharmaceutical issues and policy
*www.kaisernetwork.org*
**Pharmaceutical Industry News**—information on the pharmaceutical industry
*www.cpspharm.com/pharmanews*

## REFERENCES

Angelmar, R. (2005). Big PhRMA: In need of treatment? *Insead Knowledge*. Retrieved December 11, 2005, from *http://knowledge.insead.edu/abstract.cfm?ct=15200*.
Bary, A. (2004, October 18). A little respect. *Barron's Online*. Retrieved February 25, 2006, from *www.google.com/search?hl=en&lr=&ie=ISO-8859-1&q=Bary+%22a+little+respect%22+%22barron%27s+online%22&btnG=Search*.
Eisenberg, D. M., Davis, R. B., Ettner, S. L., Appel, S., Wilkey, S., Van Rompay, M., & Kessler, R. C. (1998). Trends in alternative medicine use in the United States, 1990-1997. *Journal of the American Medical Association, 280*, 1569-1575.

Goldstein, R. (2005). FDA chooses drug industry health over public health. CommonDreams.org. Retrieved December 11, 2005, from *www.commondreams.org/views05/0223-35.htm*.

Herzlinger, R. (2004). *Consumer-driven health care*. San Francisco: Jossey Bass.

Hunt, M. (2002). Changing patterns of pharmaceutical innovation. National Institute for Healthcare Management Research and Educational Foundation. Retrieved December 11, 2005, from *www.nihcm.org/innovations.pdf*.

Klienke, J. D. (2001). The price of progress: Prescription drugs in the health care market. *Health Affairs, 20*(5), 43-60.

Klienke, J. D. (2005). Turning point for the health care blame cycle? *Health Affairs, 24*(1), 291-293.

Levy, R. (1992). *Emerging issues in pharmaceutical cost containment*. Reston, VA: National Pharmaceutical Council. Available through the National Pharmaceutical Council (phone: [703] 620-6390).

Maraldo, P., & Lister, E. (2002). Reframe industry's image. *Pharmaceutical Executive, 22*(9), 92-98. Retrieved December 11, 2005, from *www.pharmexec.com/pharmexec/ article/articleDetail.jsp?id=29970*.

Relman, A. (2002, February 21). Presentation to the Standing Senate Committee on Social Affairs, Science and Technology looking at health reform. Retrieved February 25, 2006, from *www.healthcoalition.ca/relman.html*.

Rost, P. (2004, October 30). Medicines without borders. *New York Times*, A19.

Steinbrook, R. (2004). Registration of clinical trials—Voluntary or mandatory? *New England Journal of Medicine, 351*(18), 1820-1822.

Strunk, B., Ginsburg, P., & Cookson, J. (2005, January-June). Tracking health care costs: Declining growth trend pauses in 2004. *Health Affairs*, suppl, W5-286-W5-295. Retrieved December 11, 2005, from *http://content.healthaffairs.org/ cgi/content/full/hlthaff.w5.286/DC1*.

# chapter 14

# A Primer on Health Economics

Lynn Unruh & Joanne Spetz

*"All models are wrong, but some are useful."*

GEORGE BOX

It would be great if we could provide all the health care we wanted to anyone needing it at any time. It is becoming clearer and clearer, however, that health care resources are limited and that choices must be made—and *are* being made—with regard to *what* health care is to be provided, *who* will get health care, and *how much* health care will be received.

The scarcity of resources, and the choices that must be made, are not always obvious, but they can be seen from the following facts about our system: The United States spends more than any other nation on health care—more than $1.6 trillion per year, and more than $5000 per person (Bodenheimer, 2005). Yet approximately 16% of our population goes without regular care because of lack of health insurance (Kaiser Family Foundation [KFF], 2004), primary care is often difficult to obtain (Schoen et al., 2004), and many of our health outcomes are worse than those of other developed countries (Commonwealth Fund, 2004).

What makes our health care system more expensive, yet less accessible and less efficacious than those of other countries? Can we continue along this path, or should changes be made in how we produce and distribute health care?

These realities and policy issues of our health care system are important to *consumers* of health care, yet they also affect nurses as *providers* of health care. First, they affect the health of patients for whom nurses care. For example, when someone goes without preventive care because she does not have insurance and cannot pay for the services, she may enter the health care system sicker than if she had received the needed care to begin with (Miller, Vigdor, & Manning, 2004).

Second, the choices that are made affect the types of nursing services that are provided. Over the past few decades public and private payers in health care have altered demand for services away from inpatient hospital care toward outpatient care such as home care, same-day surgery, and urgent care centers. Care also has shifted to nursing homes, rehabilitation centers, and other subacute care centers. As a result, demand for nurses has shifted away from inpatient hospital care. Third, the choices affect the quality of care, as issues of adequate nursing skill mix, staffing, and educational levels and other structural factors are known to affect patient outcomes (Aiken, Clarke, Cheung, Sloane, & Silber, 2003; Aiken, Clarke, Sloane, Sochalski, & Silber, 2002; Needleman, Buerhaus, Mattke, Stewart, & Zelevinsky, 2002; Unruh, 2003a).

Health economics helps us make decisions about what and how much health care to produce, how to provide it, and to whom to provide it. Health economics strives to provide insight into how our health care system operates and ways to make it operate better. It assists in quantifying and evaluating the pros and cons of the multiple potential uses of limited resources. Although it is useful as an input in decision-making, it should not be seen as the "last word." Many other considerations are involved, such as cultural, social, and political concerns.

This chapter covers the theories and methods of health economics as it examines aspects of the

U.S. health care system. The chapter begins with a discussion about economic theory and its application to health care. Next, the chapter delves into the demand for health care, in which insurance and managed care play big roles. Following that, supply of health care is covered, including the roles of hospitals, physicians, and nurses. Supply and demand are combined in two sections that discuss the market for hospitals and the market for nurses.

Evaluation of costs and benefits of specific health care projects forms the topic of the next to the last section. The last section discusses the future health care system as it applies to nurses. The interaction between the broader health care system and nursing is emphasized.

## ECONOMIC THEORY AND REALITY IN HEALTH CARE

Economic theory addresses the question of how communities allocate scarce resources. Individuals have different preferences for goods, services, time, and other things of value. Moreover, individuals have different abilities to produce things that people need, such as food, equipment, and services. As a result of these two types of differences, opportunities for trade abound. A highly productive farmer can trade food she will not eat for a doctor's services, and a carpenter can trade her construction work for clothing.

In a freely competitive economy, prices can adjust as needed to ensure that the supply and demand for goods and services are balanced. When the demand for a product is greater than supply, purchasers bid up the price of the scarce product. As the price rises, fewer purchasers are interested in the product, because its cost becomes greater than its value to some buyers. Therefore the demand drops. At the same time, the higher price that can be received for the product causes suppliers to increase their supply, because they can receive greater profit for each item sold. The combined effect of the decrease in demand and increase in supply caused by the free-market change in price is that the market will reach an equilibrium point at which supply and demand are equal. When supply exceeds demand, a similar story can be told, with the price falling so that more

buyers are interested in the product and sellers want to offer less of it.

A freely competitive market, often called a "perfectly competitive" market, never faces a shortage or surplus of a product. Several conditions must be met for a market to be perfectly competitive, the most important of which are that there must be many buyers and sellers, there is no cost to becoming a seller or buyer, the products must be uniform ("homogenous"), and buyers and sellers must have perfect information about the qualities of products. Some markets exhibit many of these characteristics. For example, the low-wage labor market has many buyers (employers) and sellers (workers), job attributes are generally well known, employers can assess that workers have few skills, and employers and workers can enter the labor market easily.

It requires little analysis to recognize that health care markets violate all the basic requirements of perfectly competitive markets. For many types of health care markets, there are not many, but instead few sellers. Hospital or nursing home markets, for example, are closer to "monopolies" or "oligopolies" (characterized by one or only a few sellers in the market, respectively) than to competitive markets. Similarly, health care professionals such as physicians or nurses cannot enter the market freely; most professionals are licensed by state or professional organizations. The health care "product" is not uniform; each physician or hospital provides slightly to significantly different care compared with another. Given these noncompetitive characteristics, these health care providers have some degree of market power over the *sale* of their product. This can lead to shortages and higher prices for care than would exist in a competitive environment. Market power can also extend to the *buying* of inputs such as labor ("monopsony" or "oligopsony") and lead to shortages in the labor force because wages and benefits stay below equilibrium levels.

Perhaps more importantly, buyers and sellers do not have perfect information about patients' need for health care or the quality of health care products. Patients do not know whether or when they will need health care in the future. They may not even be sure that they are ill, nor will they know how to treat their ailments. Providers often do not know what a patient's ailment is until further tests are conducted. Moreover, providers do not know how effective a course of treatment is for an individual patient.

Most economists agree that policy intervention can be used to address problems in markets that are not perfectly competitive. Some regulations are widely accepted, such as the licensure of health professionals and hospitals so patients have assurance of the quality of their providers. Government provision of health insurance for certain populations—the elderly and poor—is designed to address the fact that these populations cannot obtain insurance otherwise and is generally accepted. But there is also much debate about the appropriate role of government. Should governments regulate health care prices? To what extent should governments invest in research that leads to new health care treatments? Should employers receive tax breaks for providing health insurance? Most debates about government intervention focus on the question of whether the health care market can be made sufficiently competitive to function with some regulation, or whether the health care market is so dysfunctional that a complete government takeover is needed.

## THE DEMAND FOR HEALTH CARE

In recent years, health policy in the United States has focused on the needs of those who demand health care services. The demand for health care is often intermediated by the purchase of health insurance. In the United States, people obtain health insurance in three general ways: their employers offer health insurance as a component of compensation for work; they purchase insurance individually from an insurance company; or they are enrolled in a government-funded program.

Once a person has insurance, she is insulated from the costs of each health care service. Apart from small payments that might be required for each service, the insurance enrollee pays only the fixed cost of the insurance, and in fact might not even pay this if insurance is provided by an employer or government entity. As a result, the enrollee tends to demand more health care than would be demanded without insurance. This is called "moral hazard."

Moral hazard leads to greater health care demand and thus greater health care expenditures than would occur in a perfectly competitive market. A fundamental issue faced by all health care systems is how to reach the socially optimal level of health care usage given the presence of health insurance.

Insurance companies try to address moral hazard in a variety of ways. Most common is the requirement that the enrollee pay some part of the cost of each health service in the form of copayment (a flat fee paid for each service) or coinsurance (a fixed percentage of the cost of each service). Many traditional insurance plans also require that the enrollee pay some amount of health care costs before the insurer pays any of the costs; this is called a *deductible*. Although the RAND Health Insurance Experiment of the 1980s found that increased out-of-pocket expenses were not associated with worse health, other studies indicate that needed health care might be neglected (Karter et al, 2003), which could lead to greater emergency room (ER) usage (Wright et al., 2005) and poorer health outcomes (Rice & Matsuoka, 2004). A recent review of studies found that cost sharing reduced appropriate usage and/or health status in nearly all of the 22 studies examined (Rice & Matsuoka, 2004). Higher usage of the ER and poorer health could lead to higher costs, the opposite of what is intended.

Since the 1940s, insurance companies have provided "managed care," in which the insurance company plays a role in directing the overall care of enrollees. One of the first managed care insurance plans was the Kaiser Foundation Health Plan, created to provide health care to employees of Henry J. Kaiser's shipyards. In the Kaiser Plan a medical group is exclusively contracted with the insurance company to provide health care services, and Kaiser Permanente operates its own hospitals. Employees pay small copayments for health services, and physicians receive extensive education and guidance about providing preventative care and evidence-based practice. A patient must be referred to a specialist by a primary care physician; self-referral is not allowed, and care received outside the Kaiser network is not covered by the insurance.

There were few other insurance companies offering managed care insurance until the past two decades, during which time numerous variants of the managed care concept have evolved. Many new health maintenance organizations (HMOs) are not "closed panel" and allow the physicians with whom they contract to treat both HMO and non-HMO patients. These HMOs maintain control over care provided to patients either directly by placing restrictions on the services offered or indirectly by providing physicians and hospitals incentives to care for patients in certain ways. Enrollees are assigned to primary health care providers, called "gatekeepers," who manage the overall care of enrollees.

Preferred provider organizations (PPOs) encourage enrollees to select certain care providers by providing lower coinsurance rates if preferred providers are chosen. They allow members to go to specialists without having to use a gatekeeper first. A point-of-service (POS) plan is a hybrid of an HMO and a PPO. Patients are assigned a primary health care provider, as they would be in an HMO, but they can seek care from other providers, albeit at a higher out-of-pocket cost.

The goal of these benefit conscriptions, in-network requirements, gatekeeper requirements, and other enrollee incentives is to control costs by better managing the care of enrollees and to reduce "moral hazard." In theory, managed care insurance plans focus on preventative health care services and try to eliminate unneeded medical care.

Because people have little information with which to judge the quality of care offered by health care providers and thus by insurance companies, they often select insurance based on price rather than quality. Moreover, a hospital that provides excellent care is usually reimbursed at the same rate as a hospital that provides mediocre care. When managed care pressures cause providers to focus on reducing costs, they often do so at the expense of quality. At a minimum, amenities are eliminated, and in some cases essential resources such as registered nurse (RN) staff are reduced.

These problems arise from the difficulty of obtaining information about health care products and are a reason for intervention by governmental regulatory or private credentialing organizations such as the Joint Commission on the Accreditation of Health Care Organizations (JCAHO). Through regulation or certification, quality can be monitored, standardized, and improved and information about quality can be conveyed to consumers.

This discussion on the demand for health care in the United States omits one important issue: the high proportion of Americans who lack adequate health insurance. Sixteen percent of the population did not have health insurance at some time in 2003, and another 5% had inadequate coverage (Schoen, Doty, Collins, & Holmgren, 2005). The uninsured tend to be poor or near-poor adults in families with at least one wage earner. Most have gone without coverage for at least 2 years. Rates of uninsurance are higher among minorities. For these people the primary issue is that they do not use primary and preventative health services as much as they should because they cannot afford the out-of-pocket costs. As a result, health problems that could be treated effectively grow into acute problems that must be treated aggressively, are more costly, and have poorer outcomes. Policymakers and the public in the United States have resisted establishing a mandatory universal health insurance program, and therefore the problem of uninsurance and underinsurance continues.

## THE SUPPLY OF HEALTH CARE

The supply of health care also has been a focus of health policy. Direct suppliers of health care are professionals (such as physicians and advanced practice nurses) and institutions of care (such as hospitals, nursing homes, home care organizations, and doctor's offices). Institutions of care, in turn, employ a number of nonprofessional and professional staff, such as the nursing staff, who enter into supply through the "derived demand" of their institutional employers.

These suppliers, or providers, of health care offer services in exchange for payment from the various demanders of health care discussed previously. Providers have experienced drastic changes in the reimbursement for their services. In general, payers have moved away from paying providers what they charge *after the service* is provided (retrospective payment) to amounts set *in advance of the service* (prospective payment). Both public and private payers have been responsible for these changes, starting with the introduction of Diagnostic Related Groups (DRGs) and Resource-Based Relative Value Scales (RBRVS) for payment under Medicare and continuing with various negotiated fees and charges under managed care. At this time, prospective payment systems (PPSs) exist for all types of health care: inpatient hospital care, nursing home care, home care, and ambulatory care.

PPSs have, in turn, prompted providers to find efficiencies in delivering care in order to be able to provide care for the agreed-on amount of money. The search for efficiencies can take the form of technology improvements that reduce the time needed to perform the services, or cost-cutting measures such as staff reductions and substitutions.

One practice that providers may engage in to compensate for reduced payment is "provider-induced demand." In this practice providers instruct patients, who generally know less about their health problem and treatment than the providers, to consume health care services that are not needed or that could be more efficiently provided. Demand inducement is not necessarily a malicious phenomenon; care providers might encourage patients to seek every medical intervention or test that could have any benefit, even if the benefit is so small that the costs exceed the benefits. Neither patients nor care providers pay the full cost of health services in most cases, so they do not make cost-benefit comparisons. Demand inducement is an example of how the health care market is not perfectly competitive. It is a problem because it leads to greater overall health care spending and can lead to iatrogenic illnesses among the patients who receive "too much" or inappropriate health care.

One set of health care providers—physicians—play a central role in the provision of medical care services and therefore make many of the demand decisions for their patients. They act as *agents* for their patients. When physicians are able to induce demand for health care, it is called "physician-induced demand." Whether physicians or other providers can actually induce demand for health care has been an area of research and debate in health care economics. Evidence exists both ways (Reinhardt, 1985). Some agreement seems to be

developing that because of managed care practices, physicians are not able to induce demand very much at this time.

In the previous section we discussed how managed care attempts to reduce "moral hazard." Managed care also attempts to reduce supplier tendencies to induce demand. One of the most drastic ways has been to capitate the payment to providers. Capitated reimbursement means that providers are paid a fixed amount per patient per year, regardless of how much care the person requires. Providers' incentives are to keep the use of resources down—for example, the number of office visits or the use of tests and procedures. The use of capitation to control health care usage is currently in decline because of consumer and provider backlash.

Managed care uses other methods to reduce provider-induced demand. Per diem and DRG-based reimbursements to hospitals limit the amount of reimbursement hospitals may receive for each patient's stay. Under these systems, greater use of resources by providers may lead to financial losses. In some cases bonuses are paid to physicians who keep resource use down, and physician reimbursement for overuse may be withheld. Case management, utilization management, disease management, the use of second opinions, and the use of practice guidelines also are aimed at reducing unnecessary medical care.

Do these managed care methods reduce health care use? In early studies, physician reimbursement mechanisms such as capitation were associated with shorter physician visits and fewer hospitalizations (Hillman, Pauly, & Kerstein, 1989; Jordan, 2001). Utilization management was found to reduce hospital admissions, lengths of stay, and use of services (Robinson, 1996; Wickizer, 1992). More recent research finds less of a difference between managed care and traditional insurance practices (Luft, 1999), possibly because managed care has influenced and changed all provider relationships from what they were prior to its rise.

## THE MARKET FOR HOSPITAL SERVICES

Hospitals are an important part of the U.S. health care system. They provide emergency care, surgeries, highly technical tests and treatments, and institutional care for those too sick to be cared for at home. Although hospitals in 2002 received 31% of all health care dollars, demand for their services fell during the1990s, primarily because of managed care influence (Cowan, Catlin, Smith, & Sensenig, 2004). The proportion of health care spending on hospital care fell throughout the 1990s. Also, the number of annual admissions fell 14% from 1980 to 1995 and has not yet returned to the 1980 level (Centers for Disease Control and Prevention [CDC], 2004). Much of this health care moved to the outpatient setting, as indicated by an 85% increase in outpatient visits from 1990 to 2002 (CDC, 2004).

Hospitals are classified according to length of stay, type of service, and type of ownership. Short-term hospitals are those with average lengths of stay less than 30 days. Community hospitals are short-stay hospitals that offer general services and some also provide specialty care and rehabilitation. They may be owned by state or local governments, nonprofit voluntary organizations, or for-profit organizations.

Hospital ownership can be private not-for-profit, private for-profit, or governmental. The most prominent form of ownership of hospitals is private not-for-profit (60% of all hospitals). However, for-profit ownership grew in the 1980s and 1990s and in 2003 included 15.4% of community hospitals and 13.2% of community hospital beds.

For-profit ownership of hospitals has been controversial. Some believe that the quality of care in nonprofit hospitals must be better because such hospitals do not focus on the "bottom line." Actually, not-for-profit hospitals have had to be just as conscious of costs and revenues as for-profits. Both for-profit and not-for-profit hospitals can generate surplus revenue. Where they differ is that for-profits can distribute the surplus in the form of profit to stockholders or owners, whereas not-for-profits must maintain the surplus within the institution or use it to provide some benefit to the community. Also, for-profits can raise capital through stock offerings, whereas not-for-profits must look toward donations, grants, and other forms of equity. Both for-profits and not-for-profits can issue bonds, and not-for-profit hospital bonds are tax exempt. Finally, for-profit net revenues are taxed, whereas not-for-profit surpluses are not.

So is quality better at not-for-profit hospitals? The research record is mixed. Sloan (2000) found that patients did better in teaching hospitals but that there was no difference between nonteaching not-for-profit and for-profit hospitals. On the other hand, McClellan and Staiger (2000) found that for-profit hospitals have higher mortality and that the difference from not-for-profit hospitals was growing.

Because of the reimbursement and managed care pressures described earlier, hospital organization, finances, services, and employment patterns underwent dramatic change in the past decades. At the beginning of the 1990s, hospitals found themselves having to negotiate unfavorable contracts with managed care companies because those companies had power on the buyer's side of the market. In response to this pressure, hospitals merged and formed multihospital systems in the 1990s. Some hospitals merged or expanded vertically by adding noninpatient types of health care such as home care, nursing home care, rehabilitation, or ambulatory care. Some hospitals closed.

These changes provided integrated hospital systems with greater market power to counter that of managed care, greater economies of scale (efficiencies resulting from size), and greater economies of scope (efficiencies resulting from the production of many different types of products). It also produced hospital markets that are classically "monopolistic" or "oligopolic" as sellers— that is, one or a handful of hospital systems have carved out the market for hospital care in each geographic area. Managed care plans must negotiate with these few sellers of hospital services. It is interesting to note that the cost savings that managed care was wringing out of the health care system in the 1980s and early 1990s began to dissipate in the late 1990s as the hospital oligopolies arrived on the scene.

It is thought that hospitals respond to reduced public reimbursement by shifting costs to patients with higher-paying insurance plans by charging privately insured patients higher prices. Since the 1980s, Medicare and Medicaid have underpaid hospitals by as much as 30% of costs (Lee et al., 2003; Medicare Payment Advisory Committee [MedPac], 2002). If hospitals are able to shift costs, they should be able to make up the difference by charging private payers more for the same services. Those who believe that hospitals cost-shift point to the fact that the payment-to-cost ratios of private payers rose throughout the 1980s and early 1990s (as Medicare and Medicaid ratios fell), peaking at 130 in 1992. However, with the rise of managed care, the payment differential has declined significantly to around 112 (Lee et al., 2003).

Internally, in response to lower demand and reduced public and private payments, hospitals downsized and restructured. Professional and nonprofessional, nursing and non-nursing staff were affected. We discuss the changes and their impact on nursing staff in the next section. In addition, hospitals reorganized care so that patients complete their hospital stays in a shorter amount of time. Average lengths of stay in nonfederal, short-stay hospitals fell from 7.5 days in 1980 to 4.9 in 2001, a drop of 35% (CDC, 2004). Because hospitals are often paid a fixed or maximum amount per patient stay, length-of-stay reductions allows them to provide care at costs lower than the fixed reimbursements and therefore maintain financial viability.

## THE MARKET FOR NURSES

The term *nurse* means different things to different people. By *nurse* we refer to both licensed nurses, such as RNs and licensed practical nurses (LPNs), and unlicensed staff, such as nursing assistants. We focus primarily on the market for RNs.

Because most nurses are employees of health care institutions, the demand for their employment is derived from their employers, who employ nurses based on the demand and prices for their services, and the productivity and prices (wages, salaries, and benefits) of the nurses being hired. As reimbursement changed to prospective systems and as managed care practices grew, the growth in demand for inpatient care slowed and the prices paid for care were constrained. Hospitals were heavily affected by these trends in the 1980s and 1990s. As a consequence, it is believed that hospital

demand for licensed nurses fell. Surveys of RNs reported reductions in staff, substitutions of nursing assistants for licensed staff, and increases in workload (Shindul-Rothschild, Berry, & Long-Middleton, 1996). Primary nursing models were replaced with team nursing, which enabled skill-mix substitutions. Recent studies "counting nurses" indicate that nurses' perceptions were correct (Unruh, 2002; Unruh, 2003b).

On the other hand, the demand for nurses in other areas such as ambulatory surgery centers and home care has grown. This growth slowed in home care after 1997, when the Balanced Budget Act (BBA) introduced a PPS for home care. With that, the demand for home care nurses plunged. In other areas, such as nursing homes and physicians' offices, demand has been more stable. Analyses of the National Sample Survey of Registered Nurses have shown that the share of RNs employed in hospitals dropped from 68% in 1984 to 59% in 2000.

So far we haven't mentioned the current nursing shortage. After reports of surpluses of nurses in the mid 1990s, a shortage of RNs reemerged in the late 1990s. At that time public reimbursement improved and managed care pressures lessened. Admissions increased, and length of stay stabilized. In addition, the typical hospitalized patient was acutely ill. Suddenly, demand for nurses, particularly RNs, rose. By 1999, hospitals began to experience RN vacancy rates of 9%, an indication of a nursing shortage (Grumbach, Ash, Seago, Spetz, & Coffman, 2001). High vacancy rates have continued at 11% to 14%, indicating continued shortages, especially in certain regions such as the South (Seago, Ash, Spetz, Coffman, & Grumbach, 2001). Nursing homes and home health agencies also are reporting shortages (Pindus, Tilly, & Weinstein 2002). By 2020 a shortage is expected to exist in nearly every state, and the gap between supply and demand is expected to climb to 29% (U.S. Department of Health and Human Services [DHHS], 2000).

The reasons for the current and future shortage are multiple on both the demand and the supply sides. On the demand side, population growth and an aging population will exert growing health care consumption pressure over the next few decades. Other factors affecting demand include levels of access afforded by public and private insurance, the efficiency of health care delivery, and regulations and accreditation requirements that involve nurse staffing. On the supply side, significant factors include a large population of older RNs who are expected to retire soon, educational bottlenecks that restrict the growth of nursing supply, and difficult work environments and low wages that discourage entry into and encourage withdrawal from the profession and nursing jobs (Buerhaus, Needleman, Mattke, & Stewart, 2002; Spetz & Given, 2003; Unruh & Fottler, 2005).

It was mentioned earlier that in a competitive market shortages would not occur. Why do we see shortages in the market for nurses? One economic theory is that the primary employers of nurses—hospitals—enjoy a monopsony over the hiring of nursing labor; they have market power in the buying of nursing labor, which they use to keep wages, benefits, and working conditions at lower-than-equilibrium levels. Even though employers would like to employ more nurses, the wages, benefits, and working conditions they offer do not attract people to their jobs. Raising wages alone may not be the answer to this problem, however, as long as working conditions remain difficult (AFT Healthcare, 2002). The many other supply and demand factors listed previously must also be addressed.

It may be that wages, benefits, and working conditions for nurses are at suboptimal levels because nursing care is not appropriately valued and priced. This can occur at several levels. First, at the societal level, market economies have tended to neglect the quantification of "caring" services, as well as "women's work," both of which are the cultural and historical legacy of nursing. Second, at the payer level, specific nursing services have generally not been included in reimbursement systems. Studies of the DRG payment system have shown that DRG values are not strongly associated with the intensity of nursing care for that category (Adams & Johnson, 1986; Mitchell, Miller, Welches, & Walker, 1984). Third, at the organizational level, health care facilities such as hospitals typically treat nursing care only as an "expense" item in their budget, not as a revenue-generating item. The price of nursing is wrapped into the room rate.

To receive adequate wages, benefits, and working conditions, these societal, financial, and organizational impediments to properly valuing and pricing nursing services need to be overcome. Ways to accomplish this include conducting and disseminating research on the following:

- What nurses do, including their caring activities, but also their intellectual, technical, managerial, and other activities
- How what they do affects health outcomes
- What the costs of adequate nursing care are, versus the costs of inadequate care

As nursing care is understood more deeply and by a broader audience, nursing advocates can work for societal, financial, and organizational change that will allow for valuing and pricing nursing services.

The monumental changes in reimbursement and the cost-consciousness of public and private payers have brought one advantage for nursing: The demand for advanced practice nurses is rising. In acute care, nurse clinicians and nurse practitioners are needed to clinically manage a more acutely ill clientele, and to provide efficiencies in care that may help alleviate the shortage of staff RNs. In ambulatory care, demand for nurse practitioners is on the rise, as community centers and managed care organizations look for lower-cost ways of providing primary care. However, the expansion of advanced practice nursing continues to face opposition by the medical establishment, and many legal barriers remain.

## CLINICAL ECONOMICS: EVALUATING HEALTH CARE PERFORMANCE

As we become more aware of the limited resources in health care, and the choices among them that we must make, methods to help us make those choices are welcome. Economics offers a set of techniques that clarify options and point to an efficient use of resources. Six types of economic techniques are used in health care decision-making:

- Cost of illness
- Cost identification
- Cost minimization
- Cost-consequence analysis

- Cost-effectiveness analysis (CEA)
- Cost-benefit analysis (CBA)

When performing *cost-of- illness* analyses, investigators look only at the total costs of one or more *illnesses* in order to ascertain whether they should be a priority for treatment and/or public health measures. Often the entire economic burden of a disease is described, including not only the medical costs but also days lost from work. The comparative costs and effectiveness of different treatments for those illnesses are not studied. A recent example is a study on the cost of prematurity (Cuevas, Silver, Brooten, Youngblut, & Bobo, 2005). It finds that charges for initial hospitalization increased as birth weight and gestational weight decreased and concludes that interventions to improve prenatal care targeted to high-risk pregnancies would reduce health care costs.

*Cost identification* looks at the costs of a health care *service*. This can be done for several different services for a given health care problem. Then, the cost of the different services can be compared, and the service with the lowest cost can be chosen. At this point, the analysis becomes a *cost-minimization* study. Cost minimization is a common evaluation method, as it is useful to compare the costs of treatments for health problems. For example, through cost-minimization analysis, the lowest-cost treatment for diagnosing pancreatic cancer can be assessed (Chen, Arguedas, Kilgore, & Eloubeidi, 2004). In both cost identification and cost minimization the effectiveness of the treatments is not studied; therefore in the example just cited the effectiveness of the lowest-cost treatment is not considered.

Several analytic strategies measure both the costs and the effectiveness of health care interventions. In *cost-consequence* analysis, one creates a comprehensive listing of all the benefits of competing interventions and lets decision-makers determine which benefits are most important. A *cost-effectiveness analysis* measures the benefits of projects with a consistent unit of measure, such as "cost per life saved" or "cost per case of breast cancer detected." A special case of this is called *cost-utility analysis*, in which a standard utility measurement of quality-adjusted life years (QALYs) is used. QALYs are developed through surveys and other methods to determine how people value the quality of life with certain illnesses, restrictions, and disabilities.

With CEA the objective is to find the treatment that has the relatively best effectiveness for the relatively best costs. Treatments that have both higher costs and less effectiveness are eliminated. If several alternative treatments are considered, more than one may turn out to be "economically rational"— that is, they are all equally reasonably cost-efficient, the main difference between them being the level of costs associated with the effectiveness. The final step is to decide among the economically rational options, usually by picking the option for which the payer is willing to pay. Although CEA enables the investigator to relatively rank treatments, a judgment about the absolute effectiveness of the treatments is not possible. In other words, in CEA, even though one or some treatments are better, all the treatments could entail high costs for few benefits. As with cost minimization, there are many examples of studies that use CEA. Box 14-1 contains an example of a study concerning sleep apnea (Mar et al., 2003).

Finally, sometimes the technique of *cost-benefit analysis* (CBA) is used. In this analysis both costs

---

**BOX 14-1**  Example of Cost Effectiveness Analysis

**Objective:** To compare the cost-effectiveness of nasal continuous positive airway pressure (nCPAP) with other treatments for those with moderate to severe obstructive sleep apnea (OSAS).

**Methods:** A Markov-type decision tree was used to diagram the possible progression of obstructive sleep apnea. The measure of effectiveness of treatments was quality adjusted life years (QALYs). Direct costs of diagnosis and treatment of OSAS as well as costs of not being treated were considered. The incremental cost-effectiveness ratio (ICER) was calculated for various scenarios.

**Results:** The ICER was similar to that of other interventions, indicating that nCPAP is a cost-effective treatment modality.

From Mar, J., Rueda, J. R., Duran-Cantolla, J., Schechter, C., & Chilcott, J. (2003). The cost-effectiveness of nCPAP treatment in patients with moderate-to-severe obstructive sleep apnea. *European Respiratory Journal, 21,* 515-522.

and benefits are placed in dollar amounts. For each treatment, the total costs are subtracted from the total benefits to find the *net benefit*. If costs are greater than benefits, the net benefit is negative. Sometimes, a ratio of benefits to costs is calculated, with ratios greater than one indicating positive benefits. The net benefits of each treatment can be compared, and the one with the greatest net benefits chosen. With CBA a judgment of both the relative and absolute effectiveness of the treatment can be made; the investigator knows not only which treatment has the best net benefit but also whether the net benefit is positive and by how much. The use of CBA in health care is controversial, however, because dollar amounts must be placed on human life and health. For this reason, it is not used nearly as much as CEA. Box 14-2 contains an example of a CBA of using bike and pedestrian trails (Wang, Macera, Scudder-Soucie, Schmid, Pratt, & Buchner, 2005).

It may be noted that these techniques form a spectrum. They go from methods requiring only

---

**BOX 14-2**   Example of Cost Benefit
               Analysis

**Objective:** To calculate the cost-benefit ratio of the medical benefits of using bike/pedestrian trails for physical activity.
   **Methods:** Construction and maintenance costs were calculated for the use of the trails, assuming a 30-year trail longevity and adjusting costs to the present value. Individual costs of using the trails were included. The direct health benefit was measured as the difference in the medical costs for active persons versus inactive persons. A cost-benefit ratio was calculated. Sensitivity analyses were conducted for worst- and best-case scenarios.
   **Results:** The cost-benefit ratio was 2.94, meaning that every $1 investment in using trails provided $2.94 in direct medical benefits. The cost-benefit ratios were greater than 1 in all scenarios.

From Wang, G., Macera, C. A., Scudder-Soucie, B., Schmid, T., Pratt, M., & Buchner, D. (2005). A cost-benefit analysis of physical activity using bike/pedestrian trails. *Health Promotion Practice, 6*(2), 174-179.

---

limited information and returning simple information about the costs of an illness, to methods requiring a high degree of information, even questionable information about the monetary worth of a life, and returning a specific picture about the net benefits of each treatment option. Which method to use should be based on the question to be answered and the available data. In practice, cost minimization and cost effectiveness are the two most often used.

## REFORM OF THE U.S. HEALTH CARE SYSTEM AND THE FUTURE OF NURSING

The U.S. health care system presents three challenges: lowering costs, improving access, and improving quality. Moreover, there is some degree of tradeoff among the three. How do we simultaneously lower costs, improve access, and improve quality? Being able to implement a reform that would do all three has been part of the difficulty. Some advocates believe that market forces can be used to solve health care problems, and the government's role is to ensure that health care markets are competitive. One market-oriented reform is medical savings accounts. Other policymakers believe a single national health care system should be established. There are many policy proposals, such as "managed competition," that seek intermediate ground.

Recently some policymakers suggested that medical savings accounts would help reduce costs without worsening access or quality. Medical savings accounts would be created for every individual either through their employer, by themselves, or through public assistance. Individuals would use the money in their savings accounts for primary health care, such as routine physician visits, medications, and tests. For larger medical expenses, including hospitalization, individuals would buy a low-cost, high-deductible insurance plan. This type of health plan is favorable to healthy and wealthy families and is generally more expensive for people with chronic illnesses. Moreover, poor families might avoid seeking primary health care services because of the out-of-pocket costs, and thereby allow problems to reach a catastrophic level before seeking care. Then they would be faced with a high insurance deductible they could not afford.

At the other extreme, advocates of a single-payer health care system believe that eliminating the multiple payers of the U.S. system and providing everyone with the same access to health care would both reduce costs and improve access. They cite that the administrative costs of our current system take away 31 cents of every health care dollar (Woolhandler, Campbell, & Himmelstein, 2003). If the system could be streamlined by creating a single governmental payer, around half of these administrative costs could disappear. The "single-payer" system could use payroll taxes and the money saved from reduced administrative costs to provide health care to all, expanding care to the underinsured and uninsured. Issues with this system involve those having to do with moral hazard and supplier-induced demand. Unless the system also maintains a managed care approach to delivering care, the easy availability of health care could lead to a rise in health care costs and to waiting periods to receive health care.

Other reform alternatives take a middle-of-the-road approach. "Managed competition" seeks to make individuals more knowledgeable about the costs and benefits of health care. Insurance companies are required to offer a standard set of health care benefits, and patients have access to information about the quality records of the health plan. Patients then can choose a health plan based on price and known quality. Managed competition could guarantee universal insurance through a government mandate that employers provide health insurance to their employees or that employers pay a tax that can be earmarked to purchase health insurance.

Why have we not been able to enact a major health care reform plan despite the obvious need? Economists believe that policy is often motivated by a combination of interest and power (Feldstein, 2003). The constituents who are most affected by a reform must be able to influence policymakers, and multiple constituents need to agree on a plan. In health care, powerful interest groups, such as insurance companies, hospitals, pharmaceuticals,

unions, and others, influence politicians to move in different directions rather than a unified one, and the group that would most benefit from reforms—the poor and uninsured—has little influence at all. As a result, politicians have been unable to find the support to enact one or another plan.

The future of nursing depends very much on the type of health care system the United States adopts or evolves into in the future. Reforms that focus on cost containment at the expense of access and/or quality could lead to continuing problems with staffing and working conditions as institutions attempt to tighten their belts even further. Reforms that do not constrain costs while providing greater access could lead to even greater shortages of nursing personnel and the possibility of more crises down the road—although, at least temporarily, the opportunities for nursing would be great. The best situation for nursing, as for health care consumers in general, will be if a solution can be found that has the fewest tradeoffs among costs, access, and quality yet improves all three. In this scenario, nurses should find increased opportunities, as well as improvements in working conditions.

It is in the interests of the nursing profession to promote change toward an efficient, equitable, and quality-focused health care system. In this process it is important for professional nurses to elucidate their value in the delivery of health care so that cost containment is not equated with reductions in nursing resources. Nurses can be instrumental in finding ways to create efficiencies other than staff reductions—for example, the increased use of computer technologies. They also can experiment with and evaluate models of nursing care that efficiently use various types of nursing personnel while providing safe, high-quality health care. Advanced practice nurses may lead the way in providing cost-effective primary care or managing complex groups of patients in the institutional setting. Because nursing is the one of the largest professions in health care—and in fact one of the largest professions in the United States—nurses should provide leadership in the development of institutional or local policies that improve health and national strategies to reform the health care system.

## Key Points

- Health care is a scarce resource, and choices must be made as to what health care is to be provided, who will get health care, and how much will be received.

- Health care markets do not operate "perfectly competitively" and may require market adjustments or government interventions.

- An increase in competition in health care markets and reduced reimbursement to providers has led to restructuring and downsizing of health care providers and has affected the demand and supply of nurses.

- Nurses play a key role in promoting an effective, efficient, and equitable health care system in the United States.

## Web Resources

**American Society of Health Economists—** an affiliate of iHEA
*www.healtheconomics.us*
**International Health Economics Association (iHEA)**
*http://healtheconomics.org*
**National Information Center on Health Services Research and Health Care Technology (NICHSR)**
*www.nlm.nih.gov/nichsr*
**NICHSR self-study course on health economics**
*www.nlm.nih.gov/nichsr/edu/healthecon*
**Office of Health Economics (OHE)—**an independent research and consultant group based in London
*www.ohe.org*
**OHE self-study course on health economics**
*www.oheschools.org/index.html*
**World Health Organization (WHO) programs in health economics**
*www.who.int/topics/health_economics/en*

## REFERENCES

Adams, R., & Johnson, B. (1986). Acuity and staffing under prospective payment. *Journal of Nursing Administration, 16*(10), 21-25.

AFT Healthcare. (2002). *The vanishing nurse ... and other disappearing healthcare workers.* Washington, DC: AFT Healthcare. Retrieved May 1, 2005, from *http://www.aft.org/pubs-reports/healthcare/Vanishing-Nurse.pdf.*

Aiken, L. H., Clarke, S. P., Cheung, R. B., Sloane, D. M., & Silber, D. H. (2003). Educational levels of hospital nurses and surgical patient mortality. *JAMA, 290,* 1617-1623.

Aiken, L. H., Clarke, S. P., Sloane, D. M., Sochalski, J., & Silber, J. H. (2002). Hospital nurse staffing and patient morality, nurse burnout, and job dissatisfaction. *JAMA, 288*(16), 1987-1993.

Bodenheimer, T. (2005). High and rising health care costs. Part 1: Seeking an explanation. *Annals of Internal Medicine, 142*(10), 847-854.

Buerhaus, P. I., Needleman, J., Mattke, S., & Stewart, M. (2002). Strengthening hospital nursing. *Health Affairs, 21*(5), 123-132.

Centers for Disease Control and Prevention (CDC). (2004). Health, United States, 2004. Tables 93, 98, 109. Retrieved April 1, 2005, from *www.cdc.gov/nchs/data/hus/hus04trend.pdf#topic.*

Chen, V. K., Arguedas, M. R., Kilgore, M. L., & Eloubeidi, M. A. (2004). A cost-minimization analysis of alternative strategies in diagnosing pancreatic cancer. *American Journal of Gastroenterology, 99*(11), 2223-2234.

Commonwealth Fund. (2004). First report and recommendations of the Commonwealth Fund's International Working Group on Quality Indicators. Retrieved April 1, 2005, from *www.cmwf.org/usr_doc/ministers_complete2004report_752.pdf.*

Cowan, C., Catlin, A., Smith, C., & Sensenig, A. (2004). National health expenditures, 2002. *Health Care Financing Review, 25*(4), 143-166.

Cuevas, K. D., Silver, D. R., Brooten, D., Youngblut, J. M., & Bobo, C. M. (2005). The cost of prematurity: Hospital charges at birth and frequency of rehospitalizations and acute care visits over the first year of life. *American Journal of Nursing, 105*(7), 56-64.

Feldstein, P. (2003). *Health policy issues: An economic perspective* (3rd ed.). Chicago, IL: Health Administration Press.

Grumbach, K., Ash, M., Seago, J. A., Spetz, J., & Coffman, J. (2001). Measuring shortages of hospital nurses: How do you know a hospital with a nursing shortage when you see one? *Medical Care Research and Review, 58*(4), 387-403.

Hillman, A., Pauly, M., & Kerstein, J. (1989). How do financial incentives affect physicians' clinical decisions and the financial performance of health maintenance organizations? *New England Journal of Medicine, 321*(2), 86-92.

Jordan, W. (2001). An early view of the impact of deregulation and managed care on hospital profitability and net worth. *Journal of Healthcare Management, 46*(3), 161-172.

Kaiser Family Foundation (KFF). (2004). Myths about the uninsured. The Kaiser Commission on Medicaid and the Uninsured. Retrieved April 1, 2005, from *www.kff.org/uninsured/upload/52996_1.pdf.*

Karter, A. J., Stevens, M. R., Herman, W. H., Ettner, S., Marrero, D. G., et al. (2003). Out-of-pocket costs and diabetes preventive services. *Diabetes Care, 26*(8), 2294-2299.

Lee, J. S., Berenson, R. A., Mayes, R., & Gauthier, A. K. (2003). Medicare payment policy: Does cost shifting matter? *Health*

*Affairs*, Web Exclusive, October 8, 2003, W3-480, 480-488. Retrieved May 15, 2005, from *http://content.healthaffairs.org/cgi/reprint/hlthaff.w3.480v1.*

Luft, H. (1999). Why are physicians so upset about managed care? *Journal of Health Politics, Policy and Law, 24*(5), 957-966.

Mar, J., Rueda, J. R., Duran-Cantolla, J., Schechter, C., & Chilcott, J. (2003). The cost-effectiveness of nCPAP treatment in patients with moderate-to-severe obstructive sleep apnoea. *European Respiratory Journal, 21*, 515-522.

McClellan, M., & Staiger, D. (2000). Comparing hospital quality at for-profit and not-for-profit hospitals. In D. Cutler (Ed.), *The changing hospital industry: Comparing not-for-profit and for-profit institutions.* Chicago: The University of Chicago Press.

Medicare Payment Advisory Committee (MedPac). (2002). Report to the Congress: Medicare Payment Policy, March 2002. Retrieved May 15, 2005, from *ww.medpac.gov/publications/congressional_reports.*

Miller, W., Vigdor, E. R., & Manning, W. G. (2004). Covering the uninsured: What is it worth? *Health Affairs*, web exclusive, March 31, 2004, W4-157, 157-167. Retrieved June 1, 2005 from *http://content.healthaffairs.org/cgi/reprint/hlthaff.w4.157v1.*

Mitchell, M., Miller, J., Welches, L., & Walker, D. D. (1984). Determining cost of direct nursing care by DRGs. *Nursing Management, 15*(4), 29-32.

Needleman, J., Buerhaus, P., Mattke, S., Stewart, M., & Zelevinsky, K. (2002). Nurse-staffing levels and the quality of care in hospitals. *New England Journal of Medicine, 346*(22), 1715-1722.

Pindus, N., Tilly, J., & Weinstein, S. (2002) *Skill shortages and mismatches in nursing related health care employment.* Report to the U.S. Department of Labor, Employment and Training Administration. Washington, DC: The Urban Institute.

Reinhardt, U. (1985). The theory of physician-induced demand: Reflections after a decade. *Journal of Health Economics, 4*(2), 190-193.

Rice, T., & Matsuoka, K. Y. (2004). The impact of cost-sharing on appropriate utilization and health status: A review of the literature on seniors. *Medical Care Research and Review, 61*(4), 415-452.

Robinson, J. (1996). Decline in hospital utilization and cost inflation under managed care in California. *JAMA, 276*(13), 1060-1064.

Schoen, C., Doty, M., Collins, S. R., & Holmgren, A.L. (2005). Insured but not protected: How many adults are underinsured? *Health Affairs*, web exclusive, June 14, 2005, W5-289, 289-302. Retrieved May 15, 2005, from *http://content.healthaffairs.org/cgi/reprint/hlthaff.w5.289v1.*

Schoen, C., Osborn, R., Trang Huynh, P., Doty, M., Davis, K., Zapert, K., & Peugh, J. (2004). Primary care and health system performance: Adults' experiences in five countries. *Health Affairs*, web exclusive, October 28, 2004, W4-487, 487-503. Retrieved May 15, 2005, from *http://content.healthaffairs.org/cgi/reprint/hlthaff.w4.487v1.*

Seago, J., Ash, M., Spetz, J., Coffman, J., & Grumbach, K. (2001). Hospital registered nurse shortages: Environmental, patient, and institutional predictors. *Health Services Research, 36*(5), 831-853.

Shindul-Rothschild, J., Berry, D., & Long-Middleton E. (1996). Where have all the nurses gone? Final results of our patient care survey. *American Journal of Nursing, 96*(11), 25-39.

Sloan, F. (2000). Not-for-profit ownership and hospital behavior. In A. J. Culyer & J. P. Newhouse (Eds.), *Handbook of Health Economics* (volume 1B). New York: North-Holland Press.

Spetz, J., & Given, R. (2003). The future of the nurse shortage: Will wage increases close the gap? *Health Affairs, 22*(6), 199-206.

Unruh, L. (2002). Nursing staff reductions in Pennsylvania hospitals: Exploring the discrepancy between perceptions and data. *Medical Care Research and Review, 59*(2), 97-214.

Unruh, L. (2003a). Licensed nurse staffing and adverse events in hospitals. *Medical Care, 41*(1), 142-152.

Unruh, L. (2003b). The effect of LPN reductions on RN patient load. *Journal of Nursing Administration, 33*(4), 201-208.

Unruh, L., & Fottler, M. (2005). Projections and trends in RN supply: What do they tell us about the nursing shortage? *Policy, Politics, & Nursing Practice, 6*(3), 171-182.

U.S. Department of Health and Human Services (DHHS). (2000). The registered nurse population: Findings from the National Sample Survey of Registered Nurses, March 2000, U.S. DHHS, HRSA, BHP, Division of Nursing. Retrieved May 1, 2005, from *http://bhpr.hrsa.gov/healthworkforce/reports/rnproject/default.htm.*

Wang, G., Macera, C. A., Scudder-Soucie, B., Schmid, T., Pratt, M., & Buchner, D. (2005). A cost-benefit analysis of physical activity using bike/pedestrian trails. *Health Promotion Practice, 6*(2), 174-179.

Wickizer, T. (1992). The effects of utilization review on hospital use and expenditures: A covariance analysis. *Health Services Research, 27*(1), 103-121.

Woolhandler, S., Campbell, T., & Himmelstein, D. U. (2003). Costs of health care administration in the United States and Canada. *New England Journal of Medicine, 349*(8), 768-775.

Wright, B. J., Carlson, M. J., Edlund, T., Devoe, J., Gallia, C., & Smith, J. (2005). The impact of increased cost sharing on Medicaid enrollees. *Health Affairs, 24*(4), 1106-1116.

# SOCIAL SECURITY: KEY TO ECONOMIC SECURITY

Shirley S. Chater

*"...it is well that we pause to celebrate one of the great peacetime achievements of the American people, namely, the enactment of the Social Security Act."*

HARRY TRUMAN

Popular stories suggest that older Americans frequently choose between buying food and buying medications. It is well known that poverty contributes to illness and poor health. Without some degree of economic security, there can be no health security. The Social Security Act, signed into law in 1935 by President Franklin Delano Roosevelt, provides a minimum "floor of protection" for retired workers. Later Social Security was broadened to provide benefits for workers and their families who face a loss of income because of disability or the death of a family wage earner. Social Security, which in 2005 covered approximately 159 million workers and paid benefits to more than 48 million people, is recognized as the most successful domestic federal program.

During the last few years, and particularly during the present Bush administration, the program has come under attack from some policymakers, selected members of Congress, and the press, with allegations that the program will be "bankrupt": that benefits paid will exceed tax revenues and that Social Security will not be there when it is needed. This argument has some merit for the long term, but the situation is not catastrophic. The financial instability has not reached a crisis level, despite what some would have us believe. It is true that fewer workers are paying into the system now than before and that benefits are being paid to more people

for longer periods of time as longevity increases. In 2005 there were 3.3 workers for each beneficiary; by 2031 that number will be reduced to about 2.1 workers for each beneficiary. There are more than 37 million Americans over the age of 65, but by 2031 there will be twice as many. Americans over the age of 85 represent the fastest-growing population group. The persuasive facts regarding the future financial status of the program come annually from the report of the trustees of the program. Therefore, although there is no "crisis," there are compelling reasons why the Social Security program should be reexamined to see what solutions will guarantee fiscal stability for the future.

During 2005, President George W. Bush promoted a change in Social Security that would "privatize" part of the program, making it an "ownership" program. Although privatization does not solve the solvency issue, the administration seems focused on this controversial change. It is likely that Congress will put forth legislation that will generate discussion, debate, and political upheaval among those who favor keeping the structure and philosophy of the program as it is and those who favor private or personal accounts.

## SOCIAL SECURITY PROGRAM

Social Security is a family program, providing monthly benefits to retirees, to survivors, and to persons who are disabled. The program is based on the simple concept that if you work, you pay taxes into the system, and when you retire or become disabled, you, your spouse, and your dependent children receive monthly benefits that are based on your earnings. Your survivors collect benefits when you die. Most people think of social security as

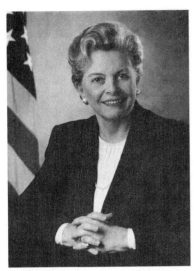

The Honorable Shirley S. Chater, Commissioner, U.S. Social Security Administration, 1993-1997.

a retirement program. Of all beneficiaries, 63% *are* retirees, but others are survivors of those who have died—a widow, widower, or child. Still others are persons with disabilities who have worked, paid into the system, and qualify under the definition of disability used by the Social Security program. Of the 47.7 million people receiving benefits from Social Security in 2005, 33 million are retired workers and family members, 6.6 million are survivors, and 6.3 million are disabled persons. It is interesting to note that owing to retirement, survivor, and disability benefits earmarked for children of American workers, more children, a total of 3.9 million, are covered by benefits from Social Security than by any other government program except the earned income tax credit.

The Social Security program is financed by a "pay as you go" system, with present-day workers paying for present-day beneficiaries. Each worker pays Social Security taxes of 7.65% (6.2% for Social Security and 1.45% for Medicare) of gross salary. The employer also pays an equal amount. For the self-employed, both parts of the payroll tax are paid by the individual, but one-half is tax-deductible as a business expense. In 2005, Social Security taxes are paid on gross salary up to $90,000. (There is no maximum limit for taxes paid for Medicare.)

The taxes are paid into the Social Security Trust Fund. According to the law, excess funds not needed for immediate payment to beneficiaries or for administrative expenses are invested with interest in U.S. government bonds. Funds are returned for Social Security purposes as needed.

> The specific rules and regulations for calculating the benefit formula and implementing the program are complex. Readers are advised to visit Social Security's website at *www.ssa.gov* for easy-to-use online benefit calculators or to seek consultation at a local Social Security office.

Eligibility for Social Security coverage is acquired by earning "credits" for working and paying into the system. People who are dependents or survivors may receive benefits based on another's work record. The worker earns one "credit" per quarter for $920 earned, up to four credits per year of $3680 (2005). Many people still refer to credits as *quarters* or *quarters of coverage.* The dollar amount required to be earned per credit is established every year. Most workers need 40 quarters to qualify for benefits, although younger people need fewer credits to qualify for disability or for family members to be eligible for survivor benefits if the worker dies. How much workers pay into the system and how long they have worked helps to determine how much they will receive in benefits. High-wage earners get higher benefits than low-wage earners. However, the benefit formula is weighted in favor of the low-wage earner by providing 53% of preretirement earnings compared with the replacement of 40% of an average wage earner's preretirement earnings.

## RETIREMENT

For people retiring in 2005, the full retirement age is 65 and 6 months, and the average monthly benefit is $955. In 1981, Congress passed a law that changed the retirement age from 65 to 67 for those born in 1938 and later. The change gradually increased from 65 to 67 beginning in 2003, so that by 2027, the full retirement age will be 67. Retirement at age 62 is still an option, but with a permanent reduction in benefits. Generally speaking, early retirement is calculated to give about the same total Social Security benefits over a lifetime but in smaller amounts. This takes into account the longer period the early retiree receives benefits. On the other hand, delaying retirement and continuing to work adds earnings to the worker's record, increasing the eventual benefit amount (Box 14-3).

During the time a worker receives retirement benefits, a spouse can also receive benefits on the worker's record if the spouse is 62 years of age or older. The spouse can also receive benefits at retirement age on his or her own work record, and Social Security pays whichever benefit is higher. At full retirement age, the spouse receives one-half of the retired worker's full benefit.

When the worker retires, other benefits may be paid to family members who meet the requirements (Social Security Administration, 2004a):

- A spouse under age 62, if caring for the worker's child who is under age 16 or disabled
- A former wife or husband age 62 or older
- Children up to age 18
- Children ages 18 or 19 if they are full-time students through grade 12
- Children over age 18 if they are disabled

There are certain limits on how much money a family may receive. First, the full amount of the worker's benefit is provided. Then, if the benefits of all other family members exceed the limit, they are adjusted proportionally, keeping the total equal to the limit set by law.

Several factors affect the amount of Social Security benefits paid monthly. First, if the worker chooses to receive benefits before reaching full retirement age and decides to work as well, there is a penalty in which $1 in benefits will be deducted for each $2 in earnings above an annual limit. The limit for 2005 is $12,000. In other words, the worker can earn $12,000 without reducing his Social Security benefits. During the months of the year in which the worker reaches full retirement age, he is penalized $1 for every $3 earned over the limit of $31,800 for the year 2005. Limits are established every year. After reaching full retirement age, the worker can work as much as he likes without penalty.

## SURVIVORS BENEFITS

Survivors of deceased workers account for 14% of total benefits paid by Social Security. When a family member who has worked and paid into Social Security dies, his survivors may qualify for benefits. Survivors include widows, widowers (as well as divorced widows and widowers), children, and dependent parents. This life insurance benefit helps to keep families together after the breadwinner dies. Widows or widowers receive full benefits at full retirement age or reduced benefits as early as age 60. Widows or widowers who are raising children under age 16 or who are disabled can get full benefits at any age. Children under age 18 are also eligible for benefits, and if they are still in school at age 19, they too qualify for survivor benefits. Dependent parents who are 62 or older also qualify.

## DISABILITY

It is interesting to note that approximately 72% of the private sector workforce has no long-term disability insurance. Social Security does provide benefits to persons who become disabled. According to the Social Security Administration, studies show that a 20-year-old worker has a 33% chance of becoming disabled before reaching retirement age. Social Security pays benefits to those who are unable to work for a year or more because of a disability.

---

**BOX 14-3** Age to Receive Full Social Security Benefits

| YEAR OF BIRTH | FULL RETIREMENT AGE |
|---|---|
| 1937 or earlier | 65 |
| 1938 | 65 and 2 months |
| 1939 | 65 and 4 months |
| 1940 | 65 and 6 months |
| 1941 | 65 and 8 months |
| 1942 | 65 and 10 months |
| 1943-1954 | 66 |
| 1955 | 66 and 2 months |
| 1956 | 66 and 4 months |
| 1957 | 66 and 6 months |
| 1958 | 66 and 8 months |
| 1959 | 66 and 10 months |
| 1960 and later | 67 |

From the Social Security Administration. Available online at *www.ssa.gov/retirement.*

Social Security uses a definition of disability different from that of other programs. For example, it does not pay for partial disability. Disability, as defined by Social Security, exists if workers cannot do the work they did before, if workers cannot adjust to other work, and if the disability is expected to last at least a year or to result in death. Certain family members may also qualify for benefits while the worker is disabled. After full retirement age, disability benefits cease, and retirement benefits begin.

## SUPPLEMENTAL SECURITY INCOME PROGRAM

Many people confuse the Social Security program with the Supplemental Security Income (SSI) program because the Social Security Administration manages both. Social Security, as previously noted, is based on the philosophy that if one works and pays taxes for the program, one will qualify for retirement, survivor, and disability benefits. The program allows older Americans and family members to remain independent and to have a degree of economic security. The SSI program is a federal and state welfare program, providing benefits to the most needy. It pays benefits to people who are age 65 and older, blind, or disabled and to children who are blind or disabled. To qualify, recipients must have little income and own very little as well. Many SSI beneficiaries also receive food stamps and Medicaid. SSI is funded from general revenue. *Money from the Social Security program is never used to pay for the SSI program.*

## SOCIAL SECURITY: A PROGRAM ESPECIALLY IMPORTANT FOR WOMEN

Social Security is a gender-neutral program. However, because women live so much longer than men, spend down their savings over time, and live on non–inflation-adjusted pensions if they are lucky enough to have them, women depend heavily on their Social Security income. Social Security benefit amounts are adjusted annually for inflation, whereas most pensions are not. Age differences between women and men show just how important Social Security is to older and oldest women (Social Security Administration, Office of Research, Evaluation and Statistics, 2005) (Box 14-4).

| BOX 14-4 | Gender Differences in Social Security Recipients | | |
|---|---|---|---|
| **AGE** | **WOMEN** | **MEN** | **TOTAL** |
| 65 and older | 19,498,570 | 14,196,869 | 33,695,439 |
| 85 and older | 3,046,768 | 1,307,912 | 4,354,680 |
| 100 and older | 35,548 | 5,734 | 41,282 |

When the Social Security program was signed into law in 1935, few women worked outside the home and the law reflected this. Women were and are covered under their husbands' work records. Now that more than 60% of women work outside the home, some believe the regulations of the program are antiquated and unrelated to present circumstances. On the other hand, some of the rules of the program are especially helpful to women and need to be retained. Important policy decisions affecting women may be made during the coming years as the future of the program is debated. Women, women's groups, nurses, and nursing organizations need to follow the debate to ensure that women's benefits are not unnecessarily reduced.

Coverage for widows and divorced women may be targets for future changes. At present, widows receive about 71% of the deceased husband's benefit amount if they take benefits at age 60, or 100% if they are age 65. Consistent with the increase in retirement age to age 67, and depending on the year of birth, this rule will change beginning in 2005 and will gradually increase to age 67 by 2029. Divorced women may receive benefits based on an ex-husband's record if he is receiving benefits (or is deceased) if she had been married for 10 years or longer, assuming she is unmarried and at least 62 years of age. If women qualify for benefits on their own work record *and* on their husbands' or former husbands' record, Social Security pays whichever benefit is higher, but not both. Personnel from the Social Security Administration will always study the individual record for each inquiry and suggest the best option, guaranteeing the highest benefit under the circumstances. For the 71% of all beneficiaries aged 85 years and older who are women, Social Security's protection is urgently important.

## FINDING FINANCIAL STABILITY FOR SOCIAL SECURITY

The Board of Trustees of the Social Security Administration reports annually to Congress about the financial stability of the program. In the 2005 report the trustees estimated that the program would be solvent until 2041, when there would be enough money to pay only approximately 74% of expected benefits (Board of Trustees of the Federal Old-Age and Survivors Insurance and Disability Trust Funds, 2005). In order to "fix" the program, many policy options have been and will continue to be suggested. These options fall into categories of either increasing revenues through taxation or reducing benefits. Neither option is easy: It seems unlikely that Congress will favor increased payroll taxes, nor will the American people readily accept major benefit reductions. Future policies will certainly be controversial. Many believe that the best solution to the long-term solvency problem is a combination of new policies that would slightly reduce benefits while also finding ways to increase revenue to the Social Security trust fund. These thoughtful suggestions for creating a "package" of minor changes in the program assume that the present structure of the program would be retained. Furthermore, the program's shortfall over 75 years (the period for creating estimates) is 1.92% of taxable payroll, an amount that could be made up with small changes in the program.

The following policy changes are the most frequently suggested remedies to solve the future fiscal problem of the Social Security program:

- *Add all new employees of state and local governments.* At present about 5% of state and local government employees do not pay into the Social Security program. Adding them or adding all new state and local employees to the program would help to increase revenues.
- *Reduce the cost-of-living adjustment (COLA).* Social Security is one of the few programs adjusted annually for the cost of living. Some believe that the COLA, determined by the federal Bureau of Labor Statistics, is too high. If research determines that the COLA should be reduced, it would cut the monthly amount of the Social Security check.
- *Increase the retirement age.* Some suggest that the retirement age should be extended to age 68 or 70 because people are living and working longer. Others suggest that the retirement age, which is scheduled to rise to 67 from 65 by 2027, be accelerated. Increasing the retirement age could adversely affect laborers and others who can no longer work at hard manual labor. Ethnic considerations need to be considered also, because some minority groups have shorter life spans.
- *Change the formula for calculating benefits from 35 years to 38 years of highest earnings.* At present, benefits are calculated by using the worker's highest 35 years of earnings, based on the assumption that the average time a worker spends in the workplace *is* 35 years. As people live and work longer, there is rationale to increase the number of years to 38. If this were changed, however, women would be adversely affected because they tend to spend less time than men in the workforce. Using 38 years to calculate the formula gives a minor reduction in benefits but saves money for the system.
- *Change the formula from wage indexing to price indexing.* Presently the formula by which benefits are determined includes wage indexing. Wages grow faster than prices (inflation) and keeps Social Security in line with the economy. Price indexing would lower benefits over time and most likely put more beneficiaries into poverty.
- *Means test to reduce benefits.* It is sometimes suggested that high earners should not receive benefits, even though they have paid into the system. This is the extreme case. Others suggest that benefits should be lower for those who earn more than a certain amount. The fear regarding means testing is that eventually those who pay into the system and get little or nothing from the system in return will want to "opt out" of what is now a universal system. Means testing is seen by some to undermine the system and its philosophy.
- *Raise the amount of earnings on which payroll taxes are paid.* In 2005, Social Security payroll taxes are paid on earnings up to $90,000 but not on

dollars earned over that amount. This cap differentiates it from Medicare taxes which are paid on total earnings. The amount of earnings on which Social Security taxes are paid is adjusted annually. Some favor removing the cap altogether; others recommend that a higher cap be established. Currently only a small percentage of workers earn more than $90,000.

- *Increase income tax paid on Social Security benefits.* Social Security benefits are taxable if income exceeds certain amounts. If one is single with a combined income between $25,000 and $34,000, 50% of benefits are subject to income tax. If one's combined income is over $34,000, 85% of benefits are taxed. For married couples filing jointly with combined income between $32,000 and $44,000, 50% of benefits are taxed. If the combined income is over $44,000, 85% of benefits are taxed. It is interesting to note that revenue generated from the 50% tax goes to the Social Security trust fund, whereas the proceeds from the difference between the 50% and 85% taxes go into the Medicare trust fund, according to law. To increase revenue, the tax received from benefits could be increased, or the portion that goes to Medicare could instead be deposited in the Social Security trust fund.
- *Invest Social Security funds in the stock market.* Present law requires that trust funds be invested in Treasury bonds, which generate about 3% interest and provide the maximum safety for investments. When the stock market is doing well, suggestions abound that part of the excess of Social Security funds should be invested by the government in the stock market. This not only raises questions about risk, but also raises questions about the role of the federal government and its potential influence on the economy. When the stock market is down, less enthusiasm is seen about those investments.

The options listed here generally maintain the current structure of the Social Security program as it was designed in the 1930s.

## PRIVATIZATION OR PERSONAL ACCOUNTS

President George W. Bush has made Social Security "reform" a central part of his domestic policy agenda for his second term. He wants young workers to have the opportunity to invest part of their payroll taxes in "private" or "personal" accounts, with reduced benefits from the regular program. He believes that if workers create personal investment accounts, retirement funds would accumulate at higher rates, making up for the reduced benefits awarded from lower contributions to Social Security. No formal legislative proposal has been put forth to date, but it has been suggested that workers under age 55 today would have the option of voluntarily choosing to create a personal account, into which 2% to 4% of payroll tax from both the worker and the employer would be deposited. The worker would manage the account, perhaps according to guidelines that would be outlined by the government, and the account would belong to the owner and later to the beneficiaries.

The president's plan, which changes the basic structure of the program, would do nothing to solve the long-term financial problem. In fact, by having some workers choose to pay less payroll tax into the system in order to create a personal account, total revenues coming into the program would be decreased, causing the solvency issue to become even more critical than it is. Most recently the President has said that he would like to accomplish *two* objectives: create personal accounts *and* solve the solvency problem, in part by using price indexing in the formula to calculate benefits rather than wage indexing. These objectives will likely be the substance of legislation during the duration of the president's term.

## ATTEMPTS TO CHANGE POLICY

A total of nine commissions and advisory panels have been formed over the past two decades, charged with finding solutions to the perceived financial crisis of Social Security. Most of the commissions' and panels' recommendations were never enacted into law, illustrating how difficult it is to change one of America's most popular domestic programs.

The most successful attempt to make changes in the program was the National Commission on Social Security Reform, created by executive order, which met from 1981 through 1983. Its recommendations included a proposal to freeze the COLA, increase the payroll tax, and raise the retirement age from 65 to 67. These recommendations were enacted into law.

In 1994, President Clinton appointed 32 members to the Bipartisan Commission on Entitlement and Tax Reform. That commission proposed an increase in the retirement age for full benefits to age 70, a reduction in the COLA, and the creation of mandatory private *supplemental* retirement accounts. No legislation was enacted. Then from 1994 to 1996 the Advisory Council on Social Security, with members named by the Secretary of Health and Human Services, met to discuss long-term remedies for the program. The Council advocated three alternative solutions, each a combination of reducing benefits and investing part of the trust funds in the stock market or in private accounts. None of the three plans was enacted into law.

In 1997 the National Commission on Retirement Policy, a private commission, proposed the creation of private accounts using part of the payroll tax paid by workers. Some benefit cuts were also recommended. Again, no legislation was enacted.

The newest Social Security Commission, appointed by President George W. Bush in May 2001, was different from past commissions because it was given a specific charge to develop a plan whereby individual personal accounts would become part of Social Security. The 16-member commission presented its report to the President in December 2001. Rather than presenting a single plan that could easily be considered for legislation, it produced three plans, each one complicated and controversial from the start. Each would allow individuals to divert a certain percentage of their payroll taxes to private accounts to be individually invested. Each plan also recommended selected benefit reductions from Social Security. Politically, the objectivity of the membership of the Commission was questioned from the beginning because all members favored private accounts. As indicated previously, the long-term cost to the Social Security program would be substantial if funds were diverted from payroll taxes to private accounts, even with benefit reductions. According to some analysts, paying for privatization will cause a multi-trillion dollar increase in federal borrowing. Likewise, the whims of investment markets will also surely influence whether it is timely to pursue individual private accounts.

## SUMMARY

It is likely that Social Security's long-term fiscal problems can be solved with a combination of some of the policy changes that have been discussed. Each has advantages and disadvantages. Each solution must be studied to see how various population groups would be affected. Women must be especially attentive to potential changes in the program that would adversely affect them. Social Security is an antipoverty program, lowering the poverty rate among the elderly from approximately 50% in 1935 to 11% today. Nurses appreciate the relationship of economic security to health security and must serve as advocates for maintaining the protective elements of the program while supporting minor changes to ensure long-term financial solvency. Nurses should become informed about the program and participate in policy discussions and proposed changes, letting Congress know what effects these changes will have on the elderly, the disabled, and children.

## *Key Points*

- Social Security is one of the most successful programs of the United States government, helping millions of retirees and their families retain their independence and their dignity as they age.
- The problem of fiscal solvency exists because we are living healthier and longer lives; at the same time families are having fewer children to work and pay payroll taxes.
- Whether the problems related to the fiscal solvency of the program are solved with a package of small legislative changes or an overhaul of the program's structure such as private accounts, it is certain to be one of the most important policy debates in Congress.

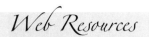

## Web Resources

**The Century Foundation**
*www.socsec.org*
**National Academy of Social Insurance**
*www.nasi.org*
**National Committee to Preserve Social
   Security and Medicare**
*www.ncpssm.org*
**Social Security Administration**
*www.ssa.gov*
**Social Security Resources**
*http://the-social-security.net*

### REFERENCES

Board of Trustees of the Federal Old-Age and Survivors Insurance and Disability Trust Funds. (2005). *Annual report.* Publication No. 20-372, March 23, 2005. Washington, DC: U.S. Government Printing Office.

Social Security Administration (SSA). (2004a). *Retirement benefits* (SSA Publication No. 05-10035).

Social Security Administration (SSA). (2004b). *Survivors benefits* (SSA Publication No. 05-10084).

Social Security Administration (SSA). (2005a). *A snapshot* (SSA Publication No. 05-10006).

Social Security Administration (SSA). (2005b). *Disability benefits* (SSA Publication No. 05-10029).

Social Security Administration (SSA). (2005c). *Supplemental Security benefits* (SSA Publication No. 05-11000).

Social Security Administration (SSA). (2005d). *The future of Social Security* (SSA Publication No. 05-10055).

Social Security Administration (SSA). (2005e). *Understanding the benefits* (SSA Publication No. 05-10024).

Social Security Administration, Office of Research, Evaluation and Statistics. (2005). *Fast facts and figures about Social Security* (SSA Publication No.13-11785).

# chapter 15

# Financing Health Care in the United States

Joyce A. Pulcini & Mary Ann Hart

*"Can anyone remember when the times were not hard and money was not scarce?"*

RALPH WALDO EMERSON

A 55-year-old man loses his job at a high-tech company after serving 25 years as a janitor. He has a pension but no health benefits because he cannot afford the payments. Soon after he leaves the job he experiences chest pains and needs triple bypass surgery. What are the prospects that this patient will receive the care he needs even if the surgery is successful with no complications? Will this man ever be able to get back on his feet financially? He is also worried about the viability of his pension in 20 to 30 years, given the fact that his older peers are having these benefits jeopardized at an unprecedented rate.

This chapter describes and analyzes the features of the health care financing system in the United States. It first presents a historical perspective to provide a basis for understanding the current system. The chapter then explores the financial and economic forces that drive the health care system and describes measures to contain costs. The health care financing system is described, including the public and private sectors. Implications for nursing and health care are discussed.

## HISTORICAL PERSPECTIVES

History reveals some dominant values underpinning the U.S. political and economic systems. From its origins, the United States has had a long history of individualism, an emphasis on freedom to choose among alternative options, and an aversion as a nation to large-scale government intervention into the private realm (Kingdon, 1999). Social programs have been the exception rather than the rule and have arisen primarily during times of great need, such as in the 1930s and 1960s. Health care in the United States had its origins in the private sector, and as a result, strong resistance has been raised to government intervention in health care, particularly by physician and hospital groups.

The Great Depression of the 1930s saw the creation of Blue Cross (an insurance plan to cover hospital care), then Blue Shield (to cover physician care). Starr (1982) describes the initial reluctance of the American Hospital Association and of the American Medical Association to adopt any form of prepaid hospital or medical expenses. But hospitals in 1933 and physicians in 1938 experienced enough bad debt to motivate them to endorse plans that laid the foundation for what is now Blue Cross and Blue Shield. The belief that persons should pay for their medical care before they actually got sick, thus ensuring some security for both providers and consumers of medical services in time of need, was the rationale behind instituting such private insurance plans. Starr (1982) points out that the development of these plans effectively defused a strong political movement toward legislating a compulsory health insurance plan. The Social Security Act of 1935, a comprehensive piece of social legislation, is striking for its failure to include health care. After an attempt by President Truman in the late 1940s, a national health program did not reach the national agenda again until the 1960s.

Blue Cross and Blue Shield continued to dominate the health insurance industry until the 1950s, when commercial insurance companies entered the market. These insurance companies had been discouraged from entry partially because of discounted room rates negotiated with hospitals by Blue Cross. Moreover, state regulations required Blue Cross/Blue Shield to use *community rating*, or rates based on the total usage of health care services across a whole population or community. Commercial insurance companies were able to compete with Blue Cross/Blue Shield by using *experience rating*, targeted to a select, low-risk population or community. Experience rating decreases the price of health insurance because high-risk individuals are more likely to be excluded from the plan. The distinction between Blue Cross/Blue Shield and commercial insurance companies has become increasingly blurred over the past 10 years, and many Blue Cross/Blue Shield plans have converted to for-profit status and established companion nonprofit foundations. Blue Cross/Blue Shield has evolved to offer the same range of managed care products as commercial insurance companies as it competes in the current health care marketplace (Jonas & Kovner, 2005). The United States in the 1960s enjoyed relative prosperity, along with a burgeoning social conscience that led to a heightened concern for poor and elderly people in this country. Another issue at this time was the failure of health insurance to protect persons who had catastrophic illness. The catalyst for a governmental solution to the lack of health care for these populations was the framing of these issues as a series of "crises" that garnered public support and created an atmosphere for change (Alford, 1975). As a result of these forces, Medicaid and Medicare, two separate but related programs, were created in 1965 by amendments to the Social Security Act. Medicare, or Title XVIII, is a federal program for the aged and disabled, and Medicaid, or Title XIX, is a program jointly funded by both federal and state governments, with eligibility determined by income and resources (U.S. Department of Health and Human Services [USDHHS], Centers for Medicare and Medicaid Services [CMS], 2005b).

Within a few years of the passage of Medicare and Medicaid, it became clear that these programs were contributing greatly to escalating costs of health care. The government and society's inability to control the escalation of health care costs is one of the root causes of our fiscal crises in health care. In fact, it was within a decade after the passage of Medicare and Medicaid that cost began increasingly to dominate all policy decisions in health care.

The health care field has evolved from rather small and disorganized private and public enterprises to a large, multifaceted business affected by interrelated forces. The role of third-party payers in the financing of the health care industry has grown tremendously in the past 40 to 50 years. Historically, the majority of payments for health services came from first- or second-party payers (from the patients or their families, respectively). In 1940, 81.3% of health care was paid for by the individual or family and 18.7% was financed by third-party, or intermediary, payers. By 1980 these figures had reversed themselves, with 32.9% of costs borne by the patient or family and 67.1% of these costs by third-party or public payers (Gibson & Waldo, 1982). Figure 15-1

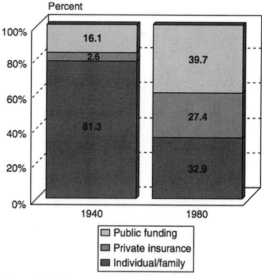

**Figure 15-1** Changes in payers over time: 1940 to 1980. (From Pulcini, J., Neary, S., & Mahoney, D. [2002]. Health care financing. In D. Mason, J. Leavitt, & M. Chaffee [Eds.]. *Policy & politics in nursing and health care* [4th ed.]. St. Louis: Saunders, p. 243.)

shows the change in payers in 1940 versus 1980 (USDHHS, Health Care Financing Administration [HCFA], Office of the Actuary [OA], 2001). Figure 15-2 shows changes in payers from 1980 to 2003 (Kaiser Family Foundation [KFF], 2005a).

Since the 1970s, cost escalation in health care has created a powerful incentive to alter the system. Figure 15-3 provides a graphic picture of the costs of health care from 1960 to 2003 (2005b). As costs rose in the 1970s and 1980s, the balance of power

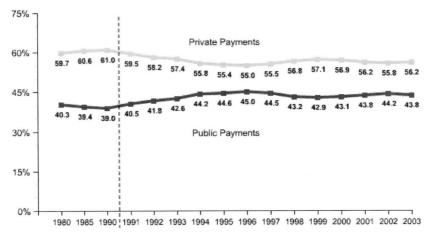

**Figure 15-2** Trend in personal health expenditures by source of payment: 1980 to 2003. (Reprinted with permission from The Henry J. Kaiser Family Foundation. [2005, February]. *Trends and indicators in the changing health care marketplace*, #7031.*)

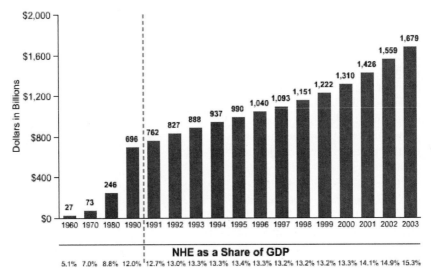

**Figure 15-3** National health expenditures and their share of the gross domestic product: 1960 to 2003. (Reprinted with permission from The Henry J. Kaiser Family Foundation. [2005, February]. *Trends and indicators in the changing health care marketplace*, #7031.)

*For Figures 15-2, 15-3, 15-4, 15-5, 15-8, and 15-9, the Kaiser Family Foundation, based in Menlo Park, California, is a nonprofit, independent national health care philanthropy and is not associated with Kaiser Permanente or Kaiser Industries.

changed in the health care field. More and more groups outside the health field became involved in attempts to contain costs. Leaders from business, large corporations, and labor offered solutions to the problems because they were purchasing or negotiating for health care benefits. Patients also became disillusioned, initially with the quality of health care that they were receiving and later with the high cost of this care. Physicians who had traditionally managed hospitals and health care facilities were increasingly replaced with business executives who focused on cost-containment efforts. By the 1990s, health care had undergone radical changes that ultimately revolutionized the financing and delivery of health care to include a deep penetration of managed care plans.

Managed care dominated the health care market in 2005, with the majority of people in the United States covered by employer-based health insurance. About 95% of employees with health care benefits are enrolled in some form of a managed care organization (MCO) (KFF & Health Research and Educational Trust [HRET], 2004). Yet many full-time jobs with benefits have been replaced with part-time positions without benefits. This phenomenon is occurring particularly in lower-paid positions in the service sectors of the economy. Others who do not have health insurance available through the

workplace must attempt to obtain private insurance if they can afford it or government-supported care through Medicare or Medicaid if they qualify. Most employers require some portion of the monthly premiums to be paid by the individual. Two decades ago most employers offered 100% payment as a fringe benefit; however, the sharp escalation of health care costs has brought a drive to share these costs with employees or to shift the cost of health care to government programs. Wal-Mart is an example of a large corporation in which 5% of its employees were on Medicaid and 46% of the children of Wal-Mart's 1.3 million employees were uninsured or on Medicaid. Even with insurance, 38% of Wal-Mart workers spent more than one sixth of their income on health care in 2004 (Greenhouse & Barbaro, 2005).

In 2000, persons with incomes below $20,000 spent 15.2% of their income on health care compared with 2.6% for those with incomes above $470,000. Those over 65 spent 12.9% of their income on health care. This inequity continues today (USDHHS, CMS, 2005a). According to the KFF and the HRET (2004), about 80% of covered workers with single coverage and over 90% of those with family coverage contributed toward health insurance premiums. Employee contributions in particular have also gone up, as seen in Figures 15-4 and 15-5 (KFF, 2005c, 2005d). In 2004, workers on average contributed

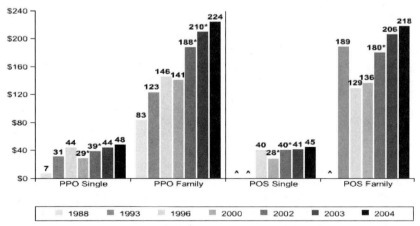

**Figure 15-4** Monthly worker contributions for single and family coverage in PPO and POS plans: 1988 to 2004. (Reprinted with permission from The Henry J. Kaiser Family Foundation. [2005, February]. *Trends and indicators in the changing health care marketplace*, #7031.)

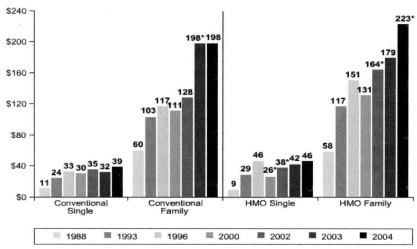

**Figure 15-5** Monthly worker contributions for single and family coverage in conventional and HMO plans: 1988 to 2004. (Reprinted with permission from The Henry J. Kaiser Family Foundation. [2005, February]. *Trends and indicators in the changing health care marketplace,* #7031.)

$558 of the $3695 annual cost of single coverage and $2661 of the $9950 annual coast of family coverage (KFF & HRET, p. 3). After 4 years of declining costs in insurance premiums, largely a result of the proliferation of managed care, premiums rose steadily from 1988 to 2004. In 2005 the average cost of an insurance premium for single coverage was $4024 and for family coverage was $10,880 (Gabel et al., 2005). But only 61% of all workers received health coverage from their employers in 2004, a 4% drop since 2001, accounting for about 5 million fewer jobs with health insurance (KFF & HRET, 2004).

Another vulnerable group consists of the 55- to 65-year-old individuals who either have taken an early retirement or have been laid off from their jobs. During the Clinton years, several proposals were introduced to allow people ages 62 to 65 and displaced workers ages 55 to 65 to buy into Medicare (USDHHS, HCFA, 2000). But health care costs are projected to rise incrementally as the average life expectancy is extended and the "baby boomers" age, leading to alternative proposals for a delay in the time when Medicare Part A benefits can be accessed. With the current focus on implementation of the Medicare prescription drug benefit, these proposals have not received great attention.

## COST CONTAINMENT IN HEALTH CARE

Efforts toward cost containment have taken many forms as providers, insurers, employers, unions, and individuals have become alarmed about the current and long-term economic consequences of the escalating costs of health care. A range of strategies has been used to curb these costs over the last 40 years.

**Health Care Expenditures.** Health care expenditures as a percentage of the gross domestic product (GDP) had increased steadily from the passage of Medicare and Medicaid in 1965 to 1993, when it was 13.4%. By 2000, health care expenditures had declined slightly to 13.1% of the GDP but rose again to 15.3% in 2003, or $1.7 trillion, and are projected to be about 18% by 2013 (USDHHS, HCFA, OA, 2001; Heffler et al., 2004; Smith, Cowan, Sensenig, Catlin, & the Health Accounts Team, 2005). Overall health care spending rose 8.5% in 2001; 9.3% in 2002; and 7.7% in 2003 (Levit et al., 2004; Smith et al., 2005). The growth stabilization experienced until 2001 was due in part to some of the aforementioned cost-containment measures but also may be accounted for by major upward revisions of the GDP resulting from a booming U.S. economy (Heffler et al., 2001). One important factor in this equation is the fact that the private share of health care spending grew rapidly between 1997 and 1999, caused in part by rapid increases in spending on prescription drugs. Prescription drugs will be covered by Medicare in 2006 as a result of the Medicare Prescription Drug Improvement and Modernization Act of 2003.

Also, cost-containment strategies of managed care plans may have produced a one-time cost-cutting effect in the 1990s (Heffler et al., 2001). Since the turn of the twenty-first century, real health care spending has been increasing. Between 1967 and 1998, Medicare spending for inpatient hospital services declined from 70% to 49%. Figure 15-6 illustrates trends in Medicare spending for hospitals, home health care, and nursing homes from 1992 to 2002 (Cowan, Catlin, Smith & Sensenig, 2004). Costs for skilled nursing facilities (SNFs) and home care have been increasing rapidly, especially for the most elderly (Lubitz, Greenbery, Gorina, Wartzman, & Gibson, 2001). The average price paid for SNFs in 2004 reached a 10-year high of $44,600 per bed, according to Levin, Irving, and Associates (2005). This represented an increase of more than 40% compared with 2003, when the average price per bed hit a 10-year low. The median price per bed increased by 34% to $36,000 per bed in 2004.

Economic solvency has an important effect on the relative strength of the health care economy. For example, from 1995 to 2001 the United States experienced a booming economy and an unprecedented budget surplus after years of budget deficits. This surplus was projected to be $5.6 trillion over the first decade of the twenty-first century. Of that amount, just under $2.5 trillion would come from excess Social Security revenue, which the Congressional delegations from both the Republican and Democratic parties pledged would be used to reduce the $3.1 trillion national debt or to strengthen the retirement system (Stevenson, 2001a, 2001b). In May of 2001, Congress passed a $1.35 trillion tax cut to be implemented over the next decade (Stevenson, 2001a, 2001b). Subsequently with changes in policy and the terrorist attacks of September 11, 2001, the country experienced another recession, which led to unprecedented budget deficits and a weakening of the U.S. economy. With this budget deficit came renewed concerns regarding the solvency of Medicare and the Social Security system, which will be discussed later.

## REGULATION VERSUS COMPETITION

In the 1970s the preferred solution to the escalating cost of health care was government regulation.

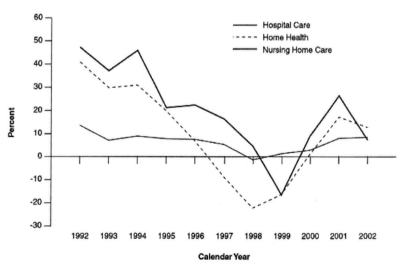

**Figure 15-6** Growth in Medicare spending for hospitals, home health, and nursing homes: 1992 to 2002.

Regulation took the form of health planning at all levels of government and included Certificate of Need programs, which were administered by health systems agencies (HSAs) at the federal, state, and local levels. These programs were intended to avoid duplication of new technologies and certain health care services, limit capital expansion, and ultimately cut unnecessary costs. Professional groups, such as physicians, responded to cost containment through self-regulation mechanisms such as professional standards review organizations (PSROs). PSROs were created by the 1972 Medicare amendments to monitor the quality of federally funded care and to ensure its delivery in the most efficient and economic manner (Davis, Anderson, Rowland, & Steinberg, 1990). In 1983, peer review organizations were created and placed under contract to the HCFA for utilization review and quality-of-care assessments of hospitals, health maintenance organizations (HMOs), and some office practices.

Many of the regulatory efforts of the 1970s and 1980s went by the wayside because they did not significantly reduce costs. Although regulation did involve consumers and community agencies in the process of thinking about cost containment, the solution to the problem was beyond its grasp. Local health planning agencies were often controlled by provider groups or consumers with vested interests, who were unwilling or unable to curb expanding health care costs. Professional groups, while discussing cost reduction, continued to respond to the overwhelming economic incentives inherent in the health care system, and as a result HSAs disappeared or lost much of their influence during the 1980s.

The 1980s saw an emphasis on competition as a mechanism to cut costs. Competition is based on the premise that the health care system has enough similarities to the free market that cost would be controlled by the entry of a large number of competing elements. The problem lies in the fact that, at least at the level of the patient, the health care system does not act like a free market system and, indeed, has few similarities to a fully competitive market in economic terms (Pulcini, 1984). Chapter 14, which focuses on economics, more fully describes the mechanisms underlying the market system.

Although it is not a perfect solution, competition is based on the economic assumption of scarcity; that is, health care is not an unlimited resource, so choices must be made as to how care will be allocated. Competition forced the public to more directly experience the effect of market forces in health care. The 1980s saw attempts to change the existing incentives in health care so that providers and patients could begin to understand the financial effects of high-cost care. Competition has been used effectively at the health plan level, especially with the entry of many new MCOs that do compete vigorously with one another. In this realm the purchasers of health insurance tend to be large corporations, businesses, or unions that buy health benefits for their employees or members. The major impetus for cost containment in the 1980s came from these groups, which are indeed the ultimate buyers of health insurance.

Other examples of cost-containment mechanisms are copayments, deductibles, and coinsurance, which not only discourage unnecessary use but also may increase pressures on low wage earners who cannot afford these extra direct costs. Some argue that although these efforts have had some effect, they have tended to discourage early identification of health problems. One can question whether these efforts have, in effect, decreased access to primary prevention and increased the overall cost of care initiated at later stages in an illness episode. By the end of the 1980s there was a realization that neither pure competition nor regulation would be effective as a solution but that some combination would be needed. Managed competition, as put forth by President Clinton's Health Security Act, was an example of this concept. At the level of the individual patient, care received is dependent to a great extent on what will be reimbursed by insurance companies and covered by managed care plans.

## PROSPECTIVE PAYMENT VERSUS FEE-FOR-SERVICE FINANCING

Pressure on the government from corporations and business groups to change financing from fee-for-service, or retrospective, reimbursement to prospective modalities increased in the 1980s. Because the federal government has direct control only of its own programs, it targeted Medicare Part A by developing in 1983 a prospective payment system (PPS) for hospital care, establishing payment based on diagnosis-related groups (DRGs). DRGs set a payment level for each of 503 diagnostic categories typically used in inpatient care. The goal was to place a cap on escalating hospital costs. Prospective payment measures have helped to slow the rate of growth of hospital expenditures and had a major impact on length of stay (Fuchs, 1988; Heffler et al., 2001). Initially, DRG rates were allowed to increase each year, and payment rates were also adjusted for geographic differences in wage levels. Certain services (such as outpatient and long-term care services) and certain hospitals (such as children's hospitals, psychiatric facilities, and rehabilitation hospitals) were originally excluded from the PPS, but many of these (such as long-term care) are now subject to PPS. Capital and training expenses were reimbursed at cost. Since its initial passage, PPS has undergone some changes, but generally the payment received per hospital discharge is based on what is called the DRG "relative weight" and a national average cost per discharge.

Before the mid 1990s, the enormous federal budget deficit led to political pressure to decrease outlay by cost-saving measures aimed at Medicare Part B, which primarily covers outpatient care. In March of 1992, physician payment reform was initiated by means of the resource-based relative value scale (RBRVS). Its goal was not only cost savings but also a redistribution of physician services to increase primary care services and decrease the use of highly specialized physician care. The RBRVS was developed by William Hsiao and his colleagues (1988) to establish comparable fees for medical services based on time and intensity of effort, with consideration of typical overhead and malpractice costs. Other Medicare Part B cost-saving measures are limitation of home health care services and institution of fixed payments for outpatient care. Medicaid and more recently Medicare are using managed care arrangements to contain costs. Prospective payment has also been extended to long-term care facilities. These will be discussed in the federal programs sections on Medicare and Medicaid, later in this chapter.

The PPS contributed to significantly increased patient acuity in inpatient settings, and resulting gaps and problems still exist. Decreased length of hospital stay caused a ripple effect in the home care industry, which has had to care for more acutely ill persons in the home. Costs then shifted to home care as a result of patients being discharged quickly after a hospital stay.

## MANAGED CARE

**Overview.** Managed care had its origins in early prepaid health plans that have been in existence in the United States since at least the 1920s. A managed care system shifts the emphasis of the provision of health care away from the fee-for-service mode toward a system in which the provider is a "gatekeeper," or manager, of the client's health care. In a managed care system, the provider or insurance company assumes some degree of financial responsibility for the care that is given. According to Curtiss (1989), managed care implies not only that spending will be controlled but also that other aspects of care will be controlled and managed, such as price, quality, and accessibility.

In managed care systems, the primary care provider was traditionally the gatekeeper, deciding what specialty services are appropriate and where these services can be obtained at the lowest cost. In the 1990s, insurance companies themselves became involved in patient care decisions in their attempts to control authorization of payment for less-expensive procedures. Many providers questioned this type of intervention in direct patient care and started their own plans that leave more of the decisions to the providers themselves.

Around the year 2000, enrollment in managed care plans peaked with 165.4 million persons enrolled or more than triple the 51.1 million persons who were enrolled in HMOs in 1994 and a 600% increase from enrollments in 1988 (Bodenheimer & Grumbach, 2005; Kongstvedt, 2001; Managed Care On-Line, 2001). Although managed care is well integrated as the dominant health care financing and delivery system in the United States, its prevalence has begun to decrease in many sectors of the health care system.

Managed care systems have clearly moved in the direction of cost containment but have grown in recent years to a predominance of the less-restrictive plans, which limit the gatekeeper function and give consumers more freedom of choice to choose providers. Before 2001 there was a proliferation of health plans with low copayments for coverage of drugs. This phenomenon occurred as a temporary solution because of a tight labor market, leading employers to offer broader employee benefits in their attempt to attract and retain more workers (Heffler et al., 2001). Cost sharing did go up after 2001 but has leveled off in the last 2 years (Gabel et al., 2005).

**Types of Plans.** Many types of managed health care plans exist. They range from models that have increased control, accountability, and operating complexity to plans that incorporate some aspects of managed care but not all. Kongstvedt (2001) places these on a continuum from closed-panel HMOs to managed indemnity plans (Figure 15-7). HMOs assume responsibility for organizing and providing comprehensive health care services for members in return for a monthly set payment. HMOs incorporate four key concepts:

- An enrolled population
- A prepayment of premiums
- Coverage of comprehensive medical services
- Centralization of medical and hospital services

*Closed-panel HMOs* include staff model HMOs, in which physicians or providers are salaried employees, and group model HMOs, which contract with multi-specialty physician group practices to provide all physician services to their members.

*Open-panel HMOs* include network HMOs, which contract with more than one group practice, and the individual practice association (IPA) type

of HMOs, which contract with an association of physicians to provide services to members.

In *point-of-service* (POS) plans and in *preferred provider organizations* (PPOs) patients are allowed to self-refer to a specialist but must pay higher premiums if they do so. The POS plan is distinguished from the PPO in that the enrollee belongs to an HMO and must have a designated primary care provider, or gatekeeper, but can opt to see a provider outside of the HMO at a greater cost to the enrollee. PPOs are entities through which employer health plans and insurers contract to purchase health care services for covered beneficiaries from a selected group of participating providers. PPOs guarantee a certain volume of business to hospitals and physicians in return for a discounted fee. PPOs benefit physicians, hospitals, and consumers. Physicians do not share in any financial risk, and they are paid on a fee-for-service basis, which many prefer. Hospitals can plan on a certain volume, an important benefit in an environment of declining occupancy rates. Members benefit by paying typically lower premiums. The popularity of PPOs has grown. In 2005, PPOs enrolled 61% of all the people covered by managed care plans, whereas POS plans enrolled 15% and HMOs enrolled 21% (Gabel et al., 2005).

The managed indemnity plan is the most traditional model and uses only some managed care mechanisms, such as precertification of elective admissions and case management of catastrophic cases. The service plan may, in addition, have minimal contractual relationships with providers regarding allowable fees (Kongstvedt, 2001).

**Medicare, Medicaid, and Managed Care.** Government health insurance programs such as Medicaid and Medicare also have incorporated managed care to cut costs. All 50 states offer some type of Medicaid managed care plan, and states can decide if participation is voluntary or mandatory. Some states have created state-run Medicaid-only plans, but others enroll Medicaid recipients in private MCOs. As of 2000 55.8% of the total Medicaid population, or 18.8 million persons, were enrolled in managed care plans (KFF, 2001). From 1996 to 2000 alone there was a 40.1% increase in Medicaid managed care recipients (USDHHS,

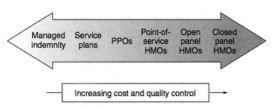

**Figure 15-7** Continuum of managed care. (From Kongetvedt, P. [2001]. *Essentials of managed care* [4th ed.]. Gaithersburg, MD: Aspen.)

HCFA, OA, 2001). By 2003, 60.2% of the Medicaid population was enrolled in Medicaid managed care, and this number is still increasing (KFF, 2005e).

Medicare managed care plans have not been as successful. Under the Tax Equity and Fiscal Responsibility Act (TEFRA) of 1982, Medicare beneficiaries were given the option of remaining in traditional fee-for-service Medicare or enrolling in an MCO. Many elders took advantage of the choice of this option through Medicare + Choice (now known as Medicare Part C or Medicare Advantage plans). Between 1996 and 2000, enrollment in managed care increased 12% to 17%. Although the intent of the Medicare + Choice program within the Balanced Budget Act (BBA) of 1997 was to increase enrollment in Medicare managed care, the same legislation cut reimbursement to MCOs. As a result, when MCOs dropped out of the Medicare managed care program, 800,000 beneficiaries lost their health coverage between 2000 and 2001. As of 2005, 12% of Medicare enrollees were enrolled in Medicare Advantage Plans (Medicare Part C) such as HMOs or PPOs and 88% had traditional fee-for-service Medicare coverage (KFF, 2005f). This number has decreased from 17.2%, or by 1.7 million beneficiaries, since 2000 (ManagedCare On-Line, 2001). The Medicare Modernization Act of 2003 significantly changed the Medicare program, offering beneficiaries more plans to choose from, including a fee-for-service option. This is covered extensively in *Reforming Medicare*, later in this chapter.

**Costs, Enrollment, and Quality.** Cost increases may be a result of higher prescription drug costs and usage, consumer demand for more choice and better access to services through less-restrictive plans, higher reimbursement rates charged by providers, and increased pressure to improve profits (Sultz & Young, 2004). When premiums go up, people tend to drop their coverage and businesses curtail their coverage of employee health care. It is estimated that for every 1% increase in premiums, 300,000 people lose their health coverage (National Coalition on Health Care, 2000). Managed care enrollment has continued to grow despite a "backlash" against managed care in the media and though public perception. Concerns have been raised about the

degree to which the financial incentives of managed care have caused withholding of needed services and compromised quality of care. However, these concerns are not supported by available evidence. Hoffman (2002) found that quality of care in MCOs has improved over time. Numerous other studies show either improvement in access to care or little difference between managed care and fee-for-service medicine. Most managed care legislation is at the state level and has been directed at limiting financial incentives for physicians to curb usage, has promoted continuity of care, and has set minimum hospital maternity stays. State and federal laws that further regulate managed care plans encompass a variety of areas such as grievance procedures, confidentiality of health information, requirements that patients are fully informed of the benefits they will receive under a managed care plan, antidiscrimination clauses, and assurances that various quality assurance mechanisms are in place so that patient satisfaction is measured and efforts to control costs do not curtail needed care.

In the 1990s the quality of care in MCOs became a major issue. Many states and the U.S. Congress passed regulatory legislation in the form of health plan accountability laws to further regulate managed care plans (Kongstvedt, 2001). These laws encompassed a variety of areas such as grievance procedures, confidentiality of health information, requirements that patients are fully informed of the benefits they will receive under a managed care plan, antidiscrimination clauses, and assurances that various quality assurance mechanisms are in place so that patient satisfaction is measured and efforts to control costs do not curtail needed care.

Most states have adopted policies giving health plan enrollees a right to appeal plan determinations involving a denial of coverage to an independent medical review entity, which is often a private organization approved by the state (American Association of Health Plans, 2001). Efforts to pass into law the federal Patient's Bill of Rights, which contains many consumer protections related to managed care, have not been successful. A major controversial provision of the legislation is the right it gives individuals to bring lawsuits against their managed care plans, which are protected from such lawsuits under the

Employee Retirement Income Security Act (ERISA) of 1974. ERISA is a federal law that sets minimum standards for most voluntarily established pension and health plans in private industry to provide protection for individuals in these plans. ERISA requires plans to provide participants with *plan information* including important information about plan features and funding; provides *fiduciary responsibilities* for those who manage and control plan assets; requires plans to establish a grievance and appeals process for participants to get benefits from their plans; and gives participants the right to sue for benefits and breaches of fiduciary duty (U.S. Department of Labor, 2005).

**Social Security.** To understand public health care financing it is first necessary to understand Social Security as a social insurance program because Medicare, Medicaid, and SCHIP are part of the Social Security Act. Although America has always valued individualism, the Great Depression of the 1930s taught U.S. workers that they were financially vulnerable because of factors beyond their control. The Social Security Act of 1935 provided a base of economic security that allowed older Americans to live with dignity and independence. The act was carefully crafted to distinguish the program from welfare programs and to promote its acceptance as social insurance.

*Principles of Social Security.* Social Security was established based on the following principles (Kingson & Schulz, 1997; Schulz, 2001; Steuerle & Bakija, 2000):

*Individual equity or fairness.* This principle means that the amount a worker pays into the system determines how much he or she will earn in benefits.

*Social adequacy (horizontal equity).* According to this principle, benefits are calculated by means of a weighted formula that ensures a minimum floor of protection for workers with lower lifetime earnings. Benefits are also adjusted for inflation, which offsets financial erosion with time. The concept of social insurance and protection of individual dignity evolved from this principle. The social insurance aspect includes three important tenets. First, insurance protection

is provided not only to workers, but also to their dependents. Second, all eligible workers participate; individuals cannot opt out of the system. Exceptions to eligibility include most federal employees hired before 1984, railroad employees with more than 10 years of service, some state and local employees, and children under age 21 who work for a parent (Social Security Administration, 2001a). Third, contributors are protected against destitution by pooling the risk of lost income among all contributors.

*Economic efficiency.* This principle dictates that the highest possible benefits be provided to retirees with minimum administrative costs both to the beneficiary and to the nation.

*Individual dignity.* A belief in individual dignity dictates that there be no means test for a person to qualify for benefits and that benefits be considered a statutory right.

*Eligibility and Populations Covered.* To be eligible for Social Security, one must earn credits by working and paying taxes into Social Security for approximately 10 years, or 40 credits. The amount of Social Security benefits received is based on a formula that takes into consideration individual earnings, overall wage inflation, and retirement age (see *Social Security: Key to Economic Security* in Chapter 14).

*Current Financing.* Social Security is financed through the Federal Insurance Contributions Act (FICA), which authorizes payroll deductions for Social Security. As of 2006 the Social Security part of the tax is 6.2% of an employee's gross wages, up to $94,200 in wages (Social Security Administration, 2005a). Employers match workers' tax payments with an additional 6.2%. Self-employed persons pay taxes equal to the combined employer-employee tax, but half of this payment is deductible as a business expense. These taxes are deposited in the Social Security Trust Funds, financial accounts in the U.S. Treasury from which Social Security and Medicare benefits are paid. There are four Social Security trust funds:

- Old Age and Survivors Insurance (OASI)
- Disability Insurance (DI)
- Hospital Insurance Trust Fund (HI, or Medicare Part A)

■ Supplementary Medical Insurance (SMI, or Medicare Part B)

The "social insurance" aspect of Social Security makes the program more than just a retirement plan. The Social Security Administration has referred to Social Security as "America's Family Protection Plan" (Social Security Administration, 2000b). In addition to retirement benefits, Social Security pays survivor benefits to spouses age 60 or older (50 or older if disabled) and to spouses of any age if the spouse is caring for one child under age 16, for multiple children under age 18, or for a parent if the earner had provided more than one half of the parent's support. In addition, Social Security pays a one-time $255 lump sum death benefit to a spouse or minor children (Schulz, 2001; Social Security Administration, 2005b; Social Security Administration, 2005c).

Social Security was never designed to be the only source of retirement income. Retirement income is seen as a three-legged stool, with one leg being Social Security benefits, the second being pension income, and the third being personal savings and investments. Social Security is seen as replacing 40% of a worker's salary after retirement; it therefore provides a "safety net," but not the entire amount (approximately 70% of preretirement income) necessary to support a comfortable retirement (Social Security Administration, 2000b).

## THE HEALTH CARE FINANCING SYSTEM IN THE PUBLIC REALM

**Federal Level.** The health care financing system is composed of many interrelated parts at the federal, state, and local levels. Both government and private sectors play a role at each level. No single entity oversees or controls the entire system. At the federal level, Medicare, Medicaid, and SCHIP are financed at least in part through the CMS (formerly HCFA), an agency of the USDHHS. Federal health expenditures totaled $504.7 billion in 2003, and the federal government financed 32.5% of all health care expenditures in that year.

Medicare outlays were $280 billion in 2003 and are projected to be $325 billion in 2005 with 42 million enrollees including 35.4 million aged and 6.3 million disabled persons served (KFF, 2005b).

Medicaid outlays in 2003 were $257.3 billion, with 52.4 million people receiving care through this program (Harris, 2005; USDHHS, HCFA, OA, 2001). Enrollment of women and children in Medicaid dropped after the 1996 Personal Responsibility and Work Opportunities Act came into effect, with greater employment of this population, and a delinking of Medicaid eligibility and welfare that occurred with the passage of Temporary Assistance for Needy Families (TANF) (Heffler et al., 2001; USDDHS, HCFA, OA, 2001). This program took up 22% of the average state budget in 2005 (Harris, 2005). As the number of uninsured increased to more than 47 million persons and as the population aged, the number of Medicaid enrollees, which was relatively stable for 30 years, greatly increased (Harris, 2005). Medicaid will be covered further in the section on the state level later in this chapter.

***Medicare.*** Medicare legislation was passed in 1965 as an amendment (Title XVIII) to the Social Security Act of 1935, to enable older people to pay for their health care in retirement. Before enactment of Medicare, elders were more likely to be uninsured and more likely to be impoverished by excessive health care costs. This was particularly true for the "oldest old." According to the National Center for Health Statistics (cited in Lubitz et al., 2001), in 1962 and 1963, 61% of persons from age 65 to age 74 and only 41% of persons aged 75 years and older had hospital insurance. Before the enactment of Medicare, half of older Americans had no health insurance; as of 2000, 96% of seniors had health care coverage through Medicare (Federal Interagency Forum on Age-Related Statistics, 2000). As evidence of Medicare's beneficial economic effect, the percentage of persons over age 65 living below the poverty line decreased from 35% in 1959, when elders had the highest poverty rate of the population, to 6.5% in 2004 (Federal Interagency Forum on Age-Related Statistics, 2000; U.S. Census Bureau, 2005). Medicare has also had a beneficial effect on the health of the elderly, facilitating access to care, to medical technology, and, in 2006, to prescription drug coverage (Lubitz et al., 2001; USDHHS, CMS, 2005a).

Medicare includes Part A (hospital insurance); Part B (Supplemental Medical Insurance); Part C, or

Medicare Advantage plans (originally Medicare + Choice programs), which expand beneficiaries' options for participation in private-sector health plans; and Part D, the outpatient prescription drug benefit that began in January 2006. Individuals are eligible for Medicare Part A at age 65, the age for Social Security eligibility. Part A is financed through payroll deduction to the Hospital Insurance Trust Fund at the 2005 payroll tax rate of 2.9% of earnings paid by employers and employees (1.45% each) (KFF, 2005b). Most Americans (and their spouses) who have worked for at least 10 years and have paid Medicare taxes are automatically enrolled in Part A. Disabled persons younger than 65 who are receiving Social Security disability benefits (Supplemental Security Income [SSI]) may also enroll in Part A after a 24-month waiting period. This waiting period was waived, under the Consolidated Appropriations Act of 2001, for persons with amyotrophic lateral sclerosis (ALS). Persons with permanent renal disease who are undergoing dialysis or who have had a renal transplant are also eligible for Part A, regardless of age. (See *Reforming Medicare*, later in this chapter.)

*Current Financing.* Persons enrolled in Medicare Part A may choose to sign up for Part B, which partially covers outpatient services. Part B is funded through the SMI Trust Fund, which is supported by enrollee contributions and a share of general revenues. Enrollee contributions by law are to constitute approximately 25% of Part B costs, with the remaining 75% coming from general revenues (USDHHS, CMS, 2005b). Under the provisions of the BBA of 1997, a PPS was established for some services covered under Part B. These include outpatient services such as immunizations, casting, partial hospitalization for mental health disorders, and other services traditionally covered under Part B. Under PPS, Medicare reimburses the provider a set amount for these services. The consumer may be responsible for a co-payment (Social Security Administration, 2000a).

Individuals must apply for Part B during a 7-month enrollment period that starts 3 months before their sixty-fifth birthday. For those who delay enrollment, the cost of Part B goes up by 10% for each year that Part B could have been in place,

resulting in increased consumer lifetime costs (USDDHS, HCFA, 2001a). Part B requires a yearly $100 deductible and a monthly co-payment by enrollees ($78.20 in 2005). Covered services include 80% of the fees for physician services, outpatient medical services and supplies, home care, durable medical equipment, laboratory services, physical and occupational therapy, and outpatient mental health services (USDHHS, CMS, 2005b; USDHHS, CMS, 2005c).

*Gaps in Medicare Coverage.* Despite its success in facilitating the provision of basic health care to elders, significant gaps in Medicare coverage remain. Medicare has maintained an acute care focus that has led to inadequate coverage for preventive services, case management, vision and hearing services, and, most significantly, long-term care and catastrophic illness coverage (Cassel, Besdine, & Siegel, 1999). *Custodial* long-term care is not covered under Part B, an omission that shifts provision of care for the approximately 10 million Americans who need long-term care to families and to the Medicaid program (Feder, Komisar, & Niefeld, 2000). Another gap in Part B coverage is reimbursement for certain preventive services. Although Medicare has expanded Part B reimbursement for preventive care to cover mammogram screening, Pap smears, prostate and colorectal cancer screening, diabetes monitoring, and immunizations, important preventive services such as vision care other than glaucoma tests, dental care and dentures, routine foot care, and routine annual physical examinations are not covered beyond a physical in the first 6 months after coverage begins (USDHHS, CMS, 2005a).

*Fee-for-Service Versus Managed Care Medicare.* At its inception in 1965, Medicare was modeled after private employer-provided fee-for-service insurance plans (Atherly, 2001). With passage of the 1997 BBA, Medicare enrollees, under the Medicare + Choice program, were given a choice of three Medicare plans. These include the original Medicare fee-for-service coverage, Medicare managed care, and the privately insured fee-for-service. The Medicare Advantage Plan replaced Medicare + Choice under the Medicare Prescription Drug, Improvement, and Modernization Act and was renamed and modified to expand beneficiaries' options for participation in private-sector health plans. A second goal was to increase competition among Medicare providers and thus lower costs (Neuman & Langwell, 1999). The original Medicare fee-for-service plan, which covered 83% of Medicare beneficiaries in 2000 (Oberlander, 2000), offers the beneficiary a choice of hospital and provider. It requires, however, the payment of an annual deductible, a fee each time the service is used, and the payment of the difference between the Medicare-approved amount for the covered service and the Medicare payment (i.e., "balance billing"). Under this plan, consumers pay considerable out-of-pocket charges for health care, including charges for "Medigap" insurance to supplement services not covered under Medicare. Over the past 15 to 20 years, out-of-pocket expenses for health care have increased for elders across all income groups, with the poor paying a larger portion of their income for health care.

On a fee-for-service basis, Medicare pays fixed monthly payments to certain plans, from which beneficiaries purchase private indemnity health insurance policies. The consumer maintains choice of provider and health care setting and receives extra services such as partial prescription drug coverage, but the individual must pay deductibles and premium fees that may exceed those charged by the original Medicare. The plan, not the provider, determines the rate of provider reimbursement, and providers may be allowed to balance-bill Medicare patients 15% above the payment level set by the plan. Medicare fee-for-service is not available in all areas. Patients with end-stage renal disease, covered under Medicare, are not covered with the private fee-for-service option (USDHHS, CMS, 2005b).

Although the majority of Medicare recipients remain in the fee-for-service sector (Federal Interagency Forum on Age-Related Statistics, 2000), Medicare managed care has received increased attention as a strategy to control costs. In 1983, Congress, under TEFRA, authorized Medicare payments to qualified "risk-contract" HMOs (Social Security Administration, 2000a). In risk plans, called *coordinated care plans*, the beneficiary is required to receive all services from within the organization's network of providers. Medicare beneficiaries can also enroll in "cost plans." Under cost plans, care

may be received outside of the provider network or service area. Subscribers to Medicare HMO plans (Medicare Part C) must be enrolled in Medicare Part B and are required to pay a copayment for services. Costs not covered under fee-for-service Medicare, including preventive care and prescription drugs, may be covered under Medicare managed care plans (Social Security Administration, 2000a). Participation in a managed care plan may offer additional consumer savings by negating the need for supplemental Medigap insurance.

***Medicare Reform.*** Because the shift by some beneficiaries to Medicare managed care in the 1990s did not produce intended savings, there have been numerous proposals for insuring the solvency of Medicare. Proposals for Medicare reform include delaying the age of retirement; increasing payroll taxes for higher-income taxpayers; offering so-called "premium support" (in which Medicare prefunds premiums for individuals) to Medicare enrollees to encourage them to join HMOs; and improved risk-sharing between Medicare and HMOs (Burman et al., 1998; Dowd, Coulam & Feldman, 2000; Etheredge, 1999, 2000; Gorin, 2000; Oberlander, 2000; Seidman, 2000). The 1997 BBA attempted to modernize Medicare financing and created the National Bipartisan Commission on the Future of Medicare, with the aim of long-term structural reform. The BBA mandated demonstration projects to test the hypothesis that applying market principles could cut Medicare costs (Nichols & Reischauer, 2000). The Medicare Medical Savings Account (MSA) Plan, for example, was proposed as one premium-support model with potential cost-savings to both consumers and to Medicare.

MSAs, commonly called *health savings account* (HSA) plans, have two components: a tax-sheltered Medicare-funded savings account for health care expenses and a private catastrophic health insurance plan with a high deductible (not more than $6000) (Hall & Havighurst, 2005; Kendix & Lubitz, 1999; USDHHS, HCFA, 1998). According to CIGNA (2005), an HSA is "a consumer-driven health plan in which the plan member pays for health costs through a fully funded, tax-exempt savings account. Members or employers or both fund the account. An HSA is subject to regulations mandated by the federal government that limit coverage to IRS section 213(d) medical coverage. All unused funds carry over indefinitely during a member's lifetime." Another option is the Health Reimbursement Arrangement (HRA), which is "a consumer-driven health plan in which the plan member is reimbursed for covered health expenses by his/her employer up to a predetermined amount. Unused funds may be carried over to the next year, subject to limits set by the employer" (CIGNA, 2005). In 2005, about 4% of employers offered this type of high-deductible plan, covering about 2.4 million workers and tending to favor the young and healthy (Gabel et al., 2005). Recipients receive a capitated (capped) amount from Medicare, equal to 95% of the traditional costs of fee-for-service Medicare. From the capitated amount, Medicare pays the premium for the catastrophic insurance and deposits money into the individual's MSA or HSA. Money in the savings account is used to pay the deductible on the insurance policy, if needed. Beneficiaries who have insufficient money in the savings account must pay the balance of the deductible out of private funds. If the beneficiary does not use the money in the savings account in a given year, the money accumulates in the savings account for use in another year. MSAs or HSAs could potentially cut Medicare costs, because Medicare saves 5% on the capitated amount. Consumers would also be motivated to save health care dollars, because they would be responsible for costs incurred over the amount in the MSA up to the deductible. MSAs or HSAs would also eliminate the need for supplemental, or Medigap, coverage, again resulting in consumer savings (Kendix & Lubitz, 1999).

MSAs, HSAs, and other attempts at premium support or high-deductible plans have been criticized for moving the healthiest and wealthiest persons from traditional fee-for-service Medicare to the private insurance sector. This results in overall increased costs to the Medicare system (Baker & Weisbrot, 1999; Kendix & Lubitz, 1999; Oberlander, 2000). According to Oberlander (2000), premium-support plans actually reduce choice for many Medicare recipients, who are already overwhelmed by the options available under Medicare. These elders, many of whom will be chronically ill, frail, and financially challenged, will choose a plan according to what they can afford rather than according to what they need. Prescription drug coverage is covered extensively in *Interests, Ideology, and Institutional Dynamics in the Creation of the Medicare Prescription Drug Benefit*, later in this chapter.

Another trend is to move to Disease Management Programs (DMPs) in order to deal with the sickest of the population (Gabel et al., 2005). Berk and Monheit (2001) reported that from 1977 to 1996, a very stable 5% of the population accounted for 55% of the health care expenditures. This occurred in spite of major changes in financing, including PPSs, managed care predominance, and use of other cost-cutting mechanisms. Those in the lower 50% in health care expenditures spent 3% of the resources. Those in the top 1% in health care expenditures spent 22.3% of health care dollar in 2002, whereas those in the bottom 50% spent 3.4%, as shown in Figure 15-8 (KFF, 2005g). They also show that a majority of those in the high-expenditure group were not elderly and that costs were unaffected by enrollment in a managed care plan. Although much health services research is being conducted in this area of high-cost care, more studies are needed using nursing models of care delivery and their effect on cost outcomes.

**Balanced Budget Act of 1997.** The BBA of 1997 was signed into law on August 5, 1997, as PL 105-33. This legislation made major changes in the Medicare program, including a $116.4 billion reduction in net spending over the following 5 years until 2002 and a $393.5 billion cut over 10 years. Savings came first from reductions in payments to hospitals and then from private plan payment reductions as well as increases in Medicare Part B premiums to a projected $105 per month in 2007. Payment methods were restructured in part to control fraud and abuse activities in rehabilitation hospitals, home health agencies, SNFs, and outpatient services. This led to an abrupt slowdown in Medicare spending from 1997 to 2000 and, subsequently, costs as payments to hospitals, nursing homes, and home health agencies again began to increase (Cowan, et al., 2004).

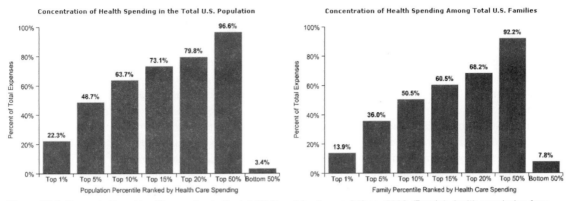

**Figure 15-8** Concentration of health spending in the total U.S. and family populations: 2002. (Reprinted with permission from The Henry J. Kaiser Family Foundation. [2005, February]. *Trends and indicators in the changing health care marketplace*, #7031.)

This law also contained the largest spending reductions for Medicaid since 1981, with a saving of $17 billion over 5 years and $61.4 billion over 10 years by greatly expanding the substantial discretion that states have in administering their Medicaid programs, by eliminating minimum payment standards, and by allowing states to require most beneficiaries to enroll in MCOs. Although it left most of the critical elements of the Medicaid program intact, it did limit Medicaid eligibility for persons who had legally immigrated since August 1996. Prospective payment schemes, managed care, and particularly the BBA of 1997 and its amendments had a significant effect in decreasing inpatient costs in the 1990s. The price of medical care and usage decreased until the year 2000, and usage in particular has been increasing since then (Cowan et al., 2004). Although hospital spending increased slightly both in 1998 and 1999, it continued to fall as a share of national health expenditures (NHEs) from 1991 to 2001, when it began to level off (Cowan et al., 2004). Medicare spending for inpatient care also fell in the 2 years after the passage of the BBA of 1997, with relative declines in inpatient case-mix intensity. This change may have been attributed to BBA provisions affecting home care, shifts to ambulatory care, and changes in hospitals' coding of admissions (Heffler et al., 2001).

*Nurse Practitioner Reimbursement and Medicare.* The Omnibus Budget and Reconciliation Act (OBRA) of 1997 extended Medicare Part B coverage of nurse practitioner (NP) and clinical nurse specialist (CNS) services. Earlier legislation (OBRA 1990) provided reimbursement for NPs and CNSs in rural areas. OBRA 1997 extended coverage of nurse-provided services, removing geographic and setting restrictions. Under this legislation, all NPs and CNSs are able to obtain a Medicare provider number and directly bill Medicare for reimbursement at 85% of the Medicare physician fee schedule for services that they are legally authorized to perform under their state practice acts. NPs or CNSs may bill for services that they provide directly or that they provide "incident to" services provided by a physician. The new regulations do not require a physician to be on site when an NP is delivering care in order for NP services to be reimbursed. Neither does the law require that physicians make an independent evaluation of all NP or CNS patients. There is a requirement, however, for physician "collaboration," loosely defined as a relationship with a physician that enables consultation on cases outside the nurse's scope of practice (Abood & Keepnews, 2000).

**Other Federal Programs.** Federal health care programs other than Medicare, Medicaid, and SCHIP exist to provide services for specific segments of the population and are funded from general tax revenues.

*Programs for Veterans.* Eligible military veterans are covered through the U.S. Department of Veterans Affairs (VA). These veterans can access a wide range of general health and medical services through the Civilian Health and Medical Program of the Veterans Administration (CHAMPVA), plus services that are specifically geared to veterans, such as the Agent Orange Health Effects and Vietnam Veterans Programs. The VA funds several notable research initiatives such as the Centers of Excellence in Hepatitis C Research and Education. Elderly veterans are afforded the full range of long-term care programs, hospice programs, home-based primary care, geriatric evaluation and management programs, adult day health care, and respite care. The Foreign Medical Program is a health care benefits program for U.S. veterans with VA-rated service-connected conditions who are residing or traveling abroad. More information is available at *www.va.gov* and in *The U.S. Veterans Administration: Policy Change for the Greater Good in an Integrated Health System* in Chapter 13.

**Military Programs.** Active duty service members in the Army, Navy, Air Force, Marine Corps, and Coast Guard and their dependent families are covered through TRICARE, formerly the Civilian Health and Medical Program of the Uniformed Services (CHAMPUS), a program within the Defense Department. This program offers three options to TRICARE-eligible beneficiaries ranging from TRICARE Standard, a benefit similar to the original CHAMPUS program, TRICARE Extra, a network of civilian preferred providers, and TRICARE Prime, which is an HMO-like program. The annual budget expenditure in the Department of Defense (DoD) Health Program is about $21 billion. The CHAMPUS program is notable because it was one of the first federal programs to reimburse nurses for their services (DoD, 2001). An evaluation of this program is available at *www.tricare.osd.mil* and in *The Department of Defense TRICARE Program: Health Care for the U.S. Military* in Chapter 13.

**Federal Employee Program.** The Federal Employees Health Benefits Program (FEHBP) is another federally administered plan that has required direct payment to NPs and physician assistants authorized to practice in their respective states. It is important to remember that just because care is reimbursed through federal policy; it doesn't mean that nurses, as providers of that care, can be covered if state laws interfere. An example is a state with nurse practice acts that limit nurses' scope of practice. For further information, see *www.opm.gov/insure/01/index.html*.

**Native American Program.** The Indian Health Service (IHS) is an agency within the USDHHS and provides direct health services to Native American populations throughout the country. The IHS is the principal federal health care provider and health advocate for Native American people, and its goal is to ensure that comprehensive, culturally acceptable personal and public health services are available and accessible to Native American and Alaska Native people. The IHS provides health services to approximately 1.5 million Native Americans and Alaska Natives who belong to more than 550 federally recognized tribes in 35 states. For further information see *www.ihs.gov*.

**Programs for Rural Populations.** The U.S. Public Health Service provides a wide range of services for rural health. One key program is the National Health Service Corps (*http://nhsc.bhpr.hrsa.gov*) and other initiatives that provide services in rural health areas and that fund rural health clinics. Important resources to be aware of are the eight rural health research centers in the nation funded by the Office of Rural Health Policy, including the Rural Health Resource Center of the University of Minnesota (*www.hsr.umn.edu/rhrc*) and the University of North Dakota Center for Rural Health (*www.med.und.nodak.edu/depts/rural*).

**Federal and State.** Some federal health programs such as Medicaid and SCHIP are administered at the state level (see *Children's Health Insurance Coverage: Medicaid and the State Children's Health Insurance Program [SCHIP]*, later in this chapter). Another example of state administration of a federal program is the Title V Maternal-Child Block Grant Program, which has as its objective the improvement of maternal, infant, and adolescent health and the development of service systems for children at risk of chronic and disabling conditions.

States also have an important role in designing health policy through health planning efforts and in regulating health care costs and insurance carriers through rate-setting efforts. States take on responsibility for ensuring quality health services through oversight of health care providers and facilities. Local government health services are also authorized at the state level.

In addition, the state insurance regulation agency has a major role in regulating insurance companies through the insurance laws. It is in this capacity that states are increasingly becoming involved in regulating the quality of care provided in health insurance plans or managed care programs.

Individual state decisions around financing for Medicaid are being driven by the overwhelming demands on health care budgets and by the continued pressure on states to decrease taxes. States are often using managed care plans to provide services for Medicaid recipients and are seeking cost-effective solutions to what has continued to be a crisis in health care at the state level as state legislators become more cost conscious.

***Medicaid.*** Medicaid is a jointly funded program of both federal and state governments, and until 1997 eligibility was determined by income and resources. Those eligible included some persons receiving Temporary Assistance to Needy Families (TANF); persons older than 65 years of age who are income eligible; blind and totally disabled persons who received cash assistance under the SSI program; pregnant women; and children born after September 1983 in families with incomes at or below the poverty line. To qualify for federal Medicaid matching grants, a state must provide a minimum set of benefits, including hospitalization, physician care, laboratory services, x-ray studies, prenatal care, and preventive services; nursing home and home health care; and medically necessary transportation. Medicaid programs are also required to pay the Medicare premiums, deductibles, and copayments for certain low-income persons (Bodenheimer & Grumbach, 2005).

***Eligibility and Populations Covered.*** In 1997, major changes began to occur in Medicaid, particularly in eligibility requirements. Public law (PL) 104-193, the Personal Responsibility and Work Opportunities Act of 1996, eliminated the AFDC cash assistance program and replaced it with the block grant program TANF. Under this welfare law, Medicaid

was delinked from AFDC and SSI so that automatic coverage is not guaranteed. By September of 1997, states were required to redetermine the Medicaid eligibility of many individuals, including children eligible for SSI and many individuals who are not U.S. citizens or who had been receiving disability cash assistance (SSI) based on alcoholism and drug addiction. Under PL 104-193, states are permitted to deny Medicaid benefits to adults and heads of household who lose TANF benefits because of refusal to work (National Center for Children in Poverty [NCCP], 2005).

As an optional service, states may continue to cover the "medically needy." These individuals are often poor or have spent enough on medical bills to bring them to poverty level after a catastrophic illness. However, they earn too much money to qualify for TANF or SSI and would be eligible for one of these programs only by virtue of being in a family with dependent children, more than 65 years of age, blind, or totally and permanently disabled. It is under this medically needy category that many elderly individuals or persons with life-threatening chronic illnesses such as acquired immunodeficiency syndrome (AIDS) may qualify for Medicaid (Bodenheimer & Grumbach, 2005).

Medicaid is increasingly becoming a long-term care program of last resort for elderly persons in nursing homes. Many elderly have to "spend down" their life savings to become eligible for Medicaid. Figure 15-9 indicates the current numbers served by category and amounts of money attributed to each group (KFF, 2005h) Family NPs, pediatric NPs, geriatric NPs, and certified nurse midwives must also be reimbursed under Medicaid if, in accordance with state regulations, they are legally authorized to provide Medicaid-covered services.

***Current Financing.*** Medicaid is funded partially by a general fund allocation of the federal budget but is a matching government program with state revenue budget allocations. Medicaid was originally intended as a dollar-for-dollar match between state and federal governments. However, the federal matching formula is calculated on a per capita income base, so many of the poorer states actually pay less than half and do not match dollar for dollar.

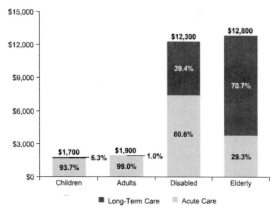

**Figure 15-9** Medicaid enrollees and expenditures on benefits (by eligibility category): 2003. (Reprinted with permission from The Henry J. Kaiser Family Foundation. [2005, February]. *Trends and indicators in the changing health care marketplace,* #7031.)

The federal match makes Medicaid an attractive payer for state governments that are committed to covering as many of their residents as possible with comprehensive health insurance. On the other hand, states are hesitant to expand Medicaid because of the rapid increase in costs.

Several alternatives to cutting spending have been proposed in the 108th Congress. Raising taxes to cover expenses is politically unpalatable. Other options include cutting benefits, charging premiums, and increasing copayments for most services. This is an approach favored by the Bush administration, the House of Representatives, and the National Governors' Association. The Senate supports keeping benefits intact and expanding Medicaid by allowing parents of severely disabled children to buy coverage. The Senate also increases efforts to get eligible people to enroll. Many advocacy groups, including the Academy of Pediatrics and the March of Dimes, favor the Senate bill. It is clear that major changes for the Medicaid program will occur through federal legislation.

Through 1115 Medicaid research and demonstration waivers granted by the federal government, most states have moved Medicaid recipients into managed care plans, but some others have creatively designed ways to expand coverage to uninsured

residents by using the federal reimbursement that comes though the Medicaid program. Lawmakers have found that expanding coverage to uninsured people through existing programs like Medicaid is more palatable because of the cost-sharing between the federal and state governments and because Medicaid already has a built-in administrative structure (McDonough, 1999). For example, in the late 1990s, Massachusetts created a new category of people eligible for Medicaid—adults without children who are the long-term unemployed—and expanded income limits for existing categories, allowing greater coverage of low-income children and families and people with disabilities. The waiver also allowed the state to pay hospitals and MCOs caring for a large number of uninsured people enhanced payments at no additional state cost. As a result of the Medicaid waiver in Massachusetts, an additional 300,000 people got their health insurance covered through Medicaid, partly paid for through federal funding (see *Massachusetts' Strategy for Financing Health Care for the Uninsured* following this chapter).

Because of the waivers, the TANF block granting process, and SCHIP, many are concerned that state Medicaid programs are so diverse that we have, in essence, 50 different Medicaid programs nationwide.

**State Level.** State governments not only administer some federal insurance programs such as Medicaid and SCHIP, they run federal and state public health programs. State health departments also administer federal block grant programs, such as the Title V Maternal-Child Block Grant Program, as well as funding and running their own public health initiatives with state dollars. Usually state health departments combine state and federal dollars to develop and implement public health initiatives around programs such as those involving maternal and child health, smoking cessation, human immunodeficiency virus (HIV) and AIDS, substance abuse, and environmental health. These initiatives are primarily population-based prevention programs in which health services and are not reimbursable by private or government insurance programs, such as Medicaid or Medicare. States also have an important role in designing health policy through health planning efforts and in regulating health care costs and insurance carriers through rate-setting efforts. States take on responsibility for ensuring high-quality health services through oversight of health care providers and facilities. Local government health services are also authorized at the state level.

In addition, the state insurance regulation agency has a major role in regulating insurance companies through the insurance laws. It is in this capacity that states are increasingly becoming involved in regulating the quality of care provided in health insurance plans or managed care programs. State health departments have assumed an increasing role in providing direct services such as Early and Periodic Screening, Diagnostic and Treatment (EPSDT) programs in schools and child care centers as well as programs for children with disabilities (see *Using Private Funds to Improve School Health*, later in this chapter).

***Local and County Level.*** Like state governments, local and county governments in many states also have the responsibility for protecting the public health and in many instances provide indigent care by funding and running public hospitals and clinics. New York City's Health and Hospitals Corporation and Chicago's Cook County Hospital are examples of this type of control. Even these hospitals, although receiving a subsidy from their local government, tend to get large amounts of operating money from Medicaid and Medicare, so public hospital care is indeed dependent on the decisions made within these two programs. In the early 1990s in many areas of the country, public hospitals were in danger of being sold or privatized or were otherwise in jeopardy because of mergers or acquisitions by larger hospitals or networks. As the costs of care have increased and more care has been performed in the home and in the community, competition among hospitals has intensified. Another problem for hospitals has been the increased supply of medical specialists and a decreased supply of primary care providers. The 1997 BBA included a nationwide expansion of a program that began in New York City and that offers financial incentives to hospitals that train fewer doctors, especially in the medical

specialties, with the idea that savings would occur with a reduction of the physician supply (One thousand hospitals, 1997). Since that time many public hospitals such as the New York Health and Hospitals Corporation hospitals have successfully begun to reduce costs and operate with decreased subsidies. In the early years of the twenty-first century that trend reversed, with increased deficits in large public hospital systems resulting in increased pressure on insurers to increase their reimbursement rates (Freudenheim, 2001; Steinhauer, 2001).

With the cost-constraint strategies of the 1980s and 1990s and the misconception that infectious diseases were no longer a major threat, population-based health services such as those originating from state and local health departments received proportionately less and less funding (Institute of Medicine [IOM], 1988). Traditional public health nursing functions to provide surveillance in this important area were minimized or eliminated in this period because they were viewed as having a lower priority than individual health (morbidity) services, which were also being cut back. The crises in the control of infectious diseases such as measles and tuberculosis have taught us important lessons about the need for strong local public health agencies (Brudney & Dobkin, 1991). The onset of AIDS greatly escalated the problem and has reinforced the need for primary prevention and basic public health strategies. When public health strategies are superseded by an emphasis on the individual, major health problems can "fall through the cracks" of the system, and the whole of society will suffer. The 1990s brought a resurgence of interest in integrating these public health strategies and reemphasizing community-based approaches. The tragedy of September 11, 2001 and a series of natural disasters also brought to light the difficulties in our public health system, especially in light of the threat of bioterrorism.

## PRIVATE HEALTH CARE SYSTEM

The private component of the health care system consists of all nongovernmental sources and, in fact, is the largest component because most health care facilities in this country are run by private for-profit or nonprofit corporations. The entire health insurance industry is also within the private system. Included as part of what has been called the "medical-industrial complex" are the pharmaceutical companies, suppliers of health care technology, and the various service industries that support the health care system (Meyers, 1970; Relman, 1980). Because so much of the industry is controlled by private sources, it is difficult for cost controls to be consistent across different sectors of the health care industry. The greatest growth in this country has come from the for-profit sector, with for-profit firms' purchase of or consolidation with private nonprofit hospitals (Lutz & Gee, 1995). In 1997 Columbia/ HCA Health Care was the nation's largest for-profit hospital system, owning 350 hospitals in 38 states and maintaining a 20% gross profit target (Herman, 1997). The health care industry has been transformed in the past 15 years by a business philosophy that has and will continue to have far-reaching effects on the overall health care system. Although this chapter has largely described the public sector in health care, one must also recognize the large role the private sector plays in today's health care system. For more information, see Chapter 14, which discusses economics.

## IMPACT OF FINANCING ON HEALTH SERVICES

### AMBULATORY CARE AND OUTPATIENT AND PRIMARY CARE SERVICES

*Outpatient care* and *ambulatory care* are terms that are often used interchangeably, but Shi and Singh (2004) argue that the term *outpatient services* is more comprehensive and precise because it refers to health care services that are not provided on the basis of an overnight stay. Outpatient services include care delivered in physician offices, which are today likely to be part of a group practice rather than a solo practice; in hospital-based facilities, usually as part of the hospital campus; and in non–hospital-based facilities, like community health centers, home care agencies, and outpatient surgery centers. Because of advances in medical technology and changes in reimbursement policies, many secondary and tertiary services are now provided in the outpatient setting. Examples include emergency and urgent

care, surgery, dialysis, chemotherapy, and rehabilitation services.

Important reimbursement changes affecting inpatient and outpatient care have accelerated the growth of outpatient care. The adoption of more restrictive reimbursement policies for inpatient care and a decrease in usage has created a "balloon effect," in which outpatient services have grown dramatically as inpatient services contract. Before the 1980s, insurance reimbursement was higher for inpatient, compared with outpatient, services. Whereas the Medicare PPS for inpatient acute care services that went into effect in the mid 1980s severely reduced payments to hospitals, no such limit was placed on payment for outpatient services. This was a powerful incentive for hospitals to expand their outpatient services, causing outpatient care to be an important source of profit for hospitals (Shi & Singh, 2004). Eventually, in 2000, Medicare responded to rapid outpatient growth by implementing some limits through the Medicare Outpatient PPS (OPPS) for hospital outpatient services and the Home Health Resources Groups (HHRGs) for home health care.

Primary care is one component of outpatient care and should be viewed as an approach to providing health care rather than as a set of specific services (Starfield, 1994). The IOM Committee on the Future of Primary Care defined primary care (Vanselow, Donaldson, & Yordy, 1995) as "The provision of integrated, accessible health care services by clinicians who are accountable for addressing a large majority of personal health care needs, developing a sustained partnership with patients, and practicing in the context of family and community." The IOM Committee also emphasized personal health promotion and disease prevention, and the definition recognized caring for the patient within the context of his community.

Primary care services are delivered in many types of outpatient settings by physicians, NPs, physician assistants, and certified nurse midwives. The demand for primary care is high. It is estimated that 75% to 85% of people require only primary care services in 1 year, whereas 10% to 12% need short-term secondary care services and 5% to 10% use tertiary services (Starfield, 1994). The financing for primary care varies according to the structural setting in which the care is delivered. Much of primary care for lower income citizens is provided in Community Health Centers, which are described in *Community Health Centers: A Successful Strategy for Improving Health Care Access* in Chapter 13.

## INNOVATIVE FINANCING AND IMPLICATIONS FOR NURSING

Nursing has a major role in creating cost-effective but viable options for patients who are in need, particularly the chronically ill and elderly who need care as well as cure. Consider the community nursing organizations that care for patients with HIV infection and chronic illness at home. Nursing organizations such as visiting nurse services are providing innovative solutions for patients who need care across a full continuum of services but with a reconsideration of patient needs and costs of care. Technology itself has been harnessed with the use of computers and "telehealth" services to reach patients at home without an actual home visit each time the patient needs a contact. Computerization supplements nursing care in a way that can actually increase the number of contacts that can be made with patients, thus increasing the chances that they will remain stable at home (Mahoney, 2000; Mahoney, Tennstedt, Friedman, & Heeren, 1999; Mahoney, Tarlow, & Sandaire, 1998). NPs and other advanced practice nurses are increasingly an important alternative for innovative care of chronically ill individuals. As the barriers to nursing practice are lifted, more opportunities will arise for these important providers.

## Key Points

- The financing of health in the United States is a complex system of public, private, and public-private funding that forces patients to be categorized into different systems of care.
- The projected large-scale retirement of the baby boomers in 2010 and growing prescription costs under the Medicare Prescription Drug Improvement and Modernization Act of 2003 will stress the system to the point that another crisis is inevitable.

- Nursing must participate in finding solutions to integrate services that enable all people to be eligible for care regardless of setting.

## *Web Resources*

**Centers for Medicare and Medicaid Services (CMS)**
*www.cms.hhs.gov*
**Institute of Medicine (IOM)**
*www.iom.edu*
**Kaiser Family Foundation (KFF)**
*www.kff.org*
**Levin, Irving, and Associates—The Senior Care Acquisition Report**
*www.levinassociates.com/pressroom/pressreleases/pr2005/pr503scar.htm*
**Social Security Administration**
*www.cms.hhs.gov*

## REFERENCES

Abood, S., & Keepnews, D. (2000). *Understanding payment for advanced practice nursing services. Vol. 1: Medicare reimbursement.* Washington, DC: American Nurses Publishing.

Alford, R. (1975). *Health care politics: Ideological and interest group barriers to reform.* Chicago: University of Chicago Press.

American Association of Health Plans. (2001). *Independent medical review of health plan coverage decisions: Empowering consumers with solutions.* Washington, DC: American Association of Health Plans.

Atherly, A. (2001). Supplemental insurance: Medicare's accidental stepchild. *Medical Care Research and Review, 58*(2), 131-161.

Baker, D., & Weisbrot, M. (1999). *Social Security: The phony crisis.* Chicago: University of Chicago Press.

Berk, M. L., & Monheit, A. C. (2001). The concentration of health care expenditures, revisited. *Health Affairs, 20*(2), 9-18.

Bodenheimer, T., & Grumbach, K. (2005). *Understanding health policy: A clinical approach* (4th ed.). New York: Lange Medical Books/McGraw Hill.

Brudney, K., & Dobkin, J. (1991). Resurgent tuberculosis in N.Y.C.: Human immunodeficiency virus, homelessness and the decline of tuberculosis control programs. *American Review of Respiratory Disease, 144*(4), 745-749.

Burman, L., Penner, R., Steuerle, G., Toder, E., Moon, M., et al. (1998). Policy challenges posed by the aging of America: A discussion briefing prepared for the Urban Institute Board of Trustees Meeting, May, 20, 1998. Washington, DC: Urban Institute Press.

Cassel, C. K., Besdine, R. W., & Siegel, L. C. (1999). Restructuring Medicare for the next century: What will beneficiaries really need? *Health Affairs, 18*(1), 118-131.

CIGNA. (2005). CIGNA Choice Fund: Glossary of terms. Retrieved October 30, 2005, from *www.cigna.com/health/ employer/medical/ccf/glossary.html#H.*

Cowan, C., Catlin, A., Smith, C., & Sensenig, A. (2004). National Health Expenditures, 2002. *Health Care Financing Review, 25*(4), 143-166.

Curtiss, F. R. (1989). Managed health care. *American Journal of Hospital Pharmacy, 46*, 742-763.

Davis, K., Anderson, G., Rowland, D., & Steinberg, E. (1990). *Health care cost containment.* Baltimore: Johns Hopkins University Press.

Department of Defense (DoD). (2001). TRICARE. Retrieved August 2, 2002, from *www.tricare.osd.mil.*

Dowd, B., Coulam, R., & Feldman, R. (2000). A tale of four cities: Medicare reform and competitive pricing. *Health Affairs, 19*(5), 9-29.

Etheredge, L. (1999). Three streams, one river: A coordinated approach to financing retirement. *Health Affairs, 18*(1), 80-91.

Etheredge, L. (2000). Medicare's governance and structure: A proposal. *Health Affairs, 19*(5), 60-71.

Feder, J., Komisar, H. L., & Niefeld, M. (2000). Long-term care in the United States: An overview. *Health Affairs, 19*(3), 40-56.

Federal Interagency Forum on Age-Related Statistics. (2000). *Older Americans 2000: Key indicators of well-being.* Hyattsville, MD: Federal Interagency Forum on Age-Related Statistics.

Freudenheim, M. (2001, May 25). Medical costs surge as hospitals force insurers to raise payments. *New York Times.* Retrieved June 4, 2001, from *www.nytimes.com.*

Fuchs, V. (1988). The "competition revolution" in health care. *Health Affairs, 7*(3), 5-24.

Gabel, J., Claxton, G., Gil, I., Pickreign, J., Whitmore, H., et al. (2005). Trends; Health benefits in 2005: Premium increases slow down, coverage continues to erode: The average yearly income of minimum wage Americans. *Health Affairs, 24*(6), 1273-1280.

Gibson, R. M., & Waldo, D. R. (1982). National health expenditures, 1981. *Health Care Financing Review, 4*(1), 1-35.

Gorin, S. (2000). A "society for all ages": Saving Social Security and Medicare. *Health & Social Work, 25*(1), 69-73.

Greenhouse, S., & Barbaro, M. (2005, October 26). Wal-Mart memo suggests ways to cut employee benefits costs. *New York Times,* C1.

Hall, M. A., & Havighurst, C. C. (2005). Reviving managed care with health savings accounts: HSAs with active benefit management by high-deductible plans could lessen patients' resistance to managed care. *Health Affairs, 24*(6), 1490-1500.

Harris, G. (2005, June 19). Gee, fixing welfare seemed like a snap. *New York Times,* 3.

Heffler, S., Levit, K., Smith, S., Smith, C., Cowan, C., et al. (2001). Health care spending growth up in 1999: Faster growth expected in the future. *Health Affairs, 20*(2), 193-203.

Heffler, S., Smith, S., Keehan, S., Clemens, M. K., Zezza, M., & Truffner, C. (2004). Health spending projections through 2013. *Health Affairs,* Web Exclusive. Retrieved October 24, 2005, from *http://content.healthaffairs.org/cgi/content/full/ hlthaff.w4.79v1/DC1.*

Herman, E. (1997). Downsizing government for principle and profit. *Dollars & Sense, 210,* 10-13.

Hoffman, M. A. (2002). Quality of health care improving. *Business Insurance, 36*(38), 1-2.

Hsiao, E., Braun, P., Dunn, D., & Becker, E. (1988). Results and policy implications of the resource-based relative value scale. *New England Journal of Medicine, 319,* 881-888.

Institute of Medicine (IOM). (1988). *The future of public health.* Washington, DC: National Academies Press.

Jonas, S., & Kovner, A. (2005). *Jonas and Kovner's Health care delivery in the United States* (7th ed.). New York: Springer.

Kaiser Family Foundation (KFF). (2001). Medicaid and managed care. Retrieved August 2, 2002 from *www.kff.org/medicaid/ 2102-budget_rep1.cfm.*

Kaiser Family Foundation (KFF). (2005a). Trend in personal health expenditures by source of payment, 1980-2003. Retrieved October 24, 2005, from *www.kff.org/insurance/ 7031/ti2004-1-9.cfm.*

Kaiser Family Foundation (KFF). (2005b). National health expenditures and their share of the gross domestic product: 1960-2003. Retrieved October 24, 2005, from *www.kff.org/ insurance/7031/ti2004-1-1.cfm.*

Kaiser Family Foundation (KFF). (2005c). Monthly worker contributions for single and family PPO and POS plans, 1988-2004. Retrieved October 24, 2005, from *www.kff.org/insurance/ 7148/sections/ehbs04-6-7.cfm.*

Kaiser Family Foundation (KFF). (2005d). Monthly worker contributions for single and family PPO and POS plans, 1988-2004. Retrieved October 24, 2005, from *www.kff.org/insurance/ 7148/sections/ehbs04-6-6.cfm.*

Kaiser Family Foundation (KFF). (2005e). Medicaid managed care enrollees as a percent of state Medicaid enrollees as of December 31, 2004. Retrieved February 10, 2006, from *http://statehealthfacts.org/cgi-bin/healthfacts.cgi?action= compare&category=Medicaid+%26+SCHIP&subcategory= Medicaid+Managed+Care&topic=MC+Enrollment+as+a+ %25+of+Medicaid+Enrollment&gsaview=1.*

Kaiser Family Foundation (KFF). (2005f). Medicare at a glance: Fact sheet. Retrieved April 16, 2005, from *www.kff.org/ medicare/1066-08.cfm.*

Kaiser Family Foundation (KFF). (2005g). Concentration of health spending among total U.S. families. Retrieved October 24, 2005, from *www.kff.org/insurance/7031/ti2004-1-11.cfm.*

Kaiser Family Foundation (KFF). (2005h). Medicaid enrollees and expenditures on benefits, by eligibility category, 2003. Retrieved March 27, 2005, from *www.kff.org/insurance/ 7031/print-sec1.cfm.*

Kaiser Family Foundation (KFF) & Health Research and Educational Trust (HRET). (2004). *Employer health benefits: 2004 summary of findings.* Retrieved June 16, 2005, from *www.kff.org/insurance/7148/index.cfm.*

Kendix, M., & Lubitz, J. D. (1999). The impact of medical savings accounts on Medicare program costs. *Inquiry, 36*(3), 280-290.

Kingdon, J. (1999). *America the unusual.* New York: Worth.

Kingson, E. R., & Schulz, J. H. (1997). *Social Security in the 21st century.* New York: Oxford University Press.

Kongstvedt, P. (2001). *The managed health care handbook* (4th ed.). Gaithersburg, MD: Aspen.

Levin, Irving, & Associates. (2005). *The senior care acquisition report* (10th ed.). Retrieved October 24, 2005, from *www.levinassociates.com/pressroom/pressreleases/pr2005/ pr503scar.htm.*

Levit, K., Smith, C., Cowan, C., Sensenig, A., Catlin, A., & the Health Care Accounts Team. (2004). Trends: Health spending rebound continues in 2002. *Health Affairs, 23*(1), 147-159.

Lubitz, J., Greenbery, L. G., Gorina, Y., Wartzman, L., & Gibson, D. (2001). Three decades of health care use by the elderly, 1965-1998. *Health Affairs, 20*(2), 19-32.

Lutz, S., & Gee, P. (1995). *The for-profit health care revolution: The growth of investor-owned health systems in America.* Chicago: Irwin Professional.

Mahoney, D. (2000). Developing technology applications for intervention research. *Computers in Nursing, 18*(6), 260-264.

Mahoney, D., Tarlow, B., & Sandaire, J. (1998). A computer-based program for Alzheimer's caregivers. *Computers in Nursing, 16*(4), 208-216.

Mahoney, D., Tennstedt, S., Friedman, R., & Heeren, T. (1999). An automated telephone system for monitoring the functional status of community-residing elders. *Gerontologist, 39*(2), 229-234.

Managed Care On-Line. (2001). Managed care national statistics. Retrieved August 2, 2002, from *www.healthplan.about.com/ industry/healthplan/GI/dynamic/offside.htm.*

McDonough, J. E. (1999). *Healthcare policy: The basics.* Boston, MA: Access Project. Retrieved August 1, 2005, from *www.accessproject.org.*

Meyers, H. (1970). The medical-industrial complex. *Fortune,* 90-91, 126.

National Center for Children in Poverty (NCCP). (2005). Temporary Assistance for Need Families (TANF) Cash Assistance. Retrieved October 30, 2005, from *www.nccp. org/policy_long_description_12.html.*

National Coalition on Health Care. (May 2000). Déjà vu all over again: The soaring cost of private health insurance and its impact on consumers and employers. Cited in H. A. Sultz, & K. M. Young. (2004). *Health Care USA: Understanding its organization and delivery.* Sudbury, MA: Jones and Bartlett.

Neuman, P., & Langwell, K. M. (1999). Medicare's choice explosion: Implications for beneficiaries. *Health Affairs, 18*(1), 150-160.

Nichols, L. M., & Reischauer, R. D. (2000). Who really wants price competition in Medicare managed care? *Health Affairs, 19*(5), 30-43.

Oberlander, J. (2000). Is premium support the right medicine for Medicare? A challenge to the emergent conventional wisdom. *Health Affairs, 19*(5), 84-99.

One thousand hospitals will be paid to reduce supply of doctors. (1997, August 25). *New York Times,* A16.

Pulcini, J. (1984). Perspectives on level of reimbursement for nursing services. *Nursing Economics, 2,* 118-123.

Relman, A. (1980). The new medical-industrial complex. *New England Journal of Medicine, 303,* 963-970.

Schulz, J. H. (2001). *The economics of aging* (7th ed.). Westport, CT: Auburn House.

Seidman, L. S. (2000). Prefunding Medicare without individual accounts. *Health Affairs, 19*(5), 72-83.

Shi, L., & Singh, D. A. (2004). *Delivering health care in America: A systems approach.* Sudbury, MA: Jones and Bartlett.

Smith, C., Cowan, C., Sensenig, A., Catlin, A., & the Health Accounts Team. (2005). Health spending growth slows in 2003. *Health Affairs, 24*(1), 185-194.

Social Security Administration. (2000a). *Annual statistical supplement to the Social Security Bulletin.* Washington, DC: Social Security Administration. Retrieved August 3, 2002, from at *www.ssa.gov/statistics/supplement/2000.*

Social Security Administration. (2000b). The future of Social Security. Publication No. 05-10055. Retrieved August 2, 2002, from *www.ssa.gov/pubs/10055.html.*

Social Security Administration. (2001a). How you earn credits. Publication No. 05-10072. Retrieved August 2, 2002, from *www.ssa.gov/pubs/ 10072.html.*

Social Security Administration. (2005a). Social Security announces 4.1% benefit increase for 2006 (press release). Retrieved on November 1, 2005, from *www.ssa.gov/pressoffice/ pr/2006cola-pr.htm.*

Social Security Administration. (2005b). A special lump sum death benefit. Retrieved October 30, 2005, from *www.ssa.gov/ survivorplan/ifyou7.htm.*

Social Security Administration. (2005c). 2005 Social Security changes. Retrieved October 30, 2005, from *www.ssa.gov/cola/ colafacts2005.htm.*

Starfield, B. (1994). Is primary care essential? *The Lancet, 344*(8930),1129-1133.

Starr, P. (1982). *The social transformation of American medicine.* New York: Basic Books.

Steinhauer, J. (2001, May 23). New York public hospital system faces $210 million deficit. *New York Times,* A25.

Steuerle, C. E., & Bakija, J. M. (2000). *Retooling Social Security for the 21st century.* Washington, DC: Urban Institute Press. Retrieved August 2, 2002, from *www.urban.org/pubs/retooling/ chapter2.html.*

Stevenson, R. W. (2001a, May 27). Congress passes tax cut, with rebates this summer. *New York Times,* A1.

Stevenson, R. W. (2001b, May 27). Still uncertain, budget surplus is gobbled up. *New York Times,* A1.

Sultz, H. A., & Young, K. M. (2004). *Health Care USA: Understanding its organization and delivery.* Sudbury, MA: Jones and Bartlett.

U.S. Census Bureau. (2005). Poverty statistics. Retrieved October 30, 2005, from *http://pubdb3.census.gov/macro/032005/pov/ new04_100_01.htm.*

U.S. Department of Health and Human Services (USDHHS), Centers for Medicare and Medicaid Services (CMS). (2005a). Medicare and you. Retrieved October 24, 2005, from *www.medicare.gov/publications/pubs/pdf/10050.pdf.*

U.S. Department of Health and Human Services (USDHHS), Centers for Medicare and Medicaid Services (CMS). (2005b). *Medicare information resource.* Washington, DC: USDHHS, CMS. Retrieved June 16, 2005, from *www.cms.hhs.gov/ medicare.*

U.S. Department of Health and Human Services (USDHHS), Centers for Medicare and Medicaid Services (CMS). (2005c). Medicare premiums and deductibles for 2006. Retrieved October 30, 2005, from *www.cms.hhs.gov/media/press/release. asp?Counter=1557.*

U.S. Department of Health and Human Services (USDHHS), Health Care Financing Administration (HCFA). (1998). *Your guide to Medicare medical savings accounts.* Publication No. HCFA-02137. Baltimore, MD: USDHHS.

U.S. Department of Health and Human Services (USDHHS), Health Care Financing Administration (HCFA). (2000). *Your Medicare benefits.* Publication No. HCFA-10116. Baltimore, MD: USDHHS.

U.S. Department of Health and Human Services (USDHHS), Health Care Financing Administration (HCFA). (2001a). Medicare basics: What is Medicare? Retrieved August 2, 2002, from *www.medicare.gov/basics/whatis.asp.*

U.S. Department of Health and Human Services (USDHHS), Health Care Financing Administration (HCFA), Office of the Actuary (OA). (2001). *HCFA data and statistics.* Hyattsville, MD: USDHHS, HCFA, OA. Retrieved August 6, 2002, from *www.hcfa.gov/stats/nhe.oact.*

U.S. Department of Labor. (2005). Health plans and benefits: ERISA. Retrieved October 24, 2005, from *www.dol.gov.*

Vanselow, N. A., Donaldson, D., & Yordy, K. (1995). From the Institute of Medicine (IOM). *Journal of the American Medical Association, 273*(3), 192.

# *Taking Action*    Mary Ann Hart

## Massachusetts' Strategy for Financing Health Care for the Uninsured

*"This has been a time of dramatic transformation, and you have risen to every new challenge."*

PRESIDENT BILL CLINTON

How does a public policy problem get on the agenda of lawmakers, advocates, and stake-holders such as doctors, nurses, hospitals, labor leaders, and the business community? How does significant public policy change happen? This section provides an account of "three waves" of heath care reform in Massachusetts over the last 20 years and my firsthand experience as a nurse in government and as an advocate, participating in those efforts.

As a nurse and the Director of the Office of Health Policy within the administration of Massachusetts Governor Michael Dukakis (who later unsuccessfully ran for president in 1988), I participated directly in Massachusetts' "first wave" of health care reform efforts in the mid 1980s. The centerpiece of that initiative was both reforming hospital rate regulation in Massachusetts and providing health insurance to the rising number of uninsured Massachusetts residents. During the "second wave" of reform in the mid 1990s, which expanded health insurance coverage for children, and during the current "third wave," which seeks to cover more of the uninsured, I have been a nurse-lobbyist. I have represented nonprofit provider, advocacy, and professional

groups, including two advanced practice nurse groups with a stake in the outcome of Massachusetts health reform efforts.

McDonough (2000) uses two useful models to analyze the emergence and recession of issues from the public policy agenda, and specifically the three waves of health reform efforts in Massachusetts. The first model—punctuated equilibrium—originally constructed by Kuhn and first applied to political change by Baumgartner and Jones, can be used to

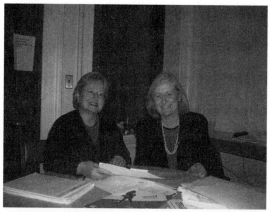

Rep. Kay Khan (D-MA), RN, MS (sixth term in Massachusetts House of Representatives) *(left)* and Mary Ann Hart, RN and lobbyist.

explain the process of revolutionary versus incremental change in political systems. According to the model, conflict and instability are the driving forces behind change and a way that new ideas are advanced to topple existing regulatory and institutional structures. The conflict arises through competing public policy ideas, and one set of ideas must be replaced by another. Some political and social scientists argue that slow incremental change dominates and is more successful in American politics, whereas others argue that destabilizing a previously stable situation is more effective. The second model, proposed by Kingdon (1995), says that change can happen only when three dynamic processes come together at around the same time to open up a "window of opportunity." The first stream is the *problem stream*, which occurs when those with the power to act believe that a genuine problem exists and needs to be addressed. The second is the *political stream*, which occurs when those with the power to act believe that the timing is right in relation to public sentiment and other public policy objectives. The third is the *policy stream*, which occurs when the existence of an implemental policy that fits the scope of the problem is understandable to those who need to understand it and can attain sufficient support.

## THE FIRST WAVE OF HEALTH CARE REFORM IN MASSACHUSETTS

During the first wave of health care reform, an important health care financing issue—how to control costs through regulating what Massachusetts hospitals were paid—gave rise to Governor's Dukakis' 1988 so-called "Universal Health Care" proposal. How did this major public policy issue, which became one of the public policy centerpieces of Dukakis' 1988 presidential campaign, spring from one state's attempt to change the way that hospitals got paid?

Conflict and instability—the first element of the punctuated equilibrium model—were evident through the widespread dissatisfaction in Massachusetts with the old fee-for-service model, which failed to hold down rising health care costs and no longer met the needs of the major stakeholders in health care—legislators, the governor, insurers, providers, labor, the business community, and consumers. Although there was agreement that the old model wasn't working and needed to be replaced by a new idea, there was initially no agreement on what would replace the old system. The second feature of the model—competition between policy ideas—occurred in a pitched battle between the major stakeholders in the early 1980s over how and how much hospitals should be paid. In 1982 a new all-payer regulatory system went into effect, designed to control the growth of all inpatient hospital spending, and Medicaid, Blue Cross, the commercial insurers, and even Medicare fell under the new regulatory scheme. Only health maintenance organizations (HMOs), then a small part of the insurance market, were left outside the new rules and were allowed to negotiate their own special payment rates with hospitals. The change to an all-payer system for inpatient costs was considered by some to be incremental change, and by others to be somewhat revolutionary in nature.

While the debate regarding how hospitals should be paid and how health care costs could be controlled raged, policymakers kept bumping up against the seemingly intractable problem of the ultimate cost the uninsured represented to the system both in poorer health outcomes and in uncompensated hospital costs. In 1982 a section of the new law addressed the financial responsibility of insurers in helping hospitals pay for "uncompensated care" through the creation of an uncompensated care pool (UCP). However, both Governor Dukakis and legislative leaders agreed that the creation of the UCP, which would pay only hospitals for the inpatient costs of the uninsured, did not go far enough.

From the beginning of this early health care reform debate, which initially focused on how to pay hospitals, the problem stream, as visualized through Kingdon's model, was escalating health care costs. Once the problem of rising hospital costs was addressed through agreement on an all-payer system, policymakers turned their attention to another part of the health care cost dilemma—the cost of the uninsured to the health care system.

Over a period of months the problem and political streams were moving forward as the governor and legislative leaders worked with the major stakeholders on a plan to provide health insurance to the uninsured. The third component of the Kingdon model that is necessary for change to occur—the policy stream—was in development. In 1987, Governor Dukakis announced a plan for "universal health care" in Massachusetts. The centerpiece of the Dukakis' plan was a mandate for employers with more than six employees to pay 80% of the cost of health insurance for their employees, or $1680 per worker, as a kind of annual tax to the state to purchase coverage. As a concession to small business, which opposed the proposal, the implementation of the employer mandate would not go into effect until January 1, 1992. The legislation, which also contained other important provisions such as a requirement that all college students have health insurance and extended health insurance coverage for the unemployed, was signed into law with much fanfare.

The Massachusetts plan took the national stage when Dukakis ran for and won the Democratic nomination for president. The issue also figured predominantly in the next presidential election, and when Bill Clinton took office in January 1993, the problem and political streams were moving with terrific force toward reforming the U.S. health care system. The window of opportunity for health care reform and major public policy change on the uninsured had opened both in Massachusetts and nationally.

Meanwhile, in Massachusetts, several critical events between 1988 and 1992 derailed the employer mandate—the most controversial provision of the Dukakis plan. First, Massachusetts plunged into an economic recession, and the concern about the financial burden of the employer mandate on struggling small business grew. Second, Michael Dukakis lost the 1988 presidential election and was replaced by William Weld, a Republican governor who opposed the employer mandate and who pledged to repeal it as quickly as possible. Third, the number of Republicans in the Massachusetts senate increased, enough to sustain a governor's veto with the support of some conservative Democrats. The problem and political streams had changed. The problem stream became less about the uninsured and more about the financial challenges a recession

posed for small business; those with the power to act increasingly felt that the employer mandate was a burden to small business and did not have the support of the general public. The political stream had also changed: The governor opposed the employer mandate; more Republicans had been elected to the state legislature, making it less likely the legislature could override the governor's vetoes; and legislators began to hear from small businesses in their districts that were opposed to the new law. To avert an outright repeal, House leaders passed a delay in implementation of the employer mandate to January 1995, in hopes that the governor would lose a bid for reelection and be replaced by a Democrat who supported the mandate.

On the national level, by 1994 Clinton's health care reform efforts had failed, derailed by opposing special interests, especially the small business community and the commercial health insurers. The Clinton administration had faltered in its development of the policy stream, moving too slowly to develop an understandable plan that would be acceptable in its scope with the public (McDonough, 2000). Nationally, the window of opportunity was also closing.

## THE SECOND WAVE OF HEALTH CARE REFORM IN MASSACHUSETTS

When Governor Weld was reelected in November 1994, a repeal of the Dukakis employer mandate seemed inevitable. However, legislative leaders and advocates supporting reform turned this threat of retrenchment to their advantage by tying the repeal of the mandate they supported to the adoption of another package of reforms being worked on by Weld administration officials, which needed the legislature's approval. To keep the mandate as leverage and buy more time, the legislature once again extended the date for implementation of the mandate to January 1996.

Some of the reforms being proposed by the Weld administration in the spring of 1994 were in response to the federal government's invitation to states to redesign their Medicaid programs to expand access through a federal Medicaid waiver. Expanding eligibility to all families below 133% of the poverty level ($20,000 for a family of four), instead of limiting eligibility to certain categories of people such as those in the Aid to Families with Dependent Children (AFDC) or Supplemental Security Income (SSI) programs, and providing tax credits to employers who provide their employees with health insurance and workers with subsidies to purchase insurance were two major components of the Massachusetts Medicaid waiver application. In addition, Weld administration officials also proposed diverting $200 million from the $315 million hospital UCP to their program to provide tax credits and employee subsidies; urged the legislature to reform non-group insurance for people who could not obtain group insurance through their employers; proposed allowing funds to be set aside in tax-deferred Medical Savings Accounts, a popular Republican proposal nationally; and finally, proposed repeal of the 1988 employer mandate. All these measures needed approval by the legislature.

When President Clinton's health care reform package was defeated and William Weld was reelected governor of Massachusetts, the push for reform in Massachusetts lost important momentum. Nationally the debate over reform began to center around curtailing the growth in Medicare expenditures and turning the Medicaid program into a block grant program administered by the states. How should advocates and legislative leaders refocus the problem on the uninsured and move forward again?

The executive and legislative branches had wildly differing estimates of the number of uninsured people in Massachusetts. Numbers can be both tools and weapons in politics, and they should be used in a specific context with a political purpose in mind. Legislative leaders found funding for the Weld administration to contract with an independent, respected researcher to document the number of uninsured in Massachusetts. Results of that research showed that the uninsured had risen from 455,000 in 1989 to 683,000 in 1995 and the number of uninsured children had risen from 90,000 to 160,000 in that same period.

While the Weld administration sought to downplay the new numbers, legislative leaders and advocates spoke eloquently at every meeting and forum across the state about the most recent data—the uninsured were growing in number in Massachusetts.

Once again the problem and policy streams began to build momentum for tackling the problem of the uninsured. Legislative leaders cobbled together a complex legislative package with many provisions that included a 25-cent increase in the cigarette tax to expand health insurance coverage for uninsured children through the Children's Medical Security Plan and for medications for senior citizens through the Senior Pharmacy Program, as well as the governor' proposal to restructure Medicaid through the Medicaid waiver to open eligibility to all families with incomes below 133% of the poverty level. The legislation also repealed the employer mandate, which had become so despised by small business.

Many lawmakers were wary of raising taxes—even taxes on cigarettes. Governor Weld had also taken a "no new taxes" pledge, and he opposed the new cigarette tax proposal. To attempt to address concerns about a new tax, legislative leaders commissioned a poll that asked the public their opinion. A whopping 77% of respondents agreed with raising the cigarette tax by 25 cents to fund health insurance for children, and only 19% were opposed. Even 73% of Republicans agreed with raising the cigarette tax to expand health insurance.

This second wave of health care reform was dubbed the "Campaign for Children" because its focus was expanding insurance coverage for children and poor families. The consumer advocacy group, Health Care for All, led the effort with legislative leaders to win the support of key players—the Massachusetts Medical Society, Harvard Pilgrim Health Care, the Massachusetts' Teachers Association, Blue Cross, the American Cancer Society, and Children's Hospital Boston. After a considerable effort by legislative leaders to woo the business community with a promise to repeal the employer mandate, the major players in the business community got on board. In spite of a well-funded effort to kill the proposal by the tobacco industry, the legislature approved the health care reform package by a wide margin and was able to comfortably override Governor Weld's veto by the required two-thirds vote.

Although the employer mandate enacted during the Dukakis administration was repealed, it had given birth to a new effort. Advocates pushed open the window of opportunity that was closing and achieved important incremental but significant change—providing health care coverage to more of the Commonwealth's uninsured children and families. As a result, the numbers of uninsured dropped from 680,000 to 365,000 and enrollment in Medicaid increased from 670,000 to nearly one million. This successful effort to expand health insurance coverage was also to have larger ramifications. At the end of 1996, health care advocates and key legislative leaders from Massachusetts met with U.S. Senator Edward M. Kennedy (D-MA) to share their experience raising the cigarette tax in Massachusetts to expand health insurance coverage for children. In early 1997, Senator Kennedy and Republican Senator Orin Hatch (R-UT) announced their own federal legislation to raise the cigarette tax by 43 cents and dedicate most of that revenue to expanding health insurance coverage for children. In July 1997 that bill was signed into law as the State Children's Health Insurance Program (SCHIP), which provides $24 billion to states to provide health insurance to children.

## THE THIRD WAVE OF HEALTH CARE REFORM IN MASSACHUSETTS

In spite of important gains during the "second wave" in providing coverage to the uninsured, the numbers of people without health insurance in Massachusetts began to swell once again. In November 2004, the Blue Cross Blue Shield of Massachusetts (BC/BS) Foundation released a report that said that there were 450,000 to 650,000 uninsured people in Massachusetts (Holahan, Bovbjerg, & Hadley, 2004). The study found that employers were providing less coverage or dropping coverage as health care cost continued to rise, higher insurance premiums were putting health care out of reach for many people who were not covered through an employer, and Medicaid state budget cuts in the middle of a severe recession had resulted in thousands of low-income people losing their health insurance coverage. The BC/BS Foundation released the study to the media and public at a conference that featured the president of the Massachusetts Senate, Robert Travaglini, as a keynote speaker.

In his remarks, President Travaglini committed to reduce the number of uninsured by half in 2 years—from 460,000 to 230,000. Not to be upstaged, the next day Governor Mitt Romney promised to soon release the details of his own plan for health care reform. The Speaker of the Massachusetts House, joining in, said that health care reform and covering the uninsured would be a top legislative priority for the 2005-2006 legislative session. Health Care for All, the consumer advocacy group that led the Campaign for Children in the mid 1990s, announced the details of its own bill, launching an initiative called the "Affordable Care Today! Campaign" (see the Web Resources). The BC/BS Foundation study had ignited the problem, and political streams and the window of opportunity for health care reform began to open once again for the state of Massachusetts.

The policy stream, which according to the Kingdon model is the final critical component needed to keep the window of opportunity open until success is achieved, is in its development stage. Policymakers and advocates used the BC/BS Foundation study to launch four major health reform bills, sponsored by Governor Romney, the Massachusetts State Senate, the Massachusetts House of Representatives, and Health Care for All. All sought to provide health insurance for the uninsured, but they had significantly differing proposals for how to structure and pay for that coverage. Governor Romney proposes to offer a scaled-down health plan, called "Commonwealth Care," with lower monthly premiums. The Senate's bill proposed to make health insurance more accessible for individuals and the small business market through certain insurance market reforms and to charge larger companies a fee for their uninsured employees who use the hospital UCP. Both the House legislation and the legislation proposed by Health Care for All expand Medicaid coverage significantly and contain provisions that require employers to provide insurance for their employees ("employer mandate"). In addition, the House bill contained an "individual mandate," a requirement that all state residents have health insurance. In November of 2005, a conference committee was appointed to hammer out the differences between the House and

Senate bills and propose a final piece of health care reform legislation.

Advocates used another strategy to reform the health care system in Massachusetts by threatening to go to the voters directly through the initiative petition process. The ballot, sponsored by the Health Care for Massachusetts Campaign, proposed an amendment to the Massachusetts Constitution that would ensure that every Massachusetts resident has access to affordable, comprehensive, and equitably financed coverage for medically necessary health and mental health care services.

On April 4, 2006, the Massachusetts legislature, overwhelmingly approved the Health Care Access and Affordability Act, legislation that reformed the Massachusetts health care system and will insure 90% to 95% of the state's uninsured in 3 years (515,000 people by 2009). The key elements of the plan include:

- **Establishing employer and individual responsibility:** Employers with 11 or more employees must contribute to insurance coverage for their employees and all residents must carry health insurance.
- **Establishing the Commonwealth Care Health Insurance Program:** Low-income people can purchase insurance on a sliding fee scale basis or obtain it at no cost.
- **Expanding Medical eligibility and outreach:** An additional 92,500 children and adults are covered.
- **Establishing market-based reforms:** Insurers have incentives to offer affordable health insurance benefits to small businesses.

The sweeping Massachusetts plan will undoubtedly reignite the sagging health care reform debate nationally and serve as a model for other states seeking to improve access to care for their citizens though the expansion of health insurance. (For continued updates, see *www.hcfama.org*.)

## HEALTH CARE REFORM AND NURSING

What was the role of nursing in Massachusetts during these efforts at health care reform? Individual nurses were actively involved in advocacy efforts through the various groups pressing for change, such as Health Care for All, and nursing organizations for

the first and second waves of health reform played a supporting role. For this reason organized nursing was never considered a major stakeholder in the debate, and it had little impact on the political process or in the final policy package that was approved. In contrast, the Massachusetts Medical Society was one of the most powerful advocates in the push to provide health insurance for children in the mid 1990s.

In the third wave of health reform, the Massachusetts Nurses Association (MNA) has taken a strong position in favor of legislation for a single-payer health care system and has been critical of the current effort to expand health insurance coverage to the uninsured, arguing that the incremental approach of current efforts are insufficient. Although many individuals and organizations working on health reform support the idea of a Canadian-like single-payer system, it is not being considered seriously in Massachusetts, nor is it likely to be in the near future. MNA, although supporting the single-payer approach, is focusing its advocacy on passing its "safe staffing" legislation. Organized nursing is once again a marginal player in the current debate on health care reform in Massachusetts. Strong political leadership in nursing is needed to ensure that nursing is not only part of the most important public policy debates, but that nursing has a key role in the development of public policy around health care reform in the future.

## *Web Resources*

Groups that are advocating for health care reform through proposed health care legislation, the Massachusetts Quality Affordable Health Care Act are:

**Health Care for All**—the advocacy group that filed legislation, called the Massachusetts Quality Affordable Health Care Act, which expands Medicaid coverage to many uninsured and requires employers to insure their employees.

*www.hcfama.org*

*Continued*

## *Web Resources — cont'd*

**Health Care for Massachusetts Campaign**—a campaign pushing for a November 2006 ballot initiative for a Health Care Constitutional Amendment ensuring that every Massachusetts resident has access to affordable, comprehensive, and equitably financed coverage for medically necessary health and mental health care services.
*www.healthcareformass.org/about/fact-sheet.shtml*

**Massachusetts Nurses Association (MNA)**—the MNA is supporting single-payer health care in Massachusetts and the Health Care for Massachusetts Campaign.
*www.massnurses.org*

**MassAct Campaign**—this is a coalition of groups including Health Care for All that is working to ensure that legislation is implemented fairly and is fully funded.
*http://massact.org/index.asp*

Other groups that are advocating for health care reform:

**MassCare**—a group pushing for legislation, An Act to Establish a Massachusetts Health Care Trust, that would establish single-payer health care in Massachusetts.
*www.masscare.org*
**MNA Single-Payer Health Care Campaign**
*www.massnurses.org/single_payer/index.htm*
**MNA Health Care for Massachusetts Campaign**
*www.massnurses.org/News/2004/02/univhealth.htm*

### REFERENCES

Holahan, J., Bovbjerg, R., & Hadley, J. (2004) Caring for the uninsured in Massachusetts: What does it cost, who pays, and what would full coverage add to medical spending? The Urban Institute for the Blue Cross Blue Shield of Massachusetts Foundation. Retrieved September 26, 2005, from *www.bcbsmafoundation.org/foundationroot/en_US/documents/roadmapReport.pdf.*

Kingdon, J. (1995). *Agendas, alternatives and public policies.* New York: HarperCollins College.

McDonough, J. E. (2000). *Experiencing politics: A legislator's stories of government and health care.* Berkeley: University of California Press.

# **POLICY**SPOTLIGHT

## REFORMING MEDICARE

Susan C. Reinhard

*"Medicare costs are taking up an increasing portion of the overall federal budget, and the program could become part of the growing problem of funding the U.S. health care system. ...If there's one thing that could bankrupt the country, it's health care. It's out of control."*

U.S. COMPTROLLER GENERAL DAVID WALKER, MAY, 2005

### THE ISSUE

Forty years ago, President Lyndon Johnson proclaimed that one of our most important social mandates was to protect the elderly from the financial hardships associated with illness. Medicare was the solution. Today, some economists and policymakers say Medicare is the problem, causing financial hardships for the nonelderly. The sociopolitical-economic context has changed the debate about how we will manage the demands for financing health care for older adults and certain people with disabilities. As a major provider of health care for people on Medicare, the nursing profession should be a substantive part of this debate.

## INITIAL INTENT AND EVOLUTION OF THE MEDICARE PROGRAM

Before 1965, over half of the U.S. population age 65 years and older had inadequate or no health insurance coverage. After years of debate, modification, and compromise, Medicare was established with the signing of HR 6675, the Social Security Amendments of 1965, by President Lyndon Johnson. As a core element of the Johnson administration's "Great Society Initiative," the initial intent of the Medicare program was to improve the availability of health care for the elderly and disabled (Gluck & Sorian, 2004). The program became operational in 1966, providing millions of seniors with access to health care services.

Since its inception this complex social program has gone through periodic reform. Currently the program is embarking on one of the most radical changes since its inception, the addition of a prescription drug benefit. Addition of the outpatient drug benefit comes at a time when many are questioning the financial vitality of the Medicare program. The eligible population is increasing, and the costs to provide services under the program as currently structured are growing at a rate faster than the payroll taxes that are funding the program. Many argue that the program structure is flawed and unsound. Some contend that the program offers too few services. Others assert that the program is too generous. A brief look at the program's evolution may shed some light on this ongoing dialogue and the policy options that nurses should consider.

In its initial form in the 1960s, Medicare offered compulsory hospital insurance (Part A) for persons over the age of 65 and an optional program of government assistance in covering doctors' fees (Part B). Under Part B, participants could opt not to participate in the government-assisted insurance program. These provisions established a substantive role for the private sector, because participants would purchase health care services in the open fee-for-service market and the federal government would pay the bills.

President Nixon signed amendments to Medicare in 1972, extending benefits to certain individuals under the age of 65 with disabilities. These amendments also included provisions to review the quality of patient care and encourage the use of health maintenance organizations (HMOs) (Kaiser Family Foundation [KFF], 2005a).

In 1980, Congress expanded coverage of home health services and established major hospital reimbursement reform. The prospective payment system (PPS) and diagnostic-related groups (DRG) methodology for hospital payment radically altered the hospital industry by replacing the cost-based ("open checkbook") payment method and financially discouraging long hospital stays. In the later half of the 1980s the Medicare Catastrophic Coverage Act added a drug benefit to Medicare. It was repealed almost immediately in 1989 when older adults complained that their personal contribution to this program was too high (KFF, 2005a).

The Balanced Budget Act (BBA) of 1997 again reformed Medicare payment policies by adding a PPS for five services: home health services; skilled nursing facilities (nursing homes); hospital outpatient services; outpatient rehabilitation services; and inpatient rehabilitation hospitals. It also created the Medicare + Choice program, which promised to increase Medicare enrollment in managed care by offering beneficiaries more private sector, managed care choices.

The Medicare + Choice program did increase enrollment in private managed care plans for a brief period, reaching a maximum enrollment of 6.3 million in 2000 (Gold, Achman, Mittler, & Stevens, 2004). As Medicare entered the new millennium, however, the number of plans participating in Medicare + Choice began dropping significantly, from 309 in 1999 to 151 in 2000 (Gold et al., 2004). As plans dropped out, more than 2 million beneficiaries were left to find other options. Beneficiaries and providers became upset and confused, and their confidence in the managed care alternative eroded.

Disappointed by the failure of Medicare + Choice to dramatically alter Medicare, President George W. Bush advocated more changes to the Medicare program. Many other advocates and policymakers were also pushing for an expansion of benefits and various Medicare reforms. After years of debate, on December 8, 2003 the Medicare Prescription Drug Improvement and Modernization Act (PL 108-173) established the Medicare Advantage program (previously called Medicare + Choice) and a voluntary prescription drug benefit. Known by its shorter name, the Medicare Modernization Act (MMA), this legislation represents the most profound change that has been made to the Medicare program since its inception nearly four decades ago. Although it will take many years for the full impact of all of the provisions of this historic legislation to be realized, its most significant component took effect in January of 2006 when the Medicare "Part D" Prescription Drug Benefit program unfolded. About 29 million Medicare beneficiaries are expected to enroll in Medicare Part D in 2006.

The MMA offers a Medicare Part D program that combines two policy goals. First, it offers voluntary coverage for outpatient pharmacy benefits with "extra help" (a subsidy) for low-income Medicare beneficiaries. Second, it relies on the use of market forces to provide this complicated governmental benefit. Within the structure of a government contract overseen by the Centers for Medicare & Medicaid Services (CMS), and governed by numerous regulations, private companies will develop their products, assume financial risk, and compete for market share (Golub, 2005).

## THE MEDICARE PROGRAM TODAY

Medicare is a popular and trusted national social program. Fundamentally, Medicare is a government-run health insurance program for America's older adults and certain people with disabilities. The original policy intent was to ensure that all older adults have access to medically necessary acute care services (Part A), regardless of where they live, their health status, or their income. Current Medicare policy continues this entitlement status for older adults (KFF, 2005b). Coverage starts the first day of the month an individual turns 65. People with

end-stage renal disease are also entitled to Medicare Part A, regardless of their age. Individuals who are under the age of 65 and become disabled receive Medicare benefits after having received Social Security benefits for 2 years. The number of Medicare beneficiaries has more than doubled since 1970. Currently there are over 35 million seniors in the program and 6 million younger persons with disabilities.

Contrary to popular belief, Medicare does not cover all of beneficiaries' health care costs; it covers about half of their total health care expenses (Scala-Foley, Caruso, Ramos, & Reinhard, 2004). That's because Medicare does not cover all health care services and because it is not a free program. Medicare is covering more prevention services, such as immunizations, mammograms, pelvic examinations, bone mass measurement, colorectal and prostate cancer screenings, glaucoma screenings, and nutrition therapy for people with diabetes (Scala-Foley, Caruso, Archer, & Reinhard, 2004). But it does not cover routine vision and hearing care, dental care, or long-term care. Medicare beneficiaries pay 25% of the cost of the Medicare program through premiums and copayments; taxpayers pay the other 75%. Over the past 40 years the cost to Medicare beneficiaries has risen, with double-digit premium hikes in the last several years. In 1965 the Medicare Part A deductible was $40 annually; it was $912 per year in 2005. The Part B premium grew from $3 per month in 1965 to $78.20 per month in 2005 and $87.70 a month in 2006 (Boards of Trustees, 2005). These higher premiums reflect the rising costs of health care provided to beneficiaries and new preventive benefits.

Low-income Medicare beneficiaries can get help paying these costs through the Medicare Savings programs, which are administered by the states through Medicaid funding (Reinhard, Scala-Foley, Caruso, & Archer, 2004). Unfortunately, only about half of those who are entitled to receive this help actually apply for it.

## MEDICARE A, B, C, Ds

Medicare pays for health care for the elderly and some people with disabilities, although it does not pay for all acute and long-term care. As the program has evolved, it has become more complex. Currently, Medicare has four "parts" and is administered by the CMS (CMS, 2005a; KFF, 2005b).

## Part A (the Hospital Insurance Program)

Part A helps to cover medically necessary costs for hospital stays, skilled nursing facility care, home health care, and hospice care. It accounts for 45% of Medicare spending.

## Part B (Supplemental Medical Insurance)

Part B assists in the coverage of outpatient care and services from physicians and advanced practice nurses. It also covers some services not included in Part A, such as physical and occupational therapists and home health care when medically necessary. Part B also covers some clinical laboratory services and preventive services, such as cardiovascular screening and blood tests. It accounts for 35% of Medicare spending. Participation is voluntary (95% of those enrolled in Part A also enroll in Part B), and the program has deductibles and premiums.

## Part C (Formerly Medicare + Choice)

This part of Medicare offers choices for a variety of managed care plans to provide Part A and B benefits. Part C was originally called "Medicare + Choice." It has been renamed "Medicare Advantage." Under Part C plans, beneficiaries may have lower copayments and get added benefits. In 2005, about 5 million Medicare beneficiaries were enrolled in these plans, which account for 15% of Medicare spending. By 2013, enrollment is expected to double, a midrange estimate between those provided by the Congressional Budget Office (CBO) and the U.S. Department of Health and Human Services (USDHHS) (KFF, 2005b).

## Part D (Prescription Drug Benefit Program)

Part D refers to the voluntary coverage of outpatient prescription drugs that began in January 2006. The government-sponsored drug benefit programs are offered by private companies and require payment of a premium, copayments, and deductibles. Plans can establish their own premiums, subject to CMS approval; therefore the cost of premiums varies from plan to plan. In addition to covering monthly premiums of about $37 in 2006, beneficiaries who choose to enroll in Part D must pay the following (KFF, 2005d):

- The first $250 in drug expenses (the deductible)
- 25% of total medication costs between $250 and $2250
- 100% of drug expenses between $2250 and $5100 (the so-called "doughnut hole" amounts to $2850 in 2006)
- The greater of $2 for generic drugs, $5 for brand drugs, or 5% coinsurance after the $3600 out-of-pocket limit is reached ($5100 catastrophic threshold)

Medicare beneficiaries with low incomes and limited assets can get "extra help" with their Part D drug benefit (CMS, 2005b). In a major departure from traditional Medicare policy, the MMA imposes asset and income tests on people seeking a low-income subsidy to receive federal assistance with their Medicare Part D coverage. One in three Medicare beneficiaries is eligible for this extra help. An estimated 14.4 million people who are eligible for both Medicare and Medicaid (dual eligibles) and beneficiaries living below 150% of the poverty level need additional assistance to cover their prescription drug needs. About half of those who are eligible for this extra help (about 7 million people) are "deemed eligibles" who do not have to apply; the remaining 7 million have to apply for the extra help.

Many advocates are concerned about how well Medicare beneficiaries understand their options and enroll. Low enrollments in the Medicare Savings programs and Medicare Advantage plans are evidence that age and various disabilities often make it difficult for some people to act on complex Medicare choices (Biles, Dallek, & Nicholas, 2004). Beneficiaries often need individual counseling to guide them through the intricacies of Medicare coverage.

## PROGRAM STRENGTHS AND WEAKNESSES

Medicare is part of America's social fabric. It has succeeded in its initial promise of lifting the elderly out of the ranks of the uninsured. It has changed over the last 40 years, and it is likely to change in the decades ahead. Various stakeholders push for change based on their differing perspectives.

- Most older adults have a favorable view of Medicare, think it is well run, and prefer reforms that build on the existing Medicare program rather than those that favor privatization and competition (KFF & Harvard School of Public Health, 2003). Many are disappointed that Medicare does not cover long-term care and are concerned about their ability to pay for it. They also worry about their ability to pay their increasing copayments for care, and they remain skeptical about managed care plans and the new pharmacy benefit.

- Younger Americans differ in significant ways from older adults about their views on Medicare. They are less likely to think Medicare is a well-run program and have a more favorable attitude about private plans (KFF & Harvard School of Public Health, 2003).

- The business community claims the rising health care costs of covering retirees lead to higher prices for their products, which reduces their competitive edge in a global marketplace. They want Medicare to pay for better coverage so they can drop their retiree coverage. The share of retiree coverage is dropping fast, from 66% in 1998 to 38% in 2003 (KFF & Health Research and Educational Trust [HRET], 2003) and is likely to drop further now that Medicare is covering prescription drugs (Wellner, 2005).

- Members of the health care industry, including hospitals, nursing homes, and the pharmaceutical industry, among others, advocate for or against Medicare policy changes that affect their specific interests.

- Health care professionals (including nurses) want better access for the people they serve and policies that promote high-quality care that is based on research evidence, such as adequate staffing in hospitals and more efficient care of persons with multiple chronic illnesses.

- Federal policymakers, particularly those who must run for office, may see the need for far-reaching Medicare reform but view it as a "third rail"—touching it is potentially fatal for an elected official's career.

## FORCES FOR CHANGE IN MEDICARE

Stakeholders' varying perspectives shape the debate for changes to Medicare and there may be generation differences in preferred policy approaches. But the greatest driving force for change in Medicare is the growing cost of funding it. More than half of those surveyed in 2003 agree that Medicare has major financial problems (KFF & Harvard School of Public Health, 2003). Total Medicare spending exceeded $300 billion in 2004 and will grow significantly in the coming years, to $444 billion in 2010 (CBO, 2005). Medicare now accounts for 2.6% of the gross domestic product (GDP). Currently medical costs are growing at a rate faster than the economy. Medicare started paying out more in benefits than it receives in taxes in 2004, a situation that is called a "structural deficit" because the current design (structure) of the program is resulting in spending that is not supported by its financial base. Medicare's trustees have indicated that the program could grow to 13.6% of GDP by 2079 (Boards of Trustees, 2005).

These escalating costs and demands for an increasing share of the nation's budgetary resources as America ages are stimulating debate over the future solvency of Medicare. The number of Medicare beneficiaries is increasing, with an accelerated pace starting in 2011 when the country's "baby boomers" will reach retirement age. Between 2010 and 2030, the number of older adults will double, reaching 71.5 million (USDHHS, 2004). The number of elderly and disabled Medicare beneficiaries is projected to rise from 40 million in 2000 to 78 million in 2030. During the same period the ratio of younger workers per Medicare beneficiary will decline from 4.0 to 2.4 workers per beneficiary (KFF, 2005c).

In addition to these demographic and cost pressures for change, many health care professionals and policymakers seek Medicare reforms to introduce more innovations and promote quality. For example, the Medicare Payment Advisory Commission (MedPAC), which was created as an independent federal body to advise Congress, is advocating the diffusion of health care information technology to promote improvements in care coordination and quality (MedPAC, 2004). The MMA includes provisions for several pilots that may lead to Medicare reforms. The Voluntary Chronic Care Improvement program seeks to improve self-care among beneficiaries with diabetes, congestive heart failure, and chronic obstructive pulmonary disease. This program will test different models of care coordination across health care settings and service providers to see if better management of patient information can reduce program costs and improve quality of care. The Care Management Performance pilot encourages the use of health information technology among physicians as a way of reducing the hospitalization of chronically ill patients (MedPAC, 2004; Super, 2004).

## OPTIONS FOR CHANGES IN THE MEDICARE PROGRAM

Over the years, policymakers have considered several options for slowing the growth of Medicare spending, including enhancing provider competition in delivering services and increasing the share of spending paid by beneficiaries (CBO, 2005). Other options that have been offered include:

- Raising the age of eligibility for Medicare to 67, which will become the age of entitlement for Social Security
- Reduction in payments to providers
- Reducing coverage
- Targeting changes in the care of high-cost Medicare beneficiaries
- Improving efficiency

### More Managed Care?

The current emphasis on promoting the Medicare Advantage managed care plans is a preferred policy option for market-oriented policymakers. This has been a controversial policy direction with mixed public support. According to a 2003 national public opinion survey by the KFF and Harvard School of Public Health, the public does support policy changes that provide more choices in Medicare (KFF & Harvard School of Public Health, 2003). However, there is a significant difference in opinions based on age. Older adults want more choices among health care professionals and hospitals than among managed care plans. Younger adults are more favorably inclined toward private plans.

### Change Entitlement?

Regardless of their age, a majority of those surveyed by the KFF and Harvard School of Public Health support having higher-income seniors pay higher Medicare premiums, but two thirds oppose raising the Medicare entitlement age to 67 (KFF & Harvard School of Public Health, 2003). Indeed, the political pressure is to make Medicare available sooner to those who retire before the age of 65.

### Reduce Provider Payments?

Policy options to constrain Medicare's costs without reducing quality or access to care are limited. Over the last two decades, Congress has reduced payments to providers, but it has also increased provider payments, most recently to managed care organizations. Imposing significant cost-savings limits on health care for older adults would result in a political backlash. Medicare now covers all "reasonable and necessary" medical treatments, regardless of costs. In fact, Congress has been more likely to increase coverage than to reduce it. The addition of a pharmacy benefit will add $700 million over 10 years to the cost of Medicare.

### Spending Based on Research Evidence?

Despite the "third rail" concern of examining the basic structure of Medicare, there may be strong evidence to closely examine the underlying Medicare policy of paying for all treatments regardless of cost. Research findings indicate that Medicare spending does not necessarily translate into better care or improved health (Fisher et al., 2003a; Fisher et al., 2003b). There are dramatic regional differences in Medicare spending. People on Medicare who live in higher spending regions of the country receive 60% more care than those who live in lower spending regions. But that spending difference does not lead to better health outcomes. It might be possible to reduce Medicare spending by 30% without negatively affecting the health of Medicare beneficiaries, but more research is needed to determine how to do that safely.

This kind of research might lead to evidence-based policymaking that nurses and other health care professionals could support with more enthusiasm than ideologic battles between policymakers who purport that market-based competition is the answer and those who claim that a stronger government role is the better solution. One intriguing area for exploring this kind of evidence-based approach is to target high-cost Medicare beneficiaries and work on ways to improve the efficiency and cost-effectiveness of care in a more strategic way than has been accomplished in the past. A small fraction of Medicare beneficiaries account for a large share of the program's spending in any given year, suggesting the possibility of targeting this group of potentially high-cost beneficiaries and finding effective interventions to reduce their spending. If successful, even a small percentage reduction in the spending of this group could lead to substantial Medicare savings. Ultimately the extent to which these beneficiaries reduced their spending would rest on the ability to devise and implement effective clinical and administrative intervention strategies to change the use of services (CBO, 2005).

The focus on discovery of the most efficient and effective treatment methodologies, and elimination of those that do not meet these standards, could improve the quality of care and financial status of the nation's entire health care system. We also need to weigh Americans' thirst for unlimited care with societal needs for equitable care. These are not easy discussions at a family dinner table. They are even more difficult in the halls of Congress in the transparent, political contexts in which our society operates. Nurses need to be part of this complex, critical discussion. The health of the people that nurses serve depends on it.

## Key Points

- The eligible Medicare population is increasing, and the costs to provide services as the program is currently structured are growing at a rate faster than the payroll taxes that fund the program.
- Stakeholders' varying perspectives shape the debate for changes to Medicare and preferred policy approaches.
- The current emphasis on promoting the Medicare Advantage managed care plans is a controversial policy direction with mixed public support.
- There is little public support for raising the Medicare entitlement age to 67, but there is interest in having higher-income seniors pay higher Medicare premiums.
- One promising area for Medicare reform comes from research that finds dramatic differences in

Medicare spending do not necessarily translate into dramatic differences in health outcomes; aligning spending with evidence-based practice holds some promise for more efficient, high-quality care, particularly for those with multiple chronic illnesses.

## Web Resources

**Henry J. Kaiser Family Foundation**—funds nonpartisan research on Medicare policy and broadly disseminates findings to policymakers, researchers, professionals, and the public
*www.kff.org*

**Medicare Payment Advisory Commission (MedPAC)**—established in 1997 by federal law to act as an independent body in advising Congress on issues related to the Medicare program
*www.medpac.gov*

**Official Government Website on Medicare**—administered by the U.S. Department of Health and Human Services (USDHHS), it includes information from the Centers for Medicare & Medicaid Services (CMS), the USDHHS agency responsible for Medicare and Medicaid
*www.Medicare.gov*

**The Commonwealth Fund**—a philanthropic organization that supports research on Medicare and other health-related topics
*www.cmwf.org*

## REFERENCES

Biles, B., Dallek, G., & Nicholas, L. H. (2004). Medicare Advantage: déjà vu all over again? *Health Affairs 23*(Suppl 2), W4-586-597.

Boards of Trustees of the Federal Hospital Insurance and Federal Supplementary Insurance Trust Funds. (2005). *2005 annual report*. Washington, DC: Boards of Trustees. Retrieved July 15, 2005, from *http://cms.hhs.gov/publications/trusteesreport/tr2005.pdf*.

Centers for Medicare & Medicaid Services (CMS). (2005a). *Medicare and you: 2005 national Medicare handbook*. Baltimore, MD: CMS. Retrieved July 15, 2005, from *www.medicare.gov*.

Centers for Medicare & Medicaid Services (CMS). (2005b). Guidance to states on the low-income subsidy. Retrieved June 15, 2005, from *www.cms.hhs.gov.*

Congressional Budget Office (CBO). (2005). *High cost Medicare beneficiaries.* Washington, DC: CBO.

Fisher, E. S., Wennberg, D. E., Stukel, T. A., Gottlieb, D. J., Lucas, F. L., & Pinder, E. L. (2003a). The implications of regional variations in Medicare spending: Part 1: The content, quality, and accessibility of care. *Annals of Internal Medicine, 138*(4), 273-287.

Fisher, E. S., Wennberg, D. E., Stukel, T. A., Gottlieb, D. J., Lucas, F. L., & Pinder, E. L. (2003b). The implications of regional variations in Medicare spending: Part 2: Health outcomes and satisfaction with care. *Annals of Internal Medicine, 138*(4), 288-299.

Gluck, M. E., & Sorian, R. (2004). *Administrative challenges in managing the Medicare program.* Washington, DC: American Association of Retired Persons (AARP) Public Policy Institute.

Gold, M., Achman, L., Mittler, J., & Stevens, B. (2004). *Monitoring Medicare + Choice: What have we learned?* Washington, DC: Mathematica Policy Research.

Golub, B. B. (2005). *A Guide to the Medicare drug benefit.* Washington, DC: Atlantic Information Services. Retrieved July 15, 2005, from *www.aishealth.com/Products/dben.html.*

Kaiser Family Foundation (KFF). (2005a). Medicare: A timeline of key developments. Retrieved July 15, 2005, from *www.kff.org.*

Kaiser Family Foundation (KFF). (2005b). Medicare fact sheet: Medicare at a glance. Retrieved July 15, 2005, from *www.kff.org.*

Kaiser Family Foundation (KFF). (2005c). Medicare spending and financing. Retrieved June 15, 2005, from *www.kff.org.*

Kaiser Family Foundation (KFF). (2005d). The Medicare prescription drug benefit. Retrieved June 15, 2005, from *www.kff.org.*

Kaiser Family Foundation (KFF) & Harvard School of Public Health. (2003). *National survey of the public's view on Medicare.* Menlo Park, CA: KFF & Harvard School of Public Health.

Kaiser Family Foundation (KFF) and the Health Research and Educational Trust (HRET). (2003). *Employer health benefits 2003 annual survey.* Retrieved June 15, 2005, from *www.kff.org.*

Medicare Payment Advisory Commission (MedPAC). (2004). *Report to the Congress: New approaches in Medicare.* Washington, DC: MedPAC.

Reinhard, S. C., Scala-Foley, M. A., Caruso, J. T., & Archer, D. (2004). Medicare Savings programs. *American Journal of Nursing, 104*(6), 62-64.

Scala-Foley, M. A., Caruso, J. T., Archer, D., & Reinhard, S. C. (2004). Medicare's preventive services. *American Journal of Nursing, 104*(4), 73-75.

Scala-Foley, M. A., Caruso, J. T., Ramos, R., & Reinhard, S. C. (2004). Making sense of Medicare: The top 10 myths about Medicare. *American Journal of Nursing, 104*(1), 34-37.

Super, N. (2004). Medicare's chronic care improvement pilot program: What is its potential? *National Health Policy Forum Issue Brief* (No. 797). Washington, DC: George Washington University.

U.S. Department of Health and Human Services (USDHHS) Administration on Aging. (2004). A profile of older Americans 2003. Retrieved April 28, 2005, from *www.aoa.gov/prof/ Statistics/profile/profiles2002.asp.*

Wellner, A. S. (2005). Decision time for retiree Rx coverage. *HR Magazine, 49*(8), 67-76.

# POLICYSPOTLIGHT

# INTERESTS, IDEOLOGY, AND INSTITUTIONAL DYNAMICS IN THE CREATION OF THE MEDICARE PRESCRIPTION DRUG BENEFIT

Thomas R. Oliver, Philip R. Lee, & Tanisha Cariño

*"Politics is not an exact science."*
PRINCE OTTO VON BISMARCK

On December 8, 2003, President George W. Bush (R) signed the Medicare Prescription Drug Improvement and Modernization Act (PL 108-173), which authorizes Medicare coverage of outpatient prescription drugs as well as a host of other changes to the program. The new drug benefits represent a major new federal entitlement for Medicare beneficiaries, who now spend an average of $2864 per year on prescription drugs. It is projected to cost taxpayers $724 billion from 2006 to 2015 (Kaiser Family Foundation [KFF], 2005).

During a 2-year transition beginning in 2004, the federal government authorized privately sponsored cards to obtain price discounts on prescription drug purchases and offered a $600 credit to certain low-income beneficiaries. As of mid 2005, 6.3 million beneficiaries had enrolled in the Medicare-approved discount card programs, and 1.9 million were receiving the transitional financial assistance (Centers for Medicare and Medicaid Services [CMS], 2005b).

In 2006 a full-fledged Medicare Part D program began. As of that time, nearly 42 million beneficiaries have the following options: maintain any private prescription drug coverage they currently have; enroll in a new, free-standing prescription drug plan; or obtain drug coverage by enrolling in a Medicare managed care plan. The government projects that about 29 million beneficiaries will opt to join the new Part D program. Medicare will subsidize the cost of coverage for about 14 million low-income beneficiaries. Other beneficiaries will face significant gaps in coverage and as a result will still be liable for up to $3600 or more in annual expenses.

This chapter analyzes the political conditions and maneuvers behind the creation of the new Medicare Part D program. It explains how political leaders finally agreed to provide Medicare coverage for this critical component of modern medicine and why that agreement was so fraught with controversy. It summarizes the financing and organization of the new program and shows how it was necessary to build a legislative package of other reforms to attract sufficient support from a variety of constituencies. Finally, it identifies some of the preliminary challenges involved in implementing the drug benefits, focusing on the development of Part D drug formularies, as the start of the new program drew near.

## EARLIER EFFORTS TO ESTABLISH MEDICARE PRESCRIPTION DRUG COVERAGE

In 1951 the idea of a health insurance program for the elderly was initially proposed by Oscar Ewing, head of the Federal Security Administration. Only after the 1964 election produced a landslide victory for President Lyndon Johnson (D) and the largest Democratic majorities in both houses of Congress since the 1936 election, however, was enactment of new medical assistance for the aged assured (Marmor, 2000).

The main Democratic proposal supported by the Johnson administration, the King-Anderson Bill, aimed only to cover much of the costs of hospitalization through a universal social insurance mechanism. The counterproposal put forward by Republicans, the Byrnes Bill, called for voluntary enrollment in a health insurance program financed by premiums paid by beneficiaries and subsidized by general revenues. It included an expanded set of benefits, including physician services and prescription drugs. In addition, the AMA proposed a state-based, means-tested program of comprehensive benefits to expand the Kerr-Mills program for impoverished seniors first enacted in 1960.

Representative Wilbur Mills (D-AR), chairman of the House Ways and Means Committee, made the surprise suggestion that the Democratic and Republican proposals essentially be combined into Title XVIII of the Social Security Act, a new Medicare program with both Part A (Hospital Insurance) and Part B (Supplementary Medical Insurance). President Johnson supported this proposal. As the Ways and Means Committee marked up the combined bill in March 1965 (and also added what would become Medicaid), the outpatient prescription drug benefit for Part B was dropped "on the grounds of unpredictable and potentially high costs" (Marmor, 2000, p. 49).

Therefore, in spite of overwhelming Democratic majorities in both the House of Representatives and the Senate as well as nominal Republican support for such a benefit, the first of many opportunities to cover Medicare beneficiaries for the costs of outpatient prescription drugs ended in failure. The Medicaid program, enacted as Title XIX of the Social Security Act, ended up providing far more comprehensive coverage for the indigent elderly, blind, and disabled, as well as families with dependent children. It included outpatient prescription drug coverage as an optional benefit, which all states elected to provide when they set up their Medicaid programs.

The omission of outpatient prescription drugs from the initial package of Medicare benefits prompted the development of other sources of coverage—employer retirement programs, privately purchased supplemental benefits ("Medigap"), Medicaid, and managed care plans—that generally deterred subsequent efforts to integrate prescription drugs into Medicare. The ensuing history of initiatives to develop Medicare prescription drug benefits includes administrative actions in the Johnson and Nixon administrations, the enactment and repeal of the 1988 Medicare Catastrophic Coverage Act (MCCA), President Clinton's proposals for national health care reform, the deliberations of the National Bipartisan Commission on the Future of Medicare, proposals before and after the 2000 presidential election, and finally the adoption of prescription drug coverage and other reforms in late 2003. Throughout the program's history, action to add this basic element of modern medicine has been hampered by divided government, federal budget deficits, and ideological conflict between those seeking to expand the traditional Medicare program and those preferring a greater role for private health care companies. From the late 1960s to the late 1990s, prescription drug coverage for Medicare beneficiaries was always linked to the fate of other proposals for health care reform, and only at the end of the Clinton administration did the issue take on a life of its own (Oliver, Lee, & Lipton, 2004).

## BREAKING A LONG-STANDING POLITICAL DEADLOCK

In his initial budget for fiscal year (FY) 2002, submitted to Congress in February 2001, President Bush proposed that $153 billion be allocated over 10 years for "Medicare modernization," including prescription drug assistance (to put this in perspective, Medicare spent a total of $238 billion in FY 2001 with no outpatient drug coverage). The president proposed creating a block grant to the states to help provide drug coverage for Medicare beneficiaries with household incomes below 175% of the poverty level and to provide catastrophic coverage to limit annual out-of-pocket spending to $6000 for beneficiaries at all income levels. In July 2001 the Bush administration added a plan for Medicare beneficiaries

to purchase prescription drugs at discounted prices through private pharmacy benefit managers (U.S. Department of Health and Human Services [USDHHS], 2001).

The initiatives stalled when the courts found that the administration had no legal authority for the drug discount program, and Congress failed to endorse any form of drug assistance (Pear & Bumiller, 2003). Legislators in both parties opposed the concept of block grants, wary that Medicare beneficiaries would resent means-testing, state-by-state variation in benefits, and especially the need for beneficiaries to go through welfare agencies to enroll in state Medicaid programs. Another reason for the deadlock was that the amount proposed in the president's budget was only one tenth of the amount that the Congressional Budget Office (CBO) projected the Medicare population would spend on prescription drugs during that period.

A final reason for the deadlock was that Democrats briefly gained majority control of the Senate when James Jeffords of Vermont left the Republican Party to become an independent. Therefore Senate Democrats were able to stop Republican leaders in Congress from working out a plan with the White House and claiming victory before the 2002 election. The switch in the Senate only increased partisan tensions that remained from the controversial election of President Bush and the subsequent shift of his administration from moderate to conservative rhetoric and policies.

The congressional elections in November 2002 produced a political alignment not seen since the 1950s: Republicans were now in charge of the White House, the House of Representatives, and the Senate. In addition, two of the Republicans most interested in Medicare reform—new Senate Majority Leader Bill Frist and House Ways and Means Committee chair Bill Thomas—were in a position to give the issue priority and exert considerable control over the legislative process.

In March 2003 the president announced his new "Framework to Modernize and Improve Medicare." Relaxing his previously stated concerns over expanding the federal budget deficit, he offered $400 billion in new spending over 10 years—not all of it devoted to prescription drug assistance.

Low-income beneficiaries would be eligible for $600 credit toward their drug spending. All beneficiaries would receive a drug discount card, and those enrolled in the traditional fee-for-service Medicare program would receive "catastrophic" coverage for annual prescription drug costs above an unspecified amount, most likely $5500 to $7000. The president's proposal would openly encourage Medicare beneficiaries to leave the traditional fee-for-service program, in which 89% are currently enrolled, by offering additional prescription drug coverage to those who joined private, Medicare-approved health plans (California Healthline, 2003; White House, 2003). Thus, there would be considerable variation in coverage among beneficiaries, and access to the benefits would depend on the availability of a private plan in a beneficiary's locale.

With the distraction created by the war against Iraq in the spring of 2003, many observers believed that Medicare reform would once again be caught up in partisan politics and, without a significant investment of political capital by the president, would languish as in prior years (Toner, 2003a). In June 2003, however, the Senate Finance Committee came forward with a "bipartisan" agreement that helped break the 4-year old deadlock over Medicare prescription drug coverage. The committee chair, Charles Grassley (R-IA), and ranking minority member, Max Baucus (D-MT), announced the agreement with great fanfare and hoped to move the legislation to the Senate floor with little delay. With increasing encouragement from outsiders—including the White House and the leading Democratic voice on health issues, Senator Kennedy—it took only 7 days to go from the announcement of a skeletal two-page agreement to markup and committee approval of the 90-plus pages of S.1, the Prescription Drug and Medicare Improvement Act (Pear & Toner, 2003d).

The Finance Committee's approach deviated considerably from the Bush Administration's proposal and from legislation previously passed in the House. Medicare beneficiaries would be offered two basic options, starting in 2006: they could join new single-state or multistate preferred provider organizations, which would offer not only enhanced prescription drug benefits but also specialized disease management services for individuals with chronic conditions; or they could remain in the traditional Medicare program and, if they elected, receive prescription drug benefits comparable to those offered by private plans. Significantly, the Senate provided that if multiple private plans were not available in a geographic region, the CMS would step in and provide coverage under a "fallback" plan (Toner, 2003b). On June 27, 2003 the full Senate passed S.1 by a margin of 76 to 21. The bill passed with substantial bipartisan support, as key Democrats such as Kennedy and Minority Leader Tom Daschle (D-SD) believed it was best to accept the new $400 billion commitment as "money in the bank" toward a more comprehensive program (Toner & Pear, 2003).

The week after senators unveiled their tentative plan, House Republicans in the two committees with jurisdiction over Medicare—the Ways and Means Committee and the Energy and Commerce Committee—announced an agreement on HR 1, their version of a drug benefit and other elements of Medicare "modernization." They, too, rejected the Bush administration's proposal to provide significant benefits only to beneficiaries who enrolled in private health plans. The House bill introduced substantial new subsidies for low-income beneficiaries, as the Senate had done, but made them subject to income and asset tests. These provisions reintroduced the type of income-related financing that proved so controversial in the MCCA (Himelfarb, 1995). An even more controversial provision injected a modified form of "premium support" into the overall Medicare program: It linked future increases in beneficiaries' premiums to cost increases in whichever part of Medicare they were enrolled, in effect creating explicit competition between private health plans and the traditional fee-for-service program (Pear & Toner, 2003d).

The House proposal prompted "an impassioned partisan debate over the proper roles of government and private industry in delivering health care to the elderly" (Toner & Pear, 2003). Despite strong resistance from Democrats and some Republicans, the full House narrowly passed HR 1 216-215 on the same day as the Senate, June 27, but only after an abnormally long roll-call vote. House leaders had to persuade several Republican representatives to switch their votes at the last moment to save the measure. Many conservatives were reluctant to commit such large sums to a new federal entitlement and also believed that the bill did not go far enough in creating incentives for beneficiaries to switch from the traditional fee-for-service program to private health plans. To hold some conservative votes, House leaders attached a provision to expand tax-exempt health savings accounts for uninsured or self-insured individuals and families, a move that was projected to add $174 billion more to the federal deficit over 10 years (CBO, 2003; Toner & Pear, 2003).

House and Senate leaders convened a conference committee in August of 2003 and heavily stacked it in favor of Republican priorities. The chair, Thomas, allowed only two Democratic senators to participate in all the day-to-day discussions—Baucus, who was working side by side with Finance Committee chair Grassley, and John Breaux, who had long supported market-oriented reforms with Frist and Thomas. Minority Leader Daschle, who voted for the original Senate bill, was excluded entirely from the discussions. The three Democratic conferees from the House were also excluded, which reduced their participation to signing or not signing the conference committee report (Carey, 2003a; Pear & Toner, 2003c).

This "hardball" approach did not assure a smooth process, however, and it took 4 months of negotiations to craft a package that might attract the number of votes needed to get a bill to the president's desk. Given the real possibility that private drug plans would not develop or would prove unsustainable in some areas, policymakers needed a way to assure universal availability of the drug benefits. Conservatives, however, fiercely resisted the Senate requirement for the federal government itself to provide "fallback" drug coverage.

There were also emerging budgetary constraints. After tax cuts and a sluggish economy eliminated the surplus revenues that could have funded new Medicare benefits, the federal government faced record budget deficits of $375 billion for FY 2003 and $477 for FY 2004, exacerbated further by the invasion and occupation of Iraq and hundreds of billions of dollars in additional tax cuts (CBO, 2004a;

Weisman, 2003). Many conservative Republicans were growing anxious about further expanding commitments for mandatory federal spending (Grier, 2003).

Yet the $400 billion devoted to prescription drug coverage would scarcely cover one fifth of the estimated $1.85 trillion that Medicare beneficiaries were expected to spend on drugs over the next decade. The new benefits, therefore, would be costly to the government but of marginal value to many beneficiaries who did not qualify for additional low-income subsidies (Pear & Toner, 2003b). Only 33% of seniors agreed with the argument that "something is better than nothing. Congress should pass this bill now, even though it would leave many seniors paying a substantial share of their drug costs, and work to improve benefits in the future" (KFF & Harvard School of Public Health, 2003). If "sweeteners" were added in the conference committee negotiations to assuage particular constituencies and gain votes, the cost of the overall package might exceed the $400 billion ceiling and the legislation could be ruled out of order.

Passage was also more difficult because Republican leaders chose not to pursue an omnibus budget reconciliation bill in 2003. Budget reconciliation has an important advantage in the Senate: it cannot be filibustered and requires a simple majority to pass. That both houses proceeded with independent legislation suggests that even though Republicans may have had the power to enact Medicare reforms of their choosing, they feared that a nearly straight party line vote would leave them and President Bush vulnerable to a voter backlash in 2004 if beneficiaries were disappointed with the financial value, the workability, or the timing of the new prescription drug benefits, which would not fully kick in until 2006.

## THE MEDICARE PRESCRIPTION DRUG IMPROVEMENT AND MODERNIZATION ACT OF 2003

At several points, participants close to the conference committee negotiations believed that the opportunity for reform would be missed. On November 15, however, the conferees reached agreement on a new version of HR 1, the Medicare Prescription Drug

Improvement and Modernization Act of 2003. The 678-page conference report included many of the features that had come to be widely accepted in earlier proposals, such as the discount card, additional assistance for low-income beneficiaries, a substantial gap in benefits for individuals with high drug costs ("doughnut hole"), and the use of private pharmacy benefit managers in lieu of direct governmental regulation. Yet the bill reflected "concession" more than "compromise," with the final provisions on some of the most controversial issues watered down so as to become almost meaningless to their proponents. This deepened rather than resolved cleavages that pitted Democrats against Republicans and, at times, Republicans against Republicans (Goldstein, 2003a; Rapp, 2003).

The final product included the following major provisions (CBO, 2004a; Health Policy Alternatives, 2003; KFF, 2004):

- It offered Medicare beneficiaries relatively immediate, if modest, financial relief in the form of drug discount cards sponsored by private firms with federal approval. The voluntary interim program would begin in mid 2004. Medicare would pay the $30 enrollment fee and provide a $600 credit for beneficiaries with household incomes below 135% of poverty (in 2003, $12,123 for an individual and $16,362 for a couple) who do not qualify for Medicaid or have other coverage. Beneficiaries would be allowed to enroll in only one discount program.

- It required most beneficiaries to choose whether to maintain any existing prescription drug coverage or to join a new Medicare Part D program, beginning in January 2006. The Part D drug benefits would be offered through stand-alone drug plans or through comprehensive plans under Part C, renamed the *Medicare Advantage* program. The standard Part D benefits would have an initial premium of approximately $35 per month and a $250 annual deductible. Medicare would pay 75% of annual expenses between $250 and $2250 for approved prescription drugs, nothing for expenses between $2250 and $5100, and 95% of expenses above $5100. Including $420 in premiums, beneficiaries would need to spend $1590 out of pocket to reach an initial

break-even point, and they would be responsible for $4020 of the first $5100 (79%) in annual drug expenses. Private plans could alter the specific benefits as long as they remained actuarially equivalent to the standard benefits.

- It mandated that all individuals who are eligible for both Medicare and Medicaid would now receive their drug coverage through Medicare. The government would cover the premiums, deductible, and coinsurance for beneficiaries who are eligible for Medicaid or who have incomes below 135% of poverty and meet an asset test of $6000 per individual or $9000 per couple. Beneficiaries under 150% of poverty and who meet an asset test of $10,000 per individual or $20,000 per couple would be eligible for sliding scale premiums, a $50 deductible, and 15% coinsurance. All beneficiaries would be required to make small copayments for each prescription. States would be required to pass back to the federal government $88 billion of the estimated $115 billion they would save on Medicaid drug coverage.

- It prohibited beneficiaries who enroll in Part D from purchasing supplemental benefits to insure against prescription drug expenses not covered in the program. Thus, they would not be able to enroll in Part D and convert existing retiree benefits or Medigap policies into "wrap around" coverage to pay the Part D premiums, deductible, and coinsurance. Also, a late enrollment penalty would increase Part D premiums at least 1% per month of delayed enrollment (for beneficiaries who switch out of preexisting coverage or fail to enroll in Part D when they first become eligible).

- It required that at least two options for Part D benefits from different entities be available to beneficiaries. Medicare could assume financial risk and contract with private entities to establish regional "fallback" plans where necessary, but it could not establish a national fallback plan.

- It provided over $86 billion in subsidies for employers and unions to encourage them to maintain their prescription drug coverage for retirees. This addressed one of the key concerns of AARP and earlier estimates by the CBO (2003)

that approximately one quarter of Medicare beneficiaries with current employer-sponsored drug coverage would lose it once the benefit was enacted.

■ It allowed new Part D prescription drug plans to use formularies approved by the government and to negotiate independently with drug manufacturers, but it prohibited any direct governmental price negotiation.

■ It maintained the current ban on reimportation of prescription drugs from other countries and authorized the Food and Drug Administration to study the potential effects of reimportation from Canada.

■ It abandoned the House plan to establish price competition between the traditional fee-for-service program and the managed care program and replaced it with a demonstration project in up to six metropolitan areas, not to begin until 2010.

■ It significantly scaled back the scope and expected use of health savings accounts, reducing the estimated cost from $174 billion to $6 billion in lost tax revenue.

■ It committed $14 billion to boost payments to managed care plans in the Medicare Advantage program. At least temporarily, managed care plans would for the first time be paid more per enrollee than the average cost per enrollee in the traditional fee-for-service program.

■ It provided $21 billion to increase Medicare fee-for-service payments to health care providers in rural areas.

The most direct benefits of the legislation went to low-income Medicare beneficiaries who had no supplemental source of insurance coverage through retiree benefits, Medigap plans, or Medicaid. But there were other clear winners as well: Pharmaceutical manufacturers could now expect higher demand among their best customers and prevailed on all three of their priority issues—avoiding direct federal administration of benefits, explicit cost control measures, and legalization of drug reimportation (Connolly, 2003; Harris, 2003). Employers, managed care plans, rural health care providers, and teaching hospitals would receive over $125 billion in short-term subsidies (Goldstein, 2003b; Biles, Nicholas, &

Cooper, 2004). In the eyes of one analyst it was "a classic election-year giveaway, a year early" (Abelson & Freudenheim, 2003). Each of the major and minor subsidies inserted into the final version of HR 1 might help achieve a given policy objective, but more important, they could help attract the votes of legislators who would otherwise oppose the bill for partisan or ideologic reasons (Abelson, 2003; Lee, 2003; Samuelson, 2003). They also helped to mobilize support from a number of major interest groups, including the American Association of Health Plans, American Medical Association, American Hospital Association, the U.S. Chamber of Commerce, General Motors, and, most importantly, the Pharmaceutical Research and Manufacturers of America (PhRMA) (Goldstein, 2003b; Pear & Toner, 2003c).

The prospects for reform increased dramatically when, on November 17, AARP appeared to go against the tide of public opinion and announced its support: "The endorsement provides a seal of approval from an organization with 35 million members. Republicans also hope it provides political cover against charges by some Democrats that the bill would undermine the federal insurance program for the elderly and disabled" (Pear & Toner, 2003e). The AARP endorsement, in turn, infuriated its usual allies in the Democratic leadership, labor, and consumer groups and cost it 60,000 members who resigned or chose not to renew their membership in protest (Broder, 2004; Broder & Goldstein, 2003; Carey, 2003b; Pear & Toner, 2003e; Stolberg, 2003; Vaida, 2004).

Despite the AARP "defection," the outcome was still very much in doubt as congressional leaders laid plans for the final debate and votes on the reform package. Liberal opponents such as the AFL-CIO; Association of Federal, State, County, and Municipal Employees; Consumers Union; Families USA; and the American Nurses Association criticized the inadequacy of the drug benefits, the threat to retiree benefit programs, the boost it gave to private health plans, and the lack of any meaningful price controls. Key Democrats who supported the original Senate bill, particularly Daschle and Kennedy, came out strongly against HR 1 when it increased Part B premiums for high-income beneficiaries and did not allow the government itself to directly offer drug benefits when private options were unavailable (Dionne, 2003; Pear & Toner, 2003a; Pear & Toner, 2003c). A few Republicans planned to vote against the bill because it failed to include provisions allowing seniors and other Americans to buy lower-priced drugs from other countries—a proposal that the general public supported by a three-to-one margin (KFF & Harvard School of Public Health, 2003). At least one Republican, Senator John McCain of Arizona, found it "outrageous" that HR 1 prohibited the federal government from using its purchasing power to negotiate better prices for Medicare beneficiaries (Pear & Hulse, 2003).

On the other hand, conservative groups such as the Heritage Foundation and the National Taxpayers Union attacked the new benefits as a burden to taxpayers and the economy. They criticized what they regarded as an inevitable replacement of employer-sponsored retiree coverage with a massive new public prescription drug program (notwithstanding its administration through private contractors). They also opposed any Medicare legislation that did not establish direct price competition between the managed care and fee-for-service programs (Agan, 2003; Butler et al., 2003; Chen, 2003). Conservative Republicans in the House had earlier warned the leadership they would vote against the final bill if it eliminated or scaled back the main market-oriented reforms: premium support and health savings accounts (Goldstein, 2003a).

Trying to quell a rebellion in his own party, House Speaker Hastert recognized that the upcoming vote was tenuous. He went ahead because members were anxious to break for the Thanksgiving holiday and the bill could not realistically be revived during the upcoming presidential election campaign (Koszczuk & Allen, 2003). The House vote on the conference report came at 3:00 AM on November 22. The reforms appeared to be dead when, at the end of the normal 15 minutes allowed for voting, the bill was losing by 15 votes. At that point, Hastert and the rest of the Republican leadership went into action and eventually reduced it to a razor-edge margin of 216 to 218. It stuck there while USDHHS Secretary Thompson, defying

House custom, moved onto the floor and the leaders roused President Bush to make another half-dozen calls to convince a handful of their colleagues to change their votes. A Republican who was retiring in 2004 claimed he was offered $100,000 to help his son run for his seat on the condition that he switch his vote (Schuler & Carey, 2004). After the vote was held open for nearly 3 hours—by far the longest known roll call vote in the history of the House—HR 1 passed by a margin of 220 to 215. The vote closely followed party lines: only 16 Democrats supported the final package, whereas 25 Republicans opposed it (Broder, 2003; Carey, 2003b; Koszczuk & Allen, 2003).

On November 25 the Senate leadership brought up HR 1 for final action, and again the outcome was far from certain for many hours. A vote to close off debate prevailed by a wide margin, but it appeared that opponents would succeed in blocking the legislation on a budgetary point of order. The CBO officially projected a net cost of $395 billion for the reform package. Democrats, however, contended that the budgetary impact of the tax-free health savings accounts was not fully counted and, if it was, the cost of the full package would exceed the $400 billion limit allowed by the Senate budget resolution several months earlier. After colleagues beseeched him to support the president and his party, former Republican majority leader Trent Lott (R-MS) gave in and cast the deciding vote to waive the budget rules and proceed to an up or down vote on the Medicare bill itself. He then voted against the bill along with eight other Republican senators, but 11 Democrats and one independent (Jeffords) voted in favor of the reforms, and the final version of HR 1 was approved by a margin of 54 to 44 (Carey, 2003a; Koszczuk & Allen, 2003). Some of the supporters felt it was best to help out low-income beneficiaries, even if the financial assistance was inadequate for the majority of beneficiaries. Plus, the congressional budget resolution for FY 2004 set aside $400 billion in future spending for augmenting Medicare before the war and a second round of tax cuts; so if Congress did not act now, it would become difficult to set aside anything close to that amount in future budgets (Carey, 2003b).

Senator Daschle and House Minority Leader Nancy Pelosi (D-CA) protested the extraordinary moves that the Republican majority took to secure passage of the new law. They predicted that this was not the end of the process and promised to introduce legislation to repeal parts of the legislation (Bettelheim, 2003; Carey, 2003a; Pear, 2004). Several controversies over Medicare and prescription drug coverage continued as the policy process moved from enactment to implementation in 2004.

One issue was the affordability of drugs. The head of a prominent consumer group, Families USA, argued that the price of drugs was the "No. 1, 2, and 3 concern" of beneficiaries and said the provision barring the federal government from directly negotiating prices for Medicare was a "lightning rod" in the new law (Toner, 2004). Of greatest concern is that the coverage itself will prove inadequate for large numbers of beneficiaries, particularly those who have no current source of supplemental drug coverage. The vast majority of the elderly have limited financial resources: 39% have household incomes below 200% of poverty, and 44% have assets under $5000 (KFF, 2005). Yet the new law requires hundreds or thousands of dollars in cost sharing every year except for beneficiaries with very low incomes, and even they will still need to make out-of-pocket copayments for each prescription. This problem will be exacerbated if, as the CBO and other analysts expect, large numbers of employers who currently provide retiree benefits attempt to drop them once the Medicare benefits become available (CBO, 2003; Freudenheim, 2003). Any effort to improve the benefits, however, will almost certainly be stymied in the short run by fiscal concerns.

Another issue was the failure to legalize the reimportation of drugs. Many states and local governments developed plans to directly purchase or enable their residents to purchase prescription drugs from Canadian companies, directly challenging the federal ban on such practices (Belluck, 2003; *Washington Post*, 2004b).

Further controversy arose in January 2004 when the president's Office of Management and Budget projected the new law would cost the federal government $534 billion over 10 years—30% higher than the estimate of $395 billion that lawmakers had relied on when they voted on the final package just a few weeks earlier (CBO, 2004b; Pear, 2004). In March 2004 the chief actuary of the CMS revealed that, as early as the previous summer, his office had estimated much higher costs for the proposed reforms than the congressional budget analysts. His superiors in the Bush administration, however, had ordered him to withhold the estimates from members of Congress and warned him that "the consequences for insubordination are extremely severe" (Goldstein, 2004; Stolberg, 2004). Members of both parties acknowledged that if the administration's estimates had been known to legislators and the public, significant changes would likely have been required in the final provisions of HR 1. Otherwise, it would have faced even stronger opposition from conservatives in the House, and opponents in the Senate may well have succeeded in blocking the bill on a budgetary point of order (Schuler & Carey, 2004; Stolberg & Pear, 2004; *Washington Post*, 2004a).

## CHALLENGES IN IMPLEMENTATION: DEVELOPMENT OF FORMULARIES FOR THE MEDICARE PART D PROGRAM

There are numerous challenges ahead to implement an effective policy that meets the actual needs of Medicare beneficiaries. Although the issue of prescription drug coverage is highly specialized, almost every aspect of implementing the Medicare Part D benefits involves not only technical skill but also political negotiation among a large, diverse set of stakeholders. In 2004 alone, the health care industry spent $325 million on lobbying—far more than defense contractors, the banking industry, or any other sector—attempting to influence rules for the drug benefits and other provisions of the new law, with hundreds of billions of dollars at stake (Pear, 2005).

The task of developing and approving Part D drug formularies illustrates the ongoing politics of policy implementation. It highlights the critical interdependence of government and private actors in program development; the tension created by multiple, often competing policy objectives; and the difficulty of meeting the needs of "special populations" in a general regulatory framework.

At the center of the implementation process for formulary development was CMS. The other stakeholders in the development of Part D formularies included pharmaceutical manufacturers, health plans, pharmacy benefit managers, retail pharmacies, employers and unions with drug benefits for retirees, state governments in their capacities as insurers as well as purchasers, pharmacists and other health professionals, groups representing beneficiaries in general, groups representing patients with specific diseases, and of course Congress, the White House, and numerous executive branch agencies apart from CMS (Box 15-1).

The challenge for CMS was to balance the objective of ensuring access to current medications against the objective of cost containment and the objective of promoting market choice through variations in coverage. Bowing to industry concerns, Congress expressly prohibited CMS from making binding coverage determinations for specific drugs under Part D. Both Medicare Advantage plans and private drug plans participating in the Part D

---

**BOX 15-1** Stakeholders in Medicare Part D Implementation

**PHARMACEUTICAL INDUSTRY**

Biotechnology Industry Organization
Pharmaceutical Research and Manufacturers of
America (PhRMA)
Individual drug manufacturers (Pfizer, Merck,
Sanofi-Aventis, GlaxoSmithKline, Amgen, and
Johnson & Johnson)

**HEALTH PLANS**

America's Health Insurance Plans
Individual insurers (Aetna, Blue Cross Blue Shield
Association, Kaiser, United Healthcare)

**PHARMACY BENEFITS MANAGERS**

Pharmaceutical Care Management Association
Individual pharmacy benefits managers
(Caremark, Medco)

**STATES**

National Association of State Medicaid Directors
National Conference of State Legislatures
National Governors' Association
State Pharmaceutical Assistance Transition
Commission

**EMPLOYERS AND UNIONS**

AFL-CIO and National Education Association
American Benefits Council and the U.S. Chamber of
Commerce
Business Roundtable
National Business Group on Health

**PATIENT GROUPS**

AARP (formerly American Association of Retired
Persons)

National Patient Advocate Foundation
Access to Benefits Coalition
Families USA

**RETAIL PHARMACY**

National Community Pharmacists Association
Individual pharmacies (Rite Aid, CVS, Walgreens)

**PROVIDERS**

American Society of Consultant Pharmacists
Academy of Managed Care Pharmacy
American Society of Health-System Pharmacists
Long Term Care Pharmacy Alliance
American Medical Association
American Psychiatric Association
American Society of Clinical Oncologists

**DISEASE GROUPS**

National Alliance for the Mentally Ill
National Mental Health Association
American Cancer Society
Cancer Leadership Council
National Breast Cancer Coalition

**GOVERNMENT**

Congress and Medicare Payment Advisory
Commission
Executive Branch (White House)
Centers for Medicare and Medicaid Services
National Institutes of Health
Health Resources and Services Administration

From Avalere Health, LLC.

program would therefore have some degree of flexibility in developing formularies and management tools for cost and quality control.

Section 1860(D)(4) of the statute established the general standard for beneficiary protection: "The formulary must include drugs within each therapeutic category and class of covered Part D drugs, although not necessarily all drugs within such categories and classes." The statute also directed the Secretary of Health and Human Services to request that a private entity, the United States Pharmacopeia (USP), develop and periodically revise model guidelines for the list of covered drugs in consultation with pharmacy benefit managers and other interested parties. USP historically has established manufacturing standards for pharmaceutical products and information on ingredients, clinical uses, and dosing. Its standards are ordinarily developed by a council of experts and committees composed of over 600 elected scientists and practitioners from academia, drug companies, government, consumer organizations, and professional associations (USP, 2005).

As requested, USP took the lead in developing model guidelines. From May through December 2004, a 17-member expert committee oversaw a process that also included advisory forums representing manufacturers, health plans, providers, and beneficiaries, a contentious public meeting for review and comment on draft model guidelines, and informal consultations. After releasing the draft guidelines in August of 2004, USP received over 1300 public comments from interested parties (USP, 2004b). After minor adjustments, the final list released in January 2005 included 43 therapeutic categories, 138 pharmacologic classes, and 146 unique classifications (USP, 2004a). Plans participating in the Part D program are not required to use the USP model guidelines—they can, for example, follow the American Hospital Formulary Service classification instead—but the USP guidelines offer a "safe harbor" when plans are submitted to CMS for review and approval (CMS, 2005a).

With the model guidelines completed, the implementation process and political pressure shifted back to CMS. The agency was responsible for final approval of proposed drug formularies, and it could withhold approval during the bidding process between the plans and the agency if it found that the choice of drugs, cost-sharing tiers, or history of appeals substantially discouraged enrollment of certain types of beneficiaries. Various stakeholders, especially manufacturers and consumer groups, requested that CMS designate individuals with mental health conditions, cancer, human immunodeficiency virus (HIV) infection or acquired immunodeficiency syndrome (AIDS), dual Medicare and Medicaid eligibility, or residence in long-term care facilities as "special populations" in weighing whether a formulary design was potentially discriminatory. They argued that those groups should have some or all of the following protections to assure access: open formularies, alternative formularies specially designed for them, limits on cost sharing, expedited appeals, or coverage of off-label uses.

In its final regulations released in late January 2005, CMS did not identify any special populations or make special provisions for particular disease groups. Instead, it elected to provide less formal "guidance" on how it would review Part D formularies—a practice that could send clear signals to stakeholders but would presumably not have the same force of law as the final rule (CMS, 2005a).

The CMS guidance specified that the agency would review proposed Part D formularies based on "best practices" from employer-sponsored health plans, Medicaid, and plans participating in the Federal Employee Health Benefits Program. The agency would stress access to medically necessary drugs but also allow flexibility in benefits that "promote real beneficiary choice while protecting beneficiaries from discrimination." The review of formularies would focus on inclusion of a range of drugs in a broad distribution of therapeutic categories and classes; consideration of specific drugs; and analysis of tiered cost sharing and utilization management techniques.

CMS did establish some highly detailed parameters to steer formulary design: It identified 26 specific conditions for which it would compare formulary design with widely accepted national treatment guidelines (Box 15-2). In addition, CMS planned to analyze availability and cost-sharing for 40 drug

---

**BOX 15-2**   CMS Review of Conditions with Widely Accepted National Treatment Guidelines

Asthma
Atrial fibrillation
Benign prostatic hyperplasia
Bipolar disorder
Chronic obstructive pulmonary disease
Chronic stable angina
Community-acquired pneumonia
Dementia
Depression
Diabetes
End-stage renal disease
Epilepsy
Gastroesophageal reflux disease
Heart failure
Hepatitis
HIV
Hypertension
Lipid disorders
Migraine
Multiple sclerosis
Osteoporosis
Parkinson's disease
Rheumatoid arthritis
Schizophrenia
Thrombosis
Tuberculosis

From Centers for Medicare and Medicaid Services (CMS). (2005). *Medicare Modernization Act final guidelines— Formularies: CMS strategy for affordable access to comprehensive drug coverage.* Accessed March 2, 2006, at *www.cms.hhs.gov/PrescriptionDrugCovContra/Downloads/ FormularyGuidance.pdf.*

---

**BOX 15-3**   Centers for Medicare and Medicaid Services Review of Top 40 Drug Classes by Cost and Usage

Alpha blockers
Angiotensin-converting enzyme (ACE) inhibitors
Angiotensin receptor blockers
Anticoagulants
Antigout medications
Atypical antipsychotics
Beta blockers
Biguanides
Bisphosphonates
Calcium channel blockers
Calcium channel blockers/ACE inhibitors
Cardiac inotropes
Cholinesterase inhibitors
Corticosteroids
Cyclooxygenase (COX)-2 inhibitors
Estrogen replacement
γ-Aminobutyric acid (GABA) agents
Leukotriene modifiers
Long-acting beta agonists/inhaled corticosteroids
Loop diuretics
Nitrates
Nonsedating antihistamines
Ophthalmic prostaglandins
Opioids
Opioids/analgesics
Platelet aggregation inhibitors
Potassium
Potassium-sparing diuretics/thiazide diuretics
Proton pump inhibitors
Quinolones
Sedatives
Selective estrogen receptor modifiers
Selective serotonin reuptake inhibitors (SSRIs)
Short-acting beta agonists
Statins
Sulfonylureas
Thiazide diuretics
Thiazolidinediones
Thyroid replacement
Tricyclic antidepressants

From Centers for Medicare and Medicaid Services (CMS). (2005). *Medicare Modernization Act final guidelines— Formularies: CMS strategy for affordable access to comprehensive drug coverage.* Accessed March 2, 2006, at *www.cms.hhs.gov/PrescriptionDrugCovContra/Downloads/ FormularyGuidance.pdf.*

---

classes commonly prescribed for the Medicare population (Box 15-3). Finally, it expected that formularies conforming to best practices would include a majority of drugs in the classes of antidepressants, antipsychotics, anticonvulsants, antiretrovirals, immunosuppressants, and antineo-plastics. Deviations from common benefits management practices would require written clinical justification by Part D plans.

Despite the circuitous regulatory process, it can be argued that CMS has done everything it can within the constraints of the legislation to fulfill its principal role of protecting and promoting the well-being of Medicare beneficiaries. Neither the process, particularly the privacy of USP decision-making, nor the remaining ambiguity in the final regulations satisfies manufacturers concerned about coverage of their individual drugs and advocates concerned about the efficacy and stability of therapeutic options for the mentally ill and other patient groups. The outcomes depend in large part on the capacity of CMS to conduct its initial reviews of proposed Part D formularies in a careful manner despite limited time and available personnel; to provide beneficiaries sufficiently accurate and complete information about formulary coverage and cost-sharing to ensure fairness and real choice; and to monitor formulary operations, especially changes in coverage, and correct problems as they emerge in the new program.

## SUMMARY

In 2003, policymakers seized a historic opportunity to integrate prescription drug benefits into a program that 42 million older and disabled Americans admire and rely on. Despite this opportunity, the effort to establish Medicare drug benefits was boxed in by current sources of coverage, by ideologic insistence on market "solutions" for a massive social problem, by arbitrary budgetary constraints, and by the failure of managed care in rural America. The resulting program design makes it more difficult for Medicare administrators and private organizations to successfully implement the policy, satisfy the expectations of millions of Medicare beneficiaries, and protect the public purse.

If the patterns of policymaking in the past hold true, the action that Congress and President Bush began in 2003 will be only the first step in a serial process of reform. Nearly every episode of Medicare reform, whether it involves adding new benefits, controlling costs, or developing new delivery systems, requires several years of legislation and regulatory development before those elements become routine parts of the program (Oliver & Lee, 2000). Much work remains, therefore, before political leaders can claim to have solved the problems that pushed this issue to the top of the nation's domestic agenda.

## Key Points

- In 2003, policymakers overcame a number of political, ideologic, and fiscal obstacles that had stopped many prior efforts to add outpatient prescription drug coverage to the Medicare program.
- The Medicare prescription drug benefit represents a major new federal entitlement that is expected to cost taxpayers over $700 billion in its first 10 years.
- The legislation enacting the benefit requires beneficiaries to choose whether to maintain any existing drug coverage or join a new Medicare Part D program beginning in January 2006.
- The new law requires all individuals who are eligible for both Medicare and Medicaid to receive their drug coverage through Medicare and requires states to reimburse the federal government for most of the cost savings in their Medicaid programs.
- Political controversy followed the passage of the act creating the Medicare prescription drug benefit, stemming from Office of Management and Budget estimates that the new law would cost 30% more than the estimate previously given to lawmakers and from the failure of the legislation to allow either governmental negotiation of drug prices or legal reimportation of lower-cost drugs from other countries.

## Web Resources

**Centers for Medicare and Medicaid Services**
*www.cms.hhs.gov*
**Medicare Drug Benefit Calculator**
*www.kff.org/medicare/rxdrugscalculator.cfm*
**Medicare Prescription Drug Benefit Website**
*www.medicare.gov/medicarereform/drugbenefit.asp*
**Medicare Rights Center**
*www.medicarerights.org*

## REFERENCES

Abelson, R. (2003, September 4). Narrow interest in a broad measure. *New York Times*, C6.

Abelson, R., & Freudenheim, M. (2003, November 18). Medicare compromise plan won't cut costs, critics say. *New York Times*, A18.

Agan, T. (2003, August 26). Dangerous interaction: How mixing a drug benefit with Medicare could mean an overdose of federal spending. *National Taxpayers Union Foundation Policy Paper*, 143. Retrieved March 8, 2004, from *www.ntu.org/main/press_papers.php?PressID=164&org_name=NTUF*.

Belluck, P. (2003, December 11). Boldly crossing the line for cheaper drugs. *New York Times*, A38.

Bettelheim, A. (2003, November 29). Medicare plan faces rough ride through the reality mill. *CQ Weekly*, 2952.

Biles, B., Nicholas L. H., & Cooper, B. S. (2004). *The cost of privatization: Extra payments to Medicare Advantage plans.* New York: Commonwealth Fund Issue Brief.

Broder, D. S. (2003, November 23). Time was GOP's ally on the vote. *Washington Post*, A1.

Broder, D. S. (2004, March 18). AARP's tough selling job. *Washington Post*, A31.

Broder, D. S., & Goldstein, A. (2003, November 20). AARP decision followed a long courtship. *Washington Post*, A1.

Butler, S. M., Moffit, R. E., & Riedl, B. M. (2003, November 10). Cost control in the Medicare drug bill needs premium support, not a 'trigger.' *The Heritage Foundation, Backgrounder No. 1704.*

California Healthline. (2003). President Bush unveils Medicare reform framework in speech to American Medical Association. Oakland: California Healthcare Foundation.

Carey, M. A. (2003a, November 29). GOP wins battle, not war. *CQ Weekly*, 2956.

Carey, M. A. (2003b, November 22). Medicare deal goes to wire in late-night House vote. *CQ Weekly*, 2879.

Centers for Medicare and Medicaid Services (CMS). (2005a). *Medicare Modernization Act final guidelines—Formularies: CMS strategy for affordable access to comprehensive drug coverage.* Accessed March 2, 2006, at *www.cms.hhs.gov/PrescriptionDrugCovContra/Downloads/FormularyGuidance.pdf.*

Centers for Medicare and Medicaid Services (CMS). (2005b, July 25). *Open door forum on low income health access* (online question and answer forum).

Chen, L. J. (2003, 26 August). What seniors will lose with a universal Medicare drug entitlement. *The Heritage Foundation, Backgrounder No. 1680.*

Congressional Budget Office (CBO). (2003, July 22). *Cost estimate for HR 1, Medicare Prescription Drug and Modernization Act of 2003, as passed by the House of Representatives on June 27, 2003 and S 1, Prescription Drug and Medicare Improvement Act of 2003, as passed by the Senate on June 27, 2003 with a modification requested by Senate conferees.*

Congressional Budget Office (CBO). (2004a). *The budget and economic outlook: Fiscal years 2005 to 2014.* Washington, DC: CBO.

Congressional Budget Office (CBO). (2004b). Letter from Douglas Holtz-Eakin, Director, Congressional Budget Office to the Honorable Jim Nussle, Chairman, House Budget Committee regarding the comparison of CBO and administration estimates of the effect of HR 1 on direct spending, 2 February. Retrieved March 8, 2004, from *www.cbo.gov/showdoc.cfm?index=4995&sequence=0.*

Connolly, C. (2003, November 21). Drugmakers protect their turf. *Washington Post*, A4.

Dionne, E. J., Jr. (2003, November 18). Medicare monstrosity. *Washington Post*, A25.

Freudenheim, M. (2003, July 2). Employers seek to shift costs of drugs to U.S. *New York Times*, A1.

Goldstein, A. (2003a, November 30). For GOP leaders, battles and bruises produce Medicare bill. *Washington Post*, A8.

Goldstein, A. (2003b, November 24). Medicare bill would enrich companies. *Washington Post*, A1.

Goldstein, A. (2004, March 19). Foster: White House had role in withholding Medicare data. *Washington Post*, A2.

Grier, P. (2003, September 25). Shift against drug benefits in Medicare. *Christian Science Monitor*, 1.

Harris, G. (2003, November 25). Drug makers move closer to big victory. *New York Times*, A20.

Health Policy Alternatives. (2003). *Prescription drug coverage for Medicare beneficiaries: A summary of the Medicare prescription drug, improvement, and modernization act of 2003.* Prepared for the Henry J. Kaiser Family Foundation.

Himelfarb, R. (1995). *Catastrophic politics: The rise and fall of the Medicare Catastrophic Coverage Act of 1988.* University Park, PA: Pennsylvania State University Press.

Kaiser Family Foundation (KFF). (2004). *The Medicare prescription drug law.* Menlo Park, CA: KFF.

Kaiser Family Foundation (KFF). (2005). *Medicare Chartbook* (3rd ed.). Menlo Park, CA: KFF.

Kaiser Family Foundation (KFF) & Harvard School of Public Health. (2003). *Medicare prescription drug survey.* Menlo Park, CA: KFF.

Koszczuk, J., & Allen, J. (2003, November 29). Late-night Medicare vote triggers some unexpected alliances. *CQ Weekly*, 2958.

Lee, C. (2003, November 23). Medicare bill partly a special interest care package. *Washington Post*, A11.

Marmor, T. R. (2000). *The politics of Medicare* (2nd ed.). New York: Aldine de Gruyter.

Oliver, T. R., & Lee, P. R. (2000). *Understanding the evolution of Medicare: Patterns of policy making and their consequences* (unpublished manuscript). Johns Hopkins University.

Oliver, T. R., Lee, P. R., & Lipton, H. L. (2004). A political history of Medicare and prescription drug coverage. *Milbank Quarterly 82*, 283-354.

Pear, R. (2004, January 30). Bush's aides put higher price tag on Medicare law. *New York Times*, A1.

Pear, R. (2005, August 23). Medicare law prompts a rush for lobbyists. *New York Times.*

Pear, R., & Bumiller, E. (2003, January 30). Doubts are emerging as Bush pushes his Medicare plan. *New York Times*, A18.

Pear, R., & Hulse, C. (2003, November 25). Senate removes two roadblocks to drug benefit. *New York Times*, A1.

Pear, R., & Toner, R. (2003a, November 20). Counting votes and attacks in final push for Medicare bill. *New York Times*, A25.

Pear, R., & Toner, R. (2003b, June 22). Criticism of drug benefit is simple: It's bewildering. *New York Times*, A22.

Pear, R., & Toner, R. (2003c, November 17). GOP begins push for Medicare bill. *New York Times*, A18.

Pear, R., & Toner, R. (2003d, June 18). House Committee approves drug benefits for Medicare. *New York Times*, A19.

Pear, R., & Toner, R. (2003e, November 18). Medicare plan covering drugs backed by AARP. *New York Times*, A1.

Rapp, D. (2003, November 22). Editor's notebook: An imperfect art. *CQ Weekly*, 2870.

Samuelson, R. J. (2003, November 24). Medicare as pork barrel. *Washington Post*, A21.

Schuler, K., & Carey, M. A. (2004, March 20). Estimates, ethics, and ads tarnish Medicare Overhaul. *CQ Weekly*, 699.

Stolberg, S. G. (2003, November 23). An 800-pound gorilla changes partners over Medicare. *New York Times*, D5.

Stolberg, S. (2004, March 19). Senate Democrats claim Medicare chief broke law. *New York Times*, A14.

Stolberg, S. G., & Pear, R. (2004, March 18). Mysterious fax adds to intrigue over the Medicare bill's cost. *New York Times*, A1.

Toner, R. (2003a, January 11). Political memo. Weapon in health wars: Frist's role as a doctor. *New York Times*, A12.

Toner, R. (2003b, June 2). Reshaping Medicare, rural roots in mind. *New York Times*, A14.

Toner, R. (2004, March 17). Seems the last word on Medicare wasn't. *New York Times*, A16.

Toner, R., & Pear, R. (2003, June 27). House and Senate pass measures for broad overhaul of Medicare. *New York Times*, A1.

United States Pharmacopeia (USP). (2004a). *Medicare prescription drug benefit model guidelines: Drug categories and classes in Part D*. Rockville, MD: USP.

United States Pharmacopeia (USP). (2004b). *Summary of USP approach and methodology to the model guidelines*. Rockville, MD: USP.

United States Pharmacopeia (USP). (2005). About USP—An overview. Retrieved September 2, 2005, from *www.usp.org/aboutUSP*.

U.S. Department of Health and Human Services (USDHHS). (2001, July 12). *HHS fact sheet: Medicare Rx discount card*.

Vaida, B. (2004). Lobbying—AARP's big bet. *National Journal*, 13 March. Retrieved March 17, 2004, from *http://nationaljournal.com*.

*Washington Post*. (2004a, March 18). Contempt for Congress (editorial), A30.

*Washington Post*. (2004b, March 15). Dealing drugs (editorial), A24.

Weisman, J. (2003, July 15). Budget deficit may surpass $450 billion: War costs, tax cut, slow economy are key factors. *Washington Post*, A1.

White House. (2003). Framework to modernize and improve Medicare fact sheet. Retrieved March 13, 2003, from *www.whitehouse.gov/news/releases/2003/03/print/20030304-1.html*.

# **POLICY**SPOTLIGHT

## Children's Health Insurance Coverage: Medicaid and the State Children's Health Insurance Program (SCHIP)

Kathleen M. White

*"It was once said that the moral test of government is how that government treats those who are in the dawn of life, the children; those who are in the twilight of life, the elderly; and those who are in the shadows of life—the sick, the needy, and the handicapped."*

Hubert H. Humphrey

### HEALTH INSURANCE COVERAGE FOR LOW-INCOME CHILDREN

Health insurance coverage for the children of the United States has improved over the last 25 years. However, in 2005 there were 9 million children under age 19 in the United States who were uninsured. Nearly three quarters of uninsured children live in families with household incomes below 200% of the federal poverty level (FPL) (Kaiser Commission on Medicaid and the Uninsured, 2004). This trend began in the early 1980s as the country saw an increase in child poverty resulting from the stagnating economic situation and an increase in single-parent families. The uninsurance rates increased from 20.9% to a high of 30.8% between 1977 and 1987 (Cunningham & Kirby, 2004; Selden, Hudson, & Banthin, 2004; Wise, 2004). During the same period, there was also a steady decline in the percentage of private insurance coverage for children. The Medicaid program was not able to address this worsening situation, as many of the children came from homes that did not meet Medicaid eligibility criteria. An expansion of public coverage was needed, and the State Children's Health Insurance Program (SCHIP) was the answer.

## PUBLIC HEALTH INSURANCE COVERAGE FOR CHILDREN

### Medicaid

Medicaid is a federal entitlement program enacted in 1965 that guarantees eligible children access to a health care benefit package with little or no cost to them or their families. It is jointly financed and administered by the federal and state governments. The federal government has established minimum standards for the Medicaid program, including eligibility requirements and the minimum benefit package, and the states administer the program within those parameters. The states may vary their programs if they receive permission in the form of a "waiver" to depart from the federal standards, which has resulted in significant variation among the states.

Because of the increasing uninsurance rates between 1984 and 1990, which reached a high of 30%, the Medicaid program implemented several poverty-related expansions to include many poor and near-poor children who were not eligible for welfare, the traditional pathway to receive Medicaid coverage (Selden et al., 2004). States were required to cover children 6 years of age and under from families earning up to 133% of the FPL and were allowed to expand coverage to include families earning up to 185% of the FPL and still receive federal matching funds (Lo Sasso & Buchmueller, 2004). "From 1988 to 1998, the proportion of children insured through Medicaid increased from 15.6% to 19.8%. At the same time, the percentage of children without health insurance increased from 13.1% to 15.4%, mostly as a result of fewer children being covered by employer-sponsored health insurance" (Centers for Medicare and Medicaid Services [CMS], 2005). However, many low-income children who were above the poverty level were still not eligible for these Medicaid expansion programs, and it was widely recognized that

something else was needed to address the coverage gap for low-income children not eligible for Medicaid.

### SCHIP

After the defeat of President Bill Clinton's universal health insurance plan, many in Congress still felt that it was time to expand health care coverage to the most vulnerable in the population; children became a likely choice. In 1997, SCHIP was enacted as part of Title XXI of the Social Security Act (Balanced Budget Act of 1997, PL 105-33). This legislation provided health insurance coverage to children, up to age 19, in low-income families that were not eligible for Medicaid because the family income was too high to qualify for Medicaid or that were not covered by private health insurance, often because the family income was too low for them to afford the private coverage. The SCHIP legislation apportioned $40 billion in federal matching funds over a 10-year period to allow participating states to receive federal contributions to expand Medicaid eligibility, to create a new health care coverage program under the SCHIP legislation, or to develop a program that combined Medicaid with a new program. Under SCHIP the states could provide health care coverage to children in families earning up to 200% of the FPL. The SCHIP program provided the funds to the states, not to the individual as in Medicaid, and the states could design the program to meet their own needs (Table 15-1).

The procedure for the development of the SCHIP programs was similar to that of Medicaid. The state must develop a program plan and submit it to CMS for approval. CMS must approve or disapprove the plan within 90 days of submission. States are allowed to modify the state plan by again submitting it to CMS for approval. The amount of federal funding for each state participating in SCHIP is defined in the statute appropriation, with annual allotments determined by a statutory formula based on the number of children and the state cost factor. The state cost factor is a geographic factor based on the annual wages in the health care industry for that state. The state plan must address eligibility standards, enrollment caps, disenrollment policies, type of health benefits covered, basic

**TABLE 15-1** Federal Poverty Level Percentages: 2005 Poverty Level Guidelines, All States (Except Alaska and Hawaii) and the District of Columbia

| FAMILY SIZE | PERCENT OF POVERTY | | | | | | | | |
|---|---|---|---|---|---|---|---|---|---|
| | 100% | 120% | 133% | 135% | 150% | 175% | 185% | 200% | 250% |
| **ANNUAL GUIDELINES** | | | | | | | | | |
| 1 | 9,570.00 | 11,484.00 | 12,728.10 | 12,919.50 | 14,355.00 | 16,747.50 | 17,704.50 | 19,140.00 | 23,925.00 |
| 2 | 12,830.00 | 15,396.00 | 17,063.90 | 17,320.50 | 19,245.00 | 22,452.50 | 23,735.50 | 25,660.00 | 32,075.00 |
| 3 | 16,090.00 | 19,308.00 | 21,399.70 | 21,721.50 | 24,135.00 | 28,157.50 | 29,766.50 | 32,180.00 | 40,225.00 |
| 4 | 19,350.00 | 23,220.00 | 25,735.50 | 26,122.50 | 29,025.00 | 33,862.50 | 35,797.50 | 38,700.00 | 48,375.00 |
| 5 | 22,610.00 | 27,132.00 | 30,071.30 | 30,523.50 | 33,915.00 | 39,567.50 | 41,828.50 | 45,220.00 | 56,525.00 |
| 6 | 25,870.00 | 31,044.00 | 34,407.10 | 34,924.50 | 38,805.00 | 45,272.50 | 47,859.50 | 51,740.00 | 64,675.00 |
| 7 | 29,130.00 | 34,956.00 | 38,742.90 | 39,325.50 | 43,695.00 | 50,977.50 | 53,890.50 | 58,260.00 | 72,825.00 |
| 8* | 32,390.00 | 38,868.00 | 43,078.70 | 43,726.50 | 48,585.00 | 56,682.50 | 59,921.50 | 64,780.00 | 80,975.00 |
| **MONTHLY GUIDELINES** | | | | | | | | | |
| 1 | 797.50 | 957.00 | 1,060.68 | 1,076.63 | 1,196.25 | 1,395.63 | 1,475.38 | 1,595.00 | 1,993.75 |
| 2 | 1,069.17 | 1,283.00 | 1,421.99 | 1,443.38 | 1,603.75 | 1,871.04 | 1,977.96 | 2,138.33 | 2,672.92 |
| 3 | 1,340.83 | 1,609.00 | 1,783.31 | 1,810.13 | 2,011.25 | 2,346.46 | 2,480.54 | 2,681.67 | 3,352.08 |
| 4 | 1,612.50 | 1,935.00 | 2,144.63 | 2,176.88 | 2,418.75 | 2,821.88 | 2,983.13 | 3,225.00 | 4,031.25 |
| 5 | 1,884.17 | 2,261.00 | 2,505.94 | 2,543.63 | 2,826.25 | 3,297.29 | 3,485.71 | 3,768.33 | 4,710.42 |
| 6 | 2,155.83 | 2,587.00 | 2,867.26 | 2,910.38 | 3,233.75 | 3,772.71 | 3,988.29 | 4,311.67 | 5,389.58 |
| 7 | 2,427.50 | 2,913.00 | 3,228.58 | 3,277.13 | 3,641.25 | 4,248.13 | 4,490.88 | 4,855.00 | 6,068.75 |
| 8 | 2,699.17 | 3,239.00 | 3,589.89 | 3,643.88 | 4,048.75 | 4,723.54 | 4,993.46 | 5,398.33 | 6,747.92 |

From Income guidelines. (2005). *Federal Register*. Retrieved February 21, 2005, from *www.dhs.ri.gov/DHS/whatnew/pov_guidelines_05.pdf*.

*For family units of more than eight members, add $3260 for each additional member.

delivery system approach, cost sharing, and screening and enrollment procedures.

SCHIP had several important goals: to expand health insurance for children whose families earn too much money to be eligible for Medicaid but not enough money to purchase private health insurance; to provide access to quality medical care without dependence on cost; to develop a system that establishes a medical home for clients; to simplify the enrollment process for a public insurance program; and finally, to provide flexibility and innovation for the states to design a program that met the needs of their population, such as cost sharing different benefit packages in order to cover a wider segment of the population.

The states have different SCHIP eligibility criteria, but in most states, uninsured children whose family income is at 185% to 200% of the FPL are eligible for the program with little or no cost to the family.

The coverage under SCHIP also varies depending on the state plan. Generally, all plans are required to cover well-baby and well-child care, immunizations, hospitalization, and emergency room visits. For states that opt for a Medicaid expansion, the services provided under SCHIP mirror the Medicaid services provided by that state. For states that opt for a separate child health program, there are four options for determining coverage:

1. *Benchmark coverage:* This is a coverage package that is substantially equal to either the Federal Employee Health Benefits Program Blue Cross/Blue Shield Standard Option Service Benefit Plan; a health benefits plan that the state offers and makes generally available to its own employees; or a plan offered by a Health Maintenance Organization that has the largest insured commercial, non-Medicaid enrollment of any such organization in the state.

2. *Benchmark equivalent coverage:* In this instance the state must provide coverage with an aggregate actuarial value at least equal to that of one of the benchmark plans. States must cover inpatient and outpatient hospital services, physicians' surgical and medical services, laboratory and x-ray services, and well-baby and well-child care, include age-appropriate immunizations.

3. *Existing state-based comprehensive coverage:* In the states where existing state-based comprehensive coverage existed before the enactment of SCHIP (i.e., New York, Pennsylvania, and Florida), the existing health benefits package is deemed to be meeting the coverage requirements of the SCHIP program.

4. *Secretary approved coverage:* This may include coverage that is the same as the state's Medicaid program; comprehensive coverage for children offered by the state under a Medicaid demonstration project approved by the Secretary; coverage that either includes full Early and Periodic Screening, Diagnosis, and Treatment (EPSDT) benefits or has been extended by the state to the entire Medicaid population in the state; coverage that includes benchmark coverage plus any additional coverage; coverage that is the same as the coverage provided by New York, Florida, or Pennsylvania; or coverage purchased by the state that is substantially equal to coverage under one of the benchmark plans through the use of benefit-by-benefit comparison (see CMS website for more information).

By the fall of 1999 all states had adopted some type of SCHIP program. Initially, in all but 12 states the coverage was given to children in families with incomes of least 200% of the FPL, allowing more near-poor families to meet the states' eligibility criteria. As of March 2001, 19 states had expanded Medicaid, 15 states had created a separate SCHIP program, and 17 states had implemented some type of combination program (Lo Sasso & Buchmueller, 2004). By 2002, SCHIP covered 3.8 million children and uninsurance rates among children had decreased to 18.6% (Selden et al., 2004).

## COMPARISON OF SCHIP TO MEDICAID

Medicaid and SCHIP are both joint federal- and state-funded programs. The Medicaid program is an open-ended entitlement program to the individual. Under SCHIP, each state is funded as a block capped grant to the state, with the amount of funding determined by a formula set by Congress. Federal matching money is about 30% higher under SCHIP than under Medicaid.

The SCHIP legislation prevented children who were already enrolled in Medicaid from enrolling in the SCHIP program, preventing the states from shifting children from Medicaid to SCHIP and taking advantage of the more generous matching funds under SCHIP. The legislation set up a procedure that required all SCHIP applicants to be screened for Medicaid eligibility as part of the SCHIP application process. It has been noted that this screening requirement has had an indirect effect on increasing the numbers eligible for and enrolled in Medicaid (Government Accountability Office [GAO], 2000). The increased number of children covered by Medicaid because of SCHIP has been important in reducing the total number of uninsured children in the United States. The innovation allowed in the application procedures for the SCHIP program has also been credited for better enrollment and reenrollment procedures for Medicaid.

SCHIP also offers states more flexibility in designing the program that meets their needs, including eligibility criteria and benefits. Income eligibility levels have remained relatively stable over recent years (Kaiser Commission on Medicaid and the Uninsured, 2005). As of July 2004, 38 states and the District of Columbia had set their Medicaid and SCHIP income eligibility levels at or above the 200% of the poverty level (Kaiser Commission on Medicaid and the Uninsured, 2005). Also as of July 2004, 33 states charged premiums or enrollment fees for SCHIP but were restricted from charging in Medicaid (Kaiser Commission on Medicaid and the Uninsured, 2005).

With the implementation of SCHIP, innovations in outreach and enrollment have been the hallmark of the program's success. Unlike Medicaid, SCHIP required states to include outreach efforts as part of their expansion program. The outreach campaigns were designed to get the word out to eligible families and have included mass media campaigns and community-based efforts. Many states created television, radio, and print media campaigns to educate the public and increase awareness of the new program. Toll-free numbers were used; the public could call in to get enrollment information.

The new SCHIP programs have also included reforms to the application process, making it simpler. The most important enrollment innovation has been the adoption of an electronic submission application that is a short, joint application for both Medicaid and SCHIP, eliminating the face-to-face interviews that had previously been required of all Medicaid applications. In addition, the resource and asset tests were also eliminated, which allowed applicants to self-declare their income. The final innovation relies on passive renewal so that 12-month continuous eligibility for SCHIP has been established (Figure 15-10).

## EVALUATION OF SCHIP

The SCHIP legislation required the states to complete an evaluation by March 31, 2000. The evaluation was to include an assessment of the effectiveness of the state plan in increasing the number of children with creditable health coverage; describe and analyze the effectiveness of elements of the state plan, including the characteristics of the children and families assisted under the state plan including age of the children, family income, and the assisted child's access to or coverage by other health insurance before the state plan and after eligibility for the state plan ends; the quality of health coverage provided, including the types of benefits provided; the amount and level (including payment of part or all of any premium) of assistance provided by the state; the service area of the plan; the time limits for coverage of a child under the state plan; the state's choice of health benefits coverage and other methods used for providing child health assistance; and the sources of nonfederal funding used in the state plan. In addition, the states were required to assess the effectiveness of other public and private programs in the state in increasing the availability of affordable quality individual and family health insurance for children; review and assess state activities to coordinate the plan under this title with other public and private programs providing health care and health care financing, including Medicaid and maternal and child health services; analyze changes and trends in the state that affect the provision of accessible, affordable,

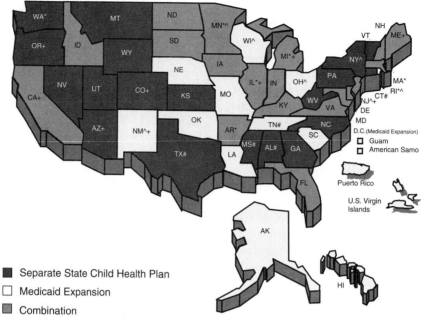

Separate State Child Health Plan

Medicaid Expansion

Combination

*Approved Unborn State Plan Amendment.
^Approved SCHIP 1115 Demonstration.
+Approved HIFA Demonstration.
#No longer has a Medicaid expansion program as of September 30, 2002, due to the aging out of the children phased into the Medicaid program under OBRA '90.

**Figure 15-10** State Children's Health Plan activity map (plan activity as of August 9, 2005).

high-quality health insurance and health care to children; describe any plans the state has for improving the availability of health insurance and health care for children; and make recommendations for improving the program. These evaluation plans were submitted to CMS. Enrollment data continue to be required for annual reporting to CMS *(www.cms.hhs.gov/schip/annualreport)*.

## THE CURRENT SCHIP ENVIRONMENT

The Kaiser Commission on Medicaid and the Uninsured (2004) found that between 1997 and 2003 the percentage of poor children who were uninsured declined from 22.4% to 15.4% and that uninsurance rates have declined even more dramatically for the group of slightly higher income children who were the main target of SCHIP—those with family incomes of 100% to 200% of the FPL. Uninsurance rates for that group fell from 22.8% to 14.7% in 2003,

a decline of more than one third (36%). However, participation in public coverage for health care is still a problem. The number of children eligible for public coverage who remain uninsured is estimated to be about 21%. An estimated 5.6 million children are eligible but not enrolled.

As of December 2003, SCHIP provided coverage to 3,927,000 children, a decline of roughly 37,000 from June 2003, when enrollment peaked at 3,964,000 (Kaiser Commission on Medicaid and the Uninsured, 2004). Declines were seen in 11 states and the District of Columbia, with Texas accounting for the largest decreases; however, 37 states continued to have modest increases. SCHIP has also seen enrollment as a substitution of public coverage for private insurance coverage, when eligible children with access to private insurance enroll in the free or low-cost public program (GAO, 2000).

## "The SCHIP Dip"

The original budget allocations for SCHIP included $40 billion over 10 years, with stable dollar allocations over the first 4 years. However, because of early projected budget shortfalls, the allocations for 2002 to 2004 were over $1 billion less annually to the SCHIP program than in the previous 4 years. States that had not spent their full allocations in previous years could use that unused portion to help during these lower-funded years because the legislation allowed them to carry over unspent funds to the next budget year in the early years of the program. However, the dip in available funds for SCHIP also came at a time when many states were beginning to experience budget constraints or shortfalls and has led most states to make cuts in their Medicaid and SCHIP program budgets. Some of the cutbacks have included reduction in the eligibility requirements, enrollment caps or freezes on enrollment, increased premiums, increased cost-sharing amounts, and limited outreach and marketing efforts. The Kaiser Commission on Medicaid and the Uninsured (2004) found that in most states outreach funds were cut in 2002 and not restored in 2003. In addition, four states cut eligibility levels, one state imposed an enrollment cap, several states increased premiums, and nine states cut or restricted the benefits (Kaiser Commission on Medicaid and the Uninsured, 2004). The return of double-digit health care inflation, causing increases in health insurance costs, rising unemployment, and increased child poverty rates, has contributed to continued decreases in private insurance coverage since 2000 (Cunningham & Kirby, 2004).

## Successes in the SCHIP Programs

After the passage of SCHIP in 1997 the Massachusetts state plan for SCHIP took advantage of an allowance to use SCHIP dollars with the federal match to subsidize employer-sponsored insurance premiums (Mitchell & Osber, 2002). These employer-sponsored plans must meet the various federal criteria regarding eligibility, benefit package, and cost sharing, and the legislation required employers to contribute at least 60% toward the cost of the premium. In addition, the states have to demonstrate that subsidizing the employer-sponsored health insurance is cost effective, meaning that the cost of the subsidy is no more than what it would have cost Medicaid to cover the children in the family. Maryland, Mississippi, New Jersey, Virginia, and Wisconsin have also gained approval to use SCHIP dollars for premium assistance. However, the Massachusetts program is unique in that it offers this premium assistance also to small employers, thereby increasing the number of employers offering health insurance coverage as well as the number of employees receiving the coverage (see *Massachusetts' Strategy for Financing Care for the Uninsured*, earlier in this chapter).

New York's SCHIP program was developed from an existing statewide health insurance program called Child Health Plus. The New York SCHIP program expanded the age eligibility from 13 to 19 years, included an expanded benefit package, changed the family premium structure, and introduced a facilitated and combined enrollment procedure for SCHIP and Medicaid. The new program was provided by an expanded network of managed care providers throughout the state, and vigorous marketing and outreach policies were used. The New York SCHIP program increased the number of children being covered by the state's public program from 70,000 in 1994 to 590,000 in 2001, making it the nation's largest SCHIP program (Dick et al., 2005). The SCHIP program included black and Hispanic children, more New York City residents, more children from lower income families, and more children from families with parents not working. Word of mouth was the most common means by which families heard about the program, but a greater proportion of SCHIP enrollees heard about SCHIP from the marketing or outreach sources. In addition, enrollment in the SCHIP program was associated with improved access as measured by a decrease in difficulty getting a medical care appointment and a decrease in difficulty getting a medical person by telephone; a decrease in the proportion of children with unmet health needs; an increase in the proportion of children with a preventive care visit; and an increase in the proportion of children who used their usual source of care for most or all visits from 47% to 89% (Dick et al., 2004; Szilagyi et al., 2004). These improvements occurred even in children who had been insured through other systems, both public and private, pointing to the importance of coordination and continuity of care (Szilagyi et al., 2004).

### SCHIP Program Difficulties

Although successful in improving access to and satisfaction with health care for its enrollees (Dick et al., 2004) the SCHIP program in Florida, along with six other states, implemented a freeze on enrollment in July 2003 and started a waiting list for the program. In March of 2004, funds were allocated to enroll the children that were on the waiting list as of March 11, 2004, and families that had joined the waiting list after that date were informed that they must reapply during some future open enrollment period. In addition, there are new rules and procedure changes for Florida SCHIP: children are no longer eligible for the program if they have access to health insurance through a family member's group health plan or employer health plan unless the cost is more than 5% of the family's income; new verification of income requirements are imposed for renewal, including pay stubs, written documents, wage and earning statements, and federal tax returns; dental benefits were reduced; and finally, children whose families are late with premium payments will be barred from the program for 6 months. The biggest effect of the freeze on enrollment is that it is likely to deter families who are Medicaid-eligible from submitting an application, because they do not understand that their application will still be screened for Medicaid coverage and they will be enrolled in Medicaid if eligible (Ross, 2004).

Texas, facing a budget shortfall in 2003, reduced budget allocations for its Medicaid and SCHIP programs at a time when Texas had one of the nation's lowest rates of employer-sponsored coverage and the highest rate of uninsured (Dunkelberg & O'Malley, 2004). These budget cuts have resulted in significant policy changes to eligibility for and benefits of the programs. The SCHIP eligibility changes were designed to reduce continued or new coverage by reducing continuous coverage from 12 months to 6 months, establishing a 90-day waiting period, require higher premiums for families with incomes between 101% and 150% of the FPL, including new

income and asset tests for eligibility, and increasing the cost sharing. The benefit reductions included elimination of dental, hospice, and skilled nursing care, tobacco cessation, and vision care and eyeglasses and a reduction of 50% in coverage of mental health and substance abuse services (Dunkelberg & O'Malley, 2004). The data show that the Florida SCHIP enrollment has dropped by more than 149,000, or 29%, in response to the changes, with the biggest net reduction among children in families with incomes below the 150% FPL.

### FUTURE POLICY IMPLICATIONS

The SCHIP program has become an important source of health care for many children in the United States. As of 2003, the SCHIP program had enrolled almost 4 million children. In the same year more than 25 million children were enrolled in Medicaid. The goal of providing health insurance for the nation's children is widely shared by policymakers. Despite substantial gains in health insurance coverage through SCHIP, it is still estimated that only half of all children eligible for SCHIP are enrolled.

The SCHIP program had a remarkable beginning. It was enacted in 1997 with federal funds appropriated and available within 2 months of legislative approval. However, that meant the federal rules governing the program had not been written, but states still were required to submit their plans in order to get the funding. So during that early time, the policy rules were being written as states were planning and implementing programs, which in the end required modifications to be made.

Despite the accomplishments of the SCHIP program and the Medicaid expansion, there are still shortcomings of the SCHIP program that need to be addressed. For instance, there is variation in state eligibility criteria, with income caps ranging from 133% to 400% or higher of the FPL. If uniform eligibility requirements were implemented, it has been estimated that many more children would be covered and that the rates of uninsurance overall could be dramatically reduced.

The SCHIP program also lacks a uniform information management system that can produce data to assess the ongoing effect of the program or the evidence to show that certain enrollment procedures or outreach efforts produce greater results.

Another big concern is the potential shortfall in federal funding at a time when states are experiencing their own fiscal constraints and limited budgets. The state response to date has been to cut outreach efforts, change renewal criteria, and increase cost sharing. These are all efforts that were associated with the initial successes of the program. The ramifications of these changes are uncertain at present but may increase the number of children leaving the program.

The "crowd out" provision of the SCHIP legislation and the rules that followed were developed to ensure that SCHIP did not crowd out or substitute for existing employer-sponsored coverage. However, this created inequities across the program. Some states permitted children to be enrolled if they met the eligibility criteria. Other states developed policies to exempt children from SCHIP if they had access to employer-sponsored coverage, even if the family met the income thresholds. This was especially difficult for families with children with special health care needs, who were often carrying a high-cost catastrophic insurance plan.

Several provisions of the SCHIP program, such as the simplified enrollment procedures, the lack of a resource or asset test, and the longer eligibility for coverage, have contributed to reducing the stigma associated with a public assistance program. This occurred at a time when the Medicaid program distanced itself from the Aid to Families of Dependent Children program, which also had the stigma of welfare and which was very restrictive. These have had positive results in getting those children and families most needing the program to apply and to get the appropriate coverage. SCHIP was originally funded as a 10-year block grant and is scheduled to be up for reauthorization in 2007.

The program has had many successes. The evaluations have shown that improvements have occurred in different states and under different types of programs, reinforcing the conclusion that SCHIP is having a positive impact on the lives of children who enroll and their families (Kenney & Chang, 2004). There is strong evidence to show that insurance improves access to health care and health outcomes. The system needs to focus on what is most needed to keep our children healthy and on programs that meet the needs of children. However, there has been a lack of focus on quality. Critics have suggested that Congress needs to develop a core set of quality measures as part of the reauthorization. However, policymakers are constrained by fiscal realities that require them to balance the budget. This creates an uncertain future for SCHIP. The federal and state government partnership of SCHIP may have to develop other creative policy options in order to take care of the health of our children while retaining the flexibility of SCHIP across states, resisting temptations to define a standard benefit package, considering options to extend SCHIP to currently excluded children, and enhancing coordination with Medicaid.

## *Key Points*

- SCHIP, as a partner to Medicaid, has resulted in a significant increase in health care coverage for near-poor children.
- The number of uninsured Americans is likely to increase again in the next couple of years because of the continuing increase in costs of private health insurance and the erosion of employer-based health insurance.
- During the 2007 reauthorization of SCHIP, it will be important to preserve the flexibility of the current SCHIP program, allowing states to meet the local and regional health care needs of their children.

## *Web Resources*

**Commonwealth Fund**
*www.cmwf.org*
**Kaiser Family Foundation**
*www.kff.org*
**Medicaid—Centers for Medicare and Medicaid Services**
*www.cms.hhs.gov/medicaid*
**SCHIP—Centers for Medicare and Medicaid Services**
*www.cms.hhs.gov/schip*

## REFERENCES

Centers for Medicare and Medicaid Services (CMS). (2005). State Children's Health Insurance Program. Retrieved October 1, 2005, from *www.cms.hhs.gov/schip.*

Cunningham, P., & Kirby, J. (2004). Children's health coverage: A quarter-century of change. *Health Affairs 23*(5), 27-38.

Dick, A. W., Brach, C., Allison, A., Shenkman, E., Shone, L. R., et al. (2004). SCHIP's impact in three states: How do the most vulnerable children fare? *Health Affairs 23*(5), 63-75.

Dick, A. W., Klein, J. D., Shone, L. P., Zwanziger, J., Yu, H., & Szilagyi, P. G. (2005). The evolution of the state children's health insurance program (SCHIP) in New York: Changing program features and enrollee characteristics. *Pediatrics, 116*(6), e542-e550.

Dunkelberg, A., & O'Malley, M. (2004). *Children's Medicaid and SCHIP in Texas: Tracking the impact of budget cuts.* Washington, DC: The Kaiser Commission on Medicaid and the Uninsured.

Government Accountability Office (GAO). (2000). *Medicaid and SCHIP: Comparison of outreach, enrollment practices and benefits.* GAO/HEHO-00-86. Washington, DC: GAO.

Kaiser Commission on Medicaid and the Uninsured. (2004). *SCHIP program enrollment: December 2003 update.* Washington, DC: Kaiser Commission.

Kaiser Commission on Medicaid and the Uninsured. (2005). Enrolling uninsured low-income children in Medicaid and SCHIP. Washington, DC: Kaiser Commission.

Kenney, G., & Chang, D. (2004). The state children's health insurance program: Successes, shortcomings, and challenges. *Health Affairs 23*(5), 51-62.

Lo Sasso, A. T., & Buchmueller, T. C. (2004). The effect of the state children's health insurance program on health insurance coverage. *Journal of Health Economics 23*(8), 1059-1082.

Mitchell, J. B., & Osber, D. S. (2002). Using Medicaid/SCHIP to insure working families: The Massachusetts experience. *Health Care Financing Review, 23*(3), 35-45.

Ross, D. C. (2004). *Update on the Florida SCHIP enrollment freeze.* Washington, DC: The Kaiser Commission on Medicaid and the Uninsured.

Selden, T. M., Hudson, J. L., & Banthin, J. S. (2004). Tracking changes in eligibility and coverage among children, 1996-2002. *Health Affairs 23*(5), 39-50.

Szilagyi, P. G., Dick, A. W., Klein, J. D., Shone, L. P., Zwanziger, J., & McInerny, T. (2004). Improved access and quality of care after enrollment in the New York state children's health insurance program (SCHIP). *Pediatrics 113*(5), e395-e404.

Wise, P. H. (2004). The transformation of child health in the United States. *Health Affairs 23*(5), 9-25.

# *Taking Action*  Kaye Bender

## Using Private Funds to Improve School Health

*"Small opportunities are often the beginning of great enterprises."*

DEMOSTHENES

Called yet again to an impromptu meeting of state agency representatives, I was not looking forward to one more tedious discussion about the health needs of our state and the creative ways in which we might address them. This is a cynical-sounding statement, perhaps, but a realistic one nonetheless. I have lived in Mississippi and have worked in state government long enough that my expectations about the long-term outcomes of impromptu meetings of this nature are typically skeptical. However, as the meeting progressed, I became intrigued with the private foundation representative who had requested the audience. She asked one simple question of the group: "If you had $1 million in private funds to leverage federal resources, what would you do to significantly alter local health policy and health systems in our state?" Now, that is a question I could get my arms around. So, I said simply, "I would invest that money in school nurses, and I would assure their placement with a sustainable resource." Almost simultaneously the Medicaid Director said, "I would improve the health of our school-aged Medicaid population." Viola! We had a policy match!

## IDENTIFICATION OF A COMMON GOAL FOR FOUR STATE AGENCIES

It isn't a new idea that school nurses significantly contribute to improving the health status of school-aged children (Adams & Johnson, 2000). Even Mississippi has a strong history of using school health nurses for students, especially those with special health care needs. Our state has also produced evidence that school health nurses are an influential factor in reducing teen pregnancy, drug and alcohol use, tobacco use, and school dropout rates (Baird et al., 2000). At the time of the initiation of this project in 2001, four basic models of school nursing existed in the state:

- An individual school nurse model whereby school nurses are funded by various funding sources with varying job descriptions
- School nurses funded for the specific purpose of providing services to children with special health care needs, such as Title I
- School nurses funded to provide specific health education and health promotion aimed at reducing or eliminating tobacco use by the school-aged population
- School-based clinics staffed with nurses, nurse practitioners, and other school health personnel as part of a comprehensive team

While advocates for each of these models often point to anecdotal successes of the project, none of the models has a sustainable resource to ensure long-term viability beyond the life of the specific grants or local discretionary funds that support it. Historically, school health nursing services have been the first to be cut in times of tight public funding and related budget constraints.

The Medicaid Director had identified the percentage of children who received annual health screenings under the provisions of the Early Periodic Screening, Diagnosis, and Treatment (EPSDT) program, a well-child screening program for children at or below the applicable federal poverty level for their Medicaid eligibility age group. According to the 2000 census report, Mississippi's population is 2,933,216. The latest economic studies at the time identified 25.5% of Mississippi's population as being under 100% of the Federal Poverty Level (approximately 643,304). There are 835,021 children

under age 19 in Mississippi (Mississippi Census Report, 2000). At the time of the initiation of the project, less than 30% of the eligible school-aged children received annual health screenings (*Division of Medicaid Annual Report,* 1999). Searching for the evidence for this policy to be considered was not difficult; multiple examples of the relationship between healthy children and educational achievement exist in the literature. In a state in which the educational level of the population has been historically low, it seemed reasonable to consider any policy that might positively affect educational outcomes. Three state agencies found mutual ground in this proposed policy change: the Division of Medicaid, the Department of Health, and the Department of Education. Ultimately, a fourth agency was added when the University of Mississippi Medical Center School of Nursing became the grant administrator. The grant program was aimed at providing funding for a school health nurse who would be hired to administer and provide EPSDT services, basic nursing care, and general health education. The nurse would work with the local medical community to establish the screening program and a definitive link to the child's medical home. The policymakers were also excited to know that not one state dollar would be requested for this program. The matching funds were provided by the Bower Foundation, a nonprofit private corporation that provides grants to other exempt organizations for the purpose of promoting fundamental improvements in the health status of all Mississippians through the creation, expansion, and support of high-quality health care initiatives. These private funds would leverage the federal Medicaid dollars for the program. Mississippi's federal match ratio is 4:1, meaning that for every private dollar identified by the state, the federal government matches it four times.

## COMMITMENT BY STATE AGENCY PARTNERS TO CHANGE THE EXISTING SYSTEMS

The School Health Nurse EPSDT project was developed in accordance with state and federal law, rules, and regulations and clinical standards of practice. A Request for Proposals (RFP) process was developed to identify public schools willing to actively participate in the establishment of a school health nurse EPSDT clinic program in their local school or school district. The four partner state agencies agreed not to charge one another any administrative fees or indirect cost rates (the first of several policy concessions implemented to make this program work). Parameters for the applications were as follows:

- One school nurse per application would be funded.
- Each application would target children in a public school in Mississippi with age-appropriate nursing intervention referrals and outreach services.
- Applicants would be public schools representing a team of school personnel and local medical and health providers committed to participating actively in the establishment and implementation of a school health nurse EPSDT program in the school setting.
- Priority would be given to schools or school districts initiating new school health services.

Then the real negotiations began. For the project to work, a strong commitment from the state agencies had to exist, and there had to be a monitor, a conscience in a way, to ensure that the commitment remained strong through the project. Initial policy level commitment from the state agency partners are summarized as follows:

- *The Division of Medicaid* agreed to ensure the establishment of an auditable billing process; to assist schools receiving grants under the grant program in establishing that billing process; to coordinate with and assist the participating schools in billing processes for EPSDT; to monitor and audit EPSDT sites of service for compliance with Medicaid; to coordinate with other partners to remedy any compliance failures; to maintain data on the administration of the EPSDT service; to provide specific data as needed for monitoring and evaluating the effectiveness of the grant program; and to consult with and advise the development of applications for the grant program.
- *The University of Mississippi Medical Center School of Nursing* agreed to receive grant funds from the grant program and distribute the funds

to participating schools; to coordinate the development, distribution, and review of applications for the grant program; to provide technical assistance to participating schools regarding nursing protocol and practice and referral criteria; to coordinate all evaluation data and reports and prepare an end-of-grant report containing information on the distribution of funds, participating schools, and effectiveness of the grant program; and to provide the specifications for the area or building to be used as a clinic in the participating schools and the list of equipment required for the clinic to be certified.

- *The Mississippi State Department of Education* agreed to consult with the grant administrator in developing applications for the grant program; to assist in the identification of schools and notification about the grant program opportunity; to act as a liaison between the grant administrator and participating schools on all matters associated with the grant program; and to serve as the lead agency for selected educational billing components.
- *The Mississippi State Department of Health* offered to consult with and advise the development of applications for the grant program; to assist in the identification of schools and notification about the grant program opportunity; and to act as a liaison between the local county health departments and the participating schools for all public health matters associated with the grant program.
- *The local public schools and school districts* who submitted successful proposals were expected to agree to do the following as a condition for participation in the grant program: to prepare a grant application for submission within the RFP time frames; to provide the appropriate consents from primary care physicians, community health centers, and rural health clinics as part of the grant application; to designate space and renovate as needed for the clinic area; to hire a full-time equivalent registered nurse; and to ensure the maintenance of the on-site clinic and supervise the nurse. In addition, the applicant schools agreed to become providers of Medicaid-billable services

and to sustain those services after the close of the grant period.

The Bower Foundation, as the facilitator and funding source, agreed to provide the funding for the grants; to separately fund the development and beta-testing of registered nurse (RN)–specific billing software and to serve as the monitor (the conscience) for the overall process. A memorandum of understanding (MOU) incorporating the responsibilities of the statewide partnerships was signed by each of the Executive Directors of the state agencies. With the signing of the MOU, state and local funding challenges were matched with the goals of the foundation. We were on our way to changing health systems policy in the state.

## POLICY ISSUES ADDRESSED THROUGH THE DEVELOPMENT OF THE PROJECT

The project has been in place since 2001. Through the implementation of three phases of the project, 39 school districts from varied geographic areas in the state are engaged in the project. Eleven of these schools have sustained their programs 2 years past the end of the grant period. As the nurses are hired and the clinics are renovated and equipped for their Medicaid certification, training programs are developed and implemented in order to ensure that the nurses are knowledgeable about the EPSDT process, Medicaid requirements, software billing management, standards of school health nursing practice, and general well-child health care. Required training sessions are held on each of these topics, with speakers provided by each of the statewide partnership agencies, as well as other knowledgeable faculty. This cycle of the project is completed in approximately 9 months. In order for the initial segment of the project to get the program started in a timely manner, each partner state agency has to make the program activities a priority, with no interruptions delaying the time line. Otherwise, the first year of the project does not lay the needed foundation for a productive second year of screenings under the grant funding. The Bower Foundation has continued to be the inspiration in monitoring the progress of the grants and therefore also monitoring the ongoing commitment of the state agencies to the project.

## FACTORS IN SUSTAINING HEALTH SERVICES IN AN EDUCATIONAL SETTING

The initial report of the formal evaluation process was completed in December of 2005. Recommendations based on that evaluation define the project for the future and include the following key points:

- Administrative support for the program at the school level is paramount in the sustainability of the program; therefore turnover in education system administrative personnel was identified as a major variable in the sustainability of the program past the grant period. The future sustainability of the program depends on the organizational placement of the program inside the state educational system in which other education-related grants are administered.

- Turnover in administrative personnel in the partner state agencies, especially at the executive level, has not yet proven to affect sustainability as much as had been anticipated. The degree to which state agency personnel interact to support the project as a priority was identified as another major success factor. No changes are being recommended in the statewide agency relationships.

- Transition of an educational system to a health services system is a major change. Although several of the schools had previously participated in grant-funded or state-supported school nurse programs, participation in this project constituted the first time that schools had been providers of health services involving billing. There is a philosophical difference in managing a billing-based health system and in managing a more simple school nurse program. It has been a challenge for the schools to change their administrative focus. Ongoing training will be required.

- Productivity of the school nurse is the primary factor in sustainability of the program. Given the multiple needs of the children in the public schools in our state, there are always competing activities for the school nurse. Maintaining focus on the average number of children to be screened in a given time frame is often difficult for the nurse when other needs are also evident. The schools will need to make this program a priority if sustainability is dependent on third-party earnings.

- Accurate data on the number of free and reduced school lunches in any school are a strong predictor of Medicaid status. Schools that have access to solid data have been better able to plan for the number of children to be screened.

## *Lessons Learned*

Multiple lessons learned from this project hold relevance for potential replication in any public school setting:

- School readiness (the entire local educational system) for implementing a health services project should be a major consideration as the project is being developed. We identified this factor to be as important as the training and orientation of the school nurse.
- Invoice payments for the grant period should reflect performance indicators that are similar in nature to the final performance indicators with which the schools will need to comply in order to assist the schools with a smoother transition from the grant period to "solo" operations.
- Strong, clear, ongoing communication among all state agencies is a vital factor in the success of the project.
- Clear lines of connection between health outcomes and educational outcomes must be articulated early and often to school personnel.
- Communication about the project with local medical providers of EPSDT and other well-child services is necessary in order to avoid communication gaps that may become barriers to the link with a "medical home" philosophy.
- Performance criteria must be established early and consensus built on the evaluation parameters in order for the initial goals to be sustained throughout the project time frame.
- Flexibility among the key partners is critical to the success of the program. Throughout this project, roles have changed as the needs have changed.

The need for school health nursing services in the public school system has been a policy issue of consensus for multiple state agencies and child health advocacy groups. A method for providing a sustainable funding source for these services has not been as easily identified. Leveraging private foundation dollars to provide the matching funds for federal dollars has removed the argument about the identification of scarce state money for this purpose. Partnering with relevant state agencies that can provide the nonfiscal resources to support a program such as the one described in this Taking Action creates the infrastructure needed to remove policy and procedural barriers that may otherwise hinder the program's progress. Flexibility to respond to political and other environmental changes retains the creativity needed to keep the program moving.

## *Web Resources*

| The Bower Foundation |
| --- |
| *www.bowerfoundation.org* |

### REFERENCES

Adams, E. K., & Johnson, V. (2000). An elementary school-based health clinic: Can it reduce Medicaid costs? *Pediatrics, 105*(4), 780-788.

Baird, C., Southward, L., Dunaway, G., Haug, R., Green, E., et al. (2000; November 14). *Evaluation of the School Health Nurses for a Tobacco-Free Mississippi* (oral report of technical research paper). American Public Health Association.

*Division of Medicaid annual reports.* (1999). Office of the Governor, Mississippi State Government. Retrieved December 12, 2005, from *www.medicaid.state.ms.us./Annual_Reports/AR1999.pdf.*

Mississippi Census Report. (2000). Washington, DC: United States Bureau of the Census.

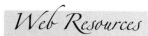

# 16 Contemporary Issues in the Health Care Workplace

Pamela Thompson, Laura Caramanica, Elaine Cohen, Veronica Hychalk,
Pat Reid Ponte, Kristin Schmidt, & Rose Sherman

*"Far and away the best prize that life offers is the chance to work hard at work worth doing."*

THEODORE ROOSEVELT

The current practice environment is creating an unprecedented challenge for leaders and clinicians as we try to align policy with the issues that we must address. There is no single framework for the discussion and analysis of the multiple factors that must be dealt with as we try to manage these complex health care institutions and systems. Health care institutions function as complex systems, and it is important that we consider the policy issues from this systems perspective. There are five key policy areas. They include the essential elements of the practice environment, education and practice partnerships, the impact of technology, regulation and legislation governing quality and safety, and the current and future models for delivery of care.

## ESSENTIAL ELEMENTS OF THE PRACTICE ENVIRONMENT THAT AFFECT POLICY

### EVIDENCE-BASED PRACTICE

At the turn of this century the Institute of Medicine (IOM) Committee on Quality signaled that there is not enough safety in the American health care system for patients and health care workers.

Alarming statistics on medical errors shocked the nation and left health care workers embarrassed and dismayed. This has resulted in greater emphasis being placed on achieving higher levels of safety through evidence-based practice (EBP). EBP is a process by which scientific evidence is systematically used to improve health care and specific patient outcomes and to determine the appropriate deployment of resources. The rise of EBP is partially a result of the fact that the use of scientific evidence as to what constitutes best practice in medicine is the standard of practice to ensure patient and staff safety. It is also gaining popularity because consumers are becoming more distrustful and concerned with personal risk, and they will no longer rely on expert professional opinion alone. The transfer of scientific evidence into practice, however, is a complex process. Changing provider behavior can be a real challenge, even when relative advantages of change are strong.

### PATIENT SAFETY

The first two IOM Reports, "To Err Is Human" (1999) and "Crossing the Quality Chasm" (2002), explain why an alarming number of medical errors do occur in America's health care system, citing three primary reasons: the health care environment acts in a compartmentalized way; there is a proliferation of complex medical technology; and health care workers are slow to accept the fact that they can and do make mistakes. The third IOM Report,

"Keeping Patients Safe" (2004), offers guidance on how to design the workplace of nurses so that safe, high-quality patient care can be achieved. It does so by explaining how an organization can implement the key recommendations made in the previous two reports (see *Health Services Research: Shaping Patient Safety Policy,* following this chapter). Although the same interventions will assist all health care workers, emphasis is placed on nursing because of the key role that nurses play in hospitals and health care systems. Patients are at risk when there are not enough qualified staff equipped with the appropriate information and when staff are not working in a way that promotes effective communication, collaboration, and the continuous striving for improvement. To achieve these, leaders and staff must be willing to acknowledge that mistakes can happen, learn from them, and set up a means to support patients and staff who are affected by medical errors.

The third IOM report also lays out the necessary patient safeguards for high-quality care that begins with leadership; governing boards and administrators must focus on safety and become knowledgeable about the link between management practices and patient safety.

Patient safety is also being addressed through accreditation standards of the Joint Commission Accreditation for Hospital and Organizations (JCAHO) and national initiatives such as the Institute for Healthcare Improvement's "Saving 100,000 Patient Lives Campaign" *(www.ihi.org).* This initiative seeks to improve care at the bedside and at a system level. The six changes that are identified are:

1. The use of "Rapid Response Teams." These teams of clinicians, known as the "Emergency Medical Teams," bring critical care expertise to the patient's bedside. Similar to resuscitation or code teams, they are activated by the nurse when a patient's condition warrants medical attention so as to prevent the patient from coding.
2. Care standards for acute myocardial infarction.
3. Reduction in ventilator-acquired pneumonia.
4. Decreased central line infections.
5. Decreased surgical site infections.
6. Medication reconciliation to prevent adverse drug events.

Hospitals are encouraged to join the campaign as a way to initiate large-scale, national improvements in care, quality, and safety.

Quality processes from other industries, such as Failure Mode and Effect Analysis (FEMA), a proactive risk analysis that seeks to find the source of problems before they occur, is being adopted by many health care organizations (see JCAHO Website). For example, a FEMA can be done on the hospital's medication system to determine what part of the system (prescription, transcription, administration, or documentation) is weak, resulting in a risk for errors. Public accountability is further spurred by activist groups like Leapfrog, a group of Fortune 500 employers who started looking at the quality of health care to understand better what they were negotiating as they were contracting and paying for health care services (see Web Resources). This group is striving to make physician and hospital performance measures more publicly known, and it is anticipated that this may well be followed by a systematic way for "paying for performance" by all payers.

## NURSING WORKFORCE

In 2002, the Robert Wood Johnson Foundation published the results of a study on the nursing shortage in the United States, "Health Care's Human Crisis: The American Nursing Shortage." The report provided strong evidence that the current nursing shortage sharply differs from those in the past and noted that previous failures to address underlying issues underscore the current crisis. The report describes the confluence of several environmental factors that have brought about today's shortage such as the aging population of nurses, the fact that there are fewer young people in the general workforce and a tandem generation gap in which nursing is not perceived as appealing, the rise of consumer activism especially pertaining to medical errors, racial disparity, and a ballooning health care system that increases the pressures of financing our current health care system as we know it.

In addition to working under the pressures of this shortage, nurses are challenged by violence in the workplace, downsizing, long working hours, the lack of enough technologic support to assist with safe patient handling, the need for improvement in the prevention of workplace injuries such as needle sticks and back and neck injuries, undue fatigue, and burdensome documentation processes and requirements that take so much time away from the bedside. Although there is hope that computerized information systems are being designed to support clinical decision-making and corresponding documentation requirements, the reality is that these systems either do not yet have the capacity to perform in a way that is easy and functional for the nurse or their impact has yet to be realized on a grand scale.

## PROFESSIONAL PRACTICE ENVIRONMENTS

Achieving a milieu that supports professional nursing practice is the shared responsibility of the health care system and nursing. Elements of professional nursing practice include autonomy, empowerment, respect, responsibility, peer review, accountability, and the continuous striving for excellence. Knowledge and skill of the nurse must be synchronized with effective teamwork, communication, and collaboration. Governance structures that nurses work in should employ their full contribution and active involvement in decisions that affect professional practice and patient care. Evidence-based practice should influence policy and practice in addition to providing for improved patient care outcomes. The prominence of the role that the nurse plays in health care should be more widely known. This is a shared responsibility of the nurse, who must demonstrate excellence, and the organization, which must promote practice environments that are designed to assure accountability for excellence.

## COLLECTIVE BARGAINING AND WORKPLACE ADVOCACY

Collective bargaining is again emerging as a solution to the nursing shortage. Over the past decade organizations have decreased nurse staffing and redesigned whole work systems, creating poor practice environments. This is different from the past shortage issues, which were mostly centered on wages. Today's unions are much different from their predecessors. The organizers are graduates of business schools trained in typical business school curricula such as sales, marketing, organizational behavior, and communication. They are intelligent and personable and have an evangelic flare.

Health care leaders are using organizational strategies to address some of these practice environment issues. These include shared governance structures, career pathways, educational incentives, increased visibility of nursing contributions, strengthening of nursing leadership, and education of the public and lawmakers about practice issues. Achieving accreditation as a Magnet Hospital affords a reputation for quality and professionalism, which attracts nurses. Partnerships between schools and hospitals are coming back as a solution for increasing capacity for new nurse graduates.

One of the core values of nursing is to keep patients safe through high-quality care. Nurses have expressed concern over being unappreciated and disenchanted in their jobs. They want to practice in a safe environment in which they have a voice in decisions. They desire control over their own practice. Leadership can support these efforts by learning about collective bargaining, routinely reviewing staffing patterns and work conditions, practicing management by walking around, communicating often, and building relationships with employees.

## PRINCIPLES OF HEALTHFUL PRACTICE AND WORK ENVIRONMENTS

The Nursing Organizations Alliance *(www.nursing-alliance.org)*, an alliance of over sixty professional nursing associations, supported the following nine principles and elements of a healthful practice and work environment in 2004. The Alliance asked each of the sixty associations to take the document through their internal endorsement procedure. As of November, 2005, forty-eight association boards had endorsed the Principles and were actively promoting them to their membership.

1. Collaborative practice culture
2. Communication-rich culture
3. A culture of accountability
4. The presence of adequate numbers of qualified nurses
5. The presence of expert, competent, credible, and visible leadership

6. Shared decision-making at all levels
7. The encouragement of professional practice and continued growth and development
8. Recognition of the value of nursing's contribution
9. Recognition by nurses for their meaningful contribution to practice

It is the joint responsibility of leadership and nursing to provide practice-rich environments that incorporate these elements. This builds the strength to trust and respect each other, provide high-quality care, and have balance between work and home while giving options for career advancement and continuing education.

## GROWTH OF THE MAGNET RECOGNITION PROGRAM

Achieving the coveted distinction of Magnet Status from the American Nursing Credentialing Center is a statement about the excellence of nursing. Organizations that have achieved this status have fewer problems with recruitment and retention of nurses because they provide good places to practice nursing, subsequently increasing job satisfaction. Some of the characteristics of this environment include greater levels of empowerment and control over practice, strong physician relations and support, and opportunity for learning and advancement. Magnet hospital leaders have greater visibility and responsiveness and support participatory management for a professional nursing climate. These facilities strongly support a self-managed and governed operation. High-quality nursing leadership, a clear organizational structure, an interactive management style, clear organizational policies, defined models of care, and opportunity for professional development are key elements of magnetism.

## LEADERSHIP COMPETENCY

There are many opportunities for nurses to lead. Some leaders seem to demonstrate their expertise as though they were born with the skills, and others must study to learn the skills. Nurse leaders used to have the time to prepare, experience, and adjust to change. Today, that luxury does not exist, and therefore a new set of leadership skills is required. Leaders today are faced with highly political environments, shifting economics, increasing business

challenges, and rapidly evolving technologies. Leadership education is critical for all leaders, whether in academia, in administration, or at the bedside (see Chapter 17).

In the IOM report, "Keeping Patients Safe: Transforming the Work Environment of Nurses," the facts refer to a safety strategy in leadership. The report states that leadership and management should be evidence based and that the precursor to evidence-based leadership is transformational leadership. Key characteristics of transformational leaders are their ability to see and guide others toward a vision that inspires those around them. Evidence-based leadership, then, is the transformational use of management theory and research for the purpose of making decisions, affecting change, and creating vision.

One of the unique aspects of being a nurse leader is the emotional side of the practice. The emotional side of leadership requires that leaders have the ability to perceive, facilitate, understand, and manage emotions. This is also called *emotional intelligence* (EI). Leaders with high EI have a strong awareness of self and others. They lead with the heart and manage the emotional aspects of the job. This is another key for the future success of nursing.

Nursing professional organizations are a great way to develop leadership skills. Membership and participation link nurses to better understanding, content, and opportunity through networks of mentors and peers. The Robert Wood Johnson Foundation, the Wharton School of the University of Pennsylvania, and many others have developed leadership programs focusing on critical thinking, negotiation, finance, management, and executive coaching.

## EDUCATION AND PRACTICE PARTNERSHIPS AND THE POLICY IMPLICATIONS

The persistent nursing shortage over the past decade, with no end in sight, has resulted in a focus on the need to build capacity for increased enrollments in our nation's nursing programs. Several organizations have worked to improve the image of nursing through campaigns like Johnson and Johnson's "Dare to Care," which uses television commercials targeted to recruit young people into nursing, and the nursing coalition Nurses for a Healthier Tomorrow. In addition, there have been a number of hospital and state workforce and professional organizational efforts. These efforts, coupled with a downturn in the booming economy of the 1990s, have led to increased enrollments in nursing programs and an inability to accept all qualified candidates; thousands of qualified applicants are being turned away (American Association of Colleges of Nursing, 2005). Major issues in building capacity in our nursing programs include a widespread nursing faculty shortage, clinical site availability for student training, and adequate financial resources to expand nursing programs. Nursing education in the United States is currently funded by three public sources: Medicare, the Nurse Education Act (NEA), and state appropriations (Thies & Harper, 2004, p. 297).

Over the past decade, nursing education programs have become more reliant on resources from local health care agencies to help build their programs because of inadequate funding for nursing education at the federal level, accompanied by reduced state resources. This trend will be difficult to sustain with the declining reimbursement for patient care services and health care access issues. To adequately address current and future nursing workforce needs and avoid a health care crisis, a federal policy response of increased nursing education funding will be needed (Thies & Harper, 2004).

Although no one disputes the need to produce many more nurses in response to the growing needs of our health care system, recent reports have highlighted the importance of nursing education and nursing service working together to produce high-quality graduates who are prepared to work in today's complex health care environments. The JCAHO (2002) in *Health Care at the Crossroads: Strategies for Addressing the Evolving Nursing Crisis* discussed the urgent need for nursing education and practice to work together to reduce the "continental divide" between the two settings. The IOM (2003), in a report on health professions education, recommended an increased emphasis on interdisciplinary education and development of core competencies to deliver evidenced-based, patient-centered care focused on quality improvement.

## EDUCATION AND PRACTICE PARTNERSHIPS

The need for collaborative partnerships will become more critical with a looming shortage of up to 800,000 registered nurses (RNs) by the year 2020 (Buerhaus, Staiger, & Auerbach, 2003). Recent research linking increased nursing education with improved patient outcomes (e.g., Aiken, Clarke, Cheung, Sloane, & Silber, 2003; Estabrooks, Midodzi, Cummings, Ricker, & Giovannetti, 2005) suggest that a smaller but better educated nursing workforce should be the direction of workforce planning. Innovative ideas that are emerging in this direction include the Clinical Nurse Leader Project, a nationwide project to prepare nurses with a generalist master's degree to provide clinical leadership at the point of care. A unique feature of this project is that the role, curriculum, and redesign of nursing care delivery systems is a joint effort between academic and clinical practice partners (Bartels & Bednash, 2005).

The current RN workforce is aging faster than other occupational groups. Over the next decade, significant numbers of experienced RNs will either be retiring or reducing their work hours (Buerhaus, Staiger, & Auerbach, 2000). There is widespread recognition that without significantly expanding the timeframe of nursing education, current nursing curriculums are unable to adequately prepare new graduates to transition into high-acuity and high–patient turnover environments without considerable orientation and mentorship. Results from structured nursing residency programs indicate that this is a promising future direction to ensure the smooth transition and workforce retention of new graduates (Rosenfeld, Smith, Iervolino, & Bowar-Ferres, 2004).

## CLINICAL SITE AVAILABILITY

The expansion of health professional programs including those for nursing has resulted in increased competition for clinical training sites. Lack of available clinical sites is a major limitation to nursing program expansion. Health care agencies are sensitive to the needs of educational programs but also must weigh the work demands that the supervision and coaching of students place on staff. Acute care rotations in clinical specialty areas such as obstetrics and gynecology, pediatrics, and psychiatry and mental health are required in nursing curricula today but are also in short supply. State boards of nursing are reviewing the potential that technologic simulation may have for replacing on-site experiences in areas with specialty shortages. Furthermore, the expansion of electronic medical records and medication bar coding are introducing new challenges into nursing education as health care agencies consider the security and privacy issues of granting students and faculty access to new technologies.

## TECHNOLOGY AND ITS IMPACT ON POLICY

Health care organizations have lagged behind other industries in the implementation of information technologies. The health care information technology structure as currently designed is not interconnected, resulting in considerable information duplication and unnecessary health care expenditures. Large health care systems with strong leadership, a relatively favorable payer mix, and access to capital have been able to finance technology more effectively than inner city, rural, or public systems (Larkin, 2005).

The slow adoption of technologies such as the electronic medical record, physician order entry, and medication bar coding, which have the potential to significantly improve patient safety and efficiency, led to a presidential pledge in 2004 to make interoperable health records available for most Americans within 10 years (Larkin, 2005). Reimbursement for technology investments continues to be a major policy issue. Well-designed electronic documentation systems have the capability to capture information from other systems such as the laboratory and pharmacy and equipment such as cardiac monitors and intravenous smart pumps. With a reduced nursing workforce, the need to explore the potential for technologic advances to improve patient safety and reduce workload demands will be critical.

### THE ELECTRONIC HEALTH RECORD

As health care organizations slowly shift to electronic health records (EHRs), there is now widespread recognition that EHR implementation is a major change for an aging nursing workforce and requires careful planning and staff education. Nursing leaders recognize that their involvement in the selection, design, and implementation of the EHR is a critical success factor (Cato, 2005). The efficiencies of the electronic medical record have been widely reported, but the impact of the change in work processes has received less attention. Nursing Informatics, a specialty that combines computer science, information management, and nursing science, has emerged as a key specialty to provide support for clinical information systems (Meadows, 2002). Although the shift to the electronic medical record may be difficult for some, technologically savvy younger nurses who grew up in a digital age are surprised to learn as they enter the profession that health care is not further ahead in the information age. Investments made in the level of an organization's technology may become a significant recruitment and retention factor in the future (Case, Mowry, & Welebob, 2002).

### TECHNOLOGY AND PATIENT SAFETY

Technology can be effectively used in health care to improve processes, standards, and protocols to result in better patient outcomes and enhanced patient safety. Organizations such as the Leapfrog Group and the IOM have strongly advocated the adoption of computerized physician order entry (CPOE). Movement toward CPOE on a national level has been slow as organizations evaluate the best practice strategies to implement this transformational technology (Cato, 2005). A revision of Medicare reimbursement guidelines to include a requirement for CPOE is one recommendation that has been suggested to expedite implementation (Lambrew, Podesta, & Shaw, 2005).

Medication bar coding, pioneered by the Department of Veterans Affairs on a national level, has resulted in a decrease in the number of incorrect medication administrations at the point of care. A challenging aspect of implementation has been the availability of unit-dose, bar-coded medications. Federal regulations will soon require that drug manufacturers apply bar codes to single-dose units of almost all drugs dispensed in hospitals (Smaling & Holt, 2005).

Current patient safety initiatives from the JCAHO (2004) include a requirement to improve the safety of using infusion pumps. "Smart pump" technology uses clinically tested software with algorithms embedded in intravenous pumps that can alert nurses to errors before they occur. This technology is providing organizations with an opportunity to improve patient outcomes by evaluating both actual and potential adverse event information around the administration of intravenous medications (Steingass, 2004). Remote intensive care management, better known as the electronic intensive care unit (eICU), is a growing trend in the nation's hospitals, which are struggling to improve care in ICUs while coping with a severe shortage of intensive care medical specialists. Preliminary studies done with patients who are hospitalized in eICUs have found a decline in mortality and in lengths of stay in critical care units where the bedside care is supplemented by remote staff (Breslow et al., 2004). The future work of nurses will be in a high-technology environment. Parker (2005) predicts that we are at the dawn of the digital hospital. Integrated EHRs, telehealth, robotics, "cyber" home visits, and smart equipment with decision support will be commonplace. A challenge for nursing will be to provide care in this high-technology environment without losing the focus of the humanistic side of patient care.

# REGULATION AND LEGISLATION GOVERNING QUALITY AND SAFETY

Consumers, employers, regulators, providers, insurers, and private and public health plans have prioritized the work of defining, measuring, and demonstrating health care quality and safety. Over the past decade, robust and sophisticated indicators of the quality of care and concomitant reporting systems have been developed. Public and private organizations and agencies have created both voluntary and mandatory reporting of quality and safety measures. Financial incentives and rewards are more routinely offered to provider groups and health care institutions for demonstrating higher standards of quality and safety. To ensure that

health data are protected during the provision of care or reporting about it, the Health Insurance Portability and Accountability Act (HIPAA) mandates systems of data security and integrity of personal health care information.

## HOW QUALITY IS MEASURED

**Accreditation.** Accreditation is a "seal of approval" given by a private independent group. Health care organizations must meet national standards of quality and safety to be accredited. Accreditation is offered by a number of groups including the National Committee for Quality Assurance (NCQA), which accredits managed care plans; JCAHO, which evaluates and accredits hospitals, health care networks, managed care plans, home care programs, long-term care programs, behavioral health programs, laboratories, and ambulatory practices; the American Accreditation Healthcare Commission, which accredits managed care plans; and the Community Health Accreditation Program (CHAP), which evaluates and accredits home health care organizations. Providers and insurers have criticized these organizations and accrediting processes because of the planned nature of the review process. They claim that these processes can result in an artificial or contrived compliance with standards. To improve the process and to assure "regulatory readiness" at all times, the JCAHO has moved to unannounced visits starting in 2005. This approach will assure constant attention, vigilance, and compliance with the regulatory standards.

**Clinical Performance Measures.** In an attempt to focus attention on the most critical issue in health care—the safety and quality of patient care and the measurement of outcomes of care, private and public agencies and organizations have developed systems of data collection and reporting of indicators that demonstrate clinical quality.

*Nursing-Sensitive Quality Indicators for Acute Care Settings and the National Database of Nursing Quality Indicators.* In 1994 the American Nurses Association (ANA) launched a multiphase initiative to investigate the impact of health care restructuring on the quality of nursing care. This project resulted in the creation of a national database of nursing-sensitive quality indicators known to be related to the provision of nursing care. The National Quality forum (NQF), a membership organization created to develop and implement a national strategy for health care quality measurement and improvement, underwent further consensus building to add to the initial list, resulting in NQF-endorsed national voluntary consensus standards for nursing-sensitive outcomes. The NQF's primary purpose of measuring nursing care is to achieve the highest levels of patient safety and health care outcomes in acute care hospitals. These indicators capture care or its outcomes most affected by nursing practice and are categorized into three groups. The patient-centered outcome measures include death among surgical inpatients with treatable serious complications (failure to rescue); pressure ulcer prevalence; prevalence of falls; falls with injury; restraint prevalence; urinary catheter–associated urinary tract infection for ICU patients; central line catheter–associated blood stream infection rate for ICU and high-risk nursery (HRN) patients; and ventilator-associated pneumonia for ICU and HRN patients. The nursing-centered interventions include smoking cessation counseling for acute myocardial infarction; smoking cessation counseling for heart failure; and smoking cessation counseling for pneumonia. The system-centered measures include skill mix (RN, licensed practical nurse [LPN], and unlicensed assistive personnel [UAP]); Practice Environment Scale—Nursing Work Index; and voluntary turnover.

**Medicare Pay-for-Performance Initiatives.** The Centers for Medicare and Medicaid Services (CMS) has collaborated with a wide range of public and private agencies and organizations that have a common goal of improving health care quality and decreasing unnecessary costs. These include the NQF, JCAHO, NCQA, Agency for Healthcare Research and Quality (AHRQ), and American Medical Association (AMA). ANA, AONE, the American Association of Critical Care Nurses, and other nursing associations, as well as individual nurse leaders, have been active participants in this work, aimed at improving health care quality and safety through standard setting, research, education, and public reporting. The development and implementation of pay-for-performance initiatives to support quality improvement and improved patient outcomes involve approaches that reduce variation in care and utilization by using evidenced-based best practice guidelines, shared decision-making with patients and families, and culturally and ethnically appropriate care. By linking the reporting of the quality indicators for each discharge, hospitals that submit the required data receive full payments for each Medicare diagnostic-related group (DRG). There is a broad range of programs that include disease management, physician group practice, and hospital initiatives. Many of these pay-for-performance initiatives are currently being piloted to determine feasibility of approach for reporting and the reliability of metrics. For instance, a pilot program is currently underway to test a population-based model of disease management, in which participating organizations are paid monthly per beneficiary fee for managing a population of chronically ill beneficiaries with advanced congestive heart failure and/or complex diabetes. The disease management groups and insurance companies must guarantee CMS a savings of at least 5% plus the cost of the monthly fees compared with similar populations of beneficiaries (see CMS Website).

## THE HEALTH PLAN EMPLOYER DATA AND INFORMATION SET

The Health Plan Employer Data and Information Set (HEIDIS) is a set of standardized performance measures designed to ensure that purchasers and consumers have the information they need to reliably compare the performance of managed health care plans. These performance measures are directly related to major public health issues such as heart disease, cancer, tobacco use, asthma, and diabetes.

HEIDIS is a set of standardized performance measures designed to ensure that purchasers and consumers have the information they need to make informed choices about their health care.

There is a groundswell of support by providers, insurers, employers, and advocacy groups to provide consumers with information about the quality of the health care that they seek. Quality reports include consumer ratings, clinical performance measures, or both. These reports are often referred to as "report cards" or "performance reports." These reports are often available through employers, health plans, hospitals, nursing homes, and community health clinics.

## CONSUMER ASSESSMENT OF HEALTH PLANS SURVEY

The Health Care Financing Administration (HCFA), which restructured into the CMS in 2001, is using Consumer Assessment of Health Plans (CAHPS) to report on consumers' assessment of their Medicare managed care plans. CAHPS was developed by the AHRQ, an arm of the National Institutes of Health. The CAHPS survey asks members of a particular health plan about the quality of care of their own plans. Their answers are reported and used by consumers to help them decide which plans to choose.

## THE LEAPFROG GROUP: A PRIVATE ORGANIZATION

The Leapfrog Group is composed of over 170 companies and organizations that buy health care. This organization also focuses on providing data to consumers and employers in order to improve the quality and safety of health care, decrease medical errors, increase public reporting, reward and recognize hospitals that demonstrate best practices and drive improvement, and help consumers make decisions about where to receive their health care. The Leapfrog Group most recently partnered with the Institute for Healthcare Improvement (IHI), a quality improvement organization, in a campaign to "Save 100,000 Lives" through implementing best practices based on evidence that are known to reduce variation in care and improve overall patient outcomes.

## CURRENT AND FUTURE DELIVERY MODEL CHALLENGES

### PATIENT-CENTERED CARE

Patient-centered and integrated care focuses on the delivery of health services across the continuum of all systems and settings. As we witness the emergence of collaborative models in health care, we realize how new generations of nursing care exemplify care of individuals and communities. To establish accountability and guarantee value, nursing care must embrace the panorama of health care processes and retain a broader, more global, political, public, and social systems perspective. The challenges of health care disparity, access, generational differences, chronic and disease management, and cultural diversity all affect the delivery of health care services and inform our practice as nurses (Cohen & Cesta, 2005).

## CARE MANAGEMENT: CHRONIC AND DISEASE MANAGEMENT

Shifts in the nation's demographics are causing substantial changes in the delivery of health care. The prevalence of chronic illness and disability associated with the demographic changes is influencing public health policy as we shift our resources from acute to chronic care. Although chronic illnesses are present across all age cohorts, the elderly consume a large share of our nation's health care products and services. By 2025 they are expected to consume one third of health care resources (Hospitals & Health Networks/IDX, 2003). State and federal health budgets will be profoundly affected as health care demands increase for the elderly.

As chronicity represents the fastest growing, most expensive segment in health care today, alternatives to the traditional approaches of acute patient care have fostered the growth of integrative models such as disease management. Disease management is defined as a system of coordinated health care interventions and communications for populations with conditions in which patient self-care efforts are significant (Disease Management Association of America, 2003). Disease management has been highly successful with disease states such as asthma, heart failure, and diabetes and is being used by insurers and employers in the treatment of depression, tobacco addiction, and obesity.

Key success factors for disease management include understanding the course of the disease; targeting patients likely to benefit from the intervention; focusing on prevention and resolution; increasing patient compliance through education;

providing full-care continuity across health care settings; establishing integrated data management systems; and aligning incentives (Todd & Nash, 1997).

Disease management is evolving from simply targeting those members most at risk for the disease to encompass educating populations about prevention and health promotion. This evolution cannot occur without the integration of nursing knowledge and practice into all elements of the program, from the planning phase and throughout evaluation and data analysis (Lind, 2005). The next generation of disease management will expand to a total population management approach through customized resources for risk identification and stratification, wellness programs, disease and case management, and end-of life care (Edlin, 2002).

Emerging technologies such as e–disease management have promoted applications of telehealth in the management of chronic illnesses without the challenges posed by geographic and time boundaries. It is defined as any application of Internet-based technologies to organize disease management (LeGrow & Metzger, 2001). These tools allow nurses to augment their practice, extend their reach into communities, and collaborate and partner with clients and health care professionals (Skiba, Sorensen, McCarthy, Brownrigg, 2005). E–disease management supports patient risk screening; population screening; guidelines and protocols; decision support at point-of-care; patient empowerment; outreach care management; cross-continuum coordination; team-based care; alternate encounters; and performance feedback (LeGrow and Metzger, 2001; Skiba et al., 2005). It has successfully been applied in the treatment of diabetes (Whitlock et al., 2000), cardiovascular monitoring and counseling (Friedman et al., 1996), congestive heart failure (Baer, DiSalvo, Cail, Noyes, & Kvedar, 1999), asthma (Finkelstein, Hripcsak, & Cabrera, 1998), and videophone "reassurance visits" for Veterans Administration patients with posttraumatic stress syndrome, schizophrenia, and clinical depression (Kleyman, 2001).

## AONE GUIDING PRINCIPLES FOR THE DELIVERY MODEL FOR THE FUTURE

Nursing leaders are helping to conceptualize and reshape the emerging health care system of the future.

To this end AONE has defined the primary question, "What are the principles that can guide us as we define future patient care delivery models and the nurse who will be providing care to our patients and populations in the future?"

AONE developed guiding principles to provide a framework for and help inform and position future nursing practice. These principles are grounded in the following assumptions:

- There will not be enough health care workers in the future to deliver care using the same models that define current practice.
- The work of the future requires definition with subsequent interpretation of that future work as it relates to role specification, competency, and education.
- The delivery of high-quality and safe patient care will be dependent on emerging technology.
- As leaders, we must not wait until we have all the answers, instead taking proactive, measured, and meaningful action.
- Our planning and implementation are grounded in the science of complex adaptive systems, with an emphasis on systems thinking.
- Dramatic change and revolutionary thinking are imperative to be successful.
- The delivery models of the future will require collaborative, multidisciplinary, and intradisciplinary approaches to care.

*Guiding Principles* outlines seven tenants to guide the dialogue:

1. *The core of nursing is knowledge and caring.* The actual work that nurses do in the future will change, but core values will remain.
2. *Care is user based.* Care will be directed in partnership with the patient, client, and family or population or community needs and will be respectful of the diversity of health belief models of all users.
3. *Knowledge is access based.* The knowledge base of the nurse will shift from "knowing" a specific body of information to "knowing how to access" the evolving knowledge base to support the needs of those for whom care is managed.
4. *Knowledge is synthesized.* The processing of accessed knowledge will shift the work of the nurse from critical thinking to "critical synthesis."

Synthesis occurs as care is coordinated across multiple levels, disciplines, and settings.

5. *Relationships of care.* Our knowledge and the care provided are grounded in the relationships with our patients, clients, and populations. The relationship will be multidisciplinary and include the full societal scope of generations, diversity, and interdependency.

6. *The "virtual" and the "presence" relationship of care.* The relationships will be dramatically changed by the increased application of technology, causing us to further define the relationship context as being "virtual" or "physical presence" and to know when each is required.

7. *Managing the journey.* The work of the nurse in the future will be to partner with patients, clients, and families to manage their journey in accordance with their needs and desires and available resources.

These principles are now being used to guide a dialogue among nurse leaders and staff to recraft current models of care to encompass a new direction for the delivery of service. The work environment with all its challenges serves as the backdrop for this dialogue and provides the depth and breadth to proactively drive policy development and implementation that foster improvements in our health care system. AONE's guiding principles are reality-based strategies that position nursing at the center of work environment transformation in order to meet the needs of our future health care providers and the demands of our patients (see *www.aone.org*).

## Key Points

- The current and future work and practice environments contain multiple challenges to the ability to deliver safe, high-quality care.

- The need to partner with education to create policy to support educational initiatives will only increase as the shortage of nurses presses us to produce more in a world lacking students, faculty, and preceptors.

- Emerging innovational use of technology holds promise and emphasizes the need to increase the role of nursing in the future policy decisions.

## Web Resources

**Agency for Healthcare Research and Quality**
*www.ahcpr.gov*
**American Organization of Nurse Executives (AONE)**
*www.aone.org*
**Centers for Medicare and Medicaid Services (CMS)**
*www.cms.hhs.gov*
**Institute for Healthcare Improvement (IHI)**
*www.ihi.org/ihi*
**Joint Commission on Accreditation of Healthcare Organizations (JCAHO)**
*www.jcaho.org*
**Leapfrog Group**
*www.leapfroggroup.org*
**Nursing Organization Alliance**
*www.nursing-alliance.org*

## REFERENCES

Aiken, L. H., Clarke, S. P., Cheung, R. B., Sloane, D. M., & Silber, J. H. (2003). Educational levels of hospital nurses and surgical patient mortality. *JAMA, 290*(12), 1617-1623.

American Association of Colleges of Nursing. (2005). New data confirms shortage of nursing school faculty, hinders efforts to address the nation's nursing shortage. News release. Retrieved May 16, 2005, from *www.aacn.nche.edu/Media/NewsRelease/2005/Enrollments05.htm*.

American Organization of Nurse Executives (AONE). (2004). *AONE Guiding principles for future patient care delivery.* Chicago: AONE.

Baer, C., DiSalvo, T., Cail, M., Noyes, D., & Kvedar, J. (1999). Electronic home monitoring of congestive heart failure patients: Design and feasibility. *Congestive Heart Failure, 5*(3), 105-113.

Bartels, J. E., & Bednash, G. (2005). Answering the call for quality nursing care and patient safety: A new model for nursing education. *Nursing Administration Quarterly, 29*(1), 5-13.

Breslow, M. J., Rosenfeld, B. A., Doerfler, M., Burke, G., Yates, G., et al. (2004). Effect of a multiple-site intensive care unit telemedicine program on clinical and economic outcomes: An alternative paradigm for intensivist staffing. *Critical Care Medicine, 32*(1):31-38.

Buerhaus, P., Staiger, D. O., & Auerbach, D. I. (2000). Implications of an aging registered nurse workforce. *JAMA, 283*(22), 2948-2954.

Buerhaus, P., Staiger, D. O., & Auerbach, D. I. (2003). Is the current shortage of hospital nurses ending? *Health Affairs, 22*(6), 191-198.

Case, J., Mowry, M., & Welebob, E. (2002). The nursing shortage: Can technology help? Retrieved May 15, 2005, from *www.chcf.org/documents/hospitals/nursingshortagetechnology.pdf*.

Cato, J. (2005). Winning support for a clinical information solution that meets nurses' needs. *Nurse Leader, 3*(1), 42-45.

Cohen, E. L., & Cesta, T. G. (Eds.). (2005). *Nursing case management: From essentials to advanced practice applications* (4th ed.). St. Louis: Elsevier.

Disease Management Association of America. (2003). A definition of disease management. Retrieved February 15, 2006, from *www.dmaa.org*.

Edlin, M. (2002). Total population management reduces future treatment costs. *Managed Healthcare Executive, 12*(11), 46-47.

Estabrooks, C. A., Midodzi, W. K., Cummings, G. G., Ricker, K. L., & Giovannetti, P. (2005). The impact of hospital nursing characteristics on 30-day mortality. *Nursing Research, 54*(2), 74-84.

Finkelstein, J., Hripcsak, G., & Cabrera, M. (1998). Patients' acceptance of Internet-based home asthma telemonitoring. In C. Chute (Ed.), *AMIA '98 Annual Symposium Proceedings*. Philadelphia: Hanley & Belfus.

Friedman, R., Kazis, L., Jette, A., Smith, M., Stollerman, J., et al. (1996). A telecommunications system for monitoring and counseling patients with hypertension. *American Journal of Hypertension, 9*, 285-292.

Hospitals & Health Networks/IDX. (2003). *Digest of health care's future*. Chicago: Health Forum.

Institute of Medicine (IOM). (1999). *To err is human: Building a safer health system*. Washington, DC: National Academies Press.

Institute of Medicine (IOM). (2001). *Crossing the quality chasm: A new health system for the 21st century*. Washington, DC: National Academies Press.

Institute of Medicine (IOM). (2004). *Keeping patients safe: Transforming the work environment of nurses*. Washington, DC: National Academies Press.

Joint Commission on Accreditation of Healthcare Organizations (JCAHO). (2002). *Health care at the crossroads: Strategies for addressing the evolving nursing crisis*. Chicago: JCAHO.

Joint Commission on Accreditation of Healthcare Organizations (JCAHO). (2004). 2004 National hospitals patient safety goals. Retrieved May 15, 2005, from *www.jcaho.org/general+public/patient+safety/04_npsg.htm*.

Kleymann, P. (2001, November-December). VA sunshine network test five technologies. *Aging Today* [Electronic version]. Accessed July 1, 2006, from *www.asaging.org/at/at-226/infocus_vasunshine.html*.

Lambrew, J. M., Podesta, J. D., & Shaw, T. L. (2005). *Health Affairs*. Retrieved February 23, 2005, from *http://content.healthaffairs.org/cgi/content/full/hlthaff.w5.119/DC1*.

Larkin, H. (2005). Uncle Sam wants your EHR: Will America's 'can do' spirit conquer IT's continental divides? *Hospitals & Health Networks, 78*(2), 38-53.

LeGrow, G., & Metzger, J. (2001). E-disease management. *California Healthcare Foundation*. Retrieved February 15, 2006, from *www.chcf.org/topics/view.cfm?itemID= 12864*.

Lind, P. H. (2005). Disease management: Applying systems thinking to quality patient care delivery. In E. L. Cohen & T. G. Cesta (Eds.), *Nursing case management: From essentials to advanced practice applications* (4th ed.). St. Louis: Elsevier.

Meadows, G. (2002). Nursing informatics: An evolving specialty. *Nursing Economics, 20*(6), 300-301.

Parker, P. J. (2005). Technology in the crystal ball. *Nursing Administration Quarterly, 29*(2), 123-124.

Rosenfeld, P., Smith, M. O., Iervolino, L., & Bowar-Ferres, S. (2004). Nursing residency program. *Journal of Nursing Administration, 34*(4), 188-194.

Skiba, D. J., Sorensen, L., McCarthy, M. B., & Brownrigg, V. J. (2005). Telehealth applications for case management. In E. L. Cohen & T. G. Cesta (Eds.), *Nursing case management: From essentials to advanced practice applications* (4th ed.). St. Louis: Elsevier.

Smaling, J., & Holt, M. A. (2005, April). Integration and automation transform medication administration safety. *Health Management Technology Online*. Retrieved May 15, 2005, from *www.healthmgttech.com/*.

Steingass, S. K. (2004, December). *Preventing harm with high-risk medications: The role of infusion technologies*. Orlando, FL: American Society of Health System Pharmacists Meeting.

Thies, K. M., & Harper, D. (2004). Medicare funding for nursing education: Proposal for a coherent policy agenda. *Nursing Outlook, 52*, 297-303.

Todd, W. E., & Nash, D. (1997). *Disease management: A systems approach to improving patient outcomes*. Chicago: American Hospital Publishing.

Whitlock, W., Brown, A., Moore, K., Pavliscsak, H., Dingbaum, A., et al. (2000). Telemedicine improved diabetic management. *Military Medicine, 165*, 579-584.

# How Magnet Status Drives Change in Health Care Institutions

Carolyn K. Lewis & Jan Jones Schenk

*"The quality of a person's life is in direct proportion to their commitment to excellence, regardless of their chosen field of endeavor."*

VINCENT T. LOMBARDI

The public is inundated with media coverage on the quality of care in hospitals, and consumers are asking questions such as "Who provides the care?" "How much does it cost?" and "How does the nursing shortage affect quality?" Many variables can influence patient quality outcomes, such as nurse staffing, nurse autonomy, control over the practice environment, effective communication between nurses and physicians, and a positive, supportive, educational work environment.

The American Nurses Credentialing Center (ANCC), a subsidiary of the American Nurses Association, has a formal recognition program for hospitals that recognizes excellence in nursing services. This program looks at outcomes from two perspectives. First, what are the results of the leadership and advocacy of the chief nurse executive for the nursing service administration and for the nurses providing the direct care? Second, are the nurses able to provide the care they do because of the value placed by the hospital on the nurse as related to the 14 forces of magnetism (Lewis & Matthews, 1998)? This chapter discusses the Magnet program and some of the organizational policy issues that have evolved from its implementation.

## HISTORY OF THE MAGNET PROGRAM

The Magnet Recognition Program for Excellence in Nursing Services is the most prestigious credentialing program for nursing services in hospitals, both nationally and internationally. The program was first developed to recognize facilities that provide excellent nursing care and was called the Magnet Hospital Program—formally initiated in 1992, with the first ANCC hospital receiving the recognition in May, 1994. The Magnet Hospital Program was identified as a method of developing nursing service organizations in hospitals in the early 1980s during a severe nursing shortage. The American Academy of Nursing commissioned a research study to explore work environments with high nurse retention rates and those able to recruit nurses during a time when most organizations had significant shortages (McClure, Poulin, Sovie, & Wandelt, 1983).

Academy members were asked to submit the names of hospitals from their designated regions that were exemplars of excellent practice environments. Of the 165 nominated hospitals, 41 emerged as magnets for professional nurses. These 41 hospitals shared seven core organizational attributes (Aiken, Havens, & Sloane, 2002):

- The chief nurse executive was a representative on the highest decision-making body.
- Nursing service represented a flat organizational structure.
- Decision-making was decentralized to patient care units.

**461**

- Administration supported nurses' decisions related to patient care.
- Good communication was identified between nurses and physicians.
- Units had self-governance.
- Management encouraged continuing education.

These 41 hospitals demonstrated excellence in nurse recruitment and retention by having uncommonly low nurse turnover. In addition, an intensive analysis of these 41 organizations revealed a set of shared characteristics and attributes, which became known as "the forces of Magnetism" (Box 16-1).

The forces of magnetism are the concepts underlying the recognition program. The program focuses on recruitment, retention, quality indicators, and standards of nursing practice, as well as these 14 forces, which serve as the magnet standards.

From the inception of the program, ANCC carefully monitored and evaluated the program and its recognized hospitals to ensure the integrity of the Magnet Recognition. Approximately 2 years after the program was officially launched, ANCC commissioned an extensive evaluation of the program. It was determined that additional requirements would need to be implemented to ensure compliance with quality and regulatory standards and an ongoing commitment from the hospital organization.

---

**BOX 16-1  Forces of Magnetism**

- Quality of nursing leadership
- Organizational structure
- Management style
- Personnel policies and programs
- Professional models of care
- Quality of care
- Quality improvement
- Consultation and resources
- Nurse autonomy
- Community and the hospital
- Nurses as teachers
- Image of nursing
- Collegial nurse-physician relationships
- Professional development

From McClure, M., Poulin, M., Sovie, M., & Wandelt, M. (1983). *American Academy of Nursing, Task Force on Nursing Practice in Hospitals. Magnet hospitals: Attraction and retention of professional nurses.* Kansas City: American Nurses Association.

---

A new component included a formal public review process and public testimony from community members during the Magnet Site Visit. This public input assured a 360-degree review of the organization from unit staff to community stakeholders. Applicants had to demonstrate through documentation and site visits that the forces of magnetism had been in place for at least 12 months before the recognition was sought, which ensured that the hospital had a longstanding commitment to sustain a magnet environment. It discouraged organizations from using the recognition program only to recruit and retain nurses instead of emphasizing excellence in nursing practice and high-quality patient care.

In 1996, ANCC released new standards and additional requirements for documentation and a public review process that moved the policy issues from organizational policy to public policy. In essence the implementation of the public process and the requirement for submission of information related to regulatory, legal, and labor findings against the hospital signaled a new and higher level of transparency. Candidate hospitals were subject to more extensive scrutiny, and only those meeting the highest standards would become recognized. This was consistent with the goal of ensuring designation for those organizations with the highest standards of corporate integrity, clinical quality, and community commitment. The name was also changed from the Magnet Hospital Program to the Magnet Recognition Program for Excellence in Nursing Services.

## FROM A NATIONAL MODEL TO AN INTERNATIONAL DESIGNATION

The first international pilot project evolved from the work of the international Magnet Modifications Task Force, which included participants from the United Kingdom, Canada, Latin America, and others. The group was tasked to identify and clarify what aspects of the program, if any, would require modification in order to make the program applicable in other health care delivery systems. Because the magnet program was designed from findings in U.S. hospitals, the international representatives were specifically asked to review the standards in detail and identify any aspects that would not transcend international boundaries. This work stimulated the international dialogue resulting in Credentialing International, a new service, in the fall of 1999 to assist international colleagues in pursuing credentialing goals. In partnership with Rochdale National Health Trust (NHS) in Rochdale, England, representatives from the Royal College of Nursing and ANCC and nurse researchers from the United Kingdom and United States convened an international project board to study and facilitate the application of Magnet principles in non-U.S. hospitals. Subsequently Rochdale applied and completed the magnet review process, and in 2001 Rochdale NHS became the first internationally recognized Magnet hospital.

## MAGNET RECOGNITION: VOLUNTARY OR REGULATORY

During the late 1990s the Magnet program was beginning to influence the hospital industry. The number of Magnet hospitals was small (Magnet-designated hospitals didn't reach double digits until 2000) (Figure 16-1), but nurse executives and Magnet advocates were beginning to discuss the possibility of a collaborative relationship between the Joint Commission on Accreditation of Healthcare Organizations (JCAHO) and Magnet designation.

During this time JCAHO began to use a survey rating system that recognized levels of quality. JCAHO accreditation with commendation was the

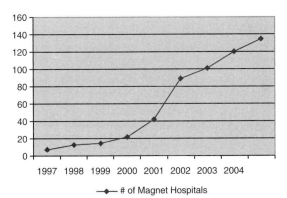

**Figure 16-1** Growth in the number of Magnet hospitals. (From The PRINE Group, LLC, 2005.)

highest level. Magnet-recognized hospitals consistently achieved this level of accreditation. It therefore seemed a logical next step to consider how JCAHO and Magnet might develop a collaborative recognition program. In these early discussions, the concept was thought to be one of "deemed status." In other words, Magnet-recognized hospitals would be "deemed" as having met (in fact exceeded) the JCAHO standards for nursing service. In addition, Magnet researchers were beginning to demonstrate that environments that supported nurses practicing at a high professional level, through the provision of shared governance strategies and commitment to professional development, achieved better patient outcomes as well.

There were two different perspectives about required accreditation through a regulatory body (JCAHO) versus voluntary recognition through ANCC. One group held that Magnet should be recognized for accreditation purposes and that efforts should be made to facilitate such a dialogue with JCAHO. In fact, by 2000 public dialogue had started both in the United States and internationally. The other perspective held that once a program received deemed status it was less able to act as a leader in raising new issues and standards. Deemed status in this case means the Magnet program would be recognized for regulatory purposes, much as JCAHO accreditation is recognized by the federal government and therefore hospitals achieving JCAHO accreditation are eligible for federal reimbursement through Medicare. JCAHO has deemed status from the Centers for Medicare and Medicaid Services (CMS) to serve as a quasi-regulatory agency. If Magnet received deemed status, it too would have regulatory clout but would also have to comply with whatever requirements these regulators would impose. The regulatory mantle would bring with it additional bureaucracy and expense associated with paperwork and potentially compliance with standards set by others outside of nursing. If Magnet remained a voluntary program, the ongoing program improvement focus would be more responsive to issues from nurses and the nursing community at large. Responsiveness is essential for the program to provide true leadership in improving nurse practice environments.

Moving from the realm of a voluntary recognition program into a formal regulatory accreditation program was not without its issues. ANCC had experienced these implications previously when its advanced practice certification examinations were recognized by the National Council of State Boards of Nursing for the purpose of licensure (see *The Politics of Nursing Regulation and Licensure* in Chapter 24). This transition from certification to a regulated examination clarified the limitations and controls that the regulatory body could impose on the process. If Magnet was to remain free to grow and provide leadership for nursing care quality in hospitals, perhaps deemed status wasn't such a good idea after all.

JCAHO was also experiencing some issues and challenges about the accreditation process (Office of Inspector General [OIG], 1999) The OIG of the Health Care Finance Administration (HCFA, now CMS) was increasingly critical of JCAHO's accreditation process and issued a report calling for significant reforms (JCAHO, 2002). Hospitals were also questioning the value of JCAHO as an accrediting entity as well as the cost required to support the process. The burden of the JCAHO accreditation process had significant impact on dwindling hospital resources, and some hospitals were considering using their state Medicaid survey process instead of JCAHO to qualify for Medicare funding.

Other institutions were troubled by the lack of information from the JCAHO survey about the quality of the hospital environment. This group viewed Magnet recognition as providing a better indication of their organizations' commitment to high-quality outcomes and preferred to use state surveys as the way to comply with federal regulatory requirements for reimbursement. State surveys were a known quantity and were much less expensive and intensive than JCAHO surveys. In the past JCAHO accreditation was assumed to be necessary for regulatory purposes and to satisfy the organization's public reputation. With Magnet as a viable option for quality review, hospital organizations would have more flexibility in achieving both accreditation and regulation standards.

Fundamental issues related to accreditation versus recognition continue to evolve. The Magnet program has always included a direct review of quality processes as experienced by both patients and nurses. While patient satisfaction measures have become standard in the JCAHO accreditation process, the issue remains that patients experience satisfaction primarily because of high-quality nursing care. The Magnet program recognizes that outstanding nursing practice environments assure high-quality care and thus attract and retain the best nurses. The Magnet program remains an influential player in achieving patient care quality, not through a regulated accreditation system but through a system of data collection know as *performance indicators,* which are institutionally driven.

Magnet, without becoming a regulator of hospitals, has had a significant influence on how hospitals function and compete. One example of the reach of the program's impact is illustrated in the penetration of Magnet-recognized hospitals on *U.S. News and World Report*'s Best Hospitals list *(www.usnews.com/usnews/health/best-hospitals/tophosp.htm).* In 2005 the list of 176 best hospitals by service category also included an honor role of 16 hospitals whose organizations were identified as having significant breadth of excellence in at least six specialties. Thirty-seven percent of the "Honor Role" hospitals are Magnets.

Voluntary commitment and compliance are key to the Magnet program and other quality-recognition programs like the Malcolm Baldridge National Quality Award (MBNQA). The MBNQA has long been recognized as the hallmark of organizational quality in the business world. A health care category was instituted in 2002, and the first health care recipient of the MBNQA was Sisters of Saint Mary Healthcare (SSM), a national not-for-profit Catholic health care system. St. Mary's Hospital Medical Center, a member of SSM, was also awarded Magnet recognition that year (Smith, 2003). By 2004 only three hospitals (two of which are Magnets) nationally had received this quality recognition. The most recent is Robert Wood Johnson Hospital, a Magnet facility in New Brunswick, New Jersey.

## MAGNET RECOGNITION: NOT JUST FOR NURSES

When organizations begin to deliberate about seeking Magnet recognition, many questions come from administrators, physicians, and other departments.

Is this a program just for nurses? Dr. Linda Aiken, one of Magnet's most well-known researchers, often says, "Magnet is *about* nurses but not *for* nurses. Magnet is *for* patients". Despite the research data about Magnet's positive impact on patient care outcomes, the internal selling of the Magnet concept to administrators and physicians can be challenging. How do these groups understand a concept that is primarily focused on nurses' work environment? How does Magnet have meaning (in the early stages) for key organizational policymakers?

The challenges that health care systems currently encounter can be mediated by achievement of Magnet status because of the focus on quality. In fact, the federal legislation known as the Nurse Reinvestment Act incorporates funding to help organizations achieve Magnet status. In addition, Magnet has proven to be a significant factor in physician recruitment and in retaining other key hospital personnel.

Institutions with Magnet status create competition with others for a qualified workforce. For those markets that do not have Magnet hospitals within a region or state, the first such designated facility will have an enormous advantage. Historically the first Magnet in a market has expended considerable resources in marketing and advertising the designation as a market differentiation strategy. The number of designated Magnets has been growing exponentially, by 600% between 2000 and 2004 (Figure 16-2). As of 2006, there were 180 Magnets in 37 states and two foreign countries.

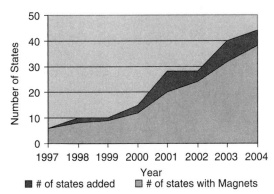

**Figure 16-2** Growth in state penetration of magnet hospitals. (From The PRINE Group, LLC, 2005.)

As the number of Magnet hospitals grows, competition revolves around organizational culture and quality improvement. At one time, hospitals were required to provide care based on "prevailing community standards." Now there are national standards based on quality-improvement outcomes; however, achievement of standards is determined by clear and appropriate institutional policies. Passive dissemination of knowledge to individual practitioners has not proven to be an effective strategy for changing practice. The stimulus for changing practice is the presence of peer hospitals with an imbedded culture focused on improvement. Magnet hospitals raise the bar in the markets in which they are present and compete with non-Magnets.

## MAGNET'S EFFECT ON ORGANIZATIONAL POLICY

Magnet hospitals provide significant data as a result of the voluntary reporting requirements of the program. The data about nurse retention and improved patient outcomes have resulted in a number of noticeable changes in the U.S. health care policy landscape.

Magnet serves as an impetus for facilities to develop policies on shared governance models, with decision-making at the staff nurse level. Magnet principles drive the facility to collect data and submit these to the National Data for Nursing Quality Indicators (NDNQI) for national benchmarking. Within shared governance models, nurses are represented at the unit level and serve on hospital-wide committees, which enables them to affect institutional policy.

### Nursing Involvement in Governance

Nurse decision-making is not an accidental or a casual process in Magnet hospitals. It is supported by an infrastructure for nurse involvement in decision-making at all levels of the organization. Organizations that formalize nurse self-governance processes in policy and practice benefit from the expertise of those who are closest to and have the most interaction with and opportunity to observe their patients. Formal systems of governance that are truly authoritative influence policy throughout the hospital organization. In their most advanced states, governance systems are interdisciplinary and have authority over all aspects of clinical nursing practice, even those traditionally viewed as the purview of management, such as staffing, budgeting, and scheduling. The development of governance systems requires organizations to recognize the patient bedside as a locus of control. Effective governance systems balance the nurses, teams, units, patient care groups, and organizational needs in their decision-making but also provide mechanisms for involvement and influence that are streamlined to reduce bureaucracy as much as possible. Complex models that do not deliver results are not tolerated, but there must be tolerance for the evolution of skills in group decision-making and group process. Evolved governance systems are interdisciplinary, with nurses playing a key role.

The key policy implication for such systems is the devolution of authority to governance groups. Not only are nurse managers and nurse leaders required to participate differently as coaches and facilitators, but program administrators, directors, and human resource professionals must be willing to seek and use advice and input from nurses. This can be a difficult task for organizations with entrenched, traditional management structures and philosophies. Although most organizations can easily adapt to supporting clinical decision-making by nurses, such as in nursing policy, procedure, and unit-based issues, the real challenge comes when the scope of authority expands to include budgeting. Because the budgeting process is traditionally the exclusive domain of nurse managers and directors, nurse input may be viewed as threatening. However, in Magnet environments this becomes shared decision-making.

### Patient-Centered Culture

Culture is described as a set of values, ideals, and belief systems that are shared among a group or organization. Nursing culture emerges over time. The nurse's cultural values influence the extent of the patient's involvement in the care and the quality of care. Behaviors for the various roles in the organization are culturally prescribed and affect the manner in which the nurse cares for the patient. An organization has a unique set of values, norms, and beliefs that are collectively held by its employees and that are passed on to new employees; this constitutes the organizational culture. This culture directly affects the nurse's set of values, norms, and beliefs. The relevance of organizational culture in a Magnet environment is that it influences performance and it reflects the vision, mission, and goals of the facility.

Nursing leadership must be sensitive to the "degree of fit" between the organizational culture and the goals of nursing. A good match in how the organization views its mission, philosophy, beliefs, and values is of utmost importance to the success of nursing. The organizational culture that has a supportive environment and that empowers nurses at the bedside encourages autonomous feelings of control over the practice setting. This organizational culture increases respect, improves problem solving, increases creativity and ideas, improves the quality and retention of nurses, and directly affects the quality of care.

### How Nurses Affect Policy

Policy is both internal and external to an organization. External influences include governmental regulations, marketing pressures, accrediting bodies, labor and professional groups, community and consumer advocacy groups, and economic and political trends. Magnet hospitals have realized significant improvement in patient outcomes, reduced patient lengths of stay, and improved nurse retention and recruitment. These result in significant financial benefits, as well as improved patient care.

In addition, because of "intensity of presence," nurses have a unique opportunity not only to observe the patient's (and family's) responses to the care experience but also to have a firsthand perspective of what system barriers and issues exist to impede the care process. Thus, nurses can be instrumental in effecting policy changes within the facility.

The knowledge nurses gain through their daily encounters with patients, families, and organizational operations is a valuable resource. Organizations that can effectively tap into this resource realize significant benefits. Magnet hospitals model nurse decision-making and have evolved systems for nurse involvement in institutional policy. Effective nurse decision-making systems share these common features:

- Unit-level governance
- Recognized scope of authority
- Visible governance systems that are recognized and consulted
- Governance outputs (decisions) that are systematically integrated into the organization's policy-making process
- Nurses as part of policy decisions, as evidenced by representation on hospital-wide committees

Nurses are "resource mobilizers" who are empowered in Magnet environments to exert control over that environment. Nurses have effected policy changes in staffing, collecting data on performance indicators and setting institutional benchmarks, budget processes, delivery of care models, safety policies, funds for higher education, recognition of specialty certification, and integrating evidenced-based research into the practice setting and have had input in creating hospital-wide information systems, such as the e-chart. The Magnet Recognition Program for Excellence in Nursing Services will continue to promote excellence of nursing care and the high standards of the nursing profession, as well as providing a mechanism for involvement in institutional policy.

## Key Points

- The Magnet Recognition Program is built on empirical findings about what is required to create a professional, supportive practice environment that attracts and retains nurses.
- Magnet recognition is a voluntary program that recognizes excellence in creation of a practice environment. This is not the same as accreditation or other mandatory standards hospitals must achieve in order to be deemed "safe." Hospitals seeking Magnet status must demonstrate a five-star level of nursing services.
- The impact of Magnet status on hospital markets and in consumer-focused media has grown significantly as data have increasingly shown how patients also benefit from Magnet environments.

- The key policy implication for Magnet environments is the devolution of authority to direct-care nurses. Moving patient care decision-making as close as possible to the bedside is the most significant factor in achieving both nurse and patient satisfaction as well as improved patient outcomes.

## Web Resources

**American Federation of State, County and Municipal Employees**—comparison of Magnet hospitals on 15 different measures including staffing (both day and evening), vacancy rates, and availability of continuing education
*www.afscme.org/una/sns12.htm*

**American Nurses Credentialing Center**— official Magnet site, including information about how to pursue Magnet status, publications, and a full listing of all current Magnet facilities
*www.nursingworld.org/ancc/magnet/index.html*

**Arizona Nurses Association**—article discussing Magnet status and a report analyzing the current state of Arizona hospitals
*www.aznurse.org/news_feature.asp?story=120*

**Ireland Office for Health Management**— article summarizing the Magnet master class presented by Dr. Linda Aiken and Jan Jones-Schenk
*www.tohm.ie/newsandevents/newsletter/20010702145313.html*

**Nursing Spectrum**—article on Magnets that includes a U.S. map illustrating the penetration of Magnet hospitals across the United States
*http://community.nursingspectrum.com/magazinearticles/article.cfm?aid=18469*

**PRINE Group: Why Magnet?**—a white paper for Sr. Hospital Executives on how Magnet recognition is changing the competitive environment
*www.theprinegroup.com*

**U.S. News and World Report—Best Hospitals in 2005**

*Continued*

## REFERENCES

Aiken, L. H., Havens D. S., & Sloane, D. M. (2002). The Magnet Nursing Services Recognition program: A comparison of two groups of Magnet hospitals. *American Journal of Nursing, 100,* 26-35.

Joint Commission on Accreditation of Healthcare Organizations (JCAHO). (2002). Healthcare at the Crossroads: Strategies for addressing the evolving nursing crisis. Retrieved on December 12, 2005, from *www.jcaho.org/about+us/public+ policy+initiatives/public+policy+initiatives.htm.*

Lewis, C. L., & Matthews, J. (1998). Magnet program designates exceptional nursing service. *American Journal of Nursing, 98*(12), 51-52.

McClure, M., Poulin, M., Sovie, M., & Wandelt, M. (1983). *American Academy of Nursing, Task Force on Nursing Practice in Hospitals. Magnet hospitals: Attraction and retention of professional nurses.* Kansas City: American Nurses Association.

Office of Inspector General (OIG). (1999). *The external review of hospital quality: Holding the reviewers accountable.* OEI-01-97-00053. Retrieved January 12, 2006, from *http://oig.hhs.gov/ oei/reports/oei-01-97-00053.pdf.*

Smith, A. P. (2003). Magnet and Baldridge: SSM Health Care's Journey for Excellence (part II of II). *Nursing Economics, 21*(3), 127-129, 139.

# POLICYSPOTLIGHT

## WHEN A HURRICANE STRIKES: THE CHALLENGE OF CRAFTING WORKPLACE POLICY

Janice M. McCoy & Susan McDonough Stackpoole

*"The smart thing is to prepare for the unexpected."*
CHINESE FORTUNE COOKIE

At Cape Canaveral Hospital the television announcers are relentless in their continuous coverage of the approaching hurricane. Every TV in every patient's room is blaring the same message: "Leave now!" The nursing staff is hearing the message, but their first responsibility is to ensure the safety of their patients as they are loaded into waiting ambulances for the trip to our sister hospital in Melbourne, Florida, 35 miles to the south. The wind is picking up, and anxiety is increasing as the staff hurry to finish their tasks, secure their areas, and evacuate to a safe location to wait out the approaching storm.

Hurricanes are a force of nature that challenge many states along the east and gulf coasts of the United States. Florida is especially vulnerable, and every community must be ready to respond quickly to protect its citizens and their property during violent weather. Cape Canaveral Hospital, one of three hospitals in Health First, Inc., is located 1 mile from the Atlantic Ocean in Cocoa Beach, Florida, and is under mandatory evacuation orders when a hurricane approaches (Figure 16-3). Coordinating

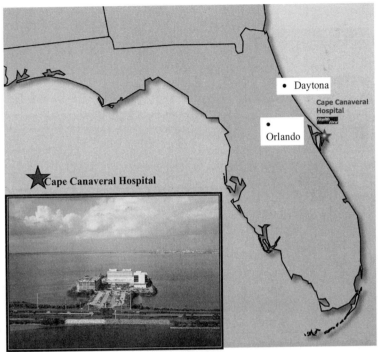

**Figure 16-3** Map of Cape Canaveral Hospital. (Courtesy of Cape Canaveral Hospital.)

the evacuation process is a challenge, as patient safety and well-being are a primary concern. Time is a critical factor to ensure that the patients are relocated, the hospital is secured, and employees also have adequate time to prepare their homes and their families for evacuation. All of these things must be completed before the causeways are closed and travel to safety is no longer possible.

Several hurricane evacuations in recent years highlighted problems and led to the development of policies to address nursing staff expectations and responsibilities and to define the consequences of failure to adhere to these policies. The ultimate goal is to hold employees accountable for their job responsibilities, at a time when the community depends on them, without risking the safety of the employees and their families.

## ANNUAL PREPARATION AND PLANNING

Hurricane season begins each June 1, but hospital planning and preparations begin every January. Health First has a Hurricane Task Force that is composed of representatives from all of the Health First entities. This interdisciplinary team meets to review the experiences from the previous year and to ensure that all of the policies address any issues that were identified. May is designated as Hurricane Preparedness Month, and all educational activities for staff and physicians are completed during the month.

### Before the Storm

Because of the nature of the preparation process, three planning phases have been defined: prestorm, during storm, and poststorm. The prestorm team includes all of the employees who are on duty at the time the evacuation is ordered. Hospital department evacuation plans have been developed that clearly define expectations of the employees. When this plan is activated, discharge or transfer orders for patients are obtained, patients and their medical records are prepared for transfer, and the nursing units are secured and closed down as the patients are discharged or transported to other facilities.

Once the unit or department is closed, employees are allowed to leave. All staff members are expected to tell their directors where they will be and how they can be contacted.

### During the Storm

The "during storm" team is composed of those employees who are scheduled to work during the shifts when the hospital is closed. This may be from 1 to 4 or 5 days or more, depending on the extent of the damage that occurs at the hospital. The expectation is that employees will report to work at another facility to which the patients have been transferred to assist the staff with the extra workload. It is also expected that employees will report to the facility in advance of the storm to ensure that they are able to reach their destination safely. They are to bring enough food, clothes, and personal care items to last for several days.

### After the Storm

The poststorm team includes employees who are able to return to the hospital as soon as the roads are passable to assess the damage and begin to prepare the facility to reopen. Certain departments arrive first, including security, administration, environmental services, food services, and plant operations, to begin the cleanup and ensure that the hospital is safe for staff and patients. Staff members involved in patient care are notified as soon as it is safe to return to reopen their units and begin the process of returning patients to the facility.

### EMPLOYEE EXPECTATIONS

A brochure that is updated and distributed each year clearly explains the expectations for the employees, and meetings are held to review the information. Flyers entitled "Hurricane Preparedness Tips" are distributed monthly during hurricane season to all employees to reinforce the information in the brochure.

Health First developed a number of forms to clearly communicate the expectations for each individual employee, depending on their family situation.

The most important form is the employee During Hurricane Exemption Form (Figure 16-4). This form is used by staff to request an exemption from working before, during, or after the storm. The eligible exemptions include the following:

- Providing care on a routine basis for an elderly immediate family member who does not qualify for a special needs shelter and for whom no other care provider is available
- Providing care on a routine basis for an immediate relative who is handicapped or has a chronic illness
- Sole care provider for a child less than 2 years old
- Both parents of a child under 2 years old work for emergency service providers (e.g., hospital, law enforcement, fire and rescue) and are required to work during the storm simultaneously; the Health First employee is exempt
- Both parents of a child under 2 years old work for the Health First Corporation and have simultaneous roles during a storm; one is exempt

The employee signs the exemption form, which must be approved by his or her direct supervisor and forwarded to the Employment Manager. The form is completed at the time of hiring and annually in May and is updated as necessary throughout the year.

### Child Care Services

For employees who volunteer or are required to work during or after the storm, Health First provides childcare for children through age 20. Older children (over age 16) may be permitted to volunteer in the hospital in appropriate areas. A childcare enrollment form must be completed on hire and annually in May. If schools and daycare facilities are unable to open poststorm, working employees who have no other childcare options may bring their children to Health First designated childcare facilities.

### COMMUNICATION ISSUES

Health First uses numerous methods of communication to ensure that information is available to all employees throughout the entire disaster situation. Every employee is to provide contact information, including cell phone numbers or phone numbers where they can be reached if they are evacuating to another location. The corporation also sets up a hotline, which is updated on an ongoing basis and is accessible to all employees at any time.

*(By June 1, send completed form to the Employment Manager and place a copy in your department Disaster Manual. Associates meeting any of the following exemptions must complete this form annually in May, and update as necessary throughout the hurricane season.)*

Associate name: _____ Dept: _____

Facility: _____

    I am requesting exemption from working at any Health First facility **during** a hurricane or other severe weather incident because I meet one of the following criteria:

☐ I provide care for an elderly immediate relative who cannot care for himself or herself on a routine basis. There are no other adult family members to provide this care. This person would not otherwise qualify for a special needs shelter.

☐ I provide care that cannot otherwise be delivered for an immediate relative who is handicapped or has a chronic illness.

☐ I am a sole caregiver with a child less than 2 years of age.

☐ When both parents of a child less than 2 years old, one of whom works for another emergency services employer (i.e., nursing, other hospital, law enforcement, fire and rescue, city employee), are required to work and have simultaneous roles during a storm, associate is exempt.

☐ When both parents of a child less than 2 years old work at Health First and normally would have simultaneous roles during a storm, one is exempt.

**I certify that the above checked statement is true. I also understand that untrue statements may subject me to disciplinary action.**

Associate signature: _____ Date: _____

    Based on the above statement, I am in agreement that this associate be granted exemption from working during a hurricane or other severe weather incident.

Director's signature: _____ Date: _____

**Figure 16-4** Cape Canaveral Hospital During Hurricane Exemption Form.

Announcements are also sent out via the media as appropriate. It is important to use as many options as possible, because many of them may not be accessible as a result of power outages and overloaded phone lines.

## PERSONAL IMPACT

One of the most difficult things to deal with is the stress on the employees who are trying to balance their personal needs with the job expectations. Health First encourages employees to make preparations at home at the beginning of the hurricane season so that supplies are available at a moment's notice. When a storm is approaching, personnel are expected to secure their property, make arrangements for their family members and pets, and pack the essentials that they will need during and after the storm. Depending on their previously agreed-on assignment, they will report to the appropriate facility to provide assistance during and after the storm.

Post-hurricane critiques are done by every nursing unit as well as hospital-wide to identify areas for improvement of the disaster processes as well as to address the needs of the nurses and other staff members. A study by Cohan and Cole (2002) found that "There is robust evidence community-wide disasters lead to mental health problems." In addition, they identified that "posttraumatic stress disorder increases following natural disasters, including hurricanes" (Ironson et al., 1997). The hospital's Pastoral Services department provides multiple opportunities for the employees to attend counseling sessions. This enables the employees to share their experiences and receive further treatment if needed. The Employee Assistance Program (EAP) is also available to all employees to assist with personal crises. Short-term counseling, identification of resources, and referrals for long-term services are included in the free sessions.

## RECENT HOSPITAL DISASTER EXPERIENCES

Cape Canaveral Hospital was founded in 1963, and until 1995 had evacuated only once. Since 1996, with the improvement in storm predictions and warning systems, the accuracy of the information has improved considerably, resulting in a total of five evacuations in the past 9 years. In the early evacuations, the policies and expectations were very casual and not clearly defined. Employees volunteered to assist as necessary, and the evacuation process was completed without incident. However, as the corporation grew to include three hospitals and various other entities, it became increasingly important to more clearly define the responsibilities and expectations. During the evacuation in 1999 for Hurricane Floyd, approximately 100 associates failed to fulfill their obligations, and as a result 30 were terminated. Some personnel had evacuated to other states and were unable or unwilling to return for duty in a timely manner. Others simply abandoned their positions and quit. During the poststorm critique, it was apparent that the expectations were not clearly defined, and after careful review of individual circumstances, several employees were reinstated to their positions.

In 2004, a total of four hurricanes struck the state of Florida, with three of them hitting the east coast of central Florida. Cape Canaveral Hospital was ordered to evacuate twice in 3 weeks, which placed an incredible burden on the staff and available resources. Unfortunately, a number of employees had sustained significant damage to their homes and personal property during the first storm, which added to their stress in responding to the second. However, most employees rose to the occasion and provided the support needed to accomplish the task a second time.

Unfortunately, there were still a few employees who failed to meet their obligations and were terminated. It was a much better process than in 1999,

because the policies were more clearly defined and communicated. Fellow employees also reinforced their obligations and expectations to their peers, and several made the statement when told that their co-workers were evacuating outside the immediate area, "You know you could lose your job if you do that, don't you?"

## PERTINENT POLICIES

It became clear after the problems related to the Hurricane Floyd evacuation in 1999 that Health First would benefit from improved policies to guide both employee and hospital actions and better define responsibilities. Policies that have been defined include:

- *Hurricane and Severe Weather Policy:* This clearly defines what is expected of each employee and employees' responsibilities in a hurricane.
- *Positive Discipline and Corrective Action Guide:* This includes "failure to report to work when scheduled during a hurricane or other community crisis or disaster" in the list of violations that result in disciplinary action.
- *Department-specific plans:* These plans are guides for each hospital department for evacuation and staffing during a hurricane.

## LESSONS LEARNED

### Clear Expectations Are Critical

The most important lesson learned from these disaster experiences is the need to clearly define organizational expectations in writing and communicate them to every employee in the organization. The employees' signatures on the forms indicate that they have reviewed and understand the information and agree to the expectations as defined. It is critical to inform employees that failure to meet their obligation may result in disciplinary action, up to and including termination, depending on the circumstances. After the 2004 hurricanes an appeal process was also defined and implemented in which employees had a formal mechanism to tell their story and appeal their situation before executive leadership. The severity of infractions was defined, with corresponding disciplinary actions outlined, to ensure consistency across the entire system

(Box 16-2). A detailed review was conducted to ensure that the follow-through was equal and consistent depending on the circumstances. Most of the original decisions were upheld after the appeal process. This was a critical factor for those employees who sacrificed their own needs to ensure that the needs of the patients and their fellow employees were met.

---

**BOX 16-2** Types of Disciplinary Action for Noncompliance with Hurricane Policies at Cape Canaveral Hospital

- **Nondisciplinary action:** Miscommunication (includes instances of staff evacuating too far away and not being able to get back in time to meet their assignments so they arranged to "trade" with other staff and instances when phone messages were left but the phones were out of service).
- Hospital action: Written documentation and explanation to file.
- **Level 1:** Poststorm employees with extenuating circumstances (running out of gas, traffic backups, cleaning up from damage to their homes).
- Hospital action: Nonpaid decision day (a day for the employees to consider their own desire to remain within the organization based on the expectations for them to continue in their roles).
- **Level 2:** Negligence on behalf of employee for defined storm responsibilities; effort made to return as soon as possible for poststorm duties.
- Hospital action: 24- to 40-hour employee suspension; loss of annual team bonus for failure to support the team.
- **Level 3:** Flagrant disregard for responsibilities before, during, or after for one of the storms; either not scheduled or fulfilled scheduled shift before, during, or after second storm.
- Hospital action: 40- to 80-hour suspension; loss of annual team bonus, for failure to support the team.
- **Level 4:** Flagrant disregard for responsibilities before, during, or after, for both storms; understood consequences as explained to and/or by their manager; no-call, no-show at any time.
- Hospital action: Termination of employment.

---

### Safe Evacuation Plans Are Needed

Another lesson learned is that evacuation from coastal areas does not necessarily need to be a long distance to be safe. In the past, people were encouraged to move at least 2 hours away from the projected path of a storm, but experience has shown that 2 hours may be too far because of the huge traffic delays when trying to return home. As storms can be unpredictable in their direction and severity, it is now recommended that people remain as close to home as safely possible, as directed by local emergency authorities.

### EMPLOYEE NEEDS

French, Sole, & Byers (2002), in a study on nurses' needs following Hurricane Floyd, identified that the primary concerns of nurses were family safety, pet care, and personal safety while at work. Secondary concerns were basic needs such as food, water, sleep, shelter, and rest.

Health First recognized these employee concerns and addressed them. Before, during, and after the storms, they identified numerous ways to assist the employees to meet their personal needs. Cash advances were made available to assist with evacuation expenses (hotels, gas, and food). Transportation between facilities was provided to ensure that staffing was adequate but that the employees did not have to drive their own vehicles during the storm. The action that was most appreciated by those in need was that after the storms a roofing crew was made available to provide temporary repairs to the homes of employees who suffered damage to protect their property as much as possible until permanent repairs could be made.

Counseling was offered to employees who had suffered great loss and anxiety as a result of the storms. According to the Florida Coalition Against Domestic Violence, "It's not the wind and the floods. It's about the aftermath, a lessening of a standard of living that is very disruptive to families" (Lapidario, 2005). Other issues that remain to be resolved include accommodations for employee family members and employee pets that need a secure facility for shelter (Box 16-3).

**BOX 16-3** Health Care Worker Needs during Emergencies (in Order of Priority)

- Security at work
- Training
- Shelter for self
- Medical care
- Shelter for family
- Clarification of role
- Food
- Scheduled relief
- Compensation
- Security at home
- Stress debriefing
- Transportation
- Childcare, pet care, and elder care

From Martens, K. A., Hantsch, C. E., & Stake, C. E. (2003). Emergency preparedness survey: Personnel availability and support needs. *Annals of Emergency Medicine, 42*(4), S105.

## FINAL THOUGHTS

Clearly defined policies, and communication of these policies and expectations to every employee of the organization, are essential to ensure that the needs of the hospital, its patients, and its employees

are met in a fair and consistent manner. Health First implemented policy changes that clarified what was expected of the employees and the consequences that would ensue if the policies were not followed. All of these efforts ensure that we have adequate staffing during a disaster to meet the needs of our hospitalized patients while also protecting the individual needs of the employees.

## REFERENCES

Cohan, C. L., & Cole, S. W. (2002). Life course transitions and natural disaster: Marriage, birth, and divorce following Hurricane Hugo. *Journal of Family Psychology, 16*(1), 14-25.

French, E. D., Sole, M. L., & Byers, J. F. (2002). A comparison of nurses' needs/concerns and hospital disaster plans following Florida's Hurricane Floyd. *Journal of Emergency Nursing, (28)*2, 111-117.

Historic hurricanes. Retrieved May 9, 2005, from *www.hurricaneville.com/historic.html.*

Ironson, G., Wynings, C., Schneiderman, N., Baum, A., Rodriguez, M., et al. (1997). Posttraumatic stress symptoms, intrusive thoughts, loss, and immune function after Hurricane Andrew. *Psychosomatic Medicine, 59,* 128-141.

Lapidario, M. (2005, February 5). Domestic abuse rises after storms. *Daytona Beach News Journal,* 3C.

Martens, K. A., Hantsch, C. E., & Stake, C. E. (2003). Emergency preparedness survey: Personnel availability and support needs. *Annals of Emergency Medicine, 42*(4), S105.

# *Taking Action*    Ronda Hughes

## *Health Services Research: Shaping Patient Safety Policy*

*"The safety of the people shall be the highest law."*
                                        CICERO

Health services research goes beyond clinically based research by assessing the structures, processes, and outcomes of health care delivery organizations. It is through health services research that the impact of organizations on the safety of care afforded patients is uncovered. The environment

of and the culture within an organization have a significant influence on the delivery of health care. Findings from health services research can be effectively used to effect changes in practice, thereby improving the care experience and subsequent health outcomes for patients.

## WHAT IS HEALTH SERVICES RESEARCH?

Health services research is where social science and policy decision-makers come together (Lomas, 2000).

The field of health services research assesses the impact of health care on the organizations that provide or finance it and the people who receive it. Health services research is defined as "the multidisciplinary field of scientific investigation that studies how social factors, financing systems, organizational structures and process, health technologies, and personal behaviors affect access to health care, the quality and cost of health care, and ultimately our health and well-being. Its research domains are individuals, families, organizations, institutions, communities, and populations" (Lohr & Steinwachs, 2002, p. 8). It entails assessing the nature of the problem, the degree to which implementation or change can occur, and the impact of the change.

From a simplistic standpoint, it assesses health care associated with the structure, process, and outcomes of care. *Structure* of health care systems includes access to care, type of health insurance coverage, and number of hospital beds. Key components of assessing the *process* of care delivery include patient acuity, quality of care, length of hospital stay, and number of hospitalizations. For each component it is important to stratify groups to ascertain the possible presence of differences by race, type of clinician, type of organization, and other factors that could influence outcomes of care, because there continues to be large, unjustifiable variation in the quality of care delivered throughout the United States (Jencks, Huff, & Cuerdon, 2003; Leatherman & McCarthy, 2002).

In assessing the nature of the problem and what services ought to be delivered, health services research seeks to determine what is known and where gaps in knowledge exist. When assessing organizations' ability to change and the potential obstacles to changing norms and practices, research topics could include the following:

- How are specific services used?
- What are the effects and benefits of process change?
- What are the barriers and costs associated with implementation of change?

Finally, health services research focuses on *outcomes;* patient outcomes are examined and evaluated ultimately to determine best practices for care delivery. In assessing the impact and outcomes of the change, health services research considers the following:

- The policy impact resulting from clinical and organizational research
- Differences from existing policies or procedures

All told, resources for health services research are growing though federal and private funders. In the United States, millions of dollars are invested in health services research, predominately by the following federal agencies:

- U.S. Department of Health and Human Services:
  - U.S. Federal Agency for Healthcare Research and Quality (AHRQ)
  - Centers for Disease Control and Prevention
  - Centers for Medicare and Medicaid Services
  - Health Resources and Services Administration
  - National Institutes of Health
- U.S. Department of Defense
- U.S. Department of Veterans Affairs

Millions are also invested by private organizations such as the Robert Wood Johnson Foundation, the Kaiser Family Foundation, and the Commonwealth Fund. Yet the overall amount of research dollars directed specifically toward health services research continues to be almost insignificant given the magnitude of funds directed toward basic biomedical research (e.g., the budget for the National Institutes of Health is over $28 billion).

## INDICATORS OF QUALITY HEALTH SERVICES RESEARCH

Research that should be used to effect change should be of high quality with a measurable impact and benefit. There are certain basic indicators of high-quality research. The key indicators of high-quality health services research are that it is methodologically rigorous, carefully conducted, generalizable, and timely.

Realistically, not all health services research meets these criteria. Generalizability is key to moving findings to practice, in that if the study population does not represent the population of interest as a whole, the intervention studied cannot be duplicated in other settings with the expectation of achieving the same results.

Many nonresearchers do not know (and many researchers ignore) the following aspects of policy-relevant research that could inform policy and does not:

- Studies of interventions that have negative results (e.g., the intervention makes health worse or has no effect) are not publishable (DeAngelis et al., 2004) and therefore cannot guide the development of future interventions.
- Some research that is published is of poor quality, generally because of substandard methodology.
- Sometimes the focus of the research is not on the most important issues or the research fails to provide full analysis of these issues because of limited resources.
- Quality improvement efforts may be too focused (e.g., only on patients with one type of disease) and often are not considered as a basis for informing research, leaving key findings inaccessible to others who could benefit.

These issues limit the information that is needed to inform change and policy.

Findings from health services research are available from a variety of sources, including peer-reviewed journals, professional publications and presentations, continuing education programs, and systematic reviews of the literature—Evidence-Based Practice Center (EPC) reports and the Cochrane library (see the Web Resources). These findings convey single research project findings as well as evaluations and synthesis of research. Research synthesis and systematic comparative summaries of research can provide the foundation for the delivery of evidence-based health care and improved health care quality.

## THE NUANCES OF ORGANIZATIONS

Although individual skill and knowledge affect how health care is delivered to patients, the environment and culture of organizations are the true determinants of patient outcomes. The environment in which nurses work can affect their physical and cognitive functioning, limiting their ability to ensure that the health care being delivered is of high quality (Miles & Snow, 2003). The organizational culture denotes the organization's shared values, character, norms, and approach or adaptation to change, thereby reflecting the way in which health

care is delivered. Culture reflects the behavior of the individuals within health care settings (Scott, Mannion, Davies, & Marshal, 2003).

Perfectionism taught in clinical schools and implied with punishment for errors may instill a drive for high performance but fails to recognize human vulnerabilities in every clinician and system flaws in every health care organization. Human factors research looks at how systems can be redesigned to minimize human error and decrease injury while increasing efficiency.

## USING RESEARCH TO INFORM AND DRIVE ORGANIZATIONAL CHANGE

Health services research generates knowledge and evidence that can compel organizational action to improve care delivery and decision-making (Cabana et al., 1999; Silverman & Yetman, 2001), effectively changing current practices and processes. Factors that influence the use of clinical and organizational research to change processes of care include the following (Ferguson, 1995; Rogers, 1995):

- Economic factors such as reimbursement, regulations, insurance, and the business case for change
- Pressure from external sources demanding comparison, quality measurement, and accountability
- Stakeholder involvement

It is important to begin by understanding the nature and scope of the problem, including whether the problem is new, has been around for a long time (e.g., is it a continuing problem because there have been other unsuccessful attempts to resolve it?), or is resolvable by a new intervention.

Health services research has led to a variety of change and management strategies that have been and can be used to structure improvement process. Two of the proven strategies are continuous quality improvement (CQI) and clinical practice improvement (CPI). The key components of CQI, the health care version of the non–health care industry's total quality management approach, are organizational strategic goals, leadership involvement, team-based actions, staff training, and improvement decision-assisting tools (McLaughlin & Kaluzny, 1999).

CPI is a data-driven approach to assessing the impact of care processes on patient outcomes. Examples of how CPI can be used include the following:

- Examining the contribution of clinicians' actions to patient outcomes
- Determining if the proposed change or innovation improves patient outcomes
- Assessing whether the change would be required or optional
- Calculating if the improvement would save the organization money or cost patients more

Although there are critiques of the merits and shortcomings of CQI and CPI, what makes these processes effective is the use of performance measures that are valid and accurate, using benchmarks, and ensuring timely and ongoing feedback.

Modifying practice requires organizational change that must employ a combination of evidence-based, short-term, and long-term components that can have a visible impact both immediately and over time. Change that is both meaningful and effective and has a longer-term focus (where the results are not immediately visible) requires patience and endurance to adopt strategies that seek longer-term results. Change takes time because it is difficult to revise habits of thought and action. But the time required for change to occur can be accelerated when one of the key drivers of process changes in health care organizations is external organizations that regulate practice (e.g., Joint Commission on Accreditation of Healthcare Organization [JCAHO], professional organizations, the federal government).

## BARRIERS TO USING RESEARCH IN PRACTICE

Even the best research will not be used or will not have an impact on practice unless the following barriers are overcome.

### Gaps in What Is Known from Research

The significance of research findings needs to be understood by all involved, from organizational leaders to clinicians to patients. When knowledge is restricted, it can reflect limited dissemination of effective practices based on tested evidence. This also reflects the paucity of evidence supporting care delivery improvements.

### Ambiguity

Findings from research can support a range of responses, from a "laissez-faire" attitude (doing nothing) to active interventions resulting in significant change. Research is often associated with ambiguity, particularly regarding how research findings can be used in clinical practice, what the associated cost would be, what the effect will likely be on the quality of patient care and on nursing staff. Research needs to be presented and discussed in ways that can lead to clear and appropriate policy and procedural responses (Lomas, Fulop, Gagnon, & Allen, 2003).

### Meaning of Change

The process of change and the degree to which change is required can be powerful repellants to valid improvements. For change to occur, it is important to understand the status quo, the degree of resistance (both active and passive), and who is and who should be involved (Kingdon, 1995). Change reflects adaptive behavior toward desirable outcomes, is often a slow process, and is more successful if it is minimal (Langley, Nolan, Nolan, Norman, & Provost, 1996).

### Lack of Consensus

Implementing research findings is more likely to occur when there is consensus on the findings and the magnitude of the change that is needed. In implementing any form of change, there needs to be frequent and timely feedback on the impact of the program changes. It is also important to have leadership commitment and support, motivating actions to support change; if leadership support is absent, the new process can easily be disregarded and used inconsistently (Davis & Howden-Chapman, 1996).

### Independence

Independence (autonomy) and self-monitoring, as well as interdependence and collaboration, are parts of the roles and responsibilities exercised by both physicians and nurses. Lack of standardization encourages misuse, underuse, and overuse of interventions. Benchmarking and setting minimal thresholds can facilitate progression of clinicians' understanding of the change or intervention over time and as processes change, to further minimize errors.

### Level of Complexity and Lack of Transparency

Changing the processes of health care delivery involves a complex set of relationships, making it difficult to identify factors that can dilute the effectiveness of research implementation. Everyone involved needs to understand his or her role, indicators of successes and failures, and the impact that the new process is having at the macrolevel (e.g., the organization) as well as the microlevel (e.g., the patients) (Roos & Shapiro, 1999).

### A NATIONAL CRISIS: MEDICAL ERRORS

Each of the four patient safety–related Institute of Medicine (IOM) reports ("To Error Is Human: Building a Safer Health System" [IOM, 1999]; "Crossing the Quality Chasm: A New Health System for the 21st Century" [IOM, 2001]; "Keeping Patients Safe: Transforming the Work Environment of Nurses" [IOM, 2004a]; and "Patient Safety: Achieving a New Standard for Care" [IOM, 2004b]) calls for a "fundamental change" in health care delivery. As noted in the second report, "patients, physicians, nurses, and health care leaders are concerned that the care delivered is not the care we should receive" (IOM, 2001, p. 1). Even when evidence for change is well documented, the highly fragmented U.S. health care system thwarts a coordinated approach to improving health care delivery (McGlynn & Brook, 2001; Newhouse, 2002). "Crossing the Quality Chasm: A New Health System for the 21st Century" (IOM, 2001) put forth a framework for the redesign of the culture of the health care system that would ensure care that is safe, patient centered, timely, effective, efficient, and without disparities.

For decades the negative consequences of health care delivery were most visible through malpractice claims and payouts (Brennan et al., 1991; Leape et al., 1991). Research eventually indicated that there were systemic causes and consequences of poor-quality care. In 1998 the Presidential Advisory Commission on Consumer Protection and Quality in the Health Care Industry, led by health care quality improvement leader Donald Berwick, recommended strategies such as having a shared vision of health care delivery undergoing CQI and measuring quality in a systematic way to improve the quality of health care (Berwick, 1989, 1993). Research indicated that throughout health care organizations, the quality of care was inextricably linked to the knowledge, behavior, and actions of clinicians.

Following the release of the first IOM report, "To Err is Human: Building a Safer Health System" (IOM, 1999), the verbiage used to describe the problem changed from *quality* to *safety*. This report quantified the magnitude of the negative impact of our nations' dysfunctional health care delivery systems and framed many of the issues threatening patient safety. After this report was released there was extensive media coverage of the issue that generated national outrage at the awareness that errors in health care were the eighth leading cause of death in this country. Patient safety became and today remains a top health policy issue. The report precipitated immediate change by triggering an array of patient safety–driven activities that show no sign of ending. Up to this point the problem had been recognized but was not a priority (Blendon et al., 2002).

Continuing pressure from the media forced health care leaders and managers to develop strategies to promote patient safety (Millenson, 2002). Even though the report presented evidence from health services research that patient safety threats were the direct result of system failures, both the public and physicians believed that errors result from individual failures and that individual accountability would improve patient safety (Blendon et al., 2002).

### The Patient Safety Movement

Health services research has provided the evidence base driving today's focus on improving patient safety. In responding to one of the recommendations in "To Err Is Human" (IOM, 1999), AHRQ evaluated the clinical and health services research literature to identify evidence supporting patient safety practices. "Making Health Care Safer"

(Shojania, Duncan, McDonald, & Wachter, 2001) presented the best available evidence regarding those aspects of patient safety that had been studied. Several issues became clear. First, many aspects of potentially harmful practices (e.g., clinician fatigue) and solutions to patient safety problems (e.g., health information technology) still needed to be studied using health services research, not clinically based research trials. Second, the evidence on the role and impact of nursing on patient safety was, at best, sparse. And third, it was also clear that many evidence-based approaches to patient safety practices were not being practiced throughout our nation's health care system, but more sporadically.

To improve the quality and the safety of health care, significant change in the process of care delivery is needed, especially in such areas as medication administration and surgical procedures on the right patient at the right time. Changes in the structure of health care organizations, influenced by reimbursement policies such as managed care (Miller & Luft, 1997), have alone not succeeded in improving the quality of health care (Shortell, Bennett, & Byck, 1998). The evolution of patient safety research is relatively new and expanding. In just 5 years the data and tools to improve health care safety and quality have become widely available, but the gains in safety and quality are thought to be only modest (Leape & Berwick, 2005). The government, private health care insurers, and consumers want care practices to be monitored and quality improvements rewarded (Epstein, Lee, & Hamel, 2004).

Efforts to improve safety should not be limited to those issues that have been studied and have documented evidence (Leape, Berwick, & Bates, 2002). Using root cause analysis, the U.S. Department of Veterans Affairs (VA) has instituted an objective basis for deciding which problems need to be addressed urgently, and the CEO is then required to support the specific recommendations. Problems identified though this process must be addressed (Bagian et al., 2001). This process depends on the availability and accessibility of data and information. The largest contributors of data on errors include patient records, voluntary or mandatory reports, and administrative data. To encourage voluntary reporting of errors, there needs to be a nonpunitive or safe environment, simplicity in reporting, and timely, valuable feedback (Leape, 2002).

### Transitioning to a Patient Safety Environment

Nurses must be fully involved in the process of improving patient safety. Without nurses there would be no patient safety. There must be a clear leadership position regarding decisions; unambiguous decisions must be continually reinforced to ensure consistent understanding. It is important to use planning and implementation processes that rely on collaboration and consensus building horizontally as well as vertically within an organization (e.g., hospital) and to use organizational and management consultants to facilitate the hospital planning team's ability to envision new models of nursing and patient care.

Improving patient safety will be a continual process. Governments and organizations are moving forward with serious change efforts, in large part based on evidence from health services research. The Leapfrog Group, a coalition of more than 170 businesses concerned with health care safety and improving the cost and outcomes of care, has identified safety standards for computerized physician order entry, referrals, and round-the-clock coverage in intensive care units. Florida and Connecticut have used patient safety research to form state legislation and are launching near-miss reporting systems. Florida held consensus conferences with leading patient safety researchers to formulate a comprehensive state plan. Minnesota also used extensive input from research programs to formulate their program. States and professional organizations are using AHRQ-funded research on fatigue to set boundaries for the number of hours worked by residents and nurses. The JCAHO is using patient safety research as the basis for its patient safety goals.

The IOM patient safety reports provided the window of opportunity (Kingdon, 1995) to drive changes in clinical practice and the organization of health care. The path to patient safety improvement across health care organizations is not clear. How do organizations take what works and put it into daily action? The question is whether or not research supporting evidence-based health care delivery is sufficient. To improve the process of how health care is delivered, it is important to understand the following (Deming, 1993):

- The health care system and what patient outcomes result from the care
- Why variation and disparities exist
- What motivates change, and how care is delivered
- How research findings can be incorporated into practice

To effect change and continually be engaged in improvements for patient safety, key stakeholders, the best evidence, and commitment need to come together.

## NURSES AND HEALTH SERVICES RESEARCH

More emphasis on funding and conducting health services research is required to meet the changing needs of patients. For now, the field of health services research, which owes its beginnings to Florence Nightingale (Dossey, 2000), is dominated by physicians and social scientist that are, with few exceptions, non-nurse researchers. But there is a growing cadre of nurses engaged in this research in recognition of its importance to advancing nursing care and policy that affects that care. The delivery of safe, high-quality health care hinges on informed nurses.

*Web Resources*

### Agency for Healthcare Research and Quality (AHRQ)—twelve Evidence-Based Practice Centers (EPCs), based primarily on funding from AHRQ, develop systematic reviews of peer-reviewed literature on nominated topics, informing both policy and practice
*www.ahcpr.gov/clinic/epc*
### Cochrane Collaboration—provides systematic and other reviews on topics related to the delivery of health care
*www.cochrane.org/reviews/clibintro.htm*
### Practice Guidelines—practice guidelines based on systematic reviews, expert opinion, and other evidence, are collected by AHRQ
*www.guidelines.gov*

## REFERENCES

Bagian, J. P., Lee. C., Gosbee, J., DeRosier, J., Stalhandske, E., et al. (2001). Developing and deploying a patient safety program in a large health care delivery system: You can't fix up what you don't know about. *Joint Commission Journal on Quality Improvement, 27*, 522-532.

Berwick, D. M. (1989). Continuous improvement as an ideal in health care. *New England Journal of Medicine, 320*(1), 53-56.

Berwick, D. M. (1993). Do we really need a framework in order to improve? *Joint Commission Journal on Quality Improvement, 19*(10), 449-450.

Blendon, R. J., DesRoches, C. M., Brodie, M., Benson, J. M., Rosen, A. B., et al. (2002). Views of practicing physicians and the public on medical errors. *New England Journal of Medicine, 347*(24), 1933-1940.

Brennan, T. A., Leape, L. L., Laird, N. M., Hebert, L., Localio, A. R., et al. (1991). Incidence of adverse events and negligence in hospitalized patients: Results from the Harvard Medical Practice Study I. *New England Journal of Medicine, 324*, 370-376.

Cabana, M. D., Rand, C. S., Powe, N. R., Wu, A. W., Wilson, M. H., et al. (1999). Why don't physicians follow clinical practice guidelines? *Journal of the American Medical Association, 282*, 1458-1465.

Davis, P., & Howden-Chapman, P. (1996). Translating research findings into health policy. *Social Science & Medicine, 43*, 865-872.

DeAngelis, C. D., Drazen, J. M., Frizelle, F. A., Haug, C., Hoey, J., et. al. (2004). Clinical trial registration. *JAMA, 292*, 1363-1364.

Deming, W. E. (1993). *The new economics for industry, education, government.* Cambridge, MA: MIT Press.

Dossey, B. M. (2000). *Florence Nightingale: Mystic, visionary, healer.* Springhouse, PA: Springhouse.

Epstein, A. M., Lee, T. H., & Hamel, M. B. (2004). Paying physicians for high-quality care. *New England Journal of Medicine, 350*, 406-410.

Ferguson, J. H. (1995). Technology transfer: Consensus and participation—the NIH Consensus Development Program. *Joint Commission Journal on Quality Improvement, 21*(7), 332-336.

Institute of Medicine (IOM). (1999). *To err is human: Building a safer health system.* Washington, DC: National Academies Press.

Institute of Medicine (IOM). (2001). *Crossing the quality chasm: A new health system for the 21st century.* Washington, DC: National Academies Press.

Institute of Medicine (IOM). (2004a). *Keeping patients safe: Transforming the work environment of nurses.* Washington, DC: National Academies Press.

Institute of Medicine (IOM). (2004b). *Patient safety: Achieving a new standard for care.* Washington, DC: National Academies Press.

Jencks, S., Huff, E., & Cuerdon, T. (2003). Change in the quality of care delivered to Medicare beneficiaries, 1998-1999 to 2000-2001. *Journal of the American Medical Association, 289*(3), 305-312.

Kingdon, J. W. (1995). *Agendas, alternatives and public policies.* New York: HarperCollins College.

Langley, G. J., Nolan, K. M., Nolan, T. W., Norman, C. L., & Provost, L. P. (1996). *The improvement guide: A practical* approach to enhancing organizational performance. San Francisco: Jossey-Bass.

Leape, L. L. (2002). Reporting of adverse events. *New England Journal of Medicine, 347,* 1633-1638.

Leape, L. L., & Berwick, D. M. (2005). Five years after *To Err Is Human*: what have we learned? *Journal of the American Medical Association, 293,* 2384-2390.

Leape, L. L., Berwick, D. M., & Bates, D. W. (2002). What practices will most improve safety? Evidence-based medicine meets patient safety (editorial). *Journal of the American Medical Association, 288,* 501-507.

Leape, L. L., Brennan, T. A., Laird, N., Lawthers, A. G., Localio, A. R., et al. (1991). The nature of adverse events in hospitalized patients: Results from the Harvard Medical Practice Study II. *New England Journal Medicine, 324,* 377-384.

Leatherman, S., & McCarthy, D. (2002). *Quality of healthcare in the United States: A Chartbook.* New York: Commonwealth Fund.

Lohr, K. N., & Steinwachs, D. M. (2002). Health services research: An evolving definition of the field. *Health Services Research, 37*(1), 7-9.

Lomas, J. (2000). Health services research: A domain where disciplines and decision makers meet. In W. Sibbald & J. Bion (Eds.), *Evaluating critical care: Using health services research to improve quality.* Amsterdam: Springer-Verlag.

Lomas, J., Fulop, N., Gagnon, D., & Allen, P. (2003). On being a good listener: Setting priorities for applied health services research. *Milbank Quarterly, 81*(3), 363-388.

McGlynn, E. A. & Brook, R. H. (2001). Keeping quality on the policy agenda. *Health Affairs, 20*(3), 82-90.

McLaughlin, C. P., & Kaluzny, A. D. (1999). *Continuous Quality improvement in health care: Theory, implementation, and applications* (2nd ed.). Gaithersburg, MD: Aspen.

Miles, R. E., & Snow, C. C. (2003). *Organizational strategy, structure, and process.* Stanford, CA: Stanford Business Books.

Millenson, M. L. (2002). Pushing the profession: How the new media turned patient safety into a priority. *Quality & Safety in Health Care, 11,* 57-63.

Miller, R., & Luft, H. (1997). Does managed care lead to better or worse quality of care? *Health Affairs, 16*(5), 7-25.

Newhouse, J. P. (2002). Why is there a quality chasm? *Health Affairs, 21*(4), 13-25.

Rogers, E. M. (1995). Lessons for guidelines from the diffusion of innovations. *Joint Commission Journal on Quality Improvement, 21*(7), 324-328.

Roos, N. P., & Shapiro, E. (1999). From research to policy: What have we learned? *Medical Care, 37,* JS291-JS305.

Scott, T., Mannion, R., Davies, H., & Marshal, M. (2003). The quantitative measurement of organizational culture in health care: A review of the available instruments. *Health Services Research, 38*(3), 923-945.

Shojania, K. G., Duncan, B. W., McDonald, K. M., & Wachter, R. M. (Eds.). (2001). *Making health care safer: A critical analysis of patient safety practices.* Evidence Report/Technology Assessment, No. 43. AHRQ publication 01-E058. Rockville, MD: Agency for Healthcare Research and Quality.

Shortell, S. M., Bennett, S. L., & Byck, G. R. (1998). Assessing the impact of continuous quality improvement on clinical practice: What it will take to accelerate progress? *Milbank Quarterly, 76*(4), 593-624.

Silverman, D. C., & Yetman, R. J. (2001). The care path not taken: The paradox of underused proven treatments. *Journal of Clinical Outcomes Management, 8,* 39-51.

# chapter 17

# Ten Keys to Unlocking Policy Change in the Workplace

Karlene M. Kerfoot & Mary W. Chaffee

*"For us who Nurse, our Nursing is a thing, which, unless in it we are making progress every year, every month, every week, take my word for it, we are going backward."*

FLORENCE NIGHTINGALE

Influencing policy in any environment is about influencing change. Policies and procedures are the blueprints for how an organization behaves. Policies explain how goals will be reached and serve to guide the behavior of leaders and their teams. Policies serve as the basis for action and decisions, guide planning, and encourage organizational consistency because different leaders faced with decisions have a framework to work within (Tomey, 2004).

Changing a workplace policy can be a complex leadership task—just as influencing policy in a legislature or city hall can be. The workplace environment is somewhat different from other environments where policy is made, such as a legislature. In a workplace an organizational structure exists, personnel are relatively stable, and it would be unusual for advocates outside the organization to be involved in influencing policy (as lobbyists do when influencing policy in government).

The workplace can be a very difficult place to influence the development of new policy or the revision of current policy. The same forces that support and inhibit policy development in legislatures are at work in workplaces also. Not recognizing the political forces that reside in the workplace,

when attempting to influence policy, can take a toll on the leader and result in stagnant workplace policy.

Workplace policy is developed at all levels. Nurses who serve in middle management and executive positions will be influential policymakers on a regular basis. However, many other nurses will have the opportunity to influence policy on clinical units, when serving on committees, in designing education programs, and in other activities. Once the policy process is understood, every nurse can take advantage of opportunities to revise, update, and craft policy.

## TYPES OF WORKPLACE CHANGE

In the workplace, nurses are confronted with three kinds of change, as described by Black and Gregersen (2002).

### ANTICIPATORY CHANGE

Anticipatory change is vital to a long-range policy success. It is based on the ability to recognize weak signals in the environment early and to respond quickly and appropriately. Change that is anticipated and effected early is the least costly in human angst and financial resources but also the most difficult kind of change to initiate. Crafting policy to guide change that addresses subtleties in the environment is difficult. People who are happy with the status quo will not see the storm clouds on the horizon and may operate in a state of denial. For example, before every serious nursing shortage that has occurred there were obvious signs on the horizon that an impending shortage was inevitable. But organizations and society have not been able to make the necessary changes to avoid the next cycle of shortages. Consequently, we continually face shortages, react, and respond to each crisis.

## REACTIVE CHANGE

Reactive change is possible when the signals are stronger and people can sense an impending crisis. This kind of change is easier to generate, because people can see the need for it. However, the costs of reactive change are greater. Often, expensive processes must be put in place quickly to avoid the impending crisis. Reactive leadership is appropriate in workplace situations when the signals in the environment are not clear enough to decipher. People and organizations do not tolerate continual reactive change. For example, when appropriate policies are not in place to retain nurses, a reactive leader will respond to the loss of nurses with interventions such as retention bonuses. These do little except irritate the nurses who do not get the bonuses. A successful long-term anticipatory strategy will trump reactive leadership every time, but it is much more difficult to accomplish.

## CRISIS CHANGE

Even with sound policies and planning, organizations encounter crises. Crisis change is, in a way, the easiest to lead because the need for change is visible and undeniable, and the organizational survival machinery kicks into gear. However, this kind of change is the most expensive, leaves casualties in its wake, and can cause unintended consequences. When the continual mode of the operation is crisis, there is little energy left to work on the building blocks of a solid organization, such as strategic planning. For example, when nursing shortages become severe enough, employers of nurses pull out very expensive solutions such as international recruiting, reducing hours of care, and other costly measures that do not solve the problem. Magnet-designated hospitals are recognized for having implemented long-range anticipatory change strategies that make

them more immune to cyclic nursing shortages and put them less at risk during crisis.

## TEN KEYS TO INFLUENCING POLICY CHANGE

The practice of leading policy change in a workplace is exciting and complicated. The following 10 key activities are the building blocks of influencing change in any environment.

### 1. SPARK A PASSION

Change happens only when you believe in what you are doing. People know when you believe in your vision. They catch your passion, and they feed on the energy it creates. That "fire in your belly" will sustain you and your organization through difficult times. At times you will need to create a "burning platform" for yourself and others to ignite that passion, especially when you are focusing on anticipatory change. It's not easy to ignite your passion when all is going well. When you are passionate about your plans, you will be able to continually keep your torch lit.

### 2. READ THE CULTURE

Culture dictates what people do. There are workplaces where people welcome change and see it as a wonderful opportunity for creative destruction and the birthing of new policies that are more effective than the old ones. Other cultures sabotage even the most effective plans for change because the forces that fear change are stronger. Bossiday and Charan (2002) make the case that "The culture of the company is the behavior of its leaders. You change the culture of the company by changing the behavior of the leaders." Leaders who can model excitement and positive change create culture when continual evolution is welcomed. People watch leaders and follow their lead.

### 3. CRAFT POLICY THAT CREATES A ROADMAP (IT'S THAT 'VISION' THING!)

The story of two bricklayers illustrates this concept. When asked what they were doing, the first of two bricklayers said he was laying bricks. The second said he was building a cathedral for everyone to enjoy and marvel at for generations. We can never be about just laying bricks.

Many leaders do not achieve success because they cannot communicate their policies in a way that would make people want to sign on for the ride. It's one thing to have the vision, but along with that must come the roadmap. The purpose and goals of a proposed policy change must be explained to those who will be affected by it. Effective change requires both the vision and the roadmap.

## 4. GET THE RIGHT PEOPLE ON THE BUS

Collins (2001) in *Good to Great* makes a case for building the infrastructure right. His message is that first you have get the right people on the bus, assign people to the right seat, and tell them where the bus is going, then you invite people who are not interested in that direction to get off the bus. Once this is clear for all, the ride can begin. This is a convenient analogy for ensuring that you have done your homework, have thought through the strengths and weaknesses of your team, and have identified the first- and second-string players who can get the job done. When designing any policy, it is essential to determine who will be the natural supporters (likely those who will benefit in some way) as well as who will obstruct the change overtly or covertly.

## 5. HAND THE WORK OFF TO CHAMPIONS

Successful policy change comes from within the people of the organization. Wheatley (2005) indicates leaders should move from hero to host. A leader invites people to participate in change and hosts the process that brings people together to make the necessary changes. Leaders know that unless you create believers and hand the work over to them, change won't be sustained. Unless there are champions of change on the front lines and throughout the organization, the change will likely not work. Politicians win elections by enlisting many champions who believe in the politician's agenda and can reach out and touch large numbers of people. Clarian Health Partners has used unit-based champions for many of its major policy initiatives.

## 6. VALUES DRIVE POLICY

Values underlie all policy decisions. A policy means that an organization believes a certain course is the right direction. It serves as the compass that points all workplace activity in a certain direction. It's essential for new policies to be aligned with the organization's values; if not, conflict and dissonance will likely ensue.

Values drive your internal ethical standards. They function like a rudder to keep you on the right course. Refusing to act in a way that is in conflict with your ethics may be difficult at the time, but in the long run, those ethical standards will keep your life, and your professional decisions, on course (Neuhauser, Bender, & Stromberg, 2004).

## 7. CHANGE DOESN'T HAPPEN IF YOU GIVE UP

When you are attempting to design or implement a new policy, you will sometimes be stressed, be tired, and want to give up. Winston Churchill is known to have given one of the shortest graduation speeches ever. He told the graduates to "Never give up" and promptly sat down. It's easy to throw up your hands in the middle of a frustrating initiative and declare defeat. But when you do that, you break a promise.

## 8. ORGANIZATIONS DON'T CHANGE UNLESS PEOPLE DO

Organizations don't change. Instead, people change, then organizations evolve. New policies and procedures are only as good as the people who now believe in the new way of getting the work done. Gaining support for a new policy can require "marketing"—literally selling people on why the change is the right thing to do.

## 9. PEOPLE ARE WHAT MATTERS

Wheatley (2005) wrote that the only thing we can rely on is human goodness. In her view people can be incredibly resourceful and imaginative and want to help, contribute, and create value. However, she goes on to say that many organizations continue to keep people in boxes, police people into good behavior, and do not invite people to participate and contribute. As a result, we create organizations where people feel rebellious, hostile, and cynical and are deadened by apathy. It is impossible to make policy change without capturing the human spirit and enrolling people in the significance of the outcomes the policy change will create.

## 10. FILL YOUR TANK

Leaders who design and influence policy in the workplace can feel like a perpetual motion machine. Although success can refuel leaders, there is more to sustaining the energy needed for progress. Our brains need to relax just as muscles do after a workout. We can be rejuvenated with things such as appreciative inquiry, practicing gratitude, or challenging dancing, yoga, Tai Chi, music, art, and other interests. Machines that are in a constant production mode fail just as do our brains and our bodies if we can't relax and recharge our batteries.

Maintaining a healthy balance in life, and avoiding the virulent disease "burnout" is a challenge for many people with demanding careers, but there are ways to do it. The authors of *I Should Be Burnt Out by Now...So How Come I'm Not?* point out important and realistic actions that can help keep your tank filled. They include:

- Watch your thoughts, because optimism works!
- Get a grip on what really matters.
- Keep your options open.
- Develop healthy rituals.
- Defend yourself from toxic people (Neuhauser, Bender, & Stromberg, 2004).

## SUMMARY

Workplace policies chart the course for an organization's activities. Policies outline what the goals of the organization are, underscore what the organization values, and define how the people who work there will go about achieving the goals. Policies let employees know what is important and what they can expect. Understanding the role of policy in the workplace can help leaders craft and implement policies designed to achieve a specific purpose without causing unforeseen complications.

## Web Resources

**Harvard Business School Working Knowledge**
*http://hbswk.hbs.edu*
**Leadership and Change Books**
*www.leadershipandchangebooks.com*
**National Academies Press:** *Academic Health Centers: Leading Change in the 21st Century*
*www.nap.edu/openbook/0309088933/html*

### REFERENCES

Black, J. S., & Gregersen, H. (2002). *Leading strategic change.* New York: Prentice-Hall.

Bossiday, L., & Charan, R. (2002). *Execution: The discipline of getting things done.* New York: Crown Business.

Collins, J. (2001). *Good to great.* New York: Harper Business.

Neuhauser, P., Bender, R., & Stromberg, K. (2004). *I should be burnt out by now...so how come I'm not? How you can survive and thrive in today's uncertain world.* Canada: Wiley.

Tomey, A. M. (2004). *Guide to nursing management and leadership* (7th ed.). St. Louis: Mosby.

Wheatley, M. (2005). *Finding our way. Leadership for an uncertain future.* San Francisco: Berett-Koehler.

# *Vignette*   Karen A. Daley

## Needlestick Injuries in the Workplace: Implications for Public Policy

*"Never doubt that a small group of thoughtful, committed citizens can change the world; indeed it is the only thing that ever has."*

MARGARET MEAD

By July 1998 my clinical nursing career had spanned more than 25 years. For 22 of those years, emergency nursing was my chosen specialty. My entire nursing career had been spent in the same large Boston-area teaching hospital where, over many years, my professional practice and growth had been nurtured. I always felt fortunate and proud to be a nurse there. It was also the place where, in a split second, I was thrust into an unknown world—a world for which nothing in my previous experience could have prepared me.

In this world I have been forced to deal with uncertainties that have threatened every aspect of my life—my health, my career, my financial security, my self-image, and my relationships with others. Now, almost 3 years later, as I think back to my injury and its life-altering consequences, I see how easily it could have been prevented. Like so many injuries in the workplace, it did not have to happen.

### MY INJURY

There was nothing unusual about that shift in July of 1998. Like many others, it was busy. That particular day I was assigned to perform triage. With a little more than an hour left in my 12-hour shift, a colleague asked if I would try to draw blood from one of her patients. I had someone cover triage and I went to see the patient—a frail, elderly man with dementia. I drew the blood and while holding pressure on the puncture site, I turned to dispose of the needle I had used. As I introduced the needle into

the sharps container on the wall behind me, I felt a sudden, sharp sting. A second needle wedged inside the needle box had stuck my index finger.

I have often been asked since then how I felt at that moment. I remember my first reaction was anger—the needle box had been a source of complaints in our unit. The second reaction was a strong impulse to ignore what had just happened. I remember thinking that I didn't want to deal with what would follow once I reported my exposure: staying beyond the end of my scheduled shift to be evaluated, coming in on my days off for follow-up lab tests, and the anxiety of thinking about what I might have been exposed to while waiting for results. I simply wanted to return to triage, finish what was left of my shift, and pretend it had never happened.

Fortunately, the nurse who had asked me to draw the blood was there when my injury occurred and must have sensed what I was thinking, because she insisted I sign in to be seen as a patient. As required by policy, 2 days later I returned to the hospital's occupational health clinic for baseline lab work and counseling. In the weeks and months that followed, I worked hard to put my injury out of my mind. I was largely successful in that effort—in fact, too successful.

Within 6 to 8 weeks, I began to experience a number of vague symptoms that I couldn't account for: weight loss, fatigue, insomnia, episodic nausea, and abdominal pain, among others. I just didn't feel well. Initially, I related my symptoms to the first anniversary of my closest brother's sudden death in a car crash. His death had been one of the most profound losses I had ever suffered, and it seemed a logical explanation for my symptoms.

However, my symptoms persisted, and by the time I finally scheduled an appointment with my primary care physician, I had lost about 12 pounds. An unremarkable examination and negative results from lab tests failed to identify the underlying problem. Because it never occurred to me that my needlestick injury could in any way be related to my symptoms, I never thought to mention it.

After one more visit to my primary care physician, almost 5 months after my exposure, blood tests performed as part of routine occupational health clinic follow-up revealed incomprehensible news: my needlestick had infected me with both the human immunodeficiency virus (HIV) and hepatitis C virus (HCV).

## NEEDLESTICK INJURIES AND WORKPLACE SAFETY

It is estimated that 400,000 to 600,000 needlestick injuries occur each year in the United States. There is also evidence to suggest that more than 80% of those injuries could be prevented through the use of safe needle technology available for more than three decades. Based on existing data at the time of my injury, and despite widespread and long-standing accessibility, it also appeared that less than 15% of employers were providing their employees with one or more types of these safer devices within their practice setting (American Nurses Association [ANA], 2000a).

As soon as it happened, I knew my injury could easily have been prevented, either by a safer disposal box or by some type of protective needle design. Such is the case for a large majority of needlestick injuries that occur every year in the United States. In the weeks that followed my injury, I learned more about the scope of the problem and the preventable nature and emotional toll of these injuries—before I ever knew the personal toll of my needlestick—and I asked legislative staff at the Massachusetts Nurses Association (MNA) to file and lobby for a needlestick prevention bill. It would be the first such bill introduced in Massachusetts.

## THE PERSONAL BECOMES PUBLIC

After the initial shock of learning that I was infected with two potentially life-threatening viruses, I kept the news largely to myself. I learned pretty quickly how emotionally draining it was for me to share the news with others. I also knew I needed to conserve emotional energy to deal with what had happened to me. For the first few weeks, I told only my closest friends and family. I also asked the occupational health staff not to disclose my identity to anyone else in the hospital. They respected my request.

It soon became apparent there were a number of decisions I would need to make, but initially I felt so overwhelmed that I focused only on those I actually had to make at that time, such as choosing a new primary care physician, one whose practice was not based in the setting where I had practiced for more than 25 years. I was referred to an infectious disease physician who specialized in the care of HIV-infected patients.

Almost immediately after learning about the infections that resulted from my needlestick, I decided not to return to clinical nursing in the emergency department where I had practiced since 1977, an emotional and extremely difficult loss for me. I left behind a practice that I loved and many close friends and colleagues, but within just a few weeks of beginning treatment, the debilitating effects of the drugs to combat the HIV and HCV would make it a physical impossibility for me to return to such a demanding setting.

A short time later, after returning from a trip to North Carolina to tell my younger sister the devastating news in person, I began to see my new primary care physician. For the first couple of months, I made almost weekly visits to see him because of the difficulty in stabilizing my care and treatment regimen. At the same time, I was learning about both viruses and focused on coming to terms with what had happened to me. Absolutely nothing in my world was the same as it had been just a few months before.

I then began a slow, deliberate process of disclosing my illnesses. First, I met face to face with several key hospital executives and shared with them the profound personal and physical effects of my injury: how preventable I realized it was; the uncertainties I was now facing as a result; and the importance of doing what they could to prevent similar injuries. I left that meeting with the assurance that they were committed to doing what was possible to prevent this from happening to others within the institution. To this day, they continue to meet that commitment.

Safety sharps devices were introduced in a pilot program in the year after my injury and are now in use throughout the institution.

Once I had met with the hospital administration, I knew it wouldn't take long for the news to reach other hospital and MNA staff, so I decided to meet with my colleagues from the emergency department. Many were beginning to ask why I had been out of work so long. That meeting, although difficult, allowed me to tell them in person what had happened while reassuring them by my presence that I was doing well. I also asked the MNA's executive director to read a letter on my behalf that I had written to the staff sharing with them what had happened.

In the months that followed, I underwent aggressive medical therapy to reduce my viral loads and prevent further damage to my immune system and liver. It's impossible for me to describe what this ordeal has been like for me: the physical toll of the drugs; the energy they stole, leaving me with numbing fatigue; the fear and uncertainty I experienced at times; and the moments when it actually seemed to me that the effects and toxicities associated with the treatments might be worse than to simply allow damage from the viruses to progress unchallenged over time. Looking back over the time since my injury, sometimes I'm amazed I was able to get through it. The support of friends and family helped so much. Today I feel extremely grateful, more than anything else.

## PUTTING A FACE ON THE ISSUE

I struggled for some time to come to terms with the anger I felt and to understand why this had happened to me. But I've also always believed that things happen for a reason, regardless of whether it appears to make sense at the time. Once I moved beyond the anger, I was able to see more clearly that although I couldn't do anything to change what had happened to me, I could perhaps use my experience and position within the nursing community to prevent an injury like mine from happening to others.

Beyond my work setting, the first real opportunity I had to put a face on this issue was at a legislative hearing before the Massachusetts Joint Health Care Committee in April 1999. At that hearing, I spoke

publicly for the first time about my injury and the infections I suffered as a result, and I offered testimony on the needlestick prevention bill MNA had endorsed the previous November. Following my testimony and that of other health care community representatives, the committee voted unanimously that same afternoon to report the bill favorably. As a result of the hearing testimony and the attention paid to it by statewide print and television media, the commissioner of public health also called for the immediate formation of a Needlestick Prevention Advisory Committee under the Department of Public Health (DPH). He charged the committee with examining regulatory approaches to reduce needlestick injuries to health care workers across the state.

By April 1999, there was evidence of a burgeoning movement across the United States to prevent needlestick injuries among health care workers. The previous July, California had become the first state to enact legislation mandating use of safer devices. Tennessee followed in early 1999, becoming the second state to pass such a bill, one that called for state health officials to review available safer technologies and make further recommendations. In 1999, needlestick prevention legislation was introduced in a total of 22 states; by the end of the year, five had enacted it (ANA, 2000b).

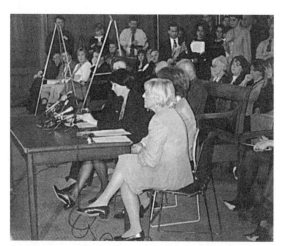

**Figure 17-1** Karen Daley reads testimony before the Massachusetts Health Care Committee in support of the needlestick injury prevention bill in April 1999. The bill passed in that same legislative session.

Since 1982 the ANA had been at the forefront of the issue, advocating federal legislation to mandate the use of safer devices through amendment of the Occupational Safety and Health Administration (OSHA) Bloodborne Pathogen Standard (BPS). Senator Harry Reid (D-NV) was the first to champion the cause in Congress, sponsoring a needlestick prevention bill in every session since 1997 but having little success despite the consistent support of the ANA and other health care worker unions.

Following my testimony on the MNA bill, I attended the spring 1999 ANA Constituent Assembly, a 2-day meeting of state association presidents and executive directors held in Washington, DC. I expected some colleagues at the meeting would have heard about my situation. With the permission of the ANA president and Constituent Assembly chair, I addressed the assembly shortly after the meeting opened. I shared with them what had happened to me as a result of a needlestick and my willingness to do whatever I could to raise awareness among nurses and help move legislation within their individual states. That moment became the catalyst for a whirlwind of activism on local, state, and national levels, and I began to speak around the country. Over the next 2 years, I traveled to more than 15 states to assist in an ongoing campaign to educate nurses and legislators on the importance of needlestick injury prevention.

## A COMING TOGETHER OF INTERVENING FACTORS

The time was right for serious reform to occur for several reasons. Safer needle systems and technologies had evolved to the point where many products were clearly demonstrating their effectiveness in the settings where they were in use. The pioneering spirit and courage of a Pennsylvania nurse named Lynda Arnold, who had contracted HIV several years before from a needlestick, laid important groundwork and brought attention to the issue as she waged a campaign to encourage hospitals to voluntarily commit to using safer devices. In the spring of 1999, OSHA was also engaged in a process of collecting data from hospitals to assess the overall effectiveness of engineered sharps protection devices in preventing needlesticks (OSHA, U.S. Department of Labor, 1999). That request for information would subsequently provide unequivocal evidence of the effectiveness of safer needle devices. Every one of the more than 300 responding hospitals using safer devices in their work settings reported a reduction in the number of needlestick injuries.

Several other factors brought about a shift in the political environment. An expanded coalition of powerful stakeholders, including the ANA, the American Hospital Association (AHA), specialty nursing organizations, other health care worker unions, and manufacturers were working together to educate employers and workers as well as to put pressure on legislators.

Hepatitis C, now considered the greatest health risk faced by health care workers resulting from needlesticks, and the primary reason for liver transplants in the United States, was gaining widespread attention in the media. Finally—and most unfortunately—stories like Lynda Arnold's and mine were becoming all too familiar and were viewed as a serious wake-up call for the health care industry and policymakers who had the power to bring about needed reform.

## REGULATORY AND LEGISLATIVE ACTIVITY

In May of 1999, Representatives Pete Stark (D-CA) and Marge Roukema (R-NJ) cosponsored House Resolution (HR) 1899, also known as the Health Care Worker Needlestick Prevention Act of 1999, to amend OSHA's BPS by requiring health care facilities to use safer sharps devices and systems. An identical bill sponsored by Senators Barbara Boxer (D-CA) and Harry Reid (D-NV) was introduced in the Senate 6 days later. At a press conference held at the U.S. Capitol before the National Press Corps to announce the introduction of the House bill, I offered a statement on behalf of the ANA, along with Representative Stark, the vice president of Kaiser Permanente in California, and the president of the Service Employees International Union (SEIU).

In June of the same year the ANA launched a new "Safe Needles Save Lives" campaign in an effort to coordinate all the needlestick injury prevention professional advocacy activities—including federal and state regulatory, workplace, and collective bargaining strategies—within ANA and its constituent member state associations (ANA, 1999a). As part of the campaign over the next year the ANA cosponsored educational conferences in a number of states to train nurses in the evaluation, selection, and implementation of safer devices in the workplace.

In September, I traveled on two separate occasions to Washington, DC, again at the invitation of the ANA. The first event was an educational briefing hosted by the Congressional Women's Caucus, where I shared my story to educate congressional staff who wanted to learn more about needlestick injuries. By the time the briefing was held, HR 1899 had gained the bipartisan support of 120 sponsors in the House as well as the support of more than 30 organizations representing a coalition of health care workers, nurses, physicians, public health associations, consumer advocacy groups, and manufacturers (ANA, 1999b). It had been hoped beforehand that the briefing would attract additional House sponsors; afterward, the entire Caucus membership signed on in support of the bill.

I returned to Washington for the second time in September on a 2-day visit. My mission this time was a bit more challenging. The Senate bill, although identical to the House version, was not garnering as much support—and little, if any, support from Senate Republican members, who controlled the majority vote at the time. It was clear that without bipartisan support in both the Senate and the House, the bill was unlikely to pass.

My goal was to meet with the staff of key Senate Republican leaders to solicit additional sponsors for the bill. Over those 2 days an ANA legislative staff member and I met with top-level staff of 11 Republican leaders, among them Representative Cass Ballenger (R-NC), who would later play a pivotal role in moving the federal legislation forward.

Resistance to bill sponsorship related to several areas of concern expressed by the Republican leadership of the time:

■ The increased cost of safer devices
■ The widespread perception that employer investment in safer needle systems was not cost-effective

and that it would add an undue financial burden, particularly in rural settings
■ Lack of willingness to support any legislation that created new OSHA mandates for constituents
■ A clear reluctance to offer support for the legislation if it meant standing alone or apart from other Republican senators

During those meetings, the most common questions I heard from legislative staff, often even before they requested any background or information on the bill, were "What will this bill cost?" and "Who else is supporting it?" Staff resistance seemed to lessen, however, as I shared my own personal experience and provided evidence that these devices were demonstrating effectiveness in preventing needlestick injuries, thereby reducing follow-up costs. Most legislative staff members were also initially unaware of the fact that once safer devices became the norm within the industry, market costs would approach the amount currently being spent on conventional devices.

In October, Senate floor debate began on the bill. Cosponsors included Senators Reid (D-NV), Kennedy (D-MA), Boxer (D-CA), and Jeffords (R-VT), chairman of the powerful Health, Education, Labor, and Pension Committee.

## REGULATORY AND LEGISLATIVE VICTORIES

In November of 1999, two major victories occurred. First, OSHA issued a revised BPS Compliance Directive that, for the first time and based on the experience reported by over 300 hospitals, recognized safer devices as the primary line of defense against needlestick injuries. The directive instructed OSHA compliance officers who inspect health care facilities to fine employers for failing to use engineering and work practice controls to reduce needlestick injuries. Second, the National Institute of Occupational Safety and Health (NIOSH) published an alert called "Preventing Needlestick Injuries in Health Care Settings," which focused additional media attention on the importance of frontline health care worker involvement in needlestick injury prevention efforts (NIOSH, Department of Health and Human Services, 2000).

Although a welcome step forward, the compliance directive fell short of providing assurance that employers under federal jurisdiction would comply with new OSHA recommendations requiring the use of safer devices for several reasons. First, enforcement required a site visit by an OSHA compliance officer to a facility, which was triggered only by an employee complaint. Second, despite its new directive, OSHA had been provided no additional resources for enforcement and at its current funding level was budgeted to make a spontaneous inspection visit to any facility only about once every 75 years. Finally, amendment of the actual BPS (originally adopted in 1991) through normal channels and processes could reasonably be expected to take up to 10 years. In the meantime, many more hundreds of thousands of preventable needlestick injuries to health care workers could be expected to occur.

By May of 2000, HR 1899 had 177 sponsors in the House. Although the number of Democratic sponsors on the Senate side had grown considerably, Republican sponsorship had not. In states across the country, however, the issue was gaining visibility and legislative support. Since California first enacted legislation in 1998, 10 more states—New Jersey, Tennessee, Texas, West Virginia, Maine, Hawaii, Maryland, Georgia, Indiana, and Minnesota—had enacted legislation of one kind or another. Legislation had been introduced for consideration in the 2000 session in another 20 states (ANA, 2000c). The message to Congress should have been clear at that point—that the need for such health and safety legislation crossed all geographic, regional, and political boundaries. Instead, it appeared the groundswell of state activity was having little effect on the Republican leadership in Congress.

Less than a month later, in June, a congressional hearing was convened before the Subcommittee on Workforce Protections of the House Committee on Education and the Workforce. The hearing was scheduled by Representative Ballenger's chief legal counsel, and its purpose was to receive testimony on the adequacy of the OSHA compliance directive in addressing health and safety needs of providers with respect to needlestick injury prevention.

Once again I had the opportunity to provide testimony on behalf of the ANA, along with the four others invited to speak by the committee chair, among them OSHA Secretary Charles Jeffress.

In my testimony, I shared the ANA's position on why it was so important for Congress to take action beyond the OSHA directive and amend the 1991 BPS through federal statute.

By the time the 2-hour hearing concluded, subcommittee chair Ballenger and ranking member Major Owens (D-NY) voiced a new appreciation for the serious and preventable nature of health risks from needlesticks and a clearer understanding of the limitations of the 1999 OSHA compliance directive. Most important, both expressed interest in moving needlestick prevention legislation through their subcommittee and Congress before the session was scheduled to adjourn in October.

In the weeks after the hearing, under Representative Ballenger's leadership, meetings were convened with the major stakeholders involved in the issue, including the ANA and AHA, device manufacturers, key legislative leadership, and other health care worker unions. On October 4, a new bill, entitled the Needlestick Prevention and Safety Act (HR 5178), built on changes reflected in the November 1999 OSHA compliance directive, was introduced on the House floor by Representative Ballenger. In the absence of any dissenting debate the bill passed the same day by unanimous consent. On October 24 an identical Senate version also passed by unanimous consent. Senator Kennedy was kind enough to call me shortly after its passage to inform me personally that the bill was now on its way to President Clinton's desk for his signature.

On November 6, 2000, I was honored to be among about 20 individuals invited to the Oval Office to witness President Clinton sign the Needlestick Safety and Prevention Act into law (Figure 17-2). That moment represented the culmination of years of effort by individuals across the country, many of them nurses, who worked tirelessly to educate policymakers and build coalitions in order to bring about needed reform.

A few months earlier, in August of 2000, my home state Massachusetts became the eighteenth state to enact needlestick prevention. The Act Relative to Needlestick Injury Prevention extends the requirement for use of safer devices to all hospitals licensed by the Massachusetts DPH. Compliance with the provisions contained in the new state law

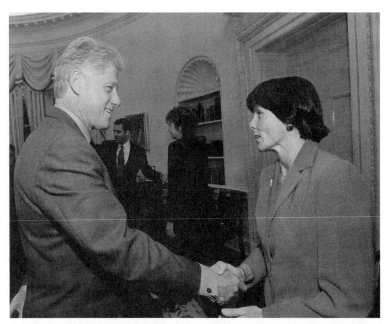

**Figure 17-2** Karen A. Daley, RN, MPH, was a leader in the development and passage of legislation to protect nurses from needlestick injuries. Her instrumental role was recognized when she was invited to the White House Oval Office to witness President Bill Clinton sign the Needlestick Safety and Prevention Act into law on November 6, 2000. The signing represented the culmination of years of effort by individuals across the country, many of them nurses, who worked tirelessly to educate policymakers and build coalitions to bring about needed reform.

is tied to hospital licensure in Massachusetts, creating an exceptionally strong incentive for employers. Of note is the fact that, with passage of this legislation, Massachusetts became the first and only state to date with mandated hospital reporting of annual sharps injury log data.

## DEVELOPMENTS SINCE PASSAGE OF THE FEDERAL NEEDLESTICK SAFETY AND PREVENTION ACT

### Occupational Safety and Health Administration Implementation and Enforcement

On the day he signed the 2000 Needlestick Safety and Prevention Act into law, President Clinton made this public statement: "The Needlestick Safety Act makes clearer the responsibility of employers to lessen the risk of injuries to workers from contaminated sharp devices. It also encourages manufacturers of medical sharps to increase the number of safer devices on the market. This legislation will help to make health care occupations safer."

The bill's passage directed changes to the 1991 OSHA BPS through legislative mandate. Under provisions of the new law OSHA requires employers to provide safety-engineered sharp devices "where appropriate." No specific devices are recommended; rather, employers "must implement the safer devices that are appropriate, commercially available, and effective" by conducting evaluation of available safety products. One of the most critical requirements of the new federal law is that employers demonstrate evidence of front-line health care worker involvement in the selection and evaluation of these devices (OSHA, U.S. Department of Labor, 2001).

Exceptions to the requirement that employers provide engineered safety devices are granted only in cases in which the technology is shown to be not yet advanced enough to meet a specialized need, as in the case of small children or certain medical procedures. Also explicitly mandated is routine HCV follow-up testing for health care workers with bloodborne pathogen exposures, as well as the collection of device-specific information on all injuries, including manufacturer.

In January of 2001, the BPS was revised as required, and in April of 2001, those changes became effective. The legislation extends unprecedented protections to at-risk health care workers employed within the private sector. One limitation of the new law at the time it passed in 2000 was exclusion of public sector (state and municipal) employees from access to these same protections in the 20 states covered only by federal OSHA. In the 27 states in which individual state OSHA plans existed, statutory protections extended to both private and public sector employees. In July of 2004, an amendment was passed as part of the Medicare Prescription Drug Act that finally afforded these same protections to state and municipal employees in all federal OSHA states.

Guidelines for employers and OSHA compliance enforcement officers are issued by OSHA in the form of compliance directives. In November of 2001, federal OSHA issued an updated version of the BPS compliance directive (the previous update was in 1999) that reflected the new requirements. Newly added language contained in the directive includes prohibition of removal of contaminated phlebotomy needles from reusable Vacutainers (used to draw blood into tubes); exclusion of safety needles for purposes not involving blood contamination (such as needles used simply to draw medications from vials); interviews of frontline employees by compliance officers to ascertain solicitation of employee input in device evaluation and selection; and a prohibition of needle unwinders provided in some sharps containers to separate contaminated needles from reusable syringes and Vacutainers.

### Benchmarks for Evaluating Progress in Needlestick Injury Prevention

Between the time of enactment and implementation of any new law, evidence of substantive change takes time to accumulate. Demonstration of a positive impact resulting from the new law will require monitoring of key indicators such as:

- A reduced incidence of preventable needlesticks
- Increased market saturation of engineered safety devices and ongoing innovation in product design
- Frontline worker involvement in institutional needlestick prevention committees, with evidence of their participation in device evaluation and selection
- Routine worker education and training programs, with proper use of safety devices and injury prevention best practices

In conjunction with the most recent revision of the BPS, OSHA has increased the number of targeted inspections of health care facilities in an effort to assure compliance, particularly among those facilities with the highest average injury rates. The major impetus for OSHA inspections, however, continues to be employee-generated complaints of employer noncompliance.

Since passage of the 2000 federal Needlestick Prevention Act, one major source of available injury trend data for periods before and after passage of the new federal statute is the International Healthcare Worker Safety Center located at the University of Virginia. Table 17-1 depicts EPINet percutaneous injury rates for 1999, 2001, 2002, and 2003 for reporting hospitals categorized according to average daily census and teaching hospital status. Findings from these studies indicate that between 1999 and 2001 there was a 35% decline in the overall annual percutaneous injury rate among EPINet hospitals (Perry, Parker & Jagger, 2003). A combination of factors is likely to account for this appreciable decline in injuries, including improved access to safer devices, improved staff education and training, more widespread use of needleless systems, and an overall reduction in use of sharps. Less appreciable differences in injury rates between teaching and nonteaching hospitals are evident in the period between 2001 and 2003. In 2001, 2002, and 2003, annual rate reductions are demonstrated by EPINet hospitals with an average daily census below 100 and between 100 and 300. Injury rates for larger EPINet hospitals increased during the same period (Perry et al., 2003; Perry, Parker, & Jagger, 2004; Perry, Parker, & Jagger, 2005).

**TABLE 17-1** EPINet Percutaneous Injury Rates (per 100 Occupied Beds): 1999-2003*

| | 1999 (21 HOSPITALS) | 2001 (58 HOSPITALS) | 2002 (47 HOSPITALS) | 2003 (48 HOSPITALS) |
|---|---|---|---|---|
| Teaching hospitals | 40 | 26 | 27.1 | 26.8 |
| Non-teaching hospitals | 34 | 18 | 17.7 | 18.7 |
| Hospitals with ADC <100 | NA | 22.8 | 19.1 | 18 |
| Hospitals with ADC 100-300 | NA | 25.8 | 22.5 | 21.5 |
| Hospitals with ADC >300 | NA | 19.8 | 22.9 | 24.8 |

Source: Perry, J., Parker, G., & Jagger, J. (2003, 2004, 2005). EPINet report: 2001 Percutaneous injury rates. *Advances in Exposure Prevention, 6*(3), 1-5.
*2000 EPINet data not available.
ADC, Average daily census.

Small sample size, wide variation in rates among individual facilities, and restricted geographic distribution of reporting hospitals in the EPINet dataset may limit generalizability of these data.

Although more recent data suggest improvements over previously reported rates, opportunities exist for continued progress in needlestick injury reduction. Operating rooms remain a predominant site of injury and concern, with little change in reported rates (Perry et al., 2003, 2004, 2005) despite the growing availability of increasingly innovative and effective engineered safety devices and sharpless surgery techniques (Perry & Jagger, 2005). Future studies are needed to evaluate broader systems impact of the Needlestick Prevention and Safety Act, including rates of safety device utilization. One recent California study found inconsistent implementation of safety device adoption across all settings in the state (Gillen et al., 2003). It is important to include nonhospital care settings in outcome evaluation studies. Future studies might also include:

- Collection of institutional data to ascertain prevalence of injury prevention task forces as part of annual injury control plans
- Monitoring of manufacturing trends to determine level of market product saturation and innovation
- Randomized surveys of frontline nurses to provide an additional key indicator as to current needs related to OSHA BPS enforcement

### Challenges Ahead

The political strategies illustrated by the regulatory and legislative successes related to needlestick injury prevention are ones used successfully throughout public policy arenas to influence change. Whether working for change in the workplace, the community, or the government, effective strategies are likely to include coalition building, identification of obstacles and solutions, seeking out those who have the power to influence and create change, and active participation in the political process.

I wish it were possible to say that the reform necessary to prevent the majority of future needlestick injuries occurred with recent passage of state and federal legislation. Although there is no question that those reforms represent important progress, the changes health care workers will experience as a result—most notably, improved access to safer devices—are simply initial steps toward creating a safer environment for health care workers.

Challenges remain with regard to every aspect of health and safety in the workplace. For employers, it means making a firm commitment to create a culture of safety. Injury prevention, not treatment, should be the true priority. Occupational health systems must be designed to both support and facilitate care of employees. Routine sharing of best practices needs to become the norm in all health care organizations.

For health care workers, the challenge means knowing your rights and no longer tolerating unacceptable health and safety risks in the workplace. It means observing health and safety precautions, reporting injuries when they occur, and getting actively involved on safety committees. As opportunities arise to offer input into the selection and evaluation of safer needle devices in a nursing unit, it means being willing to participate in pilot testing of new safety devices and provide feedback on device effectiveness. It also means identifying existing obstacles to safety and working with colleagues and management to identify and implement strategies to overcome them. Collective action is one of the most valuable tools for addressing health and safety issues in the workplace.

Perhaps one of the most important things to remember is that when it comes to creating needed change in your workplace or practice, you are the expert. Legislators and policymakers depend on shared personal experience and professional expertise to make informed decisions and formulate sound public policy.

It is time for the health care industry and nurses across the country to adopt a culture in which the health and safety of those who provide the care should be at least as important as that of the patients we provide care for—a radical but timely concept,

and one necessary for the health and survival of our profession. Finally, our efforts on behalf of those who provide care must extend to the larger international community of health care workers, particularly those in developing countries who face an unimaginable and unacceptable risk of illness and death because of lack of resources and education (Box 17-1).

## *Lessons Learned*

- Don't underestimate the power of your own voice, and remember that a collective voice is stronger than a lone one. Collectively our voices and votes represent political power and influence.
- You are the expert on nursing practice and health care. Nurses are generally considered credible and

---

**BOX 17-1**   Needlestick Protections for Workers in Developing Countries

Because even the most basic needs related to health care are difficult to meet in developing countries, protection of health care workers remains an even more daunting challenge. Procurement of disposable sterile injection equipment, access to protective equipment and vaccines, and postexposure prophylaxis and treatment pose particular difficulties for countries in which access to such resources is severely limited or virtually nonexistent. The risk of transmission of life-threatening bloodborne pathogens including hepatitis B virus (HBV), hepatitis C virus (HCV), and human immunodeficiency virus (HIV) continues to pose serious threats for health care workers in developing countries—in large part because of their prevalence in poorer and less developed areas of the world. For example, bloodborne pathogens such as HIV, HBV, and HCV are endemic to sub-Saharan African countries. Other bloodborne pathogens of serious concern are endemic to many tropical regions, including Ebola virus and other viruses that cause other hemorrhagic fevers. Of the world's population infected with HIV, about 70% live in sub-Saharan African countries, compared with 4% who live in North America and Western Europe (Sagoe-Moses, Jagger, Perry, & Pearson, 2001). Approximately 50% of patients in sub-Saharan Africa are HIV positive.

Popular belief in developing countries that medication administration via injection represents

a more effective treatment modality contributes to the number of unnecessary injections. Of the 12 billion injections administered annually around the world, more than 50% are estimated to be unsafe. Administration of unnecessary injections, reuse and excessive handling of contaminated equipment, inadequate sterilization procedures, and improper disposal of medical waste are common practices in developing countries that contribute to the high rate of unsafe injections. According to the World Health Organization (WHO), approximately 33% of new HBV cases, 40% of new HCV cases, and 5% of new HIV cases are annually attributable to unsafe injections (Wilburn, 2005). Untrained and ill-equipped health care workers in developing countries often unknowingly place themselves and others at risk of bloodborne pathogen transmission.

WHO and International Council of Nurses (ICN) priorities related to needlestick injury prevention in many developing countries include elimination of unnecessary injections, preventing reuse of contaminated needles, educational outreach and training, provision of necessary protective equipment for health care workers, and widespread adoption of best (not perfect) practices. Needleless airjet injection and autodisable needle systems are currently being trialed in a number of countries in sub-Saharan Africa. Efforts are also underway to provide health care worker access to hepatitis B vaccine and postexposure prophylaxis.

trustworthy, and legislators rely on our experience and expertise for information and guidance on many health policy issues.

- It's not enough to file a bill. Vision, strategic planning, and persistence are necessary. Passage of any bill involves a multistep process and the ability to overcome numerous obstacles. Strategies for success include identification of key legislators on both sides of an issue and mobilizing a broad base of support.

- On average it takes 5 to 7 years to pass a piece of legislation. The process of passage and enactment is a purposefully difficult process designed to ensure good laws.

- Just because a law is passed doesn't mean the intended change occurs. Resources are needed to implement, oversee, and enforce laws. Unfunded mandates hold no promise for change or implementation.

- Politics is not simply about passing legislation. Sometimes bills are filed to give a voice and visibility to an issue. The primary goal can be to foster change through increasing dialogue and awareness rather than by creating a new law.

- Timing and synergy around an issue are critically important in politics and public policy. The lack of visible or vocal support for changing public policy or passage of legislation represents sure death for the issue in the political arena.

### REFERENCES

American Nurses Association (ANA). (1999a). Needlestick prevention bill introduced in the Senate: ANA announces "Safe Needles Save Lives" campaign. *Capitol Update, 17*(10), 1.

American Nurses Association. (1999b). Congressional briefing on needlestick protections. *Capitol Update, 17*(15), 3.

American Nurses Association (ANA). (2000a). ANA testifies on needlestick prevention legislation. *Capitol Update, 18*(11), 2.

American Nurses Association (ANA). (2000b). *Needlestick injury prevention legislation: Department of Government Relations chart, January 5.* Washington, DC: ANA.

American Nurses Association (ANA). (2000c). *Needlestick injury prevention legislation: Department of Government Relations chart, May 4.* Washington, DC: ANA.

Gillen, M., McNary, J., Lewis, J., Davis, M., Boyd, A., et al. (2003). Sharps-related injuries in California healthcare facilities: Pilot study results from the Sharps Injury Surveillance Registry. *Infection Control and Hospital Epidemiology, 24*(2), 113-121.

National Institute of Occupational Safety and Health (NIOSH), Department of Health and Human Services. (2000). Preventing needlestick injuries in health care settings. Publication No. 2000-108. Retrieved May 15, 2005, from *www.cdc.gov/niosh/2000-108.html.*

Occupational Safety and Health Administration (OSHA), U.S. Department of Labor. (1999). OSHA report: Record summary of the request for information on occupational exposure to bloodborne pathogens due to percutaneous injury. Retrieved May 15, 2005, from *www.osha-slc.gov/sltc/needlestick.*

Occupational Safety and Health Administration (OSHA), U.S. Department of Labor. (2001). *Revision to OSHA's Bloodborne Pathogens Standard: Technical background and summary.* Retrieved May 15, 2005, from *www.osha-sic.gov/needlesticks/needlefact.html.*

Perry, J., & Jagger, J. (2005). The benefits of sharpless surgery: An interview with Martin Makary, MD, MPH. *Advances in Exposure Prevention, 7*(3), 29-31.

Perry, J., Parker, G., & Jagger, J. (2003). EPINet report: 2001 percutaneous injury rates. *Advances in Exposure Prevention, 6*(3), 32-36.

Perry, J., Parker, G., & Jagger, J. (2004). EPINet report: 2002 Percutaneous injury rates. *Advances in Exposure Prevention, 7*(2), 18-21.

Perry, J., Parker, G., & Jagger, J. (2005). EPINet report: 2003 Percutaneous injury rates. *Advances in Exposure Prevention, 7*(4), 42-45.

Sagoe-Moses, C., Jagger, J., Perry, J., & Pearson, R. D. (2001). Risks to health care workers in developing countries. *New England Journal of Medicine, 345*(7), 538-541.

Wilburn, S. (2005). Strategies for needlestick injury prevention. Paper presented at the annual meeting of the International Council of Nurses Conference, Taipei, Taiwan.

# *Taking Action*  Tamra E. Merryman & Elizabeth B. Concordia

## Transforming Care at the Bedside: Shadyside Hospital's Code Red

*"No problem can be solved from the same level of thinking that created it."*

ALBERT EINSTEIN

What would seem to be one of the simplest and most effective techniques to improve safety in health care today would be to empower nurses at the bedside. Although you would think that these professionals, who have spent years being the safety net for patients, would easily jump to new systems that will enable them to control their work environment, the story of Code Red at the University Of Pittsburgh Medical Center's Shadyside Hospital (UPMC Shadyside) will share a different perspective (Box 17-2). Code Red is a bedside tool for the clinical staff to provide them the authority to manage the flow of patients through their patient care units.

Although we know it was never an intentional design, health care is full of broken systems that produce significant waste and do not always have all the right properties of safety. Over the last 8 years, UPMC Shadyside has been on a journey to build systems that would improve the work at the bedside for all nurses. We began this journey by creating a

program known as our Clinical Design Initiative. The goals of the Clinical Design Initiative were threefold:

- Eliminate waste in systems.
- Provide clinical staff more time with patients.
- Improve patient and employee satisfaction in our care environments.

The Clinical Design Initiative began over the course of a summer in which we brought existing staff throughout our 521-bed organization to a vacant nursing unit and asked them one simple question. "What gets in your way of taking care of your patients?" After a 3-month period, 15 significant organizational improvements were identified and implemented that saved our organization $696,000. One innovation was the addition of noncellular telephones for the staff. The implementation of this technology allowed us to invest over $200,000 back into direct patient care. In addition, an admission team was created to assure the accurate and complete processing of all new patients. The staff involved was so energized by these changes they asked, "What are we were going to do next?"

At that point, we recognized that creating a culture of improvement was going to be a passion for UPMC Shadyside. It has evolved from that summer over a course of the past 8 years to where we are today. After the first year, the Clinical Design Initiative expanded to the emergency department; employee satisfaction initiatives and the development of simplistic technologies were instituted, all aimed at our goals.

### TRANSFORMING CARE

Approximately 2 years ago our efforts were recognized by the Institute for Healthcare Improvement (IHI) and the Robert Wood Johnson Foundation (RWJF). IHI and RWJF were launching a new

---

**BOX 17-2    UPMC SHADYSIDE**

- 521-bed campus of UPMC Presbyterian Shadyside
- Home of Hillman Cancer Center—National Cancer Institute–designated Comprehensive Cancer Center
- 24,000 admissions per year
- 38,000 emergency department visits per year
- Average length of stay: 5.3 days

---

program known as "Transforming Care at the Bedside" (TCAB). TCAB is the first national initiative that was designed to target nurse's work on a medical-surgical unit. This program was in perfect alignment with our history of Clinical Design at UPMC Shadyside. We were selected as one of three hospitals in the United States to begin this initiative. The goals come from the aims set from the Institute of Medicine report, "Crossing the Quality Chasm." The timing was perfect to gain appropriate local and national attention for the important work that needed to be accomplished. Eighty-five percent of patient care at UPMC Shadyside is provided in a medical-surgical environment. Many improvement initiatives nationally have focused on emergency departments, critical care environments, and physician-driven topics. The problems of medical-surgical units have become more acute because of the recent nursing shortages. The number of nurses leaving the medical-surgical environment for other work environments is a true concern. Nurses have grown frustrated and angry with how difficult it is for them to perform their job in the existing environment. Our goals are to transform the environment to retain the nurses at the bedside.

The initial three TCAB sites were Seton Northwest (Ascension Health System), Kaiser Roseville (Kaiser Health System), and UPMC Shadyside (UPMC Health System). Each of the three selected a medical-surgical nursing unit and began to look at small tests of change based on a brainstorming exercise on the unit and asking staff "What gets in your way of providing excellent care?"

### RED, YELLOW, AND GREEN—THE NEW STOP SIGN

At the end of the brainstorming, one of the big issues that came to the surface was the frequency, timing, and volume of new admissions to the nursing unit. These decisions were made remotely by a bed flow coordinator, leaving the staff nurse feeling extremely unempowered and at times unsafe because of the inability to control this flow. The staff identified an issue that is squarely between the financial goal of admitting and caring for as many patients as possible and the safety goal of ensuring that we are

caring for the patients safely. A delicate balance of new systems would be necessary to solve the problem.

The clinical design staff and the front line staff nurses sat down and began to talk about what type of solutions would be necessary to solve this problem. Before too many discussions, they clearly settled on the fact that there were certain situations that occur on the floor that led staff nurses to feel they were unsafe and affected their ability to observe their patients. They decided quickly that there were several levels of work that should be treated differently. There were times when they just needed a short break from new work and times when everything was chaotic and they not only needed a break but also needed more staff to assist in patient care. At the end of the discussions a draft prototype was put together (Box 17-3) for initial criteria for medical-surgical units.

We labeled our solution as "Code Red." This code was applied to situations when the nurse needed a pause to prevent new work for a period of time and additional support staff. Once the prototype was drafted, we tested this on a 24-bed medical-surgical unit by empowering each of the charge nurses to use the criteria as appropriate. In addition to educating the charge nurses and staff on the unit, the hospital bed flow coordinators were also trained on our new system.

For example, within 60 minutes the charge nurse on 4 East receives three new admissions, a patient becomes critical, and the staff calls for a rapid response team. The charge nurse would be able to contact the bed flow coordinator and put the unit on Code Red status. As noted in the table, the unit would not receive any new patients for a minimum of 45 to 60 minutes, and other support interventions would occur.

One of the earliest and most amazing findings was the fact we had to constantly remind the charge nurses they had this new tool at their disposal. When a nurse was having a difficult shift and we asked, "Did you put your unit on yellow or red?" the response was, "I forgot!" After 2 weeks of reinforcement the staff began to naturally gravitate toward the system. This was a very important learning point for the team in that we had assumed that

---

> **BOX 17-3**  **UPMC Shadyside Code System for Emergency Department and Direct Admissions to Nursing Units**
>
> **CODE GREEN**
> - All conditions normal
> - Bed assignments should be made within 15 minutes of page
>
> **CODE YELLOW**
> - >2 patients with deteriorating condition
> - RN off the unit with a patient
> - 1 Condition A/C/M* in progress
> - Maximum time 30 minutes
> - Only 1 additional patient may be assigned
> - Administrative Nursing Coordinator (supervisor) will contact unit after 30 minutes
> - Unit Director/Charge RN may extend an additional 15 minutes
> - If still no resolution, Clinical Director contacted
>
> **CODE RED**
> - >3 transfers within 1 hour
> - >2 admissions within 1 hour on night shift
> - RN leaves unit unexpectedly for >1 hour, increasing the nurse: patient ratio
> - >1 Condition A/C/M* in progress
> - Maximum time 45 minutes
> - No additional patients accepted during this time period
> - Administrative Nursing Coordinator (supervisor) will contact unit after 45 minutes
> - Unit Director/Charge RN may extend an additional 15 minutes
> - If still no resolution, Clinical Director contacted
> - If Clinical Director decision to remain on Red, Vice President approval needed

*Condition A is a full cardiac and respiratory arrest; Condition C is patient is getting critical; and Condition M is a psychiatric patient outburst needing to be managed.

nurses would engage easily in empowerment, especially after our 7-year history of clinical design and the hundreds of changes we had made to their environment. This was not the case. We needed to provide significant reinforcement.

We made several modest revisions to the prototype. We began then to deal with the delicate balance between the other areas of the hospital and nursing unit in relationship to patient flow.

Criteria were developed for the catheterization laboratory and other key procedural areas including the emergency department. Again we discovered the same issue: staff didn't quite believe they were empowered. There was one department that went on Code Red every day. This unit had traditionally received many admissions—up to 15 on an evening shift. It was important that leadership support the decision of the staff. It took 30 days for the staff to settle down and use the criteria appropriately.

## OUTCOMES AND IMPLICATIONS

The biggest outcome of the new system was the sense from the charge nurses throughout the organization that their assessment of patient situations and opinions mattered. Their sense of control over practice and patient outcomes also improved.

Politically, Code Red caused concern with our emergency department and postanesthesia recovery unit. Empowering nurses to slow throughput was unheard of in our organization. Sending a steady message that patient safety is the goal helped us to gain acceptance over time.

Excellence in health care is created through cultural transformation and system designs. Designs such as Code Red are key simple solutions that empower nurses and create a safer environment. Core to fixing health care is making it safer.

Building the hospital of the future where every patient received the right care, at the right time, in the right way, every time is the vision for UPMC Shadyside. We hope that our sharing of this solution will help you to join our journey.

## *Lessons Learned*

- Empowering nurses at the bedside to control admission to their departments can add significant safety on a patient unit.
- Diligence is required to assure the system is successfully implemented, as staff nurses need constant reinforcement.
- Overall, Code Red can be a great nurse satisfier and assist in retention.

*Taking Action*

Angela P. Clark, Cathie E. Guzzetta, Michael Aldridge, Theresa A. Meyers, Dezra J. Eichhorn, & Wayne Voelmeck

## Family Presence at the Bedside: Changing Hospital Policy

*"Here in America we are descended in blood and spirit from revolutionists and rebels—men and women who dared to dissent from accepted doctrine."*

DWIGHT D. EISENHOWER

Nurses who are committed to meeting the needs of their patients and families inevitably will be confronted with difficult clinical problems and decisions. Such a situation confronted Theresa Meyers, a trauma case manager in the emergency department (ED), the day that she encountered a critically ill 14-year-old trauma patient and his family. The patient had sustained a grade IV liver laceration after falling from a tree. After surgery he had been in and out of cardiopulmonary arrest. The staff caring for the patient notified Theresa and the family that it was "okay to come in now." When they reached his room, they were told "it's not a good time." As the door closed in their face,

Theresa correctly assumed the patient had arrested again. The patient's mother looked at Theresa and said she understood what was going on but wanted to be with her son. Theresa explained what was happening, but the mother was insistent that she needed to be at her son's side. Instead of escorting them back to the waiting room, Theresa went into the trauma room. She explained the situation to the team and asked whether she could bring the parents in. Although reluctant, the physician in charge agreed, and the parents were escorted to the bedside. Here they had the opportunity to talk to their son, coach him in the fight to keep going, and tell him how much they loved him before he died.

After this incident, some members of the health care team criticized Theresa's actions. There was talk that she might lose her job. One physician told her "pigs would fly" before family members would be allowed again at the bedside during resuscitation. Theresa defended her actions in subsequent "on-the-carpet" meetings by stating that the family had made their needs perfectly clear and that in this situation, the right thing had been done. They wanted to be at their son's bedside during his last moments of life. Later, his mother said had they not been allowed in to be with their son, they would have always wondered if his hearing their voices might have made a difference. She said that a kind of peace came to them by knowing they were there comforting him at the end of his short life.

In the days that followed, Theresa agonized over the incident. Such reflection caused her to move from an analysis of the incident to a more general examination of the rationale directing traditional practice. Then the clinical problem emerged. Theresa asked a simple question: Why do we ban all family members from the bedside during cardiopulmonary resuscitation (CPR)? Convinced that some families had a strong need to be with their loved ones during resuscitative efforts, Theresa set out on a path to change practice.

## STRATEGIES USED TO CHANGE PRACTICE

Resolving a clinical problem often can be accomplished using one of several strategies: changing a policy or procedure; using administrative decision-making; taking educational approaches; or conducting scientific research (Granger & Chulay, 1999). Theresa set out on her path believing that the unwritten hospital policy of banning all families from CPR could be resolved using the first strategy or by creating a new policy that permitted families at the bedside in the ED during CPR.

Theresa teamed with her trauma department director and the trauma psychosocial clinical nurse specialist to begin the change. They met with nurses and physicians in management positions to discuss creating a written family presence policy. It became apparent from the many personal issues and legitimate concerns voiced that the environment was not ready for an immediate change by instituting a written family presence policy. Many health care practitioners understood the desires of family members to be at the bedside but felt that the potential risks for the medical team outweighed the benefits for the patient and the family.

As the family presence team gathered the data from opponents who cited their reasons why family presence should not be permitted, it became clear that most of the arguments against family presence were based on opinions and beliefs not supported by research or experience with the event. For example, colleagues stated several problems they thought could happen if families were brought to the bedside during CPR and several reasons for not doing so, such as the following:

- Family members might lose control or faint.
- Family members might disrupt or interfere with patient care.
- The team did not have time to take care of anxious family members because patient care came first.
- The event would be too traumatic for family.
- The risk of liability might increase.

Although opposition to family presence was great and attempts to create a family presence policy were unsuccessful at this stage, the discussion provided a forum by which nurses and physicians could voice their concerns. These discussions were important in the process of change and also were productive in gathering the data about the issues and fears involved. Considering the strong opposition encountered, the family presence team consulted the hospital's nursing research consultant, who recommended seeking administrative support and educating the health care providers about the existing research on family presence.

Believing that practice might be changed by an administrative decision, the family presence team set out to gain the support of key administrative players. They met with the president and chief executive officer of the hospital and with the senior vice president of nursing. They discussed the issues regarding the first family presence case, the problems that confronted them, and their intent to change practice, and they asked for support. Although the team received unanimous support from these key individuals, they learned that any administrative decision to change the existing policy banning families from the bedside needed to be initiated by the ED.

Over time the team became aware that educational efforts would be ineffective in changing practice because there was little clinical or research documentation on family presence. However, team members distributed some of the clinical and research articles that did exist (Doyle et al., 1987; Hanson & Strawser, 1992) to their colleagues. These educational efforts were assisted when the Emergency Nurses Association (ENA) published an 84-page guideline on implementing family presence programs during invasive procedures and CPR (ENA, 1995).

## CHANGING PRACTICE THROUGH RESEARCH INVESTIGATION

Because the family presence team was unable to change practice by developing a family presence policy, by achieving administrative decision-making, or by conducting staff development, and because little research had been conducted on family presence, the group determined that the best strategy for changing practice was to examine the issue through research investigation. Doing this made the issue of family presence scientific instead of emotional, allowing agreement among even some of the strongest opponents that scientific investigation was warranted. Thus, a series of systematic studies were conducted.

### Designing the Survey

In earlier discussions, opponents told the family presence team that the family members of patients admitted to their county, regional, level-I trauma center probably would not want to be present at the bedside with their loved one during CPR. To determine the validity of this belief, the family presence team worked closely with the hospital's nursing research consultant (Dr. Guzzetta) to conduct a retrospective survey of family members of patients who had died in the ED in the prior year to determine whether they would have wanted to be present during their loved one's CPR. With her direction, the team developed a retrospective survey on family presence and collected data from 25 family members within a few months.

The findings supported what the team surmised from clinical experience: 80% of families said they would have wanted to be in the room during CPR had they been given the opportunity and believed it would have been helpful to them and to the patient if they had been at the bedside (Meyers, Eichhorn, & Guzzetta, 1998). In fact, these findings were later found to be consistent with the cumulative results from national and local surveys and polls, which have revealed that between 60% and 80% of families would want to be present in the ED with a loved one who is undergoing emergency procedures (Baucher, Vinci, Waring, 1989; Baucher, Vinci, Bak, Pearson, Corwin, 1996; Boie, Moore, Brommett, & Nelson, 1999; Klein et al., 1998; Redley & Hood, 1996; Taylor, Bonilla, Silver, & Sagy, 1996; *USA Today,* 2000).

### Another Study

After determining that the majority of the families wanted to be at the bedside, the team developed a second research proposal using both qualitative and quantitative approaches to identify the problems and benefits of family presence during invasive procedures and CPR. Additional nurse researchers were added to the team, blending the resources of academic and clinical expertise. The family presence protocol used in this study was adapted from the 1995 ENA guidelines on family presence (ENA, 1995), which had been updated in 2001 (ENA, 2001). Two additional elements were added to the existing ENA protocol: use of a family facilitator and an on-site screening of the family member to assess suitability for the family presence experience. In our protocol, a nurse or chaplain was designated as the family facilitator who determined whether family members were suitable family presence candidates by assessing individuals for appropriate levels of coping and the absence of combative behaviors, extreme emotional instability, or behaviors consistent with an altered mental state. (In a later study, we added suspected child abusers as not qualifying to be offered the family presence experience.) Agreement to bring a family member to the bedside was sought from conscious patients and the attending physician. Appropriate family members were then offered the family presence option and prepared for the visit with an explanation of the patient's appearance, what they would see and hear in the room, and the importance of their supportive role. The family facilitator brought the family members to bedside, stayed with them, and guided them through the experience.

Surveys were developed to identify the problems and benefits of family presence from the perspectives of the patient, family member, and health care provider (e.g., nurses, physicians). During the proposal and development phase of the research study, the family presence team also consulted with the chief of emergency medicine, chief of surgery, trauma surgeons, the hospital and medical school attorneys, and individuals in risk management, infection control, and psychiatry to garner advice and incorporate their recommendations into the research study. The study was approved by the hospital and Institutional Review Board and was funded by a grant from the national Emergency Medicine Foundation and Emergency Nurses Foundation.

## Study Findings

The study, completed in the ED over a 16-month period, included 43 cases of family presence (24 invasive procedures, 19 CPRs). The overall patient mortality was 56%. A total of 39 family members, 9 patients, 60 nurses, and 36 physicians were surveyed. Complete findings of this study have been published previously (Eichhorn, Meyers, Guzzetta, Clark, Klein, et al., 2001; Meyers, Eichhorn, Guzzetta, Clark, Klein, et al., 2000). For families, family presence was perceived as a right, as a family obligation, and as a natural event that they described as a positive experience. All family members said it was helpful to them to see and hear what was going on and said it helped them to understand the seriousness of the situation and to understand that everything possible had been done to help their loved one. While at the bedside, family members had a job and a meaningful role. They were emotional supporters who provided comfort and prevented aloneness. They touched, kissed, calmed, and prayed with the patient. They were staff helpers who provided information about the patient. Their presence also served as a reminder that the patient was a person and part of a family. For dying patients, family presence gave family members a chance to say goodbye and come to closure on a shared life. All families said that given a similar situation, they would do it again (Meyers et al., 2000).

The patient experiences with family presence were also positive. Patients related that family members provided them comfort and help and were a reminder of "personhood" to the health care providers. The following are a few examples of patients' comments about having a family member at the bedside (Eichhorn et al., 2001, p. 30):

- "It makes the stress easier on the patient."
- "You know somebody is there that cares about you."
- "They could help me communicate because it was a little difficult for me to do that…in that much pain."
- "I think there is a lot more compassion from the doctors and nurses if a family member is standing there."

Most (85%) of the nurses and physicians surveyed felt comfortable with families at bedside during the emergency. Likewise, most supported family presence during CPR (76%) and invasive procedures (73%) and wanted the family presence program continued at the institution (88%). The majority thought the experience helped meet the family's (78%) and patient's (73%) emotional and spiritual needs. Many nurses and physicians thought family presence made them more mindful of the patient's dignity, emphasized the need for privacy and pain management, and encouraged more professional behavior and conversations at the bedside (Meyers et al., 2000).

For many health care providers, the rather dismal outcomes from CPR provide an important context for the family presence experience as a necessary one for family members (Clark et al., 2005). The majority of patients who undergo resuscitation do not survive, with statistics reported to be less than 17% for in-hospital arrests (Peberdy, Kaye, Ornato, Larkin, Nadkarni, et al., 2003) and 1% to 20% for out-of-hospital arrests (Stiell et al., 1999). Providers recognize that it is often the last chance for families to be together in life. Some providers report that the family presence experience facilitates the grief process and acceptance of the loved one's death (Meyers et al., 2000). In a qualitative study of six family members whose loved ones underwent resuscitation, Wagner (2004) found that family members were permitted to "break the rules" and enter the room, but only after patients were stabilized. They were "kept from their loved ones during the time of CPR, just when both families and patients are extremely vulnerable" (p. 419). Poignant family responses of gratitude for being able to experience family presence during resuscitation can be found in the literature (Clark, Aldridge, Guzzetta, Nyquist-Heise, & Norris, 2005). Kirchhoff and colleagues (2002) studied family members' experiences with death in the ICU and found they spoke of the importance of having a chance to say good-bye, and regrets lingered with them about missed opportunities. Berger and other physician colleagues (2004) noted that "CPR is unique: the patient dies more often than not" (p. 241) and that the interval between the intervention of CPR and knowing the outcome is brief, usually minutes. They suggest that the benefit to families stems from the opportunity to share a loved one's last minutes of life. Notably, studies of family presence always provided family members with the option to go into the room; they were never forced or expected to do so. We believe this is one of the cardinal principles of family presence practice.

## CHANGING CLINICAL PRACTICE BASED ON EVIDENCE

Resolving a clinical problem can be accomplished by research investigation. The results of an isolated study, however, often provide insufficient evidence to change clinical practice. Therefore, when changing clinical practice, nurses will need to arm themselves with the data from published investigations.

After completion of the study, for example, the family presence team revisited the literature and found additional outcome studies on family presence that consistently documented the multiple benefits of this practice. For the families, these benefits include knowing that everything possible was done and removing the family's doubt about what was happening to the patient (Anderson, McCall, Leversha, & Webster, 1994; Doyle et al., 1987; Hanson & Strawser, 1992; Robinson, Mackenzie-Ross, Campbell-Hewson, Egleston, & Prevost, 1998; Timmermans, 1997); reducing their own anxiety and fear (Powers & Rubenstein, 1999; Robinson et al., 1998; Shapira & Tamir, 1996); feeling they had supported and helped the patient (Doyle et al., 1987; Hanson & Strawser, 1992; Powers &

Rubenstein, 1999; Sacchetti, Carraccio, Leva, Harris, & Lichenstein, 2000; Shapira & Tamir, 1996; Wolfram & Turner, 1996); achieving closure on a life shared together (Hanson & Strawser, 1992); and facilitating their grieving (Anderson et al., 1994; Belanger & Reed, 1997; Doyle et al., 1987; Hanson & Strawser, 1992; Powers & Rubenstein, 1999; Robinson et al., 1998; Sacchetti, Lichenstein, Carraccio, Harris, 1996; Timmermans, 1997).

In addition, research findings reveal that given a similar event, nearly all family members would do it again (Belanger & Reed, 1997; Doyle et al., 1987; Powers & Rubenstein, 1999). Investigators have found no disruptions in the operations of the medical team during family presence events (Anderson et al., 1994; Baucher et al., 1996; Belanger & Reed, 1997; Doyle et al., 1987; Hanson & Strawser, 1992; Robinson et al., 1998; Sacchetti et al, 1996; Mangurten, et al., 2005; Mangurten, Scott, Guzzetta, Clark, Vinson, et al., 2006; Sacchetti, Paston, & Carraccio, 2005), and no adverse psychologic effects among family members who participated in bedside visitation (Belanger & Reed, 1997; Mangurten et al., 2006; Robinson et al., 1998). Based on analyses of 193 videotaped interactions in three level-I trauma centers in the United States, researchers found that no family members lost control or interfered with medical care (Morse & Pooler, 2002). They reported a variety of emotional responses (speaking consoling words, crying, remaining silent) and noted that reactions between the patient and family member tended to occur in opposite directions (Morse & Pooler, 2002). For example, if a patient became emotional, then the family member tended to become silent or stoic. The reasons for this pattern are unclear, but it may partly explain why the emotional levels rarely escalate when family members are brought into the room.

After completion of our study, the family presence team presented the results to the staff. Because of the positive experience with family presence over a 16-month period and the findings that emerged not only from our study but also from others, a family presence policy was developed using the ENA guidelines and was later approved by the hospital's policy and procedure committee for hospital-wide use (Parkland Health and Hospital System, 1999). This practice continues today.

Evidence supporting family presence continues to mount, and this evidence is bringing about practice changes, in part as a result of support from national professional organizations. It is likely that the family presence movement will continue to grow because of the cumulative results of research demonstrating that the benefits of family presence for patients and families outweigh the risks. Endorsements of family presence by several professional organizations have been a strong influence on the movement. Family presence has recently been incorporated into the Trauma Nursing Core Course (*ENA*, 2002) and the Emergency Nursing Pediatric Course (*ENA*, 2004). Moreover, the American Heart Association recommends in its Guidelines 2005 for Cardiopulmonary Resuscitation and Emergency Cardiovascular Care (American Heart Association & International Liaison Committee on Resuscitation, 2005) and in its Pediatric Advanced Life Support course (American Academy of Pediatrics & American Heart Association, 2002) that whenever possible, health care providers should offer family members the option to remain with their loved ones during resuscitation efforts (American Heart Association & International Liaison Committee on Resuscitation, 2005). More recently the American Association of Critical Care Nurses (AACN) has published a Practice Alert on Family Presence recommending that family members of all patients undergoing CPR and invasive procedures be given the option of being present at the bedside and that all patient care units have a written practice document for family presence (AACN, 2004). In addition, the AACN journal published a critical review of the studies and evidence to date compiled by Halm (2005). The arguments for implementing a family presence program can become even more powerful when the need to comply with such guidelines is included in the dialogue.

Despite the evidence supporting family presence, a recent survey of both AACN and ENA members found that only 5% of units have a written policy allowing family presence (MacLean, Guzzetta, White, Fontaine, Eichhorn, et al., 2003). However, nearly half of the nurses surveyed reported that family presence was allowed in their unit despite the lack of a formal policy. A policy serves as a foundation for the organization's support of family presence and also identifies barriers that may be present.

## PIGS DO FLY

So it seems that pigs do fly! Our own experiences have taught us valuable lessons about how to develop institutional policies to allow family presence to occur. Many individuals from other hospitals have contacted us about their plans to start a family presence program. In personal communication, colleagues report fewer obstacles to overcome than we encountered. They attribute their success to having research findings available. They have said that instituting a family presence protocol in their hospitals has been a fairly simple process involving educating staff and implementing a policy. Theresa Meyers experienced this simplified process when she became the ED nurse manager in a private hospital a few years after she had the initial family presence case. When she presented a packet of the research findings to the health care provider team, they readily agreed to offer the option of family presence to their patients and patients' families. The team agreed that their core philosophy of care was to provide care that addresses the emotional needs as well as the physical needs of their patients.

### Finding a Champion

When we encountered opposition to our ideas, we learned that a project needs a champion. A champion is an effective leader who creates a new vision, articulates it to others, and then moves to institutionalize that vision (Ulschak & SnowAntle, 1995). Moreover, a team effort is needed to accomplish the task. Both a physician advocate and administrative support are imperative. Allowing colleagues to voice their opinions and discuss potential barriers is essential in the change process. Providing staff with research-based articles and current documentation supporting family presence not only raises awareness but also provides the solid evidence with which to counter emotional, fact-free arguments. A baseline survey for staff can help identify support for the policy as well as pinpoint misconceptions staff may have about family presence. The results of the survey can be used to help develop an educational plan. Staff surveys and interviews are available for measuring baseline attitudes about family presence (ENA, 2001; Mangurten et al., 2005).

### Drafting a Policy

Preparing a draft family presence policy using ENA guidelines and adapting it to meet the needs of the institution can lay the foundation for discussing and resolving conflicts and incorporating essential recommendations from the hospital community. Consultation with colleagues in nursing, medicine, surgery, trauma, risk management, psychiatry, social work, pastoral care, law, and infection control will ensure that various legal, ethical, and biopsychosocial concerns have been addressed in the policy. Several family presence protocols have been published that can be adapted for use (ENA, 2001; Meyers et al., 2000; Mangurten et al., 2005).

### Piloting the Policy

The role of family facilitator cannot be overlooked in the process. In particular, the staff must know who to call when the usual daytime staff is not present; otherwise, family presence may not be offered if resuscitation occurs in the middle of the night. Developing an algorithm with contact information in conjunction with support personnel may address this gap. Piloting the policy as a demonstration project allows staff and administration to learn the issues, gain experience with the practice, and embrace the concept (Guzzetta, Clark, & Wright, 2006). For those readers who might be interested in setting up a family presence program, a roadmap using the steps outlined here for developing, implementing, and evaluating a family presence policy in a pediatric ED has recently been published (Mangurten et al., 2005).

### Turning Opponents and Others into Advocates

Our research findings and those of others have demonstrated that health care providers who initially oppose family presence often become advocates for the practice after experiencing its many benefits for patients and families (Meyers et al., 2000; Robinson

et al., 1998; Sacchetti et al., 2000). Ellison (2003) reported that nurses who were certified as emergency nurses or had a bachelor's or master's degree had more positive attitudes about family presence. Over a decade of research can now be found describing trends about health care providers and family presence (Clark et al., 2005).

### Using a Team

We strongly believe that the successful results we achieved were solely possible because of our joint effort and the varied resources and talents each team member contributed to the project. For all the multiple times we were ready to give up, we have been rewarded repeatedly as families continue to share their powerful stories about family presence and the impact the event has had on their lives.

## *Lessons Learned*

- Gathering the facts about family presence and other potential changes in practice provides the necessary evidence for institutional support of the change.
- Having the research and facts is not sufficient to change policy; piloting the policy encourages buy-in from individuals and the institution.
- A significant change in institutional policy is a team effort but requires a champion to keep the change targeted and moving.
- Never forget: Pigs do fly when you're persistent, strategic, and thoughtful about making change.

### REFERENCES

American Academy of Pediatrics & American Heart Association. (2002). *PALS Provider Manual*. Dallas: American Heart Association.

American Association of Critical Care Nurses (AACN). (2004). Practice Alert: Family presence during CPR and invasive procedures. *AACN News, 21*(11), 4. Retrieved February 10, 2006, from *www.aacn.org*.

American Heart Association. (2005). American Heart Association guidelines for cardiopulmonary resuscitation and emergency cardiovascular care. *Circulation 112*(24, suppl), 1-211.

Anderson, B., McCall, E., Leversha, A., & Webster, T. (1994). A review of children's dying in a paediatric intensive care unit. *New Zealand Medical Journal, 107*(985), 345-347.

Baucher, H., Vinci, R., Bak, S., Pearson, C., & Corwin, M. (1996). Parents and procedures: A randomized control trial. *Pediatrics, 98,* 861-867.

Baucher, H., Vinci, R., & Waring, C. (1989). Pediatric procedures: Do parents want to watch? *Pediatrics, 84,* 907-909.

Belanger, M. A., & Reed, S. (1997). A rural community hospital's experience with family-witnessed resuscitation. *Journal of Emergency Nursing, 23*(3), 238-239.

Berger, J. T., Brody, G., Eisenstein, L., & Pollack, M. (2004). Do potential recipients of a cardiopulmonary resuscitation want their family members to attend? A survey of public preferences. *Journal of Clinical Ethics, 15*(3), 237-242.

Boie, E. T., Moore, G. P., Brommett, C., & Nelson, D. R. (1999). Do parents want to be present during invasive procedures performed on their children in the emergency department? A survey of 400 parents. *Annals of Emergency Medicine, 34*(1), 70-74.

Clark, A. P., Aldridge, M. D., Guzzetta, C. E., Nyquist-Heise, P., Norris, M., et al. (2005). Family presence during cardiopulmonary resuscitation. *Critical Care Nursing Clinics of North America, 17,* 23-32.

Doyle, C. J., Post, H., Burney, R. E., Maino, J., Keefe, M., & Rhee, K. J. (1987). Family participation during resuscitation: An option. *Annals of Emergency Medicine, 16*(6), 673-675.

Eichhorn, D. J., Meyers, T. A., Guzzetta, C. E., Clark, A. P., Klein, J. D., et al. (2001). Family presence during invasive procedures and resuscitation: Hearing the voice of the patient. *American Journal of Nursing, 101*(5), 26-33.

Ellison, S. (2003). Nurses' attitudes toward family presence during resuscitative efforts and invasive procedures. *Journal of Emergency Nursing, 29,* 515-521.

Emergency Nurses Association (ENA). (1995). *Presenting the option for family presence* (program educational booklet) (2nd ed.). Park Ridge, IL: ENA.

Emergency Nurses Association (ENA). (2001). *Presenting the option of family presence* (2nd ed.). Des Plaines, IL: ENA. Retrieved July 20, 2005, from *www.ena.org.*

Emergency Nurses Association. (2002). *Trauma nursing core course.* Park Ridge, IL: Emergency Nurses Association.

Emergency Nurses Association. (2004). *Emergency nursing pediatric course* (3rd ed.). Des Plaines, IL: Emergency Nurses Association.

Granger, B. B., & Chulay, M. (1999). *Research strategies for clinicians.* Stamford, CT: Appleton & Lange.

Guzzetta, C. E., Clark, A. P., & Wright, J. L. (2006). Family presence in emergency medical services for children. *Clinical Pediatric Emergency Medicine, 7*(1), in press.

Halm, M. A. (2005). Family presence during resuscitation: A critical review of the literature. *American Journal of Critical Care, 14*(6), 494-512.

Hanson, C., & Strawser, D. (1992). Family presence during cardiopulmonary resuscitation: Foote hospital emergency department's nine-year perspective. *Journal of Emergency Nursing, 18*(2), 104-106.

Kirchhoff, K., Walker, L., Hutton, A., Spuhler, V., Cole, B. V., & Clemmer, T. (2002). The vortex: Families' experience with death in the intensive care unit. *American Journal of Critical Care, 11*(3), 200-209.

Klein, J. D., Taliaferro, E., Meyers, T. A., Eichhorn, D. J., Guzzetta, C. E., et al. (1998). *Family presence during invasive procedures/resuscitation: Final report submitted to the Emergency Medicine Foundation and the Emergency Nursing Foundation.* Irving, TX. Unpublished manuscript.

MacLean, S. L., Guzzetta, C. E., White, C., Fontaine, D., Eichhorn, D. J., et al. (2003). Family presence during cardiopulmonary resuscitation and invasive procedures: Practices of critical care and emergency nurses. Simultaneously published in *American Journal of Critical Care, 12,* 246-257 and *Journal of Emergency Nursing, 29,* 32-42.

Mangurten, J., Scott, S. H., Guzzetta, C. E., Clark, A. P., Vinson, L., et al. (2006). Effects of family presence during resuscitation and invasive procedures in a pediatric emergency department. *Journal of Emergency Nursing,* submitted for publication.

Mangurten J., Scott, S., Guzzetta, C. E, Sperry, J. U., Vinson, L., et al. (2005). Family presence: Making room. *American Journal of Nursing, 105*(5), 40-48.

Meyers, T. A., Eichhorn, D. J., & Guzzetta, C. E. (1998). Do families want to be present during CPR? A retrospective survey. *Journal of Emergency Nursing, 24,* 400-405.

Meyers, T. A., Eichhorn, D. J., Guzzetta, C. E., Clark, A. P., Klein, J. D., et al. (2000). Family presence during invasive procedures and resuscitation. *American Journal of Nursing, 100*(2), 32-42.

Morse, J. M., & Pooler, C. (2002). Patient-family-nurse interactions in the trauma-resuscitation room. *American Journal of Critical Care, 11,* 240-249.

Parkland Health and Hospital System. (1999). *Protocol for family presence during invasive procedure and resuscitation.* Available on request from Parkland Hospital, Dallas, Texas.

Peberdy, M. A., Kaye, W., Ornato, J. P., Larkin, G. L., Nadkarni, V., et al. (2003). Cardiopulmonary resuscitation of adults in the hospital: A report of 14,720 cardiac arrests from the National Registry of Cardiopulmonary Resuscitation. *Resuscitation, 58,* 297-308.

Powers, K. S., & Rubenstein, J. S. (1999). Family presence during invasive procedures in the pediatric intensive care unit. *Archives of Pediatrics & Adolescent Medicine, 153,* 955-958.

Redley, B., & Hood, K. (1996). Staff attitudes towards family presence during resuscitation. *Accident and Emergency Nursing, 4*(3),145-151.

Robinson, S. M., Mackenzie-Ross, S., Campbell-Hewson, G. L., Egleston, C. V., & Prevost, A. T. (1998). Psychological effect of witnessed resuscitation on bereaved relatives. *Lancet, 352,* 614-617.

Sacchetti, A., Carraccio, C., Leva, E., Harris, R. H., and Lichenstein, R. (2000). Acceptance of family member presence during pediatric resuscitation in the emergency department: Effects of personal experience. *Pediatric Emergency Care, 16*(2), 85-87.

Sacchetti, A., Lichenstein, R., Carraccio, C. A., & Harris, R. H. (1996). Family member presence during pediatric emergency department procedures. *Pediatric Emergency Care, 12*(4), 268-271.

Sacchetti, A., Paston, C., & Carraccio, C. (2005). Family members do not disrupt care when present during invasive procedures. *Academic Emergency Medicine, 12,* 477-479.

Shapira, M., & Tamir, A. (1996). Presence of family member during upper endoscopy. *Journal of Clinical Gastroenterology, 22,* 272-274.

Stiell, I. G., Wells, G. A., Field, B. J., Spaite, K. W., De Maio, V. J., et al. (1999). Improved out of hospital cardiac arrest survival through the inexpensive optimization of an existing defibrillation program. OPALS study phase II. *Journal of the American Medical Association, 281*(13), 1175-1181.

Taylor, N., Bonilla, L., Silver, P., & Sagy, M. (1996). Pediatric procedures: Do parents want to be present? *Critical Care Medicine, 24*(Suppl), 131.

Timmermans, S. (1997). High touch in high tech: The presence of relatives and friends during resuscitation efforts. *Scholarly Inquiry for Nursing Practice, 11*(2), 153-168.

Ulschak, F. L., & SnowAntle, S. M. (1995). *Team architecture: The manager's guide to designing effective work teams.* Ann Arbor, MI: Health Administration Press.

*USA Today.* (2000, March 7). Would you want to be in the ED while doctors worked on a family member? Retrieved June 21, 2000, from *www.usatoday.com.*

Wagner, J. M. (2004). Lived experience of critically ill patients' family members during cardiopulmonary resuscitation. *American Journal of Critical Care, 13*(5), 416-420.

Wolfram, R. W., & Turner, E. D. (1996). Effects of parental presence during children's venipuncture. *Academic Emergency Medicine, 3*(1), 58-63.

# chapter 18

# The Nursing Workforce: Supply and Demand

Kim Welch Hoover

*"We face the challenge of increasing capacity to meet demand, while managing a tight supply chain."*

JOHN HANSON

The political dynamics affecting the health care workforce in the United States have become more significant as we face current and predicted shortages in many employment categories. Increasing demands for health care as our population ages, coupled with stiff competition for scarce resources, have pushed workforce issues to the forefront of political debates across the country. This chapter explores how economic, political, and demographic issues affect the future of the nursing workforce.

## DEMOGRAPHICS

In the United States, registered nurses (RNs) make up the largest number of health care professionals (Peterson, 2001). The current supply of over 2.5 million RNs is predicted to decrease as nurses retire and fewer graduate from U.S. nursing programs. Various scenarios presented by Biviano, Fritz, Spencer, and Dall (2004) indicate that increases in the number of new graduates, increases in wages relative to alternative occupations, and delays in retirement will have a modest to substantial effect on alleviating the RN shortfall predicted by 2020.

Although the nursing crisis has somewhat overshadowed the shortage of workers in allied health professions, providers such as occupational therapists, physical therapists, and pharmacists face many of the same dynamics that affect the nursing shortage. Because there are over 200 allied health professions that include an estimated 11 million workers, understanding these shortages is best accomplished by considering the issues in the context of the entire health care workforce (O'Neil, 2005).

Estimating the supply and demand for allied health workers if those workers are either unlicensed or uncertified is difficult. Those who choose not to be credentialed are often left uncounted in available data sets. The impact of broad health worker shortages is intensified as programs are susceptible to budget shortfalls, leading them to vie for competing and often scarce resources. Rather than simultaneously building educational capacities, the focus often hinges on closure of programs because of lack of funding. Many programs housed in public education settings are susceptible to state budget shortfalls. Charging higher tuition is often not an option in public institutions, and therefore there is limited ability to withstand budget cuts (O'Neil, 2005; Southeast Regional Center for Health Workforce Studies, 2005).

## EFFECT OF WORKFORCE SHORTAGES

### IMPACT ON QUALITY

As the largest group of health care professionals in the United States, RNs are crucial to the provision of high-quality health care. Yet many health care organizations have decreased nursing staff as they reduce costs to raise profits. An unintentional effect may have been compromised quality of care. However, McCue, Mark, and Harless (2003) found no decrease in profit when RN staff levels were increased.

Researchers have identified several effects of shortages in the nursing workforce. Hospitals with a higher nurse/patient ratio ran an increased risk of higher patient mortality as well as job dissatisfaction and burnout among the nurses (Aiken, Clarke, & Sloane, 2000; Aiken, Clarke, Sloane, Sochalski, & Silber, 2002b). In addition, hospitals with higher proportions of nurses with baccalaureate or higher degrees had a decrease in mortality and failure to rescue after common surgical procedures (Aiken, 2005; Aiken, Clarke, Cheung, Sloane, & Silber, 2003; Clarke & Aiken, 2003). A study using an international sample of hospitals revealed that nurses who worked in settings with low staffing were three times as likely to report lower quality of care as nurses who reported working in areas with perceived adequate staffing and support (Aiken, Clarke, & Sloane, 2002a) (see *Nurse Staffing Impact on Organizational Outcomes*, later in this chapter).

## ACCESS TO CARE

Because rural communities rely on fewer health care professionals than urban areas, shortages in health care providers usually result in greater difficulty ensuring equity in access to care. In contrast to statistics for other health care providers, the percentage of nurse practitioners providing care in rural communities is equivalent to the population distribution (Ricketts, 2005). Workforce shortages in rural areas compound the problems of recruiting and retaining health care providers. Policies likely to continue to influence access to care include those targeting required practice in underserved areas for educational loan forgiveness, reimbursement at higher levels for practitioners, the establishment of more federally funded health centers, and innovative multidisciplinary health professional training programs (National Rural Health Association, 2003; Ricketts, 2005).

## ECONOMICS ISSUES

The health care industry has a significant impact on the local, state, and national economy. For example, in Mississippi, the health industry generates over 17% of the entire workforce payroll (Mississippi Hospital Association [MHA], 2004). Economic issues around the shortage include costs to society and institutions and the cost of increasing programs. Growth in medical costs has outpaced growth in wages for the past 8 years and has shown no signs of slowing (Bradley, Ginsburg, & Cookson, 2005).

With increasing public attention on quality, errors, and the escalating costs of health care, health care professionals are searching for means of identifying cost-effective methods of providing the highest quality of care. Health care quality ratings are generated by private and public companies in the form of health care report cards available to consumers. Health Grades (*www.healthgrades.com*) provides ratings for hospitals based on how well the hospital is predicted to perform versus how well it actually performed.

Understanding how workforce shortages affect health care costs can lead policymakers to make decisions that may result in savings over the long term. Hospital care is the most significant driver of health care spending growth. Many internal and external factors affect hospital costs, but wages and salaries account for the majority of growth in costs. Workforce shortages require that hospitals increase compensation to retain a highly skilled RN workforce. As our population grows and ages, each person uses more health care services, requiring more health care workers. Consequently, workforce shortages during times of increased demand for services results in increased cost pressures on institutions providing care. Organizations such as the American Hospital Association stress the need for policymakers to include factors driving increased spending in their discussions of rising health care expenditures. Understanding how shortages of RNs, pharmacists, technicians, and other health care providers affect those expenditures is critical to salient policy decision-making (Lewin Group, 2005).

## THE IMPORTANCE OF RELIABLE AND VALID DATA

In the 1990s the nursing community spoke out about the exponential increase in the practice of replacing RNs with unlicensed assistive personnel as endangering the lives and care of patients. The Institute of Medicine (IOM) (Wunderlich, Sloane, & Davis, 1996) responded to these outcries with an analysis of the relationship between RN staffing and patient outcomes. The IOM concluded that there was not enough evidence in the form of research to support this relationship. The nursing community responded with well-designed studies of this relationship, providing policymakers, health care administrators, and others with the data documenting that RN care resulted in lower rates of mortality and morbidity.

Abundant literature exists describing the health care workforce and issues surrounding that workforce. Nursing workforce literature has centered around two themes:

- Nursing workforce analyzed and described (Auerbach, Buerhaus, & Staiger, 2000; Buerhaus, 2001; Buerhaus, 2002; Buerhaus & Auerbach, 1999; Buerhaus & Staiger, 1999; Buerhaus, Staiger, & Auerbach, 2000; Buerhaus, Staiger, & Auerbach, 2003)
- Relationship of the nursing workforce and outcomes (Aiken et al., 2002a; Aiken et al., 2002b; Aiken et al., 2003; Clarke, Sloane, & Aiken, 2002; Mark, Salyer, & Wan, 2000; McCue, Mark, & Harless, 2003; Mark, Hughes, & Jones, 2004; Mattke, Needleman, Buerhaus, Stewart, & Zelevinsky, 2004; Needleman & Buerhaus, 2003; Needleman, Buerhaus, Mattke, Stewart, & Zelevinsky, 2002; Sochalski & Aiken, 1999)

National reports have been generated at a rapid rate in the past 5 years. Reports relevant to the politics of the nursing workforce are included in Web Resources.

Policymakers, legislators, and those hoping to influence legislation are increasingly reliant on data provided in these reports and the interpretation of those data. Experts and organizations such as the Centers for Health Workforce Studies in California, as well as other groups in Illinois, New York, North Carolina, and Texas, provide analyses to assist health care professionals, health professions schools, care delivery organizations, and public policymakers in the interpretation and use of these reports.

Bleich and colleagues (2003) published an integrative review of 15 reports on the health care workforce shortage to examine characteristics and commonalities among the reports. The authors concluded that a lack of comprehensive solutions to workforce problems existed and a comprehensive plan would require a collaborative solution by federal and state governments, national industry, professional organizations, and the private sector.

## CURRENT INITIATIVES IN WORKFORCE PLANNING

### FUNDING OPPORTUNITIES

Health care workforce shortages are being examined and addressed by public and private entities, particularly around funding issues. Creative regional coalitions are bringing industry and education together to seek funding for collaborative projects.

The bulk of public workforce funding at the federal level comes from the Health Resources and Services Administration (HRSA) appropriations. HRSA funds workforce initiatives through grants focused on six key program areas (HRSA, 2005). Although the key program area for health professions is specific to the recruitment and education of health care professionals, the other five areas do have funding opportunities that include the health care workforce. HRSA offers a variety of funding for health care education, including, but not limited to, traineeships, fellowships, education centers, and loan repayment scholarships. HRSA's budget for 2005 totaled $7.37 billion, a $181 million increase over 2004 (*www.hrsa.gov/grants.htm*). These funds are distributed to support education in medicine and nursing, Area Health Education Centers (AHECs), public health, and other areas such as geriatrics, health education, rural health, and allied health.

President Bush's 2006 agenda for HRSA is to make Health Centers available in poor counties in an effort to expand direct health care to those who most need it. To that end, HRSA plans to increase funding for health centers by over $300 million. The emphasis on health profession recruitment and education appears to be waning as actual and requested funding for the support of health care provider education has been decreased from approximately $606 million to $287 million, a decrease of over 50% from the 2005 budget (HRSA, 2005).

The Department of Labor (DOL) is the second largest distributor of federal workforce funds. Funding is available through federal grants and through state development authorities or departments of labor. In 2005, approximately $25 million in community-based job training grants was announced. Workforce Investment Area (WIA) funds are accessible for health care workforce projects if they involve displaced workers or enhancement of workers' economic status or for those who are considered at risk for not being successful in a college or training program.

Private grant-making foundations have been critical in funding for the health care workforce for years. In fact, major funders, such as the Robert Wood Johnson Foundation (RWJF), have had substantial impact on health policy through their choice of funding initiatives. As a direct result of the RWJF Colleagues in Caring funding initiative, nursing workforce data collection and analysis processes had already been in place in some states for several years before nursing shortages occurred. These states were able to proactively address nursing workforce issues and provide models of data collection and analysis for other states to replicate (see Chapter 8). Today, numerous state centers are funded through a combination of self-generated, federal, state, industry, and private grant funding. Other examples of private health care workforce funders include the Kellogg Foundation, the Heritage Foundation, and the Helene Fuld Trust Foundation.

Private industry involvement in workforce issues has become more prevalent. None has been more obvious than the Johnson & Johnson nursing campaign. Johnson & Johnson, in conjunction with national nursing organizations, launched a national media campaign in 2002. The media blitz included television and print ads, as well as free promotional material touting nursing and nursing education as desirable careers. As a result of this campaign, Johnson & Johnson reported a heightened awareness of the issues surrounding recruitment of potential students into the nursing profession and nurses into faculty positions.

Grant seekers often reshape or redefine goals and objectives to better reflect the focus of private funders, thereby placing themselves in a better position for funding. However, most private foundations must rely on the information given them rather than expertise in the area to set funding priorities. Health care leaders have an obligation to ensure that foundations have adequate information about the need to increase the nursing workforce to make favorable decisions.

Finally, many health care organizations are funding workforce initiatives. Hospitals are addressing problems in the workplace environment, and many are continuing to fund scholarships for nursing students. Academic and service partnerships are being developed for faculty exchanges, internship and externship programs, and a variety of creative clinical experiences aimed at increasing the capacity of nursing schools (Buerhaus et al., 2003). The success of these initiatives indicates that these partnerships not only should continue, but should be expanded to include other organizations and stakeholders, such as civic organizations and private corporations.

## RACIAL, ETHNIC, AND GENDER BALANCE

No health care workforce issue has received more attention than the push to achieve a culturally competent workforce capable of representing our diverse population and cultures. Statements reflective of this goal are found in national and state policies. Funding initiatives are often given priority if the grant seeker identifies a method or process of moving toward ethnic or cultural equity in the workforce.

As noted in Table 18-1, the national RN population does not mirror the diversity of the national population. The majority of the 2000 U.S. population was white.

Many categories of allied health workers also have a higher proportion that is white. Males are underrepresented in the nursing workforce, but Buerhaus, Staiger, and Auerbach (2003) report that this number rose considerably between 2002 and 2003. It is surprising to note that this increase included a significant number of older men, possibly looking for more stable employment or economic security. Policymakers would be wise to determine the reasons older men are entering nursing and direct attention toward increasing that potential pool of RNs.

**TABLE 18-1** Comparison of U.S. Population to RN Population

| | U.S. POPULATION (2000) | RN POPULATION (2000) |
|---|---|---|
| White | 75.1% | 86.6% |
| Nonwhite | 24.9% | 13.4% |

Data from United States Census Bureau. (2005). United States census 2000. Retrieved August 1, 2005, from *www.census.gov/main/www/cen2000.html;* and Spratley, E., Johnson, A., Sochalski, J., Fritz, M., & Spencer, W. (2000). *The registered nurse population: Findings from the national sample survey of registered nurses.* Washington, DC: U.S. Department of Health and Human Services, Health Resources and Services Administration, Bureau of Health Professions. Retrieved January 10, 2005, from *http://bhpr.hrsa.gov/healthworkforce/reports/rnsurvey/rnss1.htm.*

## USE OF FOREIGN-TRAINED WORKFORCE

The use of foreign-trained health care workers has become a politically volatile issue as other countries are faced with minimal and substandard health care. Standards set for nurses who choose to work in the United States include first passing a national licensing examination as well as an English proficiency examination (Lee, 2004). Recruiters have been actively seeking foreign graduates from countries such as the Philippines, India, South Korea, Nigeria, and Mexico. Although foreign-trained nurses cited the promise of a better life as their primary reason for coming to the United States, nursing and world leaders have expressed concern about draining already strained health care systems in developing countries (see *Global Nurse Migration: Policies for Managing a Scarce Resource* in Chapter 34).

The analysis by Buerhaus and colleagues (2004) revealed that foreign-born RNs are increasingly being employed. The employment of foreign-born RNs accounted for almost one third of the total RN employment growth from 2001 to 2003. Although this employment growth has brought relief to many hospitals and other health care organizations, U.S. policymakers are faced with political, ethical, economic, and regulatory issues surrounding the use of this workforce. For instance, U.S. nursing leaders argue that the use of foreign nurse may have a negative impact on U.S. wages. On the other hand, the recruitment of Hispanic nurses would create more ethnic balance in a population that is predicted

to be the largest minority group in the country (Buerhaus et al., 2004). Some countries, such as Great Britain and Ireland, have set ethical guidelines for recruiting nurses from poorer countries (Lee, 2004).

Buchan and Sochalski (2004) reported that dialogue regarding the international migration of nurses has resulted in the recognition of the inadequacy of information that might inform policy analysis and policymaking. They raised several issues to be addressed by source and destination countries: regulation of recruitment agencies, development of an international professional registration database, and cost-effectiveness of recruiting foreign nurses in comparison with other strategies of increasing the nursing workforce. The International Council of Nurses commissioned a study of the trends and policy implications of the international migration of nurses. The authors concluded that although international recruitment was a short-term solution for developed countries, its cost-effectiveness as a solution remained unclear. Some of the recommendations included the collection of accurate data to monitor international flow, more policy attention to nursing workforces in all countries, continued and expanded research and evaluation to ensure that migrant nurses are not exploited and abused, and the development of ethical codes to support a more-effective approach to recruiting international nurses (Buchan, Kingma, & Lorenzo, 2005).

## REGIONAL WORKFORCE CENTERS

Many states do not have accurate, reliable health care workforce supply-and-demand data collection systems; therefore policymakers must rely heavily on federally reported workforce data. The National Center for Health Workforce Analysis was established under the auspices of the HRSA Bureau of Health Professions to facilitate the collection, analysis, and dissemination of national, state, and local workforce information to aid health workforce planning efforts. Current research activities within this center include supply-and-demand trends for 30 health professions and education, practice, and policy of the health care workforce (HRSA, 2005).

Over the past 8 years, six regional centers have been established in public universities and supported through the national center. The first center was launched in 1997 at the University of California San Francisco. These centers conduct research examining critical issues in the distribution, diversity, and supply of the health care workforce in the center's home state and surrounding states. Each regional center maintains a website for updates, research project dissemination, publication, and other health workforce resources. The centers and their corresponding websites are found in Web Resources.

Although each center is located within specific regions of the country, projects are generally related to issues of national importance. Funding for these projects is primarily through the National Center, and supplemental projects are carried out with state, local, and private support.

## LEGISLATIVE INITIATIVES

The increased need for nursing services, coupled with the widening gap in supply and demand, causes concern about the provision of quality nursing care. Cost containment, downsizing, increasing acuity of patients, and the shift to community nursing are only a few of the issues affecting demand for nursing services (Peterson, 2001). Historically, during times of shortages, provision of care has been enhanced by substituting unlicensed providers. After the publication of the IOM report "To Err Is Human" (Kohn, Corrigan, & Donaldson, 2000) drawing attention to patient safety and the potential for errors in an unhealthy work environment, health care leaders found themselves engaged in public debate and subjected to public scrutiny. Reductions in nursing budgets and nursing shortages have resulted in fewer nurses working more hours caring for more acutely ill patients (American Nurses Association [ANA], 2005).

Patient safety and quality of care are complex but directly related to adequate staffing. The ANA supports and promotes legislation holding hospitals accountable to a minimum standard. California was the first state to address nursing staffing through legislation mandating specific nurse/patient ratios. Regulations were to be developed and adopted by all nursing units in California. However, Governor

Schwarzenegger suspended the law before 2005, the year it was to take effect but his emergency suspension was overturned and regulations have been put into effect (see *California Nurse Staffing Ratios*, later in this chapter). Little research evidence exists to show that specific nurse/patient ratios guarantee safety and quality of patient care (ANA, 2005). The ANA worked with Congress to introduce the Registered Nurse Safe Staffing Act of 2005 (S 71) and the Quality Nursing Care Act of 2005 (HR 1372). These bills seek to require the development of staffing systems with input from RNs who are direct care providers. Public reporting of staffing information would also be required. Legislative initiatives involving staffing plans have been enacted in 10 states by the end of 2005. In 2005, Oregon passed legislation that strengthened 2001 legislation that required hospitals to implement a hospital-wide nurse staffing plan and establish internal reviews. This legislation mandated that hospitals had to include the staffing mix and the staffing plan must be developed with the participation of RNs who were providing direct care. Hospitals in violation of this law are subject to civil penalties (ANA, 2005).

The anticipated increase in demand for health care as our nation continues to age has changed the debate of using unlicensed health care providers to perform care typically rendered by licensed personnel to one of how to balance the appropriate and adequate mix of licensed and unlicensed providers. Demand for aides in long term care facilities and community-based organizations is expected to grow, as they predominately provide care to the elderly.

Given the predicted shortage of over 1 million RNs by 2020, increased pressure to use substitute providers rather than complementary providers may be great. However, the assurance of patient safety will necessitate evidence-based approaches to care delivery models that result in an effective multidisciplinary mix of health care providers. If one assumes unlicensed health care workers are interested in health care careers, this pool of providers can be tapped as potential licensed personnel through creative educational mobility plans.

## FUTURE POLICY AGENDA

Health care workforce issues are multifaceted, requiring informed and creative policy response. As health care providers and educators vie for shrinking resources, it becomes increasingly important that all stakeholders are involved in planning for the health care workforce. Just as important is the accessibility of the information needed to make competent and visionary decisions regarding the allocation of those resources. Data indicate that factors such as wage increases, private-sector initiatives, and a high national unemployment rate have resulted in strong employment growth among RNs (Buerhaus et al., 2003). Because this growth is evident in all health care professions, successful current initiatives may be duplicated and expanded across professions.

Key challenges include attracting new students to replace those lost to the workforce. This will require improving wages and benefits for all health care workers and maintaining a safe and desirable work environment. Forming partnerships between providers and high schools and universities is critical to the success of attracting students and retaining the current workforce (Chapman et al., 2004).

At the community level, health care leaders should be exploring community-based partnerships among health care providers, consumer organizations, private industry, and educational entities. Working through coalitions of diverse stakeholders is the most effective strategy to influence legislators to fund workforce initiatives. In addition, public funders are seeking initiatives that have widespread support with potential for sustainability. Communities no longer have the luxury of waiting for Congress to develop solutions for potentially dwindling health care resources (Healthcare Leadership Council, 2005).

Regional and state policy agendas should include data collection and analysis of the workforce to strengthen arguments for strategic planning and ultimately funding initiatives (Cleary et al., 2005). Nursing has received the bulk of attention, yet recruitment and retention of all health care providers is necessary for increased access and quality of care.

Of particular importance at the regional and state levels are the recruitment of a culturally competent health care workforce. Legislation to increase the recruitment and success of ethnically diverse persons in the health care professions is vital. Efforts to increase the supply of minority members must include economic, cultural, and language considerations (National Center for Health Workforce Analysis, 2003). Collection of data to begin to identify differences in demand and use of health care is central to determining the appropriate health care workforce needed. This collection of data must be supported at the state and regional levels to maintain databases for trending and comparisons across regions.

As we struggle to increase the nursing workforce in the United States, the health care workforce of other countries must be considered. The recruitment of foreign nurses is regarded by many as harmful to the health of developing countries. The United States will have to follow suit as other countries develop ethical and regulatory policies for the migration of nurses. The World Health Organization issued a policy brief in 2001 outlining the worsening nursing shortages in many countries. Questions of ethical behavior regarding recruitment methods and the assurance of equitable treatment once nurses are recruited to the United States are additional concerns that must be addressed. The United States can ill afford to be seen as jeopardizing the health of other countries to bolster its own health care workforce.

## Key Points

■ RN workforce shortages affect the quality of, access to, and cost of health care.
■ Health leaders must ensure the collection of reliable data to inform policy decisions.
■ Policy initiatives must include consideration of achieving gender and ethnic balance, incorporate changes in the workplace environment, and respect the international problem of nursing shortages.

■ A combination of public policy strategies and private sector coalitions is necessary to develop multiple solutions to a long-term and complex problem.

## *Web Resources*

**American Hospital Association (AHA)—** In Our Hands: How Hospital Leaders Can Build a Thriving Workforce (2002)
*www.hospitalconnect.com/aha/key_issues/ workforce/commission/inourhands.html*

**American Hospital Association (AHA)—** Workforce Ideas in Action: Series 2-5 (2004; 2005)
*www.healthcareworkforce.org/ healthcareworkforce/index.jsp*

**American Nurses Association (ANA)—** Nursing's Agenda for the Future: A Call to the Nation (2002)
*www.nursingworld.org/naf*

**Bureau of Health Professions, Health and Human Resources Services Administration—**Projected Supply, Demand, and Shortages of Registered Nurses: 2000-2020 (2002)
*http://bhpr.hrsa.gov/healthworkforce/reports/ rnproject/report.htm*

**Institute of Medicine (IOM)—**Keeping Patients Safe: Transforming the Work Environment (2003)
*www.iom.edu/report.asp?id=16173*

**Institute of Medicine (IOM)—**Health Professions Education: A Bridge to Quality (2003)
*www.iom.edu/report.asp?id=5914*

**Institute of Medicine (IOM)—**In the Nation's Compelling Interest: Ensuring Diversity in the Health Care Workforce (2004)
*www.iom.edu/report.asp?id=18287*

**Joint Commission for the Accreditation of Healthcare Organizations (JCAHO)—** Health Care at the Crossroads: Strategies for Addressing the Evolving Nursing Crisis (2002)
*www.jcaho.org/about+us/public+policy+ initiatives/health_care_at_the_crossroads.pdf*

**National Center for Health Workforce Analysis—**What Is Behind HRSA's Projected Supply, Demand, and Shortage of Registered Nurses? (2004)
*http://tcn01.centerfornursing.org/ nursemanpower/ Projected%20Supply% 20Demand%20Shortage%20of%20RNs.pdf*

**U.S. Department of Labor—**The Nursing Shortage (Alexander, 2002)
*www.bmcc.cuny.edu/business_partnerships/ trends-analysis/reports/pdfs/nursing %20shortage.pdf*

*Region Center Sites:*

**State University of New York at Albany—** Northeast
*http://chws.albany.edu*

**University of North Carolina at Chapel Hill—** Southeast
*www.healthworkforce.unc.edu*

**University of Illinois at Chicago—**North Central
*www.uic.edu/sph/ichws*

**University of Texas Health Science Center at San Antonio—**South Central
*www.uthscsa.edu/rchws/index.asp*

**University of Washington—**Northwest
*www.fammed.washington.edu/chws/index.html*

**University of California at San Francisco—** Southwest
*http://futurehealth.ucsf.edu/cchws.html*

## REFERENCES

Aiken, L. (2005). *Improving patient safety: The link between nursing and quality of care.* New Brunswick, NJ: Robert Wood Johnson Foundation.

Aiken, L., Clarke, S., Cheung, R., Sloane, D., & Silber, J. (2003). Educational levels of hospital nurses and surgical patient mortality. *Journal of the American Medical Association, 290*(12), 1617-1623.

Aiken, L., Clarke, S., & Sloane, D. (2000). Hospital restructuring: Does it adversely affect care and outcomes? *Journal of Nursing Administration.*

Aiken, L., Clarke, S., & Sloane, D., for the International Hospital Outcomes Research Consortium. (2002a). Hospital staffing, organization, and quality of care: Cross-national findings. *International Journal for Quality in Health Care, 14*(1), 5-13.

Aiken, L., Clarke, S., Sloane, D., Sochalski, J., & Silber, J. (2002b). Hospital nurse staffing and patient mortality, nurse burnout, and job dissatisfaction. *JAMA, 288*(16), 1987-1993.

American Nurses Association (ANA). (2005). ANA state government relations, 2005 legislation: Staffing plans and ratios. Retrieved August 16, 2005, from *www.nursingworld.org/gova/state/2005/staffing.htm*.

Auerbach, D., Buerhaus, P., & Staiger, D. (2000). Associate degree graduates and the rapidly aging RN workforce. *Nursing Economic$, 18*(4), 178-184.

Biviano, M., Fritz, M., Spencer, W., & Dall, T. (2004). *What is behind HRSA's projected supply, demand, and shortage of registered nurses?* Rockville, MD: Health Resources and Services Administration.

Bleich, M., Hewlett, P., Santos, S., Rice, R., Cox, K., & Richmeier, S. (2003). Analysis of the nursing workforce crisis: A call to action. *American Journal of Nursing, 103*(4), 66-74.

Bradley, S., Ginsburg, P., & Cookson, J. (2005). Tracking health care costs: Declining growth trend pauses in 2004. *Health Affairs: The Policy Journal of the Health Sphere.* Retrieved September 7, 2005, from *http://content.healthaffairs.org/cgi/content/abstract/hlthaff.w5.286v1*.

Buchan, J., Kingma, M., & Lorenzo, M. (2005). *International migration of nurses: Trends and policy implications.* Geneva, Switzerland: International Council of Nurses. Retrieved September 7, 2005, from *www.icn.ch/global/issue5migration.pdf*.

Buchan, J., & Sochalski, J. (2004). The migration of nurses: Trends and policies. *Bulletin of the World Health Organization, 82*, 587-594.

Buerhaus, P. (2001). Aging nurses in an aging society: Long-term implications. *Reflections on Nursing Leadership, 27*(1), 35-36, 46.

Buerhaus, P. (2002). Shortages of hospital registered nurses: Causes and perspectives on public and private sector actions. *Nursing Outlook, 50*(1), 4-6.

Buerhaus, P., & Auerbach, D. (1999). Slow growth in the United States of the number of minorities in the RN workforce. *Image: Journal of Nursing Scholarship, 31*(2), 179-183.

Buerhaus, P., & Staiger, D. (1999). Trouble in the nurse labor market? Recent trends and future outlook. *Health Affairs, 18*(1), 214-222.

Buerhaus, P., Staiger, D., & Auerbach, D. (2000). Implications of an aging registered nurse workforce. *JAMA, 283*(22), 2948-2954.

Buerhaus, P., Staiger, D., & Auerbach, D. (2003). Is the current shortage of hospital nurses ending? *Health Affairs, 22*(6), 191-198.

Buerhaus, P., Staiger, D., & Auerbach, D. (2004). New signs of a strengthening U.S. nurse labor market? *Health Affairs, 23*, 526-533.

Chapman, S., Showstack, J., Morrison, E., Franks, P., Woo, L., & O'Neill, E. (2004). *Allied health workforce: Innovations for the 21st century.* San Francisco: Center for the Health Professions at the University of California.

Clarke, S., & Aiken, L. (2003). Failure to rescue: Needless deaths are prime examples of the need for more nurses at the bedside. *American Journal of Nursing, 103*(1), 42-47.

Clarke, S., Sloane, D., & Aiken, L. (2002). Effects of hospital staffing and organizational climate on needlestick injuries to nurses. *American Journal of Public Health, 92*(7), 1115-1119.

Cleary, B., Rice R., Brunell, M., Dickson, G., Gloor, E., et al. (2005). Strategic state-level nursing workforce initiatives: Taking the long view. *Nursing Administration Quarterly, 29*, 162-170.

Healthcare Leadership Council. (2005). *Healthcare workforce shortage background.* Retrieved June 15, 2005, from *www.hlc.org*.

Health Resources and Services Administration (HRSA). (2005). Fiscal year 2006 congressional budget justification of estimates for appropriations committee. Retrieved June 28, 2005, from *www.hrsa.gov/about/budgetjust06.htm*.

Kohn, L., Corrigan, J., & Donaldson, M. (Eds.). (2000). *Institute of Medicine report. To err is human: Building a safer health system.* Washington, DC: National Academies Press.

Lee, M. (2004, June 29). Foreign nurses sought to fill void. *CBS News.* Retrieved June 26, 2005, from *www.cbsnews.com*.

Lewin Group. (2005). *The cost of caring: Sources of growth in spending for hospital care.* Washington, DC: American Hospital Association. Retrieved June 28, 2005, from *www.aha.org/aha/press-room-info/content/costcaring.pdf*.

Mark, B., Hughes, L., & Jones, C. (2004). The role of theory in improving patient safety and quality health care. *Nursing Outlook, 52*(1), 11-16.

Mark, B., Salyer, J., & Wan, T. (2000). Market, hospital, and nursing unit characteristics as predictors of nursing unit skill mix: A contextual analysis. *Journal of Nursing Administration, 30*(11), 552-560.

Mattke, S., Needleman, J., Buerhaus, P., Stewart, M., & Zelevinsky, K. (2004). Evaluating the role of patient sample definitions for quality indicators sensitive to nurse staffing patterns. *Medical Care, 42*(Suppl 2), II21-II33.

McCue, M., Mark, B., & Harless, D. (2003). Nurse staffing, quality, and financial performance. *Journal of Health Care Finance, 29*(4), 54-76.

Mississippi Hospital Association (MHA). (2004). *The business of caring: The economic impact of Mississippi's hospitals on the state's economy.* Jackson, MS: MHA.

National Center for Health Workforce Analysis. (2003). *Changing demographics: Implications for physicians, nurses and other health workers.* Washington, DC: U.S. Department of Health and Human Services, Health Resources and Services Administration, Bureau of Health Professions.

National Rural Health Association. (2003). *Health care workforce distribution and shortage issues in rural America.* Kansas City, MO: National Rural Health Association.

Needleman, J., & Buerhaus, P. (2003). Nurse staffing and patient safety: Current knowledge and implications for action. *International Journal for Quality in Health Care, 15*(4), 275-277.

Needleman, J., Buerhaus, P., Mattke, S., Stewart, M., & Zelevinsky, K. (2002). Nurse-staffing levels and the quality of care in hospitals. *New England Journal of Medicine, 346*(22), 1715-1722.

O'Neil, E. (2005). *Centering on the stealth health care workforce crisis.* San Francisco: Center for the Health Professions.

Peterson, C. (2001). Nursing shortage: Not a simple problem—no easy answers. *Online Journal of Issues in Nursing, 6*(1). Retrieved February 16, 2005, from *http://nursingworld.org/ojin/topic14/tpc14_1.htm*.

Ricketts, T. (2005). Workforce issues in rural areas: A focus on policy equity. *American Journal of Public Heath, 95*(1), 42-48.

Sochalski, J., & Aiken, L. (1999). Accounting for variation in hospital outcomes: A cross-national study. *Health Affairs, 18*(3), 256-259.

Southeast Regional Center for Health Workforce Studies. (2005). *Technical assistance network to improve health workforce data collection and reporting in southeast states.* Chapel Hill, NC: Cecil G. Sheps Center for Health Services Research.

Spratley, E., Johnson, A., Sochalski, J., Fritz, M., & Spencer, W. (2000). *The registered nurse population: Findings from the national sample survey of registered nurses.* Washington, DC: U.S. Department of Health and Human Services, Health

Resources and Services Administration, Bureau of Health Professions. Retrieved January 10, 2005, from *http://bhpr.hrsa.gov/healthworkforce/reports/rnsurvey/rnss1.htm*.

United States Census Bureau. (2005). United States census 2000. Retrieved August 1, 2005, from *www.census.gov/main/www/cen2000.html*.

Wunderlich, G., Sloan, F., & Davis, C. (1996). *Institute of Medicine Report: Nursing staff in hospitals and nursing homes: Is it adequate?* Washington, DC: National Academies Press.

# **POLICY**SPOTLIGHT

## CALIFORNIA NURSE STAFFING RATIOS

Joanne Spetz

*"The problems of the world cannot possibly be solved by skeptics or cynics whose horizons are limited by the obvious realities."*

JOHN F. KENNEDY

The importance of nursing to the delivery of high-quality health care has been recognized since the inception of the practice of nursing. Various factors contribute to the quality of nursing care, including the expertise of nursing staff, good nurse-physician communication, availability of supportive personnel and other health professionals, and the nurse/patient ratio. The relative importance of each of these has been debated over the decades, and it was not until recently that high-quality empirical research demonstrated consistent relationships between licensed nurse staffing and the quality of patient care (Lang, Hodge, Olson, Romano, & Kravitz, 2004).

Concerns about the effects of changes in nurse staffing in the 1990s, combined with the increasing influence of nursing unions, resulted in the passage of California Assembly Bill (AB) 394 in 1999—the first comprehensive legislation in the United States to establish minimum staffing levels for registered nurses (RNs) and licensed vocational nurses working in hospitals. This bill did not establish specific staffing ratios, but rather required that the California Department of Health Services (DHS) determine the appropriate ratios. These were announced in 2002 and implemented beginning in 2004.

This Policy Spotlight briefly reviews the history of minimum nurse/patient ratio requirements in California, with a focus on the positions of stakeholders and the reasons the legislation was passed in 1999 after a decade of effort by proponents. I then examine the effects of the ratios in their first 18 months of implementation. The first known effects of the ratios have been political maneuvering and legal actions. As of August 2005, data were not available to learn whether the staffing requirements achieved their intended purpose: to improve the quality of patient care in hospitals. I conclude with a review of key issues that must be addressed by researchers, nursing leaders, and policymakers in future years.

### THE CONTEXT IN WHICH RATIOS WERE IMPLEMENTED

Over the past 15 years, there has been substantial debate about changes that occurred in hospital staffing in the 1990s and the effects of such changes on the quality of care. In response to the financial pressures caused by the growth of managed care insurance and the introduction of Medicare's

Prospective Payment System, many hospitals reportedly reduced employment levels of RNs (Rosenthal, 1996; Shuit, 1996). It is not clear whether these changes merely reflected coincident declines in patient censuses or represented real declines in RN hours per patient day (Aiken, Sochalski, & Anderson, 1996; Hoover, 1998; Spetz, 1998). Enough concern was raised about the observed changes to lead the Institute of Medicine to examine whether changes in nurse staffing might have negative effects on the quality of care (Wunderlich, Sloan, & Davis, 1996).

## Legislation

In some states, legislators and regulatory agencies considered staffing requirements. In 1993, the California Nurses Association (CNA) and Service Employees International Union (SEIU) supported legislation that would have established fixed minimum nurse/patient ratios; one bill passed in the legislature but was vetoed by the governor. In 1996, California's DHS implemented regulations that require hospitals to use patient classification systems (PCSs) to measure the acuity of patients and determine nurse staffing needs for inpatient units on a shift-by-shift basis. These regulations augmented regulations implemented in the 1976-1977 fiscal year that required hospitals to staff a minimum of one licensed nurse per two patients in intensive and coronary care units.

The PCS requirements did not satisfy some nursing advocates, and the CNA and SEIU continued to press for fixed staffing ratios in both ballot propositions and legislation (Spetz, 1996). The PCS requirements did not provide specific criteria for determining the acceptability of a system, and therefore many hospitals developed their own systems. Nurse unions alleged that hospitals created PCSs to meet budget requirements rather than patient needs and that compliance with PCSs was low (Spetz, Seago, Coffman, Rosenoff, & O'Neil, 2000). Enforcement of the PCS requirements was limited to the regular licensing inspection process, and violations did not result in a fine or penalty. At the same time there was widespread agreement that the fixed minimum staffing requirements that applied to intensive and coronary care units were successful in ensuring adequate nursing care.

As the 1990s ended, there emerged a shortage of RNs, and concern about poor staffing in hospitals continued (Kilborn, 1999). It was in this environment that AB 394 was passed by the legislature and signed by former Governor Gray Davis. Previous Republican governors had vetoed similar legislation; union-friendly Democratic Governor Davis satisfied the union efforts to pass minimum-ratio legislation. AB 394 charged the California DHS with determining specific unit-by-unit nurse/patient ratios.

## Regulations

DHS launched an extensive effort to determine the new minimum nurse staffing ratios. At the time there was relatively little research that linked nurse staffing to the quality of patient care (Spetz et al., 2000); this legislation preceded the influential studies of Needleman and colleagues (2002) and Aiken and colleagues (2002). Moreover, none of the studies that had been published identified an ideal staffing ratio for hospitals (Lang et al., 2004). Although some analysts suggested that DHS consider creative strategies to implement the staffing requirements, such as establishing individualized ratios for each hospital (Seago, 2002), DHS determined that it must codify a set of unit-specific minimum ratios that would apply to all hospitals.

DHS received recommendations about the ratios from stakeholders. The California Healthcare Association (CHA), which represents hospitals, proposed a ratio of one nurse per 10 patients (1:10) in medical-surgical units and somewhat richer ratios in other units. The CNA recommended a ratio of one RN per three patients (1:3) in medical-surgical units and richer ratios in other units. SEIU recommended a ratio of one nurse per four patients (1:4) in medical-surgical units. This wide range of proposals reflects both the lack of scientific consensus about appropriate nurse staffing and the high level of disagreement between hospital leaders and nurse unions. Distrust between unions and hospital management was an ongoing problem, and the perceived failure of the PCS requirements to improve nurse staffing only heightened tensions.

DHS commissioned a study by researchers at the University of California, Davis, which was released with the ratios proposed by DHS (Kravitz et al., 2002).

**TABLE 18-2** California Minimum Licensed Nurse/Patient Ratios

| TYPE OF UNIT | RATIO IN 2004 | RATIO IN 2005 | RATIO IN 2008 |
|---|---|---|---|
| Intensive or critical care | 1:2 | 1:2 | 1:2 |
| Neonatal intensive care | 1:2 | 1:2 | 1:2 |
| Operating room | 1:1 | 1:1 | 1:1 |
| Postanesthesia recovery | 1:2 | 1:2 | 1:2 |
| Labor and delivery | 1:2 | 1:2 | 1:2 |
| Antepartum | 1:4 | 1:4 | 1:4 |
| Postpartum couplets | 1:4 | 1:4 | 1:4 |
| Postpartum women only | 1:6 | 1:6 | 1:6 |
| Pediatrics | 1:4 | 1:4 | 1:4 |
| Emergency room | 1:4 | 1:4 | 1:4 |
| ICU patients in the ER | 1:2 | 1:2 | 1:2 |
| Trauma patients in the ER | 1:1 | 1:1 | 1:1 |
| Step-down | 1:4 | 1:4 | 1:3 |
| Telemetry | 1:5 | 1:5 | 1:4 |
| Medical-surgical | 1:6 | 1:5 | 1:5 |
| Other specialty care | 1:5 | 1:5 | 1:4 |
| Psychiatric | 1:6 | 1:6 | 1:6 |

Sources: California Nurses Association, *http://www.calnurses.org/nursing-practice/ratios/ratios_index.html*; and Spetz, J. (2004). California's minimum nurse-to-patient ratios: The first few months. *Journal of Nursing Administration,* 34(12), 571-578.

The proposed ratios were between those recommended by the CHA and the unions, with a 1:6 ratio in medical-surgical units starting January 1, 2004, and a 1:5 ratio in medical-surgical units commencing in January, 2005. Other units have richer minimum-ratio requirements, as presented in Table 18-2. These minimum ratios do not replace the requirement that hospitals staff according to a PCS; if a hospital's PCS indicates that richer staffing is needed, the hospital should staff accordingly. However, the problems with the PCS requirements have not been remedied; legislation that would have closed loopholes in the PCS requirements and required unannounced inspections of hospitals was vetoed by Governor Davis in 2000.

## WHAT HAS HAPPENED AS A RESULT OF THE RATIOS?

The two most obvious effects of California's nurse/patient ratios have been the development of an acrimonious legal battle and the launching of an aggressive public relations war.

### Legal Challenges

The first legal salvo was the filing of a lawsuit against the state by the CHA two days before the ratios went into effect. The CHA suit argued that the regulatory phrase "at all times" should not require that nurses must cover any time a nurse leaves the work environment, such as during a break or restroom visit. DHS contended that if the ratios were to have any meaning, they must be effective "at all times." The judge hearing the case agreed with the DHS in a May 2004 ruling (Berestein, 2004).

The second major legal challenge to the ratio regulations came from Governor Schwarzenegger. Although the governor's administration allowed the ratios to be implemented in January of 2004, after Governor Davis was recalled, the new administration sought to delay the implementation of the stricter one-nurse-to-five-patient ratio scheduled for January of 2005. DHS stated that the severe shortage of licensed nurses made it overly onerous for hospitals to meet stricter staffing requirements and therefore issued an emergency regulation suspending the change 2 months before it was to have occurred. The DHS also proposed changes to the regulations for emergency departments (Rapaport, 2004).

The CNA filed suit against DHS in December 2004, alleging that the emergency order had illegally bypassed the legislature. A series of large protests by nurses was conducted in early 2005 (LaMar, 2005).

In early March a Superior Court judge tentatively ruled that DHS indeed had not followed the law when issuing the emergency regulation (Salladay & Chong, 2005). That same day the governor's administration issued another emergency order to delay the stricter ratios (California Healthline, 2005b), but the judge directed that the stricter one-nurse-to-five-patients regulation was effective the Monday after the tentative ruling. Shortly thereafter the judge signed court orders barring the Schwarzenegger administration from suspending the hospital workload rules while the court challenge continued (Benson, 2005c). The judge's initial ruling was finalized in May (Benson, 2005a). The judge's ruling in March forced hospitals to scramble to meet the new requirements; many had delayed their plans to recruit more nurses when the governor had issued the emergency regulation in November 2004. It has been reported that "most" facilities have not been able to meet the ratios (California Healthline, 2005c).

As expected, the administration appealed the judge's ruling. In April the Third District Court of Appeals denied a request to delay the stricter ratios while the court considered an appeal (Gledhill, 2005). It should be noted that this court case applies only to the issuance of emergency regulations to suspend the stricter ratios, not efforts to change the regulations through standard process. DHS also is working to enact standard regulatory changes that would amend the ratios.

The legal wrangling over the ratios has added to controversy over the Schwarzenegger administration's policies. In July the judge who ruled in the initial case scheduled a hearing to determine whether the governor and two aides should be held in contempt of court for repeatedly issuing holds on the stricter staffing ratios despite the judge's rulings. The hearing was cancelled 2 days later. At the same time, a hospital memo claimed that DHS had told hospital officials that DHS would not aggressively enforce the new ratios (Berthelsen, 2005). This revelation infuriated advocates of the ratios.

To assist hospitals in meeting the staffing ratio requirements, both former Governor Davis and current Governor Schwarzenegger dedicated funds to expanding nursing education and reducing attrition from nursing programs. Davis allocated $60 million to this effort, approximately $34 million of which was granted before the recall election. Governor Schwarzenegger's first announcement was made in March of 2005, shortly after the emergency regulation suspension was overturned. At that time, $13 million of Workforce Investment Act funds were directed toward 18 nursing programs (Benson, 2005b). A month later, Schwarzenegger announced a $90 million, 5-year initiative, in addition to the $13 million already announced. However, the $90 million initiative involves only $30 million of Workforce Investment Act funds; the rest of the money is expected to come through matching grants and donations from industry (Skidmore, 2005).

## Public Relations

Unions have sought to persuade the public that the ratios have successfully improved patient care in hospitals, and hospitals have pushed the idea that the ratios are undermining the financial stability of hospitals and access to health care. This public relations war over the ratios has been occurring at the same time many California-based unions have continued an aggressive public relations campaign against the Schwarzenegger administration. Schwarzenegger has sought to enact regulations, legislation, and propositions that limit the influence of unions, and in response unions representing teachers, prison guards, public employees, and nurses have been allied in an effort to undermine Schwarzenegger's policies and popularity.

The CNA conducted a survey of RNs in 111 hospitals across the state and in February 2004 reported that "staffing conditions are improved at 68% of the hospitals surveyed by CNA, and 59% were generally in compliance with the requirements of the law" (CNA, 2004). The CNA has reported that they are generally satisfied with hospital compliance (Robertson, 2004). However, they and other unions have drawn attention to hospitals that they believe are out of compliance with the ratios.

The CHA countered the CNA survey with one of its own. They stated that 89% of 300 hospitals have been out of compliance with the ratios at some times (Goldeen, 2004). They argue that California's severe nursing shortage makes it impossible to meet the ratios at all times without restricting access to care. They also report that the cost of the ratios has been much higher than estimated by DHS, resulting in up to $422 million in additional staffing just for 2004 (Berestein, 2004). California previously faced serious concerns about access to care for its large uninsured population, and in 1999 over half of hospitals had negative operating margins (Harrison & Montalvo, 2002).

### Are Hospitals Meeting the Ratios?

At the end of the first year of the ratios, it was reported that more than half of the hospitals inspected for alleged violations of state nurse/patient staffing ratio rules by state officials were out of compliance (Chong, 2004b). More recently it was reported that 30% of hospitals inspected for regular licensing review in the first 10 months of 2004 were in compliance with the ratios (Chong, 2005). These data have been called into question, however, because few hospitals have been inspected to determine whether they are following the nurse staffing regulations (Chong, 2004d).

Reports of DHS inspections reveal a significant problem with the minimum-ratio regulations: The enforcement mechanisms are relatively weak. DHS does not have the authority to impose any fines or monetary penalties on hospitals that are found to violate the ratios. Citations must be responded to with a specific plan to remedy the problem, and DHS monitors hospitals to ensure they are following their plans. The ability of DHS to conduct inspections is hindered by ongoing state budget shortfalls. In this context, it seems that the claim that DHS would not aggressively enforce the ratios may reflect the reality of the state government budget and the ability to impose fines rather than an administration strategy to undermine the ratios.

Other mechanisms exist to ensure that hospitals adhere to the ratios. First, government payers such as Medicare and Medi-Cal (the state Medicaid program) require that hospitals meet all state and federal regulations, and can deny payment to violators. Second, California's cap on malpractice awards does not apply in cases of negligence. It is theoretically possible that a hospital could be determined negligent if it consistently did not adhere to minimum nurse

staffing regulations, in which case the hospital could face substantial financial penalties (Robertson, 2004).

Third, unions have been drawing public attention to hospitals that were not meeting the staffing requirements, resulting in negative publicity for hospitals and increased scrutiny from DHS inspectors. One union distributed a document to the Los Angeles County Board of Supervisors criticizing the county's hospitals for failing to meet the minimum-ratio standards (California Healthline, 2004). The union subsequently filed a lawsuit against the county (Chong, 2004c). In San Diego, nurses who were in contract negotiations with Sharp HealthCare hospitals filed complaints with DHS, and subsequent DHS inspections revealed that three of these hospitals failed to meet regulatory requirements. The hospital was required to submit a detailed plan to remedy the problem (Freeman, 2004).

The only data available on unit-by-unit nurse staffing are from the California Nursing Outcomes Coalition (CalNOC) (Donaldson et al., 2005). Their analysis of 68 hospitals from 2002 to 2004 found that overall nurse hours per patient day increased by 7.4% and RN hours per patient day increased by 20.8%. These data are from a convenience sample of hospitals and might not represent the experience of other hospitals; however, they are consistent with the likelihood that hospitals are trying to comply with the minimum staffing regulations. In 2006 the California Office of Statewide Health Planning and Development (OSHPD) will release public-use hospital data that will provide some indication of whether hospitals increased staffing because of the ratio requirements. However, these data do not provide information on a unit-by-unit basis, and the data are not limited to nurses who work directly with patients. Researchers and policymakers will need to survey hospitals directly to fully understand how hospital staffing has changed as a result of the minimum nurse/patient ratios.

### Affirming Ratios in Union Contracts

Labor organizations that represent nurses, such as the CNA and SEIU, have sought to incorporate staffing standards in their contract negotiations. The first post-AB394 case of this was when Kaiser Permanente, a large integrated health maintenance organization, reached an agreement with its SEIU-represented nursing staff for a minimum ratio of one nurse for every four acute care patients at its hospitals even if the ratios established by DHS were not as stringent (Shinkman, 2001). Kaiser enjoyed a large increase in RN job applicants after this announcement, and there was substantial positive press about their effort to improve nurse staffing.

More recent contractual agreements regarding nurse/patient ratios have come through standard contract negotiations. In 2005, San Francisco officials and SEIU leaders agreed to a broad contract that included nurse/patient staffing ratios higher than those mandated by the state in the city's public hospitals and public health clinics (Gordon, 2005). Shortly thereafter the not-for-profit Catholic Healthcare West system agreed to adopt minimum nurse staffing standards that would be followed even if the governor successfully delayed or eliminated the state regulation (Osterman, 2005). The CNA has threatened a strike against University of California hospitals over a variety of issues, including the system's unwillingness to agree to nurse/patient ratio guarantees (Rapaport, 2005).

### Has the Mix of Staff Changed?

There has been concern about the possibility that hospitals eliminate support staff positions because of the minimum licensed nurse staffing requirements (Spetz, 2001). Anecdotal evidence suggests this is occurring, at least among some hospitals. SEIU filed a grievance against Stanford University Medical Center when that hospital issued layoff notices to 113 nursing aides in advance of the implementation of the ratios. The hospital planned to replace those positions with RNs. SEIU charged that the elimination of the nursing aide positions was contrary to the spirit of the minimum ratios (Ostrov, 2003). The CalNOC analysis of staffing data suggests that the substitution of licensed nurses for unlicensed staff might be widespread; the increase in RN staffing was much larger than the overall staffing increase among their hospitals (Donaldson et al., 2005).

Some analysts have suggested that hospitals could meet the ratios by moving day-shift staff to evening and night shifts, which traditionally are staffed at lower levels (Berliner, Kovner, & Zhu, 2002). Minimum staffing requirements raise the possibility that the minimum requirement will become the average observed, because hospitals will see no reason to exceed the minimum. Labor leaders argue that PCS requirements still in place will require that hospitals staff more nurses than the minimum if needed. Intensive care units have had minimum staffing requirements for 30 years, and the data suggest that hospitals staff more richly when needed. However, failure to staff appropriately in intensive care is more likely to result in a patient's death than in a medical-surgical unit, and thus hospitals have less motivation to attend to PCSs outside the intensive care unit. The PCS's shortcomings have not yet been addressed by DHS or legislation; a reexamination of the role of PCS regulations may be needed in the future.

### Have Hospitals Reduced Services?

The California Hospital Association has warned that strict minimum nurse/patient ratio requirements will force hospitals to reduce their services. To maintain the minimum ratios, hospitals might reschedule procedures, close selected units and beds, or shut their doors entirely. These fears seemed warranted when in January 2004, it was announced that Santa Teresita Hospital in Duarte, California, was closing its 39-bed inpatient department and emergency room because of its inability to meet the minimum ratios (Chavez, 2004). However, newspapers subsequently reported that nurses who had worked at the hospital said they were meeting the ratios without difficulty (Allen, 2004), and an analysis of financial data reported by the hospital to OSHPD revealed that the hospital had been suffering severe financial distress for several years before it closed (Spetz, 2004). Given this information, it seems unlikely that the ratios were the primary reason for the hospital's closure.

Thus far there have been few verified reports of the minimum nurse/patient ratios causing permanent closures of inpatient hospital units or beds. In August of 2004, a representative of the CHA stated that approximately four psychiatric units had closed, and a few other unspecified units.

Their survey data indicated that of approximately 240 hospitals, between 30% and 40% of them had temporarily closed inpatient beds during at least 1 week between January 5 and July 6 (personal communication, Dorel Harms, August 17, 2004). Emergency room diversions rose in three counties in the first quarter 2004 relative to 2003, and for one county the diversion rate had not returned to 2003 levels by April (Appleby, 2004; Ostrov, 2004). Whether these temporary service limitations have affected access to care for or the health of Californians is unknown.

### Have Hospitals Suffered Financial Losses?

In November 2004, the DHS stated that catastrophic financial losses that would result from implementing more stringent ratios in 2005 justified the issuance of an emergency order to delay ratios. This concern about hospital costs was echoed in a report released by the CHA (2004). The tenuous financial environment in which California hospitals operate has been highlighted by recent hospital closures. At the end of 2004 the Robert F. Kennedy Medical Center in Hawthorne closed because of financial problems. Hospital leadership cited expenses associated with treating uninsured patients, meeting seismic retrofitting requirements, and minimum nurse/patient ratios as reasons for ongoing financial losses. This hospital operated an emergency room, which was the sixth emergency department to close in 2004 in Los Angeles County (Chong, 2004a).

### ISSUES THAT NEED TO BE ADDRESSED

Two issues central to the success of minimum nurse/patient ratios have not been addressed: have the ratios improved the quality of patient care, and can the ratios be sustained when severe nursing shortages are projected to continue?

### Did the Ratios Improve Quality of Care?

To date, only one published study examines the effect of the minimum ratios on the quality of patient care. The California Nursing Outcomes Coalition analyzed rates of patient falls and hospital-acquired pressure ulcers between 2002 and 2004 in their sample of 68 hospitals and found that there was no statistically significant change that could be attributed to the ratios (Donaldson et al., 2005). Although this study suggests that the ratios have not improved quality of care, there are several reasons this paper does not provide a definitive verdict on the ratios. First, as noted above, only a convenience sample of California hospitals was analyzed. Second, the study extended only through the first half of 2004. During the first 6 months of the ratios, hospitals may have been in a transitional stage and therefore the positive benefits of increased nurse staffing were not fully realized. Third, the outcomes examined might not be sensitive to changes in licensed nurse staffing. Research studies that examine whether nurse staffing affects rates of hospital-acquired pressure ulcers and postoperative hip fractures (which would be caused by a patient fall) have produced mixed findings (Agency for Healthcare Research and Quality, 2005). Finally, these outcomes might be more sensitive to total staffing than to licensed nurse staffing. In this case, replacement of unlicensed staff with licensed nurses may have no net positive or negative effect.

There is a pressing need for more research on the effects of minimum ratios on patient care. Researchers should examine a variety of patient outcomes and sources of data, using various statistical methods. The first statewide studies are likely to use the OSHPD Patient Discharge Data, which are collected annually for all nonfederal hospitals in the state. These data can be linked to OSHPD's hospital-level financial and staffing data to explicitly examine changes in nurse staffing, staffing of other personnel, and patient outcomes. Data from single hospitals and prospectively collected data from organizations such as CalNOC also will be important in future research, particularly because such data can allow researchers to make comparisons across patient care units.

### Nursing Shortage

The introduction and tightening of minimum nurse/patient ratios has occurred in the midst of a significant national shortage of RNs. California's shortage has been estimated to be worse than the national average (National Center for Health Workforce Analysis, 2002), and recent forecasts indicate that the shortage is likely to worsen substantially because of future retirements of RNs (Spetz & Dyer, 2005). DHS estimated that the stricter ratios implemented in 2005 would increase RN demand by 7230 (Kravitz et al., 2002), thus worsening the projected shortage by 39% (National Center for Health Workforce Analysis, 2002).

Some proponents of the ratios believe that the improved working conditions that will result from the ratios will draw larger numbers of nurses to the hospital workforce. Recent data suggest that RN supply in California has grown more rapidly than anticipated (Spetz & Dyer, 2005), but it is not known whether the minimum ratios can receive credit for this change. It is likely that expansion of nursing education programs accounts for the bulk of the growth in supply. Most licensed nurses already work in nursing, and therefore only relatively small gains in supply could be obtained from the previously licensed population (Fletcher, Guzley, Barnhill, & Philhour, 2004).

In the long term, it is possible that improved working conditions will increase interest in entry into the profession and delay retirement rates of older nurses. But California does not have sufficient educational capacity to offer nursing education to everybody who wants to enter the profession. At this time, nearly all of California's nursing schools are now oversubscribed and have waiting lists for admission. Unless the educational pipeline can be expanded, California hospitals will continue to rely on foreign nurse recruitment, recruitment from other states, and traveling nurses.

**What Next?**

Even if the governor succeeds in eliminating California's minimum nurse/patient staffing regulation, the changes set in motion by AB 394 will persist. Many hospitals will maintain higher nurse staffing, both because recent research demonstrates the importance of nurse staffing to quality of care and because union contracts demand better staffing. Broader trends toward improving health care quality will lead hospitals nationwide to focus on staffing. Medicare's pay-for-performance system has shown promise to improve patient outcomes (California Healthline, 2005a), and recent research

suggests that the ratio of costs per life saved associated with increasing nurse staffing is favorable as compared with many other health interventions (Rothberg, Abraham, Lindenauer, & Rose, 2005). However, even if more studies demonstrate that nurse staffing is a cost-effective means to producing better health, the effectiveness of a minimum staffing mandate needs to be examined by researchers. If California's regulation succeeded in increasing nurse staffing, and if this staffing change can be shown to have improved patient outcomes, it will be easy for other states to follow in California's footsteps.

## Key Points

- Minimum nurse/patient ratio legislation led to an acrimonious battle between interest groups and government agencies.
- Preliminary data suggest that nurse staffing indeed increased after the minimum staffing regulations were implemented, but there may have been substitution of licensed nurses for unlicensed personnel.
- One study found no change in rates of hospital-acquired pressure ulcers and falls with injury after the minimum ratios were established, but this finding should be viewed as preliminary. Much more research is needed to determine whether the ratio legislation met the goal of improving quality of care.

## Web Resources

**California Hospital Association**
*www.calhealth.org*
**California Nurses Association**
*www.calnurses.org*
**Center for California Health Workforce Studies**
*http://futurehealth.ucsf.edu/cchws.html*
**U.S. Bureau of the Health Professions**
*http://bhpr.hrsa.gov*

## REFERENCES

Agency for Healthcare Research and Quality. (2005). *AHRQ Quality Indicators—Guide to Patient Safety Indicators, Version 2.1, Revision 3.* AHRQ Publication No. 03-R203. Rockville, MD: Agency for Healthcare Research and Quality.

Aiken, L. H., Clarke, S. F., Sloane, D. M., Sochalski, J., & Silber, J. H. (2002). Hospital nurse staffing and patient mortality, nurse burnout, and job dissatisfaction. *Journal of the American Medical Association, 288*(16), 1987-1993.

Aiken, L. H., Sochalski, J., & Anderson, G. F. (1996). Downsizing the hospital nursing workforce. *Health Affairs, 15*(4), 88-92.

Allen, M. (2004, January 10). Former Santa Teresita nurses speak out. *Pasadena Star-News,* A1.

Appleby, J. (2004, July 25). Cutting nurses' patient loads boosts care, costs. *USA Today,* B1.

Benson, C. (2005a, June 8). Final ruling backs higher nurse ratio. *Sacramento Bee,* A5.

Benson, C. (2005b, March 19). Governor adds funds for nurses. *Sacramento Bee,* A3.

Benson, C. (2005c, March 15). Judge orders launch of nurse staffing rule. *Sacramento Bee,* A4.

Berestein, L. (2004, May 27). Industry group contends measure may hurt patients. *San Diego Union-Tribune,* C3.

Berliner, J., Kovner, C., & Zhu, C. (2002). *Nurse staffing ratios in California: A critique of the final report on hospital nursing staff ratios and quality of care.* Washington, DC: Service Employees International Union Nurse Alliance.

Berthelsen, C. (2005, July 20). Judge threatens state officials with contempt of court: Governor, aides put nurse-patient ratios in jeopardy—Jurist. *San Francisco Chronicle,* B2.

California Healthcare Association (CHA). (2004). *California Hospitals' financial condition: On life support.* Sacramento: CHA.

California Healthline. (2004, July 15). Los Angeles county not complying with nurse staffing rules, union says. Washington, DC: Advisory Board Company. Retrieved September 9, 2005, from *www.californiahealthline.org/index.cfm?Action=dspItem&itemID=104301&classcd=CL350.*

California Healthline. (2005a, April 15). *New York Times* examines Medicare pay-for-performance pilot programs. Washington, DC: Advisory Board Company. Retrieved September 9, 2005, from *www.californiahealthline.org/index.cfm?Action=dspItem&itemID=111228&classcd=CL351.*

California Healthline. (2005b, March 9). Schwarzenegger issues new emergency order to delay nurse staffing rule change. Washington, DC: Advisory Board Company. Retrieved September 9, 2005, from *www.californiahealthline.org/index.cfm?Action=dspItem&itemID=113793&classcd=CL353.*

California Healthline. (2005c, March 27). Some California hospitals seek additional nurses to help comply with staffing law. Washington, DC: Advisory Board Company. Retrieved September 9, 2005, from *www.californiahealthline.org/index.cfm?Action=dspItem&itemID=110426&classcd=CL350.*

California Nurses Association (CNA). (2004, February 4). Press release: Staffing improved at nearly 70% of California hospitals, safe RN staffing law 'off to a good start,' says CNA. Retrieved September 9, 2005, from the *www.calnurse.org/index.php?Action=Content&id=325.*

Chavez, S. (2004, January 9). Duarte hospital to close its ER. *Los Angeles Times,* B4.

Chong, J.-R. (2004a, September 24). Hawthorne hospital to shut doors. *Los Angeles Times,* B1.

Chong, J.-R. (2004b, December 31). Hospitals fail nurse head count. *Los Angeles Times,* B1.

Chong, J.-R. (2004c, October 26). Hospitals need 25% more nurses. *Los Angeles Times,* B1.

Chong, J.-R. (2004d, November 6). Nurse ratio checks rarely done. *Los Angeles Times,* B1.

Chong, J.-R. (2005, February 6). Some hospitals met nurse ratios. *Los Angeles Times,* B1.

Donaldson, N., Bolton, L. B., Aydin, C., Brown, D., Elashoff, J., & Sandhu, M. (2005). Impact of California's licensed nurse-patient ratios on unit-level nurse staffing and patient outcomes. *Policy, Politics, & Nursing Practice, 6*(3), 1-12.

Fletcher, J. E., Guzley, R. M., Barnhill, J., & Philhour, D. (2004). *Survey of registered nurses in California 2004.* Sacramento: California Board of Registered Nursing.

Freeman, M. (2004, August 11). Sharp faulted on nurse staffing at 3 S.D. hospitals. *San Diego Union-Tribune,* C1.

Gledhill, L. (2005, March 4). Governor loses to nurses in ruling He illegally blocked law that set staffing ratios, judge says. *San Francisco Chronicle,* A1.

Goldeen, J. (2004, March 28). RN shortage in critical condition: Hospital staff ratios lacking. *Stockton Record,* G1.

Gordon, R. (2005, June 22). Nurses pact ready for vote: Plan would raise pay, offer higher signing bonus. *San Francisco Chronicle,* B4.

Harms, D. (2004). Vice President, Quality and Professional Services, California Healthcare Association. Personal communication, August 17, 2004.

Harrison, M. G., & Montalvo, C. C. (2002). The financial health of California hospitals: A looming crisis. *Health Affairs, 21*(1), 15-23.

Hoover, K. W. (1998). Nursing work redesign in response to managed care. *Journal of Nursing Administration, 28*(11), 9-18.

Kilborn, P. T. (1999, March 23). Current nursing shortage more serious than those of the past. *New York Times,* A14.

Kravitz, R., Sauve, M. J., Hodge, M., Romano, P. S., Maher, M., et al. (2002). *Hospital nursing staff ratios and quality of care.* Davis, CA: University of California, Davis.

LaMar, A. (2005, January 19). Nurses protest delay of lower patient ratio, 1500 rally at capitol to fight 3-year wait. *San Jose Mercury News,* B2.

Lang, T. A., Hodge, M., Olson, V., Romano, P. S., & Kravitz, R. L. (2004). Nurse-patient ratios: A systematic review on the effects of nurse staffing on patient, nurse employee, and hospital outcomes. *Journal of Nursing Administration, 34*(7-8), 326-337.

National Center for Health Workforce Analysis. (2002). *Projected supply, demand, and shortages of registered nurses: 2000-2020.* Rockville, MD: Bureau of Health Professions, Health Resources and Services Administration, U.S. Department of Health and Human Services.

Needleman, J., Buerhaus, P. I., Mattke, S., Stewart, M., & Zelevinsky, K. (2002). Nurse-staffing levels and the quality of care in hospitals. *New England Journal of Medicine, 346,* 1719-1722.

Osterman, R. (2005, July 13). Hospitals accept nursing ratios. *Sacramento Bee,* D1.

Ostrov, B. F. (2003, October 18). Stanford nursing levels studied. *San Jose Mercury News,* B3.

Ostrov, B. F. (2004, January 28). New rules force hospitals to turn away ambulances. *San Jose Mercury News,* 1B.

Rapaport, L. (2004, November 5). State eases nurse-staffing law until 2008—Hospital closings and delays in patient care prompt move. *Sacramento Bee*, A1.

Rapaport, L. (2005, July 19). Med Center strike plan limits care. *Sacramento Bee*, A1.

Robertson, K. (2004). New nurse law fails to cause emergency. *Sacramento Business Journal*, 21(9), 1.

Rosenthal, E. (1996, August 19). Once in big demand, nurses are now targets for hospital cutbacks. *New York Times*, A16.

Rothberg, M. B., Abraham, I., Lindenauer, P. K., & Rose, D. N. (2005). Improving nurse-to-patient staffing ratios as a cost-effective safety intervention. *Medical Care*, 43(8), 785-791.

Salladay, R., & Chong, J.-R. (2005, March 4). Judge backs nurses over staffing. *Los Angeles Times*, B1.

Seago, J. A. (2002). The California experiment. Minimum nurse to patient ratios: Are there alternatives? *Journal of Nursing Administration*, 32(1), 48-58.

Shinkman, R. (2001, September 19). Numbers game. *Nurseweek*. Retrieved September 9, 2005, from *www.nurseweek.com/ news/features/01-09/ratios.html*.

Shuit, D. P. (1996, July 1). Hospital nurses feel pain of health system's restructuring. *Los Angeles Times*, A1, A17.

Skidmore, S. (2005, April 14). Governor has plans to fill nursing void. *San Diego Union-Tribune*, C1.

Spetz, J. (1996). *Nursing staff trends in California hospitals: 1977 through 1995*. San Francisco: Public Policy Institute of California.

Spetz, J. (1998). Hospital use of nursing personnel: Has there really been a decline? *Journal of Nursing Administration*, 28(3), 20-27.

Spetz, J. (2001). What should we expect from California's minimum nurse staffing legislation? *Journal of Nursing Administration*, 31(3), 132-140.

Spetz, J. (2004). California's minimum nurse-to-patient ratios: The first few months. *Journal of Nursing Administration*, 34(12), 571-578.

Spetz, J., & Dyer, W. T. (2005). *Forecasts of the registered nurse workforce in California*. Sacramento: California Board of Registered Nursing.

Spetz, J., Seago, J. A., Coffman, J., Rosenoff, E., & O'Neil, E. (2000). *Minimum nurse staffing ratios in California acute care hospitals*. San Francisco: California HealthCare Foundation.

Wunderlich, G. S., Sloan, F. A., & Davis, C. K. (Eds.). (1996). *Nursing staff in hospitals and nursing homes: Is it adequate?* Washington, DC: National Academies Press.

# POLICYSPOTLIGHT

## Mandatory Staffing: Australia's Experience

Virginia Plummer

*"The problems that exist in the world today cannot be solved by the level of thinking that created them."*
                                        Albert Einstein

The allocation of nursing staff in acute-care hospitals is a major policy issue, and there are controversies about whether a system based on nurse/patient ratios or one based on measurement of patient acuity is more reliable. Examples of ratio policies include the introduction of mandated nurse/patient ratios in Victoria, Australia's second most populated state, and the Safe Staffing Law governing hospitals and nurse/patient ratios in California.

There is a keen interest in the outcome of these policies by observers in other Australian states, New Zealand, the United States, and various other international settings, because many of the difficulties of accounting for nursing resource consumption and ensuring a fair and equitable staffing system remain unresolved. The introduction of mandated nurse/patient ratios in Victorian public hospitals in 2000 was a world first. This is the story of Australia's mandatory staffing experience (Table 18-3).

### BACKGROUND

In Australia there is a vast amount of expertise in data management and data analysis in the health system.

**TABLE 18-3**    Comparison of Ratio Allocation Rules in California and Victoria

| | CALIFORNIA, UNITED STATES | VICTORIA, AUSTRALIA |
|---|---|---|
| Ratio rules | Ratios are the same for all shifts, 24 hours per day, 7 days per week. Charge nurse or nurse manager is additional and must relieve all nurses during their breaks or when they leave the ward such as for patient transport. Linked to hospital license to operate. | Ratios are variable according to hospital level, ward type, and shift type. Meal and toilet breaks and other reasons for nurses leaving the floor are not adjusted for. At those times ratios fall below the minimum recommended level. Linked to budgets. |
| Medical-surgical units | 1:6 prior to 2005 1:5 in 2005 | Range from 1:4 plus charge nurse on morning shift of level 1 hospital to 1:10 (no additional charge nurse) on night shift on level 3, 3A hospitals |
| Pediatrics | 1:4 | 1:4 plus charge nurse morning shift to 1:4 on night shift |
| Emergency | 1:4 1:2 ICU patients in ER 1:1 Trauma patients | 1:3 plus triage nurse, plus charge nurse, all shifts for level 1 hospitals; others according to number of annual presentations historically |
| Coronary care | 1:2 | 1:2 plus charge nurse |
| Midwifery | 1:6 (mothers only) 1:4 (postpartum couplets) | 1:5 plus charge nurse morning shifts to 1:8 on night shifts. |
| Labor unit | 1:2 | 2 midwives per shift where births <2 per day on average |
| Oncology | 1:5 | 1:4 plus charge nurse |

Australia has a national minimum data set, national coding standards, standard charts of accounts, and a national diagnosis, procedure, and diagnosis-related group (DRG) classification system. These are supported by ongoing monitoring and analysis by federal and state health departments, the Australian Institute of Health and Welfare (AIHW, an independent health and welfare statistics and information agency), the Australian Bureau of Statistics (ABS), the Commonwealth Department of Veteran's Affairs, various compensation and insurance organizations, the Health Insurance Commission, and the Private Health Insurance Administrative Council. Yet there is little that speaks to nursing, the care for which people are admitted to the hospital and that is central to the operations of hospitals.

Most Australian public and private hospitals measure nursing costs on a per diem basis. Hospital managers simply divide the costs of nurses' wages and sometimes other associated nursing costs by the number of occupied bed days. Many public hospitals include associated unit costs in their standard chart of accounts for nursing. Included, for example, may be the costs of ward consumables such as dressings, syringes, needles, patient meals, and ward clerk wages. In these hospitals the per diem cost for nursing is blurred by the inclusion of other ward costs. Costs determined in this way are often the only data available for the allocation of nursing staff. This is neither a new problem nor one that is unique to Australian hospitals. Diers (2004) comments on the apparent deficiency in reliable data, saying "Nursing remains buried in the brooms, breakfast and building mortgage" (p. 225).

## THE INFLUENCE OF PROSPECTIVE PAYMENT SYSTEMS

As a result of these accounting practices there are few reliable, comparable, or useful data available about the actual nursing care provided to individual patients, as there are for other health professions. There is little data available on the actual nursing care requirements per patient type—such as medical, surgical, postnatal, oncology, or pediatric patient types—or by DRG. DRGs are an element of the prospective payment system (PPS) and also known as *case mix*. Case-mix funding was introduced in Victoria in 1993, followed by most other Australian states under the Commonwealth Casemix Development Program, approximately 10 years after it was introduced in the United States. This prompted significant research on costing and resource allocation in acute-care hospitals by Australian nurses, who generally embraced the system.

Attempts were made to establish and refine nursing cost weights at both state and federal levels and in both the public and private hospital sectors for the purpose of allocating nursing costs by DRG. In Australia there have been three major nursing service weight studies with the specific objective of deriving Australian nursing service weights. However, the weights were always based on retrospective wage information and occupied bed day data from previous years. Case-mix funding is unlikely to have reflected the actual nursing resources allocated by DRG, despite the cost weight studies. As a result, those accountable for managing the budgets of the nation's hospitals had scant reliable and "real time" data to quantify and predict nursing care requirements and costs and allocate staff in acute-care hospitals.

## RATIOS: EVOLUTION, REVOLUTION, OR SIMPLY GOING AROUND IN CIRCLES

In the absence of reliable data, the solution for both hospital managers and nurses has been to apply nurse/patient ratios for the allocation of staff in the case-mix environment. Nurse/patient ratio systems have evolved according to a range of influences, most of which were financial. The ratios were determined by dividing the number of patients by the number of nurses available and typically allocating an equal number of patients to the care of each nurse.

In Australia, as in other countries, the use of nurse/patient ratios differs among states and between public and private hospital sectors. There are no regulations governing nurse/patient ratios in Australian private hospitals, or public hospitals in all Australian states except Victoria, where mandated ratios were introduced in 2000. In Australia and internationally, hospital managers have used a range of ratio practices in order to comply with the intent

of hospital regulations, budgets, and laws. Some ratio practices employed are:

- Informal ratios—established by precedent
- Formal ratios—set by hospital or funder policies
- Mandated ratios—established by legally enforceable policy
- Acuity-based ratios—flexible ratios according to changes in patient acuity

Whether established by precedent or policy, most applications of nurse/patient ratios are largely inflexible. This inflexibility is a popular feature for some and unpopular with others. It is popular with those determining the nursing budget based on occupancy and for nurses who in the past worked with workloads unfairly manipulated by hospital managers without consultation. Ratios are not so popular with nurses in other settings because ratios are not sensitive to the range of patient requirements. Giovanetti observed that nurse/patient ratios were derived "from the dual forces of precedent and pressure; historical budget allocations served as the precedence, and existing budget constraints and market conditions exerted the pressure" (1994, p. 332).

The practice of allocating workload by nurse/patient ratios has existed in both formal and informal arrangements for a long time. Perhaps by continuing to use this method, nurses have simply been going around in circles and have been unable to advance workload management practices. Other health service observers would say that the introduction of mandated nurse/patient ratios in Victorian public hospitals marked the beginning of a revolution in nurse staffing. When mandated ratios are in place, there is a perceived measure of control over executive management by nurses at all levels.

## A NURSING CRISIS IN VICTORIA

In 1992 the Victorian government established policy to reduce the health budget by 10% in 2 years and supported case-mix funding to achieve that goal (Patera, 2004). Over the next decade, Victorian public hospitals and funders gained an increasingly sophisticated understanding of hospital costs in most areas of health service delivery. During the same period the Liberal Victorian government of Jeffrey Kennett simultaneously cut approximately 2000 nursing positions, which forced hospitals to rely on agency nurses to staff wards and departments. Some of the agency nurses had regular jobs and worked the extra hours with an agency to meet the demand. Other nurses left permanent jobs to work full time or part time with an agency for higher rates of pay, flexible scheduling, and the absence of pressure to work unpaid overtime or to undertake additional often unpaid duties such as the requirement to attend meetings in nonscheduled time. Nurses in Australia believed not only that using agency staff in public hospitals was more expensive but also that these nurses were less efficient, leading to an increase in the workload of regular nurses (Australian Nursing Federation [ANF], 1999).

The burgeoning demand of the higher wages of agency nurses was an unpredicted and unsustainable expense for hospitals in the Victorian public health sector. As a result of the unsustainable financial position they faced, hospital managers arrived at three common solutions to the shortage: they strongly encouraged nurses to work double shifts and/or overtime, increased the use of non-nursing staff, and recruited nurses from developing countries. None of these solutions was ethically sound, if indeed financially viable. Nurses were becoming increasingly dissatisfied with their working conditions and began lobbying governments for workloads that were manageable and fair. The public and the media strongly supported nurses, who were considered essential to a viable health system. Public reaction to these solutions was not favorable. The crisis in the health system unfolded as falling nurse staffing levels resulted in bed closures and extensions in hospitals' surgery waiting lists. The Kennett government was not subsequently reelected.

## THE AUSTRALIAN NURSING FEDERATION CAMPAIGNS FOR RATIOS

The Nursing Labor Force 1998 Report conducted by AIHW found that the number of effective full-time (EFT) nurses had fallen 11.8% in 3 years. After months of trying to convince the government about the severity of the problem, the nurses union, ANF, undertook two further surveys, which were conducted in early 1999:

- The first of these was the Nursing Workforce Survey, which was conducted in conjunction with

the Australian College of Nurse Management and the Victorian Deans of Nursing. Its purpose was to establish the extent of the nursing shortage where significant numbers of nursing vacancies were found, especially in the areas of midwifery, critical care, operating room, and medical-surgical wards.

- The second survey was the ANF Work, Time, and Life Survey. Its purpose was to determine how the shortage was affecting nurses and their ability to maintain standards of care.

The results were then analyzed by the Australian Centre for Industrial Relations Research and Training at the University of Sydney (ACIRRT). The results demonstrated concern by nurses about workloads, declining care standards, increased stress, and reduced morale (Buchanan, Bearfield, & Jackson, 2004).

In response to the results of both surveys, the ANF (Victorian Branch) served a log of claims on the state government in August 2000 on behalf of public sector members. This action was the first step in establishing a legal agreement among the Victorian State Government, hospitals, and nurses. The state government opposed all components of the claim. After negotiations failed, the ANF (Victorian Branch) took the claim to the Australian Industrial Relations Commission (AIRC—the equivalent of the National Labor Relations Board in the United States). Ten days later, on August 31, 2000, a decision was handed down in favor of the ANF claim and included the introduction of mandated minimum nurse/patient ratios. The actual ratios were determined by the expert nurse opinion of ANF members. Commissioner Wayne Blair accepted that there was a crisis in the Victorian public health system and that the exodus of nurses had to be addressed, saying:

Those who choose to say that there is not a nursing crisis, in the Commission's view are in a state of denial…therefore the Commission cannot ignore the issue of nurse/patient ratio mix. It is obvious to the Commission that whatever measures (if any) have been put in place by the hospital networks to address the recruitment and retention issues, have failed…there was ample opportunity for the hospital networks to provide alternatives to the nurse/patient ratio mix proposed by the ANF and this did not eventuate. (Blair, 2000)

The Commission report suggested that hospitals should have made better progress with alternatives for measuring nursing workloads. Mandated ratios were supported by government agreement to provide funding for nurse staffing, enabling Victorian public hospitals to meet the minimum ratios under an agreement called the *Nurses (Victorian Public Sector) Multi-Employer Agreement 2000-2004*. This provided directors of nursing, nurse unit managers, and staff nurses with the autonomy to close beds, control their own staffing, and provide safe staffing levels. The introduction of mandated nurse/patient ratios was a significant reversal in circumstances. For the first time, nurses were successful in driving workload policy, rather than hospital managers.

## THE 2000 AGREEMENT

Hospital managers retained tight control over the provision in the agreement for ratio flexibility. The Victorian ratio agreement stipulated minimum staffing levels (or the maximum number of patients per nurse), as they did later in California. Under the agreement the ratios could be lowered to meet the needs of patients with higher acuity if necessary. Lower ratios would require more nurses, which were not commonly provided by Victorian public hospital managers. If provided, there was an associated higher

cost which could not be counterbalanced by allocating fewer nurses in other, less-acute clinical settings. The one-way flexibility was not embraced by hospital managers, most of whom budgeted on minimum mandated ratios and were reluctant to provide flexibility that would potentially increase costs. Therefore the minimum ratios were in reality maximum ratios in most Victorian hospitals, despite the position of the ANF that ratios provided for flexibility and accounted for the range of patient needs and nursing skill mix.

The hospitals were required to schedule staff according to agreed-on ratios or close beds. Nurses were able to control their workloads under hospital managements that had previously applied pressure on them to work with unfair workloads and at times potentially unsafe conditions. This was an effective and highly significant political strategy. The ratios were phased in between December 2000 and August 2001. The agreement did not apply to nonacute hospital care or other states or territories of Australia. The agreement also did not apply to private hospitals, and the private sector does not have mandated nurse/patient ratios, although the ANF continues to negotiate fixed ratios with employers. This is in contrast to the later decision in California by which the mandated nurse/patient ratios applied to all public and private hospitals in that state.

In associated developments, in 2000 the AIRC determined that agency staff could not be employed in a hospital or network in which they had other employment. This changed the Victorian nursing landscape significantly, as less agency work was available and many nurses sought out permanent positions with hospital employers once again. Subsequent to this decision, agency nurses could be used only for unplanned vacancies for a percentage of EFT positions, as agreed on by the hospital and the state health department (the Department of Human Services [DHS]). This was lawfully binding on the ANF, state government, nursing agencies, and public hospitals. The state government applied to the Australian Competition and Consumer Commission for permission to award a tender to one nursing agency to provide nurses on a casual basis to Melbourne metropolitan hospitals and Barwon Health, and this was successful. This had

### Chronology of Key Events in Victoria

| Year | Event |
|---|---|
| 1990 | Two thousand nursing positions made redundant. |
| 1999 | ANF and AIHW survey nursing shortage. |
| 2000 | AIRC determines nursing shortage and introduces mandated nurse/patient ratios. |
| | AIRC rules that agency nurses may be used only for unplanned vacancies. |
| 2001 | Ratios phased in over 12 months to December. |
| | Dispute regarding the staffing of emergency departments. |
| 2003 | ANF begins lobbying for improved ratios for next Enterprise Bargaining Agreement. |
| | Patient dependency system trial. |
| 2004 | 2004-2007 agreement (Enterprise Bargaining Agreement). |

*AIHW,* Australian Institute of Health and Welfare; *AIRC,* Australian Industrial Relations Commission; *ANF,* Australian Nursing Federation.

an immediate effect on controlling the escalating growth of the nursing agency industry in Victoria, and the availability of fewer agency shifts meant that significant numbers of nurses returned to permanent positions.

During 2001 the state government supported the agreement by funding an intensive media campaign promoting nursing as a career and Victorian nurses as caring professionals with a wide range of skills and expertise. The state government also funded refresher programs for nurses who had been out of clinical practice for more than 5 years and nurses transferring from aged care to public acute-care settings. Reentry programs for nurses who had lapsed registration for more than 5 years were also state government funded. These associated decisions are considered likely to have contributed to the successful recruitment of nurses back to Victorian public hospitals at that time, in addition to mandated nurse/patient ratios.

Victorian universities began seeing an increase in popularity in nursing courses, and demand for places in undergraduate degrees increased 26.5% (ANF, 2002a). Public approval for the state government was on the increase and the Labor Bracks government was reelected on November 30, 2002. It is reasonable to assume that the mandated ratios themselves were not the only factor in recruiting nurses back to hospitals. The strategies for management of nursing agency staff, support of those wishing to reenter the acute-care nursing workforce, and a successful media campaign are likely to have also contributed. Perhaps the most influential element of success was not the practice of nurse/patient ratios but nurses' satisfaction about the security in having the allocation method incorporated into the agreement (i.e., legally enforceable). This means that nurses may close beds or employers risk losing state government funding. The ANF had a different view.

## NURSES RETURN TO WORK IN VICTORIAN PUBLIC HOSPITALS

The ANF considered the implementation of mandated nurse/patient ratios to have been the key factor in retaining registered nurses and attracting them to the public health system in Victoria

(ANF, 2004b). Before the AIRC decision in July 2001, the Victorian public sector was closing 400 beds per day because of the nurse shortage. The ANF (Victorian Branch) estimates that more than 3300 nurses returned to the Victorian public hospital system as a direct result of the introduction of nurse/patient ratios. Supporters of mandated nurse/patient ratios in both Victoria and California claim that the initiative is directly responsible for improvement in recruitment and retention of nurses in those states, when compared with other states in Australia and the United States, which are still struggling with staffing shortages.

The experience in Victoria and California indicates a link between nursing resource allocation by mandated nurse/patient ratios and recruitment and retention, but not necessarily a cause-and-effect relationship. A causal relationship between the two variables is possible but outside the scope of this paper. The political context of these developments saw directors of nursing responding favorably to the agreement. Although seen to be negotiating with CEOs as part of the Victorian Hospitals Industrial Association, in reality directors of nursing were supporting an agreement that would contribute to recruitment and retention of nurses to provide a quality nursing service.

## CHALLENGE TO THE AGREEMENT

The dispute between nurses and the state government was not over. The agreement reached between the ANF (Victorian Branch), DHS, and Victorian Hospitals Industrial Association was threatened on several occasions. In December 2001 the management of the Geelong Hospital in Victoria advised that they intended to reduce nursing staff numbers in the emergency department, as they believed that this was permitted under the flexibility clause in the agreement. Recommendations were made by Senior Deputy President (SDP) Watson on December 13, 2001 and concerned the Public Sector Heads of Agreement Monitoring Committee, established in response to the Geelong Hospital action. SDP Watson recommended that the methodology used to apply the nurse/patient ratio should be consistent and ensure that the number of nurses available correlates with the number of patients requiring care.

He observed that average occupancy is unlikely to reflect actual patient numbers all the time, especially in an emergency department, and that the nurse/patient ratios should be calculated on actual patient numbers in a given unit. Watson's ruling was that the ratios apply to the number of occupied beds and that the occupancy of additional beds is subject to additional nurses being available.

As a result of this decision, it was indisputable that the nurse/patient ratios were now to be calculated on actual patient numbers in a given ward or unit. Variation in the demands on emergency departments was acknowledged, and the departments were subsequently grouped according to throughput. Emergency departments were classified in three groups. A provision was also made for adjustment for seasonal fluctuations for part of each year. If a hospital has a particular ward of 30 beds and only 26 beds are usually occupied, then the four "unoccupied" beds can be used only when additional staff are available to meet the ratio requirements. On some night duty shifts and in shifts on acute-care hospital geriatric wards, it was considered appropriate to appoint what the commission understood to be called a "floater" to make up the part ratio. For example, in two wards, each with 22 beds, five nurses could be appointed to each ward, plus a nurse "floating" between the two wards.

The agreement also allowed for different models of care such as is provided at the midwifery units of some hospitals. Nurses in some Victorian rural public hospitals requested the agreement to include staffing by TrendCare hours per patient day (a computerized patient dependency or acuity system used widely throughout Australia and New Zealand). The nurses proposed the use of TrendCare for staffing instead of mandated ratios because they felt a system based on acuity rather than occupancy would provide more realistic ratios for rural hospitals that had previously attempted to negotiate up from level 3 to level 2 without success. For example, Hamilton Hospital in Victoria requested an agreement with ratios by patient type using TrendCare rather than ward type using the ANF-designed mandated ratios. The modified agreements were agreed on for some of the hospitals, and although mandated nurse/patient ratios did not apply to those

sites, ratio equivalence was monitored by the DHS. There was a successful outcome in these special cases, and they continue to use TrendCare.

## RATIOS GAIN INCREASING POPULARITY IN VICTORIA

The benefits of mandated nurse/patient ratios for direct care nurses include a minimum safe staffing level, staff satisfaction, retention of staff and an elementary principle of fairness among wards and among hospitals. The introduction of mandated ratios was also popularly reported in the media. Nurses had strong public support during their campaign, and the ratio agreement was seen to be the solution to ensuring fair workloads and encouraging nurses back to the public hospitals. Public opinion was that a fair deal for nurses meant that the public health system could restore its acute-care services. The initiative was expected to address the public confidence in two main areas of concern:

- Lengthening waiting lists for elective surgery
- Prolonged patient care on stretchers in emergency departments because of lack of staffed ward beds, some of which were closed to maintain nurse/patient ratios

Mandated nurse/patient ratios have the benefit of requiring little consultation; no technology; no costly infrastructure, maintenance, or training; and little documentation. Ratios are therefore highly attractive to hospital managers who have historically provided little or no financial support to nurses for information technology and nursing research, including workload studies. They have not been particularly interested in paying for the collection of evidence that would potentially identify that a nursing budget was inadequate. Hospital managers are also aware that sophisticated and computerized systems require regular updating and interfacing with other hospital systems. The introduction of such a computerized system that incorporates a patient acuity system would imply an ongoing financial commitment and greater management transparency associated with links to other systems such as payroll.

Patient acuity systems have historically been considered by many hospital managers to be unreliable and easily manipulated and therefore more difficult for budget decision support. In fact, ratios are potentially just as unreliable given that they have evolved without a supporting base of evidence and that they rely on expert nurse opinion of individuals. It is interesting to note that parallel ratio research related to outcomes of care, as opposed to ratio research for budget and financial purposes, has had evidence-based results. For example, nurse skill mix and staffing ratios have been reported as being "significant predicators of mortality" according to a review by University of Pennsylvania researchers Aiken, Sloane, and Sochalski (1998). Interactions between skill-mix ratios and outcomes may be examined in future studies.

## THE 2004 CAMPAIGN

There was surprise among Victorian nurses and Australian and international observers that the successful outcome of 2001 was required to be renegotiated when there was evidence that Victoria was one of the few places in the world that had experienced a reversal of the trend in increased nursing shortages. Nurses who had reentered the public hospital workforce because of the introduction of mandated ratios and those who had stayed through the industrial campaign did not want to experience a repeat of their hard-won battle of 2000. They did not want to rely once again on any system that was not mandated, and they saw no reason for change or for trials of another system. The following view was held by 80% of ANF members interviewed during the 2004 campaign: "Few nurses in the Victorian public health system trust management to get the issue of shift staffing levels correct and almost all believe the nurse to patient ratios are essential for an effective long term solution to the systems' problems" (Buchanan et al., 2004, p. 7).

A reasonable workload can reasonably be expected to ensure nurses' job satisfaction, patient satisfaction and quality care. The potential loss of already established ratios threatened the confidence of nurses, who were likely to leave the hospital workforce and not reenter a second time (Morieson, 2004). Nurses believed that existing conditions established in 2001 were threatened by the pilot of an acuity system, referred to in the Victorian agreement as a

"dependency system." They favored ratios but wanted to improve some of the allocations in the 2004-2007 agreement. In the 2004 campaign, nurses lobbied for improved ratios, such as 1:4 plus a charge nurse for both day and evening shifts in medical-surgical wards and 1:1 in labor and delivery for all shifts plus a charge nurse for day and evening shifts. In a further example, at the Royal Children's Hospital, the ratio on night duty was proposed to be reduced from 1:5 to 1:4. Nurses compared their ratios with the night ratio of 1:4 for a childcare center caring for well children and observed that this was lower than the ratio initially mandated for sick children. Lobbying began for the incorporation of other changes in the next agreement, even though it was supported by scant empiric evidence. Since that time there has developed a body of evidence about the correlation between patient dependency and nurse/patient ratios in Victorian public hospitals (Plummer, 2005).

During the 2004 Victorian Nurses public sector campaign, the ANF (Victorian Branch) claimed that the introduction of nurse/patient ratios was a positive change in nurse workload management and that the introduction of ratios was a simple and critical decision that addressed the nurse shortage. The ANF also claimed that if nurse/patient ratios stayed, nurses would stay and work in hospitals, but if ratios were abolished, nurses would resign. This claim may have had some merit but promoted a somewhat ill-founded confidence among nurses that understaffing could not occur with mandated minimum nurse/patient ratios. The ANF (Victorian Branch) promoted their ratio policy with a strong media campaign using a simple message to promote the ratio of five nurses for 20 patients for medical-surgical wards (i.e., 5-4-20).

## AGREEMENT TO PILOT A PATIENT DEPENDENCY SYSTEM

While the ANF (Victorian Branch) was preparing for the 2004-2007 agreement, one part of the previous agreement remained unfulfilled. This was the agreement between the parties to pilot a patient dependency system in 20 Victorian public hospitals for the purposes of collecting patient dependency data. The dependency data were to be compared with ratio data for the same period. The objective of the pilot was to "provide a robust clinical decision support system that was effective, easy to use and that would assist in the management of resources by providing clinical information technology tools that engaged nurses and enabled them to utilize evidence based guidelines in planning and provision of care" (Monash University, 2004, p. 7). The pilot was managed by the Nurse Policy Branch of the DHS (the Victorian State Health Department) and supported by the Pilot Advisory Committee. The dependency system selected was TrendCare, and it was evaluated under tender to the DHS by the School of Nursing and Midwifery at Monash University.

The pilot was actively supported by the DHS and Victorian Hospitals Industrial Association. The ANF (Victorian Branch) supported the pilot while actively maintaining its position of "no support for patient dependency systems." The conflicting standpoints of the ANF meant that a genuine pilot of any dependency system was going to be extremely difficult. The outcome of the pilot was preempted by the ANF (Victorian Branch) and its membership by an extensive media campaign that supported ratios and criticized the piloted TrendCare dependency system. The ANF distributed various written and verbal directives to members on how to complete evaluation survey forms and threaten bed closures if ratios were not maintained.

Although the ANF (Victorian Branch) was highly cognizant of the capacity of the preferred system for the agreed pilot, they remained philosophically opposed to dependency systems. The government described TrendCare, the agreed system for the pilot, as more sophisticated and transparent than nurse/patient ratios. Ratios were considered by DHS to be the first step along the path of achieving manageable workloads. The next step was to look to a system that was able to produce data for the formulation of a favorable funding policy for nursing services in Victorian public hospitals. A dependency system was promoted by DHS as a system that would provide empiric evidence for support for staffing requirements and that protected individual nurses from excessive workloads (and

equally from too light a load). For example, a dependency system may address the variability in dependency occurring in the winter demand period or among sites with case-mix differences.

DHS conducted the pilot in 2003 in 20 of its 114 public hospitals, with data collection from April 1 to December 31, 2003 and evaluation in December 2003 and January 2004. There was a strong emphasis by DHS on evaluating dependency systems generally rather than specific emphasis on piloting the TrendCare system. DHS reported being oversubscribed with hospitals interested in participating in the pilot. Many hospital managers demonstrated a keen interest in understanding nursing workloads, but this enthusiasm was not matched by the nurses on the wards, who felt disenchanted at the lack of consultation with them. Nurses were also concerned that in the United States computerized systems equated to supporting systems of corporate financing, verification of care, and benchmarking (Gordon, 2004). The notion of managed care, using computerized systems, gave rise to concern among nurses that they would have little influence over their own workloads and ability to meet their patient care requirements. DHS finally selected 10 expert TrendCare user sites and 10 new user sites from a range of hospitals across the metropolitan and rural sectors of the state. The hospitals in the pilot agreed to record and submit data to DHS from TrendCare.

The pilot involved nurses recording patient care in TrendCare. Staffing throughout the pilot in Victorian public hospitals continued to be by ratio allocation as in the previous 3 years. For most nurses, compliance with the requirements of the pilot was pointless in an environment where ratios were in place and actively used for workload allocation. The pilot was seen by nurses on the wards as an additional and unnecessarily time-consuming exercise in an already busy work environment. Nurses at participating hospitals perceived that TrendCare data recorded during the pilot were for high-level management and government purposes only. Nurses were not sympathetic to the real or perceived cost-cutting agendas of the government or to the threat of losing their hard-won political victory in achieving mandated nurse/patient ratios 3 years earlier. The lack of support of the pilot by nurses raised suspicion among observers about the quality and quantity of data recorded by TrendCare.

At the time of 2004 negotiations, the DHS vision for nursing in Victoria was promoted by the "Right nurse, Right place, Right time" campaign. The campaign was used to promote a workload system that could be responsive to the changing needs of patients and allow nurses "time to care." The campaign itself began at the "wrong time." It was launched in December 2003. The timing of the launch was too late for nurses because many had already made up their minds that ratios were the only successful method of workload allocation. The ANF had already begun a campaign for the 2004 Enterprise Bargaining Agreement and claimed that the improvement in nurse recruitments in Victoria was a result of the successful incorporation of mandated nurse/patient ratios in the previous agreement (ANF, 2004a). The ANF successfully renegotiated for a second 3-year term under the 2004-2007 Enterprise Bargaining Agreement after the completion of the dependency system pilot (Monash University, 2004).

Whatever views some experts had, the role of ratios in stabilizing the nursing industrial or labor climate in Victoria was acknowledged by many stakeholders, including the public and the media. Ratios had their place in rescuing failing health systems in Victoria; they were simple, were inexpensive, and required no training or technology.

## AUSTRALIAN NURSING FEDERATION SUCCESS IN NEGOTIATIONS

Negotiations with government are difficult when one political party dominates both Houses of Parliament, as was the case in Victoria in the two previous state elections. The success of the ANF (Victorian Branch) at the negotiating table during this time was remarkable. This resulted in the renegotiation of ratios for a further 3 years for the 2004-2007 Enterprise Bargaining Agreement. Indeed, the success was achieved without evidence such as patient care data. A widely held view within the ANF membership is that nursing evidence of practice, such as that recorded in association with dependency systems, is irrelevant for workplace agreements. A common argument is that such evidence is not required for any other heath professional group.

They claim that no other health professional has a dependency-driven formula for workload allocation. The membership considers that the power and strength of the ANF is far more relevant for the achievement of improved wages and conditions than any evidence-of-practice system. The ANF claimed that successful outcomes occur using the only useful instrument—industrial action such as a strike or restriction of services. Industrial action by nurses is always considered a last resort, because the ANF never gets 100% support for industrial action from nurses and the public. The ANF's view is that if industrial action is so successful, then there is little point in recording data for nursing services, as historical data are useless and nursing care requirements of today are delivered in the same way as medical treatment is delivered by doctors.

## POSTPILOT TRENDS

The pilot had an ongoing influence on work practices at the sites, and although it officially ceased on December 31, 2003, some further funding was provided by DHS to any of the participants who indicated a willingness to continue contributing data. By April of 2004, all acute-care hospital sites continued to use TrendCare and contribute data to DHS, while still maintaining workload allocation by the mandated ratio method. Morieson's view of industrial action as the most successful method of negotiating policy for nurses' conditions and wages appeared to be a reality. The 2004-2007 agreement included maintenance of existing nurse/patient ratios but provided some flexibility by permitting negotiation at local hospital level using committees and decision by staff ballot. Variation up or down could be made on the basis of, but not limited to, the following:

- Clinical nursing assessment of patient needs
- Demands of the environment, such as layout
- Statutory obligations, including workplace safety and health legislation
- The requirements of nurse regulatory legislation and professional standards
- Workloads
- Occupancy

The use of a dependency system had apparently modified the previously inflexible practice of mandated nurse/patient ratios in Victorian public hospitals. The ratio agreement was a hybrid of both practices.

In Victoria, the following are now present:

- Compulsory, mandated but now flexible nurse/patient ratios for most Victorian public hospitals
- Flexibility in workloads by protracted negotiation processes except where patient care may be compromised

## NURSES DEVELOP THE FLEXIBLE USE OF RATIOS

After the 2004-2007 Enterprise Bargaining Agreement was agreed on, the ANF (Victorian Branch) was dissatisfied with the evaluation of the pilot and prepared and circulated to its members an alternative Executive Summary to the Monash University Patient Nurse Dependency Evaluation Report. The alternative Executive Summary suggested that an accurate evaluation of TrendCare should entail a direct comparison with ratios. In fact, such a study had been underway since 2001 and was completed in early 2005 (Plummer, 2005).

Several observations can be made about the evolution of ratios from informal or formal arrangements to mandated nurse/patient ratios that are enforceable by law. The first is that any method of allocation that is mandated is likely to succeed because it is an enforceable agreement between stakeholders. Since the ANF (Victorian Branch) and later the California Nurses Association (CNA) successfully negotiated ratios for the purpose of establishing a policy to ensure fair and equitable workloads in preference to a patient-dependency system, the ratio system had established an unprecedented popularity with nurses. The second is that any system that contributes to stabilization and improvement of recruitment and retention in the current shortage of working nurses is also likely to maintain ongoing public popularity. Third, industrial action is currently more effective for influencing government funding and hospital management resource allocation policies than any data nurses currently record. It is evident that nurses were beginning to use ratios in the Victorian public

sector in a sophisticated way to gain improvements to working conditions.

Subsequently, the 2004-2007 Enterprise Bargaining Agreement for nurses in Victorian public hospitals includes provision for ratio variation according to the clinical assessment of patient needs, environmental demands such as ward layout, occupational health and safety, workloads, and occupancy. The Enterprise Bargaining Agreement includes provision for the use of dependency, skill mix, DRGs, or length of stay (LOS) to determine these variations. Short shift provision (4- to 6-hour shifts) has been reintroduced, which is an indicator of acknowledgement of peaks and troughs in workload by the ANF. After the agreement was finalized, the DHS then conducted a series of meetings with managers of Victorian public hospitals and advised that ratios such as 1:4 can be averaged over a 4-week roster period (e.g., 1:6 on Sunday or public holidays and 1:3.5 on "postop" shifts). It would be reasonable to suggest that TrendCare was used by DHS and hospitals to negotiate this. This means that the mandated ratios are no longer rigidly fixed. But how do nurses in Victorian public hospitals determine the variable ratios, or record and track them? Will the last of the 4 weeks be unfairly "ratioed" if that is the balance after 3 busy weeks or poor allocation practices? Mandated ratio practices in Victoria have now adopted many of the features of dependency systems and will probably need a dependency system to support decisions made within it. Perhaps it is now easier to manipulate a ratio system than dependency systems.

The projection for increasing numbers of high-dependency patients has many implications for acute-care nursing. Higher numbers of high-dependency patients will be associated with advances in complex medicine and surgery, the increasing age of patients, higher levels of co morbidities and risk of complications, and shorter LOS. Higher-dependency nursing, such as that provided in coronary care, intensive care, high-dependency units, special care nurseries, and dialysis units, is highly resource intensive. This means that more nurses with specialized skills may be required to care for the same number of patients in the future. However, this may be offset by growth in robotic and laser surgery and less-risky, less–resource-intensive surgical techniques that result in lower acuity, mortality, and morbidity, resulting in lower nurse dependency. The limitation on beds available in these units means that many patients who cannot be accommodated will increasingly be accommodated in general wards. Accordingly, there will also be higher demand for more nurses with specialized skills for the general wards. The care of higher numbers of older Australians and other influences such as defensive medicine, advances in technology and communications, delayed discharge for nonacute medical reasons, and the declining health of indigenous populations are further examples of impending rise in nursing demand. The future demand for nursing is expected to be compounded by a decreased capacity to provide the nurses required, because of the aging nursing workforce. This combination of circumstances demands strong and informed nursing leadership to manage the working conditions and the distribution of current and future nursing resources.

What this means for nursing is that we must go beyond ratios and analyzing data and link workload allocation practices to clinical pathways, skill mix, variance analysis, clinical indicators, patient outcomes, and population-based care in the future. It is imperative that nurses illuminate the key concepts of acuity, dependency, and workload allocation so that we can move on to bigger agendas such as realistic nursing budgets and the achievement of sound financial and clinical outcomes within the context of existing government policy. Nurse dependency systems can provide the rudder for future policy direction.

## MANAGING FUTURE CHANGES IN THE RATIO ACUITY MIX

A federal government review predicted that by 2006 the Australian national health system would have 31,000 vacancies for nurses, with a significant majority of the 22,000 nurses leaving nursing rather than retiring (Johnson, 2002). Improved wages and conditions are at issue, and a method of fair and equitable workload allocation could be expected to stem the flow of nurses from the health system. The only Australian state in which there is now no significant nursing shortage crisis is

Victoria. The success of the nurse/patient ratio system in Victoria has most probably been the result, in part at least, of the legislated aspect of a controlled workload, which can neither be negotiated nor manipulated by management. In short, nurses returned to the workforce because they knew management could not change the ratios, rather than the actual number of patients they would be required to care for. Nevertheless, wider acceptance of ratios by nurses has not stopped them from seeking out more accurate measures or ways of determining workloads.

Nurses may be satisfied that ratios have been successful inclusions for two successive Enterprise Bargaining Agreements in Victoria. It is undeniable that there will eventually be a requirement to account for nursing workloads empirically. Governments are destined to negotiate ratios less favorably in the future in the absence of any substantiating evidence. For example, they may maintain existing ratios despite the predictable increase in age, acuity, and comorbidities of the patients in the future.

Nurses themselves are in the best position to identify patient requirements and determine how best to organize their work, but by contrast nurses at the hospital level are in a weak position to argue for a fair share of the budget and to have a strong influence on strategic planning. Arguably it is politics above all else that influences financial policy, and regrettably, in the past, nurses have been traditionally poor performers in the political environment (Prescott, 1986). In recent times an industrial strength has appeared, demonstrated by strategic negotiations, walkouts, bed closures, and restriction-of-service campaigns as methods used by nurses to demonstrate the value of their work to improve wages and conditions. Nurses have long perceived that hospital managers were not adequately recognizing their work. Nurses need data and empirical information to support their argument for fair and equitable workloads that can be used with or without withdrawing their services and threatening to compromise patient care. It is equally important for hospital managers to have data on resources and costing in order to contribute fruitfully to those negotiations. Until we get the information, nurses and nursing will remain central to cost cutting and on the periphery of policy argument (Diers, 2004).

## CONCLUSION

Success in the industrial relations setting does not equate to high-quality nursing care. Nursing cannot stand alone and claim that there is no need to record data for acuity, dependency, or workload purposes because mandated nurse/patient ratios have been successfully renegotiated. Nurses know they need to record data about their work and interface with the care systems of the rest of the multidisciplinary team. They also know they need to provide documented, publicly accountable, high-quality care. Securing fair workloads by arbitration was a logical first step and moved hospital managements "off the case" so that nurses could reestablish control of their working conditions. With that control secured, it is now time to return to the quality agenda, and research is an integral part of the process. Buchan (2004) summarized the situation very well when he said, "Ratios are a blunt instrument for achieving employer compliance, where reliance on alternative, voluntary (and often more sophisticated) methods of determining nurse staffing have not been effective" (p. 3).

Ratios and dependency hours per patient day essentially mean the same thing but are expressed differently. They are both about averages by categories. Ratios are very popular in Victoria, and the aim should be to replace the way we use them rather than replace them given that the concept is in its second Enterprise Bargaining Agreement. The need is to identify how we make a successful formula stronger and establish a database for the next round of negotiations when acuity and dependency is likely to be higher. We need to focus on developing a cooperative relationship between the two practices.

## Key Points

- Mandated nurse/patient ratios were introduced in Victorian public hospitals in 2000 and remain in place under current Enterprise Bargaining Agreements.
- There are no regulations governing nurse/patient ratios in Australian private hospitals or in public hospitals in any other Australian states.

- Mandated ratio environments provide little incentive to account for nursing workloads empirically, and governments are destined to negotiate ratios less favorably in the future in the absence of any substantiating evidence.
- Nurses need to record data about their work and interface with the care systems of the entire multidisciplinary team.
- Success in the industrial relations setting does not necessarily result in enhanced quality of care. Further research in this area is underway.

## Web Resources

**Australian Industrial Relations Commission (AIRC)**
*www.airc.gov.au/decisionssigned/html/PR912522.htm*
**Australian Nursing Federation (ANF)**
*www.anf.org.au*
**Australian Nursing Federation (Victorian Branch)**
*www.anfvic.asn.au/news_briefs/news_ratios.htm*
**Centre for Health Services Operations Management, Monash University, Australia**
*www.med.monash.edu/chsom/research.html*
**Department of Human Services (DHS) Victoria, Nurse Policy Branch**
*www.nursing.vic.gov.au*

## REFERENCES

Aiken, L., Sloan, D., & Sochalski, J. (1998). Hospital organisation and outcomes. *Quality Health Care, 7*(4), 222-226.
Australian Nursing Federation (ANF). (1999). *Work, time, life survey.* Melbourne. Retrieved November 20, 2002, from *www.anfvic.asn.au.*
Australian Nursing Federation (ANF) (Victorian Branch). (2002a). Nurse-patient ratios information summary for members. Retrieved November 20, 2002, from *www.anfvic.asn.au.*
Australian Nursing Federation (ANF) (Victorian Branch). (2002b). Nurse to patient ratios—Nursing shortage? Retrieved November 20, 2002, from *www.anfvic.asn.au.*
Australian Nursing Federation (ANF) (Victorian Branch). (2004a). *Nurse-patient ratios. ANF EBA media background information.* Melbourne: ANF.
Australian Nursing Federation (ANF) (Victorian Branch). (2004b). *For the nurses...because you're worth it. 2004 Public Sector Claim.* Melbourne: ANF.

Blair, W. (2000). Australian Industrial Relations Commission— Record of proceedings. Cited on ANF Victoria Web site. Retrieved April 6, 2004, from *www.anfvic.asn.au/news_briefs/ news_ratios.htm.*

Buchan, J. (2004). A certain ratio? The policy implications of minimum staffing ratios in nursing. *Journal of Health Services Research Policy, 10*(4), 239-344.

Buchanan, J. B., Bearfield, T., & Jackson, S. (2004). *Stable, but critical—the working conditions of Victorian Public Sector nurses in 2003.* Sydney: University of Sydney.

Diers, D. (2004). *Speaking of nursing.* Sudbury, MA: Jones and Bartlett.

Giovanetti, P. (1994). *Measurement of nursing workload.* In J. M. Hibberd & M. E. Kylie (Eds.), *Nursing management.* Toronto: Saunders.

Gordon, S. (2004, June). Will we suffer a shortage of nurses too? On the Record. *Australian Nursing Federation Victorian Branch Newsletter.*

Johnson, N. (2002, October 8). Australia's nursing crisis. ABC television report.

Monash University. (2004). *PND Pilot Evaluation Report.* Frankston, Victoria, School of Nursing.

Morieson, B. (2004). Personal interview, South Melbourne, January 15.

Patera, N. (2004). *Acute inpatient casemix funding: The status quo in Victoria and Germany* (Interim unpublished PhD results. Health Economics Unit, Monash University at the Austin Hospital).

Plummer, V. M. (2005). An analysis of patient dependency data, utilizing the TrendCare system. (Doctoral thesis, Monash University, Australia, 2005).

Prescott, P. A. (1986). DRG prospective reimbursement: The nursing intensity factor. *Nursing Management, 17,* 43-49.

Watson, I (2001). *Australian Industrial Relations Commission— Record of proceedings.* Melbourne. AG2001/7714, 23 August 2001, Heads of Agreement, December 13, 2001.

# Taking Action   Linda Burnes Bolton & Patricia Moritz

## Using Technology to Mitigate the Nursing Shortage

*"Following the light of the sun, we left the Old World."*

CHRISTOPHER COLUMBUS

As the first decade of the twenty-first century unfolds, unprecedented change is being planned that may lead to reforms in health care that are realized through technology. Recognizing the importance of achieving a well-functioning health care system, the National Coalition on Health Care (NCHC), a broad bipartisan group of organizations in all sectors of the economy committed to systemic change in health care, identified five principles for a successfully reformed health care system (NCHC, 2004):

- Health coverage for all
- Cost management
- Improvement in quality and safety

- Equitable financing
- Simplified administration

At the heart of achieving these principles is the requirement to develop and implement a national integrated and multifaceted information technology infrastructure for our health care system. Contemporaneously, President Bush released a plan for changing health information technology to achieve transformation of U.S. health care (White House, 2004a), and a new office for national coordination of health information technology was established by executive order. The leader of this Office of the National Coordinator for Health Information Technology (ONCHIT) was directed to bring about national deployment of health information technology, including a unified approach to the electronic health record, within 10 years so that substantial improvement in health care safety and efficiency could be achieved (White House, 2004b). A report from this office on possible approaches to a nationwide health information network followed within the year (U.S. Department of Health and Human Services [USDHHS], 2005), as did new legislative approaches through bills introduced in both the U.S. House of Representatives and Senate to make the ONCHIT office permanent and to establish a program of grants for innovative informatics systems. In 2005 the 109th Congress had only recently begun to consider these legislative bills, so it is too early to know which if any of these bills will be enacted into federal law.

At the same time that national approaches to enhancing health care technology and informatics systems were being initiated, there was increasing concern about the nation's health professions workforce, most especially the nursing workforce. The USDHHS Bureau of Health Professions reported that most Americans have been unaware of the severity of shortages in the health professional workforce (National Advisory Council on Nursing Education and Practice [NACNEP], 2003). Shortages will adversely affect the nation's workforce productivity and economic viability as the access to health care services is jeopardized because of a lack of workforce capacity.

Most of the funding to develop nursing and other health professions resources has been aimed at the supply side. From fiscal year 2000 to 2005 the percent increase in funds under Title VIII of the Public Health Act for nursing education and practice was 129% (Duke, 2005), enabling student enrollments to grow by 14% in entry level baccalaureate programs, almost 14% in master's specialty programs, and 73% in doctoral programs (Berlin, Wilsey, & Bednash, 2005). The increase in this source of funding stimulated a response to the shortage of nurses by increasing supply. However, the increase in the demand for nurses and other health professionals continues to grow at a rate faster than even this enhanced funding can address. Our national policy continues to focus on the number of nurses without concurrently examining what is driving the demand. This commodity model approach, as described by Kimball and O'Neil (2002), perpetuates the notion that merely expanding the numbers will

resolve the shortage and its adverse public health implications. If we continue with this approach, the gap between demand and supply will actually widen. Among the many policy implications of this situation is the need to take actions that could improve the nation's capacity to meet anticipated nursing care demand in spite of continuing limitations on the supply of personnel.

## DEMAND IN A TIME OF NURSING SHORTAGE

The demand for nurses continues to outstrip the available supply and is feared to be beyond the current capacities of the nation's schools of nursing. As of 2005 the national shortage of nurses was 7% and was projected to be 12% in 2010 and 29% in 2020 (National Center for Health Professions Workforce Analysis, 2002). The current forces driving the demand for nurses include the following:

- An aging population
- Expansion of the health disparities gap that exists between white Americans and those of other racial and ethnic populations
- The use of technology and polypharmacology that enables individuals to live longer with chronic and debilitating disease
- The growth in the U.S. populace resulting from immigration

As the shortage of nurses continues, there are now fewer nurses for several reasons, including more than a decade of limited numbers of newly graduated nurses entering the profession. This situation only recently began to change as student enrollments in nursing education programs began to slowly increase after 2000; however, graduations of new nurses continue to lag behind employer demand in most geographic areas. The average age of nurses, like that of the general population, is increasing, with many reaching retirement age at a time of an insufficient supply of younger nurses to replace them. In addition, the average age of nurse faculty is even higher, and this is occurring as the educational mix of new nurse graduates is quickly becoming problematic, because only around a third of graduates have baccalaureate degrees—the degree requirement for entry into graduate level advanced practice and faculty preparation. If this educational mix does not change, nursing may not be able to educate its own workforce.

Anecdotal and survey reports now indicate that nurses in clinical practice are reacting to chaotic and highly demanding practice environments by leaving them rather than sticking it out in the hope that the situation could be improved (Shaver & Lacey, 2003). Nurses' optimism and enthusiasm for patient care are being challenged to the breaking point. Because the current nurse shortage is occurring at the same time as initial reports of early shortages in other health professions, a solution will require new strategies (Gelinas & Bohlen, 2002; O'Neil, 1998; Sochalski, 2002).

Reports of chaotic and high-pressured practice environments were appearing at the same time that national reports on the quality and safety of health care were coming from the Institute of Medicine (IOM) of the National Academy of Sciences; the most notable of these were "To Err Is Human: Building a Safer Health Care System" and "The Quality Chasm: A New Health Care System for the 21st Century" (IOM, 2000, 2001). As these IOM reports were published, and in follow-up work that further examined their findings, there were calls for substantial change in health care and in health professions education, for the use of evidenced-based clinical and management practice (Aiken, 2001; IOM, 2003), and for increased outcomes monitoring and other aspects of clinical evaluation science. These reports set the stage for major change in policy, practice, and education and were reinforced by several factors:

- Recognition that there would not be adequate numbers of nurses in the coming decades (Buerhaus, Staiger, & Auerbach, 2000; Needleman, Buerhaus, Mattke, & Zelevinsky, 2002; Buerhaus, 2002; Buerhaus, Donelan, Ulrich, Norman, & Dittus, 2005)
- Clear indicators that practice environments required substantial change (Aiken, Clarke, & Sloan, 2002a; Aiken, Clarke, Sloan, Sochalski, & Silber, 2002b; Buerhaus, Needleman, Mattke, & Stewart, 2002; Rogers, Hwang, Scott, Aiken, & Dinges, 2004)
- New evidence that certain management approaches by nurse leaders could change an organization's internal shortage of nurses (McClure & Hinshaw, 2002; Upenieks, 2002)

- Increasing evidence that nursing education also required substantial change in approaches to all levels of nursing education (IOM, 2004a)

## ADDRESSING THE DEMAND THROUGH TECHNOLOGY

Many groups have focused considerable work on increasing the supply of nurses in the United States. However, the demand side of the nursing workforce equation is equally important, and to some it is a crucially important focus that could potentially lead to short- and long-term alleviation strategies. Factors affecting the demand for nurses include job complexity, staffing requirements, work environment, and the interaction of management and clinical work of nurses. In 2001 the American Academy of Nursing established the Nursing Workforce Commission (NWC) to address the nursing shortage; the NWC initiated an ongoing health services study to find ways of decreasing the nonessential demands on nurses' time, which could ease the demand for more nurses and consequently bring equilibrium in nurse supply and demand.

Several publications support developing, implementing, and monitoring the efficacy of improving nurses' work processes and practice environments as an effective strategy to both address the demand for care and retain nurses on the front line. The IOM's report "Keeping Patients Safe" outlined practice environment changes that should be required in order to decrease the incidence of preventable mortality and morbidity in American hospitals (IOM, 2004a). The American Hospital Association, the American Organization of Nurse Executives (AONE), the Robert Wood Johnson Foundation, and the American Nurses Association have also called for reinventing the way nurses practice and are educated to retain and attract nurses to meet projected demand. How do we get from our current state to a preferred future that allows us to provide safe, high-quality patient care despite the supply limitations?

### Framework for Assessing the Interface of Technology and Nursing Practice

The work conducted by the NWC is guided principally by the Diffusion of Innovations theory (Rogers, 2003) as informed by concepts from complexity science (Stacy, 1996). The framework identifies crucial forces, processes, and relationships in the environments and among those involved when innovations are or should be occurring. It recognizes that systems in which care is provided are complex, chaotic at times, and resistant to change. Viewed in this manner, the demand for nurses is directly influenced not only by job availability but also by the efficiency and effectiveness of their work environment—most notably the quality of technology, the extent to which it alleviates nurses' work rather than increasing it, and the extent to which it is appropriate for nursing practice. There is evidence that technologic innovations in clinical care have been developed by a variety of designers and vendors, then moved into patient care by managers who frequently lack an understanding of the factors that might lead to successful implementation of new technologies and therapies used by nurses. Diffusion-of-innovations theory suggests to us that a number of factors influence how successful the diffusion will be:

1. Perceived attributes of a technology—such as compatibility with clinical work, how technology implementation decisions are made, and what communication channels were used before, during, and after introduction of a new or revised technology
2. The nature of the clinical social system's functioning
3. The extent to which clinical change agents promote a technology or make it known that it is ineffective

In addition, complexity science also assists in interpreting the highly complex interrelationships and decision-making processes in health care systems. Such systems have within them processes, including nursing care delivery, that are highly interactive while being independent, entrepreneurial, and at the same time nonlinear. Complexity theory assists with analyzing data from nonlinear, interactive systems to reveal patterns, networks, and repeating relationships.

### Nursing Workforce Commission Assessment Strategies

A purposeful approach was used in implementing the work of the NWC to achieve a more-knowledgeable set of key informants. Phase I examined the current acute-care nursing work environment and technologies within it. Phase II used a selection of clinical settings for in-depth nested case studies (Yin, 2002) to explore the interface of technology and its impact on nurses' work in those settings. The ongoing question for this work is: Can changes in technology, including its design, introduction and use, influence and alleviate the demand for nurses? To answer this question the NWC has examined the following:

- Use and nonuse of all types of technologies, as well as their fit and success of implementation in today's patient care environment
- Gaps in technology that could enhance efficiency of nurses' work if resolved

Important in this study are the perceptions—of nurses, managers, designers, and vendors of technologies—that are explored through strategies such as focus groups, stakeholder assessments, feedback sessions, and technology-supported identification of factors associated with appropriate implementation, requirements for new technologies, and priorities for change strategies.

### Evolution of the Ongoing Assessment and Development Process

In Phase I the NWC learned the following:

- A variety of vendors have, and continue to develop, numerous clinical products.
- Effectiveness of these products vary considerably once they are used in clinical care.
- Such introductions are frequently done without consideration of best practices for their introduction and who will use them.
- Vendors believe that because a product is introduced it will be used and that the use will be appropriate for clinical practice and for nursing practice in particular.
- The end user (frontline health professionals) often misuse or underuse products or develop "work-around" processes that add to rather than reduce their workload.

Vendors and their representatives also frequently have not followed up after introduction of their products to ask evaluative questions. Such questions would have quickly identified problems with new devices such as an intravenous delivery system that was new to the hospital, involved multiple different types of programming by clinicians with visually confusing symbols that resulted in initial errors, and continuing worries about the safety of the devices.

These Phase I findings informed the development of Phase II of the NWC's assessment.

In Phase II, three in-depth field assessments have been conducted and others are planned. These field projects were conducted in acute-care hospitals and were designed to:

- Identify aspects of nurses' work that may be amenable to some form of automation
- Consider technologies that could appropriately be applied to these aspects of nurses' and other health professionals' work
- Identify new technologies that could be developed to automate components of nurses' work, including the interdisciplinary team functions carried out by all health professionals
- Evaluate the effect of work processes that improved through technology the ability of nurses to provide patient care consistent with current recommendations for safety and quality and that also reflect best-practice standards in nursing

AONE has joined the NWC as a partner to work with the technology industry to expand the work of Phase II. The findings from the initial fieldwork have led to the development of an assessment framework that uses a process matrix for further, more-focused data collection and analysis to identify requirements for new technologies. The framework will also be used for expansion of the work into strategies that clinical agencies themselves can use to conduct an in-depth examination and analysis of their use of technology and its impact on their nurses' work. This framework, which the NWC developed and called the *Technology Drill-Down Process* (TDDP), is designed from a matrix perspective in which all levels of decision-makers from executives to those who provide direct care across disciplines come together in a several-day process to identify cross-cutting issues that facilitate, hinder, or frustrate patient care processes. The TDDP is designed to be iterative with feedback loops. To ensure success, the initial discussions are designed to develop a level "playing field" so that

power differentials among participants are reduced (Figure 18-1). The TDDP will also inform clinical agencies in their development of best practices for assessment of the need for and introduction decisions for new technologies.

The TDDP has demonstrated that the previous, usual methods of technology introduction do not work well and at times fail outright, resulting in considerable expense to all organizations involved, especially the clinical agency in which they occur.

### Implications for Practice, Education, and Policy

The NWC findings to date demonstrate the ability of frontline staff, interdisciplinary teams, and technology manufacturers to envision a technology-enhanced practice environment. In Phase II the NWC field-tested the concepts using our TDDP. Although the work of the commission continues, there are already clear indicators that require change.

***Technology and the practice environments of today.*** Clinical health care and its delivery systems are changing faster than health professionals and clinical agencies can respond, as is the important ongoing requirement that all health professionals keep up their knowledge about clinical and technologic change. At a time of shortage, it is challenging to practicing nurses and their employers to allocate time and other resources to respond to growing demands. However, it is crucial that leaders, particularly those in acute-care hospitals, engage a frontline team in redesigning health care systems, because the current piecemeal approach is too costly, is redundant, and does not work for clinicians on whom we rely.

The TDDP is a thoughtful approach for transformation and change in these systems. As an interdisciplinary approach led by nurses, it has the potential to bring about lasting change. The success of this approach requires the ongoing leadership and informed advocacy of nurses. Such advocacy recognizes the pluralism of nursing, builds on the strengths of all nurses, and develops common ground and agreements for collaborative work across the health disciplines.

***Changing the work-around merry-go-round.*** Nurses who work in clinical agencies can quickly describe which technologic devices and systems in

**TD² (Technology Drill Down) Logistical Process Cycles**

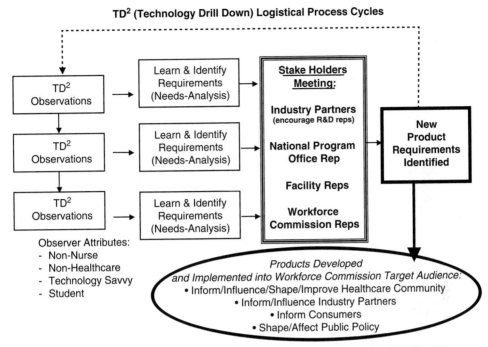

**Figure 18-1**  TD² (Technology Drill Down) Logistical Process Cycles. (Copyright AAN/AONE, 2004.)

their institutions do not work well for those who provide direct patient care, which technologies are ignored, and which they "work around"—that is, devise strategies to modify the device or how it works to make it clinically more useful or efficient, in their judgment. In these settings it is crucial that when managers and executives begin to discuss the possibility of a change in any technology, they include in the assessments and feasibility of any products those who have direct knowledge of the clinical impact.

This may seem self-evident. Airlines, for example, do not participate in the design of or purchase newly designed airplanes without the involvement of pilots who will use them and have firsthand knowledge for evaluating them. Too often in health care the obvious clinical "pilots" of care delivery are ignored. This sets up both a perceived "put down" of an important group of clinicians but also sets the stage for stress and use of work-around strategies. The TDDP has shown that existing clinical

environment factors, technologies, and systems can be assessed rather quickly and efficiently by experienced clinical professionals without compromising the achievement of reliable results. An example of this using the previous discussion of the intravenous device is that if nurses had assessed the device before purchase, the resulting problems would have been identified and solved before the devices were placed on patient units.

The results of clinical assessments of new or existing products can provide the basis for changes in the technology. The TDDP can be modified and used on a more "micro" or targeted basis than the initial hospital-wide process assessments described previously. The fact that a new product is on the market does not provide the evidence that it is needed, useful, safe, and of better quality than what is already in place, nor does it show that the product is effective in its intended purpose and hospital location.

Another aspect of changing the existing merry-go-round is accomplished through involvement of nurses in decision-making processes that affect patient care in their institutions. To achieve this there is a recognized requirement for a shared vision among health care executives, clinical managers, clinicians, and technology professionals when considering new products, seeking new product design, and asking questions about efficacy and effectiveness. Nurses must be included when such decisions are made, as their presence is crucial to quality care delivery and cost savings. To stop the costly work-around merry-go-rounds requires that nurses have lead roles in technology decision-making and change (e.g., by requiring that clinical nurses be on product assessment teams).

***Changing nursing education for twenty-first–century practice and management.*** Students in all fields, including nursing, are becoming technologically literate faster than the education programs and their faculties. Many programs and faculty are failing to meet students' expectations and to use cutting edge clinical technologies in their teaching. Clinical agencies today are demanding nurses who are highly knowledgeable, with well-honed critical thinking skills, and who are also savvy about informatics and technologies. This demand is not for rote knowledge but rather for knowledge about how to bring the complexity of what is known in a particular area together in a usable way and how to assess and find needed evidence that is missing while being comfortable with clinical and informatics technology.

AONE of the American Hospital Association took a stand in 2005 calling for the registered nurse to be educated at the baccalaureate level in the future. AONE indicated that this was done because the current proportion of nurses educated at this level is dwindling, and if this trend continues there will be few nurses for management roles in hospitals, to be educators of new nurses, or to be nurse specialists and advanced practitioners. Policymakers at all levels should heed this call because employers of nurses have already recognized that it is this level of education of nurses that yields a graduate who can effectively function in complex clinical agencies with the chronically and critically ill patients of today.

Groups that set standards for nursing education programs should consider the crucial importance of health care informatics content in curricula, and there should be an expansion of graduate programs in health care and nursing informatics so that increased numbers of these specialists are available for practice and education roles (Barton, Skiba, & Sorensen, 2004; IOM, 2003). The standard of education in undergraduate and graduate nursing programs has quickly advanced to simulation technology for student learning of complex clinical assessments and procedures, use of hand-held devices for clinical decision-making, standardized live patient models for advanced assessment, and model simulation rooms for specialty practice in such areas as critical care and perioperative nursing.

The cash-strapped hospitals and nursing schools alone cannot afford to invest the capital required to produce these technologically enhanced practice and learning environments. But, as a nation, we can't afford the status quo environments and supply-side approaches to the nursing shortage. Nurses must advocate for policy changes to assist in educating technology-proficient nurses to meet the demand for twenty-first–century nursing care.

## TECHNOLOGY, NURSING, AND THE DEMAND FOR POLICY CHANGE

The NWC strategy now requires major partners in the policy arena at all levels to join in leading changes in health care technology in the nation. The recent presidential and congressional initiatives are a step in this direction, but without a coalition of stakeholders and policymakers targeting innovative technology implementation using the TDDP framework, progress toward solutions to questions about quality and safety will be difficult.

### Where Are Hill and Burton When Health Care Needs Them?

The federal Hill-Burton Act has been well known to hospital administrators. It was initiated as part of national economic policy after World War II, when returning soldiers needed jobs in the civilian sector, and old hospital buildings throughout the country needed replacements. Formally known as the *Hospital Survey and Construction Act of 1946* (PL 79-487), but called the *Hill-Burton Act* after the major sponsors, this act set the stage for decades of health policy to assist both hospitals and indigent people who required health care but could not afford it. Its effects went on for 40 or more years through the long-term payback requirement in which a hospital that received construction, renovation, and rebuilding assistance was required to provide certain levels of indigent care for 20 years. Hospitals today need a new Hill-Burton Act targeted to supporting integrated information technology systems to bring all hospitals up to twenty-first–century standards.

Such a policy today would enable all hospitals, no matter their size, to put into place systems that facilitate safe and effective care while connecting clinical, pharmaceutical, and management systems so that there is one seamless set of data that both clinicians and administrators can use and have a common language. This policy would be designed in such a manner that key stakeholders would come together to make decisions about common technologic platforms and languages, possibly to share collective knowledge. Such an approach has been taken successfully in the software and the aviation industries.

Nurses should be advocates for such a policy and bring a voice to all debates and discussions, no matter how small or large the opportunity. Coming together through professional nursing organizations or clinical societies to consider policy initiatives at the state or national level is one way to get started. The bills already introduced in the U.S. Congress, noted earlier, would be one place to start. A collective voice can have political power.

### The Time Is Almost Beyond Ripe for a Public-Private Partnership

A public-private partnership approach would bring the changes required to achieve appropriate integrated clinical and management technologies into clinical agencies. These partnerships could take the form of agreements among the Centers for Medicare and Medicaid Services (CMS), other major funders of health care services, and national hospital associations to set standards to achieve the goals of full technologic upgrading and

reorganization by 2015. CMS should work with these partners to design a strategy that will support investment on technology in the practice arena.

In July 2005 a precedent for this was announced, in which CMS would provide to physician practices the software that hospitals use for their Medicare patient records to encourage physicians to use electronic health records in their practices. Such support is crucially important and cannot be paid for solely by the individual hospitals—nor should it be, because such investment is beyond the financial capacity of individual organizations and is a required public necessity. It should be recognized that there are enough funds in the national health care system as a whole, but more often than not, they are in the wrong place.

### Collaboration and Competition within the Health Care Technology Industry

There are multiple approaches to accomplishing this in an industry in which competition and not collaboration is the hallmark. One potential feasible strategy is for accreditors to change their scenario—for example, JACHO could change its requirements in the standards for outcomes and reporting and specify the types of data in real time. Such an approach changes the data requirement from a retrospective to a concurrent time frame for data assessment and reporting. Such an influential organization could also require that hospitals and other clinical agencies accredited by them demonstrate that they have evaluated new, revised, or replacement technologies before they are implemented in the clinical agency.

### Refocusing Evaluation Research to Include Technology in Patient Care

Clinical evaluation science must be stimulated and targeted on the interface of technology in the clinical settings and issues of health care quality and patient safety. Such technology includes not only clinical devices but also, and perhaps more importantly, clinical management applications and programs. An important question that needs to be asked is: Within and across clinical settings, do technology applications help or hinder safe patient care?

## REMAINING QUESTIONS

Health care has the highest turnover rate of any major industry in the United States and has the second highest absenteeism rate (Circadian Technologies, 2004). The issues discussed in this chapter are important factors leading to these rates. The work environment is the number one driver of dissatisfaction, turnover, and workforce shortages. Technology can help to improve the practice environment, if it is deemed relevant, useful in addressing staff-identified work process issues, and affordable.

What actions should be taken by the provider and business community to bring about changes in the current health care technology development and deployment process? How do we convince federal and state policymakers of the need to focus on this issue and to allocate resources to hospitals? How do we engage the business community, one of the largest payers for health care in the United States, to demand a more-efficient practice environment for nurses and other health care team members as a key strategy to reduce acute-care health expenditures?

All nurses must be involved in answering these questions, which are critical to health care quality and patient safety. The American Academy of Nursing's Workforce Commission is a group of nurse leaders who are working to address these and other questions. This is one approach, and it is essential to hear voices from the nursing community regarding these issues and the potential contribution a technology-enhanced practice environment may have on preventing recurrent nursing shortages. The initiatives and calls for action in this chapter can be achieved only if nurses work toward common and critical goals. A call to action is of vital importance. Become involved in a nursing organization whose goals are important to you, serve on health policy committees, and take action.

## *Lessons Learned*

- The worsening nursing shortage requires attention to nurses' work environments and ways to reduce nurses' work demands if health care is to be safe and effective.

- Technology has the potential to provide nurses with effective and efficient supports for clinical care, reducing demands on nurses' time.
- Nurses must be involved in the design, acquisition, implementation, and evaluation of clinical and information technology.
- The American Academy of Nursing's NWC has developed a tool for nurses, managers, and others to assess the use of technology in the workplace.
- Public policies that provide financial support, standard setting, and expectations for private-public partnerships are needed to stimulate the development of technology to support clinical practice that is safe and effective.

## *Web Resources*

**American Academy of Nursing, Nursing Workforce Commission (NWC)**
*www.aannet.org/committees/workforce.asp*
**U.S. Office of the National Coordinator for Health Information Technology (ONCHIT)**
*www.hhs.gov/healthit*

## REFERENCES

Aiken, L. H. (2001). Evidence-based management: Key to workforce stability. *Journal of Health Admin Education, 19*(4), 117-124.

Aiken, L. H., Clarke, S. P., Cheung, R. B., Sloane, D. M., & Silber, J. H. (2003). Educational levels of hospital nurses and surgical patient mortality. *JAMA, 290*(12), 1617-1623.

Aiken, L. H., Clarke, S. P., & Sloan, D. M. (2002a). Hospital staffing, organization and quality of care: Cross-national findings. *Nursing Outlook, 50*(5), 187-194.

Aiken, L. H., Clarke, S. P., Sloan, D. M., Sochalski, J., & Silber, J. H. (2002b). Hospital nurse staffing and patient mortality, nurse burnout, and job satisfaction. *JAMA, 288*(16), 1987-1993.

Barton, A. J., Skiba, D. J., & Sorensen, L. (2004). Preparing the next generation of advanced practice nurses. In M. Fieschi, E. Coiera, & Y. Li (Eds.), *Proceedings of the 11th World Congress on Medical Informatics: Building high performance health care organizations.* Amsterdam: IOS Press.

Berlin, L. E., Wilsey, S. J., & Bednash, G. D. (2005). *2004-2005 Enrollment and graduations in baccalaureate and graduate programs in nursing.* Washington, DC: America Association of Colleges of Nursing.

Buerhaus, P. (2002). Shortages of hospital registered nurses: Causes and perspectives on public and private sector actions. *Nursing Outlook, 50*(1), 4-6.

Buerhaus, P., Donelan, K., Ulrich, B. T., Norman, L., & Dittus, R. (2005). Is the shortage of hospital registered nurses getting better or worse? Finding from two recent national surveys. *Nursing Economics, 23*(2), 61-71.

Buerhaus, P., Needleman, J., Mattke, S., & Stewart, M. (2002). Strengthening hospital nursing. *Health Affairs, 21*(5), 123-132.

Buerhaus, P., Staiger, D. O., & Auerbach, D. I. (2000). Implications of an aging registered nurse workforce. *JAMA, 283*(22), 2948-2954.

Circadian Technologies. (2004). Absenteeism and shift work. Retrieved February 25, 2006, from *www.circadian.com/clients/absent.html.*

Duke, E. M. (2005). Remarks to the health professions all-grantee meeting, June 1, 2005. Health Resources and Services Administration, U.S. Department of Health and Human Services. Retrieved February 25, 2006, from *http://newsroom. hrsa.gov/speeches/2005/healthprofessions.htm.*

Gelinas, L., & Bohlen, C. (2002). *Tomorrow's work force: A strategic approach.* Irving, TX: VHA, Inc. Retrieved February 25, 2006, from *https://www.vha.com/portal/server.pt/ gateway/PTARGS_0_38336_0_0_18/Knowledge%20Directory/ VHA.COM/public/research/workforce/research_ tomorrowsworkforce_meth.asp.*

Institute of Medicine (IOM). (2000). *To err is human: Building a safer health system.* Washington, DC: National Academies Press.

Institute of Medicine (IOM). (2001). *Quality chasm: A new health care system for the 21st century.* Washington, DC: National Academies Press.

Institute of Medicine (IOM). (2003). *Health professions education: A bridge to quality.* Washington, DC: National Academies Press.

Institute of Medicine (IOM). (2004a). *Keeping patients safe: Transforming the work environment of nurses.* Washington, DC: National Academies Press.

Kimball, B., & O'Neil, E. (2002). *Health care's human crisis: The American nursing shortage.* Princeton: Robert Wood Johnson Foundation.

McClure, M., & Hinshaw, A. S. (2002). *Magnet hospitals revisited.* Washington, DC: American Academy of Nursing.

National Advisory Council on Nursing Education and Practice (NACNEP). (2003). *Third report to the Secretary and the Congress.* Rockville, MD: U.S. Department of Health and Human Services, Bureau of Health Professions, Division of Nursing. Retrieved February 25, 2006, from *http://bhpr.hrsa.gov/ nursing/nac/nacreport.htm.*

National Center for Health Professions Workforce Analysis. (2002). *Projected supply, demand, and shortages of registered nurses, 2002-2020.* Rockville, MD: U.S. Department of Health and Human Services, Bureau of Health Professions. Retrieved February 25, 2006, from *www.bhpr.hrsa.gov/healthworkforce/ reports/rnproject/default.htm.*

National Coalition on Health Care (NCHC). (2004). *Building a better health care system: Specifications for reform.* Washington, DC: NCHC.

Needleman, J., Buerhaus, P., Mattke, S., & Zelevinsky, K. (2002). Nurse-staffing levels and the quality of care in hospitals. *New England Journal of Medicine, 346*(22), 1715-1733.

O'Neil, E. H. (1998). *Recreating health professional practice for a new century: Fourth report.* San Francisco: Pew Health Professions Commission.

Rogers, A. E., Hwang, W. T., Scott, L. D., Aiken, L. H., & Dinges, D. F. (2004). The working hours of hospital staff nurses and patient safety. *Health Affairs, 23*(4), 202-212.

Rogers, E. M. (2003). *Diffusion of innovations.* New York: Free Press.

Sochalski, J. (2002). Nursing shortage redux: Turning the corner on an enduring problem. *Health Affairs, 21*(5), 157.

Shaver, K. H., & Lacey, L. M. (2003). Job and career satisfaction among staff nurses: Effects of job setting and environment. *Journal of Nursing Administration, 33*(3), 166-172.

Stacy, R. D. (1996). *Complexity and creativity in organizations.* San Francisco: Berrett-Koehler Publishers.

U.S. Department of Health and Human Services (USDHHS). (2005). Summary of nationwide health information network (NHIN) request for information (RFI) responses. Retrieved February 25, 2006, from *www.hhs.gov/healthit/ rfisummaryreport.pdf.*

Upenieks, V. V. (2002). Assessing differences in job satisfaction of nurses in Magnet and non magnet hospitals. *Journal of Nursing Administration, 32*(11), 564-576.

White House. (2004a). Promoting innovativeness and competitiveness. Transforming health care: The president's health information technology plan. Retrieved February 25, 2006, from *www.whitehouse.gov/infocus/technology/economic_ policy200404/chap3.html.*

White House. (2004b). Executive order: Incentives for the use of health information technology and establishing the position of the national health information technology coordinator. Retrieved February 25, 2006, from *www.whitehouse.gov/news/ releases/2004/04/print/20040427-4.html.*

Yin, R. K. (2002). *Case study research.* Thousand Oaks, CA: Sage.

# NURSE STAFFING IMPACT ON ORGANIZATIONAL OUTCOMES

Linda H. Aiken*

Nurse understaffing of hospitals is ranked by the public and by physicians as one of the most serious threats to patient safety (Blendon et al., 2002). Two thirds of hospital bedside nurses concur that there are insufficient numbers of nurses in their hospitals to provide care of high quality, and close to half score in the high-burnout range on standardized tests. Almost one in four says they intend to leave their job in a hospital within a year (Aiken et al., 2001). Federal estimates suggest the shortfall of nurses could approach 800,000 by 2020 (U.S. Department of Health and Human Services [USDHHS], 2002). Until very recently, policymakers and health care leaders have not associated hospital nurse understaffing and burnout with medical errors and adverse patient outcomes, as evidenced by the few references to nursing in the Institute of Medicine's (IOM's) first two major quality reports (IOM, 2000, 2001). The purposes of this chapter are to explicate the link between nursing and quality and to discuss the implications for the nation's quality improvement agenda.

## ROLE OF NURSES IN PROMOTING QUALITY OF CARE

Nursing is the care of the sick (and those who may become sick) and the maintenance of the environment in which care takes place (Diers, 2004). Nurses are responsible for carrying out those aspects of the

---

*Acknowledgement: Supported by a Robert Wood Johnson Foundation Investigator Award in Health Policy Research.
Reprinted with permission from Rutgers University Press. (2005). Improving quality through nursing. In D. Mechanic, L. Rogut, D. Colby, & J. Knickman (Eds.), *Policy challenges in modern health care.* Piscataway, NJ: Rutgers University Press.

medical regimen that are delegated to them by physicians (e.g., medication administration), but they are legally and professionally responsible for their own actions in carrying out delegated tasks. In the case of administering medications, nurses are responsible for ascertaining that the medication dose is correct for the age of the patient and the route of administration before they give the drug. Nurses also have a professional and legal scope of practice that is complementary to that of physicians and includes assessment and interventions within their areas of expertise, such as skin and wound care, pain management and comforting, and teaching patients and their families how to manage their care after hospital discharge, among myriad other responsibilities. Nurses are also responsible for maintaining a safe and patient-centered care environment. Thus, nurses routinely step in when non-nursing support services are not available or fail to be provided adequately in order to maintain a clean environment, ensure that patients receive adequate nourishment, enforce infection-control practices, and prevent hazards such as improper disposal of needles and sharps that could transmit bloodborne pathogens to unsuspecting staff and visitors.

Two of nurses' most important functions associated with patient safety, quality of care, and patient outcomes are surveillance for the early detection of adverse events, complications, and medical errors and mobilization of institutional resources for timely intervention and rescue. The effectiveness of nurse surveillance is potentially influenced by a number of factors, including patient-to-registered-nurse (RN) ratios, education of RNs at the bedside, and numbers of LPNs and aides relative to RNs (often referred to as *skill mix* of nursing personnel). Once a nurse detects potentially hazardous clinical signs, factors in the work environment and institutional culture can promote or impede timely and successful problem resolution. Nurses' relationships with physicians are particularly important in assuring that patients will receive the help they need. Since physicians in the United States typically combine office-based ambulatory medical practice with caring for hospitalized patients, nurses are often physicians' eyes and ears at the hospital bedside. This arrangement works best in organizations that employ well-qualified staff in sufficient numbers, in which nurses and physicians have a high degree of mutual respect and trust in one another, and where top administrators facilitate patient-centered services throughout the institution (Aiken, Clarke, & Sloane, 2002).

## NURSE STAFFING ADEQUACY

The adequacy of nurse staffing in hospitals and other health care settings is a matter of considerable debate, in large part because of the financial implications. RNs constitute the largest group of health professionals in hospitals and account for a significant share of hospitals' operating expenses. Using a conservative total compensation estimate of $60,000 a year for an RN, it would cost a hospital $3 million a year to add 50 nurses. Hospitals have many competing agendas, and, compared to the complexities of gaining savings in efficiency and productivity elsewhere in the institution, it is often easier to titrate the number of nurses employed to the available funding than to staff on the basis of objective case-mix–based standards and raise the necessary financing. At present some 1.2 million nurses are employed in the nation's hospitals.

An underappreciated aspect of the nurse staffing adequacy debate concerns the impact of understaffing on nurse turnover rates, which are estimated to average about 13% nationally, with institution-specific rates over 20% not uncommon. Aiken and associates examined the hypothesis that a minimum level of staffing is required to retain nurses and minimize turnover (Aiken, Clarke, & Sloane, 2002). They documented in a study of the outcomes of nurse staffing that each additional patient added to

the workload of a hospital bedside nurse was associated with a 23% increase in burnout and a 15% increase in job dissatisfaction, both precursors to voluntary job resignation. Forty percent of nurses who were dissatisfied and burnt out intended to leave their jobs, compared to only 10% who were satisfied and not burnt out.

### Assessing Nurse Staffing Adequacy

Nurses and hospital directors vary in their assessments of the severity of the nurse shortage in their institutions. Some 31% of U.S. hospital directors assessed the shortage of nurses in their hospitals as serious, while 66% of hospital staff nurses believed there were too few nurses to provide care of high quality (Aiken et al., 2001; Blendon et al., 2003). Hospital managers evaluate nurse shortages in terms of vacant budgeted positions and the influence of vacancies on costs and revenues, while nurses appear to use a more global measure that takes into account the illness burden and intensity of care required by their patients. Costs are affected by vacancies if hospitals elect to employ nurses on a temporary basis, which generally requires them to pay agencies more than double what they pay their own staff. It is not unusual for hospitals to be spending several million dollars a month to agencies that provide temporary nurse workers. An alternative to maintain safe patient-to-nurse ratios when vacancy rates are high is reducing the number of elective surgeries or closing units, but both of these options result in a loss of revenue. Use of temporary agency nurses also reduces the job satisfaction of full-time nurses because temporary nurses have a more limited scope of responsibility and less familiarity with personnel and procedures and higher compensation. Greater use of temporary personnel has also been associated with more adverse events including a higher rate of needlestick injuries to nurses, exposing them to bloodborne pathogens such as HIV and hepatitis (Aiken, Sloane, & Klocinski, 1997).

Measuring shortages by vacancy rates has led to the widely held belief that nurse shortages are cyclic and self-correcting in response to changing market conditions (Aiken & Mullinix, 1987; Buerhaus et al., 2002). The expectation that nurse shortages will not be of long duration has tempered efforts to address nurses' dissatisfaction or claims that quality of care is being adversely affected by inadequate investment in nursing. However, the factors associated with predictions of increased national need for nurses are not cyclic—population aging, prevalence of chronic illness, increased per capita use of health services, increase in nurse-intensive technologies—leading federal workforce planning bodies to forecast an ever-growing gap between the supply of and demand for nurses (USDHHS, 2002). And more to the point of reconciling the different perceptions of shortage held by nurses and managers is the real increase in case-mix complexity in hospitals and other health care settings that has not been fully recognized in budgeted nurse positions.

Hospitals have experienced substantial real increases in intensity of services and case-mix complexity and shorter average lengths of hospital stay since the introduction of hospital payment based upon a flat rate per patient rather than payment based on length of the stay or an itemized list of procedures. It was common until the 1980s for preoperative patients to be admitted to the hospital several days prior to surgery for tests and evaluation. Nurses used that preoperative time to develop a trusting relationship, to prepare patients and their families for what to expect following surgery, and also to assess the patient's usual physical and mental state in order to be able to evaluate abnormalities and detect possible complications postoperatively. Today nurses see patients for the first time when they are leaving the operating room still groggy from anesthesia. They do not know the extent to which the patient can see, hear, or communicate under normal circumstances or what the patient's normal color, breathing patterns, and blood pressure are. Patients often have more than one surgical site, multiple monitors, sometimes an artificial respirator, and intravenous lines, often with very powerful drugs that can result in death if the rate of infusion is not correct. On average, nurses care for five to six postoperative patients at a time. Every day about a third of the nurses' patients are coming directly from the operating room or have been admitted in an acute medical crisis; a third are in the early stages of recovery or

stabilization with many requirements for nursing time; and a third are being discharged home, often with very complicated home care requirements.

One explanation for nurse understaffing in hospitals is that hospitals have not added sufficient numbers of new budgeted RN positions to offset the substantial increase in case-mix complexity. Between 1981 and 1993 the total percentage change in full-time–equivalent nursing personnel adjusted for patient days and case-mix complexity declined by more than 7% nationally and by over 20% in some states including Massachusetts, New York, and California (Aiken, Sochalski, & Anderson, 1996). Pennsylvania hospitals experienced a 21% increase in patient acuity between 1991 and 1996 and no change in the number of employed licensed nurses (RNs and LPNs). The result was a decrease of 14% in the ratio of licensed nurses to case-mix adjusted patient days of care (Unruh, 2002).

Further evidence that at least part of the difficulty in the nurse workforce is hospital nurse understaffing relative to increases in case-mix complexity and intensity of services can be found in comparing surveys of hospital staff nurses in the United States with those of nurses in Germany, where average length of hospital stay is twice that of U.S. hospitals. For example, the average length of hospital stay for acute myocardial infarction in Germany in 1999 was 12.6 days, compared to 5.6 days in the United States (Commonwealth Fund, 2002). Over 40% of U.S. nurses are dissatisfied with their jobs and score in the high-burnout range on standardized instruments, compared with 17% of dissatisfied and 15% of burnt-out German nurses (Aiken et al., 2001). Over 80% of German nurses report being confident that their patients will be able to manage their own care after discharge, compared with only 34% of American nurses.

Real increases in case-mix complexity and faster admission-discharge cycles have placed a burden on nurses at the bedside that has not been adequately recognized in increased budgeted positions. Consequently, about 85% of nurses work longer on a daily basis than their scheduled hours. Recent research has documented a substantial increase in the rate of errors associated with nurses working more than 12 consecutive hours, and close to half of hospital staff nurses commonly work longer than 12 hours (Rogers, 2004). There are presently no policies governing safe working hours for nurses, as there are for other occupations in which vigilance is a matter of life and death, including physician residents and other occupations such as pilots. Lack of understanding by institutional management and public policymakers of how shortened length of stay and increased case-mix complexity has adversely affected the work of nurses and the safety of patients, and consequent failures to add sufficient numbers of nurse positions to make care of high quality possible, are at the heart of the ongoing nurse shortage and perceptions that hospitals are unsafe.

## Nurse Staffing and Patient Outcomes

Florence Nightingale conducted the first hospital outcome studies and used the results to establish the beginnings of modern nursing (Cohen, 1984). Indeed, hospital outcomes research has long produced findings linking nurse staffing and patient mortality, beginning with the National Halothane Study that documented a twelve-fold difference in surgical mortality nationally. Nurse staffing was found to be among the significant determinants of mortality (Moses & Mosteller, 1968). The availability of Medicare hospital mortality data for U.S. hospitals generated a series of studies on the correlates of variation in mortality (Hartz, Krakauer, & Kuhn, 1989; Shortell & Hughes, 1988; Silber et al., 2000). These studies were primarily designed to study non-nursing correlates of hospital mortality such as for-profit versus nonprofit hospital ownership status. Each study reported in passing that nurse staffing was significantly related to mortality, but not much notice was taken of these collective findings until nurse investigators began designing studies to examine the effects of nurse staffing on patient outcomes.

In 1996 the IOM published the results of its study on the adequacy of hospital nurse staffing, acknowledging the health services research evidence suggesting a link between nurse staffing and patient outcomes but concluding that insufficient evidence existed for recommending safe staffing levels for hospitals (IOM, 1996). The IOM's recommendation

for more research and research funding on the effects of nurse staffing on patient outcomes was followed by the publication of new studies reinforcing the association between nurse staffing and patient outcomes.

Aiken and colleagues, in a study of outcomes following common surgical procedures for over 230,000 patients in 168 hospitals, documented a strong association between staff nurse workloads and surgical mortality and failure to rescue patients who had developed complications (Aiken et al., 2002). Hospital nurse staffing ranged from about 4 to 8 patients per nurse; 50% of hospitals had a patient/nurse ratio of 5:1 or lower. After adjusting for over 130 patient and hospital factors, the results suggested that every additional patient in a nurses' workload increased the odds of patient mortality by 7%. Thus the risk of death and failure to rescue patients with complications was 30% higher in hospitals where nurses' average workload was eight patients compared with hospitals where nurses cared for four patients. The effect was linear, so that reducing nurses' workloads from eight to seven patients had the same 7% decline in risk of mortality that reducing the workload from five patients to four had, with the caveat that there were too few hospitals in the sample to reliably estimate the nurse staffing effect beyond eight patients per nurse.

There is a growing literature of well-designed studies documenting a variety of better patient outcomes associated with more favorable RN staffing (Blegen, Goode, & Reed, 1998; Cho, Ketefian, Barkauskas, et al., 2003; Kovner & Gergen, 1998). For example, Needleman and associates documented a significant relationship between nurse staffing and urinary tract infections, pneumonia, shock, upper gastrointestinal tract hemorrhage, and length of stay in medical patients and failure to rescue in surgical patients (Needleman, Buerhaus, Mattke, et al., 2002). Person and associates showed that the odds of dying from first-time acute myocardial infarction were significantly lower in hospitals with more favorable nurse/patient ratios (Person, Allison, Kiefe, et al., 2004). Better nurse staffing has also been shown to be associated with lower rates of medication errors and reduced needlestick injuries to nurses (Blegen et al., 1998; Clarke, Sloane, & Aiken, 2002).

## Nursing Skill Mix and Patient Outcomes

Nursing skill mix varies substantially, with some hospitals employing predominantly RNs and others a mix of RNs, licensed practical nurses (LPNs), and aides. The organization of nurses' work and the deployment of non-RNs have changed over time. In the 1960s the most common form of division of labor within hospital nursing was a team structure with RNs providing assessments, medications, and treatments to all patients and directing LPNs and aides in the performance of personal hygiene, ambulation, and other routine patient care activities. As the number of RNs employed by hospitals increased, RNs saw the value of maintaining a closer relationship with patients than team nursing allowed and the opportunity to shed the unwanted responsibility for supervising LPNs and aides. Nurses advocated returning the care of all patients to RNs under a scheme referred to as *primary nursing*. The financial incentives were right under the new Medicare prospective payment system, and hospital managers supported the transition from team to primary nursing. The result was a substantial decline in the employment of LPNs in hospitals nationally and a skill mix in which RNs represented the majority of nursing personnel. During the hospital restructuring movement to contain costs in the 1990s, many hospitals once again substituted LPNs and aides for RNs (Brannon, 1996; Norrish & Rundall, 2001). Research findings consistently support the conclusion that higher proportions of RNs are associated with better patient outcomes. Aiken and associates found no relationship between patient-to-LPN ratios or patient-to-aide ratios but a substantial effect of patient/RN ratios on surgical mortality and failure to rescue (Aiken et al., 2002). Jarman and associates found the higher the proportion of the least trained auxiliary nursing personnel in English hospitals, the higher the mortality (Jarman, Gault, Alves, et al., 1999). Person and colleagues found that patients with acute myocardial infarction were significantly more likely to die in hospitals with more LPNs after controlling for RN staffing (Person et al., 2004). Person's finding is difficult to explain and the authors speculate that the employment of large numbers of LPNs might be associated with an unmeasured characteristic of hospitals more proximally related to mortality.

## Nurses' Education

RNs in the United States receive their basic education in one of three types of programs, all of which qualify graduates to take the RN licensing examination: 3-year hospital-sponsored diploma programs, 2-year associate degree programs in community colleges, and 4-year baccalaureate nursing programs in colleges and universities. Freidson described nursing as an incompletely closed profession because of its inability to establish a minimum education requirement for entry (Freidson, 1970). In 2001, approximately 3% of new nurses graduated from hospital diploma programs, which had educated almost all nurses in the 1960s; associate degree programs replaced diploma programs, accounting for over 60% of new entrants to nursing; and about 36% of new nurses were baccalaureate graduates (National Council of State Boards of Nursing, 2001). Close to 45% of nurses nationally had a baccalaureate or higher degree in 2000, and almost one in four obtained their degree following basic education in a diploma or associate degree program (Spratley, Johnson, Sochalski, et al., 2001). Many other countries have eliminated multiple educational pathways into nursing by establishing the baccalaureate as the entry level degree for new nurses; these countries include Canada, Australia, New Zealand, Ireland, Iceland, and Cuba, among others. The United Kingdom has moved nursing education within higher education but has not yet completed the full transition to a baccalaureate degree.

There is surprisingly little research on variation in nurses' education across institutions and health care settings or on the impact of nurses' educational levels on clinical practice effectiveness and patient outcomes. A few studies have suggested that baccalaureate-prepared nurses are more likely to demonstrate professional behaviors important to patient safety such as problem solving, performance of complex functions, and effective interdisciplinary communication (Blegen, Vaughn, & Goode, 2001; Hickam, Severance, Feldstein, et al., 2003). Nurse executives in teaching hospitals have a preference for baccalaureate-prepared nurses, and aim to have at least 70% of their staff nurses trained at the baccalaureate level; community-hospital nurse executives reportedly want 50% of nurses to have BSNs (Goode, Pinkerton, McCausland, et al., 2001). There are insufficient numbers of nurses to meet these targets, with only about 43% of hospital staff nurses holding a baccalaureate degree.

Aiken and colleagues observed that the proportion of hospital staff nurses holding a baccalaureate degree ranged from none to 77% across Pennsylvania hospitals and designed a study to find out if variation of that magnitude was associated with differences in patient outcomes (Aiken, Clarke, Cheung, et al., 2003). The answer was yes. They found that hospitals with a larger proportion of baccalaureate-prepared nurses had significantly lower surgical mortality after adjusting for patient characteristics and hospital structural characteristics (size, teaching status, technology) as well as for patient-to-nurse staffing ratios, nurse experience, and whether the patient's surgeon was board certified. Every 10% increase in the proportion of nurses holding a baccalaureate degree was associated with a 5% decrease in both the likelihood of patients' dying within 30 days of admission and the odds of failure to rescue patients with complications. Moreover, effects of nurse staffing and education were found to be additive. The best outcomes were found in hospitals in which nurses took care of four or fewer patients each and 60% of staff nurses were educated at the baccalaureate level or higher, and the worst outcomes were in hospitals in which nurses cared for eight or more patients each and only 20% of nurses had baccalaureate education. The effect on mortality of a 20% increase in the percentage of baccalaureate-prepared nurses within a hospital was estimated to be roughly equivalent to the effect of adding enough additional nurses to reduce the mean nurse workload by two patients. Thus, hospitals might be able to stem the increasing need to have more nurses per 100 inpatient days by moving to a more highly educated RN workforce.

Nursing as a profession faces special challenges in raising educational requirements commensurate with trends in other health professions because of the dependency of the modern hospital on employing large numbers of nurses. Consequently the interests of hospital employers seem best served by nurses being trained quickly and inexpensively with interchangeable skills and modest career expectations. However, this scenario increasingly clashes with the aspirations of many of those attracted to nursing with hopes of upward mobility and opportunities for personally gratifying careers and reasonably remunerated work. The number of applicants to nursing schools who already have college degrees in other fields is growing rapidly, and universities have responded with programs as short as a year for college graduates to earn a BSN.

## NURSE PRACTICE ENVIRONMENTS

Flood and Scott describe hospitals as having dual bureaucratic and professional structures that represent opposing approaches to managing the performance of complex tasks (Flood & Scott, 1987). Conventional bureaucratic solutions subdivide work among many participants and control their activities through externally imposed rules and hierarchies. Organizations with professional structures support the efforts of self-regulating individuals who exercise considerable discretion in carrying out their work (Freidson, 1970). Hospital nurses are agents of a bureaucracy but hold professional values and seek peer relationships with other professionals and professional modes of organizing their work. Etzioni described professional-bureaucratic conflict as a major concern for complex health care organizations like hospitals, suggesting "the authority of knowledge and the authority of administrative hierarchy are basically incompatible" (Etzioni, 1969, p. viii). Indeed, research on hospital nurse burnout is consistent with this view, showing that organizational conflict far outweighs the psychologic and physical stress associated with caring for ill and dying patients (Aiken & Sloane, 1997).

### Impact of Nurse Work Environments on Outcomes

There are few examples of contemporary health outcomes research that integrate organizational perspectives from sociologic analyses of hospitals with advances in quantitative research methods that have made it possible to study the outcomes of thousands of patients in hundreds of hospitals.

Nursing outcomes research in particular has focused primarily on the effects of staffing on patient outcomes. Relatively little attention has been given to the impact on patient outcomes of the organizational context and culture in settings in which care takes place.

One of the first studies in nursing to integrate a sociologic perspective with a health services research focus on correlates of hospital mortality examined the outcomes of Magnet hospitals (Aiken, Smith, & Lake, 1994). The so-called "Magnet hospitals" were originally designated in the early 1980s on the basis of their success in attracting and retaining nurses when other hospitals in their local labor markets were experiencing nurse shortages (McClure & Hinshaw, 2002). Compared to other institutions, Magnet hospitals had higher nurse satisfaction, and their nurses reported more autonomy, greater control over resources required for high-quality care, and better relations with physicians than other hospitals. As a first step in exploring the effects of the constellation of common organizational features that characterized Magnet hospitals, Aiken and colleagues matched the 39 original Magnet hospitals with 195 control hospitals selected from all non-Magnet U.S. hospitals using a multivariate matched sampling procedure, propensity scoring, that controlled for 12 hospital characteristics including size, teaching status, technology, and proportion of board-certified physicians. Magnet hospitals were found to have a 4.5% lower Medicare mortality rate than matched hospitals (Aiken et al., 1994). Nurse staffing alone did not explain the lower mortality in Magnet hospitals, suggesting the possibility that the common organizational features of Magnet hospitals that devolved greater autonomy and control to nurses and established cultures promoting good relations between nurses and physicians were associated with better patient outcomes.

A subsequent program of research undertaken by Aiken and colleagues explored in a series of studies the relationship between nurses' practice environments and patient and nurse outcomes. They made use of the natural experiment in hospital organization associated with the AIDS epidemic by studying dedicated AIDS units in urban hospitals that were designed largely by nurses to represent what nurses viewed as ideal settings for nursing practice and good patient care. Dedicated AIDS units were found by Aiken and colleagues to be similar to Magnet hospitals in that nurses had greater autonomy and control over resources at the bedside and better relations with physicians than conventional medical units on which AIDS care also took place. A multiple-site study was designed, including 40 units in 20 hospitals; 10 hospitals with dedicated AIDS units were matched with comparable hospitals without dedicated AIDS units. Two Magnet hospitals without AIDS units were included for comparison purposes. Risk-adjusted 30-day from admission AIDS mortality was found to be substantially lower and patient satisfaction was significantly higher in dedicated AIDS units and in Magnet hospitals than in conventionally organized general medical units (Aiken et al., 1999). More favorable nurse staffing and improved nurse practice environments in Magnet hospitals and dedicated AIDS units were shown to be among the important explanations for better patient and nurse outcomes in these settings.

Aiken and colleagues' research has subsequently moved to the study of nurse practice environments in large representative groups of hospitals in the United States and abroad to determine the extent to which features of the nurse work environment are associated with nurse retention and patient outcomes. The international hospital outcomes study, which includes over 700 hospitals in five countries, concluded that nurses in hospitals in the United States, Canada, the United Kingdom, Germany, and New Zealand face common challenges with regard to nurse understaffing, burnout, and high levels of job dissatisfaction. Similarly, nurses in all of these countries identify deficiencies in quality of care that appear to be associated with inadequate staffing and poor nurse work environments (Aiken et al., 2001, 2002). Germany is the only country with substantially lower nurse burnout, which may be explained by its significantly longer average length of stay. Remarkably, given the many differences in culture and nurses' education across these five countries, organizational features similar to the U.S. Magnet hospitals are found in a proportion of hospitals in every country. Nurse and patient outcomes are better in those hospitals with

Magnet-like features that devolve greater autonomy and control to nurses and provide a more supportive environment for professional nurse practice. For example, the frequency of patient falls with injuries, medication errors, and hospital-acquired infections are lower in hospitals across the five countries in which nurse staffing is more favorable, the administration is reported to support nurses to provide care of high quality, career development opportunities exist for nurses, and physicians and nurses have good relations.

## NURSING AND QUALITY IMPROVEMENT

There is one area of potential discordance between the accumulating evidence base from nursing outcomes research documenting better outcomes in institutions that devolve more authority to nurses and the ongoing efforts to create safer systems of care to protect patients from medical errors. As noted in this chapter, hospitals with nurse practice environments that foster nurse autonomy and promote greater control of resources by nurses at the bedside have better patient outcomes. Much of the evolving thinking about how to reduce medical errors is leading toward the development of systems that standardize medical decision-making and minimize professional discretion. Are the aims of patient safety systems in conflict with the evidence suggesting that organizations that devolve more authority and autonomy to nurses have better outcomes in conflict? Not necessarily.

Nurses have long been responsible for many of the safeguards in hospital care, for example, counting sponges and instruments in the operating room to prevent foreign objects from being left inside patients, storing dangerous drugs in locked cabinets, having two nurses check the compatibility of blood before transfusion, and notifying physicians when a medication order seems out of the ordinary before administration. Nurses have been the de facto safety system in hospitals for over a hundred years. Indeed, recent studies confirm that of the medication errors that are detected at all in hospitals, most are detected by nurses. However, nurses understand the vulnerabilities of the people-dependent safety provisions on which hospitals rely. Indeed, a common fear of nurses contributing to their high

levels of burnout is that with their increasingly heavy workloads they will fail to detect an error committed by someone else or commit an error themselves that will go unrecognized and hurt a patient. Hence, nurses' work and mental health would be more favorably affected than any other hospital workers by more effective safety systems that minimize the opportunity for human error.

However, minimizing errors is only one of the strategies for improving quality of care in hospitals. Good nurse-patient relationships are at the heart of safe and effective hospital care. Expert clinical judgment is still required in a myriad of situations, including recognizing early signs that a patient may not be doing well and mobilizing a timely institutional response, or determining when and under what circumstances a patient can be safely discharged. Moreover, in addition to caring for patients, nurses are responsible for maintenance of the environment in which care takes place which requires the exercise of authority as well as intraorganizational status. Nurses must have some control over the resources required for meeting patients' needs, such as safe nurse staffing levels, timely responses from physicians, accessible supplies and equipment, and support departments like housekeeping, pharmacy, central supply, and the blood bank that run efficiently and effectively around the clock.

The international hospital outcomes study was challenged to show that nurse autonomy was consistent with, rather than antithetical to, effective interdisciplinary team functioning. Researchers documented that hospitals in which nurses had greater autonomy and more control over resources were more, not less, likely to have well developed and effective interdisciplinary teams (Rafferty, Ball, & Aiken, 2001). Aiken and associates' research suggests that hospitals that promote the full exercise of the professional nurse role and devolve authority to nurses in their areas of expertise are the same institutions that create effective interdisciplinary care cultures, patient-centered environments, and better patient outcomes. Such institutions will more than likely also be at the forefront of establishing new and better systems to reduce human error because of their professional culture that values clinical excellence informed by evidence-based practice.

New systems that reduce human error and an organizational practice context that enables the best performance of each health professional are both essential for ensuring safe and effective care to hospitalized patients. The evolution of the IOM's reports on quality, which began with little attention to nursing and have since moved to focus very explicitly on the need to transform the nurse work environment to keep patients safe, suggests a merging of two previously separate areas of health care concern—nurse shortages and patient safety—into a more unified approach to quality that is likely to yield important new initiatives to ameliorate both problems.

## REFERENCES

Aiken, L. H., Clarke, S. P., Cheung, R. B., et al. (2003). Education levels of hospital nurses and patient mortality. *Journal of the American Medical Association, 290,* 1617-1623.

Aiken, L. H., Clarke, S. P., & Sloane, D. M. (2002). Hospital staffing, organizational support, and quality of care: Cross-national findings. *International Journal for Quality in Health Care, 14,* 5-13.

Aiken, L. H., Clarke, S. P., Sloane, D. M., et al. (2002). Hospital nurse staffing and patient mortality, nurse burnout, and job dissatisfaction. *Journal of the American Medical Association, 288,* 1987-1993.

Aiken, L. H., Clarke, S. P., Sloane, D. M., et al. (2001). Nurses' reports of hospital quality of care and working conditions in five countries. *Health Affairs, 20,* 43-53.

Aiken, L. H., & Mullinix, C. F. (1987). The nurse shortage: Myth or reality? *New England Journal of Medicine, 317,* 641-646.

Aiken, L. H., & Sloane, D. M. (1997). Effects on organizational innovation in AIDS care on burnout among hospital nurses. *Work and Occupations, 24,* 455-479.

Aiken, L. H., Sloane, D. M., & Klocinski, J. (1997). Hospital nurses' risk of occupational exposure to blood: Prospective, retrospective, and institutional reports. *American Journal of Public Health, 87,* 103-107.

Aiken, L. H., Sloane, D. M., Lake E. T., et al. (1999). Organization and outcomes of inpatient AIDS care. *Medical Care, 37,* 760-772.

Aiken, L. H., Smith, H. L., & Lake, E. T. (1994). Lower Medicare mortality among a set of hospitals known for good nursing care. *Medical Care, 32,* 771-787.

Aiken, L., Sochalski, J., & Anderson, G. (1996). Downsizing the hospital workforce. *Health Affairs, 15,* 88-92.

Blegen, M. A., Goode C. J., & Reed, L. (1998). Nurse staffing and patient outcomes. *Nursing Research, 47,* 43-50.

Blegen, M. A., Vaughn, T., & Goode, C. J. (2001). Nurse experience and education: Effect on quality of care. *Journal of Nursing Administration, 31,* 33-39.

Blendon, R. J., et al. (2003, October 23). Results of five country survey of hospital directors. Paper presented at the Commonwealth Foundation International Symposium, Washington, DC.

Blendon, R. J., DesRoches, C. M., Brodie, M., et al. (2002). Views of practicing physicians and the public on medical errors. *New England Journal of Medicine, 347,* 1933-1940.

Brannon, R. L. (1996). Restructuring hospital nursing: Reversing the trend toward a professional work force. *International Journal of Health Services, 26,* 643-654.

Buerhaus, P. I., Needleman, J., Mattke, S., et al. (2002). Strengthening hospital nursing. *Health Affairs, 21,* 123-132.

Cho, S. H., Ketefian, S., Barkauskas, V. H., et al. (2003). The effects of nurse staffing on adverse events, morbidity, mortality, and medical costs. *Nursing Research, 52,* 71-79.

Clarke, S. P., Sloane, D. M., & Aiken, L. H. (2002). Effects of hospital staffing and organizational climate on needlestick injuries to nurses. *American Journal of Public Health, 92,* 1115-1119.

Cohen, I. B. (1984). Florence Nightingale. *Scientific American, 250,* 128-132.

Commonwealth Fund. (2002). *Multinational comparisons of health systems data, 2002.* New York: Commonwealth Fund.

Diers, D. (2004). Speaking of nursing...Narratives of practice, research, policy and the profession. Sudbury, MA: Jones and Bartlett.

Etzioni, A. (1969). *The semi-professionals and their organizations: Teachers, nurses, and social workers.* New York: Free Press.

Flood, A. B., & Scott, W. R. (Eds.) (1987). *Hospital structure and performance. Johns Hopkins series in contemporary medicine and public health.* Baltimore: Johns Hopkins University Press.

Freidson, E. (1970). Professional dominance: The social structure of medical care. New York: Atherton.

Goode, C. J., Pinkerton, S., McCausland, M. P., et al. (2001). Documenting chief nursing officers' preference for BSN-prepared nurses. *Journal of Nursing Administration, 31,* 55-59.

Hartz, A. J., Krakauer, H., & Kuhn, E. M. (1989). Hospital characteristics and mortality rates. *New England Journal of Medicine, 321,* 1720.

Hickam D. H., Severance, S., Feldstein, A., et al. (2003). *The effect of health care working conditions on patient safety.* Rockville, MD: Agency for Healthcare Research and Quality.

Institute of Medicine (IOM). (1996). *Nursing staff in hospitals and nursing homes: Is it adequate?* Washington, DC: National Academies Press.

Institute of Medicine (IOM). (2000). *To err is human: Building a safer health system.* Washington, DC: National Academies Press.

Institute of Medicine (IOM). (2001). *Crossing the quality chasm.* Washington, DC: National Academies Press.

Institute of Medicine (IOM). (2004). *Keeping patients safe: Transforming the work environment of nurses.* Washington, DC: National Academies Press.

Jarman, B., Gault, S., Alves, B., et al. (1999). Explaining differences in English hospital death rates using routinely collected data. *British Medical Journal, 318,* 1515-1520.

Kovner, C., & Gergen, P. J. (1998). Nurse staffing levels and adverse events following surgery in U.S. hospitals. *Image: Journal of Nursing Scholarship, 30,* 315-321.

McClure, M. L., & Hinshaw, A. S. (Eds.) (2002). *Magnet hospitals revisited: Attraction and retention of professional nurses.* Washington, DC: American Nurses Publishing.

Moses, L. E., & Mosteller, F. (1968). Institutional differences in postoperative death rates. *Journal of the American Medical Association, 203,* 492.

National Council of State Boards of Nursing. (2001). Annual report 2001. Retrieved May 2, 2003, from *www.ncsbn.org/public/about/res/AnnRpt_FY01.pdf.*

Needleman, J., Buerhaus, P., Mattke, S., et al. (2002). Nurse-staffing levels and the quality of care in hospitals. *New England Journal of Medicine, 346,* 1715-1722.

Norrish, B. R., & Rundall, T. G. (2001). Hospital restructuring and the work of registered nurses. *Milbank Quarterly, 79,* 55-79.

Person, S. D., Allison, J. J., Kiefe, C. I., et al. (2004). Nurse staffing and mortality for Medicare patients with acute myocardial infarction. *Medical Care, 42,* 4-12.

Rafferty, A. M., Ball, J., & Aiken, L. H. (2001). Are teamwork and professional autonomy compatible, and do they result in improved hospital care? *Quality in Health Care, 10*(Supp II), ii32-ii37.

Rogers, A. (2004). Work hour regulation in safety-sensitive industries. In A. Page (Ed.), *Keeping patients safe: Transforming the work environment of nurses,* Washington, DC: National Academies Press, 314-358.

Shortell, S. M., & Hughes, E. F. X. (1988). The effects of regulation, competition, and ownership on mortality rates among hospital inpatients. *New England Journal of Medicine, 318,* 1100.

Silber, J. H., Kennedy, S. K., Even-Shoshan, O., et al. (2000). Anesthesiologist direction and patient outcomes. *Anesthesiology, 93,* 152-163.

Spratley, E., Johnson A., Sochalski J., et al. (2001). *The registered nurse population, March 2000. Findings from the National Sample Survey of Registered Nurses.* Rockville, MD: U.S. Department of Health and Human Services.

Unruh, L. (2002). Nursing staff reductions in Pennsylvania hospitals: Exploring the discrepancy between perceptions and data. *Medical Care Research and Review, 59,* 197-214.

U.S. Department of Health and Human Services (USDHHS). (2002). *Projected supply, demand, and shortages of registered nurses: 2000-2020.* Rockville, MD: National Center for Health Workforce Analysis: Health Resources and Services Administration.

Vahey, D. C., Aiken, L. H., Sloane, D. M., et al. (2004). Nurse burnout and patient satisfaction. *Medical Care, 42,* II57-II66.

# **POLICY**SPOTLIGHT

## DIVERSITY IN NURSING: A LONG ROAD AHEAD

C. Alicia Georges

*"Without a struggle, there can be no progress."*
FREDERICK DOUGLASS

The demographics of the United States of America have changed in the last decade. Ethnic and racial minority groups are now the majority population in some states. These groups for the most part have been underrepresented in education, health, government, and the business world. Policies have been developed by government and other organizations to facilitate the movement of these ethnic and racial minority groups into the workforce. Among these policies have been those that have been developed to improve the diversity of the nursing workforce. This chapter examines some of these policies and their impact on improving diversity in the nursing workforce in the United States. The 2003 Institute of Medicine (IOM) report "Unequal Treatment Confronting Racial and Ethnic Disparities in Health Care" notes that the paucity of qualified racial and ethnic minority health professionals may be a contributing factor in the continuing disparities in health (Byrd & Clayton, 2003).

### HOW DIVERSE IS THE U.S. NURSING WORKFORCE?

The U.S. Office of Management and Budget (2006) defines five racial groups and one ethnicity classification. These designations are not based on biologic or anthropologic concepts. They usually refer to a person's place of origin, not solely their biologic characteristics.

- *American Indian or Alaska Native*—A person having origins in any of the original peoples of North America and who maintains tribal affiliation or community attachment.
- *Asian or Pacific Islander*—A person having origins in any of the original peoples of the Far East, Southeast Asia, or the Indian subcontinent including Cambodia, China, Japan, Korea, Malaysia, Pakistan, the Philippine Islands, Thailand, and Vietnam, or a person having origins in any of the original peoples of Hawaii, Guam, Samoa, or other Pacific Islands.
- *Black or African American*—A person having origins in any of the black racial groups of Africa.
- *Hispanic or Latino*—This is a designation of ethnicity not race. A person of Cuban, Mexican, Puerto Rican, Cuban, South or Central American, or other Spanish culture or origin, regardless of race.
- *Native Hawaiian or Other Pacific Islander*— A person having origins in any of the original peoples of Hawaii, Guam, Samoa, or other Pacific Islands.
- *White*—A person having origins in any of the original peoples of Europe, the Middle East, or North Africa.

The use of such defined racial groups can diminish the confusion and debate about what constitutes minority populations.

As of July of 2004, there were approximately 290 million Americans. Hispanics of any race now average about 13.7% of the population; African Americans, about 12.2%; Asians, 4.1%; American Indian or Native Alaskan, 0.8%; Native Hawaiian and other Pacific Islander, 0.1%; females, 51.1%; and males, 48.9%. States such as Texas, California, New Mexico, and the District of Columbia are now referred to as *majority minority states*, in which ethnic and racial minority groups are now the majority population. Maryland, Georgia, New York, and Arizona now have minority populations that are about 40% of the states' population (U.S. Bureau of the Census, 2005).

Figures 18-2 and 18-3 show data from the 2000 Registered Nurse Population Sample Survey (Spratley, Johnson, Sochalski, Marshall, & Spencer, 2002) and the 2004 National Sample Survey of Registered Nurses (Division of Nursing, U.S. Bureau of Health Professions, 2005) showing trends in the diversity of nurses in the United States. Although racial and ethnic minorities constituted almost a third of the U.S. population in the 2000 census and in the 2005 updated data, the data on the 2000 and 2004 registered nurse population in the United States indicate that the racial, ethnic and gender disparities continue. What has contributed to this ongoing disparity within nursing?

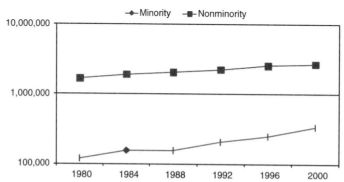

**Figure 18-2**  Trend in the number of racial or ethnic minority and nonminority registered nurses, 1980-2000. (From Bureau of Health Professions. [2002]. The registered nurse population: Findings from The National Sample Survey Of Registered Nurses. Retrieved March 25, 2006, from *http://bhpr.hrsa.gov/healthworkforce/reports/rnsurvey/rnss1.htm#Chap2*.)

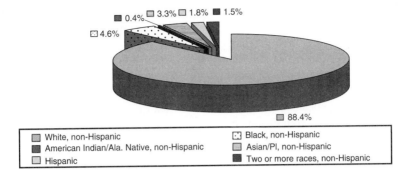

■ 0.4%  □ 3.3%  □ 1.8%  ■ 1.5%

⊡ 4.6%

□ 88.4%

| □ White, non-Hispanic | ⊡ Black, non-Hispanic |
|---|---|
| ■ American Indian/Ala. Native, non-Hispanic | ▤ Asian/PI, non-Hispanic |
| □ Hispanic | ■ Two or more races, non-Hispanic |

### U.S Population

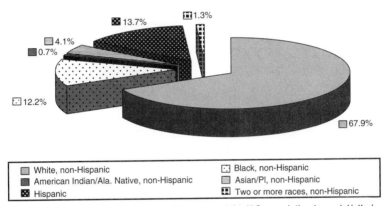

▩ 13.7%  ⊞ 1.3%

▤ 4.1%

■ 0.7%

⊡ 12.2%

□ 67.9%

| □ White, non-Hispanic | ⊡ Black, non-Hispanic |
|---|---|
| ■ American Indian/Ala. Native, non-Hispanic | ▤ Asian/PI, non-Hispanic |
| ▩ Hispanic | ⊞ Two or more races, non-Hispanic |

**Figure 18-3**  Distribution of registered nurses and the U.S. population by racial/ethnic background in 2004. (From Bureau of Health Professions. [2005]. Preliminary findings: 2004 National Sample Survey of Registered Nurses. Retrieved March 25, 2006, from *http://bhpr.hrsa.gov/healthworkforce/reports/rnpopulation/preliminaryfindings. htm#racial.*)

## SEXISM AND RACISM

Nursing has always been viewed as a profession in which women who wanted to nurture and care for others could satisfy this wish. It has not been seen as a profession for men for a number of reasons, including the fact that nurses are a female-dominated group, salaries were low, and public image was poor. As some of these conditions—particularly low salaries—changed, men have sought out nursing as a profession and a career (American Assembly for Men in Nursing, 2004).

However, numerous studies validate that sexism and racism continue to exist in the United States. Holt (2000), in his analysis of the role of race,

reminds us that race is a construct that first became useful in the sixteenth century as Europe expanded into the global market. Race has been used as a political designation, as we saw with apartheid in South Africa. He suggests that biologic and cultural definitions of race that we have used for the past two centuries should be discontinued. The use of these definitions, he purports, has added to some of the racial and discriminatory practices and problems that now exist. People sharing certain physical characteristics are treated differently based on stereotypic thinking, discriminatory institutions, social structures, and social myths. This is coupled with the nullification of human rights, equal footing, and fundamental freedoms in the political, economic, social, cultural, and public arenas (Byrd & Clayton, 2003; International Convention on the Elimination of All Forms of Racial Discrimination [ICERD], 2005). Sexism has the same outcomes. In sexism the discriminatory behaviors occur because of one's gender.

The groups affected by these belief systems have remained marginalized in society and in the nursing workforce. These two factors—racism and sexism— have contributed to the insufficient recruitment, admissions, retention, and graduation of persons from racial and ethnic minority groups in this country and the male population.

## DIVERSITY IN NURSING EDUCATION

In 1878, Mary Eliza Mahoney was the first African American to be admitted to a school of nursing in the United States. She graduated in 1879 and became the first African-American registered nurse at 34 years of age. She had worked in a variety of positions in hospitals in New England before being admitted to the New England Hospital for Women and Children. It was segregation policies that excluded Mary Eliza Mahoney and other African Americans from nursing programs and professional nursing organizations for many decades. These policies existed well into the 1960s.

Historically, Black Hospitals Schools of Nursing and Historically Black Colleges and Universities in the United States were founded because of these exclusionary policies. These schools and hospitals were concentrated mostly in the southeastern part of the United States and were responsible for the education of a large number of African-American nurse graduates from baccalaureate and diploma programs (Carnegie, 1995). Today, the Historically Black Colleges and Universities continue to produce a large number of the baccalaureate-prepared, African-American nurses. In the 2004-2005 academic year, Hampton University School of Nursing had 600 students, including 30 doctoral students, and a 100% pass rate on the NCLEX-RN (Hendricks, 2005). The same pattern has existed for Southern University in Baton Rogue, which also has a doctoral program and a high pass rate on the NCLEX-RN examination (Rami, 2003). These two Historically Black Universities Schools of Nursing have produced more doctoral-prepared nurses in a few short years than some universities with long-standing doctoral programs in cities with high racial minority nurse populations.

There has been an increase in the number of persons from racial and ethnic minority groups in baccalaureate schools of nursing throughout the United States. As of 2003, in 552 baccalaureate programs reporting to the American Association of Colleges of Nursing (AACN), the data indicate that of the students in baccalaureate nursing programs, 12.4% were African American; 5.5% were Asian, Hawaiian, or Pacific Islander; 5.5% were Hispanic or Latino; and 0.7% were American Indian or Alaskan Native. The majority of students, 76%, were white. The male enrollment remained small at about 4.5% (AACN, 2004).

The schools in which minority students are enrolled should identify what recruitment strategies may have contributed to the increase in enrollment. Graduation rates and acquisition of licensure should be evaluated. Community colleges remain a frequent choice for students from African-American and Hispanic or Latino communities. These students may be advised by their counselors or may seek this form of preparation because of the cost, length of time, and ability to earn a salary sooner.

## DIVERSITY IN THE NURSING WORKFORCE

The nursing shortages experienced in the United States and the subsequent recruitment of internationally educated nurses have contributed to an increased number of nurses from countries such as the Philippines, India, and Nigeria (Commission on Graduates of Foreign Nursing Schools [CGFNS], 2003; Organization for Economic Cooperation and Development [OECD], 2002). Although there has been an increase in the number of racial and ethnic minority nurses in the workforce since 1980, the actual impact has not been felt since the overall registered nurse workforce also increased.

Understanding racism and its historical impact is important in dissecting the variables that hinder the inclusion of racial and ethnic minorities in the registered nurse workforce. Patterns, ideologies, or infrastructures that exist in institutions and policies and practices that are inflexible are factors contributing to the historic exclusion of racial and ethnic minorities to schools of nursing in the United States. The use of the SAT or ACT by some colleges and universities as an entry into undergraduate programs in nursing has been known to exclude persons from certain racial and ethnic groups. Data support that the discrepancy that might exist in disparate scores, especially between those of African Americans and whites, is related to the systems in which the students were educated (Sullivan Commission, 2004).

Among its many responsibilities, the Division of Nursing at the United States Department of Health and Human Services is charged with increasing diversity in the nursing workforce. In the last decade the Division of Nursing has reported to the Congress about the progress in achieving the goal of increasing diversity in the nursing workforce. This responsibility is not new. Public law (PL) 9-75, the Allied Health Professions Training Act of 1966, included an authorization for Nursing Educational Opportunity grants (National Advisory Council on Nursing Education, 2000). The language of this Act did not refer to racial or ethnic groups but rather to financially needy students. There have been a number of iterations of this legislation in the last 35 years, including change of language in Title VIII reauthorization, but stagnation remains in changing the diversity in the registered nurse workforce (Sullivan Commission, 2004).

Government has not been the only stakeholder in increasing the diversity in the nursing workforce. Professional nursing organizations have developed programs to increase the number of nurses from ethnic and racial backgrounds in basic nursing programs, graduate programs including doctoral programs, and research fellowships. The Breakthrough to Nursing of the National Student Nurses Association (NSNA), the Ethnic Minority Fellowship Program of the American Nurses Association (ANA), and most recently the National Coalition of Ethnic Minority Nursing Associations offer or have offered programs to recruit, retain, and graduate persons from racial and ethnic minority groups interested in nursing as a career. The Breakthrough to Nursing, established in 1965 by the NSNA, has worked to consistently increase the number of men

and minorities in the nursing profession (NSNA, 2005). Funding for minority students in doctoral programs is the objective of the ANA Ethnic Minority Fellowship program. It has increased the number of doctoral-prepared nurses from racial and ethnic minority groups. The program started in 1974, and approximately 200 persons have participated. Although this program may not increase the number of nurses from racial and ethnic minority groups in prelicensure programs, it has increased the number of persons prepared to be researchers and faculty. The programs of the NSNA and ANA have all been supported through grants from government or corporations. They are part of their organizations' programs of service, but some have been dependent on grant funding. The National Association of Ethnic Minority Nurses Associations (NCEMNA) provides scholarships for baccalaureate, masters, and doctoral students through the Aetna health insurance company. In 2004, NCEMNA received over a million dollars from the National Institutes of Health to increase the number of nurses from ethnic and racial minority groups interested in enhancing their research skills and developing a research agenda.

The designation of institutions as Historically Black Colleges and Universities and Hispanic Serving Institutions is contained in the Higher Education Act of 1965 and its subsequent amendments. To be designated as a Historically Black College or University, a college or university must have been founded before 1964 for the purpose of educating Black Americans. The college or university must be accredited by a nationally recognized body. Hispanic Serving Institutions must have at least 25% of the student body defined as Hispanic, and of these at least 50% must be considered low income (U.S. Department of Education, 2005). This designation allows for preferences in some funding sources from the federal government. Also, for the Historically Black Colleges and Universities, Hispanic Serving Institutions, and programs that serve American Indians and native Alaskans, there is an additional designation as Centers of Excellence. This designation allows for specific types of funding from the federal government for increasing minorities in the health professions.

Hispanic nursing leaders have been successful in having nursing included in the health professions designation. Only Native American Centers of Excellence included schools of nursing in the original designation. This designation allows for monies received from the federal government through its grant program for Centers of Excellence to be used for persons interested in nursing—not just medicine, dentistry, pharmacy, and graduate programs in behavioral or mental health. Nursing leaders in the Historically Black Colleges and Universities that have Centers of Excellence need to advocate for the inclusion of nursing, as has occurred for these Centers in Hispanic Serving Institutions. This may allow them to attain some equal standing with their colleagues in medicine, dentistry, and pharmacy for funding for students interested in nursing as a career.

## SUGGESTED POLICIES TO ASSURE A DIVERSE NURSING WORKFORCE FOR THE FUTURE

There have been many commissions and reports that have produced an abundance of recommendations to ameliorate the problem of lack of diversity in the nursing workforce. What has been missing in this recommendation is the long-term commitment to those programs that have demonstrated that they recruit, admit, retain, and graduate persons from ethnic and racial minority groups. Also, the education of nurses has not been a priority for elected and appointed officials in racial and ethnic minority communities.

What is needed? The most recent report that analyzed the issues surrounding minority participation was "Missing Persons: Minorities in the Health Professions" by the Sullivan Commission on Diversity in the Health Care Workforce. The Sullivan Commission, headed by Louis Sullivan, M.D., former Health and Human Services Secretary, was created in 2003 through a grant from the W.K. Kellogg Foundation to Duke University School of Medicine. The Commission put forth a number of recommendations that may also be useful for improving the diversity of the registered nurse workforce. Three overlying principles guided the Sullivan Commission in the development of its

recommendations (Box 18-1). The Commission strongly recommended that the culture in health professions programs change (Sullivan Commission, 2004).

The Sullivan Commission is not the first entity to recommend drastic changes in policies of recruitment, admissions, and retention policies. In 2002 and 2003, the California Endowment produced two reports about improving diversity in the health care workforce. These reports delineated some specific policies that California should use to improve its racial, ethnic, and gender diversification (Box 18-2). The implementation of these strategies will require new and innovative leadership. Leaders in schools of nursing must take risks to ensure that recruitment efforts are inclusive and seek out those students from racial and ethnic minority groups interested in nursing as a career. A number of successful models, particularly those of Historically Black Colleges and Universities, could be replicated. Southern University School of Nursing in Baton Rogue is an exemplar of a program that nurtures students from disadvantaged backgrounds who complete the program and have success on the NCLEX-RN. More information about this program can be found at *www.subr.edu/son*.

---

**BOX 18-1** Report of the Sullivan Commission

The Sullivan Commission's recommendations were developed to attract broad public support and to encourage academic and professional leadership to share the Commission's vision for a health system modeled on excellence, access, and quality for all people. Three overlying principles are essential to fulfilling that vision:

■ To increase diversity in the health professions, the culture of health professions schools must change.

■ New and nontraditional paths to the health professions should be explored.

■ Commitments must be at the highest levels.

From Sullivan Commission. (2004). *Missing persons: Minorities in the health profession. A report of the Sullivan commission on diversity in the health care workforce.* Durham, NC: Duke University.

---

BOX 18-2    Policy Goals to Achieve
            Diversity in Nursing

- K-12 academic preparedness and pipeline programs should seek to build skills among diverse youth so that they are increasingly able to pursue nursing as a career.
- Health professions education and outreach initiatives should highlight strategies to target youth who are underrepresented in the nursing field.
- Nursing education and training programs should adopt strategies to encourage and support a more diverse applicant pool and student body through such efforts as targeted recruitment, mentoring, enrichment services, and academic support.
- State and federal scholarship and loans should be available to all qualified California youth who want to pursue a nursing career.
- Nursing educational institutions should develop faculty recruitment policies that recognize faculty diversification as a means to strengthen the quality of nursing education, particularly as student diversity increases.

From California Endowment. (2002). Increasing the diversity of the nursing work force: A strategy to address the nursing shortage and improve quality of care. *Health in Brief: Policy Issues Facing a Diverse California, 1*(1), 1-5.

Schools of nursing in majority minority areas that do not demonstrate that they have recruited, admitted, and graduated persons from ethnic racial minority groups in the quantity reflective of their numbers in their areas should not be eligible for federal and state funds. Centers of Excellence should have a specific amount of money from their federal grant allocated to nursing. Continuous monitoring of schools in communities with high minority enrollments should occur to ascertain if the students have a curriculum rich in science, mathematics, and language arts. There are a number of federally funded programs such as GEAR UP (Gaining Early Awareness and Readiness for Undergraduate Programs; *www.ed.gov/programs/gearup/index.html*) throughout the country that serve as models. Professional nursing organizations should make it part of their programmatic thrusts to evaluate the

status of these programs through their state and local chapters and affiliates.

The schools of nursing should have a report card on their diversity done yearly by professional nursing organizations, sororities, fraternities, political clubs, and other civic organizations that are part of racial and ethnic communities. This is not a new approach; this has become a popular strategy in the quality care movement to rate institutions and providers of health care. However, this approach requires that these groups use their political power and negotiate with the appropriate agencies to allow for the proper dispensing of funds based on the scores on the report cards for nursing programs. Nursing programs have been funded by the Division of Nursing of the Bureau of Health Professions to increase the number of ethnic and racial minorities in nursing but are not held to any adverse consequences if they do not achieve the goal. New and different nurses and other civic and community leaders dissatisfied with the status quo must be developed to begin to assume responsibility for holding the educational facilities, government agencies, elected officials, and private funding sources accountable for the services or lack of services that they provide to support minority access to nursing education.

The role of local state and national governments must not be minimized if increasing the number of ethnic and racial minorities is to become a reality. Creating a cabinet-level chief nurse in local, state, and national governments is one strategy. One of the responsibilities of this office would be to monitor the nursing schools' and nursing services' progress in increasing ethnic and racial minorities in their institutions.

Nurse migration will continue worldwide. The current trend in migration of nurses from the Philippines, India, China, and Nigeria will continue to infuse a significant number of persons from diverse backgrounds into the registered nurse workforce in the United States. In no way should the globalization of nurse migration be seen as a barrier to increasing the registered nurse workforce with persons from within the United States. It should be seen as a complementary strategy.

## Key Points

- Although the United States demographics are rapidly changing, there continues to be little diversity in the registered nurse workforce.
- Nursing schools in the United States must be held accountable for the lack of diversity in their student bodies. Nursing schools must demonstrate their commitment to increasing diversity in the registered nurse workforce by reporting yearly data on admission, retention, and success on the NCLEX. Federal, state, and private funding should be given only to those schools that demonstrate that the number of students in their programs reflects the population in their respective cities.
- Nurse leaders in practice must voice their commitment to increasing diversity in the workplace and demonstrate this commitment by having a workforce, including senior executive staff, that reflects the nursing and patient populations in their cities.
- There are legislative programs at the national and state levels of government that have appropriated funds, ostensibly to facilitate the growth in the diversity of the registered workforce. Federal and state governments that provide the funds must institute a more rigorous process to monitor the outcomes of these funded programs and hold the programs accountable for continued disparities in the nursing workforce, including imposing sanctions if needed.

## Web Resources

**Barbara Jordan Health Policy Scholars**
*www.kff.org/about/jordanscholars.cfm*
**Bureau of Health Professions, Health Resources and Service Administration**
*www.bhpr.hrsa.gov/diversity*
**California Endowment**
*www.calendow.org*
**Center for California Health Workforce Studies**
*www.futurehealth.ucsf.edu/cchws.html*

**Ethnic Minority Fellowship Program**
*www.nursingworld.org/emfp*
**Joint Center for Political and Economic Studies**
*www.jointcenter.org*
**National Black Nurses Association**
*www.nbna.org*
**National Black Nurses Foundation**
*www.nbnfoundation.us*
**Southern University at Baton Rouge School of Nursing**
*www.subr.edu/suson*

## REFERENCES

American Assembly for Men in Nursing. (2004). About us. Retrieved August 9, 2005, from *www.aamn.org/aboutus.htm.*

American Association of Colleges of Nursing (AACN). (2004). *Annual report, 2004: Annual state of schools.* Washington, DC: AACN.

Byrd, W. M., & Clayton, L. (2003). Racial and ethnic disparities in healthcare: A background and history of unequal treatment. In Smedley, B., Stith, A., & Nelson, A. (Eds.). *Unequal treatment: Confronting racial and ethnic disparities in health care* (pp. 455-527). Washington, DC: National Academies Press.

California Endowment. (2002). Increasing the diversity of the nursing workforce. *Health in Brief: Policy Issues Facing a Diverse California, 1*(1), 1-5.

Carnegie, M. E. (1995). *The path we tread: Blacks in nursing worldwide, 1854-1994.* New York: National League for Nursing.

Commission on Graduates of Foreign Nursing Schools (CGFNS). (2003). *Characteristics of foreign nurse graduates in the U.S. workforce, 2000-2001.* Philadelphia: CGFNS.

Division of Nursing, U.S. Bureau of Health Professions. (2005). 2004 National sample survey of registered nurses. Retrieved February 26, 2006 from *http://bhpr.hrsa.gov/healthworkforce/reports/preliminaryfindings.htm.*

Hendricks, C. (2005). Personal interview, August 13.

Holt, T. (2000). The problem of race in the twenty-first century. Cambridge, MA: Harvard University Press.

International Convention on the Elimination of All Forms of Racial Discrimination. (2005). Retrieved August 9, 2005, from *www.iwtc.org/ICERD.html.*

National Advisory Council on Nurse Education and Practice. (2000). *A national agenda for nursing workforce racial and ethnic diversity.* Washington, DC: Health Resources and Services Administration.

National Student Nurses Association (NSNA). (2005). Breakthrough to nursing. Retrieved August 9, 2005, from *www.nsna.org/pubs/imprint/septoct04/BTNcollumn.pdf.*

Organization for Economic Cooperation and Development (OECD). (2002). *International migration of physicians and nurses: Causes, consequences and health policy implications.* Paris: OECD.

Rami, J. (2003, February 8). Successful models in moving students through the pipeline: Southern university school of nursing. Paper presented at the National Black Nurses Association's Gloria R. Smith Issues Forum *Minorities in the pipeline: Issues and solutions*, Washington, DC.

Spratley, E., Johnson, A., Sochalski, J., Marshall, F., & Spencer, W., (2002). *The registered nurse population, 2000*. Washington, DC: Health Resources and Service Administration.

Sullivan Commission. (2004). *Missing persons: Minorities in the health professions. A report of the Sullivan Commission on Diversity in the Healthcare Workforce*. Durham, NC: Duke University.

U.S. Bureau of the Census. (2005). Fact sheet. Retrieved August 10, 2005, from *http://factfinder.census.gov/servlet/ACSSAFFFacts?*.

U.S. Department of Education. Retrieved November 17, 2005, from *www.ed.gov*.

U.S. Office of Management and Budget. (2006). Standards for maintaining, collecting and presenting federal data on race and ethnicity. Retrived February 20, 2006, from *www.whitehouse.gov/omb/inforeg/r&e app-a-update.pdf*.

# Politics of Advanced Practice Nursing

Joyce Pulcini & Mary Ann Hart

*"I was taught that the way of progress is neither swift nor easy."*

MARIE CURIE

Political activism has always been at the heart of advanced practice nursing. As nurses in these roles carved out new and expanded scopes of practice, they honed their political skills in order to make the necessary inroads into new and evolving areas, which were previously only in the realm of physicians or other health care providers. Their political teeth were cut on such important areas as expanding nurse practice acts to include new areas of practice, obtaining third-party reimbursement and prescriptive privileges.

This process of activism unified advanced practice nurses (APNs) both within and among groups. Nurse practitioners in the various specialty organizations, for example, came together through this process by necessity to fight for common goals. Nurse practitioners (NPs), certified nurse midwives (CNMs), certified registered nurse anesthetists (CRNAs), and clinical nurse specialists (CNSs), who have at times been at odds over specific wording of legislation or regulations, have learned to work together in very sophisticated ways to advance their interests.

Although tremendous progress has been made, challenges to both nursing and other health care providers continue as a result of systemic changes in the health care marketplace. For example, participation as primary care providers (PCPs) on managed care panels and maintenance of the ability to order laboratory tests and procedures and to prescribe controlled substances have more recently dominated the agenda, particularly at the state level.

Whereas past political and regulatory efforts have been largely successful, APNs must continue to be active in "bread-and-butter" political activism. Continued pressure is needed both to maintain gains in areas such as primary care and also to successfully expand the APN role into other sectors such as long-term care and acute care. APN professional associations must continue to provide leadership on state professional, regulatory, and legislative issues, where important decisions are made regarding APN practice. New initiatives or the revision of old initiatives require great vigilance and continuity as power within the profession passes from one generation to the next. With good succession planning, seasoned leaders must eventually be replaced by new, younger ones who will take on future initiatives with great forethought and care (Pulcini, 1997, 2005a).

## ADVANCED PRACTICE NURSING DEFINED

The long-term viability of APN practice depends on the ability of the nursing profession to clearly define APN titles, educational preparation, and role to consumers, health care professionals, administrators, and policymakers.

Hamric (2005) conceptually defines Advanced Practice Nursing as "the application of an expanded range of practical, theoretical, and research-based competencies to phenomena experienced by patients within a specialized clinical area of the larger discipline of nursing" (p. 89). Three primary criteria for APN designation are graduate education, certification for practice at an advanced level within a clinical specialty, and practice focused on patients and their families. Seven core competencies of APN practice are direct clinical practice; guidance and coaching of patients, families, and other health providers; consultation; use and implementation of evidence-based practice, evaluation, and conduct; clinical and professional leadership; collaboration; and ethical decision-making skills.

States, in law and regulation, have different definitions for the APN and may differ in the way that they categorize APNs and designate their scope of practice. Categories of APNs may include CRNAs, CNMs, NPs, and CNSs. For example, some states, such as Massachusetts, only define the CNS role as the psychiatric nurse clinical specialist, and others, such as New Jersey, define it more broadly. Federal law defers to state law regarding APN qualifications, and state requirements for preparation differ widely. States also differ in APN scope of practice in the areas of diagnosis, treatment, prescriptive authority, hospital admissions, and requirements for physician collaboration or supervision.

## INTERPROFESSIONAL ISSUES

As we enter a new era for advanced practice nursing, new interprofessional arenas will dominate the agenda, including proposals to require a Doctor of Nursing Practice (DNP) degree to be an APN and designation of the CNS as an APN in states where the broad definition of the CNS is not present in legislation. Here, concepts that once were clearly articulated are again coming to the fore with new educational models and the reinvention or expansion of traditional APN roles.

### PROPOSAL FOR THE DOCTOR OF NURSING PRACTICE DEGREE

Although entry into practice discussions in nursing have been with us for more than 40 years, the new DNP degree has revived discussion on the issue. The American Association of Colleges of Nursing (AACN) in 2004 recommended that all APNs

graduating by 2015 should have the DNP degree (AACN, 2004). This move parallels the action of other professional groups such as pharmacists and physical therapists, which now have entry level clinical doctorates. For nursing the DNP creates different problems, because confusion about professional levels has been the norm rather than the exception. The AACN recommendation also potentially threatens practicing NPs, who may feel pressure to move to the DNP level even if it is not a strict requirement.

The DNP recommendation also creates potential dilemmas or conflicts in decisions regarding master's entry students, who could potentially have no clinical experience outside of an educational program and practice with a DNP. Table 19-1 shows how their numbers are rapidly growing. Many argue that these new practitioners should move quickly through the educational ranks so as to practice optimally and begin clinical research early in their careers. Master's entry nurses challenge the very educational roots of nursing. Although their skills are at a beginning competency level, master's entry nurses are eligible for state licensure and credentialing by national certification bodies as APNs. This raises the question as to whether we should reconsider the competencies of all entry level nursing programs and provide APN skills at the BS level (Pulcini, 2005b).

### CLINICAL NURSE SPECIALISTS AS ADVANCED PRACTICE NURSES

In the 1980s, as cost containment strategies took effect, clinical nurse specialists, who primarily were

**TABLE 19-1** Growth in Second Degree Students: 1990-2005

|  | 1990 | 2005 |
| --- | --- | --- |
| Accelerated Bachelor of Science programs | 31 | 168 |
| Generic master's programs | 12 | 50 |
| Planning accelerated bachelor's programs |  | 46 |

From American Association of Colleges of Nursing (AACN). (2005). Accelerated programs: The fast-track to careers in nursing. Issue bulletin. Retrieved August 12, 2005, from *www.aacn.nche.edu/ publications/issues/aug02.htm.*

**TABLE 19-2** Growth in Nurse Practitioner Programs

|  | 1992 | 1995 | 1998 | 2004 |
|---|---|---|---|---|
| Nurse practitioner programs | 119 | 202 | 325 | 353 |
| Nurse practitioner specialty tracks | 235 | 527 | 769 | 706 |

Data from Berlin, L., Bednash, G., & Hosier, K. (1998). *Enrollment and graduations in baccalaureate and graduate programs in nursing.* Washington, DC: American Association of Colleges of Nursing (AACN); Berlin, L., Stennett, J., & Bednash, G. (2004). *Enrollment and graduations in baccalaureate and graduate programs in nursing.* Washington, DC: AACN; and Harper, D. C., & Johnson, J. (1998). The new generation of nurse practitioners: Is more enough? *Health Affairs, 17*(5), 158-164.

employed in hospitals, began to lose positions in cash-strapped institutions, which were looking for places to cut positions. Many feel that the broad functions of this role and lack of third-party reimbursement for its services left it vulnerable to these cuts. In the1990s, on the other hand, the role of the NP began to reach a tipping point, when the majority of nursing programs in the country began to offer this specialty. Table 19-2 demonstrates this progress and the tripling of NP programs from 1992 to 2004.

Currently the CNS role has experienced a resurgence as patient safety issues in hospitals began to escalate and the nursing shortage brought a predominance of new nurses to hospital units nationwide. The broad functions of the CNS now fit the needs of hospitals, which are struggling to reach the standards required to provide safe patient care. Research by Aiken and others has shown the importance of the workplace environment on patient mortality, and the magnet hospitals initiative blossomed as a solution for improving work conditions in the complex hospital environment (Aiken, Smith, & Lake, 1994; Aiken, Clarke, Cheung, Sloane, & Silber, 2003; Aiken, Clarke, Sloane, Sochalski, & Silber, 2002; Rogers, Hwang, Scott, Aiken, & Dinges, 2004).

With these developments to improve the hospital environment and to alleviate the nursing shortage came increased salaries for staff nurses and CNSs alike. In many areas, NP salaries have leveled somewhat compared with rising RN salaries (Pulcini, Vampola, & Levine, 2005). With a dearth of employment opportunities for NPs in some urban areas, with a large number of PCPs, new NPs, who had previously been staff nurses in high-paying hospitals,

might in some cases take a cut in pay to practice as NPs.

State nurse practice acts will need to be updated or modernized to change entry into practice requirements and to recognize CNSs as APNs in states where they do not have this legal recognition. In addition, the struggle to increase the level of independence in practice for APNs will continue. Political activism by APNs will be critical to the success of this process.

## MACROPOLICY ISSUES

Macropolicy issues will dominate as the evolution of advanced practice roles continues over the next decade. Will APNs practice across all levels of care or just in segments of the system such as primary care or tertiary care, as in the current health care environment? Following patients throughout the entire course of illness might be the most valuable, cost-effective approach to care as well as a key patient safety variable.

Given the shortage of physicians who choose to practice in primary care, will NPs begin to win the battle for dominance in primary care practice? Although NPs are well qualified to dominate this realm, barriers to practice, such as laws and regulations that require physician collaboration or supervision in APN practice, have kept NPs from achieving their full potential in this area.

To what degree will APNs be able to achieve desired independent practice? A consistent problem has been the continued dominance of medicine in advanced nursing practice. For example, although 20 states and the District of Columbia have no requirement for physician oversight, in the form of collaboration or supervision, the majority of the remaining 30 states require physician oversight that must be documented in writing. Forty states require physician oversight through supervision or collaboration in APN prescription writing (Pearson, 2005). NPs understand the importance of collaborative practice but do not want to be mandated through legislation to consult. Other constraints, either through statute or regulation or through provider or insurance policies, may include restrictions of NPs as PCPs on managed care organization (MCO) provider panels, lack of hospital admitting privileges, and reimbursement limitations.

State nursing and APN professional associations must examine and articulate the barriers to independent practice in their states and make the elimination of those barriers a top priority. They must join together to update and strengthen their state nurse practice acts in order to eliminate burdensome and restrictive practice provisions and facilitate expansion of APN practice beyond primary care into other health care sectors.

Consumers and voters are important voices in change. Surveys, which show consumer satisfaction with APN care, and APN data showing the cost effectiveness of APN practice ought to gain support for APN practice by provider, hospital, and insurance groups. Study after study has documented the cost effectiveness of APNs, and insurance companies are beginning to notice that these nurse providers are saving the system money and delaying more costly health care services (Venning, Durie, Roland, Roberts & Leese, 2000). APNs must identify and collect the data needed to document the benefits of APN practice and to use this information to market and sell their services to health care providers and insurers.

## NEW CHALLENGES IN REIMBURSEMENT FOR ADVANCED PRACTICE NURSES

In this rapidly changing health care environment the long-term financial viability of APN practice is directly related to how APNs get paid for their services. APNs must have an understanding of the reimbursement mechanisms used in various health care settings. With the growth of managed care, they must negotiate with insurers and providers for a reasonable reimbursement rate.

APNs have made important strides in having their services recognized and reimbursed directly or indirectly through various payment mechanisms because of changes in state and federal laws and regulations. In most states, traditional indemnity insurers, such as the commercial insurers and Blue Cross Blue Shield, must reimburse APNs for their services. The Balanced Budget Act of 1997 extended Medicare reimbursement to APNs in all geographic areas and clinical settings (Haber, 1997). Previously, only APNs working in rural areas and nursing homes were reimbursed for their services (Nevidjon & Knudtson, 2005). The State Children's Health Insurance Program (SCHIP), which extends insurance to children in low-income families not eligible for Medicaid, pays many APNs. State Medicaid programs reimburse some categories of APNs, including pediatric nurse practitioners (PNPs), family nurse practitioners (FNPs), and CNMs (Johnson & Pawlson, 2005) (see Chapter 15, as well as *Children's Health Insurance Coverage: Medicaid and the State Children's Health Insurance Program [SCHIP]* following Chapter 15).

Just as important gains for APN reimbursement were made in fee-for-service reimbursement through traditional health insurance, managed care began to replace the old fee-for-service model, presenting new challenges for all health care providers. Nearly all health care models now incorporate managed care, including care paid for by government programs, such as Medicaid and Medicare. MCOs act as both providers and insurers, controlling both utilization and payment. APNs and other health care providers, including physicians, now must negotiate contracts with MCOs to be on their provider panels. The contract, not only defines many terms of employment, it specifically spells out the level of reimbursement they will receive from the insurer.

Lawmakers have been hesitant to meddle with the wide contracting ability of MCOs because the MCOs' freedom to contract with selected providers at a negotiated price is a critical feature of managed care that enables MCOs to hold down health care costs. With the old fee-for-service rules no longer applying, some health care providers have made naïve attempts through legislation to force MCOs to contract with certain groups of providers. Such "any willing provider" legislation has been largely unsuccessful. APNs and other health care providers, including physicians, need a whole new set of marketing and business skills to "sell" themselves to MCOs and be successful in the new managed care marketplace.

On the other hand, state law can specifically prohibit APNs, such as NPs, from being PCPs on the provider panels of MCOs, can be silent on the issue, or can protect NP practice by recognizing NPs as PCPs in law (Buppert, 1999). While some states designate NPs as PCPs in their Medicaid programs, most are silent on the issue as it relates to private, non-Medicaid patients in MCOs. National nursing organizations are pushing for federal legislation that would amend Medicaid law to recognize NPs and CNMs as primary care case managers, require MCOs to include NPs, CNSs, CRNAs, and CNMs on Medicaid managed care panels, and expand fee-for-service Medicaid to include direct payment for services provided by all NPs and CNSs (American Nurses Association, 2005).

Laws that prohibit NPs as PCPs need to be changed, and it may be desirable to enact state laws that specifically authorize NPs to be PCPs in states that are silent on the issue. Such a measure is currently being proposed in Massachusetts by the Massachusetts Coalition of Nurse Practitioners. However, even with the removal of specific legal prohibitions and the enactment of legislation authorizing NPs as PCPs, APNs will still need to negotiate contracts with MCOs to be PCPs and to be reimbursed by MCOs.

APNs may be inexperienced in marketing and negotiating contractual and legal relationships and may not be comfortable with self-promotion (Hodnicki & Doughty, 2005). While successful negotiation of a managed care contract is necessary to be part of an MCO, APNs are also likely to have to negotiate other types of agreements in their careers, such as employment contracts, collaborative practice agreements and service contacts (Hodnicki & Doughty, 2005). APNs' adeptness at marketing their skills and developing a collaborative practice agreement with a physician or physicians, particularly when required by state law, is key to establishing a successful practice environment to reach one's full potential as an APN.

Although the individual APN should learn how to approach MCOs and group practices to market her or his services, APN professional associations also need to take a leadership role in promoting the use of APNs with these entities. This means picking up the phone, making an appointment with senior administrators, developing appropriate marketing materials, and meeting with senior administrators to "sell" the services of the APNs the organization represents. Even more important, APN administrators must be present at the negotiating table as members of management teams of MCOs and group practices that set the policies and rates that govern what APNs are paid (Hamric, Spross, & Hanson, 2005). APNs must learn how to be comfortable with and effectively operate among insurers and other business entities. APN educators should consider the best way to develop marketing savvy and business skills among prospective APNs, either as a component of the APN curriculum or through continuing education offerings.

## Key Points

- Although important gains have been made in APN practice, future challenges include developing consistent titling and educational requirements for APNs and amending state nurse practice acts to remove barriers to practice, update educational requirements, and designate CNSs as APNs.

- APNs must develop the skills to market their services and to negotiate contractual and legal relationships with MCOs, group practices, and physician collaborators.

- Strong political leadership by APN professional associations at the state and federal levels, with an active APN member base, will be needed to ensure that advanced practice reaches its full potential.

*Web Resources*

> **American Academy of Nurse Practitioners**
> *www.aanp.org*
> **American Association of Colleges of Nursing**
> *www.aacn.nche.edu*
> **American College of Nurse Practitioners**
> *www.nurse.org/acnp*
> **American Nurses Association**
> *www.nursingworld.org*
> **National Organization of Nurse Practitioner Faculties**
> *www.nonpf.org*

## REFERENCES

Aiken, L. H., Clarke, S. P., et al. (2002). Hospital nurse staffing and patient mortality, nurse burnout, and job dissatisfaction. *JAMA, 288*(16), 1987-1993.

Aiken, L. H., Clarke, S. P., Cheung, R. B., Sloane, D.M., & Silber, J.H. (2003). Education levels of hospital nurses and surgical patient mortality. *Journal of the American Medical Association, 290*(12), 1617-1623.

Aiken, L. H., Clarke, S. P., Sloane, D. M., Sochalski, J., & Silber, J. H. (2002). Hospital nurse staffing and patient mortality, nurse burnout, and job dissatisfaction. *JAMA, 288*(16), 1987-1993.

Aiken, L. H., Smith, H. L., & Lake, E. (1994). Lower Medicare mortality among a set of hospitals known for good nursing care. *Medical Care, 32*(8), 771-787.

American Association of Colleges of Nursing (AACN). (2004). AACN position statement on the practice doctorate in nursing. Retrieved August 12, 2005, from *www.aacn.nche.edu/DNP/DNPPositionStatement.htm.*

American Association of Colleges of Nursing (AACN). (2005). Accelerated programs: The fast-track to careers in nursing. Issue bulletin. Retrieved August 12, 2005, from *www.aacn.nche.edu/Publications/issues/Aug02.htm.*

American Nurses Association. (2005). Medicaid coverage of advanced practice registered nurses. Retrieved September 25, 2005, from *http://vocusgr.vocus.com/grconvert1/webpub/ana/ProfileIssue.asp?IssueID=2913|JOINT&XSL=ProfileIssue&hidLegislatorIDs=.*

Berlin, L., Bednash, G., & Hosier, K. (1998). Enrollment and graduations in baccalaureate and graduate programs in nursing. Washington, DC: AACN.

Berlin, L., Stennett, J., & Bednash, G. (2004). *Enrollment and graduations in baccalaureate and graduate programs in nursing.* Washington, DC: AACN.

Buppert, C. (1999). *Nurse practitioner's business practice and legal guide.* Gaithersburg, MD: Aspen.

Haber, J. (1997). Medicare reimbursement: A victory of APRNs. *American Journal of Nursing, 97,* 84.

Hamric, A. B. (2005). A definition of advanced practice nursing. In A. Hamric, J. Spross, & C. Hanson (Eds.), *Advanced practice nursing: An integrative approach.* St. Louis: Elsevier.

Hamric, A., Spross, J., & Hanson, C. (2005). *Advanced practice nursing: An integrative approach.* St. Louis: Elsevier.

Harper, D. C., & Johnson, J. (1998). The new generation of nurse practitioners: Is more enough? *Health Affairs, 17*(5), 158-164.

Hodnicki, D. R., & Doughty, S. E. D. (2005). Marketing and contracting considerations. In A. Hamric, J. Spross, & C. Hanson (Eds.), *Advanced practice nursing: An integrative approach.* St. Louis: Elsevier.

Johnson, J., & Pawlson, L. G. (2005). Health policy issues in changing environments. In A. Hamric, J. Spross, & C. Hanson (Eds.), *Advanced practice nursing: An integrative approach.* St. Louis: Elsevier.

Nevidjon, B. M., & Knudtson, M. D. (2005). Strengthening advanced nursing practice in organizational structures and cultures. In A. Hamric, J. Spross, & C. Hanson (Eds.), *Advanced practice nursing: An integrative approach.* St. Louis: Elsevier.

Pearson, L. (2005). The Pearson report: A national overview of nurse practitioner legislation and healthcare issues. *American Journal of Nurse Practitioners, 9*(1), 9-136.

Pulcini, J. (1997). Succession planning: From leaders to mentors. An open letter to experienced nurse practitioner leaders. *Clinical Excellence for Nurse Practitioners, 1*(6), 405-406.

Pulcini, J. (2005a). Succession planning: Mentoring at the macro level. In L. Raukhorst (Ed.), *Mentoring: Ensuring the future of NP practice and education.* Washington, DC: National Organization of Nurse Practitioner Faculties.

Pulcini, J. (2005b). Advanced practice nursing: Moving beyond the basics. In C. L. Andrist, P. Nicholas, & K. Wolf (Eds.), *The history of nursing ideas.* Sudbury, MA: Jones and Bartlett.

Pulcini, J., Vampola, D., & Levine, J. (2005). NPACE nurse practitioner practice characteristics, salary, and benefits survey: 2003. *Clinical Excellence for Nurse Practitioners, 9*(1), 49-58.

Rogers, A., Hwang, W., Scott, L., Aiken, L., & Dinges, D. (2004). The working hours of staff nurses and patient safety: Both errors and near errors are more likely to occur when hospital staff nurses work twelve or more hours at a stretch. *Health Affairs, 23*(4), 202-212.

Venning, P., Durie, A., Roland, M., Roberts, C., & Leese, B. (2000). Randomised controlled trial comparing cost effectiveness of general practitioners and nurse practitioners in primary care. *British Medical Journal, 320*(7241), 1048-1053.

## Diminishing Reproductive Choices in New York City: The Demise of the Midwifery Model

*"There is no teacher better than adversity. Every defeat, every heartbreak, every loss, contains its own seed, its own lesson on how to improve your performance the next time."*

MALCOLM X

Beginning in 2003 the local press in New York City prominently featured midwifery in a variety of ways, but too often because of the loss of one more midwifery practice and the type of care associated with midwives. The Elizabeth Seton Childbearing Center (ESCbC) closed its doors in September 2003. The midwives of Columbia Presbyterian Medical Center (CPMC) had their birthing activities curtailed in October 2004. This reduced access to midwifery services and effectively left many women across the economic and geographic spectrum with gravely limited or non-existent choices for their reproductive experiences. All that is left to them is the obstetric model of care, which derives from a "pathological until proven otherwise" concept implemented in a hospital environment focused on the care of the sick and infirmed.

The closing of ESCbC ended a project, started in 1975, that successfully demonstrated to the nation, the health care system, and the New York City community the equivalent outcomes and economic effectiveness of the concept of out-of-hospital birth. It also provided 28 years of reproductive choice for women in the New York metropolitan area. The stripping of birthing privileges from the 25 midwives of CPMC ended choice for the large and mostly Hispanic population served by the midwives in northern Manhattan.

Analysis and review of these two events, distinct in many ways but similar in others, will provide an understanding of the complexity of the system of health care delivery and the place of the client or patient in it, as well as delineate the factors of power that influenced the decisions resulting in this reduction in choices for women.

### THE ISSUE OF CHOICE

Before examining the closure of the two midwifery practices, it is important to understand what the usual experience is for a woman in labor in the New York City area. The typical laboring women looks very much like an intensive care unit (ICU) patient, hooked up to a variety of machines including a monitor and an intravenous (IV) pump, unable to walk or help herself very well since she is probably paralyzed from the waist down with epidural anesthesia, and often left alone for long periods of time. The reasons for this standard experience are multiple. The changing landscape of the health care system, both for the delivery of services and the reimbursement of services, has resulted in the amalgamation and coalescing of many institutions for the economic benefits. Therefore the same protocols and procedures exist in multiple institutions. In addition, cuts in nursing staffs to save money or positions unfilled because of the nursing shortage, combined with the move toward using all available technology, have led to dependence on machines and scarcity of human professional interaction with patients.

The large number of medical schools in New York City has also influenced care, as each program needs to provide a steady and adequate supply of medical student and resident learning experiences, which are standardized through the medical and specialty education process. As a result, there is little to distinguish one hospital's obstetric practices from another. In these environments, women have no real choice in what procedures are imposed on them in labor. They can't choose intermittent auscultation, despite the research that indicates this type of fetal surveillance results in outcomes that are as good as those with the electronic version but results in fewer cesarean sections (American Academy of Pediatrics [AAP] & American College of Obstetricians and Gynecologists [ACOG], 2002). Rather, they will be bound to the bed by the electronic fetal monitor belt or electrode so they cannot move readily or change position to facilitate the passage of the fetus through the birth canal. They can say, "I don't want an epidural," but no real alternative is offered. In most instances they cannot use hydrotherapy for pain relief because the electronic fetal monitoring equipment prohibits its use, it is not available, or there is no nurse to aid and assist while the woman is in the tub or shower, so she is left with the epidural as the only pain relief modality. Women are also not usually allowed to eat or drink during labor, a truly amazing reality, because no athlete engaged in a marathon, a close parallel to labor, would do so without rehydrating and reenergizing her body. IV glucose water is not enough.

Although many hospitals have marketed their obstetric services with a "homelike" environment theme, they have made few substantive changes. The cosmetic changes (e.g., colored bedspreads, lovely pictures on the walls, and even the use of the term "birth center" to refer to the labor and delivery area) are basically superficial and somewhat misleading. The type of care offered and the procedures required haven't changed.

## ELIZABETH SETON CHILDBEARING CENTER

The Maternity Center Association (MCA) in 1975 founded the birth center that eventually became ESCbC, to demonstrate that out-of-hospital birth was safe and cost effective as long as the providers and the health system infrastructure resources were adequate, appropriate, and integrated. The success of this demonstration project is manifest in the following:

- The numerous birth centers that existed around the country, 96 accredited by National Association of Childbearing Centers (NACC), in 2005

- The comparable, if not better, outcomes for mothers and infants evidenced in the published data associated with these out-of-hospital services and reflected in equivalent perinatal mortality rates (1.8 per 1000 for home births versus 2.1 per 1000 hospital births) but lower cesarean section rates (4.4 versus 20 in 1989) (Rooks, Weatherby, & Ernst, 1992a, 1992b).

In the mid 1990s the MCA, whose mission is "to promote safe, effective, and satisfying maternity care for all women and their families through research, education, and advocacy," decided that they had proven the effectiveness, safety, and quality of the out-of-hospital birth concept and were ready to explore other issues in maternity care that needed to be challenged. So they began to explore with local area organizations the possibility of turning the birth center over to someone else for continuing management. They ultimately reached an agreement with St. Vincent's Medical Center in lower Manhattan and moved the MCA birth center from 92nd Street to 14th Street, into beautifully renovated but expensive space, where it became the ESCbC.

For the first few years after the birth center opened its doors on 14th Street those involved in the decision to have the birth center become associated with St. Vincent's continued to play an active role in its management. As with any major change there were some difficulties, but gradually the birth center began to grow and prosper as it became better known and the available services expanded. The Center became not only a place where women could go to receive care for pregnancy and to give birth in an environment very similar to their own homes, but also a dynamic center for learning, support, and integration of a new person into a family and the development of concomitant new family and parenting roles as well as women's health care.

However, as time passed, several critical factors that affected the center changed. Key supportive players in both upper level hospital administration and the Department of Obstetrics and Gynecology left their positions, and in most instances their replacements neither valued this type of women's health care nor supported the concept inherent in the birth center—that of out-of-hospital birth. In addition, the economic equilibrium of New York City hospitals grew more unstable, including that of the Catholic Medical System, of which St. Vincent's had become a part. Related to this, the litigious environment worsened, resulting in exorbitant malpractice insurance premiums for both practitioners and facilities. Obstetricians in some parts of the United States paid as high as $201,000 in malpractice insurance premiums. The perception of the birth center's value and place in St. Vincent's Medical Center changed.

The two most critical factors that ultimately led to the close of the center were hospital and health system economics and the strongly held belief of the obstetric department leadership that all births belonged in the hospital.

## COLUMBIA PRESBYTERIAN MEDICAL CENTER MIDWIFERY PRACTICE

On the north end of Manhattan, a different picture was unfolding, but one with results similar to those down in lower Manhattan. The Columbia Presbyterian Midwifery Practice, one of the oldest hospital practices in New York City, moved from the main hospital at 168th Street to the Allen Pavilion, a community-hospital branch of Presbyterian Hospital, in the mid 1990s. At that time the midwives provided round-the-clock care for women during labor, birth, and the postpartum period, with consultative support from the attending physician. Inherent to the midwifery presence were two confounding elements that ultimately contributed to the demise of midwifery birthing care. The midwives were administratively positioned as nursing personnel and therefore part of the bargaining unit of the New York State Nurses Association (NYSNA). As such they worked a nursing schedule of 37.5 hours a week, gaining pay increases with every contract negotiated between the bargaining unit and the hospital. Most critically, their position in the nursing infrastructure prohibited them from billing and receiving payment for services rendered to the women for whom they cared.

This long-standing administrative positioning of the midwives in the nursing infrastructure resulted in the mechanism of revenues generated by the midwives' practice being paid to the obstetric department of the hospital, which also billed for these services. This was a somewhat logical route to take, as billable services were being provided, but the providers were unable to bill in their own right because their costs were included in the facility reimbursement along with all the hospital nurses and nursing care. However, this practice led to other requirements that resulted in the demise of the hospital practice. To legitimize the obstetric department billing, the physician had to be in the room for the birth. Ostensibly the physician presence was related to billing, but in the litigious world of health care today, most physicians were concerned about the professional liability involved in being present and billing for the delivery and were very likely to dictate delivery practices to the midwives.

CPMC had been struggling with the economics of health care delivery in the previous few years. This situation became more clearly focused in the obstetric department, partly because of the billing practices related to midwifery services. The presence of two providers (the midwife and the attending physician) doing one service (the delivery or birth) in a time of major economic constraint finally led to the decision to take one of these providers out of the equation. Despite the qualitative value that midwives add to women's health care services, they are not as versatile as gynecologic surgeons who also do deliveries. Therefore they are more dispensable.

## DISTINCT ELEMENTS OF EACH

These two situations appear very distinct from one another at first glance. ESCbC is associated with but separate from St. Vincent's Medical Center. The midwifery practice functioning in the ESCbC was a private practice professional model group, employed by the ESCbC to provide care for the women who chose its services. The midwives worked an on-call schedule to provide for the 24/7 health care needs of their clients, they managed the quality-assurance program for the center and the practice, and they covered second call as needed. The birth center, as an out-of-hospital facility, was governed by Article 28, Diagnostic and Treatment Center rules and regulations of the New York State Department of Health, not by the 405 hospital regulations that govern the care of women during labor and birth in hospitals. As the name indicates, an Article 28 facility focuses on patients who are ill and therefore require a physician to be in charge and present. This concept is antithetical to the success of a birth center, the focus of which is on a physiologic process called *birthing*. There is no need for medical direction of a normal physiologic process called *pregnancy and birth*. In the event of the development of complications or pathology, midwives consult or clients are transferred into the hospital for appropriate care.

The CPMC midwifery practice, on the other hand, used a hospital model in which the midwives worked scheduled hours, as do all nursing staff, and anything beyond those hours was considered overtime. Therefore it was not in the best interests of the hospital's budget for midwives to engage in appropriate and expected professional off-hour activities such as attending grand rounds and Morbidity and Mortality (M&M) conferences or managing the practice's continuous quality improvement program.

## COMMON ELEMENTS OF BOTH SITUATIONS

Despite the apparent differences in these two midwifery practices, they are not at all different in terms of power and control. Neither midwifery group had control of the business activities of the practice. They were salaried by an organization: ESCbC for the "private practice" model and CPMC for the Allen midwives. Revenues generated by each practice were also beyond the midwives' control. The ESCbC had the debt burden of the renovations for the space they occupied, so they were always seeking to reduce it. The obstetric department of CPMC had historically received the revenues of the midwives by billing for the births they attended and receiving that reimbursement. This billing mechanism also required the physician to be present for the delivery, a reality that in cost-constrained times clearly became an unnecessary redundancy. The second element shared between the two practices was that decision-making power resided in hands other than those of the midwives. In the case of ESCbC, there were four layers of decision-making: Catholic Medical System, St. Vincent's Medical Center, the Department of Obstetrics and Gynecology, and

the ESCbC administration and Medical Director. Each of these was discrete, but all were connected in a hierarchic relationship, with the midwives on the bottom rung. For the CPMC midwives, there were three layers: the Chair of the Department of Obstetrics and Gynecology, who made the decision to take birthing privileges from the midwives; the Columbia University leadership; and the hospital administration—another hierarchy in which the midwives were on the lowest rung and without any power.

## PREVENTIVE STRATEGIES THAT MIGHT HAVE CHANGED THE OUTCOMES FOR THE BIRTH CENTERS

The factor that initiated the demise of ESCbC was the resignation of the medical director, a physician who had served in this capacity for many years despite the constant negative pressure he received from some of his peers. Ultimately he capitulated to the pressure, leaving the center without the required medical hierarchy, thereby giving the chair of the obstetrics department the means to impose a moratorium on births in the center. This initial betrayal of its clientele created the first significant crack in its foundation.

The groundwork for this possibility was laid almost 30 years ago. When the birth center demonstration project was inaugurated in 1975 there was no New York State Department of Health structure for it, so it was structured as an Article 28 Diagnostic and Treatment Facility, an inappropriate structure for a care facility whose role is to support and enhance a normal physiologic process. One way to prevent what happened at ESCbC is to help the New York State Department of Health develop or create an appropriate niche for birth centers, an infrastructure that gives credence to the nature of these facilities and the resources they need to be safe and successful. This would derive from the law governing midwifery in New York State, which recognizes midwives as licensed independent providers, competent to care for women, irrespective of location. Midwives can and should run birth centers as the sole providers and proprietors, with physicians used for consultation or referral in the event of complications.

## PROFESSIONAL PRACTICE MODEL

The issue of a professional practice model remains at the heart of midwifery success or failure. Midwives need to be more than expert clinicians. They also have to use the professional business model to frame the pragmatics of practice and assure that someone, if not themselves, has their economic interests at heart (Slager, 2004). They need to be economically successful to capitalize on their clinical success.

Allied in importance with economics is decision-making—that is, who has the power and inclination to make decisions about a particular professional practice. In today's world, few individuals are totally autonomous, and in the medically dominated health care system of the United States, the lack of credentialing as physicians places other professionals in a disadvantaged position. The challenge is to be appropriately positioned within the organization and to remain politically astute, at all levels across the organization, to be diplomatic and knowledgeable and present at the table when decisions that affect the parameters of one's clinical area are made. For midwives the most essential arena is the hospital and their place in it. All can run their office practices according to midwifery practice standards, but becoming positioned in the hospital infrastructure in an effective way presents a serious challenge. Ideally midwives should have full staff privileges through which they not only practice within midwifery standards but also serve on staff committees of importance to protect the rights of women or of midwives. Learning the infrastructure to make the greatest impact is a first step. Building alliances and coalitions while influencing those with opposing stances is the most effective strategy for negotiating a viable position.

## Lessons Learned

There are two essential lessons to be learned from the ESCbC and Allen Pavilion of CPMC midwives:

- Economics drives the health care system, and survival for all providers is based on having adequate and accurate financial information and management related to the professional practice.
- Ideally, decision-making about a practice belongs in the hands of the professionals of the practice. Lacking the ideal practice, providers have to ensure that they participate in decision-making that affects their practice.

## Web Resources

**American College of Nurse Midwives**
*www.acnm.org*
**Maternity Center Association (MCA)**
*www.maternitywise.org*
**National Association of Childbearing Centers (NACC)**
*www.birthcenters.org*

## REFERENCES

American Academy of Pediatrics (AAP) & American College of Obstetricians and Gynecologists (ACOG). (2002). *Guidelines for perinatal care* (5th ed.). Washington, DC: AAP & ACOG.

Rooks, J. P., Weatherby, N. L., & Ernst, E. K. (1992a). The National Birth Center Study: Part II—Intrapartum and immediate postpartum and neonatal care. *Journal of Nurse Midwifery, 37*(5), 301-330.

Rooks, J. P., Weatherby, N. L., & Ernst, E. K. (1992b). The National Birth Center Study: Part III—Intrapartum and immediate postpartum and neonatal complications and transfers, postpartum and neonatal care, outcomes, and client satisfaction. *Journal of Nurse Midwifery, 37*(6), 361-397.

Slager, J. (2004). *Business concepts for health care providers.* Boston: Jones and Bartlett.

# REIMBURSEMENT ISSUES FOR NURSE ANESTHETISTS: A CONTINUING CHALLENGE

Rita M. Rupp, John Garde, & Frank Purcell

*"I was taught that the way of progress is neither swift nor easy."*

MARIE CURIE

A number of federal initiatives in the last three decades have had a significant impact on the nurse anesthesia profession. Three federal reimbursement policies significantly affected the American Association of Nurse Anesthetists (AANA) and its 33,000 members. Three case studies related to federal reimbursement and payment policy are presented here to demonstrate the degree to which federal policy can affect the economics of a profession, the ability of federal rules to raise or lower barriers to practice, and the ability of federal regulations to cause or remediate inefficiencies in the delivery of anesthesia services. The cases demonstrate the politics that are generated when overlapping professions—nurse anesthesia and physician anesthesia—have high stakes in the outcome.

## THE NURSE ANESTHESIA PROFESSION

Certified registered nurse anesthetists (CRNAs) are educated in the specialty of anesthesia at the graduate level in an integrated program of academic and clinical study. CRNAs are licensed and certified to practice anesthesia. In addition, they must meet the requirement of recertification every 2 years. CRNAs are eligible to receive reimbursement for their services directly from Medicare, from nearly half of all Medicaid programs, from TRICARE (the U.S. Department of Defense health program), and from a large group of private insurers and managed care organizations.

Today CRNAs, working with anesthesiologists, surgeons, and, where authorized, podiatrists, dentists, and other health care providers, administer approximately 65% of all anesthetics given each year in the United States. CRNAs provide anesthesia for every age and type of patient using the full scope of anesthesia techniques, drugs, and technology that characterize contemporary anesthesia practice. They work in every setting in which anesthesia is delivered: tertiary care centers, community hospitals, labor and delivery rooms, ambulatory surgical centers (ASCs), diagnostic suites, and outpatient settings. CRNAs are the sole anesthesia providers in more than 70% of rural hospitals, affording anesthesia and resuscitative services to these medical facilities for surgical, obstetric, and trauma care.

## HISTORICAL PERSPECTIVE

Nurses were the first professional group to provide anesthesia services in the United States. Established in the late 1800s, nurse anesthesia has since become recognized as the first clinical nursing specialty. The discipline of nurse anesthesia developed in response to surgeon requests for a solution to the high morbidity and mortality attributed to anesthesia at that time. Surgeons saw nurses as a cadre of professionals who could give their undivided attention to patient care during surgical procedures. Serving as pioneers in anesthesia, nurse anesthetists became involved in the full range of specialty surgical procedures, as well as in the refinement of anesthesia techniques and equipment.

The earliest existing records documenting the anesthetic care of patients by nurses were those of Sister Mary Bernard, a Catholic nun who worked at

St. Vincent's Hospital in Erie, Pennsylvania, in 1887. The most famous nurse anesthetist of the nineteenth century, Alice Magaw, worked at St. Mary's Hospital (1889) in Rochester, Minnesota. That hospital, established by the Sisters of St. Francis and operated by Dr. William Worrell Mayo, later became internationally recognized as the Mayo Clinic. Dr. Charles Mayo conferred on Alice Magaw the title of "mother of anesthesia" for her many achievements in the field of anesthesiology, particularly her mastery of the open-drop inhalation technique of anesthesia using ether and chloroform and her subsequent publication of her findings. Together, Dr. Mayo and Ms. Magaw were instrumental in establishing a showcase of professional excellence in anesthesia and surgery. Hundreds of physicians and nurses from the United States and throughout the world came to observe and learn their anesthesia techniques. Alice Magaw documented the anesthesia practice outcomes at St. Mary's Hospital and reported them in various medical journals between 1899 and 1906. In 1906, one article documented more than 14,000 anesthetics being administered without a single complication attributable to anesthesia (Magaw, 1906).

In 1909, the first formal educational programs preparing nurse anesthetists were established. In 1914, Dr. George Crile and his nurse anesthetist, Agatha Hodgins, who became the founder of the AANA, went to France with the American Ambulance group to assist in planning for the establishment of hospitals that would provide for the care of the sick and wounded members of the Allied Forces. While there, Hodgins taught both physicians and nurses from England and France how to administer anesthesia.

Since World War I, nurse anesthetists have been the principal anesthesia providers in combat areas of every war in which the United States has been engaged. Although nurse anesthesia educational programs existed before World War I, the war sharply increased the demand for nurse anesthetists and consequently the need for more educational programs. Founded in 1931, the AANA is the professional association representing more than 27,000 nurse anesthetists nationwide. The AANA promulgates education and practice standards and serves as a resource to both private and governmental entities regarding nurse anesthetists and their practice. The accreditation of nurse anesthesia educational programs and the certification and recertification of nurse anesthetists is a function of the AANA autonomous multidisciplinary councils.

## NURSE ANESTHESIA REIMBURSEMENT

Nurse anesthetists gained direct Medicare reimbursement in 1986. To fully understand the history leading to this achievement, a beginning understanding of the structure of the Medicare program is important. Medicare Part A establishes the regulations by which hospitals and ambulatory care facilities are reimbursed for services, supplies, drugs, and equipment used in the care of Medicare patients. Medicare Part B sets forth the payment regulations for health care professionals who are eligible to receive direct reimbursement through the Medicare program. The requirements that must be met to receive direct reimbursement from Medicare Part B are distinct and separate from those in Medicare Part A.

With the advent of the Medicare program in 1965, payment for the anesthesia services provided by nurse anesthetists was provided through both Part A and Part B of the Medicare program. For the services provided by CRNAs who were hospital employed, the hospitals were reimbursed under Part A for "reasonable costs" of anesthesia services. For the services provided by CRNAs who were employed by anesthesiologists, the anesthesiologists who employed and supervised CRNAs could bill under Part B as if they personally had administered the anesthesia. These forms of payment were workable until 1983, when the Prospective Payment System (PPS) legislation was passed by Congress in an effort to control hospital costs to the Medicare program. The law provided that all services by providers, other than those reimbursed through Medicare Part B, would be bundled into a hospital diagnostic-related group (DRG) payment. The legislation created serious problems relative to the payment for nurse anesthesia services: (1) hospitals would have been required to pay for their CRNA employees from the fixed DRG payment, jeopardizing their ability to recoup actual costs and creating a disincentive for hospitals to employ CRNAs; and (2) because PPS precluded the unbundling of services, anesthesiologists who employed CRNAs would have been forced to contract with hospitals to get the CRNA portion of the DRG. Simply put, CRNA services were effectively nonreimbursable.

In addition, it was the hospitals that had accrued Medicare cost savings by using the services of CRNAs that stood to be hurt the most by the move to a DRG payment system. Hospitals using more physicians for such services did not need to take the costs from the DRG payment because physician services were reimbursed from Medicare Part B and were not part of the services to be paid through the DRG. This offered the prospect for hospitals to reap a so-called "windfall profit" for using more-costly providers and a strong incentive for hospitals using CRNA services to shift such services to physicians. For every $1 paid to CRNAs, anesthesiologists were being paid $3 to $4. If the substitution of anesthesiologists for CRNAs were to increase, the cost of anesthesia care to Medicare beneficiaries could be expected to escalate (Garde, 1988).

## ADVOCACY ISSUES

Because of the potential negative effect of the PPS legislation on nurse anesthetists, AANA advocated the following legislative changes:

- A provision should be established to allow a temporary pass-through of hospitals' CRNA costs for a 3-year period, which would assure hospitals of no financial loss on CRNA services.
- A single exception to the unbundling provisions of the law should be allowed for anesthesiologist-employed CRNAs, because it was questionable if anesthesiologists could bill for CRNA services under the new provision.
- The Omnibus Budget Reconciliation Act (OBRA) of 1986 should include direct reimbursement for CRNAs to become effective January 1, 1989, with extension of the two temporary provisions to the effective date of the legislation.

The mission of the AANA was to convince Congress and the Health Care Financing Administration (HCFA, renamed the Centers for Medicare and Medicaid Services [CMS] in 2001) that CRNAs were concerned about health care costs as well as equitable reimbursement for their services.

Even though the American Society of Anesthesiologists (ASA) opposed the direct reimbursement legislation, AANA's message was understood because it made financial sense. Use of CRNAs in the provision of anesthesia services represents substantial cost savings from several standpoints. On average, the income of CRNAs is one third that of anesthesiologists. Also, the educational cost of preparing CRNAs is significantly less than that needed to prepare anesthesiologists. The anesthesiologists knew these numbers, and those within their ranks that opposed direct reimbursement for nurse anesthetists had to have been concerned about the potential for increased competition that could come about if the nurse anesthetists were to have equity in the market for anesthesia services.

A convincing case was made before Congress, and legislation was passed granting CRNAs direct Medicare reimbursement. Two payment schedules were incorporated in the law: one for CRNAs not medically directed by anesthesiologists and the other for CRNAs working under anesthesiologists' medical direction (Gunn, 1997).

As a result of this legislation, all CRNAs, regardless of whether they are employed or are in independent practice, have the ability to receive reimbursement from Medicare directly or to sign over their billing rights to their employers. In addition to Medicare direct reimbursement, CRNAs are reimbursed through many health plans. Although CRNAs still face a variety of practice barriers in some facilities and health plans, they can and do serve as exclusive providers for the full range of anesthesia services at hospitals and ambulatory surgical facilities.

## TAX EQUITY AND FISCAL RESPONSIBILITY ACT OF 1982

The Tax Equity and Fiscal Responsibility Act of 1982 (TEFRA) was enacted into federal law as a means to control escalating Medicare costs for hospital-based services including anesthesiology, pathology, and radiology. Among the many cost concerns that TEFRA addressed was a need to ensure that an anesthesiologist provided specified services when billing Medicare for medical direction when a CRNA was administering the anesthesia. Before enactment of TEFRA, anesthesiologists could bill for their services in conjunction with supervision of hospital-employed CRNAs without demonstrating that they had provided specific services to qualify for such payment. The 1976 Medicare manual did require that the "physician be close by and available to provide immediate and personal assistance and direction." The Medicare manual stated that availability by telephone did not constitute direct, personal, and continuous service. In the next years, private payers began refusing to reimburse anesthesiologists for more than two concurrent procedures owing to the fact that many anesthesiologists were being paid for supervision of nurse anesthetist-administered cases in which the anesthesiologists were unavailable. At the same time that these physician payment practices were coming under increased scrutiny, AANA had been preparing its case for Congress in pursuit of direct reimbursement for CRNAs. Part of the reimbursement argument that AANA advanced related to the issue of the lack of equitable reimbursement between substitutable providers, in this case, CRNAs and anesthesiologists. As previously discussed, there were numerable instances across the country in which anesthesiologists were being paid for participation in cases in which CRNAs were the sole provider administering the anesthesia. The anesthesiologists were unavailable, yet they were billing for the case as if they had been involved.

In 1983, the HCFA published the final rules implementing TEFRA relative to payment for anesthesiology physician services. In instituting the rules, HCFA chose a 1:4 ratio for medical direction, limiting payment to an anesthesiologist to no more than four concurrent procedures administered by CRNAs. The rules implemented seven conditions that an anesthesiologist must satisfy to obtain reimbursement for the medical direction of CRNAs (U.S. Department of Health and Human Services [USDHHS], 1983). The original TEFRA conditions are listed in Box 19-1 (USDHHS, 1983).

Over time, it has been found that the TEFRA regulations that stipulate the role of anesthesiologists in anesthesia care have served to create disruptions in the overall delivery and flow of services in the operating room settings, causing needless and costly delays. The AANA believes that changes favoring less-restrictive conditions would allow

> **BOX 19-1** Original TEFRA Conditions
>
> For each patient, the physician:
> 1. Performs a pre-anesthetic examination and evaluation.
> 2. Prescribes the anesthesia plan.
> 3. Personally participates in the most demanding procedures in the anesthesia plan including induction and emergence.
> 4. Ensures that any procedures in the anesthesia plan that he or she does not perform are performed by a qualified individual as defined in program operating instructions.
> 5. Monitors the course of anesthesia at frequent intervals.
> 6. Remains physically present and available for immediate diagnosis and treatment of emergencies.
> 7. Provides indicated post-anesthesia care.

From U.S. Department of Health and Human Services (USDHHS). (1983, March 2). Federal Register, 48, FR 8928.

more flexibility in allocation of anesthesia personnel and effect a more expedient service provided to patients. For example, if CRNAs could initiate the induction of anesthesia rather than waiting for the anesthesiologist to be physically present in the room as required by TEFRA, the surgical case flow and use of personnel could be more efficiently and effectively managed.

In the early 1990s, in the course of the Physician Payment Review Commission (PPRC) study of anesthesia payments (which was intended to examine ways to reduce anesthesia team payments in cases involving both anesthesiologists and CRNAs), government-related study groups and individual research studies were reporting the need for changes in TEFRA. The 1992 Center for Health Economics Research (CHER) report to the PPRC recommended the following: "Refinements to the TEFRA provisions should be considered in view of the reductions in payments to the anesthesia care team. In particular, opportunities for increasing the flexibility of role functions should be reviewed. Considerations should also be given to the appropriateness of promulgating specific practice standards within a payment policy" (PPRC, 1993). The CHER report went on to say that "with the implication of a capped payment, the HCFA should consider whether to review the TEFRA requirements to see if modifications of the TEFRA rules would permit greater efficiencies without decreasing the quality of care" (PPRC, 1993). Even though the federal government did not initiate efforts to revise the TEFRA conditions, PPRC's report did acknowledge that there was merit to study the issue. More important, these PPRC policy deliberations on payment for the anesthesia team led the PPRC to conclude that "the use of the anesthesia care team seems to be determined by individual preferences for that practice arrangement. There appears to be no demonstrated quality of care differences between the care provided by the solo anesthesiologist, solo CRNA, and the team." No longer could anesthesiologists argue that medical direction of CRNAs by anesthesiologists and the TEFRA conditions under which medical direction is provided represent any safer or higher standard of care than the care provided by a CRNA practicing alone or an anesthesiologist practicing alone. The final conclusion reached by PPRC on anesthesia payment represented a milestone in the recognition of anesthesia services provided by nurse anesthetists. A single payment methodology for anesthesia services was recommended by PPRC and adopted by Congress, which resulted in a policy that the payment for anesthesia services—whether provided by a CRNA-anesthesiologist team or by a solo anesthesiologist or solo CRNA—would be the same. The payment to the team would be split so that each practitioner received 50% (PPRC, 1993).

In 1997, as part of its legislative agenda, the AANA initiated a congressional lobbying effort to revise the TEFRA conditions of payment for medical direction by anesthesiologists of CRNAs. In 1998 the AANA shifted its focus from legislative strategies for revision of TEFRA to revision through the regulatory process. In a joint meeting in 1998 with the ASA, AANA, and HCFA, proposals were advanced by both AANA and ASA for revisions in the seven conditions of payment for physician medical direction. The ASA and the AANA reached consensus on a revised recommended set of medical direction requirements that are listed as proposed revisions in the aforementioned table (USDHHS, 1998a). However, it came to AANA's attention in

a publication entitled *Anesthesia Answer Book—Action Alert* (1998) that ASA had second thoughts about the agreed-on revisions and indicated that it disagreed that the groups had reached a consensus on this issue. HCFA's response to the concerns posed by the ASA membership and several state anesthesiologist societies was to retain the current requirements established in 1983 (USDHHS, 1998b). HCFA did decide that the medically directing physician must be present at induction and emergence for general anesthesia and present as indicated in anesthesia cases not involving general anesthesia (USDHHS, 1998b). HCFA announced plans to study the medical direction issue further, welcomed comments, and suggested it might propose changes in the future (USDHHS, 1998b).

AANA continues to monitor the impact of the TEFRA rules for physician reimbursement for medical direction of CRNAs on operating room efficiency, patient care, and CRNA practice through anecdotal reporting from CRNA anesthesia department managers and clinical practitioners. Because it is difficult for a health care provider organization to advocate and succeed in changing another provider's mechanism of payment, changes in the TEFRA conditions for payment have to come about incrementally as more evidence supports the problematic impact these conditions have on operating room efficiency and cost.

AANA has been able to influence certain changes in the formulation of the TEFRA conditions for physician medical direction payment and reimbursement for CRNA services in the following ways:

- Adoption of a 1:4 medical direction ratio rather than a 1:2 ratio, which ASA actively proposed and lobbied for in the formulation of the physician payment schedule in 1983 and 1984
- A published statement by HCFA that the criterion for medical direction should not be considered a quality-related standard, but a payment criterion
- Adoption of 1998 revisions that facilitate some degree of increased flexibility in practice
- A published requirement that the physician document personal and inclusive involvement in satisfying the conditions for medical direction payment

- Adoption of a 50% split in payment by the anesthesiologist and CRNA for a case as long as the ratio of medical direction does not exceed 1:4
- Adoption of a 50% split in payment between the anesthesiologist and CRNA when the medical direction is 1:1. (Before this change, the physician received 100% of the payment.)

## PHYSICIAN SUPERVISION OF CERTIFIED REGISTERED NURSE ANESTHETISTS: MEDICARE CONDITIONS OF PARTICIPATION

The current Medicare regulations require physician supervision of CRNAs as a condition for hospitals, ASCs, and critical access hospitals (CAHs) to receive Medicare payment. These regulations do not require that a CRNA be supervised by an anesthesiologist.

During the 1990s, AANA pursued a revision of these Medicare conditions of participation that would remove the physician supervision requirement for CRNAs. As of February 2002, 31 states have no physician supervision or direction requirement of CRNAs in nurse practice acts, board of nursing rules, regulations, medical practice acts, board of medicine rules, or their general equivalents. Clearly this is an indication that many states, as a matter of public policy, believe it is unnecessary to require physician supervision of CRNAs.

In December of 1997, HCFA released for comment the proposed revisions in the Medicare Conditions of Participation for Hospitals, ASCs, and CAHs, which would eliminate the requirement for physician supervision of CRNAs, deferring instead to state law. HCFA's proposal to remove the physician supervision requirement was opposed by the ASA, which expressed its opposition through lobbying the administration, conducting media campaigns, soliciting its members and the public to write to the administration and Congress, and pushing for a legislatively mandated study that, if enacted, would preempt HCFA from publishing the final rule. The ASA's main message has been that patients will die if the rule is implemented. Another frequently used argument claimed that a change in this rule would be detrimental to Medicare beneficiaries. In support of their claim, ASA conducted a survey of seniors that reportedly indicated that they were not in favor of HCFA's proposed rule change. To counter the

claims the AANA commissioned a survey of Medicare patients conducted in October 1999 by an independent research firm, Wirthlin Worldwide. The survey revealed the following: 88% of Medicare beneficiaries surveyed would be comfortable if their surgeon chose a nurse anesthetist to provide their anesthesia care; 81% surveyed preferred a nurse anesthetist or had no preference between a nurse anesthetist or physician anesthesiologist when it came to their anesthesia care; and 62% of those surveyed found it acceptable for the nurse anesthetist to not be supervised by their surgeon, but to work collaboratively with the surgeon who would be present throughout the surgery (American Association of Nurse Anesthetists, 2000).

From the time that the proposed rule was announced the AANA implemented a number of key activities to advocate its position on this supervision issue. These included, but were not limited, to the following:

- AANA representatives met with many key government personnel to advocate on behalf of CRNAs on the issue of supervision. Meetings were held with HCFA analysts, the Administrator of HCFA (Nancy-Ann Min DeParle), members of Congress and their staffs, the Secretary of Health and Human Services (Donna Shalala), staff members of the White House, the staff of the Office of Management and Budget, and others.
- As ASA's opposition to the proposed rule increased, together with the delay in HCFA's announcement of the final rule, AANA called on Senator Kent Conrad (D-ND) and Representative Jim Nussle (R-IA) to introduce legislation requiring HCFA to implement the proposed regulation related to deleting physician supervision of CRNAs in the hospital, ASC, and CAH as conditions for receiving Medicare payment.
- AANA retained outside legislative consultants to assist in the promotion of its legislative initiatives.
- AANA's public relations endeavors focused on increasing the public's awareness of the issues and advocating the position of the vital role that CRNAs play in anesthesia delivery in the country. Efforts included advertising in many news publications, including Capitol Hill newspapers and *USA Today;* assisting with media training for

AANA officers and staff to increase their effectiveness on radio programs and in interviews; and developing radio advertisements in Washington, DC to garner support for AANA's position.

■ AANA retained grassroots political action consultants to assist in gaining letters of support for the new proposed regulations from key members of Congress.

■ AANA solicited a broad base of support from the nursing organization community, national hospital associations, related health professional associations, civic organizations, individual nurses, physicians, and the general public.

These advocacy efforts yielded an extensive base of support from all sectors. AANA gained support for the proposed rule changes from the American Hospital Association; VHA, Inc.; Premier, Inc.; National Rural Health Association; Federation of American Health Systems; St. Paul Fire and Marine Insurance Company; Kaiser Permanente Central Office; California and Oregon Kaiser System; and numerous rural hospitals across the country. The list of national and health professional associations, individual nurses and physicians, and the public at large that have written letters to HCFA on this issue is extensive.

On March 9, 2000, after deliberating for more than 2 years, HCFA informed ASA and AANA that the proposed rule removing the physician supervision requirement for nurse anesthetists from the Medicare conditions of payment for hospitals, ASCs, and CAHs would be forthcoming. HCFA further indicated that the final rule would be published in the *Federal Register* in June 2000. However, it was not until January 18, 2001, that HCFA published the final rule in the *Federal Register*, removing the federal physician supervision requirement for nurse anesthetists and deferring to state law on the issue. On January 20, 2001, the incoming Bush administration announced that it was placing a 60-day blanket moratorium on all regulations published in the final days of the Clinton administration. In accordance with the moratorium, the final rule was scheduled to take effect March 18, 2001. This action was not unexpected. Every new administration takes the opportunity to review pending regulations that are not yet in effect. However, this was a bipartisan issue, with members of Congress from both parties on both sides of the issue. The AANA continued to work with the Bush administration and urged supporters on Capitol Hill to communicate with administration officials to ask that the scheduled implementation of this rule be allowed.

In reviewing HCFA's final rule and the rationale for its decision, it is evident that all of the major arguments advanced by the ASA opposition were thoroughly refuted. Examples of several conclusions that HCFA reached in its study of the supervision issue are as follows:

■ States have constitutionally and traditionally acted in matters of licensure and scope-of-practice and have not been found to be negligent in their exercise of this authority.

■ There is no research in the past 10 years that conclusively demonstrates a need for this federal requirement nor demonstrates that physician or anesthesiologist supervision makes a difference in anesthesia outcomes. HCFA stated in the final rule that studies purported by the ASA to demonstrate such findings had serious limitations and did not, in fact, support such conclusions. Furthermore, HCFA stated that it cannot agree with ASA's belief that anesthesia administration is the practice of medicine and therefore can be done only after medical school training.

■ HCFA's rule noted the safety of anesthesia today as reported in a study published by the Institute of Medicine (IOM) (IOM Committee on Quality of Health Care in America, 2000). HCFA stated that the improvements in anesthesia safety reported by IOM confirm the soundness of the approach taken in the final rule, which broadens the flexibility of states and providers to make decisions about the best way to improve standards and implement best practices.

■ The flexibility resulting from the rule change would provide increased access to services in some areas and broaden the opportunity for providers to implement professional standards of practice that improve quality of care and promote more efficacious models of care delivery for anesthesia services.

This decision by HCFA supports AANA's position that CRNAs provide safe, high-quality anesthesia care and advocates states' rights over federal government regulation, which is generally the norm in health care matters. The decision is also a giant step in enabling hospitals and ASCs to exercise more latitude in the use of anesthesia providers and improve operating room efficiency without affecting quality.

The AANA took its case on supervision to Health and Human Services Secretary Tommy Thompson in February 2001 and continued to urge the 107th Congress to leave the final regulation published by HCFA on January 18, 2001, in place. Although ASA reintroduced legislation calling for continuation of the supervision requirements pending a study on supervision, AANA continued to oppose ASA legislation and urged the Bush administration to do so as well.

On July 5, 2001, CMS (formerly HCFA) published in the *Federal Register* its new proposed rule (66 FR 35395-35399), which, if implemented, would replace the January 18 rule. The AANA identified two main issues of concern with the rule:

1. *State exemption from federal supervision requirements.* The proposed rule enables states to "opt out" of (or seek an exemption from) the federal supervision requirement for CRNAs. Hospitals, ASCs, and critical access hospitals in a particular state would be exempted from the requirement if the governor submitted a letter to CMS requesting the exemption. The letter would need to attest that the governor:
   - Consulted with the boards of medicine and nursing about issues related to access to and quality of anesthesia services in the state
   - Concluded that it is in the best interests of the state's citizens to opt out of the physician supervision requirement
   - Determined that opting out was consistent with state law
2. *Prospective anesthesia outcome study.* The proposal would have the Agency for Healthcare Research and Quality (AHRQ) design and conduct a prospective study to assess *only* CRNA practices with input from CMS, anesthesiologists, and CRNAs or, alternatively, establish a registry to monitor *only* CRNA practice.

The proposed rule was considered by AANA to be a potential political nightmare that, without appropriate modifications, would allow state medical boards to dictate how nurse anesthetists would be regulated on a state-by-state basis. In addition, the governors would be the targets of intense lobbying by organized medicine, and any exemption from supervision could be removed at any time because of this political pressure, creating a constant state of legal and professional limbo for CRNAs and the facilities they serve. In communicating with other national nursing organizations, AANA noted the negative effect this rule, as written, would have for the nursing profession. In essence, it would allow organized medicine to control the practice of nursing and foster the creation of barriers to patients' access to care provided by advanced practice nurses. In AANA's view the end result would limit competition in health care markets and restrict the public's right to high-quality care provided by nursing specialists.

AANA's response to CMS in response to the July 5 proposed rule presented the following arguments and proposals:

1. Revert to the January 18, 2001 final rule and defer to state law concerning anesthesia services regarding the issue of physician supervision of CRNAs. This was the correct approach that was also reflected in HCFA's December 19, 1997 proposed rule.
2. If CMS reverts to the January 18 rule, it should consider either a scientifically valid study comparing anesthesia outcomes of patients receiving anesthesia from unsupervised CRNAs with those receiving anesthesia from anesthesiologists personally providing the service or a monitoring effort comparing anesthesia outcomes of CRNAs before and after the removal of physician supervision requirements. If outcomes are similar, then CMS should take appropriate action to eliminate entirely the federal CRNA supervision requirement.

The AANA recommended to CMS that if it did not revert to the January 18, 2001, final rule, a number of amendments to the July 5 proposed rule should be made, which included implementing automatic waivers for all states that do not require physician supervision of CRNAs and considering either a scientifically valid study or a monitoring effort to involve both nurse anesthetists and anesthesiologists, as described in the second item in the response to CMS.

Many organizations and individuals wrote to CMS in response to the July 5 rule, requesting that it revert to the January 18, 2001 rule. For example, in August of 2001 the American Hospital Association issued to its members a regulatory advisory noting that it would continue to advocate that the administration return to the HCFA standard published in the January 18, 2001 rule.

The agency ultimately adopted a final rule November 13, 2001 (66 FR 56762), closely mirroring the July 5 proposed rule. As of July of 2005, 14 states had exercised the process authorized to opt out of the Medicare physician supervision requirement for nurse anesthetists: Alaska, Idaho, Iowa, Kansas, Minnesota, Montana, Nebraska, New Hampshire, New Mexico, North Dakota, Oregon, South Dakota, Washington, and Wisconsin. To date, the AHRQ had not undertaken the study authorized by the final rule, which the agency already had authority to undertake. However, anesthesia services continued to be delivered safely as the nurse anesthesia profession had promised, as measured by trends in nurse anesthetists' medical liability premiums to the extent that such premiums are a market proxy to measure relative risk. The largest insurer of CRNAs in the summer of 2005 announced its first premium increases since 2002 for policies effective 2006. Increases averaged 8% for the 4-year period. Premium increases in states that had opted out of the Medicare physician supervision mandate were lower, averaging 6% (Fetcho, 2005). The increases approximate the consumer price index (CPI) for the period and were considerably below medical liability premium increases reported by the medical community.

## SUMMARY

The primary impetus for seeking direct reimbursement legislation was the problem created by a new Medicare payment system that had the potential for threatening the viability of the nurse anesthesia profession. However, AANA saw a clear opportunity to seek this legislation not only as a means of correcting bad legislation but also as a means of obtaining equity in payment for the services provided by nurse anesthetists, thus creating a more equitable market

in which to promote their services as fully qualified anesthesia providers.

The AANA has learned from its experience in the political and legislative arena that politics is the use of power for change. Although politics may not always be nice or fair, it is critical that health care professionals engage in the political process. As has been illustrated in the federal policy initiatives discussed in this chapter, there are generally other forces at work to attempt to influence policy decisions that can have a detrimental impact on one's profession. Therefore the choice of whether to engage should be a simple one. The achievements won in the federal policy arena by AANA could not have been possible without the commitment and dedication of its members, who provide grassroots support; participate in local and national campaigns of elected members of Congress; provide congressional testimony; participate in public relations campaigns; write letters; make phone calls; organize communications systems; meet personally with leaders of business, industry, and government agencies; and provide donations to the political action committee, CRNA-PAC. One illustration of the strength of the AANA members' support is the fact that in December of 1999, AANA was ranked for the first time on the *Fortune* magazine list of Washington's most powerful lobbying organizations. AANA was the only nursing organization and the only nonphysician health care group association to make the list of 114 associations, labor unions, and interest groups. AANA registered at 101 out of 114 on the list of influential entities (Fortune, 1999).

However, it is very rare for a single group to be able to promote legislation or to effect major policy change. In the case of the federal supervision requirement for nurse anesthetists, networking with other groups, especially with nursing organizations, has been critical to achieving support on Capitol Hill and in communications with the executive branch. When nursing speaks with one voice, it is a formidable force. In the case of the nurse anesthetists and their supervision, many have rallied and provided support. The message to legislators has been loud and clear: Remove restrictive barriers to practice when it is in the public's interest and is sound health care policy.

## Key Points

- Federal policy dramatically affects the economics of health care professions. Federal rules raise or lower barriers to practice, and cause or remediate inefficiencies in the delivery of health care services.
- The processes by which federal policy and regulations are conceived and developed may be well understood by examination of politically difficult case studies, such as those involving the profession of nurse anesthesia.
- The federal policy achievements won by health care professions are attributable to members who commit their energy to sustained effort.

## Web Resources

**American Association of Nurse Anesthetists (AANA)**
*www.aana.com*
**American Society of Anesthesiologists (ASA)**—Newsletter (June 2005), "Montana Opt In"
*www.asahq.org/Newsletters/2005/06_05/ stateBeat06_05.html*
**Certified Registered Nurse Anesthetist (CRNA) Pass-Through Payments for Critical Access Hospitals**
*www.cms.hhs.gov/MLNMattersArticles/ downloads/MM3833.pdf*

## REFERENCES

American Association of Nurse Anesthetists. (2000). Nine out of 10 Medicare patients are comfortable with nurse anesthesia care. *Roll Call.*

American Association of Nurse Anesthetists (AANA). (1997). *Providing anesthesia into the next century.* Park Ridge, IL: AANA.

Fetcho, J. (2005). CNA requests rate increases. *AANA NewsBulletin, 59*(6), 34.

Fortune. (1999). *The Fortune magazine power list.*

Garde, J. F. (1988). A case study involving prospective payment legislation, DRGs, and certified registered nurse anesthetists. *Nursing Clinics of North America, 23*(3), 521-530.

Gunn, I. P. (1997). Nurse anesthesia. In J. J. Nagelhout & K. L. Zaglaniczny (Eds.), *Nurse anesthesia.* Philadelphia: Saunders.

Institute of Medicine (IOM) Committee on Quality of Health Care in America. (2000). In L. T. Kohn, J. Corrigan, & M. S. Donaldson (Eds.), *To err is human: Building a safer health system.* Washington, DC: National Academies Press.

Magaw, A. (2000). *A review of our fourteen thousand surgical anesthesias.* American Association of Nurse Anesthetists [AANA] press release. Park Ridge, IL: AANA.

Magaw, A. (1906). A review of over fourteen thousand surgical anesthesias. *Surgery, Gynecology & Obstetrics, 3,* 795-799.

Physician Payment Review Commission (PPRC). (1993). *PPRC report to Congress. Payments for the anesthesia care team.* Washington, DC: PPRC.

U.S. Department of Health and Human Services (USDHHS). (1983, March 2). *Federal Register, 48,* FR 8928.

U.S. Department of Health and Human Services (USDHHS). (1998a, June 5). *Federal Register, 63,* FR 30818.

U.S. Department of Health and Human Services (USDHHS). (1998b, November 2). *Federal Register, 63,* FR 58813.

U.S. Department of Health and Human Services (USDHHS). (2001a, January 18). *Federal Register, 66*(12), FR 4674.

U.S. Department of Health and Human Services (USDHHS). (2001b, July 5). *Federal Register, 66*(129), FR 35395.

U.S. Department of Health and Human Services (USDHHS). (2001c, November 13). *Federal Register, 66*(219), FR 56762.

# chapter 20

# Collective Action in the Workplace: The Role of Unions

Linda Warino*

*"That is what political and economic power is all about: having a voice, being able to shape the future."*

MADELEINE KUNIN

The health care climate of the early 2000s is one in which care is delivered—or withheld—in an atmosphere dominated by financial high stakes and mergers of health care facilities into large corporations. Hospital mergers, closures, and acquisitions have transpired at dizzying rates. Serious staffing cuts have occurred nationally, and quality nursing care is jeopardized. Retaining adequate staffing, quality of care, health and safety in the workplace, job security, and an effective voice in the changing systems demands collective action. It is imperative in this climate that nurses be aware of the tools available to initiate collective action in the workplace.

Hospitals and other health care organizations do not want nurses to organize. Just as in other industries, managers do not want nonmanagerial personnel overseeing and participating in management issues. If collective bargaining is seen as a power struggle between union and management—and in many cases that *is* how it is defined and played out— the opposing parties are seen as rivals, manipulating each other in an effort to improve and

advance their respective positions. One definition of collective bargaining in the health care sector describes these broadly defined bargaining objectives (Stern, 1982, p. 11):

1. To protect the economic position and personal welfare of the worker.
2. To protect the union's integrity as an ongoing institution.
3. To recognize the limits imposed on collective bargaining outcomes by the economic conditions of the industry and of the employer, and by the climate of opinion.

Collective action strategies can range from shared governance to union representation, and many variations exist. This chapter is not meant to be a primer on achieving or administering any specific strategy; it is meant to serve as an overview and to stimulate an interest in further exploration. Each setting will be different, depending in part on the administrative structure and more so on the beliefs and style of the chief administrative staff. These factors can change with time, and strategies should be evaluated on a regular basis.

This chapter will also discuss collective bargaining for nurses from a policy perspective. Collective bargaining is a highly political and complicated legal process, and many guidelines govern the conduct of bargaining. Further, laws vary between the public and private sectors. In the public sector, laws may differ among states, and the federal system has its own regulations. For specific details, please refer to the wide range of other resources available (see References).

---

*This is a revision of the chapter originally written by Mary Foley that appeared in prior editions of this book.

## CONTROL OF PRACTICE

Specific objectives identified by professional nurses as essential for control of their practice include the following:

- To improve the practice of professional nurses and all nursing personnel.
- To recommend ways and means to improve care.
- To make recommendations to the management of the health care facility; for example, to advise when a critical nurse staffing shortage exists.
- To identify and recommend elimination of hazards in the workplace.

Mechanisms to address practice issues within the institution derive from the nurse councils, practice committees, and other practice bodies that are established and empowered by either a governance model or a contract. At the heart of each governance model is the interaction between the group and the leadership. Group problem-solving is possible in any structure that encourages participation and has a leadership that accepts the outcome of that participation. Committees are an example of group participation. Committees can be given a specific task, such as to collect data, analyze them, and make recommendations. A committee can be representative (nonspecialist membership), comprised of individuals with specialized knowledge and direct interest in the issue at hand, or both at once. The downside of this may be a prolonged process, and a compromise that fails to address the problem at hand may not really satisfy any of the participants.

Not everyone believes that the group or collective action methods are the most effective. In fact, the Center of American Nurses (CAN), an Associate Organizational Member of the American Nurses Association (ANA), organized in 2003 to assist the individual nurse. "Workplace Advocacy is an array of services, products, and programs that support individual nurses to help them address their workplace challenges through policy research and advocacy, education, and communications" (Center for American Nurses, 2005).

## NURSE COMMITTEES

Nurse committees, assisted by experts in nursing, can advocate against dangerous nurse reductions.

In this instance, a nurse committee refers to a team that includes staff nurses who actually deliver the patient care and nursing management. It is important to note that in such a collaborative decision-making or shared governance model, the nurses must have the power to influence and affect all aspects of patient care including, but not limited to, practice, patient safety, nurse education and competency, quality improvement, product analysis, and staffing. If the committee exists merely as a rubber stamp to what the management team may have decided without this valuable input, then the committee's deliberations and output will be grossly lacking in the integral insight that only the nurse caregiver can add and the nurse buy-in that would be obtained with that input. One collective bargaining unit was quick to note that:

…despite practice-related recommendations being made to management by these groups [committees], however, management never had demonstrated it felt any obligation to accept nursing recommendations. Therefore, the CBU [collective bargaining unit] suspected shared governance was proposed as a model to merely give the appearance that the employer wanted staff input. (Budd, Warino, & Patton, 2004)

New patient-care models must undergo careful analysis. When the nurse committee and management collaboratively design and implement a practice model, both nurses and the public will be better served. When layoffs are necessary, as in true downsizing, every effort should be made to ensure safe care. The talents and expertise of nurses affected by the changes should be addressed by facilitating nurses' transitions to new areas of practice. The nurse practice committee can assist in enforcing standards and competencies in the new arenas and can participate in designing and overseeing transitional learning opportunities for displaced nurses.

## MAGNET HOSPITALS

In the 1980s, the American Academy of Nursing developed the concept of "Magnet hospitals" (American Academy of Nursing, 1983). A Magnet hospital is one that has a reputation of recruiting and retaining nurses and that welcomes staff involvement in unit and hospital decision-making in a way that positively influences practice. In 1994, the American Nurses Credentialing Center, a subsidiary of the ANA, developed the Magnet Nursing Services Recognition Program for Excellence in Nursing Services (American Nurses Credentialing Center, 2005). Based on quality indicators and standards defined in ANA's *Scope and Standards for Nurse Administrators* (ANA, 1996), the program measures qualitative and quantitative aspects of nursing services. Since 1994, nearly 200 hospitals have been awarded Magnet status, and 12% of the facilities awarded this recognition have a collective bargaining agreement with the nurses (a percentage that ranks higher than the 6% to 10% of the general population of all hospitals that are unionized [C. Hagstrom, personal communication, June 6, 2005]).

The significance of this program is its recognition that an organization that has nursing as one of its highest priorities, professionally and clinically, will succeed on many planes. The resulting "forces of magnetism" have been shown to result in lower nurse turnover, higher patient satisfaction, higher nursing satisfaction, and even fewer needle stick injuries of the nursing staff (Aiken, 1994).

## SHARED GOVERNANCE

*Shared* governance is a professional practice model defined as an arrangement of nursing staff and management that attempts to emphasize principles of participatory management in areas related to the governance and practice of nursing. Also labeled variously as *self-governance*, participatory decision-making, staff bylaws, and *decentralized* nursing services, shared governance attempts to involve practitioners in the control of their practice. Shared governance is an accountability-based governance system for professional workers (Porter-O'Grady, 1987). This model works when nursing managers and practitioners create an atmosphere of joint ownership that is based on trust and not limited by structures that restrict true professional involvement. Although shared governance requires *some* structure, it requires structure that is decision based and is constructed from the center of the workplace rather than hierarchical. Authority rests in specified processes, not in identified individuals. For this

model to succeed, every nurse in the organization must believe in it. Nursing staff participants should be elected, not hand-picked favorites. Leadership of the committees may be rotated between managers and staff to be more equitable. It is not recommended that individual nursing units attempt to initiate the model unless the entire setting is committed, because this can lead to unit elitism or isolation from other units within the same facility. In some settings, once the nursing department adopts the rules or bylaws that govern them, these rules are approved by the hospital trustees. The model can also include a labor-management decision-making forum for issues that concern support of practice, such as financial and interdepartmental conflicts.

There are some serious limitations to shared-governance models in practice. Some shared-governance models make no effort to conceal the fact that, in spite of the appearance of participation, a unilateral, managerial, decision-making authority remains in the institution. Such a practice negates the intent of *shared* governance and only further distances management from nurses. Other problems arise when the shared-governance model is used to bypass, or conflicts with, an already existing structure that has participation as a component, such as a collective bargaining agreement. Shared governance *can* exist in a unionized or non-unionized setting, but care must be taken to delineate clearly those topics to be handled by the shared-governance mechanisms and those subject to collective bargaining. For example, members of the shared-governance committee could be identified by the union, much as it selects a practice committee representing all units. Another caution with collective bargaining is the legal precedent set in the academic setting, in which faculty members became so involved in the governance structure offered by the shared-governance model that their roles became indistinguishable from those of managers. This made them ineligible for representation by collective bargaining (*Yeshiva*, 1980). And perhaps the greatest risk is lack of sustained commitment. The wisdom, courage, and patience of the managers and the staff may not survive the ups and downs of implementation.

## WORK ASSIGNMENTS

Registering an objection to an inappropriate work assignment is an important professional obligation of nurses. Institutions provide staff with an internal mechanism, known as an *incident report* or *notification report*, to communicate unexpected events or to document problems; however, these forms are protected as proprietary property of the institution, and access to these data is restricted. Nurses have also filed a form called an *assignment despite objection* or *assignment under protest* while completing an objectionable assignment. If a nurse does not object to an inappropriate assignment, she or he risks charges of abandonment (see state practice laws for details). These forms are usually filed because of concerns over inadequate staff, poorly prepared staff, high patient acuity, and unsafe practice situations. The practice committee and nursing administration can then review the circumstances leading to the protest. If there is a pattern of such protests, a long-term solution should be developed. This strategy is not unique to the unionized setting and could be successful in any setting in which the channels of communication are supportive of joint problem identification and resolution. The union environment, however, ensures a more formal follow-up.

## WHISTLEBLOWER PROTECTION

Professionals who speak out about working conditions, especially about issues of patient care, may not be protected from action by their employer. Holding a professional license may necessitate that you act as an advocate, but it will not ensure employment protection if what you say is unpopular with your employer. Such protection, known as *whistleblower* protection, is not adequately in place to protect registered nurses (RNs) who are using their professional judgment and decide to speak publicly when all other steps fail. Nationally, the ANA continues to support the inclusion of whistleblower-protection language in various pieces of legislation including the Patient Safety Act and in the ANA-endorsed version of the Patient Bill of Rights. Also, through its Nationwide State Legislative Agenda, ANA works with its state nurses association members to help advance whistleblower protection at the state level. Many states have addressed this issue

in health reform, patient protection, and nurse supportive legislation (Figures 20-1 and 20-2; *www.nursingworld.org/gova/state/2004/whistle.htm*), and as of late 2004, 20 states had enacted whistleblower protection laws, with 9 more states introducing similar legislation or regulations.

## NEW MODELS OF LABOR–MANAGEMENT RELATIONS

There is some optimism that new models of labor-management relations will evolve in the coming century. Studies have been made under the auspices of the U.S. Department of Labor, and in 1994 a report was issued by the Commission on the Future of Worker-Management Relations (U.S. Department of Labor, 1994). Underlying the report was a theme of employee participation and problem solving that could enhance workplace productivity.

A nurse-specific example of new relationships is the work done under the U.S. Department of Labor Transitional Workforce Stability Provisions. More than $200 million was appropriated for retraining and other worker adjustments to assist health care workers affected by the transition to a restructured health care delivery system. The Michigan Nurses Association, a member of the ANA, participated in a 3-year grant-funded project paid for by the Department of Labor to assist acute-care nurses in making transitions to other settings.

However, any optimism is tempered by the obstacles unions have met under the present federal government and its influence through new appointments to the National Labor Relations Board (NLRB). Rulings from the NLRB since 2001 have been less than amicable for unions looking to organize (Yager, 2004).

## CONTROL OF PRACTICE THROUGH COLLECTIVE BARGAINING

Collective bargaining agreements for nurses have traditionally been used as a means to equalize the power between management and nurses. Nurses have used contracts as a form of collective action to improve working conditions, hence care. Generally, unions in the health care setting stimulate better

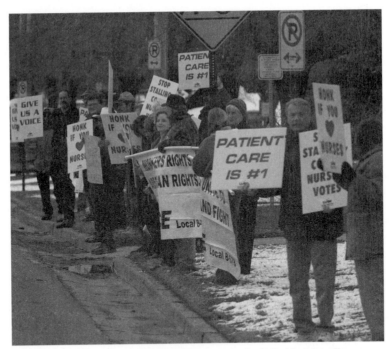

**Figure 20-1** Nurses who wanted to be organized by the United American Nurses rally outside of the Salt Lake Regional Medical Center in Utah on March 5, 2004. (Copyright Paul Montano Photographics.)

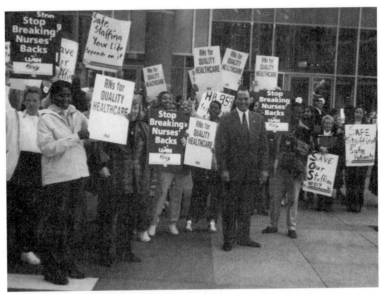

**Figure 20-2** Illinois Nurses Association members are joined by Representative Skip Saviano in a rally for safe staffing outside of the State of Illinois building on September 26, 2001.

hospital management by fostering formal, central, and consistent personnel policies with better lines of communication and lead to improvements in the workplace so that recruitment and retention become easier.

## SHOULD NURSES ORGANIZE?

In most definitions, the members of a "profession" are said to have attained expertise after a specialized education. Society grants professionals a measure of autonomy in their work in recognition of their expertise and of the value of their service to the larger community. Autonomy permits professionals to make independent judgments and decisions and to have special patient-provider relationships, such as those traditional in law and medicine. Nursing has struggled with a modified definition of *profession*. Nurses have traditionally worked as *employed professionals*—employed first by hospitals, nursing homes, and other health agencies and now by health systems. Even though nursing meets many of the other criteria of a profession (e.g., education, expertise, a value recognized by society, some autonomy in judgment, great accountability), the role of nurses as employees has compromised the patient-provider relationship. Hospitals have been organized as bureaucratic structures and have relied on hierarchical boundaries that are not congruent with the notion of a professional practice. Conflict arises when professionals believe that their professional autonomy and clinical judgment are challenged and care compromised as a result. Medicine is now facing similar conflicts, with fewer physicians in private practice and managed care plans forcing clinical decisions that erode professional autonomy. Cost containment, productivity measurements, and issues of resource utilization are the stressors that stimulate interest by health professionals in collective action. Physicians are also using collective action, including collective bargaining, to reestablish professional authority.

Nursing has also used collective bargaining to its benefit, achieving professional goals and protecting and promoting the public interest through lobbying efforts and political action. Researchers Ash and Seago (2004) illustrate this phenomenon in their work, "Do Unionized Registered Nurses Reduce AMI Mortality?" They concluded that their "study demonstrates that there is a positive relationship between patient outcomes and RN unions" (p. 19). Nurses engaged in non-union collective action face a serious limitation: They work only when all parties agree that they should. When no oversight exists to force compliance, the relationship can fail. Disappointed expectations of benevolence from an industry that was not and is not benevolent may explain why nurses have been willing to organize for collective bargaining. Nurses who support collective bargaining view it as a way to control practice by a redistribution of power within the structure of a health care organization.

What do we know about why nurses engage in collective bargaining? Two older studies suggest answers that remain relevant today. A Kansas City employee and labor relations consulting firm set out to ascertain why hospital employees and nurses join unions and how union organizers garner their support (Stickler & Velghe, 1980). The study was intended for use by hospital managers seeking to define strategies to avoid outside representation for professional nurses. Their conclusion: Hospital management widely subscribes to the myth that big powerful unions organize professional nurses, but in fact, outside unions do not organize nurses: Nurses organize themselves. They do this because administrators and nursing supervisors fail to recognize and address nurses' individual and collective needs.

Another study—this one from the University of California, Berkeley (Parlette, O'Reilly, & Bloom, 1980)—found that nurses who engage in collective bargaining do so because they believe it is the only solution to a management-employee power struggle. Parlette et al. concluded that nurses decide to unionize out of their "inability to communicate with management and their perception of authoritarian behavior on the part of management" (p. 16). The age of this study by no means diminishes its importance or accuracy, because nurses of the 2000s who are selecting collective bargaining representatives are doing so in the face of great struggles over patient-care issues with managers who appear to have lost sight of the purpose of health services.

Nursing has been unable to come to closure on the debate about whether professional nurses should organize for collective bargaining. On one side of the debate are those who want nursing to be a profession that relies on its prestige to ensure recognition. On the other side are those who view nursing as a professional or occupational group that can and should use collective action, specifically collective bargaining, to secure recognition. The disagreement has manifested itself in a variety of ways. Of particular interest is the structural change within the ANA that allowed for nurses with diametrically opposed views to continue membership with ANA while enjoying services that meet their needs. Those nurses who prefer to engage in collective bargaining now belong to the United American Nurses (UAN), Affiliate Organizational Member (AOM) of ANA. The UAN has an exclusive relationship with ANA as its only union AOM. The members have all the rights of ANA membership and enjoy a strong national union as well.

On the other hand, if nurses find a union atmosphere distasteful, they can choose to belong to the CAN, the AOM of ANA that advocates for individual nurses. They too can enjoy the whole of ANA without the union exposure.

Finally, the ANA members who value neither of the described philosophies can simply belong to ANA, taking advantage of all of its professional services without having to choose one way or the other.

The difficulties faced by RNs are acute and bode poorly for the working environment for nurses who still wish to practice in the hospital environment. Multiple surveys and publications document the stress and perceived deterioration of nurse satisfaction and, potentially, the quality of patient care.

The results of an online survey conducted by the ANA in 2000 reflect the depth of despair nurses are feeling (ANA, 2001b). One of the most discouraging findings is that 52% of nurses stated they would not recommend nursing to a relative or friend.

As the twenty-first century dawned, nurses were trying to balance an increasingly acute patient population, increasing numbers of patients per nurse, and a new stressor: mandatory overtime. Mandatory overtime was first reported in late 1999, and

by 2000 it was an epidemic. Three major strikes by state nurses associations occurred in 2000 (Worcester, Massachusetts; Nyack, New York; and Washington, DC) and one in 2001 (Youngstown, Ohio). Mandatory overtime was the primary reason for these strikes by RN collective bargaining units. RNs reject mandatory overtime for a number of reasons. It diminishes the sense of control nurses have over their work life. Nurses with families or other personal obligations found that inability to plan their work schedule added to their stress and their dissatisfaction with their work life (ANA, 2001b). From a professional practice perspective, mandatory overtime and short staffing may be contributing to the rate of medical errors documented in the Institute of Medicine report on health care errors, *To Err is Human—Building a Safer Health System* (Institute of Medicine, 1999). Also, in her study on staff nurse fatigue and patient safety, Rogers found that "the risks of making an error were significantly increased when work shifts were longer than twelve hours, when nurses worked overtime, or when they worked more than forty hours per week" (Rogers, Hwang, Aiken, & Dinges, 2004). The ANA is the lone voice recognizing these potential contributing factors and has led the way in pushing research agendas that quantify safe hours of work and how patient safety can be assured. As with the whistleblower issue, the ANA and the state nurses associations are in the lead in influencing federal and state legislative efforts to address overtime and staffing in the context of safe patient care.

A comprehensive and accurate compendium of recent changes in nursing and patient care is found in *When Care Becomes a Burden: Diminishing Access to Adequate Nursing* (Fagin, 2001), a publication funded by the Milbank Memorial Fund and edited by an esteemed nursing leader, Claire Fagin. This document, like numerous other written and spoken sources of testimony, predicts that the present hospital work environment will seriously jeopardize both recruitment and retention efforts. Attention to work environment quality will be critical to counteracting the downturn in interest in nursing as a professional choice and in retention of nurses, as many members of the current workforce age into their early and mid 50s.

Nurse health and safety have been directly affected by the restructured workplace. The combination of reduced staff, higher patient acuity, and pressure for increased productivity has led to an increase in nurse and other health worker injuries. It is important for nurse union leadership to point out the connection between practice trends and health and safety issues. Health and safety issues are potential organizing issues and appropriate subjects of bargaining.

## HISTORY OF COLLECTIVE BARGAINING IN NURSING

Nurses in the early 1900s were frustrated by their working conditions. Receiving little support from the established nursing organizations, a few thousand joined trade unions for assistance. In the 1940s, nurses in California, Ohio, and Pennsylvania were assisted in their workplaces by the ANA Constituent Member Associations (CMAs) formerly known as state nurses associations. In 1946, after considerable urging by the leaders of the state associations representing nurses, the ANA unanimously adopted a national economic security program. It was the ANA's intent to encourage the CMAs to act as the exclusive agents for nurses in the important fields of economic security and collective bargaining.

Other unions subsequently organized nurses, with more than 20 expressing an intent to solicit nurses in 1974. The competition has become more intense over the years as the stakes have gotten higher. Unions such as the Meatpackers, Paperhangers, United Food and Commercial Workers, International Longshore and Warehouse Union, Teamsters, American Federation of Teachers, United Mine Workers, Service Employees International Union (SEIU), and the American Federation of State, County and Municipal Employees (AFSCME) (all members of the American Federation of Labor-Congress of Industrial Organizations [AFL-CIO]) have competed for nurse membership among themselves and with the CMAs.

Some nurses have chosen to be organized in independent unions, unaffiliated with either an AFL-CIO union or a CMA. One well-known independent union is the Committee for the Recognition of Nursing Achievement at Stanford University in Palo Alto, California. Formed in 1964, this union has had a successful history of working closely with nursing administration to advance nursing standards and nurse recognition. Independent unions are at risk of raiding by other unions because of the difficulty and cost of providing the complex and expensive services of representation.

In the United States, the fraction of all workers represented by a labor organization is declining. Approximately 12.5% of wage and salaried workers in 2004 were unionized. This is down from 13% in 1999, 14.5% in 1996, and almost 25% in the 1970s (Union Membership and Coverage Database from the Current Population Survey, nd). As of 2003, 19.5% of all registered nurses were represented by unions, and the number is growing (United American Nurses Association). These statistics are indicative of what the Department for Professional Employees, AFL-CIO, has found overall:

These newly organized professional and related workers accounted for nearly 30% of the total number of new union members—more than 232,000—reported by 65 unions affiliated with the national AFL-CIO. This was the fastest growing occupational group within the federation, individually outpacing the transportation, manufacturing, building and construction, hospitality, and service occupations. Today, almost 50% of the AFL-CIO's membership is white collar. In fact, the professional specialty organizations now have more union members than any other occupational group. (*www.dpeaflcio.org/pdf/2003_09_risingtide.pdf*)

## WHO REPRESENTS NURSES (AND DOES IT MATTER)?

Who the bargaining representative is *does* matter to nurses. First, it is certainly going to have an effect on the public's perception of the profession. It can also determine who has the political clout in issues of legislation and regulation.

Nurses who are considering a collective bargaining agent must do some values clarification. The underlying question that must be addressed is Do nurses have identity *primarily* as nurses or as workers?

CMA collective bargaining agreements have been historically nursing-practice oriented, and their contracts are replete with references to the professional standards, codes of ethics, and professional practice committees that give nurses a voice in patient care concerns. Unions, on the other hand, are worker oriented; their expertise has been in attaining wage and benefit packages and, in some cases, advocating for health and safety issues. Yet in a paper prepared for the Albert Shanker Institute, Richard Hurd (2000) has observed that while professional associations are struggling to respond to their members' needs more like unions, many unions are attending to professional workers' needs more like professional associations.

In 1998, the ANA started to work on a two-track strategy: to explore the possibility of an affiliation with the AFL-CIO while creating a defined labor arm of the ANA. In 1999 this arm—the UAN—was created by an overwhelming vote of the delegates attending the ANA House of Delegates meeting. In 2001, the UAN became an affiliate of the AFL-CIO. In 2003, the UAN progressed from a structural unit of the ANA to an AOM with autonomy of governance and finance. This change in status also provided that the UAN would be the exclusive collective bargaining entity of the ANA. The UAN now represents nursing's voice on the AFL-CIO Executive Council. One immediate implication was a mutually respectful working relationship that ended a negative type of competition that has existed between the AFL-CIO unions and the CMAs: namely, raids (see Raids and Decertifications).

However, nurses will still have to decide whether to join the UAN or more traditional trade unions as new bargaining units are organized, because many trade unions still intend to recruit nurses, just as the UAN intends to bring more nurses into its membership.

## COLLECTIVE BARGAINING PROCESS

### ELECTING THE AGENT

When nurses decide to elect a collective bargaining representative, they are guaranteed legal protection, as all workers in the private sector are, by the National Labor Relations Act (NLRA). The employer is also ensured some protection, especially protection against disruption of the workplace during the organizing or election process. Once the nurses (or other employees) start a campaign for representation and 30% of the eligible nurses have signed cards signaling their interest in electing a representative, the employer is prohibited from engaging in certain activities defined as unfair labor practices:

- It may not fire the organizers for their union activity.
- It is prohibited from interfering with, restraining, or coercing employees who choose to organize, form, join, or assist a labor organization.
- It cannot refuse to allow dissemination of union information in the workplace.
- It cannot ignore a request for a vote of the workers for representation by the union as a collective bargaining agent.

After the campaign, a vote is conducted under the guidance of the NLRB. Other unions may enter the race at this time. A vote of 50% of those voting plus one (i.e., a simple majority) is required to select the agent.

### RAIDS AND DECERTIFICATIONS

Nurses represented by a bargaining agent have the right to drop or change (decertify) that agent by a similar campaign of signatures (30%) of the affected members, followed by a vote, again, of 50% plus one. This is an increasingly common event, particularly given the competition between trade unions and nursing unions and among trade unions themselves. When a union tries to decertify an existing union, the campaign is called a *raid*. Raids are one of the easiest ways to recruit new members, making this practice more and more attractive. It is easier and cheaper to recruit a bargaining unit that is already organized than to recruit the unorganized. Competing unions often make exaggerated promises, and the larger trade unions have resources to use on raids. Critical questions must be asked: Has the union delivered on such promises in the past? Would the services of the new bargaining agent in fact be better? Would the nurses actually be better represented?

Service Employees International Union (SEIU) believed that their services would be better and commenced an attack on the California Nurses Association (CNA). All the while, CNA was waging war on the ANA in Hawaii and in Illinois. Eventually SEIU and CNA came to an organizing agreement that allows for all the newly organized nurses to become members of CNA and all other employees to be members in SEIU. In July, 2005, however, SEIU, along with the International Brotherhood of Teamsters and the United Food and Commercial Workers, left the AFL-CIO over disagreements about a proposed new structure.

## RECOGNITION APPEALS

An employer may choose to bargain in good faith on matters concerning employee working conditions by voluntarily recognizing the bargaining agent in lieu of awaiting the outcome of an election. This may occur if the support for one union is evident and a strong majority exists. More commonly, however, the employer will appeal employee requests for representation to the NLRB. The appeal may be based on a technical distinction or definition, but the purpose behind the appeal is the desire of the employer to prevent union representation in the workplace.

During such an appeal, arguments about why, by whom, or how nurses will be represented are made before the NLRB. The net effect of the appeal may not change the outcome of the process, but it does come at a high price to the union and the nurses in staff time, resources, and often loss of focus and momentum.

## INSULATION

Early challenges to nursing unions arose when the hospitals challenged whether a state nurses association (SNA) was properly structured to be a labor union. In question was the membership of the SNAs; all RNs could belong to the association. Because RN managers could belong to the SNA, it was necessary to provide a real and substantial "insulation" of the collective bargaining program of the SNA from any potential managerial influence. This protection is required by the NLRB and prevents employers from interfering in, dominating, or discriminating in an employee's pursuit of a representative for collective bargaining. In spite of a precedent-setting case in 1979, some hospitals appealed the SNA structure, and a series of cases in the 1980s ensued. Eventually the issue was resolved successfully for the SNAs and the nurses.

Each CMA is permitted to determine its own structure for insulation and therefore there is not uniformity on how it is done. The one common factor is the expectation that it must be done. There is the structure of a collective bargaining program that is so insulated that nurse members of the CMA who are not eligible for collective bargaining would be denied the opportunity to sit on the Board of Directors for the CMA; on the other extreme is the CMA Board having oversight of the collective bargaining program despite who might sit on the Board of Directors, including managers. This variance has been the topic of many discussions and some dissension.

## UNIT DETERMINATION

Another class of challenges to nursing unions is the appeals on the issue of unit determination. When the NLRA and the subsequent 1974 amendments covering health care employees were adopted, Congress intended simultaneously to limit the number of individual bargaining units that an employer or industry would have to recognize and bargain with while allowing for distinctions among employees that may have unique issues or circumstances. Nurses have historically been organized into all-RN bargaining units because RNs were believed to have a unique "community of interest" in the way they worked within the health care system.

In 1984, a dramatic change in nurse unit determination occurred when the NLRB ruled in a case involving St. Francis Hospital (in St. Paul, Minnesota) that the nurses were no longer eligible for a distinct, all-RN bargaining unit and, instead, would have to be included in what was called an *all-professional* unit. An all-professional unit could include respiratory therapists, social workers, physical therapists, librarians, pharmacists, medical clergy, the architect, and the business officer. This determination wreaked havoc with organizing, and it coincided with the beginning of the last great national nursing shortage in the late 1980s. That shortage led to serious nurse staffing problems and working conditions that were deplorable and unsafe. As conditions worsened in hospitals, nurses all over the country were requesting organizing assistance. Despite the demand, there were very few successful elections from 1984 to 1991, mostly because of the NLRB ruling on all-professional units. First, it was difficult to organize and achieve a satisfactory election outcome among such a diverse group of health care employees. Second, though it might be possible to stimulate enough interest among employees to warrant representation, election of a single bargaining agent to represent the diverse needs of so many work classifications would be almost impossible.

The ANA and the unions representing nurses for collective bargaining decided to challenge the NLRB's decision. The major opponent in the challenge was the American Hospital Association, which worked strenuously to keep the determination in favor of the all-professional unit. After a ruling by the NLRB affirming the rights of RNs to be organized in all-RN units, the American Hospital Association challenged that ruling in a federal court and an injunction was issued. Realizing that this issue stood in the way of nurses' being represented for collective bargaining as they tried to improve working conditions and protect patient care, the ANA and the NLRB appealed the case to the Supreme Court. In May 1991, the Supreme Court confirmed that the NLRB had ruled properly and reinstated all-RN bargaining units.

## THE REGISTERED NURSE AS SUPERVISOR

Soon another employer-initiated legal strategy challenged the nursing profession and the future protection of nurses by the NLRA. In a shocking decision in May of 1994, the Supreme Court ruled that any nurse who "directs other employees" is to be classified as a supervisor and can be fired for protesting job conditions or questioning management decisions

that the nurse sees as putting the quality of patient care at risk (*NLRB v. Health Care & Retirement Corp. of America*, 1994). Nurses inevitably supervise a wide range of ancillary personnel, such as assistants, clerks, and, in the case of RNs, licensed practical/vocational nurses; it had been a 20-year policy of the NLRB that nurses' direction or assignment of others is exercised in the interest of the patient, not of the employee. The 1994 ruling overturned this policy and was a staggering setback for all nurses as they advocate for patient safety and quality in a climate of downsizing and restructuring. It is threatening to all unions, who strongly protest the "supervisory" label for nurses because it makes nurses ineligible for collective bargaining. Because of the 1994 decision and the subsequent confusion it has created, the Supreme Court instructed the NLRB to reconsider its definition of "supervisory" as it pertains to nurses and to be consistent in the use of that term throughout all industries, not treating nurses or the health care industry with any distinction. Employers have used this legal discrepancy and unsettled issue to delay or avoid bargaining with nurses. Circuit court decisions following the 1994 Supreme Court decision continued to be split on the question of RN status as employees or supervisors, so the Supreme Court considered another case in late 2000 (*NLRB v. Kentucky River Community Care Inc. et al.*, 2001). The ANA submitted an amicus curiae brief in support of the NLRB, in coordination with the four other AFL-CIO unions that represent large numbers of nurses.

The critical issue, again, revolved around the following question: When an RN exerts professional judgment in assigning and directing junior colleagues and nonprofessional assistants, are they doing so as a licensed professional or as a manager? To nurses' great disappointment, in May of 2001, the Supreme Court voted five to four to strike the NLRB interpretation of what constitutes supervisory independent judgment (ANA, 2001a). While this may further complicate which nurses will be eligible for collective bargaining, the court did note that it might be possible to distinguish employees who direct the manner of others' performance of discrete tasks from employees who direct other employees.

## JOB SECURITY OR PROFESSIONAL AND CAREER SECURITY?

The economic environment in the health care industry, coupled with rapidly advancing technological breakthroughs and a renewed interest in primary and preventive care, has dramatically shifted health care away from the inpatient hospital setting. Many nurses who previously practiced in the acute care setting have chosen to move to settings that offer a more satisfactory environment and recognize the value of the RN. In the 2000 Division of Nursing Sample Survey, the total number of nurses involved in care was found to have risen to 2.7 million RNs from 2.6 million in 1996 (Bureau of Health Professions, 2001). About 2.5 million nurses are still reported as working in nursing. Where are the 500,000 who do not report working? About 59% of nurses are now employed by acute care institutions. More acute care positions are vacant and remain vacant longer, and this trend is intensifying. Hiring incentives are commonplace, and nurses are being offered sign-on bonuses and relocation packages never seen before. Efforts to retain RNs have not had the same attention, and that is why the concept of "magnetism" and attention to the work environment are critical to keep the current expert-knowledge worker, the experienced RN, in the system. As this country's senior population grows in size and scope of health needs, inpatient censuses will remain high, and hospitals will struggle with fewer staff, busier schedules, emergency department diversions, and surgical delays.

These new paradigms have challenged nurses and their representatives to modify bargaining strategies and turn attention to maintaining the essential role of the RN in the acute care setting through bargaining agreements and workplace advocacy while simultaneously helping nurses prepare for changing settings and roles. Will nursing care be improved if we adopt fixed ratios of nurses to patients? These are professional-practice issues that continue to deserve debate and study, and which may distinguish the unions who can advocate for a profession from a traditional union. The struggle to simultaneously address current staffing shortages and safe standards of care as defined by patient load and hours of work, and to prepare to address the future nursing shortage, is a challenge for all representatives and advocates for nursing.

## Key Points

■ Collective action is an effective strategy by which RNs can achieve power in the workplace over their practice and environment equal to the level of their expertise, responsibility, and accountability.
■ There are alternative strategies to collective action for registered nurses who find the concept of union not satisfactory to meet their needs.
■ Despite the noted value of collective action, there are continual external and internal challenges for registered nurses who seek to organize or continue to be represented for collective action.

## Web Resources

**AFL-CIO**
*www.AFLCIO.ORG*
**Michigan Nurses Association's Nurse Staffing Initiative**
*www.minurses.org/spc/Legislative%20Hearings %20April%202005.htm*
**National Labor Relations Board**
*www.NLRB.gov*
**United American Nurses**
*www.UANNURSE.org*

### REFERENCES

Aiken, L. (1994). Lower Medicare mortality among a set of hospitals known for good nursing care. *Medical Care, 32*(8), 771-787.

American Academy of Nursing. (1983). *Magnet hospitals: Attraction and retention of professional nurses.* Washington, DC: American Nurses Association.

American Nurses Association (ANA). (1996). *Scope and standards for nurse administrators.* Washington, DC: ANA.

American Nurses Association (ANA). (2001a). ANA not dissuaded by Supreme Court decision on "supervisors." *The American Nurse, 33*(4), 1-2.

American Nurses Association (ANA). (2001b). ANA poll: RNs say poor working conditions affect care. *The American Nurse, 33*(2), 1-2.

American Nurses Credentialing Center. (2005). Magnet database. Retrieved September 6, 2005, from *www.nursecredentialing. org/magnet/facilities.html*.

Ash, M., & Seago, J. A. (2004). The effect of registered nurses' unions on heart-attack mortality. *Industrial and Labor Relations Review, 57*(3), 422-442.

Budd, K., Warino, L., & Patton, M. (2004, January 31). Traditional and non-traditional collective bargaining: Strategies to improve the patient care environment. *Online Journal of Issues in Nursing, 9*(1), Manuscript 5. Retrieved September 8, 2006, from *www.nursingworld.org/ojin/topic23/tpc23_5.htm*.

Bureau of Health Professions. (2001). *The registered nurse population*. Washington, DC: Health Resources and Services Administration.

Center for American Nurses. (2005). Retrieved July 13, 2005, from *www.centerforamericannurses.org/*.

Fagin, C. (2001). *When care becomes a burden: Diminishing access to adequate nursing*. New York: Milbank Memorial Fund.

Hurd, R. (2000, Summer). Professional workers, unions, and associations: Affinities and antipathies. Background paper prepared for Seminar on Unions Organizing Professionals, Albert Shanker Institute, New York.

Institute of Medicine. (1999). *To err is human—Building a safer health system*. Washington, DC: National Academy Press.

Lutz, S. (1994). Let's make a deal: Health care mergers, acquisitions take place at a dizzying pace. *Modern Healthcare, 24*(51), 47-50.

NLRB v. Health Care & Retirement Corp. of America, 114 U.S. 1778 (1994).

NLRB v. Kentucky River Community Care Inc. et al., 121 U.S. 1861 (2001).

Parlette, G. N., O'Reilly, C. A., & Bloom, J. R. (1980). The nurse and the union. *Hospital Forum, 23*(6), 16-17.

Porter-O'Grady, T. (1987). Shared governance and new organizational models. *Nursing Economics, 5*(6), 281-287.

Rogers, A., Hwang, W., Aiken, L., & Dinges, D. (2004). The working hours of hospital staff nurses and patient safety. *Health Affairs, 23*(4), 202-212.

Stern, E. (1982). Collective bargaining: A means of conflict resolution. *Nursing Administration, 6*(2), 9-20.

Stickler, F. B., & Velghe, J. C. (1980). Why nurses join unions. *Hospital Forum, 23*(2), 14-15.

Union Membership and Coverage Database from the Current Population Survey. (nd). Retrieved July 25, 2006, from *www.trinity.edu/bhirsch/unionstats*.

United American Nurses. (2005). Registered nurse unionization. Retrieved on July 25, 2006, from *www.uannurse.org/research/pdfs/unionization.pdf*.

U.S. Department of Labor. (1994, May). *Health care workforce transition*. Washington, DC: U.S. Department of Labor.

Yager, D. (2004, November 29). NLRB issues major rulings on temporary agency workers, disciplinary rules. *www.nlrbwatch.com/news/news_story.asp?ID=1892*.

Yeshiva, supra, 103 LRRM at 2553 (1980).

# *Taking Action*  Kathryn Hall

## Non-Union Collective Action in Nursing

*"Thoughts are the seed of action."*
RALPH WALDO EMERSON

### NON-UNION COLLECTIVE ACTION

Nurses work in a variety of settings. In some settings where nurses are represented by a collective bargaining contract, a labor union representing those nurses works out an employment contract with the employer that specifies many aspects of the nurses' employment, such as management and payment of overtime hours worked or under what conditions a nurse can be reassigned. In the majority of health care work settings, nurses are not represented by a labor union and the conditions of their employment are not predetermined by a collective bargaining contract. The work of nurses in these non-union settings is governed by employer-based policies and procedures or by state law and regulations. Nurses in non-union settings must advocate for themselves to make changes in the rules governing their employment.

There are many more nurses working in health care not represented by collective bargaining contracts than nurses who are. In 2004, there were 2,432,286 working registered nurses in the United States, 406,779 of whom were dues-paying members of a union with another 49,036 represented under collective bargaining contracts (Hirsch & Macpherson, 2003). Based on these figures, approximately 82% of registered nurses in the United States are not represented by a collective bargaining contract. The challenges, however, that today's nurses face in the workplace—regardless of whether a contract is in place—are very much the same: workplace safety, patient safety, and the work environment. It is the manner in which they address the issues and challenges that differs.

Non-union nurses must be able to effect change in their work settings that make the work environment safer and more appealing to nursing staff. They must also be able to effect change that will improve the safety and quality of patient care. Nurses and the patients they care for are inseparably linked. Outside of a bargaining contract, these nurses use a powerful tool for themselves that all nurses have long used in protecting the best interest for patients, that is, advocacy.

In recent years, the delivery of health care has undergone incredible change in the way services are reimbursed, in the use of life-extending and life-saving technology and in the availability of licensed staff to care for patients. A nursing shortage unlike cyclical shortages of the past has further stressed an already stressed health care delivery system. Nurses are being faced with caring for more complex, more critically ill patients, learning the use of more advanced technology, and having fewer staff with whom to share the workload. These things have frustrated nurses and forced them to use collective action to influence their work environments. The 2004 Institute of Medicine Report, *Keeping Patients Safe, Transforming the Work Environment of Nurses,* documented the many challenges nurses face. This report and other recent research have provided important tools to nurses for workplace advocacy.

## THE RIGHTS AND RESPONSIBILITIES OF THE NURSE

Every nurse in the United States practices under the guidance of a nurse practice act (NPA). While a state's practice act is designed to offer protections to the public by assuring safe and competent care by nurses, it also outlines the specific rights and

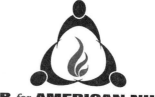

Center for American Nurses logo.

responsibilities of the nurse. Currently each state has its individual practice act and while many laws governing practice may be similar, they are not the same. It is very important that nurses review the practice acts within the states in which they practice to make sure they understand their rights and responsibilities for practice. Only nurses holding a license have the legal right to practice nursing or to delegate nursing acts. The extent to which a nurse may do this is spelled out in the NPA. When a license is issued, the nurse accepts the responsibility and accountability to practice safely and competently. Every nurse must be responsible for knowing his or her competencies and being able to communicate them to a coworker or supervisor. Understanding the law and one's own competencies allows the nurse to responsibly negotiate a work assignment. Whenever a nurse accepts assignments that are beyond his or her competencies, or when the nurse fails to meet accepted standards of practice, that individual may be disciplined by the board of nursing.

If nurses know the parameters of the NPA and within a unit or employment setting are being asked to work beyond their competencies, without the support of appropriate education and supervision, those nurses may advocate for themselves using state law governing their practice to guide them. Nurses in some states have put together an advocacy framework by jointly working with employers in their states, their board of nursing, nurse executive groups, and others to develop guidelines based on state law that more clearly spell out the responsibilities of the individual nurse, nursing supervisors, and employers in the critical areas of giving, accepting, or rejecting work assignments. Such frameworks help to hold everyone accountable for their individual practice and result in better patient care. For example, the Ohio Board of Nursing worked with nurses statewide to clarify the process of delegation of nursing acts to unlicensed assistive personnel. Their work helped guide registered nurses in delegating nursing functions based on the condition of the patient and helped to clarify the role of the unlicensed person.

Decision trees are another tool that has been developed to assist nurses in both accepting work assignments and also in their important role in delegating nursing tasks. A decision tree is a tool that guides the thought process of an individual to making a correct decision. It is designed to pose a question to which an individual must answer yes or no. The answer will then guide the individual to another level of the decision process. For example, *"Is the work assignment permitted by the state Nurse Practice Act?" If yes the nurse would proceed; if not then the nurse should stop and either not accept or delegate an assignment.* Often it is in the area of reasonability of assignments where conflict between nurses and their employers arise. Again, such decision trees must be anchored in the law governing nursing practice. Decision trees provide a logical sequence of questions that assist the nurse and/or nurse supervisor in making assignments or delegating tasks that will support the right of the patient to receive safe quality nursing care (Figure 20-3). Several states have developed decision trees that have become useful tools for nurses. The delegation work done by the Ohio Board of Nursing resulted in a *Decision Tree for Delegation.*

It is important for nurses to realize that while the NPA governs nursing practice, nurses can influence the NPA legislatively. The NPA is essentially a state law and laws can be changed through collective action either in whole or in part. Existing state statute can be modified to put in place elements that will go further to protect the practicing nurse. For example, in Maryland, where there was a concern about supervisors giving assignments that were outside of the scope of practice for some nurses, nurses worked together to put into place a regulation that holds a supervisor accountable if an inappropriate assignment is given. This was supported by employers because it was important to them in ensuring patient safety that assignments be appropriate because each group has the same responsibility to safe quality care. Many states who do not have nurses organized in collective bargaining or have only a small percentage of nurses represented by contracts often work legislatively to ensure reasonable protections for nurses. Much of the time this type of work is spearheaded by the states' nursing associations.

## WORKPLACE SAFETY

Much of the time employers will dictate policy and procedure related to ensuring safety in the workplace, but often policy is nonexistent or not enforced and nurses find themselves in situations that compromise their own personal safety and well-being. Some of the larger areas of concern around workplace safety are needlesticks, violence, and environmental hazards. How can nurses influence the workplace to put policies and procedures in place to make the work environment safer?

Transmission of blood borne pathogens, AIDS, and the impact on workplace policies have been concerns of nurses since the early 1980s. The American Nurses Association's (ANA) House of Delegates supported resolutions protecting nurses in 1988 and has continued to work in this area. The work of the ANA helped to put into place written exposure control programs, implementation of safe devices for patient care areas such as the needleless or shielded-needle IV line, and appropriate postexposure treatment, all of which were key to the passage of the Needlestick Safety and Prevention Act (PL 106-430), which became law in November 2000 (Wilburn, 2001). However, even with all of the work nationally through the ANA, Congress, the Occupational Safety and Health Administration (OSHA), and the Centers for Disease Control (CDC), nurses in some states are still struggling with many of the related issues to exposure to blood borne pathogens at a state level and in their workplaces. One of these issues is providing a nurse or health care worker with the HIV status of the source patient. This type of issue is one that is tied to state law, and not even a collective bargaining contract can help the nurse in this instance. The only way to make this level of support available to the nurse and others affected is to use collective

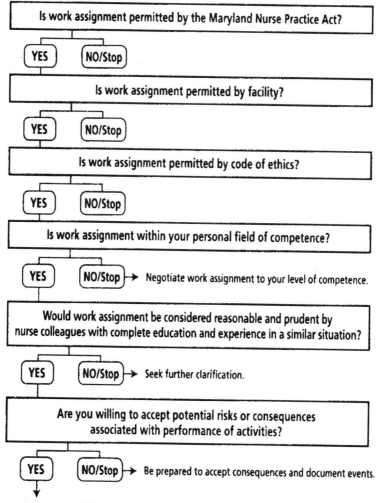

**Figure 20-3** Decision tree for registered nurse/licensed practical nurse work assignment. (From *Giving, accepting or rejecting a work assignment: A guide for nurses.* [1999]. Maryland Nurses Foundation.)

action to change state law. One of the most effective workplace advocacy tools is coalition building and collaboration. Nurses must first recognize their own power to influence change and then use their keen collaboration skills to build coalitions with other groups to make change happen. As a result of such efforts, states around the country are passing better laws that allow nurses and other providers—including emergency medical personnel, firefighters, and police—to have access to critical information

that directly affects their health. In those instances where employers support their staff to move this type of agenda, workplace allegiance is strengthened.

There are other areas where collective action may not be in lobbying to change state law but in changing existing procedures or policy within an employment area. Nurses can be successful in enhancing or changing policies or procedures by engaging themselves in decision-making committees or task forces. It appears that when a nurse is an active participant in a decision-making committee, the outcomes of that committee are better not only for the nurse but also for the institution. Often nurses do not recognize or appreciate the wealth of knowledge they have that is relevant to key decision-making in the facilities in which they work. In almost every area, from patient care to purchasing to pest management, nurses are important in helping to ensure the safety of both health care providers and patients. An example is in the area of safe patient handling. Lifting and moving patients are risky for both nurses and patients. While some professions have had lift policies defining parameters of weight to be safely lifted, nurses for centuries have moved and lifted patients of all sizes and weights. Between 1994 and 2000, nursing occupations continued to have one of the highest rates of work-related back problems, with nursing aides second and truck drivers third at risk for musculoskeletal injuries (Nelson et al., 2003). Such injuries could result in patient injury, time lost from work, need for extended medical care, and all the related costs. Patient lift devices are expensive, and time for educational sessions on lifting techniques for staff also is costly; however, nurses have done much of the work to influence both of these areas by involving themselves in educating employers and by showing the cost-benefit ratio.

In fall of 2003, the ANA, as part of their workplace focus, launched a "Handle With Care" ergonomics campaign. Collective action works best when it is based on solid data. Most often, nurses "know" what works best and what does not work best, but they fall short in providing objective documentation of that knowledge. Such objective data can support nurses in their collective action and can bring important changes such as no-lift policies to their workplace.

## THE CENTER FOR AMERICAN NURSES

The Center for American Nurses provides non–collective bargaining workplace advocacy solutions for registered nurses. The Center is an independent affiliate of the ANA established as the non–collective bargaining Associate Organizational Member by action of the ANA House of Delegates in 2003. It works to promote through its membership non-union collective action by supporting nurses in

> ### The Center for American Nurses
>
> The Center for American Nurses was established in 2003 to support the workplace advocacy efforts of American nurses. The Center is an organizational member of the ANA. Workplace advocacy is a wide variety of services, products and programs that support nurses as they address challenges in their workplaces through policy research, advocacy, and education.

their personal and professional growth and development in the practice setting in an effort to promote a positive work-related experience. The Center works to provide education to nurses on workplace issues, promote and provide leadership and mentoring in the workplace environment and to conduct, evaluate, and support workplace-related research.

The Center evolved from the collective action of a handful of state nurses associations' interest to offer a non-union focus within ANA. These efforts grew to involve more than half of the constituent members of ANA and in June 1999, the ANA House of Delegates charged a task force to develop strategies and recommendations to ensure that nurses who were not represented by collective bargaining have access to meaningful workplace advocacy strategies. The next year in 2000, the ANA House of Delegates voted overwhelmingly in support of a bylaws amendment that created The Commission on Workplace Advocacy. Three years later, in 2003, the Center for American Nurses was established and now provides a national organization for nurses not under collective bargaining contracts to obtain collective action tools to effect change in their individual work environments. In August 2003, the Center for American Nurses was incorporated as a professional association.

The Center offers workforce advocacy tools, services and strategies designed to make nurses their own best advocates in their practice environments. Its mission is to create a community of nursing organizations that serve individual, non-union nurses by providing programs, tools and policies that address challenges and opportunities in their practice environments (Center for American Nurses, 2006).

In 2005, the Center identified several key issues and related strategic objectives. Patient safety is one of the key issues where The Center plans to rapidly disseminate research findings and their meaning for working nurses. From the Institute of Medicine work, "Keeping Patients Safe, Transforming the Work Environment of Nurses," the Center prepared a 12-page call-to-action booklet for nurses outlining steps for workplace improvements in fixing error-prone work designs, maximizing workforce capacity, instilling and sustaining a culture of safety, and enhancing leadership management (Greiner, 2004). Appropriate staffing is another focus of the Center with special emphasis on the mature nurse and strategies for keeping experienced nurses in the workforce. The Mature Nurses Project was launched in 2003, when approximately 3500 nurses completed an online survey. This survey supported existing data that large numbers of experienced nurses were approaching retirement or had plans to leave nursing. The interest of The Center was to keep this experienced workforce at the bedside and to identify the support and technology that employers would need to put into place to accomplish this goal. A monograph outlining best practices for keeping the mature nursing workforce in patient care was prepared to offer ideas to others facing workforce challenges. A stakeholders roundtable was held in the summer of 2005 to discuss the challenges previously identified through the 2003 survey and to begin to develop solutions. The Center sought and received a designation of the roundtable as an independent agency agenda event under the auspices of the 2005 White House Conference on Aging. As a result of this designation, it is expected that solutions identified at this meeting will be incorporated into the policy recommendations provided to participants of the White House Conference. It is hoped that state demonstration projects will roll out in 2006. Additionally, The Center is preparing resources and tools to assist the nurse with managing conflict, persuasion and influence, and non-union negotiating strategies all directed toward improving the nurse's work environment. The Center hopes to develop rapid response systems to get pertinent information into the hands of individual nurses and their employers.

## Lessons Learned

- There are many more nurses working in health care not represented by collective bargaining contracts than nurses who are.
- The work of nurses in these non-union settings is governed by employer-based policies and procedures or by state law and regulations.
- The Center for American Nurses, an independent affiliate of the ANA, promotes non-union collective action by supporting nurses in their personal and professional growth and development in the practice setting in an effort to promote a positive work-related experience.

## Web Resources

**Center for American Nurses**
*www.centerforamericannurses.org*
**National Labor Relations Board**
*www.nlrb.gov*
**U.S. Department of Labor**
*www.dol.gov*

## REFERENCES

Center for American Nurses. (2006). About us/mission. Retrieved February 27, 2006 from *www.centerforamericannurses/can.about/mission/htm*.

Greiner, A. (2004). *The nation's quality problem and why nurses must step up to the plate.* Silver Spring, MD: Center for American Nurses.

Hirsch, B. T., & Macpherson, D. A. (2003, January). Union membership and coverage database from the Current Population Survey: Note. *Industrial and Labor Relations Review, 56*(2). Retrieved January 30, 2006, from *www.trinity.edu/bhirsch/unionstats/UnionStats.pdf*.

Maryland Nurses Foundation. (1999). Giving, accepting, or rejecting a work assignment: A guide for nurses, legal/ethical considerations. Retrieved January 30, 2006, from *www.mbon.org//practice/assignments.pdf*.

Nelson, A., Owen, B., Lloyd, J. D., Fragala, G., Matz, M., Amato, M., et al. (2003). Safe patient handling & movement. *American Journal of Nursing 103*(3), 32-43.

Wilburn, S. (2001, March). Know your rights: Ensuring your employer's compliance with federal needlestick law. *American Journal of Nursing, 101*(3), 90.

# chapter 21

# A Political Minefield: Conducting Nursing Research

Dorothy Brooten, JoAnne M. Youngblut, Deborah Donahue, & Victoria Menzies

*"Research is removed from politics—it is pure and almost holy."*

A Physician Quoted by Dorothy Brooten (1984)

*"Not hardly!"*

The Authors (2006)

Very few scientists are able to isolate themselves from the outside world to conduct their research and avoid political influences that affect the work. For those whose research involves patients, providers, health care delivery systems, and academia, politics is an ever-present part of the work. It influences all aspects of research, from the very definition of what constitutes nursing research to the choice of a topic to the dissemination of results.

## WHAT CONSTITUTES NURSING RESEARCH?

Debate on what constitutes nursing research has been going on for some time. Proponents of nursing history, for example, argue for inclusion of historical research in the definition of nursing research and in the funding mechanisms of the National Institutes of Health (NIH), especially of the National Institute of Nursing Research (NINR). Proponents of educational research—research into the most effective teaching methods, how students best learn, and so on—argue forcefully for placing such

research under the rubric of nursing science. Opponents, who view nursing as a practice discipline, argue that nursing research must build nursing knowledge for the improvement of care to patients. And indeed, the NINR's mission statement notes that it

*supports clinical and basic research to establish a scientific basis for the care of individuals across the life span—from management of patients during illness and recovery to the reduction of risks for disease and disability, the promotion of healthy lifestyles, promoting quality of life in those with chronic illness, and care for individuals at the end of life. (NINR, 2005)*

While debate continues over what constitutes nursing research, there are considerations and potential political problems inherent in each phase of the research process, beginning with choice of a research area.

## CHOICE OF RESEARCH AREA

Most researchers consider a number of factors when choosing a research area: importance or significance, scope, cost, and potential yield. The choice of research area also has potential political ramifications for the researcher's professional career, the institution in which the researcher works, the researcher's profession, and the availability of funding for the research, in addition to broader societal implications.

## INDIVIDUAL FIT

Choice of a research topic can have a long-term yield as well as potential political consequences for the researcher. Factors to consider include whether the research is important to the researcher, the organization, and society; whether it is timely now and when completed; whether it is a career enhancer that can increase professional contacts with key individuals or groups; and whether it is fundable and will lead to further studies.

In some ways, the selection of a topic is a personal statement. The choice may express the researcher's philosophy, personality characteristics, and style. Some individuals are conservative and choose relatively safe studies over which they have maximum control. Risk-taking individuals often choose topics that challenge the status quo and conventional wisdom, thus placing them in the spotlight or isolating them from the mainstream of colleagues and support (Browne, 2001; Cody & Mitchell, 2002). Others focus on the abstractions of philosophical inquiry (Fawcett, Watson, Neuman, Hinton Walker, & Fitzpatrick, 2001). Some researchers prefer to study a narrow area in depth, whereas others study broader areas in less depth. In each case, the choice of topic in some ways reflects researchers' perspectives, personality, and values.

## INSTITUTIONAL FIT

The potential fit of the research area with the institution is very important. If the research is in keeping with the stated mission and goals of the organization, it can promote the institution's image, improve care and the delivery of its services, or reduce the costs of providing those services, improve relationships among disciplines, and improve relationships between the organization and the community. Research in these directions is likely to be supported, not blocked.

In academic settings, individual schools of nursing are increasingly known for their lead in specific research areas (e.g., elder care, chronic illness, women's health, cardiac risk reduction in children, health outcomes research). Faculty recruitment for these areas and informal pressure on current faculty to fit their research within them can be substantial and can have benefits or consequences for faculty promotion and retention. A school's research focus also changes as groups of investigators move to other institutions or progress to other areas of research. In addition, what research is needed for the discipline also changes over time. In general, progression from development of grand theories of nursing to middle-range theories with more tangible application to nursing practice has occurred over several decades. What appeared to be a singular focus on physiologic research in many institutions has progressed to recognition of the need for behavioral research and research that incorporates both of these types of research.

**Potential Political Problems.**  Research topics at odds with institutional philosophy, mission, or informal priorities are not likely to be facilitated and may even be stopped because of institutional disapproval. For example, it is unlikely that a Catholic institution will provide support for work on abortifacients. Other examples may be less obvious. For instance, a study of the feasibility of earlier discharge of low-birth-weight infants may be received differently, depending on the institution. If the payer mix for the care of low-birth-weight infants is such that longer hospitalization is revenue-generating for a particular institution, the proposed research is not likely to receive much support from that institution. Alternatively, if the hospital's costs of providing care to this group exceed the charges for which it can be reimbursed, the institution is likely to support the work.

## FIT WITH THE PROFESSION AND SOCIETY

The choice of a research topic also has import for the profession and society. Research can improve health and nursing's image with the public or with policymakers, add to nursing's knowledge base, provide data on the cost-effectiveness of nursing services, and help increase future funding for nursing. Research that fits with regional or national funding or health care priorities will have greater potential yield for the profession. Alternately, the choice of a research topic can have a divisive effect on the profession. For example, studies that pit nurses against physicians rather than promote nurses and physicians working as a team can waste research energy and resources that might be better spent on ways to improve patient care.

Choice of a research area has implications also on the national scene. In 1999, Congress started a 5-year plan to double the budget of NIH in the hope that it would lead to new treatments for some of the nation's most serious diseases. The plan also aimed to distribute the money to a greater number of academic research universities and to increase funding for younger investigators. While the infusion of money increased the number of NIH research awards, the grants were still concentrated among established researchers and among a small number of the most elite research universities (Brainard, 2004e).

In addition, there has been much criticism about the focus of the awarded grants. Senator Tom Harkin, one of NIH's strongest supporters, commented, "There is a reason it's the National Institutes of Health and not the National Institutes of Science" (quoted in Brainard, 2004e). He and others are proponents of translational rather than basic research as the main focus of research at NIH. While this group understands the contribution of basic research, they want the research at NIH to "help us lead healthier lives." Others have criticized the awarding of grants focused on sexuality and funding of research centers and cooperative agreements.

E. Fuller Torrey, a long-standing critic of funding at the National Institute of Mental Health (NIMH), has criticized that institute's funding of projects, such as the examination of webpages set up by college students and objects displayed in their dorm rooms to learn about how they express their identities. He argues that practitioners and researchers in psychiatry are overly interested in treating the problems of relatively well-adjusted people at the expense of those suffering from particular serious and debilitating mental illness. He has noted that the Institute's priorities are skewed toward studies of behavior and cognition and it has become a "jobs program" for academic psychologists (Brainard, 2004c). He and others want the NIMH's research priorities to focus on improving clinical treatments and care of those with major mental health problems.

The Bush administration began evaluating federal programs for their progress toward their goals. The Government Performance and Results Act took effect in 2000. Low-scoring programs could have their funding reduced. For research programs, there is concern that examiners understand the time for research results to be realized and for the products of research to be ready for use in clinical care (Brainard, 2003). In addition, while the majority of federally funded research undergoes peer review for funding, in 2003 for example, more than $2 billion in congressional earmarks was awarded without competition.

## FUNDING

Much research requires funding. Where to apply for funding is an important consideration for researchers. Some of the issues to be addressed include What is a likely funding source, and are there politics involved in securing funding from that source? Will there be political ramifications of one or another level of indirect cost recovery (i.e., overhead, or costs above those incurred to directly conduct the study) on the grant? Will the investigator or the division or department receive any of the indirect cost recovery?

Federal funding, such as that from the NIH, carries substantially greater indirect cost recovery (now called Facilities and Administration by federal agencies) than do most private sources. Federal indirect cost recovery ranges from 40% to 65% of the money needed to actually do the work (i.e., direct costs) and is additional to it. Thus, a grant of $100,000 granted to an institution that has negotiated an indirect cost recovery rate of 55% actually costs the funding agency $155,000. This $55,000 indirect cost recovery is for the institution's maintenance of its libraries, research space, research facilities, and so forth. Although the indirect cost recovery on federal grants is continuously under review, federally funded research grants still carry much higher indirect cost recovery than do privately funded research grants or training grants, for which the rate is generally around 8% to 10%.

Some institutions and schools are reluctant to allow investigators to seek private research funding because of the small indirect cost recovery. The cost of providing the research space and support that investigators need may far exceed the indirect cost recovery provided by such grants. If private funding is needed, the investigator's next step may be to investigate the unpublished priorities and politics of the funding agency. This is usually done through informal networking and contacts.

Managed care has affected research funding, especially for clinical research. Academic medical centers for many years supported clinical research with the income generated by medical faculty practices. In addition, some clinical research costs (e.g., for tests and medications) were underwritten as patient care costs. However, managed care organizations have refused to pay such research-related costs and have forced academic medical centers to compete in the marketplace by lowering their costs for providing patient care. This has reduced both revenue for medical clinical research and the time physicians have to conduct clinical research, as physicians are forced to increase clinical practice time to maintain the same income level as before the incursion of managed care (Mechanic & Dobson, 1996).

Yet managed care may favor nursing research, and for several reasons. First, far less research conducted by nurses has been subsidized through clinical practice and patient care costs. Second, managed care organizations are interested in and supportive of research whose findings can be applied immediately to patient care. They are far less interested in basic research with findings that will benefit patients in future decades. Because patients remain in managed care plans for an average of 2 years, managed care executives are interested in findings that provide a market edge and can be used before enrollees change plans. Third, administrators of managed care plans are interested in research that prevents illness and minimizes disability, a strength of nursing research (Brooten, 1997).

## POTENTIAL POLITICAL PROBLEMS

Currently, there are a number of funding issues at the nation's largest funder of health research, NIH. They include the funding of some types of research, setting of research priorities, and the yield from investments in research over the past several decades.

One area of research under question has been research on sexual practices (Suplee, 1991). The dean of social sciences at the University of Chicago was notified that researchers at his institution had been awarded more than $1 million in federal funding to study the social patterns that govern the choice of sexual partners among adults. Several weeks later, he was informed that the funding had been delayed indefinitely because NIH grant officials were unwilling to submit the proposal request for review to the parent agency, the U.S. Department of Health and Human Services. A few years previously the same team of researchers, at the request of the federal government, had designed a major national survey of sexual behavior to provide data needed by public health officials to understand the spread of acquired immunodeficiency syndrome (AIDS) and other sexually transmitted diseases. The House Appropriations Committee killed funding for that program some months later, citing its controversial aspects (Suplee, 1991). Congressional interests and influence thus have a clear and direct effect on the direction of, and financial support for, research.

Special interest groups have a direct effect on research funding. Debate on the use of fetal tissue in research has been ongoing between anti-abortion activists, legislators who support them, and researchers. The area of stem cell research is a major focus. Stem cell research holds promise of finding treatments and cures for several diseases, including heart disease, diabetes, and Parkinson's disease. Stem cells are obtained from human embryos and can also be obtained from adults and umbilical cords. The Bush administration's policy prevents taxpayer dollars from being used to destroy human embryos. Opponents of stem cell research say the destruction of human embryos is akin to abortion and the moral equivalent of murder (Hebel, 2004). Supporters of the research point out that embryos donated from in vitro fertilization clinics would otherwise be destroyed or frozen in limbo (Brainard, 2004d). Korean investigators have now harvested stem cells from cloned human embryos (Monastersky, 2004). Clearly, the research with stem cells is proceeding. In 2004, Governor Schwartzenegger of California, signed a bill for $3 billion in state funds to be used over 10 years to advance stem cell research in the state's universities and hospitals (Brainard, 2004b). Some other states subsequently also pursued legislation to support stem cell research.

Following the September 11, 2001, attack and subsequent anthrax letter attacks, the Bush administration began investing large amounts of money in defenses against weaponizable pathogens such as anthrax, plague, botulism, and Eboli hemorrhagic fever. While the investments have brought money to colleges and universities, it has also required greater investments in the security of facilities, in personnel, and in project documentation. Some academic institutions with such projects have required laboratories working with select agents to hire full-time biosecurity officers to ensure compliance with the complex rules (Tucker, 2004). The U.S. Department of Defense now may require university laboratories with military-sponsored projects to obtain special licenses to employ foreign scholars. This policy came in response to an audit by the inspector general that found that some universities were unwittingly granting foreign researchers access to unclassified but sensitive technologies (Field, 2004a).

The winning of such projects can bring further criticism. Boston University won a national competition and $178 million from NIH to establish a biocontainment laboratory. The University has received severe criticism from the community, academics, and others over its plan to locate the laboratory in the heart of Boston. A professor from the Harvard School of Public Health warned of the real and potentially catastrophic risks to the health and safety of the people in the local and surrounding communities. Others comment that the lab represents the growing militarization of public health. Still others complain that the lab and similar bioterrorism facilities are draining money and talent from more pressing public health problems such as AIDS, malaria, and tuberculosis (Field, 2004b; Rosenstock & Lee, 2002).

Even if a study can be conducted without funding, the researcher may experience pressure to have it funded anyway. The motive may be to secure extra money for the institution or division, to use the funded research to improve the organization's image or ranking, or to establish the researcher's funding track record (Meleis, 2001). Conducting funded

pilot work also may be necessary to establish credibility to receive full-scale funding. In settings where senior faculty have not received funding for research, there may be pressure to *not* pursue funding, or disincentives when funding is received. Senior faculty, in this instance, may be threatened by the research funding successes of more junior colleagues as well as perceive pressure to increase their own research funding and productivity. As senior faculty, a greater level of funding and productivity is expected, and junior faculty successes add to the expectations in these areas for the more senior faculty.

Not all researchers approach the issue of funding in the same way. Research purists are heavily invested in a line of research—so invested that they will not change areas, no matter what, even when there are funds available to conduct the work. The work may thus never really flourish. Opportunistic researchers will conduct any type of research, so long as the funding is available; in the long run, these researchers do not develop a program of research or a body of knowledge. Research realists are invested in a program of research but are also cognizant of the reality of needing funds to conduct the work. Realists generally seek several potential funding sources and can slant a proposal to coincide with the organization's funding priorities, providing that the integrity of the research can be maintained. Some organizations that support research even have the equivalent of research czars. Unlike a developmental model, in which a senior researcher gathers junior colleagues and works with them to develop their research skills and thus their independence, research czars create a dependence model. The senior researcher writes proposals *for* junior colleagues rather than *with* them. The end result, if the proposals are funded, is a short-term increase in the organization's research funding; unfortunately, the junior colleagues are not taught by this process to conduct research or to prepare the subsequent follow-up study proposal. They become increasingly dependent on the senior researcher for the next proposal and for maintaining the status that often accompanies funded research. Ultimately the organization will suffer, as will science, because senior researchers can oversee only a limited number of people unprepared to conduct what should be their own independent work.

Unfortunately, the organization may reward its research czars well, and those who become ever more dependent on them will do the same. This method may come to be viewed, often by non-research-intensive institutions, as the only viable solution for producing grant applications, but it is shortsighted with regard to the long-term development of junior faculty and the organization.

## CONDUCT OF RESEARCH

There are as many political considerations associated with the actual conduct of a research project as there are with selection of a research topic. Some research is conducted by single investigators. Most studies today, however, are conducted by teams of investigators. NIH has acknowledged the importance of interdisciplinary research teams in the conduct of health research. The 2004 NIH Roadmap (*http://nihroadmap.nih.gov*) has established funding for programs to educate interdisciplinary research teams. Choice of research team members, the role each plays in the project, and selection of the site of data collection all also carry political considerations. The politics of the home institution too can be a significant potential source of conflict.

### SELECTION OF THE RESEARCH TEAM

Nursing alone does not control patient outcomes. Research to improve patient care involves interdisciplinary health care teams. However, who is included on the research team and who is excluded can be a political hot potato. There are issues of needed skills, access to study participants, staffing needed for data collection and data entry, and someone to manage the project on a day-to-day basis. Careful selection of members of the research team—co-investigators, project directors, specialty personnel (e.g., economists, statisticians, clinical specialists), and research assistants—is critical. When choosing team members, consider members' ability to be flexible and to work together, skills needed for success of the study, and characteristics of patience, persistence, honesty, and humor.

When physicians serve as coinvestigators, there are often benefits: added expertise and different views, access to subjects, increased subject safety, and opportunities for nurse-physician collaboration. Additionally, collaborative relationships with members of other disciplines promote a positive image of nurses as rigorous researchers and valued colleagues. Benefits to physicians and members of other disciplines from involvement in nurse-led research include money, involvement in funded research, publication, and presentations. For new physicians, this involvement often provides needed research training, research courses not being part of the required medical school curricula (Clinical Research Summit, 1999).

Nurses on staff in hospitals or health care agencies who are involved in developing research protocols generally have a clearer understanding of why a certain protocol is necessary and provide extremely valuable information concerning practical day-to-day aspects of conducting the research within their institutions. The specific role that nurses play as heads or as members of the research team is determined by a variety of factors, among which are available time, job requirements, interest, research preparation, and institutional support for these activities. Coghlan and Casey (2001) note the challenges of researchers conducting research within the hospitals in which they work. Challenges include combining their research with their regular organizational role and managing the political dynamics involved in what the institution wants from the research and what the researcher wants.

Benefits can accrue to individuals involved in research projects, such as tuition subsidy, coauthor status on publications, the opportunity to present the research, participation in additional research, and participation in a mentoring relationship with senior researchers.

**Potential Political Problems.** Research that requires nursing staff participation can be facilitated if key members of the staff are involved as coinvestigators, project directors, or research assistants. If the staff members are not compensated or do not see the value of their involvement, the result can be devastating. Feelings of frustration and outright resistance can occur when staff members believe that their time is being consumed by research tasks not clearly linked with patient care or their job responsibilities. They may also resent the fact that patients' available time is being used to meet research requirements rather than for needed care.

In some institutions, the chief executive officer or department head may not support an individual's being included on a research team. This may be due to a personal dislike or fear of the person or a wish to dismiss him in the future. Success on a study, even as a team member, might make future termination more difficult, so the individual's participation may be opposed.

Physicians can also act as gatekeepers and block access to the patient group under investigation unless they are included in the project. In one study, which examined the most effective nonpharmacologic methods for treating breast engorgement in nonlactating women, a key physician in the obstetrical department would not grant access to inpatient postpartum women because "there is a pill to treat this problem." On further investigation, it became clear that this physician felt bypassed because he had not been consulted on the research proposal before it was funded. Ego problems of this sort are not uncommon.

In some instances, physician colleagues may be reluctant to give up control of patient care in favor of testing an innovative nursing approach. In one NINR-funded project, half of the traditional prenatal care visits and management of prenatal care was provided by advanced practice nurses (APNs). Because this study involved an alternative to the approach residents were accustomed to, they initially would try to block enrollment and question the management decisions of the nurses. This challenge was met by working very closely with each resident involved, keeping in constant communication, and reaching out to educate the residents to the potential benefits for them in this research. Soon it became apparent to the residents that their job was easier with this collegial relationship. Not too far into the study, the opposite problem arose. Residents wanted to suspend the randomization process and enroll all their patients into the intervention group. In this study, the residents as well as patients benefited directly from the research, thanks to the patience and persistence of the APNs (Brooten et al., 2001).

In another study examining caffeine intake during pregnancy, a physician refused to participate as a coinvestigator if the obstetrical nursing clinical director was a member of the research team. Apparently, these two individuals had a long-standing history of problems. Avoid such problems by investigating relationships among potential team members ahead of time.

## SELECTION OF SITE FOR DATA COLLECTION

Numerous factors affect selection of the site for data collection, including the number of available subjects, the number of other studies being conducted at the site, travel to and from the site, and established connections at the potential site and cooperation with key people.

Cooperation of key people was an important issue in a study of sexual abuse of children by Roman Catholic priests conducted by John Jay College of Criminal Justice (Bollag, 2004). The U.S. Conference of Catholic Bishops had ordered the bishops to cooperate with the study. However, 2 months into data collection, a significant number of bishops refused to cooperate. After the College's president and six faculty members met in a closed door meeting with almost all of the Conference's bishops, the bishops' fears were resolved and the study proceeded. Study results indicated that accusations of child molestation had been made against 4392 priests or approximately 4% of those who served between 1950 and 2002. Results indicated 10,667 people reported being abused by priests as children during that period. Critics of the report point out that the data were entirely self report and likely suffered from underreporting as there was wide variation among dioceses, with some reporting no cases of abuse to those reporting that 24% of their priests were accused.

Researchers need to follow established institutional review guidelines, monitor the site continually for potential difficulties, and maintain lines of communications and good relationships with key individuals at the data collection site. Ongoing communication is particularly important in today's climate of institutional reorganization, restructuring, and partnering.

It is also important to determine the actual functioning of an institution's research review board.

The board is formally charged with assessing the protection of human subjects but often reviews the scientific merit of studies, though this is not its primary responsibility. It is important to know the committee members, their research knowledge and experience, and their review biases and practices. It is also important for researchers to contact or court a committee member who can champion the study.

**Potential Political Problems.** A nursing colleague who had received major NIH funding for a study on elderly persons found herself embroiled in a fight for access to adequate numbers of subjects. A physician (who had a smaller amount of funding) wanted to begin his study with the same subject population and informed the nurse researcher that she could "have" the subjects he would not be using. However, the nursing research review committee for the hospital had reviewed and approved her study several months previously, whereas the physician had not bothered to submit his study to the committee. Citing overlap with an ongoing study previously approved, the committee denied the physician access to subjects at the site. Though this was a "gutsy call" by the group, they were backed up by long-standing procedures at the institution.

The political game at the study site may be a matter of raw power—or, at the opposite extreme, only of naïveté. In a study involving children with AIDS, a nurse researcher was denied access to a data collection site (one of two in the city) unless she turned the study and its data over to a physician as principal investigator. The study was her idea, and she had already developed the proposal. She chose to seek access to the other site and was successful; however, her subject numbers would have been doubled if she had been permitted entry into both institutions.

In another example, a nurse researcher had been conducting a pilot study on caffeine and pregnancy for more than a year. She invited a toxicologist to be a coinvestigator after the study had been developed and funded. His laboratory ran the analyses of serum and salivary caffeine. His was the only laboratory doing these analyses in the city, but there was no reduction in the price of the analyses, even

though he was named as a coinvestigator. When the head of his department wanted to know what studies would be submitted for major funding within the next year in the department, the toxicologist telephoned the nurse principal investigator. He indicated what information was needed by his department head and said that if a major study were to be submitted based on the pilot, it would have to come from his department, not from the nursing school, because his department, as he informed her, needed the indirect cost recovery. Not sure whether he was naïve or attempting a power move, the nurse researcher was firm: If major funding was sought as a result of the pilot, the application would originate from the nursing school. She pointed out that she had come to him with a study already developed and funded and had asked him to join the work, that he was providing no reduction in the cost of the analyses, and that the nursing school also needed indirect cost recovery from its researchers. She concluded by saying that she hoped that her position was clear and that she had addressed his concerns, because although she would prefer not to end their work together, she would send her samples to a laboratory in another city if necessary. He not only grasped the message but gained a new perspective on nurse researchers.

In one study, a nursing clinical director stopped progress on a nurse's study for months. The clinical director, who served on the hospital nursing research review committee, would not approve this study, citing "lack of scientific merit." She claimed that the investigators were not attempting anything new and that their methods were flawed. The investigators received from her a two-page, single-spaced list of questions to be answered before the committee. Not one member of the committee had directed a funded research study, and most had never been involved in research. The principal investigator had to educate the committee about a variety of aspects of research, as well as respond to their questions. Although the study was ultimately approved, the delay of 3 months (during the summer, a time of high productivity for investigators in academia) put the study significantly behind schedule. The study under review by the hospital nursing research review committee had already been approved and funded by four national organizations.

In selecting a site for data collection, the researcher can go through the proper channels and maintain relationships and communication, but he or she often cannot counteract the behaviors of individuals who view themselves as research or practice experts in competition with the researcher. Situations like the examples cited are not uncommon. Although much progress has been made in the last 2 decades in the working of nurse-physician research teams, other problems can involve physicians who cannot comprehend why a nurse is investigating a certain problem they view as a "medical" one, or one in their perceived domain.

## HOME SITE POLITICAL ISSUES

In most institutions, there are political issues at the home site including space, release time to conduct the study, the value of research in the institution, image and understanding of research in the institution, and value placed on the type and focus of the specific research.

Research can bring substantial financial support to a school. Indeed, in fiscal year 2003, the five schools of nursing with the highest amount of NIH funding in the United States received between $6.3 million and $13.4 million for research. The total NIH funding to schools of nursing in 2003 was $144.7 million (NIH, 2005a). Proponents of funded research argue that in addition to the funds that directly support the research study, funded research provides indirect cost recovery, substantial financial support for students, enhanced educational experiences for students, and improvements in nursing practice and subsequently in patient outcomes.

In many research-intensive schools of nursing, dollars for student financial support realized through funded faculty research exceed those from all other sources of student scholarship aid combined. This is also true for schools with very large endowments. Students also benefit by participating in the faculty's research by publishing and presenting with faculty. One undergraduate group, for example, presented at the 1998 American Academy of Nursing meeting in Acapulco (Brooten, Youngblut, Donnelly, & Brown, 1998; Brooten et al., 1999). Proponents also

note that research brings indirect cost recovery dollars to the school or unit, freeing other money for new initiatives or additional faculty or as a hedge against years with decreased student enrollment. This is an especially important factor for schools of nursing in private institutions. The research dollars for direct costs pay a portion of the faculty salary of the investigator and coinvestigators as well as of the costs of conducting the research and of support for students employed on the project as research assistants, data entry people, project directors, and so on. And knowledge gained to improve nursing practice is essential to teaching "state of the art" nursing care.

Research is also critical to nursing education: Faculty research is necessary in teaching doctoral students, just as faculty practice is in teaching master's degree students. It is as sterile for doctoral students to be taught to conduct and publish research by faculty who do not conduct and publish research as it is for nurse practitioner students to be taught by faculty who do not practice. Faculty research is to doctoral education what faculty practice is to nurse practitioner education.

Issues regarding allocation of scare resources (especially space, release time, and support services) are very real for all investigators and fraught with politics. The need for space to do the research and the need for support services, such as secretarial services, are often some of the first issues to be resolved in any newly funded study (Youngblut & Brooten, 2002). Because institutional space costs money, the investigator will be far better able to negotiate space needs if the research is funded. If the institution receives indirect cost recovery from the study, the indirect costs should cover the space needs. However, indirect cost recovery may be inadequate to pay for the space needs, or there may not be any available space. Sometimes this problem can be addressed in the proposal and additional money secured for space rental for the duration of the study.

**Potential Political Problems.** Researchers always contend with political issues in their home institutions, the recipients of the money for their research. Some issues result from politics inherent in the parent organization (e.g., university, hospital), whereas others arise from school or unit politics.

***Uncovering Problems.*** Some clinical research may actually uncover some of the problems that exist in the institution where the research is being conducted. The problems may be in clinical outcomes such as exposing a very high infection rate after cesarean sections. The problems may be administrative. In a research study examining treatment modalities and outcomes in women with diabetes during pregnancy, a chart review revealed that even though this institution did almost 10,000 deliveries a year, no cases of gestational diabetes were found. Gestational diabetes is diabetes that occurs during a pregnancy and occurs in 5% to 20% of all pregnant women. The problem turned out to be miscopying of the current procedural terminology (CPT) code for gestational diabetes with the result that none of these women was identified in the medical records. This problem had huge implications for reimbursement for the hospital. Most institutions do not want problems such as this one revealed, and thus problems of this type present ethical dilemmas for researchers.

***Nursing's Place in Academia.*** At the parent-organizational level, there are many political issues. In academia for example, because nursing was the one of the last disciplines to join academia and because most nursing schools are among the smallest schools in their universities, nursing often lacks power in the university. In addition, members of the university community may not know that nurses conduct their own research and may not understand or respect the type of research that nurses conduct. Thus, in many institutions, nursing is seen as a minor player in the research arena. As a result, nurses are often excluded from forums where research issues are decided. At one university, when the search committee for a high-level institutional research official did not include a representative from nursing, the nurse administrator was told that this was because the university was looking for committee members who "knew something about research." When a meeting of the school's research deans was scheduled for a time when the nurse representative was out of town, she was told that the time was selected based on the availability of "the important people."

***Being the Lead School.*** When a funder's request for proposals specifies that only one grant can be submitted from an institution, the nursing school may not be invited to even submit a proposal for the internal competition, and if invited, the nursing proposal is often not selected because of concern on the university's selection committee's part that nursing proposals will not fare well in the external funder's competition. Selection of a nurse principal investigator for an across-school collaborative grant often requires considerable lobbying behind the scenes.

***Educator Versus Researcher.*** Political issues at the school or department level are numerous, including conflict about the value of research, the type and focus of research, and allocation of scarce resources. At one time, there was a considerable divide between nurse educators and nurses in practice. Educators often chided practicing nurses for not delivering "state of the art" care, while practicing nurses accused nurse educators of not being clinically relevant; "If you can't do, teach" was a refrain commonly heard from practicing nurses. Much of this divide has closed as educators practice, clinicians seek further education, and positions for clinician-educators increase in schools of nursing.

Currently, however, a similar divide exists between education and research in many schools of nursing. Faculty members are often divided into camps over which part of the school's mission—education or research—should get priority. Arguments are heard frequently that there is too little emphasis on teaching and students, too much on research. Other disputes center on what the operational definition of nursing research is and whether faculty research need be funded when the faculty member is being considered for promotion and tenure. Each issue is loaded with political ramifications.

***Space.*** Securing the space needed to conduct the research often requires education of the administration, money to underwrite the cost of the space, and political pull. If the conduct of funded research is a relatively new activity for the institution, the administration may not understand the investigator's need for space. One investigator was informed that because she did not have an animal colony, she did not need research space. She was expected to store her equipment, supplies, and data forms in her existing—and already overcrowded—office and to carry data and forms back and forth from her home to her office in a suitcase. The situation was eventually resolved through several discussions with the chief executive officer of the organization.

An analysis of organizations often reveals individuals who have no funding but have ample research space, whereas other, well-funded investigators have little, even inadequate, space. Sometimes this has to do with the timing of space allocation—who needed it first—and sometimes it is a statement of value and control by the head of the organization. Allocation of space sends a powerful message. In some instances, being an organization player or a confidante to the chief or to those in control of resource allocation will count far more than one's merit as a nurse researcher.

***Release Time.*** Another political issue often encountered at the home site involves the negotiation of release time to conduct the study. If the study has received major funding, a proportion of the principal investigator's salary has been included in that funding to pay for their release to conduct the study. In theory, the organization uses this money to pay someone else to conduct that portion of the investigator's regular work from which they are released. Sometimes it actually works this way, but some investigators ignore this expectation and are funded through a combination of grants for 100% or more of their salary. Obviously, the funding sources do not know that the investigator is committed for more than 100% of salaried time. This approach brings more money, resources, or power to the investigator or his or her department.

Some organizations set up disincentives to research. In these situations, the investigator may be funded for only 30% of the time that is to be allocated to the study. Rather than assisting the investigator by relieving 30% of their workload, the organization simply assumes that the individual will conduct the study in addition to the current workload—and uses the 30% salary support for other purposes. The investigator, concerned with maintaining the success of the investigation, is compelled to assume an extra-heavy workload. This is an intolerable situation, especially for junior faculty who must establish programs of research to receive tenure. The situation also causes serious problems with funding agencies.

Recently, NIH has become more concerned with effort reporting of investigators receiving federal funding for their research. When investigators in academia apply for federal grants, their colleges or universities must promise that a percentage of the investigator's time and effort will be devoted to the research study. The government then expects that the investigator will spend that amount of time and effort committed in the grant application. Documenting the time spent on the research is referred to as "effort reporting" or "salary accounting" under federal policy. Several research institutions, including Harvard, Johns Hopkins University, and Northwestern University, recently settled legal settlements of between $2.6 and $5.5 million with the federal government over allegations that they misrepresented the amount of time scientists spent on federally sponsored research. In all three cases, the researchers were accused of spending fewer hours than promised or paid for on their research projects (Brainard, 2004a). University officials complain about the required federal effort reporting, noting that effort reporting is time consuming and too inflexible to capture the diverse activities of teaching, committee work, student advising, and service activities of university researchers.

## POLITICS IN DISSEMINATION OF RESEARCH FINDINGS

There are a considerable number of issues surrounding publication and presentation of study findings, including where the findings should be disseminated, whose names should appear on the publications and in what order, and who should participate in the research presentations. Dissemination of study results has also become a national political issue.

The NIH recently announced its policy on enhancing access to publications resulting from NIH-funded research. The policy is intended to (a) create a stable archive of peer-reviewed research publications resulting from NIH-funded research; (b) secure a researchable compendium of these publications that NIH and its awardees can use to understand their research portfolios, monitor scientific productivity, and help set research priorities; and (c) make published results of NIH-funded research more readily accessible to the public, health care providers, educators, and scientists. Authors of

NIH-funded research are strongly encouraged to submit their final accepted manuscripts to the National Library of Medicines Pub Med Central within 12 months of the publisher's official date of final publication (NIH, 2005b).

The NIH policy was established for a number of reasons, including better dissemination of research findings. Dissemination of research has been challenged over the past several decades, as library subscription fees for peer-reviewed journals have risen beyond the reach of many libraries. Library subscriptions for the journal *Brain Research*, for example, costs more than $21,000, *Nuclear Physics A and B* more than $23,000, and *Biochemica et Biophysica Acta* nearly $15,000. Duke University, whose library budget for 2003 was $6.6 million, was forced to cut 525 of 1753 of the medical center's journals. Cornell also announced having to cancel more than 200 subscriptions to one publishing house alone (Guterman, 2004b).

To counteract the rising costs of library subscriptions, there has been an upsurge in new online journals that require authors to pay to have their publications put online following peer review and acceptance of the manuscript. Fees for such publication range from $500 to $1500. Advocates of these journals propose having these publication fees incorporated into research grant proposals in order to disseminate study results (Guterman, 2004b).

## POTENTIAL POLITICAL PROBLEMS

The politics involved in deciding whose names should appear on publications and in what order, and who should make presentations, is common to all studies. The principal investigator of a study has the responsibility for oversight of the rigor, integrity, and successful conduct of the study, and this includes dissemination of the study findings. Though the principal investigator is therefore first author on the main findings, coinvestigators may be first authors on secondary findings from the study. Inclusion of additional coauthors generally depends on their contributions to the manuscript. A general rule is that a coauthor must have made a significant contribution to the manuscript's development and submission. Currently, many journals (e.g., *Journal of the American Medical Association, Journal of the American Public Health Association*) now require statements indicating the role of each author in the development of the manuscript. Principal investigators should be listed as authors of all manuscripts resulting from studies they have conducted. Their authorship demonstrates oversight and agreement regarding the validity of the data presented and any conclusions drawn from work they headed.

A recent example illustrates the need for these practices. A paper published in 2001 in the *Journal of Reproductive Medicine* announced that three researchers had found that strangers' prayers could double the chances of success of women seeking to get pregnant using in vitro fertilization. The authors were Rogerio Lobo, a professor at Columbia University and lead author, Kwang Cha at Columbia, and Daniel Wirth, a lawyer and researcher into the supernatural. Shortly after the paper was published, questions arose regarding the study's procedures and methods, indicating flaws and possible fraudulence. It was also learned that women had not been informed of their participation in the experiment. The U.S. Department of Health and Human Services Office of Human Subjects Protection investigated the study and decided not to take action against Columbia University because Dr. Lobo "first learned of the study from Dr. Cha 6-12 months after the study was completed" (Guterman, 2004a, p. A20). Dr. Lobo had primarily provided editorial review and assistance with publication. Critics were amazed that someone who was the lead author had not only not participated in the study design but had not participated in the study at all. The publisher, although receiving many letters criticizing the study, did not publish the letters but subsequently published a letter from Dr. Cha defending the study. The journal did, however, remove Dr. Lobo's name from the publication at his request.

There are other issues regarding publication. The U.S. Treasury Department has now ended a policy that forbade an engineering society from editing, without a license, articles written by authors from U.S.-embargoed countries such as Cuba, Iran, Libya, and Sudan. The rationale for this policy was that such editing provided a valuable service to people living in the embargoed countries (Guterman, 2004c).

| Issues | Great/Fine | | | | Problem | |
|---|---|---|---|---|---|---|
| 1. Topic—Importance and Potential Yield to: | | | | | | |
|    a. My career & program of research | 5 | 4 | 3 | 2 | 1 | 0 |
|    b. My organization | 5 | 4 | 3 | 2 | 1 | 0 |
|    c. Profession | 5 | 4 | 3 | 2 | 1 | 0 |
|    d. Society | 5 | 4 | 3 | 2 | 1 | 0 |
| 2. Funding Possibilities | | | | | | |
|    a. Federal | 5 | 4 | 3 | 2 | 1 | 0 |
|    b. Private | 5 | 4 | 3 | 2 | 1 | 0 |
|    c. Level of indirects | 5 | 4 | 3 | 2 | 1 | 0 |
| 3. Research Team—Who, Why, Compatibility | | | | | | |
|    a. Specific skill people | | | | | | |
|       1. _____ | 5 | 4 | 3 | 2 | 1 | 0 |
|       2. _____ | 5 | 4 | 3 | 2 | 1 | 0 |
|       3. _____ | 5 | 4 | 3 | 2 | 1 | 0 |
|    b. Access people | | | | | | |
|       1. _____ | 5 | 4 | 3 | 2 | 1 | 0 |
|       2. _____ | 5 | 4 | 3 | 2 | 1 | 0 |
|    c. Students/staff | | | | | | |
|       1. _____ | 5 | 4 | 3 | 2 | 1 | 0 |
|       2. _____ | 5 | 4 | 3 | 2 | 1 | 0 |
| 4. Site for Data Collection | | | | | | |
|    a. Established connections/key people | 5 | 4 | 3 | 2 | 1 | 0 |
|    b. Available subjects | 5 | 4 | 3 | 2 | 1 | 0 |
|    c. Ongoing studies with same population | 5 | 4 | 3 | 2 | 1 | 0 |
|    d. Research review committee—facilitative? | 5 | 4 | 3 | 2 | 1 | 0 |
|    e. Travel to site | 5 | 4 | 3 | 2 | 1 | 0 |
| 5. Home site | | | | | | |
|    a. Space needs | 5 | 4 | 3 | 2 | 1 | 0 |
|    b. Release time | 5 | 4 | 3 | 2 | 1 | 0 |
|    c. Research support services | 5 | 4 | 3 | 2 | 1 | 0 |
| 6. Dissemination—Where, By Whom | | | | | | |
|    a. Main findings | | | | | | |
|       1. Interdisciplinary | 5 | 4 | 3 | 2 | 1 | 0 |
|       2. Intradisciplinary | 5 | 4 | 3 | 2 | 1 | 0 |
|       3. First author | 5 | 4 | 3 | 2 | 1 | 0 |
|       4. Coauthors—who, why | | | | | | |
|          a. _____ | 5 | 4 | 3 | 2 | 1 | 0 |
|          b. _____ | 5 | 4 | 3 | 2 | 1 | 0 |
|    b. Secondary findings | | | | | | |
|       1. Interdisciplinary | 5 | 4 | 3 | 2 | 1 | 0 |
|       2. Intradisciplinary | 5 | 4 | 3 | 2 | 1 | 0 |
|       3. First author | 5 | 4 | 3 | 2 | 1 | 0 |
|       4. Coauthors—who, why | | | | | | |
|          a. _____ | 5 | 4 | 3 | 2 | 1 | 0 |
|          b. _____ | 5 | 4 | 3 | 2 | 1 | 0 |

**Figure 21-1** Politics of research: A checklist of political health.

Each research team or each principal investigator ultimately has to decide how to handle issues regarding who appears on publications and who presents study findings. Using a team approach, the work usually receives broader dissemination, and more people can gain from the effort. The cost of inclusion is generally minimal; the cost of exclusion is generally much greater. One guiding rule for principal investigators, however, is to control their own data. It is not uncommon for associates to publish or present study results as their own, without attribution to the team or the principal investigator or the funding agency. These situations can be minimized if the rules regarding publication and presentation are established at the start of the study, agreed to, recorded, and reviewed periodically during the course of the study. Problems can also be minimized if the principal investigator is the only one with access to the most current study results. This point became clear in one situation in which a physician coinvestigator planned to present at a research conference, as his own work, the preliminary findings of a study headed by nurses. He was stymied because the principal investigator was the only member of the team with the most current findings and would share them only during the routinely held meetings of the team.

To evaluate the potential political health of your research and areas needing attention, complete the checklist in Figure 21-1. If you score 2 or less on 50% of the items in each category, you can anticipate significant challenges in the politics of conducting and disseminating this research.

## Key Points

- Politics is an ever-present part of research, from the definition of what constitutes nursing research to choice of the research topic, conduct of the work, and dissemination of the findings.
- The political context of one's home institution can make or break a program or research; things such as space, release time, funding, and independent review board approval can be barriers or facilitators to nurse researchers conducting high-quality studies.

- It behooves nurse researchers to consider the importance of dissemination of research, as it is high on the agenda of national research funders, including the National Institutes of Health.

## Web Resources

**Foundation Center**—For information on funding sources
*www.fdncenter.org*
**National Institute for Nursing Research**
*http://ninr.nih.gov/ninr/*
**National Institutes of Health**
*www.nih.gov*

## REFERENCES

Bollag, B. (2004). Pulling back the veil. *The Chronicle of Higher Education, 50*(28), A12-A13.

Brainard, J. (2003). Research-agency officials question White House's review of basic science. *The Chronicle of Higher Education, 50*(17), A25.

Brainard J. (2004a). Accounting for researcher's time. *The Chronicle of Higher Education, 50*(45), A20-A21.

Brainard, J. (2004b). California governor endorses referendum supporting stem-cell research. *The Chronicle of Higher Education, 51*(10), A26.

Brainard, J. (2004c). In mental health, a question of balance. *The Chronicle of Higher Education, 50*(32), A23-A25.

Brainard, J. (2004d). Stem-cell research moves forward. *The Chronicle of Higher Education, 51*(6), A22-A25.

Brainard, J. (2004e). What the NIH bought with double the money. *The Chronicle of Higher Education, 50*(22), A17-A20.

Brooten, D. (1997, February). *Nursing research in a managed care environment.* Paper presented to the National Institutes of Health, Washington, DC.

Brooten, D., Youngblut, J. M., Brown, L., Finkler, S. A., Neff, D. F., & Madigan, E. (2001). A randomized trial of nurse specialist home care for women with high risk pregnancies: Outcomes and costs. *American Journal of Managed Care, 7*(8), 793-803.

Brooten, D., Youngblut, J. M., Donnelly, S., & Brown, C. (1998, October). *Disseminating our breakthroughs: Enacting a strategic framework.* Paper presented at the annual conference of the American Academy of Nursing, Acapulco.

Brooten, D., Youngblut, J. M., Roberts, B. L., Montgomery, K., Standing, T. S., Hemstrom, M., et al. (1999). Disseminating our breakthroughs: Enacting a strategic framework. *Nursing Outlook, 47,* 133-137.

Browne, A. J. (2001). The influence of liberal political ideology on nursing science. *Nursing Inquiry, 11*(2), 117-121.

Clinical Research Summit. (1999). *Breaking the scientific bottleneck. Clinical research: A national call to action.* Washington, DC: Association of American Medical Colleges & American Medical Association.

Cody, W. K., & Mitchell, G. J. (2002). Nursing knowledge and human science revisited: Practical and political considerations. *Nursing Science Quarterly, 15*(1), 4-13.

Coghlan, D., & Casey, M. (2001). Action research from the inside: Issues and challenges in doing action research in your hospital. *Journal of Advanced Nursing, 35*(5), 674-682.

Fawcett, J., Watson, J., Neuman, B., Hinton Walker, P., & Fitzpatrick, J. J. (2001). On nursing theories and evidence. *Journal of Nursing Scholarship, 33*(2), 115-119.

Field, K. (2004a). Pentagon may tighten restrictions on foreign researchers. *The Chronicle of Higher Education, 50*(35), A27.

Field, K. (2004b). Residents fight Boston U.'s "biosafety" laboratory. *The Chronicle of Higher Education, 50*(42), A28-A30.

Guterman, L. (2004a). Lead author removes name from disputed prayer study. *The Chronicle of Higher Education, 51*(17), A21.

Guterman, L. (2004b). The promise and peril of open access. *The Chronicle of Higher Education, 50*(21), A10-A11.

Guterman, L. (2004c). US lifts limits on editing articles by scholars in embargoed countries. *The Chronicle of Higher Education, 50*(32), A20.

Hebel, S. (2004). Republicans hold the line on stem cells. *The Chronicle of Higher Education, 51*(3), A1, A23.

Mechanic, R., & Dobson, A. (1996). The impact of managed care on clinical research: A preliminary investigation. *Health Affairs, 15*, 72-89.

Meleis, A. (2001). Scholarship and the R01 (editorial). *Journal of Nursing Scholarship, 33*(2), 104-105.

Monastersky, R. (2004). Korean investigators harvest first stem cells from a cloned human embryo. *The Chronicle of Higher Education, 50*(24), A17.

National Institute of Nursing Research. (2005). Mission statement. Retrieved March 11, 2005, from *www.nih.gov/ninr/research/diversity/mission.html.*

National Institutes of Health. (2005a). NIH awards to health professional components, fiscal year 2003. Retrieved March 7, 2006, from *http://grants2.nih.gov/grants/award/trends/dhenrsg03.htm.*

National Institutes of Health. (2005b). Policy on enhancing public access to archived publications resulting from NIH-funded research. Retrieved March 7, 2006, from *http://grants2.nih.gov/grants/guide/notice-files/NOT-OD-05-022.html.*

Rosenstock, L., & Lee, L. J. (2002). Attacks on science: The risks to evidence-based policy. *American Journal of Public Health, 92*(1), 14-18.

Suplee, C. (1991). Sex study is scrapped due to political concerns. *Philadelphia Inquirer, 324*(88), 14A.

Tucker, J. B. (2004). Research on biodefense can get generous funds, but with strings attached. *The Chronicle Review, 1*(6), 10-11.

Youngblut, J. M., & Brooten, D. (2002). Institutional research responsibilities and needed infrastructure. *Journal of Nursing Scholarship, 34*(2), 159-164.

# chapter 22

# Contemporary Issues in Government

Deborah B. Gardner, Mary K. Wakefield, & Beth G. Gardner

*"The test of our progress is not whether we add more to the abundance of those who have much, it is whether we provide enough for those who have too little."*

FRANKLIN DELANO ROOSEVELT

At the start of the twenty-first century, tremendous fiscal pressures face national, state, and local legislators. Defense expenditures dominate budgetary concerns, and the chronic repercussions of running large deficits in times of war have returned. Potential as well as imminent public health crises, including threats of bioterrorism, flu vaccine shortages, and the swelling ranks of the uninsured, have heightened the visibility of national health care needs (Healthy Americans Organization, 2005). In spite of these and a number of other priority health needs, with limited federal dollars, increased public spending on health care is keenly scrutinized. Efforts to constrain the rate of growth in health care expenditures in the 1990s through managed care had short-term impact. In fact, national health expenditures are projected to grow at an average annual rate of 7.1% during the forecast period of 2004-2014, ultimately reaching $3.6 trillion in 2014 (Centers for Medicare and Medicaid Services [CMS], 2004).

Since 1995, these increases have been driven, in part, by price increases for prescription drugs averaging 15% per year. Marked increases in drug spending are projected beginning in 2006 with enactment of expanded drug coverage for Medicare beneficiaries. Total U.S. spending on health care currently accounts for 15% of the gross domestic product (GDP). By 2014, it is projected to account for about 18.7% of the GDP (Cover the Uninsured Week, 2004). With rising medical expenditures and the addition of the 2006 drug prescription benefits, overall U.S. health care costs are rising faster than the GDP (Reinhardt, Hussey, & Anderson, 2004). In spite of significant health care spending, in the 2004 election, 93% of voters were concerned about the availability and affordability of health care (Blendon, Brodie, Altman, Benson, & Hamel, 2004). In January of 2005, a survey by the Kaiser Family Foundation and the Harvard School of Public Health found health care on par with terrorism/ national security as the third most important priority for the administration and Congress behind the war in Iraq and the economy. Of 12 health care priorities, lowering health care costs ranked number 1. Also at the top of the list was making Medicare fiscally sound for the future and lowering the number of uninsured (Kaiser Family Foundation [KFF], 2005a).

Despite this strong public sentiment, President Bush's 2006 budget focused on overhauling Social Security and tax reform as his leading domestic initiatives. Trustees overseeing Social Security and Medicare challenged the President's focus, insisting that Medicare's financial problems far exceed Social Security's and are in urgent need of attention. Critics have also noted that Medicare problems will be harder to fix than Social Security, and partisan battles over the future of these major public programs continue (Society for Vascular Surgery, 2005). In addition to efforts to redesign major public health programs, targeted health policies also emerged. One health care proposal President Bush placed as a priority in both his bid for re-election and on his 2006 agenda was to legislate medical malpractice caps. This administration priority was shared as a top priority of the American Medical Association (AMA) while adamantly opposed by many Democrats and the American Trial Lawyers Association. In 2004, several states passed laws to cap malpractice awards. Some Republicans argue that large malpractice judgments drive up physician malpractice insurance, prompting many physicians to stop practicing medicine, thus imperiling the health care system. Conversely, Democrats argue that insurers, not jury awards, are the driving force behind rising premiums (Congressional Record, 2005).

The sheer scope and intricacy of the health care system, when coupled with the current political climate, make improving health system outcomes a formidable endeavor. This chapter focuses on the systemic interdependence of health care policy with politico-economics at federal, state, and local levels of government. The issues reviewed in this chapter are arguably some of the most threatening to the health of the largest number of Americans: caring for the growing ranks of uninsured and underinsured, bioterrorism, ongoing consequences of tobacco use, the obesity epidemic, health care quality, and consumer health literacy. These issues are linked as tangible examples of the urgency for both new health policies and funding redirected toward prevention strategies.

## HISTORICAL PERSPECTIVE

### DEFICIT CYCLES

Historically, large federal deficits have occurred during periods of war (as defense spending rises sharply) or economic downturns (Government Printing Office, 2004). Recent history arguably broke with this general pattern in the 1980s. In 1982, partly in response to the recession, large tax cuts were enacted to stimulate the economy. Instead, an economic downturn intensified between 1983 and 1992, and an unprecedented peacetime *deficit* and *debt* were incurred. These tax cuts, coupled with substantial increases in defense spending, increased

the budget deficit and shifted relationships among local, state, and federal governments significantly. Expanding federal deficits and a struggling economy marked over two decades of cramped federal funding options in every policy area including health care. In response, state governments, burdened with underfunded federal requirements and facing their own budget shortfalls, began to decrease funding to many local programs, including health care (Box 22-1).

After peaking in 1992, deficits began to decline and in 1998, during the Clinton Administration, a dramatic economic turnaround occurred. A budget surplus of 2.4% was recorded in 2000, the first budget surplus since 1969. This economic boom created huge federal revenue increases coupled with more money coming into state government coffers than predicted. Many health care advocacy groups and Democratic leaders viewed this as a window of opportunity to substantially fund priority social programs, including funding to assist low-income and uninsured citizens to obtain health insurance (Reinhardt, 2003). However, in 2000, a Republican-dominated election outcome promised "smaller government and no new taxes." Starting in 2001, President Bush proposed, and Congress enacted, three major tax cut bills in 2½ years.

Republicans argue that tax cuts spur the economy and raise incomes to bring in more revenues in the long run, a position premised on a "trickle-down"

---

**BOX 22-1**  Deficit Cycles: Terms

What is the difference between the debt and the deficit?

The national debt is the total amount of money owed by the government; the federal budget deficit is the yearly amount by which spending exceeds revenue. Add up all the deficits over the past 200 years and that is the national debt.

The fact is that the deficit is not a well-defined economic concept. The current measure of the deficit is based on arbitrary choices of how to label government receipts and payments. The government can conduct any real economic policy and simultaneously report any size deficit or surplus it wants just through its choice of words (Hall, 2005).

economic interpretation. Conversely, Democrats argue that tax cuts are a primary reason for sustained deficits and, as structured, only benefit the wealthiest taxpayers.

The conditions of economic surplus were extremely short lived. The September 11, 2001 attacks, tied with income tax cuts and an economic downturn, ended balanced-budget conditions. As tax revenue fell, spending for domestic, security and military operations in Afghanistan and Iraq grew. Despite the logical result of this equation (i.e., decrease in tax revenues plus increased spending on war equals budget deficit), even in 2002, the budget was *forecast*—by both the Bush Administration and the Congressional Budget Office—to run cumulative surpluses of $5.6 trillion between 2002 and 2011. In 2003, as the economy began weakening, the President signed the Jobs and Growth Tax Relief Reconciliation Act (JGTRRA), which accelerated many of the tax reductions passed in the 2001 Economic Growth and Tax Relief Reconciliation Act (EGTRRA) that were scheduled to take effect several years later. The 2003 "Jobs and Growth" tax cut also reduced the tax rate on dividends and capital gains, thus reducing taxes for businesses (Office of Management and Budget, 2005). Critics often refer to this policy practice as "corporate welfare." With these new policy efforts in place and ongoing military action, the federal deficit continues to grow. This deficit does not include money the government borrows from Social Security and Medicare trust funds to meet federal program expenditures. Sensitive to voter resistance to tax increases, Congress has continued to cut spending rather than raise taxes, thus pushing more of the fiscal burden onto state and local governments and creating a significant potential for subsequent generations to inherit large financial burdens from the federal debt (Public Agenda, 2004).

## STATE BUDGET CRISES

State budget crises affect the day-to-day lives of millions of Americans. States spend most of their budgets on education, health care, corrections, and transportation. Localities rely on state grants to assist in funding these services (Frontline, 2003). Despite most Americans' shared values for quality education and health care, polarized perspectives on the role and size of government help explain some of the political deadlocks preventing collaborative approaches to these issues. Traditionally, Americans have distrusted government involvement and the controls that accompany such engagement. Moreover, increasing government involvement stimulates growth in the size of government. Ideological conflicts concerning overall government size, taxation, and spending policies are further exacerbated when large budget deficits loom. These arguments have usually occurred on the federal level, but stark decreases in state revenues and increases in program expenditures have brought the debate to state and local levels as well.

State governments faced with sluggish economies, burdened by underfunded federal requirements (i.e., No Child Left Behind education initiative, special education, security/bioterrorism), and responsible for increasing Medicare and Medicaid costs, triggered larger state budget shortfalls. Therefore, local governments were sent scrambling to absorb greater social program costs. During this fiscal crisis (starting in FY 2001), states closely followed the pattern of the federal government by closing budget gaps with cuts in spending rather than enacting new taxes to support programs. While this strategy may operate well in the short term, it does not address how states will manage future cost increases or prevent the erosion of current social programs. At the forefront of these increases in state-level expenditures are Medicaid payments to care for the aging poor. Medicaid accounts for almost 20% of state budgets, making it the second largest single expense after education.

Demographic shifts compound increases in state health expenditures with the number and life expectancy of elderly poor increasing. This trend has implications for both Medicaid and Medicare, particularly related to poor elders who qualify for both programs (dual eligibility). Beginning in 2004, state revenues slowly expanded. Nevertheless, the severe fiscal problems of the previous 4 years continued to dominate the macro and micro budget picture. Furthermore, anti-tax sentiments led state budgets to their lowest spending level in 15 years and state spending is expected to continue to decline still further as a share of the GDP (Greenblatt, 2003).

Dispersing and devolving federal government programs and responsibilities, such as welfare and health care, to the budget-strapped states and to the private sector are perceived by many observers as part of the plan by Republicans to minimize federal and state government accountability. Norquist, of Americans for Tax Reform, argues that programs and responsibilities are easier to shrink at the state level, particularly when states are facing deficits. State-level pressure to cut spending is much more intense, because unlike the federal government, state governments must maintain balanced budgets (Center for Budget and Policy Priorities [CBPP], 2005). As the federal government withdraws funding support to states trying to meet federal policy priorities, the outcome may not be the reduction of federal power (smaller government), but rather increased federal encroachment/restrictions on state and local budgetary decision-making.

State and local government budgetary decision-making is further strained as the demand for public assistance increases within the larger context of shifting public services from the government sector to the private sector. Republicans argue that outsourcing social services at the state level is more effective and efficient, whereas Democrats tend to argue that privatizing traditional government services has never been shown to have the sweeping cost savings that its proponents claim. Generally, in the past, when the top level of government cuts or reduces support to the middle level (states), the middle level passes the cuts on to the bottom. Pushing problems down to the local level often creates greater difficulty for lower income communities than for higher income communities to compensate for lost resources. These types of shifts within government threaten to polarize strata differences into "the haves" and "the have-nots" (Triplett, 2003).

## EMERGING HEALTH POLICY ISSUES: BALANCING COMPETING CONCERNS AT THREE LEVELS

For the foreseeable future, health policy concerns will continue to be highly visible in state and federal public policy arenas. An array of factors, including changing demographics, increasing prevalence of chronic illness, technology breakthroughs, and many others, will continue to compete for the attention of policymakers.

Public funding of health care (i.e., Medicaid and the State Children's Health Insurance Program [SCHIP]) has increased dramatically over the past 40 years and is expected to continue to grow. This is due to increasing costs, the reduction of privately funded health care (i.e., employer-provided insurance), and the rising number of uninsured. While private funding was 75% of national health costs in 1965, public funding is expected to account for half of all health costs by 2014 (CMS, 2004). Social Security and Medicare were designed as universally applicable "entitlements" that the government is obligated by law to provide to citizens. However, congressional proposals to cut federal fiscal support of mandatory programs like Medicaid and the SCHIP over the next 5 years would increase state responsibility for domestic program funding. Many states have already cut eligibility for public health insurance (34 states), child care subsidies (23 states), and aid to school districts (34 states). Concurrently, many states across the country are cutting or at least slowing the rate of expenditures on higher education, leading to double-digit increases in college and university tuition and reduced course offerings. Cutbacks are also occurring at the local level as state aid is reduced for funding substance abuse treatment, homeless shelters, and programs for the mentally ill (CBPP, 2004). In short, services and resources that have been part of the backbone of American social mobility and minimum-standard equalizers are turning from "entitlements" to tenuous eligibility requirements masking cost-centered policies.

## THE PHARMACEUTICAL CONUNDRUM

Contributing to health care's rising costs are the workings of the American pharmaceutical industry and related high drug prices. Pharmaceuticals have made sweeping contributions to transforming health care outcomes over the past several decades by preventing, effectively managing, and sometimes curing diseases. Although the contribution of pharmaceuticals to improving health is unquestionable, the price paid for this achievement is dubious. Pharmaceutical spending has outpaced other categories of health care services. While significantly less than hospital care, drug therapy cost increases are directly felt by consumers, creating higher direct consumer impact and visibility (Reinhardt, 2003). With expanded Medicare drug coverage to some 40 million recipients in January 2006, the method used to calculate drug prices for both Medicare and Medicaid are under review by lawmakers. The central question is what, if anything, should the government do to make prescription drugs more affordable? (See *The Politics of the Pharmaceutical Industry* following Chapter 13.)

The growth in spending for prescription drugs can be attributed to four key factors: increased use of prescription drugs, higher costs for new products introduced in the market, increasing drug prices, and increased consumer awareness of new drugs as drug companies have increased their spending on direct-to-consumer marketing. These factors may be contributing to a broad consumer perception that the pharmaceutical industry prioritizes profits before people. The industry's image has also suffered because of allegations that some companies deliberately hid negative side effects of their drugs. These safety questions led to the removal of commonly used drugs such as Vioxx (rofecoxib) and Bextra (valdecoxib) and left policymakers questioning the ability of the Food and Drug Administration (FDA) to protect consumers through effective oversight (KFF, 2005b).

The pharmaceutical industry also draws scrutiny because of its financial strength reflected in having been at the top in profit-per-dollar equity since the early 1990s. Highly profitable industries are generally lauded yet certain public policies contribute to profitability. Yet when the product has to do with health care, many want the industry to act like a "good Samaritan" and lower prices. Drug companies contend that they could not survive without patent laws as an extension of private property rights. Patents affect prices by providing manufacturers who develop new products exclusive right to the drug for 20 years from the date of the patent filing. The pharmaceutical industry stance is that patents afford large drug companies, like Pfizer or Merck, the ability to increase drug prices to ensure that more can be spent on research and development.

Prices tend to drop significantly after patents expire and generic competition enters the market, however the process for generic application is back-logged. Despite patent laws and bureaucratic delays in generic approvals, without patent protection laws, pharmaceutical companies argue that they would be unable to regain their investment in product development and ultimately their investment in research would markedly decrease (Reinhardt, 2003).

Another controversial issue surrounding pharmaceuticals is price discrimination, which, in some industries, is accepted practice. For example, flying first class on an airplane is an example of accepted price discrimination; those willing to pay more get more. In the current U.S. health care context, across a range of services, including pharmaceuticals, it is not uncommon to find that those with the least amount of money often pay the highest prices (Reinhardt, 2003). Low-income elderly without supplemental health insurance often pay the highest prices. With the enactment of the Medicare Modernization Act of 2003, the federal government provided protections to the pharmaceutical industry by choosing not to negotiate drug prices and instead relying on a market-based approach to holding down costs. Yet the costs of pharmaceuticals—particularly for senior citizens with co-morbidities and multiple drug regimens—can be enormous, exceeding the coverage limits of programs such as Medicare (see *Interests, Ideology, and Institutional Dynamics in the Creation of the Medicare Prescription Drug Benefit* following Chapter 15).

A fundamental question is whether a market-based system or government intervention is the most effective way to control drug costs for seniors. Proponents argue that private health plans competing for enrollees will make drugs available at reasonable prices. Those who choose to participate in the new program will have to enroll in a Medicare drug plan. Each plan will be responsible for negotiating with drug manufacturers and pharmacies to determine the prices for medicines that will apply under the plan. These drug benefits are limited to recipients who are not low-income, thus enabling more seniors to have access to lower prices. However, they will still incur significant out-of-pocket costs for their medicines. The law prohibits the government from interfering with negotiations between plan sponsors and drug manufacturers and pharmacies. It also prohibits the establishment of any price controls or the development of any specific list of drugs. Opponents are concerned that without government intervention, there will be little competition as there are only a few large manufacturers who will basically have exclusive rights, which has historically resulted in little or no impact on price (KFF, 2005b). Ultimately, the values of a market-driven drug industry and the values of financial accessibility to drug therapy collide as policymakers struggle to decide how drug coverage can be made more affordable for those who need it most.

Another high profile issue is the re-importation of drugs and the government's role concerning drug prices in the Medicare program. Re-importation and importation are terms that refer to the purchase of drugs from other countries. It has been illegal to import prescription drugs from other countries. Only the original manufacturer may re-import a pharmaceutical product, subject to meeting certain standards on how the drugs are handled and labeled. However, in practice, the FDA does not enforce the law banning importation for personal use. Significantly lower prices for common prescription drugs in the bordering countries of Mexico and Canada have led some Americans to import drugs from those countries. Stories of seniors going to Canada to purchase their drugs are becoming more common. Politicians from both parties have proposed lifting the import ban and a number of bills were introduced before the 109th session of Congress. Impatient for congressional action, a number of states, including Illinois, Michigan, Minnesota, and Ohio, have undertaken efforts to get lower drug prices for their residents through purchases from other countries (KFF, 2004b). Some of these domestic initiatives at the individual and state level within the United States have been hindered as Canadian politicians assert control to meet domestic need within their own country before exporting beyond their borders.

Two reports released in December 2004 documented key issues in this debate. First, an analysis by the Department of Health and Human Services (HHS) Task Force on Drug Importation, chaired by the U.S. Surgeon General Vice Admiral Richard Carmon, confirmed that while drug importation is common, most of the medicines produced are not under FDA oversight. The cost of putting in an oversight system would leave consumers with only a 1% to 2% savings. The second report, released by the Department of Commerce, focused on pharmaceutical price controls in Organization for Economic Cooperation and Development (OECD) countries. The report concluded that while non-generic prescription drugs are indeed considerably cheaper in other countries—in large part due to government-imposed price controls—those reductions result in less innovation abroad (KFF, 2004b). Some are skeptical of these "findings." Ron Pollack, executive director of Families USA, criticized their purpose: "Rather than taking a year spending taxpayer dollars to write a report that simply repeats pharmaceutical industry's arguments against re-importation, the Administration should have focused on developing a system to provide Americans with access to affordable prescription drugs" (Families USA, 2004).

Health care expenditures have motivated many states to limit rising pharmaceutical costs by instituting their own plans to control prices. In a 2004 survey of state officials, 43 states reported implementing pharmacy cost controls, and 39 states reported freezing provider rates or reducing rate increases for at least one group of providers (National Conference of State Legislatures, 2005). Maine and Michigan are two examples of states that purchase drugs at a lower price for their large population of poor people. Maine enacted historical legislation that established discounted prescription drug prices for all state residents without drug coverage. Michigan directly negotiated with drug manufacturers for price discounts by purchasing in bulk for all uninsured residents (National Conference of State Legislatures, 2005).

In response, the pharmaceutical industry launched aggressive counterattacks. In California, drug makers raised $8.6 million to defeat a proposed ballot measure that would have required drug makers to provide discount prescription medications to consumers with annual incomes that do not exceed 400% of the federal poverty level. Under the measure, drug companies that did not comply with the program would be excluded from Medi-Cal, the state's Medicaid program (Health Access California, 2005).

Another cost control strategy is the establishment of discount cards. Initially, 10 drug companies partnered to establish a discount card for the uninsured. The "Together Rx Access" card was announced in January 2005. Uninsured who earn less than $30,000, with the income ceiling raised $10,000 for each additional household member, are eligible for the card and related discounts of 25% to 40% for drugs (Agovino, 2005).

## BIOTERRORISM: THE INTERNATIONAL HEALTH THREAT

*Future chemical, biological, or nuclear terrorism should be anticipated. In preparing for these attacks, we have to walk a fine line between lack of preparedness and creating undue fear in our daily lives.*

DONNA SHALALA, FORMER HHS SECRETARY
(QUOTED IN ANNAS, 2003, P. 299)

As pharmaceutical issues continue to receive almost daily focus due to their rising costs, another less visible but dangerous health threat is the possibility of future terrorism using chemical, biological, or nuclear materials and causing massive casualties. Because of its magnitude, anti-terrorism efforts compete for public health attention, time, and financial resources.

The fundamental duty of the American government is the protection of the public's health, safety, and welfare. The September 11, 2001 attacks on New York and Washington and subsequent anthrax attacks seriously challenged this federal duty. The threat to American's sense of security and public health has launched a new focus on the public health infrastructure and resources needed to effectively respond to terrorist attacks. Terrorists use bombs, explosives, and other tools for mass destruction.

Bioterrorists' weapons are infectious agents (e.g., virus, infectious substance, biological product).

These weapons are used to negatively influence the conduct of governments or intimidate populations by causing disease or death in humans (Gostin, 2001). Threats from any form of terrorist weapon demand an effective coordinated response by federal, state, and local governments. Focusing on "prevention through preparation" by investing and deploying financial, human, and technical resources is essential.

For almost 25 years, prior to the September 2001 attacks, no large-scale investments had been made in the public health infrastructure. Since then, Homeland Security programs administered by the Centers for Disease Control and Prevention (CDC) and Health Resources and Services Administration (HRSA) are intended to improve public health preparedness to respond to a terrorist attack. An additional goal is to improve the public health system's ability to address other threats as well (Lurie et al., 2004).

In response to perceived threats, the federal government has directed billions of dollars to shore up the nation's ability to prevent and respond to terrorist attacks, beginning with an infusion of, and continuing, annual appropriations of over $40 billion since 2001. How these considerable financial resources are deployed and used are critically important policy evaluation questions given the substantial magnitude of this financial investment (CQ Weekly, 2005).

Within these massive expenditures, resources are deployed and shifted toward and away from a variety of specific programs with relevance to public health. For example, expanding the public health infrastructure toward incident preparedness has been a priority at the federal, state, and local levels over recent years. Most agencies build capacity and develop response plans in preparation against both terrorist attacks and natural disasters (Alles, 2005).

Major reprogramming in federal bioterrorism preparedness funds in June 2005 resulted in about a $1 million funding decrease per state. A total of $54.9 million of 2004 funds were redirected away from state projects into activities such as upgrading quarantine abilities at the CDC and developing the Cities Readiness Initiative, to improve preparedness capacity for 21 cities. This funding shift was coupled with President Bush's $105 million cut in state and local public health preparedness funds for FY 2005. Critics perceive this move to be consistent with the government's long-time under-commitment to public health. They note that all of these programs are critical but that these decisions reflect inappropriate program and policy choices that are "either/or" choices rather than "and" propositions.

The proposed FY 2006 Homeland Security budget retargeted some preparedness resources to national or centralized resources and decreased funding to state and local government funds by 12.6%. Debate about allocation within the budgeted amount ranged from focusing on support for first responders to issues around stockpiling drugs. For example, an increase in funds for the Strategic National Stockpile (SNS) of drugs and medical supplies from $397 million in 2005 to $600 million in 2006 is a 51% increase (Center for Infectious Disease Research and Policy [CIDRP], 2004). "We're requesting $600 million to buy additional medicines, replace old ones, provide specialized storage, and get any needed medicine and supplies to any location in the United States within 12 hours," HHS Secretary Mike Leavitt said in a Feb 7, 2005 briefing. But the Association of State and Territorial Health Officials said the proposed cuts "would weaken the ability of state and local public health agencies to respond to bioterrorism, emerging infectious diseases, or other public health threats and emergencies" (CIDRP, 2004). Republicans argued that the Administration is right to restrain the amounts of funds allocated to state and local governments, in large part, because identification of national preparedness standards have not been developed which will clarify grant distribution of funds based on concrete threat and vulnerability assessments (Carafano, 2005).

The impact of regularly changing the focus of preparedness funds is thought to compromise the ability of public health workers to improve preparedness as implementation priorities change. Patrick Libby, executive director of the National Association of County and City Health officials observes, "Unfortunately, the current administration seems to be addressing public health preparedness issue by issue. What is missing is a clear sense of a systematic approach to assuring that communities are appropriately prepared" (Krisberg, 2005).

The lack of federal preparedness standards is also problematic to a cooperative planning process involving both state and local governments. A survey of health officials in 26 states found that most rural areas would not be prepared for a bioterrorist attack or have the resources to handle the surge of people fleeing urban areas under assault (Jordon, 2005).

In addition to identifying the priorities of policymakers, it is also useful to determine preferences of the American public. A January 2005, nationwide poll conducted by Trust for America's Health, found that Americans are more concerned with diseases that impact their daily lives than they are with potential disasters. About 52% believe that the country is not well prepared to respond to a terrorist emergency and 7 out of 10 Americans favor the federal government increasing spending on researching the causes and prevention of disease. In 2003, the government spent 92% of health dollars on diagnosis and treatment of disease and 8% on research (Healthy Americans Organization, 2005).

As long as the public's health is threatened through terrorist attacks causing competition in public health priorities, the challenge is to reconstitute the public health infrastructure, while shifting focus from disease control to health promotion, and addressing continuing social inequities and their impacts on health (Annas, 2003). A strong public health infrastructure can serve complementary purposes to keep the public both safe and healthy. A clear challenge is to avoid strengthening one focus at the expense of the other.

## THE UNINSURED

*Federal budgets are memoranda in which we tell God what moral trade-offs we are willing to make as a nation. Ironically, the socio-economic class we neglect in health policy happens to be the prime recruiting ground for the soldiers we ask to stand tall for America abroad.*

UWE E. REINHARDT (2004 PRESENTATION)

There are more uninsured Americans than the total population of Canada (Lambrew, Podesta, & Shaw, 2005). Conservative estimates for 2004 indicate that 41.6 million persons of all ages (14.5%) were uninsured and 51.0 million (17.7%) were uninsured for at least part of the year (Cohen, Martinez, & Hao, 2005). Projections suggest that by 2013, one in four Americans under the age of 65, nearly 56 million people, will be without health care insurance because coverage will be too expensive (CQ Healthbeat News, 2005). The United States spends more money on health care than any other nation, yet, it is the only industrialized nation that does not ensure that all citizens have health care coverage. Every year, approximately 18,000 unnecessary deaths occur because of the lack of health insurance in the United States (Institute of Medicine [IOM], 2002). Proponents of universal health care coverage view this set of problems as fixable, but only with a significant overhaul of our current insurance system. Examining the disparities in who is uninsured contributes to understanding how health treatment disparities are produced in our society and how they relate to the production of a chronically uninsured segment of the population.

### Disparities in Health Insurance Status.

The distribution of health care coverage is unequal across the U.S. population and related to a number of characteristics including race, ethnicity, socioeconomic status, and age. The enactment of Medicaid and Medicare in 1965, coupled with enforcement of the 1964 Civil Rights Act, made inroads into reducing health care divisions in the United States. In terms of race, about one in three residents of the United States self-identify as African American, American Indian/Alaska Native, Asian/Pacific American, or Hispanic. While racial/ethnic minorities comprise about a third of the U.S. population, these groups disproportionately comprise 52% of the uninsured (KFF, 2004c). The growing American Hispanic population is particularly disadvantaged in receiving health care. Based on 2004 CDC data, Hispanic persons were more likely than either white or black persons to be uninsured for more than a year. Approximately one third of the Hispanics interviewed were uninsured or had been uninsured for at least part of the year, and more than one fourth had not been covered by a health plan for more than a year (Cohen et al., 2005).

Unfortunately, the influence of race today is more subtle. There is compelling evidence that racial/ethnic disparities persist in the medical system. The IOM landmark report *Unequal Treatment: Confronting Racial and Ethnic Disparities in Care* found disparities in treatment exist when comparing individuals of similar income and insurance as well as same illness. This finding is most troubling because health insurance coverage was considered to be the "equalizer" in health care delivery (IOM, 2002).

**The Impact.** In 2000, IOM convened a Committee on the Uninsured to examine the effects of the lack of health coverage on individuals, families, communities, and society. They found that uninsured people tend to have worse health outcomes because of delayed care, are occasionally denied care, and receive negative differential treatment once in the system. In a series of five reports, the IOM Committee concluded the following:

1. The number of uninsured individuals under the age of 65 is growing and has persisted even during periods of strong economic growth.
2. Uninsured children and adults do not receive the care they need, they suffer from poorer health, and they are more likely to die that those with coverage.
3. Even one uninsured person in a family can put the financial stability and the health of the entire family at risk.
4. High numbers of uninsured people within a community can adversely affect the overall health status of the community.
5. The value gained by providing coverage across the population in healthy years is greater than the additional costs of insuring those who now lack coverage (IOM, 2004c).

From an economic perspective, it is estimated that the annualized cost from diminished health, productivity, and shorter life spans of uninsured Americans is between $65 and $130 billion each year.

Furthermore, as lack of coverage may lead to debt and personal bankruptcy, when the uninsured obtain care from hospitals, it results in billions of dollars in uncompensated care that get passed on through the health care system to taxpayers

(Reinhardt et al., 2004). In its final report, the IOM Committee outlined five principles to guide future policy strategy and dialogue. These five principles propose that health care coverage be universal, continuous, affordable, sustainable, and that the coverage provide access to quality health care that promotes the well being of all (IOM, 2004c). While the concept of universal health insurance does not have a nationally accepted definition, it implies that all Americans should have access to health care when needed, whether or not they have the ability to pay. A survey by the Pew Forum on Religion and Public Life found that more than half of all Americans consider providing universal coverage a moral issue, whereas only about a third view it as a political issue (Pew Research Center for People and the Press, 2003).

### Policy Needs and Economic Realities.
With the shifting economics of employment-based coverage expenditures necessary to maintain health care coverage and treatments are rising, but incomes themselves are not rising with these demands. In 2004, the cost of employer-based health benefits increased at a rate five times higher than that of wages (Gilmer & Kronick, 2005). Since 2000, the family share of this type of coverage has increased 60%. It is estimated that by 2006 the average family health insurance premium will exceed $14,500 a year (National Coalition on Healthcare, 2004). This strains even the middle class and limits employers' abilities to create jobs, let alone maintain them. According to an article in the *New York Times*, "high costs, job losses, and state cutbacks swelled the numbers of the uninsured...[and] the majority of the uninsured are neither poor by official standards nor unemployed." It is estimated that more than half a million middle-class families, per year, have turned to bankruptcy as a result of unpaid medical bills (Strom, 2003).

Access to health insurance increases as income rises. For example, in 2001, the total nonelderly U.S. population that lacked insurance was 17%. Of that percentage, only about 6% were in households 300% above the poverty level, 29% were in households with incomes between 100% to 199% of poverty, and 37% were in households below the federal poverty level (Frontline, 2003). With the increasing number of workers *not* offered employer-based health insurance and many finding private health coverage too expensive, the number of uninsured is growing and more people are turning to public programs for assistance. Enrollment in government health care programs increased as access to Medicaid expanded in 2000. The number of children covered under the SCHIP has risen in the United States. In 2004, 69.6% of poor children and 44.6% of near-poor children were covered by a *public* health plan. From 1999 to 2003, estimates of public coverage show increases among children coinciding with a decrease in the percentage of poor and near-poor children with private coverage (Krisberg, 2005).

Fundamental to policy solutions is the ability to quantify the cost of covering the uninsured with meaningful health benefits. Based on 2001 figures, it is estimated that $100 billion was spent to care for the uninsured. Two cost projections have been developed regarding the extension of health care to the uninsured to near-universal levels: (a) the additional costs that uninsured coverage would trigger, and (b) the additional costs that would be required to implement the policy. If insurance were provided through private coverage like that held by some middle- and low-income families, the additional costs are projected to be approximately $70 billion a year (Reinhardt, 2003). One strategy for extending health care coverage is through expansion of public insurance programs such as Medicaid and SCHIP. It is estimated that 35% of the estimated $100 billion spent on "uncompensated care" is not billed by providers. Emergency rooms have been hard hit by such uncompensated costs, as federal law requires staff to care for anyone who needs treatment with or without payment. Another 26% of the $100 billion costs are paid out of pocket by the uninsured. These two cost centers, the service provider and the consumer, would be reflected in increased government spending. Additionally, some insured might choose to drop their coverage to move into a universal coverage umbrella depending on the parameters set. Clearly, extending insurance coverage is exceedingly complex, with multiple stakeholders invested in alternative approaches to ensuring access to health care.

**Current Federal Policy Action.** Given a significant federal deficit and rapidly increasing health expenditures in the Medicaid program, and political priorities, achieving the recommendation to insure every American citizen by 2010 (IOM, 1999) will be an exceedingly difficult aim. For example, the Medicaid proposal in the Administration's 2006 budget would have led to an increase in the number of uninsured and underinsured Americans by weakening states' ability to fund health and long-term care coverage for low-income populations. While the spending cuts imposed by the Congress were not as draconian as the Administration's budget, nevertheless, Medicaid funding was reduced by $10 billion over 4 years. The Administration's budget also proposed the "modernization" of Medicaid and SCHIP, giving states more flexibility to restructure coverage, contingent on no additional federal cost. The language implies a "cap" on Medicaid funding to ensure that federal costs do not increase. Such a budget could further shift costs to the states (CBPP, 2005). Conclusions have been drawn that access to health care not only improves health status but that better health also leads to higher labor force participation and productivity. Despite the objective benefits of health and its potential positive relationship to the economy, achieving universal coverage is extremely difficult. Underscoring this point, Reinhardt asserts that the lack of proposed legislation for covering the uninsured during periods of economic surplus does not demonstrate hope that lawmakers will legislate coverage during deepening deficit cycles (Lurie et al., 2004).

**State Responses to Uninsured Health Care Needs.** States have pursued various strategies to deal with the chasm emerging between increasing health care expenses and decreasing budgets. Illustrating one strategy, Missouri Governor Matt Blunt (R) proposed health care cuts that would drop 89,000 of the state's 1 million Medicaid recipients and cut the benefits for 370,000 others, while strongly opposing tax hikes (Hanna, 2005). The largest health care cuts proposed by any state occurred in Tennessee, where Governor

Phil Bredesen (D) proposed massive cuts to deal with his state's budget crisis. TennCare, launched in 1994, was an innovative Medicaid program that tried to go beyond the federal Medicaid requirements for covering low-income children and pregnant women by providing broader coverage to more people in need. With expansion ultimately covering a quarter of the population, costs began to spiral by 15% per year soon after its implementation (Dentzer, 2005).

Exceptions to this cost-cutting trend are rare. One alternative was Democratic Kansas Governor Kathleen Sebelius' (D) proposals to raise tobacco taxes in order to fund the expansion of Medicaid to assist poor adults. Sebelius' plan to reduce the state's uninsured population would add 30,000 uninsured low-income adults to the state's Medicaid program. California approached coverage for the uninsured by considering apportioning costs of universal coverage among businesses, individuals, and government. Ideas included a mandate on employers to insure workers, a mandate on individuals to purchase insurance coverage, and a public-private partnership that would cover all children (Hanna, 2005). Clearly these two different approaches—cutting spending versus developing strategies to expand coverage—would lead to different health and economic outcomes among states.

## PREVENTION FOCUS: RHETORIC OR REALITY?

Nearly half of all causes of mortality in the United States are linked to social and behavioral factors, such as smoking, diet, alcohol use, sedentary lifestyle, and accidents. Yet, less than 5% of the approximately $1 trillion spent annually on health care is directed at reducing risks posed by these conditions. Research has established a dynamic interplay among biological, socio-behavioral, and environmental influences on health and behavior, which ultimately shape health status and outcomes. The implications of this relational perspective lead to a need for a stronger focus on illness prevention and health promotion efforts. The fact that multiple intersecting factors influence health status for individuals and populations provides a particular challenge for policymakers intent on crafting meaningful health policy.

One administrator for the CMS, Mark McClellan, stated that Medicare "must focus on prevention." McClellan noted that about 95% of the program's spending goes to treating health *problems*. Treatment of preventable illness carries significant financial burden for the Medicare and Medicaid program. For example, spending for imaging services rose over 60% from 1999 to 2003, $5.7 billion to $9.3 billion. Increased Medicare program enrollments, in addition to greater use of new and more intensive medical services, are expected to double Medicare expenditures over the next decade. To decrease the rate in growth of Medicare spending, McClellan proposed a preventative approach to diseases coupled with more effectively managing conditions (WebMD, 2005).

Maintaining a focus on prevention through public programs and policies has been particularly challenging given the political and fiscal environment. For example, the Administration's budget for 2006 included a cut of nearly 7% for the CDC's chronic disease prevention and health promotion programs and proposed eliminating the Prevention Health and Health Services Block Grant, which provided millions of dollars to states for unanticipated health emergencies. Historically, this funding was used for outbreaks such as the West Nile Virus and SARS and could be used for services such as offering mammograms to low-income women and to create programs to bridge health disparities. Federal deficits put tremendous pressure on the government to restrain spending, and the resultant choices often pit high-need programs against each other. For example, the Administration's budget proposal called for increased funding for the flu vaccine supply and proposed program cutbacks in the CDC HIV/AIDS prevention and surveillance program. Policies within specific programs are also often refashioned to link political ideology with changes in expenditures. For example, in terms of sex education, the President's budget provided funds for abstinence-only education tracks, which have been shown to puts teens at increased risk by withholding key disease prevention information (Krisberg, 2005).

## THE TOBACCO SETTLEMENT: UNDERFUNDING PUBLIC HEALTH

Tobacco use remains the number one preventable cause of death in the United States, resulting in more than 440,000 deaths each year. Also alarming is the CDC projection that more than 6.4 million children living today will die prematurely as a result of deciding to smoke cigarettes as adolescents (National Center for Chronic Disease and Prevention, 2004a). In addition to human costs, monetary costs to treat smoking-related diseases exceed $75 billion per annum. In spite of this significant toll on human and financial resources, many state policymakers have chosen not to fund smoking prevention programs or the treatment of smoke-related diseases with the $246 billion Master Settlement Agreement (MSA) that was reached with tobacco companies in 1998, instead using tobacco settlement funds for an array of non-health-related purposes, including highway and other infrastructure (Cooper, 2004).

**The Anti-Smoking Campaign.** Individual smokers with cancer, respiratory diseases, and other related illnesses unsuccessfully filed suits against the tobacco industry for 50 years. As evidence linking smoking with disease intensified, public health and taxpayer groups fought for decades (1970s-1990s) to abolish tobacco subsidies, as well as increase the regulation of tobacco. The 1960s marked a turning point for public awareness when the "Surgeon General's Report on Smoking and Health" was published and established a direct link between smoking and lung cancer. This launched a series of annual reports detailing the expanding list of dangers posed by tobacco use. It was another 30 years of slow progress before incremental holistic and ultimately systemic attempts at prevention were instituted.

In 1990, smoking was banned on interstate buses and domestic airline flights. In 1994, after tobacco-company executives testified before Congress that they did not believe nicotine was addictive, public rejection of this position served to bolster efforts to regulate the industry. Incremental regulations, that is, bans on cigarette ads, smoking bans in public transportation, and increased tobacco taxes, began to slowly impact tobacco sales. Additionally, in 1994, internal documents revealed that executives of the large tobacco company Brown & Williamson had been aware of the negative effects of smoking for years. This enabled then Food and Drug Administration Commissioner David Kessler to assert his agency's authority to regulate tobacco because of deceptive industry practices. That same year, Minnesota and Mississippi Attorneys General led the way, with Florida and Texas close behind, in suing the major cigarette firms to recover the costs of treating tobacco-related disease incurred by their state Medicaid programs. Every state in the country quickly followed suit. In 1996, negotiations began between four main tobacco companies and 46 state Attorneys General, culminating in the November 1998 MSA.

The MSA stipulated that the companies pay the states $246 billion over 25 years. From this sum, only $1.7 billion was earmarked for prevention and smoking cessation programs. In 2004, only 17% of the money paid went for health programs (Cooper, 2004). Meanwhile, federal decisions shifted national social service responsibilities to states, local governments, individuals, and private companies. With no requirements that states use the tobacco-company/industry payouts for health-related programs, the settlements became a lost opportunity. Instead, the economic climate catalyzed numerous finance-thirsty programs to vie for settlement awards. Meanwhile, other compartmentalized policy options related to smoking cessation were pursued. Patient advocacy groups, state health departments, the Partnership for Prevention (a coalition of pharmaceutical companies), and others lobbied for Medicare coverage of counseling for older Americans who wanted to quit smoking. Officials for Medicare and Medicaid agreed that evidence supported that seniors with diseases and health effects related to smoking can improve their health by quitting even if they have smoked for years. Unfortunately, critics have noted that the new counseling coverage was not designed to include payment for drugs, patches, or other products used to quit smoking (American College of Preventive Medicine, 2005).

**Current Outlook.** The ability of the tobacco industry to survive stock declines is far from threatened when a surprise, last-minute change in the request for monetary settlement damages was reduced from $130 billion to $10 billion by the Justice Department (Leonnig, 2005). Initially, the Justice Department had requested $280 billion, charging cigarette makers conspired to defraud the public about the dangers of smoking (Cooper, 2004). The government's racketeering case resumed settlement discussions in March, 2005. Lawyers for the government have aggressively pursued settlement since a federal appeals court panel decision in 2005 barred them from seeking millions of dollars in past industry profits as damages. The lawsuit was launched during the Clinton Administration, and anti-smoking groups feared that the Bush Administration would settle the case on terms favorable to the tobacco industry (Yahoo News, 2005). The survival of tobacco companies are further secured as companies, such as Philip Morris, have diversified their products to include other consumer goods (Nestle, 2002).

Meanwhile, in spite of tobacco settlement dollars and piecemeal policies and smoking prevention programs, over a quarter of American teens smoke by the time they leave high school. In fact, evidencing the power of the tobacco industry in 2004, lawmakers defeated a bill that would have authorized the FDA to regulate tobacco products. Industry critics continue to complain that cigarette ads and new products, including flavored cigarettes, continue to target minors. The push for the FDA to regulate tobacco was revived again through a bipartisan effort. Another blow to anti-smoking efforts was the passage of an overarching bill called "Class Action Fairness" by the U.S. Senate Judiciary Committee, which restricts class action law suits against tobacco companies to federal court reviews, not state courts (Tobacco Free Kids, 2005). Requiring federal court reviews makes the wait for a case even longer, allowing the case to, in some circumstances, go unheard. In effect, beyond recent smoking bans in public places and monetary awards from litigation, the tobacco industry can continue to exploit tobacco consumer dependency.

## OBESITY: HOW BIG IS THE PROBLEM?

*While data about the incidence of obesity may not be definitive, anyone with one or two of the five senses knows that obesity is not only an issue, a threat and a problem, but also an epidemic with dire physical and economic consequences.*

TED HOLLANDER (2004)

Diseases caused by diet and inactivity rival tobacco as the leading cause of preventable death in America. Currently, at least 300,000 Americans die each year from obesity-related diseases and over 30 obesity-related diseases have been identified, including heart disease, diabetes, stroke, and arthritis (Greenblatt, 2003). The National Health and Nutrition Examination Survey 1999-2000 estimated that 64% of U.S. adults aged 20 years and older were either obese or overweight (National Center for Chronic Disease Prevention and Health Promotion, 2004b). The prevalence in children is even more alarming. Over the past three decades, the rate has more than doubled for preschool children aged 2 to 5 years and adolescents aged 12 to 19 years. It has tripled for children aged 6 to 11 years. At present, approximately 9 million children over 6 years of age are considered obese (National Academy of Sciences, 2005).

In response to these alarming statistics, in 2004 and 2005 the federal government increased efforts to draw the public's attention to the problem by highlighting the extent of the problem while encouraging diet modifications and increased exercise. Unfortunately, one of the frequently cited studies sponsored and conducted by CDC researchers had flawed data that overstated the prevalence of obesity, leaving some consumers questioning accuracy of government information on obesity and the true seriousness of related problems (Center for Consumer Freedom, 2004). Despite admission by the CDC that the obesity statistics were flawed, obesity is still

---

**BOX 22-2** Obesity: Terms

What is the difference between overweight and obesity?

An individual is overweight when their body mass index (BMI) is between 25 and 29.9. An adult is considered obese if the BMI is above 30. For example, an adult with a BMI of 26 who is a 5'4" woman is considered to be 26 pounds over her healthy weight. A child considered overweight is defined as a BMI for age and sex at or above the 95th percentile of the CDC growth charts.

From www.cdc.gov/nccdphp/dnpa/obesity/defining.htm.

---

considered the fastest growing cause of illness and death in the United States (Hollander, 2004). Tom Skinner, a spokesman for the CDC, stated, "Some people are taking these numbers and saying that obesity is not a public health problem—that is simply not the case" (quoted in Egan, 2005). It is currently estimated that approximately 135 million individuals are overweight or obese. Treating obesity-related health problems are estimated to cost $117 billion annually. Given the numerous serious health effects resulting from being overweight or obese, and if current trends are sustained, the health of the nation and to the health care system are at high risk (Greenblatt, 2003, p. 2) (Box 22-2).

**Complex Environmental Factors Contribute to the Obesity Epidemic.** The reasons why so many Americans are overweight are complex, but one key factor is American eating habits. In considering the "politics of health," it is important to recognize that the food industry influences our health as it promotes what to eat. Recently, two widely recognized books have highlighted critical examples of efforts by the food industry to compromise government policy development in the areas of nutrition and health safety practices in order to benefit their own interest. The politics of food and the larger quandary of the politics of consumption within a market-driven society are challenged. Marion Nestle's book *Food Politics: How the Food Industry Influences Nutrition and Health* (2002) and Eric Schlosser's *Fast Food Nation: The Dark Side of the All-American Meal* (2001) provide astute analyses concerning the potential conflict of interest as companies competing to sell foods, regardless of their effect on nutrition, use the political processes to obtain government support for the sale of these products. The United States Department of Agriculture (USDA) is one agency both authors focus on in discussing the pressures placed on an agency with limited resources for oversight on both food production and simultaneously providing nutritional guidance to the public.

Nestle demonstrates in her book that the primary mission of food companies, like tobacco companies, is to sell products for profit. She notes that in the food industry, nutrition, or the perception of nutrition, becomes a factor in corporate thinking only when it can help sell the food product. She further contends that unlike tobacco, food is required for life and therefore is an even more complicated issue. Some nutrition advocates note that rather than taking on legal fights against the food industry, they would like to see legislation enacted to ensure that food companies cannot lie about the health effects of their products. John Banzhaf, a George Washington University law professor contends, "Legislation would be much preferable, but what happened in this area is exactly what happened in tobacco—legislators refused to legislate" (quoted in Greenblatt, 2003, p. 18).

The food industry spends $10 billion a year in direct media advertising. By comparison, little money is spent to educate consumers about healthy eating choices. The campaign highlighting the importance of fruit and vegetable consumption spends roughly $2 million a year on public education. Another $20 billion is spent by the food industry on indirect marketing, that is, "vertical integration" and marketing alliances, such as Disney movie toys with Happy Meals, Coca-Cola Barbie, and other cross merchandising opportunities. In addition to the role of marketing, there are a relatively small number of food industry giants that dominate the market:

In 2000, seven U.S. companies—Phillip Morris, ConAgra, Mars, IBP, Sara Lee, Heinz, and Tyson Foods—ranked among the ten largest food companies in the world. ... In the United States three companies—Philip Morris (Kraft Foods, Miller Brewing), ConAgra, and

RJR-Nabisco—accounted for nearly 20% of all food expenditures in 1997. (Nestle, 2002, p. 14)

This concentration of resources plays a large role in the standardization of unhealthy consumption patterns within the United States, and this pattern cannot be ignored in considering the obesity epidemic.

Another example of a powerful strategy used by restaurants to influence eating patterns is "supersizing." Serving large portions that significantly exceed normal dietary needs translates into overeating by doubling or tripling portions of food. Certain fast food chains advertise their products using this strategy but generally, average portion sizes have grown to too-large portions throughout the restaurant industry. Studies indicate that people will eat larger portions of food when put in front of them, even when the portion is out of proportion to their initial hunger. A study published in the *Journal of the American Medical Association* (Mokdad, Marks, Stroup, & Gerderding, 2003) found that this pattern is self-reinforcing, as Americans are supersizing their portions at home to match the portions they are served in restaurants. Despite these marketing practices, the fast food industry denies the connection between its products and increased obesity. Although causation is difficult to establish, it has been noted that larger portion practices started at the same time that obesity rates began to increase (Nestle, 2002).

Another factor of concern to some public and health policymakers is the education system and its growing partnership with the fast food industry. An unprecedented marketing event occurred in 1993 when, in return for much-needed capital, a Colorado school district signed a marketing contract with Burger King in a deal that helped set off a nationwide trend in public school corporate sponsorship. The same schools that were driven to save money by eliminating physical education classes turned to fund-raising through contracts with fast food companies and soft-drink vending machines. As public schools are inadequately funded, it is hard to criticize education administrators for seeking finances from wherever they can obtain them. Meanwhile, the returns on investment for corporations are manifold as these educational arrangements are fully tax deductible. Educators point out that policymakers have continued to underfund schools, while placing heavy emphasis on academic achievement at the expense of decreasing or cutting physical and nutritional education. Some contend that this situation mirrors the governments' own traditional "cheap-food" policies. For example, federal government food programs served highly processed, high fat, high salt food commodities on Indian reservations for years (Schlosser, 2001, p. 52).

The health of the U.S. population can be affected when nutrition, food safety, and health information for the public are impeded because of the structural arrangements that limit information dissemination to protect the interest of the agribusiness (Lee & Estes, 2003, p. 180). A critical health policy process question raised by these authors is which influence will be greater on Congress and federal regulators, that which allocates resources for the benefit of the population or special interests? Can both win? What would be the cost?

**Current Policy Initiatives and Funding.** Obesity is a health care issue that provides an invaluable opportunity to teach the public how lifestyle and behavior impact health as well as the value of preventative medicine. The policy question is whether systemic weight gain across a diverse population is a matter of individual responsibility or whether a society that makes it easy to get fat should hold some responsibility. Just as society slowly came to perceive and respond to the fact that the costs of treating smoking-related illnesses are too high, there is an increasing perception that individual weight gain, multiplied by millions, constitutes a national public health problem.

As usual, there is a political divide on how to best approach the issue. The Republicans want a more voluntary approach by the food industry to provide healthier choices and are focusing more on physical activity and prevention. Democrats have called for increased government regulations on the food industry. Both parties are concerned with rising health costs associated with obesity and are stepping up efforts to educate the public about the dangers of being overweight. How the causes will be addressed remains unclear. In 2000, the Physical

Education for Progress Act was authorized to award grants directly to school districts to initiate or improve physical education programs. However, the 5-year program is struggling for enough funding each year (Greenblatt, 2003, p. 16). Congress continues to reauthorize the Child Nutrition Act, which established the school breakfast program in 1966. Under the Act, lunches served in school cafeterias have to meet certain minimum nutritional standards. But food served elsewhere (e.g., vending machines) is exempt from nutritional requirements or USDA oversight (Finance Project Organization, 2005). There is an absence of oversight as to the quality of choices actually made by children in the lunch line.

**Obesity: Medicare and Medicaid.** In July 2004, the Secretary of HHS announced that Medicare was removing the phrase "Obesity is not an illness" from its regulations. Medicare, by statute, only pays for the treatment of illnesses and accidents. This vocabulary adjustment indicated that Medicare would begin paying for treatments of obesity that are "reasonable and effective" (Finance Project Organization, 2005). Effectiveness was to be decided by the established Medicare process. Critics have noted that historically Medicare has not sufficiently questioned the effectiveness of interventions being funded. The guidelines for Medicaid have been similarly restrictive.

In 1990, Congress enacted the Omnibus Budget Reconciliation Act (OBRA), which funds state programs to provide pharmaceutical products to Medicaid recipients. The policy under OBRA *excluded* coverage for drugs used for anorexia, weight loss or weight gain, or to promote smoking cessation. There seem to be loopholes, however, for some pharmaceuticals. For example, in response to the restrictions of OBRA, the HHS ordered states to cover Viagra while continuing to exclude anti-obesity and smoking cessation agents (American Obesity Association, 2005).

Medicaid still does not cover obesity. However, the need for weight loss coverage among Medicaid recipients is apparent. Women and children who are poor and members of minority groups are the primary beneficiaries of Medicaid and health disparity reports indicate that the prevalence of obesity is significantly higher in this population. Although Medicaid does not directly cover obesity, it absorbs the spiraling costs indirectly as obesity-related illnesses, like diabetes, require costly treatment. Medicare and Medicaid are financing about half of these costs (Health Affairs, 2003). Economist Eric Finkelstein of RTI International in North Carolina, who assisted the government in computing these costs, says that the findings reveal the great extent to which the public is financing obesity-related costs. He states,

There has been a debate about whether obesity is a personal or societal issue and whether the government has any business being involved. The fact that the taxpayer is financing half the economic burden of obesity suggests that the government has a clear justification to try to reduce obesity rates. (Quoted in Health Affairs, 2003)

Annual medical spending associated with being overweight or obese comprises 9% of what the United States spends on medical care, and this percentage is likely to increase in conjunction with the rising number of obese children. Currently, the least informed poor and minority adults and children are most likely to be obese and need to rely on the public health infrastructure that does not offer them quality access. Costs for them will continue to increase over the long term if the present trajectory is not changed.

## HEALTH CARE QUALITY

*There is no more pressing concern for the American health care system than improving the quality of care we provide. Improving quality of care not only enhances patient's lives, it saves patients lives.*
TOMMY G. THOMPSON, SECRETARY, DEPARTMENT OF HEALTH AND HUMAN SERVICES (AHA TRENDWATCH, 2003)

The IOM has defined quality as "the degree to which health services for individuals and populations increase the likelihood of desired health outcomes and are consistent with current professional knowledge" (IOM, 2001). The problems with the quality of health care can be categorized as overuse, underuse, and misuse (Chassin & Galvin, as cited in Bodenheimer, 2003). The movement to improve the quality of health care in the United States at a time when cost containment dominates the health care agenda could not be more critical. Improved quality can decrease costs, particularly costs due to the overuse and misuse of services. While substantial investment is needed to reduce misuse, funds are also needed for underuse, such as the care of patients with chronic disease (Bodenheimer, 2003). The infrastructure currently in place to monitor quality improvement has taken the efforts of many health professionals, policymakers, and organizations to develop and sustain. New momentum must be generated to maintain these foundations.

Historically, policy actions to ensure health care quality have been far less frequent or significant than actions designed to increase access to care or decrease health care costs. Quality has long been the least visible part of the cost-access-quality triad. Media accounts of consumer backlash against managed care and fiscal pressures on health care systems fueled concern that quality of care was being eroded and patient safety jeopardized. Consequently, in 1996, President Clinton signed an executive order creating the Presidential Advisory Commission on Consumer Protection and Quality in the Health Care Industry. The President directed the 32-member Commission to make recommendations on how to preserve and improve quality in the health care system. The Commission reached some distressing conclusions and charted needed strategies for addressing quality, some of which were immediately acted on, others of which have, to date, been ignored. Since this order, numerous quality organizations, forums, and federal agencies have emerged to sustain this quality effort.

In 1999, the IOM Committee on Quality of Health Care in America released a damning report titled *To Err Is Human—Building a Safer Health System*, which suggested that between 44,000 and 98,000 people die annually in American hospitals as a result of health care errors. Congress and the White House responded immediately, prompted no doubt in part by nationwide front-page stories reporting this startling assertion. Congress held five committee hearings between the end of 1999 and mid-2000, and a number of bills were introduced to address some of the IOM's recommendations. By the beginning of fiscal year 2001, $50 million had been appropriated to the federal Agency for Health Care Research and Quality (AHRQ) to study patient safety. Other legislation was subsequently introduced to address issues around the reporting of medical errors. In spring 2001, the same IOM committee released its final report, titled *Crossing the Quality Chasm,* which argued the need for radical systemic reform. This reform was envisioned to occur at three different levels: the environmental level, the health care organization level and the interface between clinician and patient (IOM, 2001). The IOM recommendation was to design a "patient-centered" health care system with the qualities of safety, effectiveness, equitability, efficiency, and timeliness, and it required the development of a way to promote both public accountability and quality improvement. The development of national standardized measures became the initial implementation strategy.

## AN EMERGING INFRASTRUCTURE FOR QUALITY

A national system to monitor how well health care delivery systems meet quality standards is slowly emerging. Perhaps the most visible agency supporting quality is the AHRQ, which has been directed by Congress to present an annual report on the quality of health care in the United States. The 2005 AHRQ Report, comparing states in 14 categories of health care quality, showed an average improvement across all states of around 3% over 2004. AHRQ Director Carolyn Clancy stated, "I think fundamental change is occurring." However, she also adds that the slow pace of quality care improvement should "outrage" health care professionals. In this same vein, Donald Berwick, president and CEO of the Institute for Healthcare Improvement, insists that the federal government needs to establish goals and deadlines for making improvements in areas identified in the report. Berwick said, "It is a politically correct mantra to claim that the U.S. has the best health care system in the world. It does not." (Medical News Today, 2005). Unfortunately, for all the costs related to health care we still have a lower life expectancy than 20 other countries. Likewise, the United States has a higher infant mortality rate than the United Kingdom, Canada, France, Germany, Sweden, and Japan (Lambrew et al., 2005). Medicare has been a primary leverage point for the adoption of quality health care standards and measures, but private insurers have been enticed as well.

Currently, there are 53 quality improvement organizations at the state level that are focused in improving the quality of care for Medicare beneficiaries. Health care quality organizations at a national level are increasing in number and size. For example, the National Committee for Quality Assurance (NCQA) is a not-for-profit organization established in 1991 to evaluate the performance of managed care health plans. At this time, there are over 260 commercial health care organizations that rely on NCQA accreditation program to disseminate their performance results. The NCQA uses a quality measurement tool known as the Health Plan Employer Data and Information Set (HEDIS), to determine which providers it will grant accreditation. HEDIS is used by the majority of managed health plans to measure performance on important dimensions of care and service. These outcome measures represent a type of report card for consumers to review in selecting a health care plan. NCQA uses HEDIS's more than 60 measures to audit plan-specific information on clinical performance and client/member satisfaction in order to assess performance by identifying "quality gaps." *Quality gap* is a term used by NCQA to compare the difference in performance among the top 10% of health plans and the national average. It can be applied to any industry. For example, in the airline industry the gap between the top 10% performers and the national average is less than 1%. In health care, where variation in practice is quite high and leads to a wide variation in quality, on some measures the gap can reach 20% (NCQA, 2004).

The National Quality Forum (NQF), established in late 1999, is another organization monitoring health care quality but with a somewhat different approach. Their quality focus is on developing processes to increase patient safety in hospitals. In response to a 2001 joint request from CMS and AHRQ, NQF facilitated a national forum to develop voluntary consensus standards for hospital care, quality performance measures, and to design a national reporting system for hospital care. The 30 measures presented in the NQF 2003 Consensus Report represent the first set of nationally standardized performance practices and measures to assess the quality of care provided by more than 6000 acute care hospitals (NQF, 2003). Similarly, the Leapfrog Group, composed of a large consortium of companies who purchase health care benefits, grew, in part, in response to the IOM's *To Err is Human—Building a Safer Health System* report that noted about 1 million preventable medication errors occurred annually. This group, founded with the support from the Robert Wood Johnson Foundation, identified hospital quality practices they believed would leverage large-scale changes (leaps) to dramatically increase patient safety. Computer physician order entry, intensive care unit physician staffing, evidence-based hospital referrals, and the Safe Practices Survey are currently their four quality indicators. In partnership with NQF, the survey is based on the 30 safe practices identified by NQF, and the scores are used by the hospitals to evaluate their success in implementing these practices. The Leapfrog Patient Safety Initiative recognizes, ranks, and rewards hospitals that meet NQF-endorsed safety standards. Hospitals are then ranked to enable consumers to make informed choices in their health care plans (Leapfrog Group for Patient Safety, 2004).

Other infrastructures have evolved that include a focus on federal health care delivery. For example, the Quality Interagency Coordination Task Force (QuIC) ensures that all federal agencies involved in purchasing, providing, studying, or regulating health care services are working in coordination to improve quality care. This infrastructure was established in 1998 and is chaired by the Secretary of HHS, and the Director of AHRQ serves as the chairperson for day-to-day operations. Identifying ways to reduce medical errors has been a major focus. These identified organizations are not meant to be exhaustive,

but they serve as examples of the similarities and differences in structures that have emerged to focus on quality health care.

## THE MOST RECENT QUALITY EFFORT: PAY FOR PERFORMANCE

The idea of using incentives and disincentives to alter human behavior has traditionally been popular among health care providers and politicians alike. Among the numerous methods employed to improve quality, a common policy approach is now being adapted to the health care system. Instead of practice guidelines, disease management, and decision support systems, which are examples of previous methods used to improve quality, public and private purchasers are exploring linking payment to performance. CMS, NQF, JCAHO, and NCQA are some of the stakeholders promoting a national initiative to use "pay for performance." The idea is to reward physicians and hospitals that deliver excellent preventive and chronic illness care. Health care is still purchased in units of health services (e.g., hospital stay, lab test) or by a specific amount per person, per month. Providers are generally paid the same regardless of quality of care. The movement toward paying for performance involves setting performance expectations, measuring performance, and, based on the results, rewarding providers through financial and other incentive programs. An example of a non-financial award might be a high rating on a publicly disclosed report card.

As the health care delivery system searches for new ways to promote quality, policy questions arise in relation to the pay for performance linkage and in relation to incentive-based structures. How will pay for performance perform? Do the benefits of the incentive systems merit the costs? What level of payment is required to change provider behavior? Should consumers pay more or less for high quality care? Do these programs ultimately improve the provision of care, cost-effectiveness, and outcomes? (AHA Trendwatch, 2003). These questions are being answered very differently.

In the search to provide safe and high quality care, there are critics who charge the pay for performance strategy will not be an effective approach. Berwick criticized recent proposals to tie physician reimbursements to care, saying that this concept will not motivate doctors. Providers "need payment not for performance, but to support performance" (quoted in Reichard, 2005). Others argue that the larger strategy of developing national performance practice standards and measures is the wrong path and that government is rewarding good conformance, not good performance. They contend that the "recipe" approach in which treatment is generically outlined is too rigid. Regina Herzlinger, from the Harvard Business School, states that "these standards are based on peer review, not scientific experiments to ensure evidence-based practice. The appropriate role of the government is to measure outcomes not processes" (Herzlinger, 2005). There is a risk that this concept of quality standards can invite a cookbook approach or even increased worker surveillance. Ignoring individual circumstance in favor of a one-size-fits-all approach has been the posture of many in the health care industry for years. Developing incentives to measure performance are needed. Under current reimbursement schemes, avoidable complications that require readmission may actually be more lucrative to hospitals than getting it right the first time. More research and experience are needed to inform the development of valid quality measures and to assess the prevalence and effectiveness of the current strategies.

There remains a substantial gap between the health care we could provide and the quality of health care we do provide. As long as quality issues (including discriminating treatment), high costs, and change characterize the health care delivery system, ongoing assessment and related interventions will be part of the policy equation. Policy initiatives may take many forms, including changing accreditation and licensure requirements, prohibiting payment schemes shown to put quality of care at risk, and ensuring that consumers are informed about provider performance and able to exercise choice among plans and providers. One of the fundamental ways that health care quality may be improved is through bridging the knowledge divide between providers and patients. Improving quality of the patient experience requires input from both sides of health care: care providers and recipients. Clearly, nurses

have tremendous expertise to bring to this critically important policy discussion.

## CONSUMER HEALTH LITERACY

*A two year old is diagnosed with an inner ear infection and prescribed an antibiotic. Her mother understands that her daughter should take the prescribed medication twice a day. After carefully studying the label on the bottle and deciding that it doesn't tell how to take the medicine, she fills a teaspoon and pours the antibiotic into her daughter's painful ear.*

PARKER, RATZAN, AND LURIE, 2003, P. 3

As self-management of health care increases, individuals are asked to assume new roles in seeking information, understanding rights and responsibilities, and making health decisions for themselves as well as others. These demands rest on the assumption that people have a certain level of knowledge and skill. The IOM report titled *Crossing the Quality Chasm: Safety, Patient-Centered Care, and Equitable Treatment* identifies self-management and health literacy as priorities for health-care quality and disease prevention (IOM, 2001). This report reflects why literacy need be a priority as nearly half of all American adults—90 million people—have difficulty understanding and using health information. These adults have literacy skills that test below high school level. About 40 to 44 million of these adults have difficulty finding information in unfamiliar or complex texts such as newspaper articles, medicine labels, forms, or charts. Add to these challenges the stigma and shame that is often associated with the inability to read and write (Osborne, 1998).

Over 300 studies assessing health-related materials, such as informed consent forms and medication package inserts, were assessed to exceed the reading skill of the average high school graduate. One effect is a higher rate of hospitalization and use of emergency services among patients with limited health literacy. Limited health literacy is projected to lead to billions of dollars in avoidable health care costs. For example, it is estimated that an additional $29 billion had to be spent in 1996 due to poor patient reading skills (Parker et al., 2004). In addition to general costs to the health care system, certain groups bear the majority of the literacy-gap consequences.

"Low literacy plays an important role in health disparities," said AHRQ Director Carolyn Clancy (quoted in Gardner, 2005). Certain groups have a higher prevalence of low literacy. They include people who completed only a few years of education, certain racial or ethnic groups, the elderly, income status classified as poor or near poor, and persons with low cognitive ability.

Approaches to health literacy must bring together research and practice while reframing health literacy beyond the individual obtaining information by improving information delivery. The IOM Health Literacy report also identifies key roles for the HHS as well as other public and private sector organizations to foster research to guide policy development and to stimulate the development of health literacy knowledge, measures, and approaches to this systemic problem. Using a systems approach, the interfaces between the health system, culture and society, and the education system must be examined to develop potential interventions to improve health literacy. The key recommendations from both the AHRQ and IOM reports call for additional research. It is important to note, that at this time, the federal outlay for health services research is $870 million, out of $1.4 trillion. That is 0.02% of our health spending. This reality demonstrates an incongruence between message and action (Frontline, 2003).

The health literacy issue serves as another example of the need for the health care paradigm to shift from the individual and his or her condition toward the larger public health perspective that integrates individual biological, behavioral, and societal influences. This shift emphasizes a necessary awareness that preventative medicine requires innovative strategies to address these converging health care fronts (IOM, 2004b).

## SUMMARY

The state of the nation's health results from a confluence of factors, including policies implemented years earlier. Achieving significant improvement of the public's health is thus a formidable task, in no small part because of various levels of government activity (local, state, federal), multiple players, and pervasive underlying social problems. The challenge to lawmakers and administrators is to adopt a long-term view approach to health policy and appropriately balance the many interests and needs of diverse constituencies within an increasingly complex democratic society. The current fiscal environment, which funds a health care system focused on treating the individual with acute and chronic conditions after they occur, cannot be sustained. Incremental health policy that approaches issues separately from the context of the whole health care system and the health of the whole American population can have unintended negative consequences. Furthermore, mandated improvements without sufficient and sustained funding cannot provide value over time or simply cannot be implemented, which leads to wasted dollars.

The scope of policy action needed for health care is extensive. However, what knowledge exists regarding how to solve problems in health care is often rejected because of political ideology, fiscal constraints, and power struggles. Nurses, in addition to understanding nursing's position within the health care system, must acquire a macro view of health care policy. The lesson for nurses' intent on forging solutions to our health care problems is not that the task is insurmountable; it is developing an understanding that myriad patterns and threads are woven into the health care tapestry which is a dependent part of a larger tapestry of public policy needs. Can we as citizens/voters broaden our scope of concerns to see the interdependence of health care to other policy issues, such as decreased state funding for education and local community services? We will have to make hard choices. They can be either informed or uninformed. The challenge is to recognize and develop an understanding of how policy at the local, state, and federal levels is relevant to our day-to-day lives. Only then can nursing impact society for a greater good.

## *Key Points*

- Efforts to manage a growing federal deficit in times of war, as well as keeping the promise of no new taxes, have resulted in viewing the problems of the health care system as limited to short-term cost containment rather than a long-term investment in the health of all citizens.

- As federal funding diminishes for social policy needs, state and local governments, facing their own budget shortfalls, mirror federal cost cutting measures by decreasing funding for health care programs. This is likely to exacerbate health care crises as demographics shift, chronic illnesses become more prevalent, employee-based coverage diminishes, and rising costs increase the need for public health assistance.

- The largest investments in the public health infrastructure have been made in the arena of anti-terrorism. This has resulted in resources being deployed away from programs critical to public health, such as smoking (the number one preventable cause of death in the United States) and obesity (the fastest growing cause of illness and death in the United States).

- Underpinning all health care cost concerns should be a focus on the interdependent components of quality (focusing on prevention and health literacy), availability (reducing the number of uninsured), and sustainability (making Medicare fiscally sound).

## *Web Resources*

**Agency for Healthcare Research and Quality (AHRQ)**
*www.ahrq.gov*
**American Hospital Association (in particular, AHA Trendwatch)**
*www.aha.org*
**Center for Budget and Policy Priorities**
*www.cbpp.org*
**Congressional Quarterly (CQ), CQ Healthbeat News, CQ Researcher, and CQ Weekly**
*www.cq.com*
**Cover the Uninsured Week Organization**
*http://covertheuninsuredweek.org*
**Health Affairs**
*www.healthaffairs.org*

**Institute of Medicine (IOM)**
*www.iom.edu*
**Kaiser Family Foundation (KFF)**
*www.kff.org*
**National Academy of Sciences**
*www.nas.edu*
**National Committee for Quality Assurance (NCQA)**
*www.ncqa.org*

## REFERENCES

Agovino, T. (2005, March 25). Drug firms create, promote discount card. *Associated Press.* Retrieved March 30, 2005, from *http://abcnews.go.com/Business/wireStory?id=612875&CMP=O TC-RSSFeeds0312.*

Alles, S. (2005). Perspectives on bioterrorism: Preparedness, risk communication, and psychological health. Medscape Retrieved March 27, 2005, from *www.medscape.com/ viewarticle/501726.*

American College of Preventive Medicine. (2005, January 1). Public comment on smoking and tobacco use cessation counseling (CAG00241N). Retrieved March 20, 2005, from *www. acpm.org/2005-001(G).pdf.*

American Hospital Association (AHA) Trendwatch. (2003, September). Paying for performance: Creating incentives for quality improvement. DHHS Secretary Tommy Thompson quote. Retrieved April 20, 2005, from *www.lewin.com/NR/ rdonlyres/eyzniiua4jsqz6v7patsjmd54vlkjol4ifb64 ilsanyeiphentkgkwchchwlm4shfvhojnxwo554be/Vol5No3.pdf.*

American Obesity Association. (2005, May 2). AOA fact sheets: Obesity, Medicaid and Medicare. Retrieved February 25, 2006, from *www.obesity.org/subs/fastfacts/Obesity_Medicare. shtml.*

Annas, G. J. (2003). Bioterrorism, public health and civil liberties. In P. R. Lee & C. L. Estes (Eds.), *The nation's health* (pp. 324-333). Boston: Jones and Bartlett.

Blendon, R., Brodie, M., Altman, D., Benson, J., & Hamel, E. (2004). Voters and health care in the 2004 election. *Health Affairs.* Retrieved March 1, 2005, from *http://content. healthaffairs.org/cgi/content/abstract/hlthaff.w5.86v1.*

Bodenheimer, T. S. (2003). The American health care system: The movement for improved quality in health care. In P. R. Lee & C. L. Estes (Eds.), *The nation's health* (pp. 445-453). Boston: Jones and Bartlett.

Carafano, J. J. (2005). The FY 2006 budget request for homeland security: A congressional guide for making America safer. *Heritage Foundation Backgrounder*, No. 1835. Retrieved March 18, 2005, from *www.heritage.org/research/homeland-defense/bg1835.cfm.*

Center on Budget and Policy Priorities (CBPP). (2004, September 13). A brief update on state fiscal conditions and the effects of federal policies on state budgets. Retrieved March 10, 2005, from *www.cbpp.org/9-13-04sfp.htm.*

Center on Budget and Policy Priorities (CBPP). (2005, March 3). Medicaid cuts in president's budget would harm states and unlikely increase ranks of uninsured. Retrieved March 10, 2005, from *www.cbpp.org/3-3-05health-fact.htm.*

Center for Consumer Freedom. (2004, November 24). CDC admits obesity stats flawed— Pharmaceutical and weight loss industry at fault. Retrieved April 22, 2005, from *www.news-medical.net/print_article.asp?id=6461.*

Centers for Disease Control and Prevention (2005, September 28). Overweight and obesity: Defining overweight and obesity. Retrieved February 21, 2006, from *www.cdc.gov/nccdphp/dnpa/obesity/defining.htm.*

Center for Infectious Disease Research and Policy. (2004, August 31). Bioterrorism preparedness, planning and response. Retrieved March 28, 2005, from *www.cidrap.umn.edu/cidrap/content/bt/bioprep/planning/bt-prep-planning.html.*

Centers for Medicare and Medicaid Services. (2004). National health care expenditures projections: 2004-2014. Retrieved March 13, 2005, from *www.cms.hhs.gov/statisticsnhe/projections2004/proj2004.pdf.*

Center, U.S. Department of Health and Human Services. Retrieved March 28, 2005, from *www.healthfinder.gov/news/newsstory.asp?docID=518339.*

Chassin, M. R., & Galvin, R. W. (1998). The urgent need to improve health care quality. *Journal of the American Medical Association, 280,* 1000-1005.

Cohen, R. A., Martinez, M. E., & Hao, C. (2005, March). Health insurance coverage: Estimates from the National Health Interview Survey, January-September, 2004. Centers for Disease Control. Retrieved March 30, 2005, from *www.cdc.gov/nchs/data/nhis/earlyrelease/insur200503.pdf.*

Congressional Quarterly Weekly (2005, February 14). Bush budget: Homeland security. Retrieved March 29, 2005, from *www.cq.com/display.do?dockey=/cqonline/prod/data/docs/htm/weeklyreport/109.*

Congressional Record. (2005, February 16). The federal deficit. Retrieved March 29, 2005, from *www.cq.com/display.do?dockey=/cqonline/prod/data/docs/html/news/109.*

Cooper, M. H. (2004, December 10). Tobacco industry. *Congressional Quarterly Researcher, 14*(43). Retrieved March 20, 2005, from *www.cqresearcher.com.*

Cover the Uninsured Week. (2004). Health spending predicted to double by 2014; Government to pay for half of it. *Cover the Uninsured Week: News Index.* Retrieved March 13, 2005, from *http://covertheuninsuredweek.org/factsheets/displaycovertheuninsphp?FactSheetID=120.*

Dentzer, S., (2005, March 2). "NewsHour" examines TennCare woes as costs force governor to cut program. The NewsHour with Jim Lehrer. Retrieved March 20, 2005, from *Cover the Uninsured Week Organization* at *http://covertheuninsuredweek.org.*

Egan, T. (2005, May 4). U.S. report sows confusion on weighty topic. *The New York Times.* Retrieved May 4, 2005, from *The International Herald Tribune Online* at *www.iht.com/bin/print_ipub.php?file=/articles/2005/05/03/news/fat.php.*

Families USA. (2004, December 21). Administration continues to ask Americans to pay world's highest drug prices. Retrieved March 20, 2005, from *http://familiesusa.org/site/Pageserver?pagename=Media_Statement_Drug_Reimportation_Task_Force.*

Finance Project Organization. (2005). Supporting childhood obesity prevention programs with federal funds. Retrieved April 25, 2005, from *www.financeprojectinfo.org/publications/obesityprevention.pdf.*

Frontline. (2003. November 12). The other drug war (interview with Uwe E. Reinhardt). Retrieved April 21, 2005, from *www.pbs.org/wgbh/pages/frontline/shows/other/interviews/oldreinhardt.html.*

Gardner, A. (2005, April 8). Literacy gap harms nation's health: Two studies find that millions can't understand basic information. *HealthDay/News,* a service of the National Information.

Gilmer, T., & Kronick, R. (2005, April 5). It's the premiums, stupid: Projections of the uninsured through 2013. *Health Affairs.* Retrieved April 22, 2005, from *http://content.healthaffairs.org/cgi/content/full/hlthaff.w5.143/DC1.*

Gostin, L. (2001, December, 21). The model state emergency health powers act. Paper presented at the Centers for Disease Control and Prevention Legislative Conference. Retrieved April 2, 2005, from *www.publichealthlaw.net/MSEHPA/MSEHPA2.pdf.*

Government Printing Office. (2004, July 30). Budget of the United States Government: Historical tables introduction fiscal year 2005. Retrieved March 29, 2005, from *www.gpoaccess.gov/usbudget/fy05/browse.html.*

Greenblatt, A. (2003, January 31). Obesity epidemic: Can Americans change their self-destructive habits? *Congressional Quarterly Researcher, 13*(4). Retrieved March 25, 2005, from *www.cqresearcher.com.*

Hall, E. (2005, October 28). U.S. national debt clock FAQ. Retrieved February 25, 2006, from *www.brillig.com/debt_clock/faq.html.*

Hanna, J. (2005, February 26). Kansas governor bucks national trend and proposes Medicaid expansion. Associated Press. Retrieved March 20, 2005, from *Cover the Uninsured Week Organization* at *http://covertheuninsuredweek.org.*

Health Access California. (2005, April 9). Lobby group battling state pharmaceutical industry using campaign money to target cheaper drug measures. Retrieved April 15, 2005, from *www.healthacess.org/articles/2005/insider_4_9_05.htm.*

Health Affairs Press Release. (2003, May 14). Obesity, overweight conditions contribute as much as $93 billion to national medical bill. Retrieved February 20, 2005, from *www.healthaffairs.org/press/mayjune0302.htm.*

Healthy Americans Organization. Trust for America's Health. (2005). Public policy priorities 109th Congress. Retrieved March 20, 2005, from *http://healthyamericans.org/policy/recommendations/109thCongress.pdf.*

Herzlinger, R. E. (2005, March 29). Uncle Sam is no doctor: Instead of tracking outcomes, system prescribes medical "recipes." *USA Today.* Retrieved April 21, 2005, from *www.usatoday.com/printedition/news/20050329/oppose29.art.html.*

Hollander, T. (2004, May 4). Childhood obesity expert responds to adds claiming obesity epidemic is "hype". PRWeb press release newswire. Retrieved June 20, 2005, from *http://prweb.com/id?=235842.*

Institute of Medicine (IOM). (1999). To err is human—Building a safer health system. Washington, DC: National Academies Press. Retrieved April 20, 2005, from *www.iom.edu/Object.File/Master/4/117/ToErr-8pager.pdf.*

Institute of Medicine (IOM). (2001, May). *Crossing the quality chasm: A new health system for the 21st century.* Washington, DC: National Academies Press. Retrieved abstract April 20, 2005, from *www.iom.edu/focuson.asp?id=8089.*

Institute of Medicine (IOM). (2002, March 20). Unequal treatment: Confronting racial and ethnic disparities in care. Washington, DC: National Academies Press. Retrieved abstract April 11, 2005, from *www.iom.edu/report.asp?id=4475.*

Institute of Medicine (IOM). (2004a). Focus on health communication: Placing public health in perspective. Washington, DC: National Academies Press. Retrieved abstract January 26, 2005, from *www.iom.edu/focuson/asp?id=6095.*

Institute of Medicine (IOM). (2004b, April). Health literacy: A prescription to end confusion. National Academies of Science. Retrieved January 26, 2005, from *www.iom.edu/report.asp?id= 19723.*

Institute of Medicine (IOM). (2004c). Insuring America's health: Principles and recommendations. Washington, DC: National Academies Press. Retrieved April 11, 2005, from *www.iom.edu/report.asp?id=17632.*

Jordon, L. J. (2005, March 21). Rural areas feel unprepared for attacks. *Associated Press Wired News.* Retrieved March 28, 2005, from *http://wiredservice.com.*

Kaiser Family Foundation. (2004a, September 30). Health care and the 2004 elections. Retrieved March 20, 2005, from *www.kff.org/rxdrugs/7175.cfm.*

Kaiser Family Foundation. (2004b, October 11). Race, ethnicity and healthcare. Retrieved March 25, 2005, from *www.kff.org/minorityhealth/7187.cfm.*

Kaiser Family Foundation. (2004c, December 22). Prescription drugs: Prescription drug reimportation would provide minimal savings, safety could not be assured, federal task force says. Retrieved March 30, 2005, from *www.kaisernetwork.org/daily_reports/rep_index.cfm?hint=3&DR_ID=27369.*

Kaiser Family Foundation. (2005a, January 11). Americans favor malpractice reform and drug importation, but rank them low on health priority list for the congress and president. Retrieved March 13, 2005, from *www.kff.org/kaiserpolls/pomr011105nr.cfm.*

Kaiser Family Foundation. (2005b, January/February). View on prescription drugs and the pharmaceutical companies. Retrieved March 21, 2005, from *www.kff.org/healthpollreport/feb_2005/index.cfm.*

Krisberg, K. (2005, March). Shift in preparedness funds undermines readiness efforts: States to lose about $1 million each. *The Nation's Health.* Retrieved March 28, 2005, from *www.apha.org/tnh/index.cfm?fa=Adetail&id=335.*

Lambrew, J. M., Podesta, J. D., & Shaw, T. L. (2005, March 23). Change in challenging times: A plan for extending and improving health coverage. *Health Affairs.* Retrieved March 29, 2005, from *http://content.healthaffairs.org/cgi/content/abstract/hlthaff.w5.119?ijkey=CkO5HRafD0Ms2&keytype=ref&siteid=healthaff.*

Leapfrog Group for Patient Safety. (2004, April 7). Fact sheet. Retrieved April 22, 2005, from *www.leapfroggroup.org/about_us/leapfrog-factsheet.*

Lee, P. R., & Estes, C. L. (2003). Health policy: The politics of health. In P. R. Lee & C. L. Estes (Eds.), *The nation's health* (pp. 175-181). Boston: Jones and Bartlett.

Leonnig, C. (2005, June 8). Tobacco industry escapes huge penalty. *The Washington Post.* Retrieved June 9, 2005, from *http://msnbc.msn.com/id/8136714/print/1/displaymode/1098/.*

Lurie, N., Wasserman, J., Stoto, M., Myers, S., Namkung, P., Fielding, J., et al. (2004). Local variation in public health preparedness: Lessons from California. *Health Affairs.* Retrieved March 30, 2005, from *http://content.healthaffairs.org/cgi/reprint/hlthaff.w4.341v1.pdf.*

Mokdad, A. H., Marks, J. S., Stroup, D. F., & Gerderding, J. L. (2003, January 1). Prevalence of obesity, diabetes, and obesity-related health risk factors. *Journal of the American Medical Association.* Retrieved March 20, 2005, from *http://jama.ama-assn.org/cgi/content/full/289/1/76.*

National Academy of Sciences. (2005). Preventing childhood obesity: Health in the balance (executive summary). Retrieved March 20, 2005, from *www.nap/edu/openbook/0309091969/html.*

National Center for Chronic Disease Prevention and Health Promotion. (2004a, May). Adult cigarette smoking in the United States: Current estimates. Retrieved April 15, 2004, from *www.cdc.gov/tobacco/factsheets/AdultCigaretteSmoking_FactSheet.htm.*

National Center for Chronic Disease Prevention and Health Promotion. (2004b, October 20.). Obesity trends. Retrieved April 15, 2005, from *www.cdc.gov/nchs/products/pubs/pubd/hestats/obese/obse99.htm.*

National Coalition on Health Care. (2004). Health insurance cost. Retrieved April 15, 2005, from *www.nchc.org/facts/cost.shtml.*

National Committee for Quality Assurance. (2004). What is NCQA? Retrieved April 20, 2005, from www.ncqa.org/communications/sohc2004/intro.htm.

National Conference of State Legislatures. (2005, June 16). Pharmaceutical bulk purchasing: Multi-state and inter-agency plans, 2005. Retrieved March 15, 2005, from *www.ncsl.org/programs/health/bulkrx.htm.*

National Quality Forum. (2003). National voluntary consensus standards for hospital care: An initial performance measure set. Retrieved April 20, 2005, from *www.qualityforum.org.*

Nestle, M. (2002). *Food politics: How the food industry influences nutrition and health.* Berkeley: University of California Press.

Office of Management and Budget. (2005, March 31). Management Summary Report. Retrieved March 31, 2005, from *www.whitehouse.gov/omb/budget/fy2004/summary.html.*

Osborne, H. (1998, June). The need to understand addressing issues of low literacy and health. *On Call.* Retrieved March 20, 2005, from *www.healthliteracy.com/oncalljun1998.html.*

Parker, R. M., Ratzan, S. C., & Lurie, N. (2003). Health literacy: A policy challenge for advancing high-quality health care. *Health Affairs, 22*(4), 147. Quoted in L. Nielsen-Bohlman, A. Panzer, D. Kindig, (Eds), *Health literacy: A prescription to end confusion* (p. 3). National Academy of Sciences (executive summary). Retrieved March 20, 2005, from *www.nap.edu/catalog/10883.html.*

Pew Research Center for the People and the Press. (2003, July 24). Religion in politics: Contention and consensus. Retrieved March 23, 2005, from *http://pewforum.org/publications/surveys/religion-politics.pdf.*

Public Agenda. (2004). Public agenda issue guide: The federal budget. Retrieved March 13, 2005, from *http://publicagenda.org/issues/frontdoor.cfm?issue_type=federal_budget.*

Public health groups strongly support bipartisan FDA tobacco legislation. (2004, May, 20). News-Medical.Net Retrieved March 28, 2005, from *http://news-medical.net/?id=1731.*

Quality Interagency Coordination Task Force. (n.d.). QuIC fact sheet. Retrieved April 20, 2005, from *www.quic.gov/about/quicfact.html.*

Reichard, J. (2005, April 4). Experts see 'fundamental change' in drive to improve health care quality. *Congressional Quarterly Healthbeat, 2*(4). Retrieved April 6, 2005, from *www.cq.com.*

Reinhardt, U. (2004, May 3). Why is there so little hope for America's Uninsured? Presentation to the Center for American Progress Policy Forum. Retrieved March 9, 2005 from *www.kaisernetwork.org/health_cast/uploaded_files/050304_cfap_coverage_reinhardt. pdf.*

Reinhardt, U. (2003, August 27). Is there hope for the uninsured? *Health Affairs*. Retrieved April 21, 2005, from *http://content.healthaffairs.org/cgi/content/full/ hlthaff.w3.376v1/DC1*.

Reinhardt, U., Hussey, P., & Anderson, G. (2004). U.S. health care spending in an international context. *Health Affairs, 23*(3), 10-25. Retrieved March 13, 2005, from *http://content.healthaffairs.org/cgi/content/short/23/3/10?ck=nckk*.

Schlosser, E. (2001). *Fast food nation: The dark side of the all-American meal*. New York: Houghton Mifflin.

Society for Vascular Surgery. (2005, March 3). *Medicaid may be harder to fix than social security*. Retrieved March 7, 2005, from *http://svs.vascularweb.org/_CONTRIBUTION_PAGES/ Medical_News_Reuters/Medicare_may_be_harder_to_fix_ than_Social_Security_.html*.

Strom, S. (2003, November 16). For middle class, health insurance becomes a luxury. *New York Times*. Retrieved April 5, 2005, from *www.nytimes.com*.

Study predicts uninsured will reach 56 million by 2013. (2005, April 5). *Congressional Quarterly Healthbeat News*. Retrieved April 6, 2005, from *www.cq.com/display.do?dockey=/ cqonline/prod/data/docs/html/hbnews/109/hbnews1*

Tobacco Free Kids. (2005, February 3). *"Class action fairness" legislation is a victory for big tobacco and a defeat for the legal rights of all Americans*. Statement of Matthew L. Mayers, President, Campaign for Tobacco-Free Kids. Retrieved March 28, 2005, from *http://tobaccofreekids.org/script/DisplayPressRelease. php3?Display-813*.

Triplett, W. (2003). State budget crises. *Congressional Quarterly Researcher*. Retrieved March 20, 2005, from *http://library.cqpress.com/xsite/login.php?requested=%2 2Fdochistory. 3Dcqresearcher:cqresrre2003100300.htm*.

WebMD, & AOL Health. (2005, January 25). Interview with Mark McClellan. *"Medicare Update 2005."* Retrieved June 1, 2005, from *http://aolsvc.health.webmd.aol.com/content/ Chat_transcripts/1/105396.htm*.

Yahoo News. (2005, March 22). U.S. in talks to settle with tobacco companies. Retrieved March 30, 2005, from *www.yahoonews.org*.

---

# Taking Action
Paula C. Hollinger, State Senator, Maryland

## Stem Cell Research in Maryland: A Nurse Legislator's Initiative

*"Reform is not for the shortwinded."*
ARTHUR VANDERBILT, NEW JERSEY SUPREME COURT JUSTICE

"I want to be a normal teenager." "I want to play football." "I want to dance at my daughter's wedding." None of these statements seem to be extraordinary requests. But to those who spoke them, they are. These are the words of Annie Coble, age 14; Van Brooks, age 17; and John Kellerman, age 50. They suffer from juvenile rheumatoid arthritis, a spinal cord injury, and early-onset Parkinson's disease, respectively.

I met Annie, Van, and John during the 2005 session of the Maryland General Assembly where I serve in the State Senate. They met with me several times to share the stories behind their conditions and the hope that they share for the future. Their hope lies in the promise of stem cell research.

### MY PATH

I learned the effects of chronic illness early in my life. My parents were sick throughout my childhood. Taking care of them led me to a career in nursing. As a nurse, I was able to care for people and be an advocate, two roles that fit my people-driven personality. After training at Mt. Sinai Hospital in New York, I worked in many different nursing fields. I was the head nurse at one of the first intensive care units in the country, and I worked as an emergency room nurse, a psychiatric nurse, a camp nurse, and a school nurse.

I had a natural affinity for politics. Growing up in Washington, DC, my parents followed national politics, but it was my mother who was active in many grassroots efforts. Over the years, I began to see how public service went hand in hand with health. People needed an advocate in the state legislature as much as they did in the emergency room.

I began to think that I could fill a void in politics. I thought I could bring a unique perspective to the legislature and be involved with the issue I cared about most: access to quality health care.

I was elected to the Maryland House of Delegates in 1978, where I served two terms before going to the State Senate. I concentrated on becoming a health policy expert. As the only nurse in the Senate, I became the "go-to" person on health issues and not just on policy. Senators and staffers who were not feeling well often approached me for nursing advice.

My hard work paid off when I received my biggest honor to date. After the 2002 election, I was named Chair of the Senate Education, Health, and Environmental (EHE) Affairs Committee, one of four standing committees in the Maryland Senate. Chairs have the ability to lead the public bill hearings, decide if and when a bill will be voted on in committee, and appoint floor leaders for the debate. As EHE Chair, I have the opportunity to shape the health policies developed by the Maryland Senate.

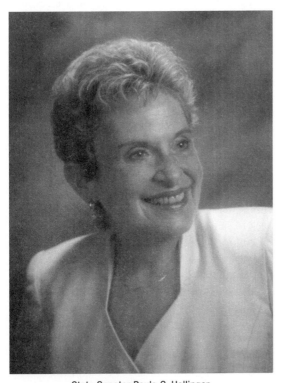

State Senator Paula C. Hollinger.

## PUBLIC AWARENESS OF STEM CELL RESEARCH

Two years into my chairmanship, stem cell research began to receive a lot of public attention with the deaths of President Ronald Reagan and actor/activist Christopher Reeve. President Reagan's body was as healthy as could be, but a 13-year struggle left his mind deteriorated to the point that he didn't know his own wife and children. Nancy Reagan and her children became public advocates for stem cell research, as did the family of Christopher Reeve. Reeve's courage became well known after a 1995 riding accident left him with a paralyzing spinal cord injury.

Stem cell research, particularly embryonic stem cell research, holds promise in the battle against Alzheimer's disease and spinal cord injury, as well as Parkinson's disease, multiple sclerosis, Lou Gehrig's disease (ALS), retinal macular degeneration, cancer, and diabetes. Most of the funding for scientific research comes from the federal government. However, in 2001, President George W. Bush limited federal funding for embryonic stem cell research to certain cells that already existed. The criteria limited research to just 71 lines worldwide (National Institutes of Health [NIH], 2005a).

Both embryonic and adult stem cells have the potential to make significant gains in the treatment of many diseases and conditions. Embryonic stem cells have the unique ability to develop into any cell type. Adult stem cells, while valuable, are less versatile. Skin stem cells can be used to reproduce skin and bone-marrow stem cells can be used to reproduce bone marrow, but researchers want to learn more about the development of embryonic stem cells. Understanding this development may allow such cells to be used for cell-based regenerative therapies that slow or stop the progression of these diseases, or even prevent them all together (NIH, 2005b).

With a significant limit on federal funding, scientists and advocates began looking to the states to support stem cell research. Across the country, states are taking action. In 2004, California voters approved a measure to use $3 billion over 10 years to build the California Institute for Regenerative Medicine and award loans to research embryonic stem cell research. New Jersey's 2005 fiscal year budget included $9.5 million for the Stem Cell Research Institute of New Jersey. A total of $750 million dollars is required to fund Governor Jim Doyle's proposal to support Wisconsin's biotechnology industry, including stem cell research. New York voters may have the opportunity to approve a measure to put $1 billion over 10 years to build the New York Stem Cell Institute and fund loans and grants to researchers (Department of Legislative Services, 2005a).

Maryland is well known for its outstanding medical community. Our biotech industry has taken off in recent years. Patients, their families, as well as the industry needed Maryland to be a leader in this field. I decided it was time for legislative action.

## MARYLAND SENATE BILL 751/ HOUSE BILL 1183

In recent years, several bills have been introduced to the Maryland General Assembly regarding stem cell research. Some bills affirmed the rights of scientists to perform such research, some included funding, and others proposed complete bans. I decided to team up with a colleague in the House of Delegates, Samuel I. "Sandy" Rosenberg to introduce SB 751/HB 1183: The Maryland Stem Cell Research Act of 2005.

Writing the bill was anything but simple. We had to measure the meaning of every word, knowing we would be attacked from all sides. After several drafts, we came up with a bill that balanced both ethical and scientific interests.

The bill provided $25 million annually for the Maryland Stem Cell Research Fund. In our original proposal, money came from the Cigarette Restitution Fund, a fund supported by a settlement with five major tobacco companies. The state will complete payments to attorneys in 2006, making $30 million extra a year available in the fund in fiscal year 2007.

The bill outlined a strict process for granting awards. The Maryland Scientific Peer Review Committee was designated to review applications for funding. Members included representatives from relevant state agencies and the medical field, who would review applications for scientific merit using guidelines set by the NIH. The Committee would

then rate and rank applications and make recommendations to the Maryland Stem Cell Research Commission for awarding funds. The bill joined representatives from state agencies with consumers and experts in the fields of science and biomedical ethics on the Commission to make awards from the Stem Cell Research Fund.

Before disbursement of awards, the grantee must submit approval to Commission from an Institutional Review Board (IRB). IRBs review research proposals to ensure ethical practices and safety.

Most importantly, the bill banned human cloning, which was defined as the replication of a human being through the production of a precise genetic copy of human DNA, or any other human molecule, cell, or tissue, in order to create a new human being (Department of Legislative Services, 2005b).

During the drafting process, I invited my colleagues to cosponsor the Maryland Stem Cell Research Act of 2005. I was able to gather 17 senators to cosponsor the bill; 57 delegates signed on in the House.

Press began long before the legislative session, with calls coming from the U.S. bureaus of international media. Support rolled in from everywhere. Calls, letters, and e-mails poured into my office from constituents who believe in the promise of stem cell research. Three former governors began working to promote the bill. Patient advocates, individuals, and professionals from the fields of medical and biotechnology formed a coalition to lobby for the bill and began meeting with key legislators.

## THE LEGISLATIVE DEBATE ON STEM CELL RESEARCH

The 90-day legislative session began the second week of January. By the first week of February, we felt comfortable enough to officially introduce the legislation. That day, we held a press conference to explain the bill to the press and the public. There were more cameras in the room than I had ever seen at a legislative press conference. Scientists explained the value of stem cell research. Ethicists and religious leaders spoke in support. People in the room were brought to tears as patients gave accounts of their illnesses and their support of stem cell research. I was overwhelmed by the support.

The bill drew attention from those with economic interests as well. Biotechnology is a key component of the Maryland economy with more than 300 biotechnology companies throughout the state. A study was also done by the Sage Policy Group regarding the economic impact stem cell research could have on the Maryland economy. States that have passed funding legislation were looking more and more attractive to our scientists. If Maryland chose to fund stem cell research, we could guarantee short-term benefits to the economy as the research dollars would attract business and increase their competitiveness. If research found successful treatments for a number of diseases, we could treat patients in a more cost-effective manner over the long term. Conservative estimates done by Sage put the state's fiscal return at 194% (Sage Policy Group, 2005).

Unfortunately, the vast support for the bill didn't mean an easy journey through the legislative process. Many opponents of the bill saw the use of embryonic stem cells as immoral. They see each embryo as a life unto itself and believe the use of an embryo for anything other than procreation is destroying a human being. This side was as determined to defeat the bill as we were to pass it.

At a press conference in Annapolis, Maryland, on February 7, 2005, Rabbi Avram Reisner, chairman of the biomedical ethics subcommittee of Conservative Judaism's Committee on Jewish Law and Standards, may have put it best when he commented that embryonic stem cells are "the stuff of life, but not life itself."

## POLITICS

Typically, each bill is assigned to a standing committee in the legislative house of origin. Each year, a handful of bills are assigned to two committees because the topic and content apply to the jurisdiction of two committees. The Senate bill was assigned to the committee I chair, Education, Health, and the Environment Affairs (EHE), due to the health policy involved, and the Senate Budget and Taxation Committee (B&T), due to the allocation of a significant amount of money in the state budget.

We thought carefully about how to make the bill more amenable to our opponents and more likely to pass through the legislature. The problem lay largely with the Senate. While the 24 votes needed for passage were coming at a sure pace, opponents were threatening to filibuster the bill. During a filibuster, debate goes on indefinitely until three fifths of the Senate, 29 members, vote for cloture to end the debate.

While 29 didn't seem far on paper, the issue was complicated by party politics. Two or three of our votes toward passage came from members of the Republican Party. With our opposition to the bill lying largely in the leadership of the Republican Party, we were unlikely to get our Republican supporters to vote for cloture, against the party line.

Hoping to make the bill more palatable, we decided to limit the source of embryonic stem cells to unused embryos and eggs created for patients being treated for infertility. With the permission of these patients, these cells could be used to help improve the lives of those suffering from debilitating conditions and prevent people from suffering in the future. Sometimes, these cells are just thrown away.

Just before committee hearings for the bill, it was reported by the media that the stem cells that were eligible for federal funding were found to be contaminated with a non-human molecule, making them no longer useful for research. Our mission became even more important (Mundell, 2005).

## COMMITTEE HEARINGS

Bill hearings can run anywhere from five minutes to five hours. A typical hearing begins with testimony from the lead bill sponsor, followed by any state agencies that have come to weigh in. From there, proponents come forward to testify, followed by opponents. Each person that speaks is subject to questions from the committee members.

Many of those interested in testifying were patients for whom traveling was a hardship. Most often, cross-filed bills are not heard on the same day. However, to save patients and their families the extra trip, we scheduled the House and Senate hearings two hours apart. I began speaking at 1:00 PM that afternoon. Physicians and researchers from Johns Hopkins University were scheduled to follow me, but when I finished presenting, the same doctors were still answering questions from House members in the hearing across the street. We continued shortly thereafter, hearing from doctors, patients, ethicists, clergy, patient advocacy groups, as well as "right-to-life" organizations and advocates.

## ON THE FENCE

With the hearings behind us, things moved quickly in the House of Delegates. The bill passed both committees and the full House with few changes, but we were still struggling for the last few cloture votes in the Senate. We began to strategize to reach out to the senators that were on the fence. Patients from their districts contacted them and asked for face-to-face meetings to explain their illnesses and how stem cells might help them. Some senators found this tough; one even refused to meet with his own constituent. An organization, "Families for Stem Cell Research," formed and conducted polls in those districts. The numbers were consistently high with 60%, 70%, and in one area, more than 90% of those polled in favor of the bill. Our Congressional delegation, county executives, and former governors made calls to urge their friends, colleagues, and representatives to support the bill. In one instance, students at the University of Maryland College Park passed a resolution in favor of the bill. They presented the resolution the next day to their senator who was still undecided.

While we worked the cloture angle, the bill passed out of EHE and later B&T. B&T removed the dedicated funding from the Cigarette Restitution Fund and inserted language leaving the program to be funded at the governor's discretion. As the primary committee, EHE accepted the new budget language and held the bill to report to the floor when we had the 29 votes for cloture.

### The Governor's Position, or Lack Thereof

After seeing the committee votes, we believed we had 27 Democratic votes to break filibuster. Two Republicans supported the bill in committee, and we presumed they would vote for the bill on the floor. However, that didn't mean they would break party ranks and vote for cloture. Our pro-choice, Republican governor remained silent on the issue, offering no indication of whether he was for or against embryonic stem cell research, for or against the bill, or if he wanted a filibuster of the bill.

We were excited to learn the governor belonged to an organization called Republican Main Street Partnership. Their Website further defines the goals of Main Street to "promote thoughtful leadership in the Republican Party, and to partner with individuals, organizations and institutions that share centrist values." Former Maine Governor John "Jock" McKernan, is quoted as best defining the message of the Partnership as "one of quiet diplomacy, rather than wedge politics."

Main Street names stem cell research as one of their top legislative priorities. Their bill of choice, HR 810, is before the United States Congress and would expand the current federal embryonic stem cell policy by funding research on new stem cell lines that are derived from discarded embryos created through infertility treatment—just like SB 751 (*www.republicanmainstreet.org/index.htm*).

With all of this in the press, as well as news that the Massachusetts legislature had passed legislation to allow embryonic stem cell research, we still heard nothing from Governor Ehrlich. Finally, with just two days left in the session, the governor finally indicated on the radio that he was in favor of embryonic stem cell research. My hope was that he would tell the Republican caucus that this was not a party vote and that they were free to vote from the heart and for their constituents.

### Sine Die

Sine Die, the 90th and final day of the legislative session, is hard to describe. Session begins that day at 10:00 AM and continues until midnight. The day is a race with the clock as you simultaneously vote on bills, field calls from interested parties, conference on bills at a stalemate, and go back to committee to vote on even more bills. Anything not voted on by both chambers by midnight is dead—no exceptions.

We began the day hopeful, and I instructed my staff to have the bill ready to report to the floor and to prepare me for the debate. Several key bills needed to come through before we could start the stem cell debate, including the final vote on the state budget.

We couldn't chance those bills being held up behind what could be a long debate. I waited for word from the Senate President that enough work was done to allow the stem cell bill to come to the floor.

Outside of the State House, an important press conference was held, featuring the Baltimore City Mayor Martin O'Malley and Montgomery County Executive Doug Duncan, two well-known Democratic rivals. Both are expected to run for governor in the 2006 election, but they came together to urge the governor to call off a Republican filibuster.

The caucus never heard from the governor. Just before the dinner break, the president commented to the full Senate that stem cell would be up after dinner. When we returned, known opponents to the bill began asking long and involved questions on otherwise simple bills. It became obvious that they were stalling in hopes that we would not be able to bring the stem cell debate to a vote. Unfortunately, their tactics worked.

The evening of Sine Die was a hard one for me. I could see the disappointment on the faces of each of the people that had stayed with me all day, hoping to see the full Senate debate this bill. At 11:30 PM, I asked to address the body. I individually thanked the crowd of supporters that was waiting in the balconies to watch the debate. Annie, Van, and John had been there all day. A five-year-old girl who has juvenile diabetes fell asleep in her mother's arms waiting for the debate. Former Governor Harry Hughes, whose own grandson has juvenile diabetes, waited with them. There was an attempt to interrupt me so we could move on, but I couldn't stop myself. I spoke louder until I had listed the more than 20 people who wanted a chance.

To them, this wasn't just another bill or political tool to make a deal. To them, it was a life or death matter; an issue of how they will live the rest of their lives. Annie wants to play sports and go out with her friends. Van wants to run down the football field and hear the crowd cheer. John simply wants to dance with his daughter. I immediately decided that I would reintroduce this bill in 2006 and would send it to the Senate floor immediately.

## DETERMINED TO DO MORE

Within a week of Sine Die, *The Baltimore Sun* reported overwhelming support for stem cell funding. In a poll conducted for the newspaper, Marylanders reported support at a rate of more than two to one (Desmon & Penn, 2005). This support was consistent across the state. A poll done for the Families for Stem Cell Research showed support at an even higher rate (Gonzales Research and Marketing Strategies, 2005).

Along with great disappointment came great determination to move forward. In the months following the legislative session, federal action and inaction has kept stem cell research in the news. Press conferences and letters to the editors have also kept people aware of what is going on. Delegate Rosenberg and I sent a letter to the governor asking him to meet with us and discuss the future of stem cell research legislation in Maryland, but we received no response. Our friends at the Families for Stem Cell Research have formalized their efforts, becoming an official non-profit organization. They joined us at a press conference recently to urge the governor to work with us. The governor has a choice to make. He can either join us or watch from the sidelines as we win this fight for the people of Maryland.

We are working on a strategy to get past the politics of this bill. Polling and constituent visits to legislators will get our message across: Funding embryonic stem cell research is the right thing to do and the people of Maryland support it.

We'll save a lot of time and effort using the language that was worked out by committees last year, but I'm not going to waste time waiting to send this bill to the floor. I know the votes for cloture are somewhere in the Senate. Therefore, no other bill will come out of my committee until both EHE and B&T have voted on this bill and it is sent to the Senate floor.

## SUMMARY

In the days following the end of the legislative session, I was amazed by the number of people, both friends and strangers, who came to me sharing their support for our work. It seemed that almost everyone I talked to personally knows at least one person who suffers from a debilitating condition that could be helped with more research in this field. If someone doesn't, I can introduce him or her to Annie, Van, and John.

## EDITOR'S NOTE

The Governor of Maryland signed legislation on April 7, 2006, that authorized $15 million in state funding for stem cell research. The legislation was passed by the 2006 Maryland General Assembly and makes Maryland the fourth state in the nation to support stem cell research.

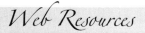

### Web Resources

---

**Coalition for the Advancement of Medical Research**
*www.camradvocacy.org/news_detail.aspx?id=080905A*
**Stem Cell Policy**
*www.healthpolitics.com*
**Stem Cell Research Foundation**
*www.stemcellresearchfoundation.org*
**Stem Cells and the Future of Regenerative Medicine (National Academies Press)**
*www.nap.edu/catalog/10195.html/*

---

## REFERENCES

Department of Legislative Services, Maryland General Assembly. (2005a). Senate Bill 751 Fiscal and Policy Note, Annapolis, Maryland. Available online at *http://mlis.state.md.us/2005rs/fnotes/bil_0001/sb0751.pdf.*

Department of Legislative Services, Maryland General Assembly. (2005b). Senate Bill 751: Maryland Stem Cell Research Act of 2005, Annapolis, Maryland. Available online at *http://mlis.state.md.us/2005rs/bills/sb/sb0751f.pdf.*

Desmon, S., & Penn, I. (2005, April 17). Support for slots down in survey; stem cell funding backed strongly. *Baltimore Sun*, A1.

Gonzales Research & Marketing Strategies. (2005, March). Poll conducted for Families for Stem Cell Research. Baltimore, Maryland.

Mundell, E. J. (2005, January 23). *U.S. embryonic stem cell lines contaminated.* Health Day, a Service of the National Health Information Center, U.S. Department of Health & Human Services. Retrieved August 26, 2005, from *www.healthfinder.gov.*

National Institutes of Health (NIH). (2005a). Information on eligibility criteria for federal funding of research on human embryonic stem cells. Retrieved August 26, 2005, from *http://stemcells.nih.gov/research/registry/eligibilitycriteria.asp.*

National Institutes of Health (NIH). (2005b). Stem cell basics. Retrieved August 26, 2005, from *http://stemcells.nih.gov/info/basics.*

Sage Policy Group, Inc. (2005). The economic impacts of funding stem cell research in Maryland.

# REEFER MADNESS: THE ILLOGICAL POLITICS OF MEDICAL MARIJUANA

Mary Lynn Mathre

"If you want to make enemies, try to change something."

WOODROW WILSON

## THE PROBLEM

It's a drug with an image problem—a drug that has been shown to help certain patients, but its use is forbidden by federal law. Most of us know it as dope, pot, reefer, grass, weed, or ganja. But in its clinical form, medical cannabis is a valuable therapeutic aid. Scientific evidence demonstrates the value of cannabis in certain clinical conditions. However, the Drug Enforcement Administration (the federal agency responsible for placing drugs in categories on the Controlled Substances Schedule) has refused to move cannabis to a less restrictive schedule, while allowing a synthetic form of the primary psychoactive substance (THC) in cannabis to be placed in a less restrictive level of the Controlled Substances. Cannabis (marijuana) and natural THC (the primary psychoactive substance in cannabis) remains in Schedule I, while dronabinol (Marinol), the synthetic form of THC, was originally placed in Schedule II but has since been reassigned to Schedule III (less control and more available) due to its safety and lack of diversion.

In 1999, at the request of the White House, the Institute of Medicine completed its 18-month study on therapeutic cannabis (Joy, Watson, & Benson, 1999). The study team found that cannabis is not highly addictive, is not a gateway drug, and has therapeutic value; the team recommended that until pharmaceutical grade products become available, cancer and AIDS patients should be allowed to smoke the crude plant material.

They also recommended that physicians should be able to conduct "n-of-1" studies on their patients whom they believe could benefit from cannabis and that research should be conducted on alternative delivery systems. This report has more or less been ignored by the federal government, but research is going forward on the therapeutic use of cannabis in the United States and other countries. Despite the barriers and seeming social bias against cannabis, 11 states have passed laws permitting the medical use of the drug. However, in June 2005, the U.S. Supreme Court ruled that federal authorities have the power to prosecute individuals for possession and use of medical marijuana even in the states that permit it (Tierney, 2005). How did this once-legal drug become socially shunned, the problem child of the pharmaceutical industry, and a political hot potato? The saga of cannabis in the U.S. health system is a story of the clash of politics, opinions, fear, emotions, and science.

## ONCE UPON A TIME, CANNABIS WAS LEGAL

Before the U.S. Congress passed the Marihuana Tax Act of 1937, cannabis was a medicine commonly used by physicians for a variety of ailments. Originally, *Cannabis sativa* and *Cannabis indica* plant material were imported to this country for use in medical products. As time went on, *Cannabis americana* was grown in the United States to provide access to fresh plant material to avoid the degradation that occurred when it was brought overseas on slow-moving ships. Cannabis tinctures, elixirs, salves, and even smokeable products were available. It was listed in the *U.S. Pharmacopoeia* until 1940 (Box 22-3).

**653**

---

**BOX 22-3** Cannabis Terms

*Cannabis*—A plant genus that is unique in the plant kingdom in that it contains a group of chemicals known as cannabinoids.

*Cannabis indica*—A species of the cannabis plant that has short, broad leaflets.

*Cannabis sativa*—A species of the cannabis plant that has long, narrow leaflets.

*Cesamet*—Synthetic derivative of THC available in Europe; manufactured by Eli Lilly.

*Marijuana/marihuana*—The Mexican name for cannabis, used by the U.S. federal government in their efforts to prohibit the use of the cannabis plant.

*Marinol*—A registered trademark of Unimed Pharmaceuticals. It is the commercial name for dronabinol (the synthetic form of delta-9-tetrahydrocannabinol) in sesame oil and encapsulated in soft gelatin capsules. When first on the market, it was a Schedule II medication for use in the treatment of nausea and vomiting caused by chemotherapy, as well as appetite loss caused by AIDS.

*Sativex*—A cannabis extract oro-mucosal spray developed by GW Pharmaceuticals in Great Britain and first on the market in Canada in 2005 for use by patients with multiple sclerosis.

*THC*—Δ-9-tetrahydrocannabinol, the primary psychoactive ingredient in cannabis/marijuana; one of 60 cannabinoids.

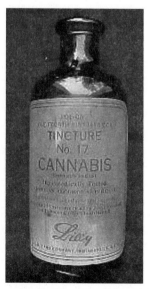

Tincture of Cannabis, No. 17, produced by Eli Lilly. *(From The Cannabis Museum, Inc., Elliston, Virginia.)*

## HOW AND WHY DID THE PROHIBITION BEGIN?

"Prohibition" (the alcohol prohibition in the United States in the 1930s) ended in failure, but the staff of The Bureau of Narcotics and Dangerous Drugs and its leader, Harry Anslinger, needed to find something for the department to do or it would be dissolved. Anslinger targeted a drug used by "negro" jazz musicians in the American South and Mexicans in the Southwest. The drug was cannabis, but was called "reefer" by the African American population and "marijuana" (alternately spelled "marihuana") by the Hispanic population.

## THE DESCENT INTO "REEFER MADNESS"

In 1936, the film *Reefer Madness* was released (a reefer being a marijuana cigarette). The film's plot involves tragic events that ensue when high school students are lured by drug pushers into using marijuana. Death, suicide, and a descent into madness are the results (Wikipedia, 2005). A "Reefer Madness" mentality was adopted by some government agencies, individuals, and media moguls like William Randolph Hearst. Few people realized at the time, that this dangerous "new" drug was the same thing as the cannabis medicine that many physicians routinely prescribed.

## MY INTRODUCTION TO THE PROBLEM OF MEDICAL CANNABIS USE

In the early 1980s, I was working in a small hospital in Washington state, when the director of nursing approached me with a problem. A cancer patient was going to be admitted who had experimental "marijuana" pills from the University of Washington. She asked what should we do? I suggested we lock it up in the narcotics cabinet and dispense it as prescribed. No problems were encountered, and I began learning about Marinol, the synthetic "marijuana" pill. About the same time, I came across a flyer about an organization called the Alliance for Cannabis Therapeutics (ACT). It was started by a glaucoma patient, Robert Randall, and his wife. In 1976, Randall had gained legal access to federally grown marijuana under the Compassionate Investigational New Drug (IND) program following a series of court battles because no other medicine could control his intraocular pressure. He formed

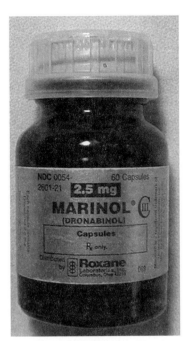

Marinol.

ACT, a nonprofit organization, to let others know about the therapeutic benefits of cannabis and how patients could get a legal, federally approved supply of it. I was drawn to the issue.

After moving to Ohio to complete graduate school at Case Western Reserve University in 1983, I conducted a survey on marijuana disclosure to health care professionals using the membership of NORML as my survey population (Mathre, 1985). The thrust of the survey was to determine if health care professionals asked patients about the use of cannabis and whether the survey subjects would disclose their use patterns. I received some surprising responses that led me to consider the therapeutic potential of cannabis. In a final question that asked the subjects to identify their concerns regarding the use of cannabis from a list of health problems, numerous respondents noted in the "other" option that they used it as medicine for stress, migraines, spasticity, pain, and other ailments (Mathre, 1988).

## AN OPPORTUNITY FOR EDUCATION

I accepted the position of director of the National Organization for the Reform of Marijuana Laws' (NORML) Council on Marijuana and Health. By 1990, there were five patients who had legal access to marijuana through the Compassionate IND program. I was serving on the planning committee for the annual NORML conference and suggested that we have all five patients present their cases in a panel presentation. The patients were eager to tell their stories and were excited to meet others in their situation. Their presentation was aired on C-SPAN and garnered national attention. Taking advantage of the opportunity, we had each patient interviewed and videotaped by a volunteer professional videographer. Over the next two years, excerpts from the interviews were used to create an 18-minute video, *Marijuana as Medicine* (Byrne & Mathre, 1992), designed to be a teaching aid. Following the airing of the patients' panel, the U.S. Food and Drug Administration (FDA) received many requests for IND access to marijuana, especially from HIV/AIDS patients. The Secretary of Health and Human Services, Dr. Louis Sullivan, responded by shutting down the IND access to marijuana in 1992. At that time, 15 patients were receiving marijuana, over 30 patients had been approved and were waiting for their medication to be delivered, and hundreds of applications were waiting for review (Randall & O'Leary, 1998). Only the 15 current patients would be allowed to continue in the program, closing the door to all others. Also during that time frame, one of the legal patient's supply of marijuana was cut off. Corinne Millet, a widow and glaucoma patient, sought help from her congressman to regain her supply of medicine, but during the six weeks she spent without her medication, she lost 80% of her peripheral vision (Byrne & Mathre, 1992).

These events made me feel it was important to end the prohibition on the use of cannabis in the United States. My perspective was that there was no justifiable reason for the marijuana prohibition. It has therapeutic value, it is safe, and patients benefit from it. Patients who might benefit from it have no knowledge of its value, health care professionals are not trained to use it, and patients are harmed by the legal consequences for their use of it.

I saw this as a problem that required patient advocacy and that had ethical implications, and I believed it to be a professional responsibility to try to end the cannabis prohibition and make this medicine legally available to patients.

The more I learned, the more determined I became. I embarked on a more than 20-year fight, met countless barriers, and often felt like David taking on the Goliath of the federal government. Colleagues have questioned me over the years why I'm still trying to change the laws, and my answer is always the same: Patients still do not have access to a safe and legal supply of this medicine.

## BARRIERS AND STRATEGIES

Over the years, I've encountered many barriers and I've tried various strategies; often the same strategies have been used under different circumstances. Barriers that I've encountered include misinformation presented as facts, censorship of information, intimidation, laws and regulations that prevent research, an image based on racism and ideology rather than science and reality, and pharmaceutical pressure to prevent potential competition. I've used strategies like finding a strong mentor, building a support system, mobilizing grassroots support, changing the image of the problem, partnering with patients, building a coalition, starting a nonprofit organization, providing continuing accredited education for health care professionals about cannabis, using the Internet effectively, playing by the government's rules, teaching others, conducting research, disseminating research findings, and educating the public through publications, the press, and the media.

## HIDING THE TRUTH

In the years following the Marihuana Tax Act of 1937, cannabis was removed from the *U.S. Pharmacopoeia*, it was no longer included in medical school curricula, and health care professionals learned about marijuana only in the context of substance *abuse*. The Controlled Substances Act of 1970 further condemned the drug when officials wrongly, in my opinion, placed marijuana in Schedule I of the Controlled Substances Schedule, the category of drugs that are highly addictive, not safe for medical use, and have no therapeutic value (Box 22-4).

By the 1960s and 1970s, the average American had little knowledge of cannabis but had been taught about the dangers of marijuana. The legal consequences for possession of marijuana became so severe (up to a life sentence for a single "joint") that people who used it medicinally kept their use a secret. Thus, the unmotivated, "stoned" teenager became the public image of a marijuana user (think Sean Penn in the film *Fast Times at Ridgemont High*).

## FINDING THE TRUTH

I knew cannabis had therapeutic value after searching for and reviewing historical records that included national studies and patient studies conducted in the late 1970s and early 1980s. For studies conducted before the Marihuana Tax Act of 1937, I had to search using the terms "cannabis" and "hemp." I initially depended on others in the field to gain access to rare copies of studies that validated the medicinal efficacy of cannabis. I found that some published reports had negative results, but on close review the studies were either flawed or not accurately reported.

## A POWERFUL MENTOR

I was lucky to meet an influential nursing leader, Melanie Dreher, PhD, RN, FAAN, who at the time was Dean of the University of Florida School of Nursing in Miami. Her doctorate was in anthropology, and her current research was on "ganja" (marijuana) use by pregnant women in Jamaica and fetal outcome (Dreher, 1997; Dreher, Nugent, & Hudgins, 1994). She taught me a great deal and validated my understanding of the benefits of cannabis.

## GAINING SUPPORT

Initially, I began collecting signatures on a petition to demand that cannabis be removed from Schedule I of the Controlled Substances to make it available for patient use. Many people agreed with the idea but were afraid to put their names on a public document. Although, together with others, I collected tens of

**BOX 22-4** Schedule of Controlled Substances in the United States

21 U.S. Code §812(b) specifies a classification system for drugs in the United States based on the purpose, safety, and effectiveness of the drug.

## SCHEDULE I DRUGS

a. The drug or other substance has a high potential for abuse.
b. The drug or other substance has no currently accepted medical use in treatment in the United States.
c. There is a lack of accepted safety for use of the drug or other substance under medical supervision.

Schedule I drugs include marijuana, heroin (Diacetylmorphine), ecstasy (MDMA), psilocybin, GHB (Gamma-hydroxybutyrate), LSD, mescaline, and peyote.

## SCHEDULE II DRUGS

a. The drug or other substance has a high potential for abuse.
b. The drug or other substance has a currently accepted medical use in treatment in the United States or a currently accepted medical use with severe restrictions.
c. Abuse of the drug or other substances may lead to severe psychological or physical dependence.

Schedule II drugs are only available by prescription, and distribution is carefully controlled and monitored by the DEA.

Schedule II drugs include cocaine, methylphenidate (Ritalin), most pure opioid agonists, meperidine, fentanyl, opium, oxycodone, morphine, short-acting barbiturates such as secobarbital, methamphetamine, and PCP.

## SCHEDULE III DRUGS

a. The drug or other substance has a potential for abuse less than the drugs or other substances in Schedules I and II.
b. The drug or other substance has a currently accepted medical use in treatment in the United States.
c. Abuse of the drug or other substance may lead to moderate or low physical dependence or high psychological dependence.

Schedule III drugs are available only by prescription, though control of wholesale distribution is somewhat less stringent than Schedule II drugs.

Schedule III drugs include Marinol, anabolic steroids, intermediate-acting barbiturates such as talbutal, preparations that combine codeine or hydrocodone with aspirin or acetaminophen, ketamine, and Paregoric.

## SCHEDULE IV DRUGS

a. The drug or other substance has a low potential for abuse relative to the drugs or other substances in Schedule III.
b. The drug or other substance has a currently accepted medical use in treatment in the United States.
c. Abuse of the drug or other substance may lead to limited physical dependence or psychological dependence relative to the drugs or other substances in Schedule III.

Schedule IV control measures are similar to Schedule III; drugs on this schedule include benzodiazepines, such as alprazolam (Xanax), chlordiazepoxide (librium), and diazepam (Valium); long-acting barbiturates, such as phenobarbital; and some partial agonist opioid analgesics, such as propoxyphene (Darvon) and pentazocine (Talwin).

## SCHEDULE V DRUGS

a. The drug or other substance has a low potential for abuse relative to the drugs or other substances in Schedule IV.
b. The drug or other substance has a currently accepted medical use in treatment in the United States.
c. Abuse of the drug or other substance may lead to limited physical dependence or psychological dependence relative to the drugs or other substances in Schedule IV.

Schedule V drugs are sometimes available without a prescription; drugs on this schedule include cough suppressants containing small amounts of codeine and preparations containing small amounts of opium, used to treat diarrhea.

From Title 21 United States Code (USC) Controlled Substances Act. Retrieved September 5, 2005, from *www.deadiversion. usdoj.gov/21cfr/21usc/802.htm#32a.*

thousands of signatures, it soon became apparent that this approach was not cost- or time-effective.

By getting the first five legal patients together, I had helped them develop a lasting bond, and they in turn trusted me. This bond empowered them to speak out about the injustice of the prohibition of cannabis use. The video, *Marijuana as Medicine* (Byrne & Mathre, 1992), has served as a powerful teaching tool for use with other health care professionals, the public, and legislators. I began to approach nursing organizations to show them the video. Following the video presentation, I urged them to pass a resolution that I had drafted in support of cannabis. My initial success began with resolutions passed by the Virginia Nurses Society on Addictions (1993), the Virginia Nurses Association (1994), and the National Nurses Society on Addictions (1995). During these presentations, the proper name for the plant, *cannabis*, was used in an attempt to change the negative image of marijuana. By getting professional organizations to formally support patient access to therapeutic cannabis, individual members had a stronger voice on the issue.

## PATIENTS OUT OF TIME

In 1995, following the deaths of a young AIDS couple who were in the IND program, my husband and I felt the need to take this issue more seriously. With the help of several legal patients and other health care professionals, we founded a national nonprofit organization, Patients Out of Time. We kept our mission simple: to educate the public and health care professionals about the therapeutic use of cannabis. Initially, we focused on getting more professional organizations to issue resolutions in support of patient access to cannabis. Next on our list was the American Public Health Association (APHA). I drafted and submitted a proposed resolution to the APHA, and it was passed at their annual meeting in California in 1995. I sent out copies of the Virginia Nurses Association's resolution and a letter to the leadership of all the state nurses associations. Colorado, Mississippi, and New York were among a few states that took action. The California Nurses Association had already passed a resolution in 1994. We posted a list of these organizations on our Website

*(www.medicalcannabis.com)*, which we continually update as more organizations join the list. We verify accuracy before placing any organization on our list. In 2002, I received a call from a New York nurse who was drafting a resolution on therapeutic cannabis to present at the American Nurses Association (ANA) 2003 House of Delegates meeting. I assisted in developing its content and went to the convention to speak on behalf of the resolution. It easily passed. I believe the ANA resolution most clearly encompasses the issues of concern regarding the marijuana prohibition. In 2005, I was appointed to the National Organization for Women's (NOW) newly created Women and Drug Policy ad hoc Committee; among other issues, I will advocate for the organization to pass a resolution supporting therapeutic cannabis.

## CHALLENGES IN DISSEMINATING INFORMATION ABOUT CANNABIS

In 1993, I sent a manuscript on the ethical and legal dilemmas for nurses related to therapeutic cannabis to the *American Journal of Nursing (AJN)* to try to increase professional awareness on this issue. I received a rejection letter from the editor of *AJN* that said it wasn't appropriate. I called Mary Mallison, the editor-in-chief, and after a discussion she suggested I submit a second article on cannabis dosing. On receipt of that manuscript, I received a letter from the editorial director, Martin DiCarlantonio, which stated: "We'd like to accept your manuscript and run it as soon as marijuana is moved to Schedule II category (if that day ever comes)."

In 1995, I was asked by Mary Gorman, RN, to write a manuscript for *AJN*'s Substance Abuse column on the medical use of marijuana. I prepared it and submitted it with the projected publication date for the fall of 1996. Again, it was considered too controversial and remained in their files for more than a year until a change in editorial staff occurred. It was published in November 1997 (Mathre, 1997b). In the May 1998 issue, several positive letters to the editor were printed. I was told that no negative letters to the editor had been received.

In 1999, I decided to submit another article to *AJN* after reading an editorial by Dr. Diana Mason,

*AJN*'s new editor-in-chief, in which she urged nurses to work to influence health policy. This manuscript was published in 2001 (Mathre, 2001), and again, only positive letters to the editor were received. In 2004, I was asked to submit a manuscript to *Nursing 2004* on therapeutic cannabis. It was accepted for publication, but in 2005 I received a letter stating it would not be published because they could not get anyone to submit an opposing view.

## BIRTH OF A BOOK AND DEATH OF A JOURNAL

In 1995, I began work on a cannabis book and began finding experts on various topics who were willing to contribute a chapter. *Cannabis in Medical Practice* was published in 1997 by McFarland, containing the work of 17 contributing authors (Mathre, 1997a). The book received great reviews. Although it wasn't a big seller, Dr. Geoffrey Guy, a physician and drug researcher from Great Britain, read my book which, per his acknowledgment, motivated him to start a pharmaceutical company to develop cannabis-based pharmaceuticals *(www.gwpharm.com)*. In large part because of my book, I was invited to serve on the editorial board of a new quarterly journal, *The Journal of Cannabis Therapeutics*, which premiered in 2001, published by Haworth Press. Unfortunately, due to the continued illegal status of cannabis, this journal was not picked up by many university libraries or individual subscriptions, and the publication ceased by 2004. I served as coeditor along with Ethan Russo, MD, and Melanie Dreher, RN, PhD, FAAN, on *Women and Cannabis: Medicine, Science and Sociology* (Russo et al., 2002), which was published as a monograph in 2002.

## RAISING AWARENESS AT PROFESSIONAL CONFERENCES

In 1995, I went to the continuing education department at the University of Virginia Health System and asked if they would host a national conference on cannabis therapeutics. My formal written proposal went to the top of the administration where it was immediately rejected. I countered with a request to limit it to a statewide nursing conference on the topic, since the 1994 Virginia Nurses Association resolution called for the "education of

Virginia Nurses on evidence-based use of cannabis." I was then informed by the director of the Continuing Education department that they wouldn't support such a conference because "it still had the same political issues." In 1996, my proposal for the 100th Anniversary Convention of the ANA to present *Therapeutic Cannabis & the Law: Ethical Dilemma for Nurses* was accepted, and in 2002 I presented "Evidence Based Support for Cannabis Therapeutics" as part of the NOLF Lecture series at the ANA convention in Philadelphia.

## THE FIRST NATIONAL CLINICAL CONFERENCE ON CANNABIS THERAPEUTICS

In 1999, Dr. Dreher, who was now the Dean of the College of Nursing at the University of Iowa (and also on the Board of Directors for Patients Out of Time), was able to gain local support to hold a national conference at the University of Iowa. Patients Out of Time managed the agenda and faculty. In 2000, Patients Out of Time held The First National Clinical Conference on Cannabis Therapeutics with the University of Iowa's Colleges of Nursing and Medicine as cosponsors. We had an international conference faculty that included researchers, clinical experts, patients, and patients' care providers, and the conference was teleconferenced to seven other sites. One of them was in Oregon sponsored by the Oregon Public Health Department, since their new law allowed patient use of cannabis under a physician's recommendation that was regulated by the Health Department. The Oregon Public Health Department broadcast the conference throughout its system, which led them to co-sponsor the second conference in Oregon with the Oregon Nurses Association in 2002. Since the first conference, we continue to hold bienniel conferences. The audience feedback has been very positive, and the faculty has been very impressed with our "nursing" approach for the conference content.

At the third conference in 2004, which was cosponsored by the University of Virginia Schools of Medicine, Nursing, and Law (persistence pays off), we applied for and received grant funding to provide scholarships to legislators and health care professionals in leadership positions to attend the conference. Some of these scholarships were nurses representing various state nurses associations. These nurses took this information back to their leadership and had articles published in their state newsletters; subsequently, the nurses from Illinois and Connecticut were able to get resolutions passed by their state associations, and the nurse representing the Virginia nurses convinced the association to reaffirm their support of the issue with the passage of a second resolution supporting therapeutic cannabis. Laurie Badzek, the director of the ANA's Center for Ethics and Human Rights was also one of the scholarship recipients and informed me that she hopes to attend our fourth conference so that she can keep the ANA up to date on the issue. Our fourth conference was in April of 2006 in Santa Barbara, California and focused on getting funding for more such scholarships. We have DVDs of all the conference proceedings available on our Website, but we also hope to broadcast the next conference live on the Internet to increase the viewing audience.

## THE NEED FOR EVIDENCE

In 2001, Patients Out of Time received grant funding from John Gilmore, Preston Parish, the Zimmer Family Foundation, and the Multidisciplinary Association for Psychedelic Studies to conduct an in-depth review of the chronic effects of cannabis on four of the surviving legal medical marijuana patients. These patients offered a unique opportunity for study because they had been receiving and using a known quality and quantity of cannabis provided by the federal government. The study was led by Ethan Russo, a pediatric neurologist and expert in cannabis therapeutics, and conducted in Missoula, Montana (Russo et al., 2002).

## TAKING ON THE U.S. DRUG ENFORCEMENT ADMINISTRATION

Attempts have been made to change the federal prohibition of cannabis and all have failed. Even the state initiatives that have been passed to allow patients to use cannabis medicinally under the recommendation of a physician have been thwarted by the federal government's prohibition. In November 2002, Jon Gettman, PhD, submitted a *Petition to Reschedule Cannabis* to the U.S. Drug Enforcement Administration (DEA) on behalf of a coalition of cannabis patients. Patients Out of Time is a leading member of that coalition and serves as the lead voice (DrugScience.org, 2005). According to the rules and regulations of the Controlled Substances Act, a drug in its natural form cannot be at a more restricted schedule than its active constituent (DrugScience.org, 2005). Synthetic THC (Marinol) was placed in Schedule II in 1980 and was approved for use as an anti-emetic and appetite stimulant. By 1989, due to a lack of diversion and its record of safety, it was moved to the less restrictive Schedule III. Following this, whole cannabis extracts should also be at a Schedule III or less restrictive category. The DEA accepted the rescheduling petition as a legitimate request and, according to protocol, passed it on to the Department of Health and Human Services (DHHS) for their review in 2004. Per protocol, they may take up to three years to review all of the new research that is available.

## PROGRESS

The public's awareness and acceptance of therapeutic cannabis has increased over the years to 70% to 80% approval per public opinion polls (Medical Marijuana ProCon.org, 2005; NORML, 2005). Despite the federal prohibition, there are now 10 states that have passed voter initiatives for patient use of therapeutic cannabis and two states that have passed similar laws through legislative action. The recent discoveries of endogenous cannabinoids and cannabinoid receptors have spawned more research. Pharmaceutical companies are now conducting research into cannabis-based products. In 2005, an oro-mucosal cannabis extract spray, Sativex, developed by GW Pharmaceuticals in Great Britain was approved as medicine in Canada and approved for clinical trials to begin in the United States in 2006 for use with terminal cancer patients.

## LOOKING INTO THE CRYSTAL BALL

International acceptance of cannabis-based medicines may help influence the United States to end its prohibition of medical cannabis. The body of science contained in the petition to reschedule cannabis hopefully will convince the DHHS about the efficacy of cannabis and get them to make a recommendation to place cannabis in Schedule III or a lower level of control. I believe that once health care professionals are familiar with this medication, it will be considered as the "drug of choice" in symptom management, because of its wide margin of safety, rather than the "last resort." Hopefully, medical cannabis will soon be on the market in the United States, and nurses are urged to increase their knowledge about how it may help their patients.

## Key Points

- Perseverance and coalition-building are essential elements in the process of changing a policy based on ideology rather than logic or science.
- Based on the evidence-based research that supports cannabis efficacy, nurses should advocate for patients to have the option of using cannabis pharmaceutical products.
- Always consider the source of your information.

## Web Resources

**Alliance for Cannabis Therapeutics**
*www.marijuana-as-medicine.org*
**International Association for Cannabis as Medicine (IACM)**
*www.cannabis-med.org*
**International Cannabinoid Research Society (ICRS)**
*www.cannabinoidsociety.org*
**National Organization for Reform of Marijuana Laws**
*www.norml.org*
**Patients Out of Time**
*www.medicalcannabis.com*
**U.S. Drug Enforcement Administration, Office of Diversion Control**
*www.deadiversion.usdoj.gov/schedules*

## REFERENCES

Byrne, A., & Mathre, M. L. (1992). *Marijuana as medicine* (video). Available at *www.medicalcannabis.com*.

Dreher, M. (1997). Cannabis and pregnancy. In M. L. Mathre, *Cannabis in medical practice: A legal, historical and pharmacological overview of the therapeutic use of marijuana*. Jefferson, NC: McFarland.

Dreher, M. C., Nugent, K., & Hudgins, R. (1994). Prenatal marijuana exposure and neonatal outcomes in Jamaica: An ethnographic study. *Pediatrics, 93*, 254-260.

DrugScience.org. (2005). Retrieved March 1, 2006, from www.drugscience.org.

Joy, J. E., Watson, S. A., & Benson, J. A., Jr. (1999). *Marijuana and medicine: Assessing the science base*. Washington, DC: Institute of Medicine, National Academy Press.

Mathre, M. L. (1985). Disclosure of marijuana use to health care professionals. Unpublished master's thesis, Case Western Reserve University, Cleveland, Ohio.

Mathre, M. L. (1988). A survey on disclosure of marijuana use to health care professionals. *Journal of Psychoactive Drugs, 20*(1), 117-120.

Mathre, M. L. (1996, June 17). Therapeutic cannabis and the law: Ethical dilemma for nurses. Presentation at the 100th Anniversary Convention of the American Nurses Association in Washington, DC.

Mathre, M. L. (Ed.). (1997a). *Cannabis in medical practice: A legal, historical and pharmacological overview of the therapeutic use of marijuana*. Jefferson, NC: McFarland.

Mathre, M. L. (1997b). Medicinal use of marijuana. *American Journal of Nursing, 97*(11), 23.

Mathre, M. L. (2001). Therapeutic cannabis: A patient advocacy issue. *American Journal of Nursing, 101*(4), 61-68.

Mathre, M. L. (2002, July 2). Evidence-based support for cannabis therapeutics. Part of the III NOLF Lecture Series at the American Nurses Association's 2002 Biennial Convention and Exposition in Philadelphia.

Medical Marijuana ProCon.org. (2005). Voting/polling on medical marijuana: 2000 to present. Retrieved October 1, 2005, from *www.medicalmarijuanaprocon.org/pop/votes2000.htm*.

National Organization for the Reform of Marijuana Laws (NORML). (2005). Favorable medical marijuana polls. Retrieved October 1, 2005, from *www.norml.org/index.cfm?Group_ID=3392*.

Randall R. C., & O'Leary A. M. (1998). *Marijuana Rx: The patient's fight for medicinal pot*. New York: Thunder's Mouth Press.

Russo, E., Dreher, M., & Mathre, M. L. (Eds.). (2003). *Women and cannabis: Medicine, science, and sociology*. Binghamton, NY: Haworth Integrative Healing Press.

Russo, E., Mathre, M. L., Byrne, A., Velin, R., Bach, P., Sanchez-Ramos, J., et al. (2002). Chronic cannabis use in the compassionate investigational new drug program: An examination of the benefits and adverse effects of legal clinical cannabis. *The Journal of Cannabis Therapeutics, 2*(1), 3-57.

Tierney, J. (2005, August 27). Marijuana pipe dreams. *New York Times*. Retrieved March 1, 2006, from *www.mapinc.org/drugnews/v05/n1394/a03.html?295921*.

Wikipedia. (2005). *Reefer madness*. Retrieved September 1, 2005, from *http://en.wikipedia.org/wiki/Reefer_Madness*.

# GENETICS, DISCRIMINATION, AND PRIVACY

Jean Jenkins & Dale Lea

*"We are the great vessel sailing around a burning
sun in the universe. But each and every one
of us is also a ship sailing through life with a cargo
of genes."*

JOSTEIN GAARDER

Mr. Norton is a 52-year-old African American who has three daughters ages 25, 27, and 32. He has a family history of early onset breast cancer in two of his four sisters. One sister died from breast cancer at age 40; his other sister, age 42, is currently undergoing treatment for breast cancer. Mr. Norton's mother died from breast cancer when she was in her 40s as well. Mr. N's 42-year-old sister has talked with him about "getting genetic testing" to see if he carries "a gene he can pass on to his daughters." Mr. Norton is very concerned about his three daughters, but he is afraid to pursue genetic testing because of a fear of insurance and employment discrimination. He has vivid memories of his father who was one of those screened for sickle cell in the 1970s and who was not able to get insurance because he tested positive as a sickle cell carrier. Mr. Norton has not shared his family history information with his health care provider because he is afraid that the family history will be documented in his chart and could lead to problems. Furthermore, Mr. Norton does not have the financial means to pay for the genetic testing "out of pocket, so it won't go on my record."

Genetic information is intensely personal information and may be available from multiple sources such as a blood sample, through a physical exam, from analysis of a relative's DNA, or in medical records (International Society of Nurses in Genetics [ISONG], 2001). Promoting the use of genetic and genomic information to maximize benefits and minimize harm requires consideration of how such information will be utilized (Collins, Green, Guttmacher, & Guyer, 2003). Indeed, the public has expressed concerns about who has access to their individual genetic information and how such information may be used against them (National Partnership for Women & Families, 2004). Of major concern is the potential for misuse of genetic information resulting in discrimination or stigmatization by health insurers, life insurers, employers, and others (Clayton, 2003). Some argue that such concerns are unwarranted and "largely reactionary to alarmist hyperbole" (Burrell, 2005). Becoming aware of the issues will facilitate nurses having an active role in policy decisions.

## ISSUES

Genetic discrimination, as defined by the National Human Genome Research Institute (NHGRI) is "prejudice against those who have or are likely to develop an inherited disorder" (NHGRI, 2005). Although new genetic testing and technologies have increased possibilities for screening, diagnosis, and intervention, many individuals fear that genetic information will be used to harm them, especially through the denial, limiting, or canceling of health insurance or through employment discrimination (Billings, 2005). This fear and the perception that genetic information will be used against an individual are preventing many people from pursuing genetic testing that could make a significant difference in health care decisions about treatment options and outcomes. This fear also is preventing individuals from becoming involved in genetic research that could improve options for those having hereditary conditions in the future (Hadley et al., 2003; Hall et al., 2005).

## HISTORY OF GENETIC TESTING AND DISCRIMINATION

Intolerance, prejudice, and discrimination are not new to the United States. The appearance of genetic discrimination—discrimination against those who have, or are likely to develop, an inherited condition—however, has compounded already existing racial and ethnic prejudice, as evidenced in the 1970s when a scientific mandate to use genetic tests to screen African Americans for sickle cell anemia was enacted. Scientists' concern was that individuals with sickle cell anemia had an increased risk from exposures to certain toxins present in the workplace. Statewide screening programs, targeting African American communities, were developed to identify individuals who had sickle cell anemia. These screening programs also identified individuals who were carriers. "A *carrier* is an individual who possesses one copy of a mutant allele that causes disease only when two copies are present. Although carriers are not affected by the disease, two carriers can produce a child who has the disease" (NHGRI, n.d.). Screening was not mandated for other groups (e.g., Mediterranean populations) also at risk for sickle cell anemia (Markel, 1997). Privacy and confidentiality of test results were not maintained, and both employers and insurers discriminated against individuals identified as carriers (who did not have sickle cell anemia).

In 1972, Congress passed the National Sickle Cell Anemia Act. The Act prevented awarding of funding to states whose sickle cell screening programs were not voluntary. Like Mr. Norton in the opening case example, the African American community has strong feelings about the way in which African Americans were discriminated against based on genetic information and the institutional racism that was allowed to occur. This influences their decisions today about whether or not to access and use potentially helpful genetic information in health care decisions.

## Other Documented Instances of Genetic Discrimination

As genetic discoveries and their clinical applications have expanded, there has been a growing fear on the part of America's public that employers and insurers will use genetic information to deny access to employment and insurance. There are now several well-documented cases of health insurance and employment discrimination based on genetic information (National Partnership for Women & Families, 2004; SACGHS, 2005a).

- For example, in 2000, the Burlington Northern Santa Fe Railroad tried to fire an employee after he refused to have a mandatory genetic test. Gary Avery, diagnosed with carpal tunnel syndrome, had taken leave in 2000 to have surgery and to recover. On returning to work, he was informed that he would have to have a mandatory medical evaluation and that refusal of the evaluation would lead to his being fired. He also learned that the Railroad was administering genetic testing to workers to identify a possible genetic predisposition to carpal tunnel syndrome secretly and without their consent as a means of refusing their compensation plans. Gary's refusal to have the medical evaluation led to disciplinary proceedings to fire him. Gary sought help from his union and the Equal Employment Opportunity Commission (EEOC). A suit was filed against Burlington Northern and was settled on Gary's behalf, allowing him to return to work ("Burlington Northern," 2001).

- In 2001, the American Management Association survey of American firms revealed a number of employers who were accessing genetic information on employees. This survey reported firms conducting genetic tests for sickle cell anemia, testing for Huntington's disease, requesting family and medical histories, and conducting susceptibility testing, which could include genetic testing (Hustead & Goldman, 2002). Susceptibility or predictive testing is targeted to healthy and presymptomatic individuals who are identified as being at high risk due to a significant family history of the condition. Results of susceptibility testing provide a probability, but not absolute certainty, of the individual's risk for developing the condition.

- Another example of employer discrimination based on genetic information occurred in the case of Terri Sergeant, who was fired from her job as office manager because she was taking expensive medication to treat her alpha-1 antitrypsin deficiency (Silvers & Stein, 2002). An individual's need for expensive health treatments and interventions is not enough reason to fire or even refuse to hire in the first place. As noted by Ellen Wright Clayton, Center for Genetics and Health Policy at Vanderbilt University, "The fact that the costs may cause the employer to go under or to decide not to provide health insurance simply underlines the inherent weakness of employment based health insurance" (Clayton, 2003, p. 566).

- Another issue for consideration concerning utilization of genetic information includes how a genetic condition might affect a person's ability to perform a job. An example is a person with a cardiac arrhythmia applying for a position as a long distance truck driver. When there is a risk to a third party, the person cannot obtain a license in many states. On the other hand, a situation in which an asymptomatic person has a genetic predisposition to a disorder (such as cardiac arrhythmia) will require specific evaluation of the nature of the condition and whether the symptoms will develop. Decisions about how predisposition genetic information is utilized will be influenced by not only the interests of the individual but also those of the employer and society (Clayton, 2003). Such individualizing of decisions, based on the information that is now available as a result of improved understanding of an individual's genomic risk, challenges current algorithms for debate and requires thoughtful consideration of many complex issues.

## PUBLIC VIEWS ABOUT GENETIC DISCRIMINATION

A number of studies have been conducted during the past decade regarding the public's views and fears about misuse of genetic information. In 1998, the National Center for Genome Resources learned that 85% of individuals surveyed did not want their employers to have access to their genetic information (i.e., genetic conditions, risks, or predispositions) (NHGRI, 2005). A public opinion survey conducted by the Virginia Commonwealth University Life Sciences division in 2001 reported that 85% were concerned that health insurance companies would deny coverage based on genetic information. Sixty-nine percent believed they would be denied employment based on genetic testing results (Virginia Commonwealth University, 2001). In 2002, a Harris Poll survey found that limited numbers of respondents thought that health insurance companies (39%) and life insurance companies (25%) should have access to and use their genetic test information (Harris Poll, 2002). A more recent study (2004) by the Johns Hopkins University Genetics and Public Policy Center revealed that 92% of individuals surveyed did not want their employers to have access to their genetic information, and 80% were against allowing health insurers to have access (Genetics and Public Policy Center, 2004).

## IMPACT OF PUBLIC FEARS

The fear of genetic discrimination is having a significant effect on individual and family health and financial well-being.

### Individual Health

As in the case of Mr. Norton, fears about genetic discrimination are preventing at-risk individuals from having genetic testing. A 2003 study of 470 individuals with a family history of colorectal cancer enrolled in the Hereditary Colorectal Cancer Registry at Johns Hopkins Hospital revealed that 50% had a high level of concern about genetic discrimination. Individuals indicating a high level of concern reported that they would be much less likely to meet with a health care professional to discuss genetic testing or undergo genetic testing. These same individuals indicated that if they were to pursue genetic testing, they would pay for it themselves or use an alias and still ask that the results not be included in their medical record (Apse, Biesecker, Giardiello, Fuller, & Bernhardt, 2004). Such concerns about insurance discrimination may be further influenced by race and other demographic factors, as determined by a recent study in a primary care population (Hall et al., 2005). African Americans and Asians were reported as more likely than Caucasians to express such concerns.

## Family Health

Genetic discrimination not only affects individual health, it also affects the health of families. As in Mr. Norton's family, a positive family history affects both the individual (his sister), and other family members (Mr. Norton and his daughters). Determining who may benefit from genetic services often requires gathering data on relatives, who are often unaware that their personal and specific information is being gathered and shared. Genetic information and the decision to pursue genetic testing can have an impact on access to insurance or employment for other family members, in Mr. Norton's case on himself and his daughters. Sometimes inadvertently, confidentiality and privacy of a family member are compromised by someone in the family only trying to improve on his or her own individual care. The potential for disruptions to family relationships is also possible. For instance, when some family members do not want to know about genetic testing, they may feel coerced by enthusiastic family members who value knowing their genetic status. Anger, denial, and anxiety may create walls between family members regarding the value of knowing genetic test results. Additionally, once a risk has been identified, failure to warn others in the family about the health risk can result in potential legal liabilities for the health care provider (Offit, Groeger, Turner, Wadsworth, & Weiser, 2004). This conflict between privacy and sharing of genetic information is influenced by the law, ethical standards, and professional responsibility.

## Financial Health

Individuals who fear genetic discrimination and avoid genetic testing may also experience an adverse financial impact (National Partnership for Women & Families, 2004). As an example, early detection and prevention offered by genetic tests could decrease the financial costs caused by untreated illnesses or treatment of an illness at a later stage. Individuals who

fear genetic discrimination and who avoid having these tests, however, may ultimately face thousands of dollars and medical debt. Those who choose to pay for genetic tests themselves to avoid having the information in their medical record feel an additional financial burden as the costs of genetic testing and counseling are significant. Many cannot afford the costs, preventing them from experiencing the health benefits of knowing their own genetic information.

Public health genetic testing and information have the potential to benefit the public's health and could lead to fewer critically ill individuals, thereby reducing the burden on America's health care system. However, the fear and concern about genetic discrimination is keeping many from pursuing genetic preventive services, driving up health care costs for employers and public health resources. (Institute of Medicine, 2004, pp. 44-45)

## POLICY RESPONSES TO THE FEAR OF GENETIC DISCRIMINATION

Genetic discrimination is not widespread at this time, but it could become more widespread as research implicates the genetic contributions to many common diseases (not only inherited conditions) that we are all at risk to experience. The public's fears about genetic discrimination are preventing people from taking advantage of the health benefits genetic testing and information can provide. There are some laws in place prohibiting genetic discrimination, but they are not uniform at this time and most have not been tested in a court of law. Federal legislation to prevent genetic discrimination is in process but has not yet been realized. A report from the Secretary's Advisory Committee on Genetics, Health and Society (SACGHS, 2005a) summarizes the status of legislation to prevent discrimination.

### State Laws

Currently, most states have some legislation to prevent genetic discrimination from health insurance and employment based on genetic information. Forty-three states have enacted legislation on genetic discrimination in health insurance (see *www.ncsl.org/programs/health/genetics/ndishlth.htm*) and thirty-three states have enacted legislation concerning the workplace (see *www.ncsl.org/ programs/health/genetics/ndiscr.htm*). The state laws do not ensure a uniform foundation of protection in employment and insurance. With health insurance, the state laws do not ensure coverage for a significant number of individuals covered by private health insurance. Fewer states restrict the use of genetic information in life, disability, and long-term care insurance. Some state laws have taken steps to safeguard other privacy concerns such as disclosure of genetic information, personal property rights, and informed consent (see *www.ncsl.org/programs/ health/genetics/prt.htm*).

### Federal Laws

There are federal laws that offer some protection against genetic discrimination. One is the Health Insurance Portability and Accountability Act of 1996 (HIPAA) (OJIN, 2005). HIPAA protects individuals with group insurance and health plans against being denied insurance, having their insurance canceled, and having their rates individually increased by virtue of having a preexisting condition. HIPAA does not prohibit an insurance company from charging an entire employer group more for coverage because of one individual's genetic information, which could discourage employers from hiring or keeping employees they suspect may have a genetic condition or predisposition. HIPAA also does not prevent insurance companies from requiring applicants to reveal whether they have undergone genetic testing in order to sign up for a particular plan, in spite of the fact that insurance companies are not allowed to utilize this genetic information to discriminate against an applicant. For those who have individual health insurance plans, HIPAA offers no protection from discrimination.

In 2000, President Clinton signed an executive order that prohibits genetic discrimination against federal employees. These individuals, therefore, have additional protection against discrimination. Additionally, in 2003 the Genetic Information Nondiscrimination Act of 2003 (S. 1053) was the first federal bipartisan legislation to propose prohibiting discrimination on the basis of genetic information with respect to health insurance and employment. The bill defines genetic information as "genetic tests of an individual or family member or occurrence of a disease or disorder in family members." Genetic services are defined as "tests, counseling, or education" (S. 1053, 2003, p. 2). The bill protects the privacy of individuals' genetic information. Employment discrimination would be enforced under the Title VII of the Civil Rights Act, while health insurance discrimination would be enforced under the Employee Retirement and Income Security Act (ERISA) or state law. Advisory committees (e.g., SACGHS) and professional organizations (Association of Women's Health, Obstetric and Neonatal Nurses [AWHONN], 2005) have offered examples of the need for such legislation and have urged Congress to address public concerns by enacting federal genetic nondiscrimination legislation. The bill was passed in the Senate by a 95 to 0 unanimous vote but stalled in the House of Representatives.

### NURSING ROLE AND GENETIC DISCRIMINATION

Nurses are responding to the public's concern about genetic discrimination on an individual patient level and at the policy level. "The challenge for clinicians will be to discuss with their patients the potential adverse social consequences of testing so that the patients can make informed choices about whether or not to proceed with testing" (Clayton, 2003, p. 566).

The International Council of Nurses Code of Ethics for Nurses identifies as a primary responsibility of nurses ensuring that patients receive sufficient information on which to base care and treatment decisions (International Council of Nurses, 2005). Nurses play an important role in the informed decision-making process about genetic testing, especially at the advanced practice level, where they review the risks, benefits, and limitations of genetic testing and information (ISONG, 2000; Oncology Nursing Society [ONS], 2002). Nurses can explain how genetic knowledge is offering new opportunities to detect, prevent, and treat many rare and common conditions with a genetic component, while keeping in mind the potential for harm and the complex ethical, legal, and social implications.

Nurses are managers of genetic information. Currently, nurses are concerned about privacy and confidentiality of all medical information, including the potential for problems when documenting genetic information (Cassels et al., 2002). There are multiple factors influencing the utilization of genetic information in health care, including coverage and reimbursement of such tests (SACGHS, 2005a). Education about the ethical, legal, and social ramifications is important to making all nurses aware of current and future issues. Informed nurses will be able to contribute to the growing need for guideline and policy discussions. In addition, nurses must be sure that when managing documentation of genetic testing and information regarding risk information, they make sound choices to protect patients' privacy and confidentiality (ISONG, 2001).

As noted by Feetham, Thomson, and Hinshaw (2005), "the genomic era provides significant opportunities for nurses to provide leadership for nursing, health care, public health, and health policy" (p. 108). Examples of nurses assuming leadership in the policy arena are currently visible, such as providing public testimony at national meetings, developing position statements, writing letters to policymakers, and informing the public about key social policy issues resulting from utilization of genetic and genomic information. Nurses have a valued perspective to contribute and are encouraged to assume an even more active role in contributing to guideline and policy discussions to further enhance and improve clinical care in the genomic era (Jenkins & Lea, 2005).

## Key Points

- The public has expressed concerns about the potential for misuse of genetic information resulting in discrimination or stigmatization by health insurers, life insurers, and employers.
- Fears and the perception that genetic information may be used against them are preventing many people from pursuing genetic services or research that could make a difference in health care decisions and outcomes.
- Current laws leave substantial gaps in coverage and offer inconsistent safeguards.
- Nurses have an important role in contributing to guideline and policy discussions.

## Web Resources

**International Society of Nurses in Genetics**
*www.isong.org*
**National Human Genome Research Institute Policy and Legislation Database**
*www.genome.gov/PolicyEthics/LegDatabase/pubsearch.cfm*
**National Partnership for Women & Families**
*www.nationalpartnership.org/portals/p3/library/GeneticDiscrimination/FacesofGenetic Discrimination.pdf*
**Secretary's Advisory Committee on Genetics, Health, and Society (SACGHS)**
*www4.od.nih.gov/oba/sacghs.htm*

## REFERENCES

Apse, K., Biesecker, B., Giardiello, F., Fuller, B., & Bernhardt, B. (2004). Perceptions of genetic discrimination among at-risk relatives of colorectal cancer patients. *Genetics in Medicine, 6*(6), 510-516.

Association of Women's Health, Obstetric and Neonatal Nurses (AWHONN). (2005, February). AWHONN sends letter to Senate urging quick action on S. 306, the Genetic Information Nondiscrimination Act of 2005. Retrieved June 7, 2005, from *www.awhonn.org/awhonn/?pg=875-7010-17040.*

Billings, P. (2005). Genetic nondiscrimination. *Nature Genetics, 37*(6), 559-560.

Burlington Northern settles suit over genetic testing. (2001, April 19). *New York Times,* C4.

Burrell, T. (2005). A note on genetic information and insurance. *American Jurist On-line.* Retrieved April 18, 2005, from *www.americanjurist.net/news/2005/04/11/Features/A.Note.On.Genetic.Information.And.Insurance-918945.shtml.*

Cassells, J., Jenkins, J., Gaul, A., Lea, D., Calzone, K., & Johnson, E. (2002). An ethical assessment framework for addressing global genetic issues in clinical practice. *Oncology Nursing Forum, 30*(3), 383-390.

Clayton, E. (2003). Ethical, legal, and social implications of genomic medicine. *New England Journal of Medicine, 349*(6), 562-569.

Collins, F., Green, E., Guttmacher, A., & Guyer, M. (2003). A vision for the future of genomics research. *Nature, 422*(6934), 835-847.

Feetham, S., Thomson, E., & Hinshaw, A. (2005). Nursing leadership in genomics for health and society. *Journal of Nursing Scholarship, 37*(2), 107-110.

Genetics and Public Policy Center. (2004). Survey, Public awareness and attitudes about genetic technologies. Retrieved June 6, 2005, from *www.dnapolicy.org.*

Hadley, D., Jenkins, J., Dimond, E., Nakahara, K., Grogan, L., Liewehr, D., et al. (2003). Genetic counseling and testing in families with hereditary non-polyposis colorectal cancer. *Archives of Internal Medicine, 163,* 573-582.

Hall, M., McEwen, J., Barton, J., Walker, A., Howe, E., Reiss, J., et al. (2005). Concerns in a primary care population about genetic discrimination by insurers. *Genetics in Medicine, 7*(5), 311-316.

Harris Poll. (2002). If genetic tests were available for diseases which could be treated or prevented, many people would pay to have them. Retrieved June 6, 2005, from *www.harrisinteractive. com/news/newsletters/healthnews/HI_HealthCareNews2002 Vol2_Iss14.pdf*.

Hustead, J., & Goldman, J. (2002). Genetics and privacy. *American Journal of Law and Medicine, 28*(2-3), 285-307.

Institute of Medicine. (2004). *Insuring America's health: Principles and recommendations*. Washington, DC: National Academies Press.

International Council of Nurses. (2005). Fact sheet: Genetics and nursing. Retrieved June 7, 2005, from *www.icn.ch/matters_ genetics.htm*.

International Society of Nurses in Genetics (ISONG). (2000). Position statement: Informed decision making and consent: The role of nursing. Retrieved June 7, 2005, from *www.isong. org/about/position_statements/index.html*.

International Society of Nurses in Genetics (ISONG). (2001). Position statement: Privacy and confidentiality of genetic information: The role of the nurse. Retrieved June 7, 2005, from *www.isong.org/about/position_statements/index.html*.

Jenkins, J., & Lea, D. (2005). *Nursing care in the genomic era: A case based approach*. Boston: Jones and Bartlett.

Markel, H. (1997). Scientific advances and social risks: Historical perspectives of genetic screening programs for sickle cell disease, Tay-Sachs disease, neural tube defects and Down syndrome, 1970-1997. National Institutes of Health. Retrieved May 12, 2005, from *www.genome.gov/10002401*.

National Human Genome Research Institute (NHGRI). (n.d.). Talking glossary of genetic terms. Retrieved June 7, 2005, from *www.genome.gov/10002096*.

National Human Genome Research Institute (NHGRI). (2005). Genetic discrimination in health insurance. Retrieved June 7, 2005, from *www.genome.gov/10002328*.

National Partnership for Women & Families. (2004). Faces of genetic discrimination. How genetic discrimination affects real people. Washington, DC: Coalition for Genetic Fairness. Retrieved April 4, 2005, from *www.nationalpartnership.org/ portals/p3/library/GeneticDiscrimination/FacesofGenetic Discrimination.pdf*.

Offit, K., Groeger, E., Turner, S., Wadsworth, E., & Weiser, M. (2004). The duty to warn a patient's family members about hereditary disease risks. *Journal of the American Medical Association, 292*(12), 1469-1473.

Oncology Nursing Society (ONS). (2002). Position statement: Cancer predisposition genetic testing and risk assessment counseling. Retrieved June 7, 2005, from *www.ons.org/ publications/positions/CancerPredisposition.shtml*.

Online Journal of Issues in Nursing (OJIN). (2005). HIPAA: How our health care world has changed. Retrieved June 9, 2005, from *www.nursingworld.org/ojin/topic27/tpc27cnews.htm*.

Privacy concerns raised by the collection and use of genetic information by employers and insurers: Hearing before the Subcommittee on the Constitution of the House Committee on Judiciary, Sept. 12, 2002 (testimony of Joanne L. Hustead, Senior Counsel, Health Privacy Project, Assistant Research Professor, Institute for Health Care Research and Policy, Georgetown University) (discussing 2001 American Management Association Survey).

S. 1053—Genetic Information Nondiscrimination Act of 2003. No. 41, Calendar No. 247. October 2, 2003.

Secretary's Advisory Committee on Genetics, Health, and Society (SACGHS). (2005a, June 15). An analysis of the adequacy of current law in protecting against genetic discrimination in health insurance and employment. Report by Robert B. Lanman. Retrieved August 2, 2005, from *www4.od.nih.gov/oba/ SACGHS/reports/legal_analysis_May2005.pdf*.

Secretary's Advisory Committee on Genetics, Health, and Society (SACGHS). (2005b). Perspectives on genetic discrimination [Video DVD]. Retrieved August 2, 2005, from *www4.od. nih.gov/oba/SACGHS/reports/reports.html*.

Silvers, A., & Stein, M. A. (2002). An equality paradigm for presenting genetic discrimination. *Vanderbilt Law Review, 55*, 1341-1395.

Virginia Commonwealth University. (2001). Americans welcome scientific advancements with caution. *Virginia Commonwealth University News*. Retrieved June 7, 2005, from *www.vcu.edu/ uns/Releases/2001/oct/100401.htm*.

## INTIMATE PARTNER VIOLENCE: A PUBLIC HEALTH AND POLICY PROBLEM

Frances E. Ashe-Goins

*"Protective Order's Dismissal Called a Mistake— A husband allegedly went to his wife's place of employment, doused her with gasoline and set her on fire."* (The Washington Post, *October 18, 2005)*

*"Domestic Violence Murder—After stabbing girlfriend 49 times, a defendant raises the 'just trying to take her knife away' defense."* (Milwaukee Journal Sentinel, *July 7, 2005)*

*"Pregnancy—In front of two children, man runs over pregnant girlfriend, police say."* (Albuquerque Journal, *July 7, 2005)*

*"I saw my father beat my mother. I remember my sister hiding under the bed when he'd come in screaming in a drunken rage."* (Los Angeles *Mayor-elect Antonio Villaraigosa on his childhood,* Newsweek, *May 30, 2005)*

Intimate partner violence (IPV) occurs in all populations, regardless of social, economic, religious, or cultural group. IPV refers to violent acts such as murder, rape, sexual assault, robbery, aggravated assault, and simple assault that are perpetuated by a current or former spouse or significant other. Physical assault is defined as behaviors that threaten, attempt, or actually inflict harm. Rape is defined as an event that occurred without the victim's consent that involved the use of or threat of force to penetrate the victim's vagina or anus by penis, tongue, fingers, or object, or the victim's mouth by penis (Rennison & Welchans, 2000).

The Centers for Disease Control and Prevention (CDC) reported in their 2003 Intimate Partner Fact Sheet that nearly 5.3 million partner victimizations occur each year in women over 18 years of age. These violent episodes result in almost 2 million injuries and nearly 1300 deaths (Box 22-5).

---

**BOX 22-5** Scope of the Problem of Intimate Partner Violence

- An estimated 1 million women and 371,000 men are stalked by intimate partners each year. (Centers for Disease and Control Prevention, 2003)
- Nearly 25% of women have been physically assaulted or raped by a partner during their lifetime, and more than 40% of them sustain a physical injury. (CDC Fact Sheet)
- 20% of all non-fatal violent crime experienced by women in 2001 was a result of intimate partner violence. (CDC Fact Sheet)
- 44% of women who were murdered had visited an emergency department within 2 years of the death, and 93% had sustained at least one injury. (CDC Fact Sheet)
- Firearms were the weapons of choice used in IPV homicides from 1981 to 1998. (CDC Fact Sheet)
- More than 324,000 pregnant women are victims of IPV each year in the USA. (CDC Safe Motherhood Report)
- Between 1993 and 1998, children under 12 years of age resided in 43% of households in which IPV was reported. (BJS 2002 Intimate Partner Violence)

Data from Rennison, C. M., & Welchans, S. (2000). Bureau of Justice Studies Special Report: Intimate partner violence. Washington, DC: U.S. Department of Justice. Retrieved April 18, 2005, from *www.cdc.gov/ncipc/factsheets/ipvfacts.htm*; Centers for Disease Control and Prevention. (2002). *Safe motherhood: Promoting health for women before, during and after pregnancy.* Washington, DC: Department of Health and Human Services. Retrieved April 18, 2005, from *www.ojp.gov/ovc/ncvrw/2005/pg5f.html*; and Centers for Disease Control and Prevention, National Center for Injury Prevention and Control. (2003). *Intimate partner violence fact sheet.* Atlanta, GA: Department of Health and Human Services. Retrieved April 18, 2005, from *www.cdc.gov/ncipc/factsheets/ipvfacts.htm.*

## CONSEQUENCES OF INTIMATE PARTNER VIOLENCE

The health consequences of IPV are significant. Women who have experienced IPV report 60% higher rates of health problems than those who have not. Reported problems include chronic pain, GI disorders like irritable bowel syndrome, depression, anxiety, low self-esteem, higher prevalence of sexually transmitted diseases, gynecological disorders, unwanted pregnancies, premature labor and birth, hysterectomy, and heart or circulatory conditions. These women and girls also display behaviors that increase risks such as substance abuse, antisocial behavior, and suicidal behavior, especially in adolescent females (CDC, 2003).

IPV has economic consequences too. The costs of IPV exceed $5.8 billion, which include $4.1 billion in direct medical and mental health care and $1.8 billion in indirect costs of loss of productivity. These victims lose nearly 8 million compensated workdays, which are more than 32,000 full-time jobs (CDC, 2003).

### Historical Perspective

Stranger violence has always been considered an outrage in the United States, yet that same violence committed against women by acquaintances or partners sometimes has been considered a criminal matter only in extreme circumstances. Sexual assault, spousal rape, spousal assault, and stalking have not been treated consistently as crimes. IPV was recognized as a serious social problem in the early 1970s. This is considered by some to be linked with the emergence of women's rights movement.

### Rape and Sexual Assault

Rape and sexual assault have been problems in the legal system. Proving criminal intent required that the victim proved her unwillingness through physical injury or incapacity. In the court, questions regarding a victim's previous sexual experience sought to weaken her credibility. Reform of rape laws in the 1970s contributed to an increase in convictions. Some states have adopted "rape shield laws" that prevent questioning victims about past sexual experience, and most states have abandoned statutes that exempt husbands from rape charges.

Physical abuse of wives was not a crime during much of U.S. history (Worden, 2000). By the 1800s, several states had enacted laws that made wife-beating a crime; however, judges only ruled on whether the abuse was excessive and cruel if this was an issue in a divorce case. Of note is that many judges decided that the abuse was not cruel or severe, and they based their judgments on whether the punishment was "deserved" (Worden, 2000).

In the 1970s, police officers, when called to a domestic violence incident, were discouraged from arresting the husband as it was considered to possibly increase marital discord. However, in the 1980s, victims were successful in suing police departments for failure to provide equal protection. Also during that time, a study was published on the deterrent effect of arrest on repeat violence (Worden, 2000). Together, these developments led to the widespread adoption of policies that promoted arrest in domestic cases.

### Stalking

Stalking is defined as a series or pattern of acts designed to frighten, annoy, or intimidate the victim. The definition of stalking used in the National Violence Against Women (NVAW) survey defines it as a course of conduct directed at a specific person that involves repeated visual or physical proximity; nonconsensual communication; verbal, written, or implied threats; or a combination thereof that would cause fear in a reasonable person (Worden, 2000).

The IPV laws that have been reformed over the years have had many objectives. In many states, those laws were enacted to facilitate prosecution of the batterer. Tougher penalties have been attached to violations of orders of protection as a deterrent factor. By 1996, the majority of states had authorized warrantless arrests in misdemeanor cases, and one in three states had adopted mandatory arrest statutes (Worden, 2000).

### Gender Role in Intimate Partner Violence

Women experienced IPV at higher rates than men between 1993 and 1998, according to a study by the Bureau of Justice Statistics (Rennison, 2003). Among women, being African American, young, divorced or separated, earning lower incomes, living in rental housing, and living in an urban area were associated with a higher rate of IPV. Women aged 20 to 24 were victimized at the highest rate, 21 per 1000 women (Rennison, 2003).

Men who were young, African American, divorced or separated, or living in rented housing had significantly higher rates of IPV than other men. The rate of IPV in African American men was 625 higher than the rate for whites. For men aged 25 to 34, the rate was 3 per 1000 men (Rennison, 2003).

Recent studies show that the number of violent crimes by an intimate partner has declined from 1993 to 2001. Women experienced about 588,490 crimes in 2001, which is down from 1.1 million in 1993. In addition, the rate for men has also declined, from 162,870 in 1993 to 103,220 in 2001 (Rennison, 2003).

The NVAW study concluded that violence against women and men is predominately male violence. All women in the study raped after age 13 were raped by a male. In addition, 91.9% of women who were physically assaulted since age 18 were assaulted by a male. Moreover, 97% of those who were stalked were stalked by a male (Rennison, 2003). Violence against men is also male dominated. Seventy percent of men who were raped since age 18 were raped by a male. Similarly, 86% were physically assaulted by a male and 65% were stalked by a male (Rennison, 2003).

Characteristics of male batterers include young age, low self-esteem, low income, low academic achievement, involvement in aggressive or delinquent behavior as a youth, alcohol and/or drug use, witnessing or experiencing violence as a child, lack of social networks, social isolation, and unemployment (CDC, 2003). Men may blame their spouse for the problems in the family and then seek to isolate the partner from family and friends who are perceived as "bad" influences. Women have an increased risk of domestic violence if they have a history of physical abuse, prior injury from the same partner, verbal abuse, economic stress, alcohol or drug use, and children in the home (CDC, 2003).

### Efforts to Address the Problem of Intimate Partner Violence

IPV is an endemic public health problem. The number of rapes, physical assaults, and stalking committed each year against women suggests that this problem needs a broad array of efforts to address it. A number of federal agencies have played a role in developing and implementing policy to reduce IPV. Additionally, several significant bills have been passed that initiated responses to the problem.

***The Violence Against Women Act.*** Congress enacted the Violence Against Women Act (VAWA) in 1994—a landmark law. This law enhanced the ability of the states and territories to respond to violence against women and created new grant programs. VAWA defined violence against women as sexual assault, stalking, and domestic violence. It outlined seven specific purpose areas that can be funded by the Services, Training, Officers, and Prosecutors (STOP) program. STOP is a formula grant program that is administered by the Violence Against Women Grants Office (VAWGO), the Office of Justice Programs (OJP), in the U.S. Department of Justice (DOJ). It required the states to allocate funds in three categories: victim services, law enforcement, and prosecution.

Building coordinated community response to violence against women is critical. The act mandated each state to develop a plan to implement the STOP program. The VAWA incorporated the key role that community-based advocates play in developing effective strategies to stop VAW. The act stipulated that each state must "consult and coordinate with non-profit, non-governmental victim services programs, including sexual assault and domestic violence victim services programs."

In 2000, Congress reauthorized VAWA, continuing these efforts, and added essential services for immigrant, rural, disabled, and older women. The VAWA was signed into law by President Bush in 2005. The new act adds a new dedicated grant program for sexual assault victims. In addition, it supports children who have been exposed to violence, strengthens the health care response to family violence, and engages men and youth in preventing violence.

***The Gun Control Act.*** In 1994 and 1996, Congress passed changes to the Gun Control Act, making it a federal crime in certain situations for batterers to possess guns. It is a federal crime to possess a firearm and/or ammunition while subject to a qualifying protection order and to possess a firearm and/or ammunition after conviction

**BOX 22-6**   Domestic Violence Victims Rights

A domestic violence victim, under 42 U.S.C. section 10606(b), has the right to:

■ Be treated with fairness and with respect for the victim's dignity and privacy
■ Be reasonably protected from the accused offender
■ Be notified of court proceedings
■ Be present at all public court proceedings related to the offense, unless the court determines that testimony by the victim would be materially affected if the victim heard other testimony at the trial
■ Confer with the attorney for the government in the case
■ Restitution
■ Information about the conviction, sentencing, imprisonment, and the release of the offender

From Arvin, M. D. (2000). *Federal domestic laws.* Retrieved April 20, 2005, from *www.usdoj.gov/usao/tnw/brochures/ federaldomesticviolencelaws.html.*

of a qualifying misdemeanor crime of domestic violence (Box 22-6).

***The Family Violence Prevention and Services Act.*** The U.S. Department of Health and Human Services (HHS) is responsible for certain provisions in the Family Violence Prevention and Services Act passed in 1984. The Administration for Children and Families (ACF) is responsible for Battered Women's Shelter Services, the National Toll-Free Hotline, the Family Preservation and Family Support Program, and five national resource centers that provide information, technical assistance, and research findings via toll-free telephone numbers.

***The Centers for Disease Control and Prevention.*** The CDC provides grants to states for rape prevention and education programs conducted by rape crisis centers or similar nongovernmental, nonprofit entities. The funds support educational seminars, the operation of hotlines, training programs, and other activities to increase awareness of and help prevent sexual assault, including programs targeted to students. In addition, CDC works to build new community programs aimed at preventing intimate partner violence and strengthening existing community intervention and prevention programs. The CDC

conducted the National Violence Against Women survey and completed a study on the cost of violence against women.

***The Personal Responsibility and Work Opportunities Reconciliation Act.*** In 1996, Congress enacted the Personal Responsibility and Work Opportunities Reconciliation Act, which included provisions to help welfare recipients who are victims of domestic violence move successfully into work. Specifically, the provisions give states the option to screen welfare recipients for domestic abuse, refer them to counseling and supportive services, and temporarily waive any program requirements that would prevent recipients from escaping violence or would unfairly penalize them.

***The National Council of Juvenile and Family Court Judges.*** Supported by HHS and DOJ funding, the National Council of Juvenile and Family Court Judges developed best practice guidelines for handling child protection cases involving domestic violence. The group published *Effective Intervention in Domestic Violence and Child Maltreatment Cases: Guidelines for Policy and Practice* in 1999. In 2000, following a competitive process, six sites were selected to demonstrate the effectiveness of community collaborations in implementing the report's recommendations.

***The Substance Abuse and Mental Health Services Administration.*** The Substance Abuse and Mental Health Services Administration (SAMHSA) supports several programs addressing substance abuse and mental health issues among victims of violence. These efforts include a five-year study designed to develop effective integrated service programs for women and their children affected by violence and co-occurring mental and addictive disorders and a multiyear grant program that focuses on the connection among domestic violence, mental illness, substance abuse, and homelessness among women and their children by assessing the effectiveness of time-limited intensive treatment, housing, support, and family preservation services to homeless mothers and their dependent children.

***The Agency for Healthcare Research and Quality.*** In 2000, the Agency for Healthcare Research and Quality (AHRQ) awarded $5.5 million to fund four comparative studies examining the effectiveness of intervention programs offered in health care settings. AHRQ and the nonprofit Family Violence Prevention Fund also jointly sponsor a Scholar in Residence, who is developing better ways to assess health system interventions.

***The National Institute of Mental Health.*** The National Institute of Mental Health (NIMH) funds a number of research studies focusing on the mental health consequences of violence, treatments for the traumatic consequences of violence, and factors that influence the initiation of physically aggressive behavior in intimate relationships.

***The Administration on Aging.*** The Administration on Aging (AoA) funds elder abuse prevention programs in all 50 states that focus on the prevention of elder abuse, neglect, and exploitation—including domestic violence.

***Other HHS programs.*** The HHS Office on Women's Health (OWH) has been instrumental in highlighting this issue for national leaders of nursing and social work organizations and institutions. OWH has developed a program targeting increased capacity building for organizations that provide services for immigrant women. In addition, many HHS programs aim to strengthen families, prevent the abuse of women and children, and help families provide a healthy and safe environment for children. These programs include the Promoting Safe and Stable Families program and Child Abuse Prevention and Treatment Act grants (U.S. Department of Health and Human Services, 2001).

## HEALTH CARE ISSUES

The National Violence Against Women survey revealed that 35.6% of the women injured during rape since age 18 received some type of health services. The most frequent treatment was hospitalization. Of the women injured during their most recent physical assault, 30.2% received some type of medical treatment; 76.1% were treated in a hospital and 61.4% of those women were treated in an emergency department (Tjaden & Thoennes, 2000). Male victims had similar rates: 37% received treatment in a hospital for physical assault and 67% of those were treated in the emergency department.

IPV is also directly related to adverse mental health effects. Unfortunately, many health care providers still do not view sexual assault, dating and domestic violence, and stalking as public health issues, and many lack the skills, knowledge, and incentives to respond appropriately. In fact, even though many health care providers favored the practice of inquiring about IPV, few made such inquiries.

Health care workers have an important role in responding to IPV. They can refer the victim to a safe place, to counseling, and to community-based resources, and refer batterers to treatment programs. Screening may be appropriate when determining the cause for the presenting symptoms. These critical questions may prevent unnecessary work-ups when the etiology is IPV.

### Policy Issues Related to Intimate Partner Violence

***Confidentiality.*** The potential for inappropriate access to, and use of, medical record information by insurance companies, employers, and law enforcement is a concern. Compliance with HIPPA laws should improve confidentiality compliance.

***Removing barriers to forensic sexual assault exams and related treatment.*** The practice of conditioning medical services to requirements that victims report to law officials or participate in court proceedings may compromise their access to emergency care services and may put them at increased risk.

***Mandatory reporting to law enforcement officials.*** There is growing evidence that mandatory reporting may not improve a patient's health and safety and may discourage some victims from seeking medical care.

***Creating reimbursement mechanisms, coding, and other incentives to provide care for victims.*** There are no specific current procedural terminology (CPT) codes for domestic violence screening or interventions exist. However, diagnostic codes (995.80-995.85) and e-codes capture additional information such as the nature of the abuse and perpetrators (National Advisory Council on Violence Against Women, 2000).

### Role of Economic Policy in Reducing Intimate Partner Violence

Women's economic security plays a role in assisting the woman to remove her family from IPV.

Efforts that can make a difference include policies and programs that provide the following:

- Job training and employment
- Safe, affordable child care in every community
- Increased availability of safe and affordable housing
- Expanded unemployment benefits, workers compensation programs, and increases in the minimum wage
- Increased educational opportunities to enhance the eligibility for permanent employment
- Elimination of insurance discrimination against IPV victims in any area of insurance—including health care, life, auto, renters, disability, home-owners, and property insurance

### Role of the Faith Community

The faith community can collaborate with existing resource organizations, become a resource for victims and families, intervene when they suspect IPV, support professional training, and address internal issues within the faith community.

### Role of Law Enforcement

Law enforcement is the entry point to the criminal justice system for both batterer and victim in IPV cases. Proactive and aggressive police response can deter further violence in many cases and can ultimately save lives. Prevention is the key, and many law enforcement agencies are promoting early intervention in domestic violence and stalking cases to protect victims.

### Critical Role of Coordinated Sexual Assault Response Team Efforts

Legislative reforms have been directed toward making testifying less intimidating, and resources have been directed to programs that support victims and improve the quality of evidence. Sexual assault response teams (SARTs) and sexual assault nurse examiners (SANEs) have been established to include specially trained personnel who work across agency lines to protect and support victims while maximizing the likelihood of successful prosecution (Worden, 2000).

A multidisciplinary response was developed to coordinate crisis intervention services and professional forensic evidence collection. For these victims, a new area of specialized health services evolved: the sexual assault examiner (SAE), the sexual assault nurse examiner (SANE), and the sexual assault forensic examiner (SAFE). SAEs are trained medical professionals who have advanced education and clinical preparation in the forensic examination of victims and who partner with local victims advocates to provide support during forensic exam and to coordinate follow-up services. When the victim wants to report an assault to law officials, existing relationships between the SAE, victim advocate, and the police department facilitate a victim-centered response.

***The Sexual Assault Nurse Examiner.*** A SANE is a registered nurse who has advanced education and clinical preparation in forensic examination and in dealing with sexual assault victims. In the 1990s, the SANE program was rapidly emerging throughout the country to address the inadequacy of the traditional model for sexual assault medical evidentiary exams. It was recognized that victims were being re-traumatized by the medical system due to long waits for examination and inexperienced workers in evidence collection, which led to failure in prosecution of the perpetrator. SANE programs have made a profound difference in the quality of care received by sexual assault victims. They preserve the patient's dignity, reduce psychological trauma, and enhance evidence collection, which leads to more effective documentation of evidence corroborating the victim's account of the incident—which in turn leads to more successful prosecutions.

In the 1970s, the first SANE programs were established in Minneapolis, Minnesota; Memphis, Tennessee; and Amarillo, Texas. By 1997, 300 programs had been established. It is important to note that SANEs are forensic nurses, but not all forensic nurses are trained to be SANEs. Forensic nurses also conduct evidentiary exams in cases of other types of IPV, public health and safety, emergencies or trauma, patient care facilities, and police and corrections custody abuse. SANEs and other forensic nurses collaborated to encourage the field to recognize this as a specialty. In 1995, the American Nurses Association recognized forensic nursing as a specialty.

Successful SANE programs operate with other members of the community sexual response system to meet the multiple needs of the victim. Other team members include, but are not limited to, advocates from a sexual assault crisis center, law enforcement officers, prosecutors, judges, other court officials, forensic lab staff, victim/witness specialists based in justice system offices, and child protective services workers. Many communities have established multidisciplinary bodies (SARTs) to oversee coordination and collaboration related to immediate response to sexual assault cares. These teams ensure a victim-centered approach to service delivery and explore strategies to prevent future victimization. In localities where SANEs exist, SANEs must be integrated to ensure a comprehensive and effective response (Littel, 2001).

## Key Points

- The Centers for Disease Control and Prevention (CDC) reported in their 2003 Intimate Partner Fact Sheet that nearly 5.3 million partner victimizations occur each year in women over 18 years of age.
- Sexual assault response teams (SARTs) and sexual assault nurse examiners (SANEs) have been established to include specially trained personnel who work across agency lines to protect and support victims while maximizing the likelihood of successful prosecution.
- Congress enacted the Violence Against Women Act (VAWA) in 1994 to enhance the ability of the states and territories to respond to violence against women.

## Web Resources

**Bureau of Justice IPV Statistics**
*www.ojp.usdoj.gov/bjs/abstract/ipv.htm*
**CDC Intimate Partner Violence Fact Sheet**
*www.cdc.gov/ncipc/factsheets/ipvfacts.htm*
**HHS Violence Against Women**
*www.4woman.gov/violence/domestic.cfm*

## REFERENCES

Arvin, M. D. (2000). *Federal domestic laws.* Retrieved April 20, 2005, from *www.usdoj.gov/usao/tnw/brochures/federaldomestic-violencelaws.html.*

Centers for Disease Control and Prevention. (2002). *Safe motherhood: Promoting health for women before, during and after pregnancy.* Washington, DC: Department of Health and Human Services. Retrieved April 18, 2005, from *www.ojp.gov/ovc/ncvrw/2005/pg5f.html.*

Centers for Disease Control and Prevention, National Center for Injury Prevention and Control. (2003). *Intimate partner violence fact sheet.* Atlanta, GA: Department of Health and Human Services. Retrieved April 18, 2005, from *www.cdc.gov/ncipc/factsheets/ipvfacts.htm.*

Littel, K. (2001, April). Sexual assault nurse examiner (SANE) programs: Improving the community response to sexual assault victims. *OVC Bulletin.* Washington, DC: U.S. Department of Justice Office of Justice Programs, Office for Victims of Crime.

Littel, K., Malefyt, M. B., Walker, A., Buel, S. M., Tucker, D. (1998). Assessing justice system response to violence against women: A tool for law enforcement, prosecution and the courts to use in developing effective responses. Washington, DC: U.S. Department of Justice, Office on Justice Programs. Retrieved April 20, 2005, from *www.vaw.umn.edu/documents/promise/pplaw/pplaw.html.*

National Advisory Council on Violence Against Women. (2000). *Ending violence against women: An agenda for the nation and toolkit to end violence against women.* Washington, DC: U.S. Department of Justice and Department of Health and Human Services.

Rennison, C. M. (2003). *Bureau of Justice Statistics Crime Data Brief: Intimate Partner Violence 1993-2001.* Washington, DC: U.S. Department of Justice.

Rennison, C. M., & Welchans, S. (2000). Bureau of Justice Studies Special Report: Intimate partner violence. Washington, DC: U.S. Department of Justice. Retrieved April 18, 2005, from *www.cdc.gov/ncipc/factsheets/ipvfacts.htm.*

Tjaden, P., & Thoennes, N. (2000). *Full report of the prevalence, incidence, and consequences of violence against women, Research Report, Findings from the National Violence Against Women Survey, November 1995-May 1996.* Washington, DC: U.S. Department of Justice, National Institute of Justice, and HHS (CDC).

U.S. Department of Health and Human Services. (2001, August). *Preventing violence against women fact sheet.* Washington, DC: Department of Health and Human Services.

Worden, A. P. (2000). *Violence against women: A synthesis of research for judges* (report submitted to Department of Justice). Washington, DC: U.S. Department of Justice.

# chapter 23

# How Government Works: What You Need to Know to Influence the Process

Karrie C. Hendrickson & Sally S. Cohen

*"What government is the best? That which teaches us to govern ourselves."*

WOLFGANG VON GOETHE

Nurses need to know how government works so that they can convince public officials to create policies that improve access to quality and affordable health care for all. This chapter provides an overview of the federal, state, and local levels of government, how each level works, and the relationships among them in a federalist system. Such information is essential to effect policy and bring nurses' unique perspective to those who make the final decisions—legislators, regulators, and staff who support them. Because budget policies underlie all health policy issues, this chapter also reviews the federal budget process and related state and local processes. All health programs require funding, and the budget process is the means by which the executive and legislative branches reconcile competing priorities and make budgetary decisions. In this chapter, we identify key access points for influencing policy at different levels and branches of government and throughout the federal budget process. We have used the issue of covering the uninsured to demonstrate why nurses need to know how government works.

## FEDERALISM: MULTIPLE LEVELS OF RESPONSIBILITY

The U.S. government was created as a federalist system. Simply stated, this means that the government consists of multiple levels, including both a centralized, national tier and at least one decentralized, subnational tier (Walker, 2000). In the case of the United States, tiers are the federal, state, and local levels of government.

Unlike a unitary state, a federalist system constitutionally divides sovereignty among the different governmental levels so that the actors at each level have final authority in some areas and can act efficiently and independently of each other. The U.S. Constitution divides governmental authority by prescribing the duties and responsibilities of the federal government and withholding both specified and unspecified powers for the states. The Tenth Amendment to the Constitution (also known as the State's Rights Amendment), ratified in 1791, helps to clarify how this authority is divided among the levels of government. It states, "The powers not delegated to the United States by the Constitution, nor prohibited by it to the States, are reserved to the States respectively, or to the people." This means that states have jurisdiction over issues that the Constitution does not explicitly grant to the

Federal government. This is a fundamental aspect of the Constitution; state policymakers often interpret their constitutional states' rights quite liberally.

Because the U.S. government is one of divided powers, citizens are accountable to three levels of authority. In a federalist system, the allocation of authority among the levels may vary over time, but typically the federal government has powers regarding defense, foreign policy, and interstate commerce (Follesdal & Zalta, 2003). The federal government may also participate in and influence local policy through government grants, sanctions, and federal mandates (federal requirements for state, local, or tribal governments to expend their own resources to achieve certain goals) (Hanson, 2004). Finally, many powers, such as taxation and law formation and enforcement, are shared equally among the levels of government and may be exercised in conjunction or independently. For more information on federalism and associated court cases, see the Stanford Encyclopedia and American Bar Association Websites listed in Web Resources.

Because governmental powers and responsibilities laid out in the Constitution are imprecise and subject to interpretation, some controversy and conflict has occurred among all the levels of government, most particularly between federal and state authorities (Hanson, 2004; Reinhard, 2002). The U.S. Supreme Court, however, works to interpret the Constitution and maintain the balance of power among the levels of government (Hanson, 2004). It is important to understand the court's stand on federalism and states' rights when designing a federally administered program and planning its implementation. Court decisions may affect when, how, and by whom your program is implemented.

## THE FEDERAL GOVERNMENT

The U.S. federal government of the United States is centered in Washington, DC, and has 10 regional offices. These regional offices are instrumental in policy implementation and enhance access to federal officials for issues concerning health and well-being. Like the three levels of government, the three branches of the federal government represent a separation of powers and work as a series of checks and balances on one another. These branches require the actors to work together to formulate policy that is acceptable to as many people as possible, and they are designed to prevent any individual or small group from making sweeping changes. For more information on the roles and powers of the federal government, see the U.S. Government's Official Web Portal Website listed in the Web Resources.

## THE EXECUTIVE BRANCH

The role of the executive branch of the federal government is to implement laws and oversee their enforcement. The executive branch is made up of the Executive Office of the President (EOP), the Executive Cabinet, and many independent agencies, boards, committees, and commissions, the staffs of which both advise the president and help to oversee the programs. Both the EOP and the Cabinet will be discussed here.

**Executive Office of the President (EOP).** The EOP consists of the president, the vice president, and related White House offices and agencies. These offices and agencies include the National Security Council, Office of Management and Budget (OMB), Office of the U.S. Trade Representative, Office of National Drug Control Policy, and Office of Homeland Security, all of which develop and implement the policy and programs of the president.

The OMB is one of the most relevant offices in the EOP to nursing. This office prepares the president's budget for presentation to Congress on the first Monday of every February. This budget reflects the president's national agenda and provides those seeking to influence a realistic picture of the likelihood of their project receiving funding. It also serves as a potential access point for policy change.

The president is the highest ranking elected federal official and serves as the head of the executive branch. The president also serves as the commander in chief of all U.S. military forces, and with the approval of the Senate, grants pardons, makes treaties, and appoints high-ranking officials such as Supreme Court justices and cabinet secretaries.

One of the president's most notable domestic powers, however, is the veto, which effectively stops (or at least delays) a newly passed piece of legislation from becoming a law. This power is not to be taken lightly because, if the president invokes the veto, it can only be overridden by a two-thirds majority vote in both houses of Congress.

Of key importance to those hoping to influence policy are the powers of the president not defined in the Constitution, including the power to set the national agenda. This is sometimes referred to as "the power of the pulpit." Newly elected presidents bring their priority issues to the forefront of the American political agenda. Even though this may not result in policy change, it does open the door for discussion and debate of some issues and closes the door on others. For example, at the beginning of his presidency, Bill Clinton's proposals for revising health policy, covering the uninsured, and revamping welfare were high on the public and policy agendas. But the election of President George W. Bush shifted emphasis away from those issues and focused on discussions regarding Social Security, Medicare prescription drug coverage, and homeland security. A savvy activist must be aware of policymakers' priorities and anticipate how changes in the political climate following an election may affect the politics of health policymaking.

White House staff is influential in setting national agendas and disseminating the president's priorities. These individuals are appointed by the president, but are not confirmed by Congress. Thus, they usually hold views similar to the president and are instrumental in White House decision-making. One can determine White House staff perspectives on health policy through newspaper and other media reports. Additional information on the federal executive branch can be found online at the U.S. Executive Branch websites listed in Web Resources.

**The Cabinet.** The Executive Cabinet is made up of the heads of 15 departments (see the President's Cabinet Websites listed in Web Resources). These departments work with the president and oversee the enforcement and administration of federal law through regulation and the appropriation of funds. Although all cabinet departments may have jurisdiction over areas of interest to nurses, the five most relevant to nursing practice are discussed next.

***The Department of Health and Human Services (DHHS).*** The DHHS is "the United States government's principal agency for protecting the health of all Americans and providing essential human services, especially for those who are least able to help themselves." To accomplish this mission, DHHS oversees more than 300 programs such as Medicare, Medicaid (Centers for Medicare and Medicaid), Head Start, the Centers for Disease Control and Prevention (CDC), the Food and Drug Administration (FDA), the Indian Health Service, and agencies involved with nursing and medical research such as the National Institutes of Health [NIH] and the Agency for Healthcare Research and Quality.

DHHS is responsible for the distribution of the second largest portion of federal budget. Most of this money goes to pay for Medicare and Medicaid claims, and the rest is distributed among the agencies. New programs or changes to existing programs advocated by health professionals will likely be overseen by the DHHS. Therefore, it is vital to understand its structure and functions. More information on DHHS can be obtained at the Websites listed in Web Resources.

***The Department of Defense (DOD).*** U.S. military spending makes up the largest portion of the federal budget, and a large part of that money goes to health care. The DOD provides care to all active duty military personnel and their families, approximately 8 million people stationed throughout the world (White, 2002). The military employs over 35,000 nurses and provides funding for nursing research. For additional information on the DOD and TRICARE, its health maintenance organization, see the DOD Website in Web Resources. (See also *The Department of Defense TRICARE Program: Health Care for the U.S. Military* following Chapter 13.)

***The Department of Veterans Affairs.*** Through the Veterans Health Administration, the Department of Veterans Affairs oversees programs to provide health care and other services to U.S. military veterans and their families. This department employs about 34,000 registered nurses (RNs) and 26,000 licensed practical nurses (LPNs) and operates 157 Veterans

Affairs (VA) hospitals and 1300 other care sites, which provide health care services to approximately 63 million eligible people (U.S. Department of Veterans Affairs, 2005) (see also *The U.S. Veterans Administration: Policy Change for the Greater Good in an Integrated Health System* following Chapter 13).

The VA also manages the largest medical education and health professions training program in the United States. Their facilities are affiliated with 107 medical schools, 55 dental schools, and more than 1200 other schools across the country. About 83,000 health professionals are trained in VA medical centers annually (U.S. Department of Veterans Affairs, 2005). The VA is also intensely involved in both nursing and medical research. It currently supports approximately 3000 researchers at 115 VA medical centers, with an estimated FY 2005 research funding level of $402 million.

***The U.S. Department of Education.*** The Department of Education provides billions of dollars in grants and loans for students to attend college and professional schools, including schools of nursing. This is highly relevant to nurses, particularly in times of nursing shortage, because the department works with hospitals and other government agencies to provide incentives such as loan repayment programs, which attract nurses to the most underserved areas (White, 2002).

***The Department of Labor (DOL).*** The Department of Labor's mission includes improving working conditions, advancing opportunities for profitable employment, protecting retirement and health care benefits, helping employers find workers, strengthening collective bargaining, and tracking measures of national economic stability such as employment. To that end, the DOL oversees enforcement of federal labor laws that are germane to nursing practice, such as those that guarantee the right to safe working conditions, fair compensation in the form of an appropriate minimum wage and/or overtime pay, and freedom from discrimination during the hiring, employment, or termination process.

One component of the DOL most relevant to health and nursing is the Occupational Safety and Health Administration (OSHA). OSHA works with states to establish protective standards for safe working conditions and oversee the enforcement of

those standards. OSHA regulations govern health care facilities, research settings, and workplaces nationwide. They affect every nurse practicing in the United States. Additional information on the DOL and OSHA is available through their Websites listed in Web Resources.

**Regulatory Functions of the Executive Branch of Government.** The executive branch of the federal government is responsible for implementing laws enacted by Congress. This task falls to staff of the relevant departments and agencies, often with input from the agencies under the EOP. Once a law is enacted, the federal agency staff develops regulations for implementation of the relevant program, which specify definitions, authority, eligibility, benefits, and standards. This step is necessary because while the laws passed by Congress express the legislators' intentions, they do not spell out the details of the new program (Smith, Greenblatt, Buntin, & Clark, 2005).

The regulations (or rules) are published in the *Federal Register*, giving interested individuals and organizations a limited opportunity to review and comment. This is an important access point for nurses interested in shaping health policy. Agency staff reviews all of the comments and then issues final regulations in the *Federal Register*. These regulations govern how agencies and individuals in states and localities are to implement the law. For additional information on regulatory functions of the federal government and the *Federal Register*, see the Federal Register Website in the Web Resources.

## THE LEGISLATIVE BRANCH

The legislative branch of the federal government consists of the Congress, which is divided into two chambers—the Senate and the House of Representatives. Members of Congress are elected by their constituents. The Senate, with two members from each state, has 100 seats. The House of Representatives has 435 seats, with each state's number of representatives based on its population size. The number of members in each state's delegation may change every 10 years based on the results of the national decennial census. Members of the Senate and House are elected for 6-year terms and 2-year terms, respectively.

The primary role of the legislative branch is the formulation of laws for recommendation to the president. The process of creating such laws can be long and arduous, and is thoroughly discussed in Chapter 24. It is key to note, however, that once a new topic or bill is introduced into a congressional chamber, it is often assigned to one of nearly 250 committees or subcommittees for further discussion and hearings. This step is critical for the nurse activist to recognize because it provides one of the primary points of entry into the policy arena.

The assignment of a bill to a committee signals to those who care about the issue that it is time to act. Although this point of entry is not without roadblocks, measures can be taken to help keep the issue salient. Successful entry requires that the policy advocate be knowledgeable about the committee with jurisdiction, its members, and their priorities. It also requires that they be prepared with both a primary and back-up policy plan, be willing and able to educate the committee members and their staff, and be capable of providing persuasive testimony before committee members. For a complete list of committees and their health-related jurisdictions, see Tables 23-1 and 23-2. A complete listing and other information is also available on the Internet on the department websites listed in the Web Resources. By following the link to each committee, one can obtain information about committee and subcommittee membership, complete jurisdiction, hearings, recent bills, and other timely health policy information. The status of all federal bills can be obtained at one of the most important Websites for congressional information: *http:// thomas.loc.gov/*. Finally, it is also important to recognize that the members of congressional staffs are accessible via phone and the Internet. Nurses should be familiar with not only representatives from their home state but also other legislators who either support their issue or sit on a committee with jurisdiction over it.

## THE FEDERAL BUDGET

Anyone involved with national health policymaking follows the federal budget process closely. The federal budget is the end result of collaboration between the executive and legislative branches. The executive

**TABLE 23-1** Standing Committees of the U.S. Senate with Jurisdiction Over Health Policy Issues

| COMMITTEE | JURISDICTION |
| --- | --- |
| Agriculture, Nutrition, and Forestry | Agricultural economics and research |
| | Food stamp programs |
| | Human nutrition |
| | School nutrition programs |
| Appropriations | Appropriation of revenue |
| Armed Services | Issues relating to national (common) defense |
| Budget | Congress's annual budget plan |
| Environment and Public Works | Air pollution and environmental policy |
| | Solid waste disposal and recycling |
| Finance | Public moneys and customs |
| | Health programs under Social Security Act |
| | Health programs financed by a specific tax or trust fund |
| Health, Education, Labor, and Pensions | Aging |
| | Biomedical research and development |
| | Domestic activities of the Red Cross |
| | Individuals with disabilities |
| | Public health |
| | Student loans |
| | Wages and hours of labor |
| Homeland Security and Government Affairs | Census and collection of statistics |
| | Studying the efficiency of government departments |
| | Evaluating the effects of enacted laws |
| | National security |
| Indian Affairs | Indian Health Service |
| Veterans Affairs | Life insurance for members of the armed forces |
| | Veterans hospitals and medical care |

branch sets the national agenda as outlined in the presidential budget, and the legislative branch, with the help of the Congressional Budget Office (CBO), reevaluates the budget and divides and allocates the available monies among the programs seeking funding.

Policy advocates need to be very familiar with the federal budget process because it sets the structure

**TABLE 23-2** Standing Committees of the U.S. House of Representatives With Jurisdiction Over Health Policy Issue

| COMMITTEE | JURISDICTION |
| --- | --- |
| Agriculture | Human nutrition and home economics |
| | Women, Infants, & Children (WIC) program and Food Stamps |
| | Rural development |
| Appropriations | Appropriation of revenue |
| Armed Services | Common defense |
| | National security |
| | Benefits of members of the armed forces (including heath care) |
| | Scientific research and development in support of the Armed Services |
| Budget | Budget resolutions and budget process |
| Education and Workforce | Child labor |
| | Gallaudet University and Howard University and Hospital |
| | Food programs for schools |
| | Education and labor generally |
| | Worker's compensation |
| Energy and Commerce | Biomedical research and development |
| | Health and health facilities (except health care supported by payroll deductions) |
| | Public health and quarantine |
| Homeland Security | National security |
| | Science and technology preparedness |
| Veterans Affairs | Veterans hospitals, medical care, and treatment |
| Ways and Means | Customs |
| | Tax exempt foundations |
| | National Social Security |

and timeline for important policy work. Its appropriation process provides key access points for nurses to educate staff members and provide testimony. The federal government's fiscal year runs from October 1 through September 30. For example, the fiscal year 2006 runs from Oct 1, 2005 to September 30, 2006. The budget process officially begins each year in early February when, after months of analysis by the OMB, the president officially presents his budget to Congress.

The House and Senate budget committees work with the CBO to create budget resolutions for their respective chambers. According to congressional rules, these are supposed to be passed during March, but due to conflicts over budget priorities, consensus is not always easily reached. Once passed, a conference committee composed of both senators and representatives works to resolve the differences between the two budget resolutions and combine them into a single resolution that should pass both houses by April 15, but again, may be delayed. Once passed, the final budget resolution lacks the power of law but is important as a blueprint for subsequent budget legislation.

After passage of the resolution, the next steps are enacting budget reconciliation legislation and enacting appropriation bills. A reconciliation bill is a piece of legislation that reconciles the amount of money coming into the government (taxes) with the amount of money the government is spending. (See Chapter 24 for more information on authorization and appropriations.) Figure 23-1 depicts some of the data that are used in calculating the reconciliation each year and shows how tax revenues compare with government spending. An appropriations bill is a piece of legislation that prescribes how much money will go to each program named in the federal budget. Figure 23-2 depicts appropriations for DHHS, DOL, and Education from FY 1998-FY 2005.

Both reconciliation and appropriation, deliberations entail hearings and opportunities for nurses to present testimonies as the legislators try to determine how best to allocate the funds for the upcoming fiscal year. Many programs such as Social Security and Medicaid receive **nondiscretionary** funds as laid out by their authorizing legislation. These programs are **entitlements**, meaning Congress is required to fund all individuals and programs that are eligible under law. The only way entitlement funding can be decreased is by changing eligibility or diminishing services through revisions in law. Such highly contentious discussions may be part of reconciliation or budget deliberations in an effort to reduce federal spending. (For trends in entitlement spending for FY 1998-FY 2004, including what it comprises, see Figure 23-3.)

Other programs, however, such as the National Institutes of Health and AIDS funding, are **discretionary** in nature, meaning that their funding is

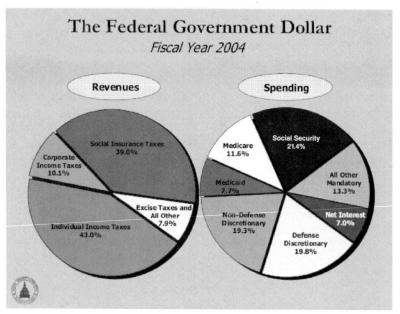

**Figure 23-1** Federal government revenues and spending for FY2004. *(Source: Budget of the U.S. Government Fiscal Year 2006.)*

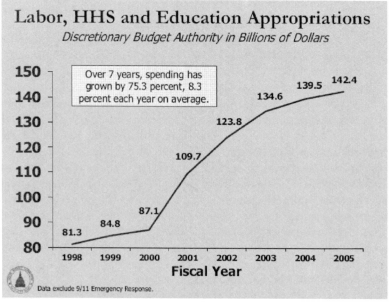

**Figure 23-2** Discretionary spending for FY1998 to FY2005. *(Source: Budget of the U.S. Government Fiscal Year 2006.)*

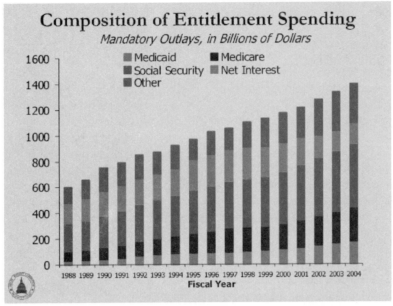

**Figure 23-3** Composition of entitlement spending for FY1998 to FY2005. *(Source: Budget of the U.S. Government Fiscal Year 2006.)* Covering the uninsured.

determined annually under the **appropriations** process. Representatives of the constituent organizations involved with these programs must, with the help of advocates, provide testimony and lobby to request annual funding from the government. (For useful budget terminology, see Box 23-1.)

**The Senate and House Committees on Appropriations.** The role of the appropriations committees is described in the U.S. Constitution, which states that before the federal government may spend any money, it must be reviewed by Congress and appropriated "by law." This power is sometimes referred to as the "power of the purse." Appropriations bills must be enacted by September 30 for the ensuing fiscal year, which begins on October 1. Failure to do so may result in a government shutdown. The appropriations access point is important because the Congress has money ready to spend and is weighing its options as to how best to spend it. Successful testimony at this point can result in money being dispersed to your program.

In sum, reconciliation and appropriations are important aspects of the budget process. Excellent information and a citizen's guide to the federal budget are available on line at the Websites of the Center on Budget and Policy Priorities and the

---

**BOX 23-1** Glossary for the Federal Budget Process

*Appropriations bill:* A piece of legislation that prescribes how much money will go to each program named in the federal budget.

*Discretionary spending:* Money for programs, the funding for which is debated annually during the appropriations process.

*Entitlement (mandatory) spending:* Money for programs which, by law, Congress must fund in full each year. Example: Medicare.

*Reconciliation bill:* A piece of legislation that balances the amount of money coming into the federal government (taxes) with the amount of money the government intends to spend in the coming year.

Government Printing Office listed in the Web Resources.

## STATE GOVERNMENTS

Each state government has its own constitution, which, similar to that of the federal constitution, defines the roles of each of the three branches of government (legislative, executive, and judicial) at the state level. Each state's constitution is unique and is based on the state's history, population, philosophy, and geography. State constitutions and individual state laws cannot, however, conflict with federal law or with the U.S. Constitution. Links to the Websites of each state along with full text of the constitutions of all 50 states can be found online through the Websites listed in Web Resources.

Although there is much variation in the structure and day-to-day functioning of different state governments, there are enough similarities for comparison. Only the basics of the state executive and legislative branches will be discussed here. For complete information on your home state, see your state government's Website.

## STATE GOVERNMENT—EXECUTIVE BRANCH

Similar to the president at the federal level is the governor at the state level. About half of the states also have a lieutenant governor, whose role is comparable to that of the vice president. The powers of these officials vary widely among the states, but they all have some common duties—the preparation of the state budget for presentation to the legislature and management of the approved budget. Also, like the president, the governors have the power to veto or approve state-level legislation along with the power to make appointments to influential positions such as the state board of health.

The governor's veto power, however, is slightly different from that of the president. Known as the "line item veto," it allows the governor to cross out or delete sections of a bill before signing it into law. This is helpful for combating "riders," legislators' favorite programs, which may be attached to bills. President Bill Clinton sought a line item veto on the federal level, but it was ultimately struck down by the Supreme Court and the president must still sign a bill in total or veto it.

## REGULATORY FUNCTION OF STATE GOVERNMENTS

Together, the 50 states employ about 5 million people in state agencies who work to translate the intentions of state legislatures, outlined in new laws, into sets of rules and regulations, which define how those intentions will become reality (Smith et al., 2005). Once a set of rules is approved, within 30 days, it has the force of law and becomes a part of the state's administrative code. Thus, laws and regulations work together to determine how public policy is implemented (Loquist, 2004).

The leaders of state agencies also work to influence policy. Many are elected officials, who attempt to keep campaign promises through the rules and regulations outlined in the agency (Smith et al., 2005). The regulatory role of the executive branch makes it a prime target for the nurse activist. Creating and maintaining relationships with both appointed and elected officials, helps to ensure that once your bill is enacted, its implementation matches the law's intent and your original vision.

**Regulation of Health Professionals.** One of the most visible roles of the state executive branch with respect to health care is the licensing and regulation of professionals, including nurses (see The Politics of Nursing Regulation and Licensure following Chapter 24). Each state sets both the educational and testing requirements for licensure and limits the scope of nursing practice through the state's nurse practice act. Even though some states have entered into compacts allowing nurses to practice in multiple states, the practice regulations continue to vary widely among states, particularly with regard to the scope of advanced nursing practice. Complete information on the regulations in your area, a list of states in the licensure compact, and links to all 50 state boards of nursing are available on the Website of the National Council of State Boards of Nursing (see Web Resources). Familiarity with your state licensing board, as well as with state agencies such as departments of public health or social services, can be very beneficial to nurses in their quest to influence policy. These agencies also serve as consultants on issues pertaining to health care to both executive and legislative branches of government. Working with staff of these agencies can help enhance your policy efforts.

## STATE LEGISLATIVE BRANCH

All 50 states have state legislatures with roles similar to that of the U.S. Congress. These groups create and pass new laws and serve as a check and balance to the executive branch by evaluating the governor's budget and appointments. Beyond this basic structure, some aspects of the state legislatures may differ. One state, Nebraska, has a legislature with a single house, whereas the other 49 states have bicameral (two-house) legislatures. While most state legislatures meet every year, six states have legislatures that meet only every other year (Box 23-2). Just as at the federal level, it is important to get to know not only the representatives from your home district but also those who support your issue, as well as members of committees with jurisdiction over your area of interest.

## LOCAL GOVERNMENT

There are many types of local governments in the United States including entities such as counties, cities, towns, villages, and school districts. Local governments often have elected executive leaders. They may be referred to as mayors, in a county, city, or town, or as superintendents in school districts. The legislative branch at the local level is often composed of an elected council or board, which works to create the laws governing the locality. These laws, of course, cannot conflict with state or national laws.

While the structure and function of local-level governments vary even more widely than the governments at the state level, they serve as vital links between the local citizens and the state and nation (Majewski & O'Brien, 2002). Billions of dollars in grant money passes from federal and state governments to local entities, which disperse funds to community health agencies. The latter often implement programs that are part of laws enacted by federal and state legislatures. In addition, in many states, local governments are also responsible for

---

**BOX 23-2** Meeting Schedules of State Legislatures

A. State Legislatures That Meet Throughout the Year
1. Illinois
2. Massachusetts
3. Michigan
4. New Jersey
5. New York
6. Ohio
7. Pennsylvania
8. Wisconsin

B. State Legislatures That Meet Annually
1. Alabama
2. Alaska
3. California
4. Colorado
5. Connecticut
6. Delaware
7. Florida
8. Georgia
9. Hawaii
10. Idaho
11. Indiana
12. Iowa
13. Kansas
14. Kentucky
15. Louisiana
16. Maine
17. Maryland
18. Minnesota
19. Mississippi
20. Missouri
21. Nebraska
22. New Hampshire
23. New Mexico
24. North Carolina
25. Oklahoma
26. Rhode Island
27. South Carolina
28. South Dakota
29. Tennessee
30. Utah
31. Vermont
32. Virginia
33. Washington
34. West Virginia
35. Wyoming

C. State Legislatures That Meet Every Other Year
1. Arkansas
2. Montana
3. Nevada
4. North Dakota
5. Oregon
6. Texas

From National Conference of State Legislature. (2005). Retrieved from *www.ncsl.org.*

many health-related services, including the county coroner's office, the medical examiner, local laboratories, public hospitals, and long-term care facilities (Majewski & O'Brien, 2002).

As local government responsibility for the health care of citizens has increased, it offers nurses increasingly accessible opportunities to influence policy. Getting to know, understand, and maintain a relationship with local officials is often much more feasible than it is with officials at the state or federal levels. In addition, addressing issues and testing proposals at the local level will allow evaluation and improvement before moving to the state or federal level.

The nurse's strategies for influence at the local level are the same as those at the state and national levels, with one possible exception. Because of the nature of localities, policy advocates and policy makers may also be neighbors, friends, or colleagues. Such informal relationships must be carefully balanced, but they may also aid the policy advocate in gaining access to influence change. Further information on local governments can be found online (see the state and local government Websites in Web Resources).

## TARGET THE APPROPRIATE LEVEL OF GOVERNMENT

The principle of divided powers is a cornerstone of our government in terms of both the levels (federal, state, and local) and the branches (executive, legislative, and judicial). The founding fathers saw this system of checks and balances as key to preventing the accumulation of power by any one group and thereby helping to maintain a democratic nation. Although this organizational structure may present challenges to nurses aiming to influence policy, it is important to understand which issues fall under the jurisdiction of each level of government and the tasks that are shared responsibilities among the levels.

When it comes to the health and health care of U.S. citizens, the preamble to Constitution addresses the government's responsibility by stating that one of the government's purposes is to "promote the general welfare." At the time of the writing in 1787, the term welfare referred to the health, happiness,

prosperity, and well-being of the people and should not be confused with the social programs it may be associated with today (Mount, 2005; White, 2002). Since that time, each level of government has addressed its responsibilities in different ways.

Today, the federal government is broadly responsible for many health policies regarding the organization, financing, and delivery of health care. More specifically, federal issues typically include programs enacted by Congress and the president, such as Medicare and Veterans Affairs, as well as the administration of programs that fall under federal jurisdiction including NIH, the CDC, the FDA, and the DHHS (White, 2002).

At the state level, governments protect the public and affect the delivery of health care through licensing of health care professionals and long-term health care facilities, and of insurance (Reinhard, 2002). Local governments oversee the provision of health care through administration and funding of safety-net programs and public hospitals and, more broadly, by addressing the public's general health by providing public education, waste management, fire and police protection, and public health initiatives (Majewski & O'Brien, 2002).

Because the process of promoting the general welfare at the national level has not always been easy, over time, the powers associated with the implementation of programs have shifted from the federal level to the state and local governments, a process called devolution. Each state and locality implements federal programs, such as those funded by block grants and those that are shared federal-state responsibilities (e.g., Medicaid), in very different ways. Despite the fact that this may or may not result in better outcomes for the program, it definitely creates challenges for the nurse activist trying to understand the policies that affect patient care. Remember that the system is murky, and any particular issue may require attention at all three levels of government. Federal laws often provide funding and overarching direction, states are often the lead funding agencies under block grants or matching federal-state programs, and local agencies may receive funding from state or federal authorities to administer programs. Each level of government also operates programs that are independent of the others.

Many health care initiatives fall to multiple levels of government for both funding and administration. For example, covering the uninsured falls under all three domains, depending on the proposal under debate. Medicaid, which provides insurance for the poorest Americans, is administered by federal and state authorities. Similarly, many education programs, although administered by local education agencies, entail some federal involvement. Laws such as the Elementary and Secondary Education Act and the No Child Left Behind Act are federal initiatives with grants to states, which in turn allocate funds to local agencies. The full text for all of these laws is available on the Internet at *http://thomas.loc.gov*.

Some public health issues, such as emergency preparedness, which is overseen by the Department of Homeland Security and executed by the Federal Emergency Management Agency (FEMA), also involve all three levels of government. Implementation of disaster response and security of mass transit has become primarily a local responsibility, resting with local public health, hospital, and crime enforcement authorities. The federal and state governments, however, retain a great deal of administrative control as well as responsibility for security of air traffic.

## PULLING IT ALL TOGETHER: COVERING THE UNINSURED

This example will demonstrate how an issue can span multiple levels (federal, state, and local) of government and the three branches of government (legislative, executive, and judicial). Addressing the issue of covering the uninsured is too broad for a single level and so has been addressed and must continue to be reformed at all three.

According to the Employee Benefit Research Institute 1998-2004, approximately 47 million Americans lack any type of health insurance for at least one year, and tens of millions of others go without health insurance for shorter periods of time (Figure 23-4). Additional information on the scope of the problem of lack of insurance in the United States can be found online at the Websites on covering the uninsured listed in the Web Resources.

Options for providing insurance coverage to the uninsured cover all three levels of government.

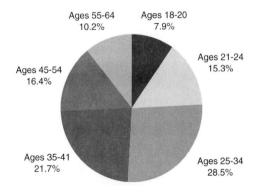

**Figure 23-4** Covering the uninsured. Uninsured nonelderly population by age (2003). (Source: *http://covertheuninsuredweek.org/factsheets/display.php?FactSheetID=102*. Reprinted with permission of the Employee Benefit Research Institute, Washington, DC.)

For example, Medicare, a federal program, can be expanded by lowering the eligibility age. Medicaid can be expanded by granting eligibility to those in families with incomes above current eligibility levels. Similarly, the State Children's Health Insurance Program (SCHIP) can be expanded by including children from families with incomes above current eligibility levels and by extending coverage to parents of SCHIP children, most of whom are uninsured. Medicaid and SCHIP expansions entail both state and federal levels of government. (See *Children's Health Insurance Coverage: Medicaid and the State Children's Health Insurance Program (SCHIP)* following Chapter 15.) Another possible solution is offering tax credits, which would allow the uninsured extra money to pay for insurance premiums. Tax credits can be administered by federal or state governments. Other options that have been suggested include insurance pools and employer mandates, both of which occur at the state level. Support for safety-net providers, school-based health centers, and community health clinics would be implemented at the local level.

## SUMMARY

Nurses must decide where to target their actions. One course is to select one of the options above and pursue legislators at the indicated levels of government, but this may require a multilevel approach. Such an approach, however, reflects the realities of the U.S. federalist structure. The nurse interested in improving coverage and care for the uninsured—or any other health policy issue—needs to know how the government works in order to know how to plan appropriate strategies.

## Key Points

- Nurses need to know how government works so that they can influence public officials to create policies that improve access to quality and affordable health care for all.
- The federalist system in the United States means that often more than one level of government is involved in any health issue, so it may be necessary to target multiple levels.
- The state and local level governments are often more accessible to nurses and may be the appropriate level to work with to influence health policy.
- The issue of covering the uninsured provides a good example of how nurses can work to influence policy. This issue involves all three levels of government, and deciding which level to target depends on the proposed solution.

## Web Resources

### STRUCTURE AND FUNCTION OF GOVERNMENT WEBSITES

**The Constitution of the United States**
*www.house.gov/Constitution/Constitution.html*
**The Federal Register**
*www.gpoaccess.gov/fr/index.html*
**Notes on the U.S. Constitution**
*www.house.gov/Constitution/Constitution.html*
**Stanford Encyclopedia of Philosophy**
*http://plato.stanford.edu/entries/federalism/*
**American Bar Association**
*www.abanet.org/publiced/preview/summary/*
  *2003-2004/f.html* (federalism and
  telecommunications)
*http://althouse.blogspot.com/2005/02/federalism-*
  *and-assisted-suicide-case.html* (federalism and
  assisted suicide in Oregon)

**U.S. Government's Official Web Portal**
*www.firstgov.gov*

### THE FEDERAL GOVERNMENT
**Complete description of all agencies of the federal government, along with links to individual Websites**
*www.loc.gov/rr/news/fedgov.html*

### U.S. EXECUTIVE BRANCH WEBSITES
**Official U.S. Executive Branch Websites (Library of Congress)**
*www.loc.gov/rr/news/fedgov.html*
**Executive Office of the President (EOP)**
*www.firstgov.gov/Agencies/Federal/Executive/*
  *EOP.shtml*
  **Office of Homeland Security**
  *www.whitehouse.gov/homeland/*
  **Office of Management and Budget (OMB)**
  *www.whitehouse.gov/omb/*
  **Office of National Drug Control Policy**
  *www.whitehousedrugpolicy.gov/*
  **Office of the United States Trade Representative**
  *www.ustr.gov/*
  **National Security Council**
  *www.whitehouse.gov/nsc/*

### THE PRESIDENT'S CABINET WEBSITES

**Department of Agriculture**
*www.usda.gov/wps/portal/usdahome*
**Department of Commerce**
*www.commerce.gov/*
**Census Bureau**
*www.census.gov/*
**Department of Defense**
*www.defenselink.mil/*
  **TRICARE**
  *www.tricareonline.com/*
**Department of Education**
*www.ed.gov/index.jhtml*
**Department of Energy**
*www.energy.gov/engine/content.do*
**Department of Health and Human Services**
*www.dhhs.gov*
  **Regional Offices of DHHS**
  *www.acf.dhhs.gov/programs/fysb/acfweb.htm*

*Continued*

*Web Resources — cont'd*

**Department of Homeland Security**
*www.dhs.gov/dhspublic*
**Federal Emergency Management Agency**
*www.fema.gov*
**Department of Housing and Urban
Development**
*www.hud.gov*
**Department of the Interior**
*www.doi.gov*
**Department of Justice**
*www.usdoj.gov*
**Department of Labor**
*www.dol.gov*
　　**OSHA**
　　*www.osha.gov/oshinfo/mission.html*
**Department of State**
*www.state.gov*
**Department of Transportation**
*www.dot.gov*
**Department of Treasury**
*www.ustreas.gov*
**Department of Veterans Affairs**
*www.va.gov*

U.S. DEPARTMENT OF HEALTH AND
HUMAN SERVICES WEBSITES

**Agency for Healthcare Research and Quality**
*www.ahrq.gov*
**Centers for Disease Control and Prevention**
*www.cdc.gov*
**Centers for Medicare and Medicaid Services**
*www.cms.hhs.gov/default.asp?*
**Food and Drug Administration**
*www.fda.gov*
**Head Start**
*www.nhsa.org*
**National Institute for Nursing Research**
*http://ninr.nih.gov/ninr*
**National Institutes of Health**
*www.nih.gov*

FEDERAL LEGISLATIVE BRANCH WEBSITES

**Congressional Budget Office**
*www.cbo.gov*

**U.S. House of Representatives**
*www.house.gov*
**U.S. Senate**
*www.senate.gov*
**Thomas: Legislative Information on the
Internet**
*http://thomas.loc.gov*

FEDERAL BUDGET PROCESS
WEBSITES

**Center on Budget and Policy Priorities**
*www.cbpp.org/pubs/fedbud.htm*
**Government Printing Office**
*www.gpoaccess.gov/usbudget*
**U.S. House Committee on the Budget,
Budget Tutorial**
*www.house.gov/budget/budgettutorial.htm*

STATE AND LOCAL GOVERNMENT
WEBSITES

**All 50 States**
*www.globalcomputing.com/states.html*
**Council of State Governments**
*www.csg.org/CSG/default.htm*
**National Council of State Boards
of Nursing**
*www.ncsbn.org/regulation/boardsofnursing_
boards_of_nursing_board.asp*
**U.S. Conference of Mayors**
*www.usmayors.org/uscm/home.asp*
**U.S. State Constitutions and Websites**
*www.constitution.org/cons/usstcons.htm*
**Links to the Websites of many local
governments**
*www.loc.gov/rr/news/stategov/
stategov.html*

COVERING THE UNINSURED WEBSITES

**Cover the Uninsured**
*http://covertheuninsuredweek.org*
**Families USA**
*www.familiesusa.org/site/PageServer?pagename=
homepage*
**Institute of Medicine: Reports on Covering
the Uninsured**
*www.iom.edu/project.asp?id=4660*

## REFERENCES

Follesdal, A., & Zalta, E. N. (2003). "Federalism" in the Stanford Encyclopedia of Philosophy. Winter 2003 Edition. Retrieved July 4, 2005, from *http://plato.stanford.edu/archives/win2003/entries/federalism/*.

Hanson, R. L. (2004). Intergovernmental relations. In V. Gray & R. L. Hanson (Eds.), *Politics in the American states: A comparative analysis* (pp. 31-60). Washington DC: CQ Press.

Loquist, R. S. (2004). Government regulation: Parallel and powerful. In J. A. Milstead (Ed.), *Health policy and politics: A nurse's guide* (pp. 89-127). Sudbury, ON: Jones and Bartlett.

Majewski, J. V., & O'Brien, M. C. (2002). Local government. In D. J. Mason, J. K. Leavitt, & M. W. Chaffee (Eds.), *Policy and politics in nursing and health care* (4th ed., pp. 479-490). St. Louis: Saunders.

Mount, S. (2005, March 18). The U.S. Constitution online. Retrieved July 4, 2005, from *www.usconstitution.net/glossary.html*.

Reinhard, S. C. (2002). State government: 50 paths to policy. In D. J. Mason, J. K. Leavitt, & M. W. Chaffee (Eds.), *Policy and politics in nursing and health care* (4th ed., pp. 491-497). St. Louis: Saunders.

Smith, K. B., Greenblatt, A., Buntin, J., & Clark, C. S. (2005). *Governing states and localities*. Washington, DC: CQ Press.

U.S. Department of Veterans Affairs. (2005). Facts about the Department of Veterans Affairs. Retrieved July 6, 2005, from *www1.va.gov/opa/fact/vafacts.html*.

Walker, D. B. (2000). The rebirth of federalism: Slouching toward Washington. New York: Chatham House.

White, K. M. (2002). The federal government. In D. J. Mason, J. K. Leavitt, & M. W. Chaffee (Eds.), *Policy and politics in nursing and health care* (4th ed., pp. 515-542). St. Louis, MO: Saunders.

# *Taking Action*
### Steven J. Wyrsch, Mary W. Chaffee, & Betty Dickson

## *Political Appointments*

*"Ask not what your country can do for you. Ask what you can do for your country."*

JOHN F. KENNEDY

The wheels of government in the United States are powered by three groups of employees: those who are elected to office, those who are career employees, and those who are appointed to serve (usually by a member of the elected contingent). All three groups have numerous opportunities to influence public policy. Despite occasional public meltdowns of less-than-optimally qualified political appointees like Michael Brown, former director of the Federal Emergency Management Agency, many political appointees bring extensive expertise and leadership skill, as well as a keen desire to serve the public, to their appointed positions.

When Lil Peters, ARNP, a psychiatric mental health nurse, got a call from the Kansas State Nurses

Association inviting her to consider an appointment to the state's Hospital Closure Commission; she accepted the challenge because she thought her patients should have a voice through her. Lil Peters was convinced that registered nurses should be involved in developing health policy and accepted the appointment. She said, "I wanted to influence the decisions that were made and to protect patients and their families. Nurses are often hesitant to get involved but, having served, I realize we need to participate in the decision-making process." Shaping policy through a political appointment constitutes a journey that runs through America's smallest towns, increases in scope at the state level, and reaches its pinnacle in federal appointments.

## WHY SEEK AN APPOINTMENT?

Although the political firestorm associated with such nominations as John Ashcroft in 2001 or John Bolton in 2005 is not the norm in the screening process, situations such as these beg the question "Why should nurses, or anyone, seek political appointments and expose themselves to such public inquiry?" Nathan (2003) identified these reasons why individuals seek political appointments:

1. Public service can produce a gratifying sense of accomplishment.
2. Public service can lead to recognition and prestige.
3. Successful leadership in public service can enhance the chances of landing a well-paid job after exiting government service.

Whatever the impetus for seeking a political appointment, there is a significant supply of appointees and a large demand. Nathan (2003) estimates 400,000 individuals serve in appointed positions in the federal, state, and local governments. In addition to recognizing their extensive numbers, Nathan tips his hat to their influence:

These (appointed) officials...do the heavy lifting of policy-making and management inside America's governments and play a significant role as change agents in the nation's political system. Yet books about American government tend to ignore them and focus instead on elected office holders.

It's important for nurses to recognize the opportunity for influencing health and public policy as a political appointee.

## WHAT MOTIVATES APPOINTEES?

Another consideration for nurses contemplating political appointment is their motivation. What motivates someone to seek a political appointment? Money, power, or personal gain might be a logical answer. However, Senator Joseph Lieberman (2000) identified a critical reason that individuals seek public service: *to make a difference.*

A political appointment places the appointee in the public spotlight. In his book *In Praise of Public Life*, Senator Joseph I. Lieberman (D-CT) provides a sound perspective about entering public life for anyone wishing to pursue a political career. He states, "I assume that everything I do in my life— *everything*—could possibly become public and therefore I should not do anything privately that I could not justify publicly" (Lieberman, 2000, p. 51).

In today's politically charged environment, it is essential that anyone seeking a politically appointed position examine his or her past closely, applying the "front page rule" to every experience that could draw public attention. The "front page rule" is a critical thinking tool. Ask yourself the question "How would this look on the front page of the *Washington Post* or *New York Times*?" Only this level of honest personal reflection will prevent embarrassing situations.

## NOMINEE SCRUTINY

The review and examination of a candidate's past is called the "vetting" process. Political vetting involves the review of financial records, personal records and relationships, tax records, business transactions and ventures, family history, and other personal credentials. Vetting can also involve the process of preparing a candidate for the nomination hearing process. Scrutiny reveals that recent federal nominations are replete with examples of defeats, withdrawals, and controversies caused by the incomplete review and examination of nominees' past experiences. Consider the circumstances surrounding the 2001 confirmation hearings for the nominee for Secretary of Labor, Linda Chavez. Chavez was forced to withdraw her nomination following the revelation that she had paid an illegal immigrant to clean her house. Other national figures such as John Bolton as the U.S. Ambassador to the United Nations and John Ashcroft to the post of Attorney General drew much more attention for political and social reasons. At the state level, scrutiny will be much less intense but still will include a thorough review of a candidate's personal and public life.

### Political Party Affiliation

Political party affiliation is essential in securing support for a political appointment. Most appointments are made as rewards for loyal support. The support could be as simple as volunteering in a local or state party office, organizing a fund-raising event for your party, or writing letters. Virginia Trotter Betts identified her political affiliation as key to her appointment as a senior-level political appointee serving the Surgeon General of the

United States. She cited a long-standing relationship with the Clinton-Gore administration after the American Nurses Association (ANA) became the first health care group to endorse the candidates in 1992. She also noted the work done on health care reform through a coalition of nursing organizations as being a major factor in her appointment. Betts was a Robert Woods Johnson fellow in the office of then-Senator Al Gore. When he ran for the position of Vice President, she worked on his campaign.

So you've decided that you are interested in a political appointment. How do you get started? Determine where your interests and experience lie. Is there something you wish to change or a service you desire in your community? Is the local school board spending a disproportionate amount of money on administrators' salaries instead of teachers' salaries? Is there no school nurse available to your child? Are nurse practitioners allowed to give physical exams to student athletes? Could your presence on the school board effect change? Is your ultimate goal to seek political office? Will serving in a political or public role enhance future advancement in your career?

Many of these questions may seem daunting and prevent one from "taking the first step" toward involvement. It can be, however, as simple as a knock on the door. Consider the experiences of Ellen Fielek Payeur, an LPN and immunizations specialist in Maine, whose story illustrates the close relationship between political activity and successfully gaining political appointments. Payeur's political experiences as a volunteer began when a Maine state senator visited her new home in Eliot, Maine. Payeur was appointed to a town committee and then was nominated for an appointment as a State Delegate to the Republican National Convention, where Gerald Ford won the nomination. While there, she met Michael Reagan, son of then-Governor Ronald Reagan. She dedicated numerous hours to fundraising and rallying local communities to support the Republican Party, culminating with her appointment as President of York County Republican Women, a grassroots organization of the state Republican Party. Although Jimmy Carter won the presidency that year, Mrs. Payeur remained a stalwart volunteer for her party. In the 1980s, she was a key player in several national campaigns, including those of Ronald Reagan, George Bush Sr., and Jack Kemp. She also ran several successful campaigns in Maine and New Hampshire for gubernatorial candidates. Her experiences illustrate the relative ease with which a person can "take the first step" toward volunteering for a political party. When asked if she would do it all over, Mrs. Payeur emphatically says, "yes." From her perspective, "If you don't get involved in what's going on in your country, then you can't sit home and complain."

## IDENTIFY OPPORTUNITIES

How does a nurse determine where the opportunities are? The types of political appointments run the gamut. For instance, a position on the state board of health affords an opportunity to develop policy, whereas an appointment to an election commission is a mechanism for carrying out state law (Box 23-3).

Most state nurses associations, specialty organizations, and other professional organizations outside of nursing offer appointment information. Organizations such as the ANA or the American Organization of Nurse Executives offer a starting place to seek information. Both organizations have recognized the opportunity to promote the collective voice of the nurses through key political appointments and offer continual updates on issues and legislative priorities.

Other sources include nonpartisan organizations such as the League of Women Voters. There may be coalitions, such as National Women's Political Caucus or Women in Government, to appoint specific persons to positions. Political parties may be responsible for some appointments.

Nurses can contribute at many levels, and the appointment doesn't necessarily have to be in health care (consider the experiences of Ms. Payeur outlined above). Beginning at the community level, nurses could serve on county health boards, task forces on redevelopment, or even a local recreation committee to address policies to prevent children from getting hurt on the playing field. Community and county appointments could

## BOX 23-3 Finding Opportunities to Serve in an Appointed Status

Although health and health care services appointments may be attractive to nurses, there are many types of appointments, not directly related to health, where nursing expertise can benefit constituents. These include the following:

*Commerce and economic development.* Tourism and industrial development appointments could benefit from nursing expertise. A nurse's knowledge of the health care system could provide industries considering relocation with valuable information about what they can expect for their employees' health care. In many states, health care is one of the top three industries.

*Conservation.* Environmental issues affect the health care of every community. For example, a nurse could provide expertise regarding hazardous waste, the value of clean water systems, or preserving green space.

*Corrections.* Nurses' expert health care knowledge could play a valuable role in policy decisions regarding the health care and education of incarcerated persons. Nurse practitioners provide much of the health care in many of today's correctional facilities, public and private.

*Education.* Nurses could offer valuable insight on policy decisions regarding school-based health care services and health curricula. A nurse's knowledge

of budgeting and cost-effective management could assist in the budget process.

*Health and human services.* A wide variety of appointments exist at the local, state, and federal levels.

*Higher education.* Policy decisions are made by state agencies and boards that have authority over colleges and universities.

*Licensure and regulatory boards.* State boards of health determine policy regarding the health of the public, including drinking water, restaurant inspections, and health care provider licensure. State boards of nursing regulate the practice of nursing and offer the opportunity to nurses to serve on their governing boards. Some state boards of medicine make decisions regarding the practice of nurse practitioners and may have seats available for a nurse appointee.

*Public safety.* Nurses can bring important perspectives to agencies and boards involved in public safety related to domestic violence, gun laws, and motor vehicle safety.

*Transportation.* Nurses have seen firsthand the effect of motor vehicle accidents and can be valuable partners in improving safety through political appointments on transportation and highway safety organizations.

---

include the zoning commission, planning commission, hospital boards, boards of education, or councils on aging or economic development.

## APPOINTEE COMPENSATION

Many political appointments offer little or no financial compensation. Federal appointments follow published compensation schedules. Potential appointees should request information in advance of an appointment about compensation—both direct compensation and reimbursement for expenses incurred before accepting an appointment. Burtless (2002) examined the adequacy and scope of pay for federal presidential appointees in a report titled "How Much Is Enough? Setting Pay for Presidential Appointees." Pay alone generally does not motivate appointees; some high-level appointees may actually receive less compensation than they could receive in the private sector.

## INFORMATION SOURCES ON POLITICAL APPOINTMENTS

### State Government Resources

Contact the offices of individual secretaries of state or check their Websites for appointment opportunities at the state level. For example, search online for "California Secretary of State." Further, with the ongoing development and population of Internet employment sites and professional organizations, postings are made available for appointment opportunities on a regular basis.

### Federal Government Resources

The federal government provides many public resources. A first stop should be the home page of the U.S. Senate Committee on Homeland Security and Government Affairs Committee at *http://hsgac.senate.gov.* Click the "Related Links" tab and find the section on Congress. There are helpful links to information about the federal appointment process, including a link to the official "Plum Book." Every four years, just after the presidential election, Congress publishes *United States Government Policy and Supporting Positions*, more commonly known as the Plum Book. (The Plum Book is so called because of the color of the book.) The Senate Committee on Homeland Security and Governmental Affairs and the House Committee on Government Reform alternate the task of review, validation, and publication of this massive document. At the end of the 108th Congress in November 2004, the Plum Book catalogued over 7000 federal civil service positions in the legislative and executive branches of the U.S. government that are potentially available for noncompetitive appointment. The electronic version of the Plum Book is actually located at the Government Printing Office's Website at *www.gpo.gov/plumbook/2004/index.html*. However, because the congressional committees oversee the publication of the document, the supporting information is located at the committee sites *(http://hsgac.senate.gov)*.

### Other Valuable Resources

There are many political sites and grassroots lobbying sites that can help provide information and assistance in seeking a nomination. Some of the most useful are the following:

- *The National Women's Political Caucus* (NWPC) *(www.nwpc.org)*. The NWPC is a grassroots membership organization that assists in the identification, recruiting, training, and support of women for elected and appointed office at all levels of the government. The NWPC is also the chair of the Coalition for Women's Appointment, a 60-member organization that assists women who seek presidential and gubernatorial appointments.
- *The National Council of Women's Organizations* (NCWO) *(www.womensorganizations.org)*. The NCWO is an organizing council of over 100 women's organizations representing more than 6 million members. Their goal is to advocate change on many issues of importance to women, including equal employment opportunity, economic equity, media equality, education, job training, women's health, and reproductive

health, as well as the specific concerns of mid-life and older women, girls and young women, women of color, business and professional women, homemakers, and retired women.

- *Brookings Institute*. The Brookings Institute provides information for those interested in pursuing a presidential nomination. *A Survivor's Guide for Presidential Nominees*, published as a component of the Presidential Appointee Initiative, provides a comprehensive summary and guide for anyone who has been asked to serve in an appointed position (available online at *www.appointee.brookings.org/survivorsguide.htm*).

### MAKING A DECISION

Seeking a political appointment, at any level, is not a decision to be taken lightly. Consider some of the following questions to gain perspective on whether this path is right for you. Some questions will be more important if you are considering a full-time federal assignment rather than a part-time community role (Box 23-4).

### PLAN YOUR STRATEGY

#### Getting Nominated

When you've identified the appointment you are interested in, the next step is getting nominated. Determine the process used for nomination and identify who will make the appointment. Having the support of more than one organization strengthens your chance for nomination.

#### Make It Easy for People to Help You

Dr. Mary Wakefield, former chief of staff to a U.S. Senator and an appointee to several federal health care commissions, states, "Expertise alone might get you a position, but frequently it won't." She emphasizes the need to have the support of nursing organizations and influential individuals that can advocate for you. Wakefield says that to successfully obtain an appointment, you must have a two-pronged approach: You need to have the expertise required by the position and a network of relationships built over time with policymakers. Wakefield highlights the importance of making it easy for people to help you. She recommends that nurses not just ask someone to write a letter of support,

---

**BOX 23-4** Considering a Political Appointment?

If you're considering seeking or accepting a political appointment, ask yourself these questions:

- Can you take time away from your job or your family to meet the demands of the position?
- How often will meetings be held? What will your time obligation be? Is this a full-time position or a group that meets occasionally?
- Will your employer support you? Will you have family support?
- Will your employer provide the time for you to serve, or will you be required to take vacation time?
- Why do you want to serve in this position? Can you articulate why you are qualified?
- What are the strengths and weaknesses you would bring to the position?
- What is your connection to your community? Do you know your neighbors? Have you served in volunteer organizations? Having a solid base of support from your neighbors, your friends, and your fellow volunteers in local organizations will enhance your chances of success.
- Where do you fit in the political spectrum? Are you registered to vote as a Democrat, Republican, or Independent? Party affiliation provides important linkages to support from individuals and groups.

- How will your education, background, and experience serve you in the desired appointment? Candidates should be able to identify aspects of each that will qualify them for the position.
- How are your health and your family's financial situation? Careful analysis should be given to each.
- Who makes the appointment? Is it the governor, the lieutenant governor, Speaker of the House of Representatives?
- Are there educational or geographic requirements? In Mississippi, the Nurse Practice Act requires a baccalaureate degree as the basic qualification for one board of nursing position and an associate degree as the basic qualification for another. One position is designated for an advanced practice nurse, and another for a nurse educator. Some appointments require certain credentials (e.g., being a physician or a nurse).
- Which stakeholders care about who gets this position? Do you have influence with them? Are there other nominees under consideration?
- Is there is a match between your qualifications and the requirements of the position? Carefully review local, state, or federal laws applicable to the appointment.
- Do you have a chance of getting the position? What connections do you have with individuals and organizations that will make the decision?

---

but that the potential nominee write the letter and provide it to the person providing the recommendation or that person's staff. If you desire, a phone call can be made on your behalf. Provide the person making the call with a brief memo about your qualifications and why you would make a great candidate.

### The Power of Networks

Patricia Montoya, another federal political appointee, echoes many of Wakefield's comments. Montoya served as a political appointee in the U.S. Department of Health and Human Services from 1998 to 2000. Following Senate confirmation, she was appointed as commissioner to the Administration on Children, Youth and Families by President Clinton. Montoya reports that she was appointed to her position because she had both the expertise and a well-developed political network. Several influential individuals who were familiar with her qualifications

advanced her name as a nominee. Montoya says that she has always mixed practice and politics in her career, and she credits her activities in the ANA for advancing her political education (Thompson, 2000).

### CONFIRMATION OR INTERVIEW

Depending on the position you aspire to, you may need to participate in confirmation hearings or interviews. It is vital to be familiar with the position and the organizational hierarchy in which it falls, as well as current issues facing the agency.

When preparing for either a hearing or interview, consider the following questions:

- What do I need to bring?
- Who will be conducting the hearing or interview?
- What questions will I be asked?
- Will I have the opportunity to ask questions?
- Should I have representation or sponsorship at the confirmation hearing?

## AFTER THE APPOINTMENT

### Relationships with Your Supporters

Once you've passed the background checks, survived interviews, and have been appointed to a challenging position, there is nothing more important than thanking all those who supported your appointment. Send letters of appreciation to recognize the efforts of others in helping you attain your appointment.

Once you are appointed, consider whom it is your duty to serve. If yours is a public appointment, your allegiance must be to your constituents. If it is to a health care organization's board of directors, your responsibility is to the patients and community. It is important that you retain your autonomy if the appointment is of a regulatory nature. If an association or other group was instrumental in your nomination and subsequent appointment, maintain open communication to keep them informed and to listen to their concerns. If your assignment is to represent a specific group on a task force where input from the organization was requested as a part of the appointment, close communication is necessary to convey the viewpoints of those you represent.

## EXPERIENCES OF NURSE APPOINTEES

### Federal Appointee: Patricia Ford-Roegner, U.S. Department of Health and Human Services Regional Director

Patricia Ford-Roegner was appointed as regional director in the U.S. Department of Health and Human Services (DHHS) by President Clinton in 1994. Because the position was a senior executive, noncareer appointment, Ford-Roegner had launched an intense lobbying effort to obtain the nomination. Her activities in the Democratic Party, her volunteer efforts on the Health Professionals Review Group, and her outstanding reputation as a clinician and entrepreneur allowed her to develop a strong network of supporters who assisted her in securing the nomination. She served in the post until 1999.

Upon her appointment, she faced immediate challenges. Although the budget for the region comprised nearly 22% of the total DHHS budget and covered eight states and nearly 50 million people, the region had not taken any significant steps to improve or coordinate health care. Also, because

her appointment occurred with the transition from a Republican to a Democratic White House, she was afforded virtually no turnover or orientation.

At first, it appeared to be a job of enormous proportion and insurmountable complexity. However, Ford-Roegner considered her appointment an excellent opportunity to develop, implement, and sustain outreach and social programs. By creating public and private partnerships throughout the region, she was able to organize collaborative efforts leading to the development of prevention and treatment programs for asthma, teen pregnancy, women's health, and children's health. Her efforts led to the first regional public dialogue on women's health and senior caregiver issues in the nation. During her tenure, the southeast region became the first in the country to implement a Medicare Beneficiaries Advisory Committee and a multiagency coalition to prevent Medicare fraud (P. A. Ford-Roegner, personal communication, March 9, 2001). Ms. Ford-Roegner had a significant impact on the health care system in the southeast United States—nearly all of the programs she initiated remain in place today.

### State Appointee: Barbara Nichols, Wisconsin Secretary of Regulation and Licensing

Barbara Nichols served as the President of the ANA from 1978 to 1982. Because of her visibility in ANA and her work as a loyal supporter of the Democratic Party, her name appeared on several lists of potential candidates for political appointments in the state of Wisconsin. When the call came from Wisconsin's governor asking if she was interested in a state political appointment, Ms. Nichols was skeptical but intrigued. She believes she was a "politically attractive" candidate for the nomination due to her reputation within the nursing community, her loyal support to the political party of the governor, and her work with minority groups. Although she was not in the governor's "inner circle" of possible political appointees, she would embody several "firsts" if nominated: the first woman, the first African American, the first health care professional, and the first nurse. This increased her attractiveness from a political perspective. By selecting Nichols, the governor could demonstrate that he was expanding his cabinet with cultural, gender, and professional diversity as operative goals.

To prepare for a successful interview with the governor, Nichols knew she must be fully primed to discuss nursing and health issues with policy implications in the state. She prepared by talking with numerous state officials, such as the district attorney, political party representatives, members of the governor's staff, and other "political insiders." She met with the American Medical Association to gain their support. The position she was to be nominated for carried the state's authority for licensing and regulation of physicians, nurses, 17 professional boards, and 57 other professions. She went into the interview confident that she could address almost any of the issues that could affect health care regulation and licensing in Wisconsin. Interestingly, there were no substantial clinical, nursing, or even health care issues brought up during the interview with the governor. About 10 days after the interview, Nichols was offered the appointment.

Because the Secretary of Regulation and Licensing required state senate confirmation, Ms. Nichols needed additional preparation for the nomination hearings. As the date approached, she employed the same strategy she used to prepare for the interview with the governor. She called local and state officials, contacted health care organizations to keep abreast of current issues, researched the questions posed to former nominees for the post, and worked with the political party to be informed of political trends. As the final measure, the Wisconsin Nurses Association sponsored a reception in her honor. She was confirmed.

Once appointed, Nichols seized the opportunity to create a level of trust within the state government that surprised even the governor. She built a reputation for honesty and sincerity in dealing with the intricacies of licensing, regulation, and policy development. Because of her excellent interpersonal skills and ability to articulate the issues, Nichols was able to create new standards for the health disciplines licensed in the state, implement regulatory standards for child boxing, and permanently put an end to the controversial "Toughman" competition in the state. She made significant strides to increase communication throughout the state on matters of licensing, regulation, and reform by publishing newsletters, distributing information to the state

legislature, and reaching out to build a strong trust throughout the executive and legislative branches of the Wisconsin government (B. L. Nichols, personal communication, March 16, 2001).

### Commission Appointee: Kaye Bender, Institute of Medicine Commission Member

Another nurse who was ready to serve was Kaye Bender, RN, PhD, FAAN, deputy state health officer, Mississippi State Department of Health. When the Committee Assuring the Health of the Public in the 21st Century was convened by the Institute of Medicine (IOM), the American nursing community saw there was no nurse appointed to the committee. Nursing represents the single largest workforce in public health. ANA sent Dr. Rita Gallagher to the first IOM committee meeting to formally inquire as to why a nurse had not been selected to the committee. The IOM was apologetic about the oversight and gave the ANA a few days to submit nominees' names and credentials. Because Bender had received the Pearl McIver Public Health Nurse award from the ANA the previous summer, her name was placed into consideration. The nursing community mobilized to support Bender's appointment, and she was selected to serve.

Bender credits her active participation in public health nursing organizations and work with the ANA and her state nurses association. Her selection for the McIver award and 24 years experience in public health helped considerably in her attaining this appointment. Bender says the quick mobilization by the nursing community was instrumental to this appointment.

### SUMMARY

When Catherine Dodd, a nurse from California, was interviewed by former Secretary of the DHHS Donna Shalala for an appointment as a regional director, Shalala commented that she had appointed three nurses to federal positions. Shalala's respect for nurses was clear in her appraisal, according to Dodd. Shalala stated, "Nurses understand health care issues, they can talk to anybody and they come prepared to work—they can hit the ground running."

Entering public life is a noble endeavor that every nurse who wishes "to make a difference" should seriously consider. Senator Lieberman provides the best insight into this motivation: "American democracy and self-government are endangered today by the American people's retreat from their government and politics. Our country's future requires that they reengage—at least to vote, at best to serve" (Lieberman, 2000, p. 161).

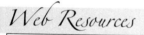

## Lessons Learned

- Government employees consist of three groups: elected officials, career employees, and political appointees.
- Accepting a political appointment can offer a significant opportunity to influence health and public policy.
- Nurses who have the correct expertise and who have developed a network of contacts through political activity should consider seeking a political appointment as a means to influence policy.

## Web Resources

**Handbook for Appointed Officials in America's Governments**
*www.rockinst.org/publications/general_institute/
gov_handbook/Handbook.pdf*
**White House Appointments**
*www.whitehouse.gov/appointments*

### REFERENCES

Burtless, G. (2002). How much is enough? Setting pay for presidential appointees. Retrieved December 4, 2005, from *www.appointee.brookings.org/events/pay.pdf*.

Lieberman, J. I. (2000). *In praise of public life*. New York: Simon & Schuster.

Nathan, R. P. (2003). Handbook for appointed officials in America's governments. Retrieved December 4, 2005, from *www.rockinst.org/publications/general_institute/gov_handbook/Handbook.pdf*.

Thompson, L. (2000). In the health policy spotlight: An interview with Commissioner Patricia Montoya. *Policy, Politics & Nursing Practice 1*(3), 189-193.

### RESOURCES

Chaffee, M. W. (2000). In the health policy spotlight: An interview with Dr. Mary Wakefield. *Policy, Politics & Nursing Practice, 1*(1), 53-59.

Coalition for Women's Appointments. (2001). *A project convened by the National Women's Political Caucus*. Washington, DC: Author.

National Women's Political Caucus (NWPC). (1997). *A guide to running a winning campaign*. Washington, DC: NWPC.

*A survivor's guide to presidential appointees*. (2000, November). Washington, DC: Brookings Institution. Available online at *www.appointee.brookings.org/survivorsguide.htm*.

United States government policy and supporting positions. (2004, November 8). Washington, DC: Committee on Governmental Affairs, United States Senate. Available online at *www.senate. gov/gov_affairs/issues.htm*.

## *Making the Most of Political Appointments: My Life as a Federal and State Official*

> *"All rising to great place is by a winding stair."*
> SIR FRANCIS BACON

Little did I know, when I accepted a position to work with the American Nurses Association Political Department in the fall of 1987, that I was beginning a journey that would change my life. My nursing background and political involvement enabled me to influence health policy at the highest levels of government at both the federal and state levels. From 1994 to 2000, I held two leadership positions in the U.S. Department of Health and Human Services under President Clinton's administration. I then served my home state of New Mexico in 2003-2004 as the Secretary of Health under Governor Bill Richardson. This is my story.

### GETTING STARTED AT THE LOCAL LEVEL

When I worked as a school nurse in the late 1970s and early 1980s, I realized that it was important to be involved politically to advocate for the many health needs of the students and their families whom I served. My ability to meet their needs and provide health services was dependent upon decisions made by the school board, city council, county commission, state legislature, and Congress. As an example, I was working with students who needed mental health counseling, and I often had no place to refer them, because they were uninsured or because of inadequate community resources. On many occasions, I remember pleading before the school board to retain a dwindling supply of school nurses. In so many situations, the nurses were the only access to health care that students had.

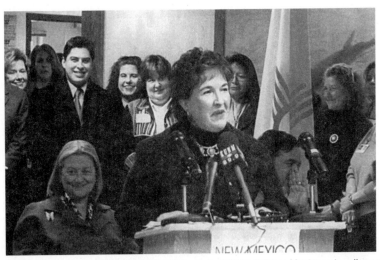

Signing the New Mexico Immunization Registry Bill in April of 2004. Patricia Montoya at podium; seated to her left, First Lady Barbara Richardson; seated to her right, Governor Bill Richardson; located behind Montoya, Department of Health staff.

During this time, I started actively working on political campaigns of people whose positions I supported. One was a friend, who was running for the state legislature. He was a teacher at the school where I was the school nurse. When I committed to working on his campaign, I shared with him why I was supporting him and let him know that I wanted him to work on nursing and health care issues if he was elected. He didn't win his first campaign but did win on the second try. He became the sponsor of the Nurse Practice Act that gave New Mexico the broadest scope of practice for nurse practitioners in the mid 1980s. I worked with the New Mexico Nurses Association to provide the technical information and assistance he needed in drafting the bill, and I lobbied for passage through the legislature. Such a successful experience early in my career hooked me into politics for life.

## THE ROAD TO WASHINGTON

In 1987, I was working at a managed care organization in Albuquerque, doing provider relations and utilization review. I continued to be involved with the New Mexico Nurses Association, working actively with their political action committee as well as volunteering with the state Democratic Party. The New Mexico Nurses Association had submitted my name to serve on the Board of the American Nurses Association Political Action Committee (ANA-PAC). When the Political Education/PAC director, Pat Ford Roegner, reviewed my resume, she called to ask me about coming to work for the organization in Washington. She wanted a nurse active in the professional organization and involved in party politics. The combination became the cornerstone for my political appointments.

## THE FIRST POLITICAL APPOINTMENT

I worked in DC for the American Nurses Association for two years but returned for family reasons to New Mexico in 1989 to become Executive Director for New Mexico Health Resources. This was a not-for-profit agency that recruited health professionals for the rural and underserved parts of the state. This job gave me much visibility as a rural health expert because I worked closely with the legislative and regulatory policymaking bodies. I honed my

management expertise by becoming a director of a family practice/urgent care facility for one of the large hospital systems. But I never stopped working on campaigns. In 1992, I focused my efforts on Bill Clinton's presidential campaign. And it paid off.

In January of 1993, I received a call from the Clinton White House to see if I would be interesting in serving in the Administration. I had just started a job with a large hospital system and felt I could not leave such an opportunity. I was honored and made it clear that I would consider a future opportunity.

In the spring of 1994, I received my second call from the White House of Personnel asking if I would consider serving as the Regional (VI) Director for the U.S. Department of Health and Human Services (DHHS), in Dallas, Texas. I said I would definitely consider it and my name was submitted, as well as that of a candidate that Governor Ann Richards was supporting for the position. This time I was ready for the job, so I immediately began to garner my political support. I asked New Mexico Governor Bruce King, U.S. Senators Bingaman and Domenici, and Congressman Bill Richardson, as well as the president of the state Senate and the speaker of the state House of Representatives, to write letters of support. I provided them with a draft and asked them to personalize their own letters. Though New Mexico is large geographically, it is small in population. My political work, as well as my professional positions, made me visible, and I felt comfortable asking those whom I supported in their campaigns to support me for a federal appointment.

It worked. I became Regional Director for the U.S. Department of Health and Human Services in September 1994 and served in that position until November 1998. It was one of the best jobs that I ever had! I was the DHHS Secretary Donna Shalala's representative in the region. In that role, I served as liaison to the state governors, legislators, other elected officials, the business community, and advocacy groups, within the five-state region. I had oversight of all of the DHHS programs and was charged with moving forward President Clinton's agenda. It was a wonderful leadership opportunity, and I was directly involved in the major federal policy initiatives, such as welfare reform and the State Children's Health

Insurance Program (SCHIP). I worked with community leaders at the state and local levels.

In early spring of 1998, the White House, DHHS Secretary Shalala, and DHHS Assistant Secretary Olivia Golden asked if I would consider moving to Washington, DC, to become the Commissioner for Children, Youth and Families in the Administration for Children Youth and Families. The position required Senate confirmation. I was to be responsible for national oversight of all Head Start, childcare, child welfare, and runaway and homeless youth programs; an approximately $13 billion budget. It was just what I had hoped: an opportunity to impact issues of children and families—my passion.

I served in that position from December of 1998 until December of 2000, the end of President Clinton's term. What did I do? One of the most significant accomplishments was working on reforming the child welfare system and crafting new regulations to improve quality outcomes in a very stressed and fragile child welfare system. It also prepared me for my next role, becoming Secretary of Health in New Mexico.

## BACK TO NEW MEXICO—THE NEW SECRETARY OF HEALTH

When Bill Richardson returned to New Mexico from serving as Secretary of Energy to run for governor in 2002, I let him know that I wanted to help him get elected. I also made it clear that if he won, I was willing to serve in his administration. I had known Bill Richardson since his early days in Congress in the mid 1980s and had been part of his Nurse Advisory Group on Health Issues. He did win and asked me to serve as Secretary of Health. I was his second Cabinet appointment.

My nursing, administrative, political, and policy experience prepared me well for the position. Because I was a native New Mexican, I was familiar with the state and its health care system. I also had developed an extensive network of policymakers, health providers, and professionals in the social service community. For the governor, my ability to work with the legislature was most critical to the success of his health agenda.

I started my position as Secretary of Health on the day Bill Richardson took the office of Governor,

January 1, 2003. The whirlwind began immediately. I was leading the largest department in state government, with 4000 employees.

My first challenge was facing the aftermath from 9/11. The threat of bioterrorism and the need for emergency preparedness were paramount. President George W. Bush charged each state to vaccinate health workers, particularly emergency first responders, against smallpox. The problem was that not everyone saw it as a threat, and the risk of taking the smallpox vaccine was well known and publicized. Many of the health professionals within the state health department, who needed to be leading the vaccination effort, were concerned and felt it was an overreaction by the Bush Administration. At the same time, a state plan was put in place to vaccinate and report on the status of getting people immunized.

How do you get staff to comply when there is so much conflict around the policy directive? My first lesson was to be a good listener, hear the concerns, and gather information to help alleviate fear. The second step was realizing that we weren't going to convince everyone to support vaccination. We had enough folks who did support the effort to begin. We created a team to coordinate the effort.

While working on the smallpox crisis, I needed to learn about the department and orient new employees. And then West Nile hit. This was a new virus-induced illness, caused by a mosquito bite, that was killing people. I needed reliable public health information about the disease and started to focus on educating all levels of the community: the public, the press, and health professionals. We created a team of experts, which included epidemiologists, public health workers, and the public information staff to clearly articulate the issues and provide education and training on how the virus was spread and what could be done for protection.

In the beginning, we were confronted daily with new cases of the disease. However, with the first deaths, we immediately began a daily press briefing to communicate with the public, educate about protection, and attempt to allay their fears. The media became our best friend and were essential in educating the public about the prevention.

While dealing with the West Nile outbreak, we began to reorganize the department. After eight months on the job, I could see what worked well and what needed improvement—without any budget increase. Governor Richardson came into office when New Mexico was one of the few states that did not have a budget deficit. To remain viable, we needed to become more efficient, not spend more money. We looked for areas where there was duplication and figured out how we could maximize resources. For instance, there were some areas of the budget where new categorical programs had been developed, and yet these populations were being served through other programs. By eliminating duplication and waste, we were able to keep our budget flat for two years.

The last challenge we faced was the flu epidemic of 2003-2004. We had a huge outbreak, and many elderly and young children died. Again, we had to coordinate vaccination delivery systems and provide good public health information. Much of the success was due to a flu consortium that was made up of the State Department of Health, health plans, and health care delivery providers that worked on tracking vaccine availability, keeping appropriate supplies on hand, and distributing supplies to where they were most needed. The members of the consortium had set up an extensive communication and tracking system to track where the flu was; they then ensured that there was enough vaccine in those areas.

The success of the program was due to expert public health professionals who had been working on this issue over many years. My job was to support them and allow them to do the job that they were trained to do.

In addition to running a department that included programs in behavioral health services, licensing and certification of health facilities, immunizations, nutrition services for women and children, and HIV/AID services, I was also helping to set the health and public policy agenda for the future.

To demonstrate to the public Governor Richardson's concern about health, we decided to focus on immunizations of children. The immunizations for children aged 0-3 had severely dropped in the state to only 62% immunization rate, ranking us 48th in the country. It was another poor indicator of the level of health of New Mexicans. The reasons were many: the high rate of poverty, the rural nature of the state, and an inadequate infrastructure. Too often it was just a lack of oversight and focus on setting appropriate health priorities.

One of the successful strategies to improve the immunization rate was to get First Lady Barbara Richardson to champion the initiative. Within two years we saw real improvement. The rate went from 62% to about 75%. In fact, New Mexico received recognition from the Centers for Disease Control and Prevention for the most improved state in immunization rates. We established a partnership between the Department of Health and the Immunization Coalition, which we located at the University of New Mexico Health Sciences Center. We worked with all the stakeholders throughout the state, including physicians, school nurses, health plans, and service organizations like the Rotary Club.

We also developed a strategic health plan to focus on prevention and early intervention. We chose four health status indicators: childhood immunizations, obesity, teen pregnancy, and youth suicide. For obesity we created the program "Get New Mexico on the Move" to encourage competition among communities to start moving by walking and encouraging physical fitness. We addressed obesity in schools by focusing on nutrition—for example, examining what was being served in the cafeteria and assessing the snack foods in vending machines, removing the bad snack foods, and replacing them with healthier choices. We also worked on reinstituting physical education programs. This would all be put in legislation for long-term sustainable change.

It has been an incredible journey from school nurse to Secretary of Health in New Mexico. I encourage many nurses to take such a journey.

## Lessons Learned

- Get involved in political campaigns and share your knowledge and skills with candidates and elected officials.
- Be clear at the beginning of a campaign about your expectations if the candidate should win.
- Be willing to take risks and follow opportunities.

# chapter 24

# An Overview of Legislation and Regulation

Yvonne Santa Anna

*"Law is order, and good law is good order."*

ARISTOTLE

## INFLUENCING THE LEGISLATIVE PROCESS

Public policy formation in the United States often appears to be indecisive and slow, and it can be difficult for the casual observer to distinguish the subtleties of the process. These nuances require that the observer select a conceptual model of policy-making to assist in understanding the specifics of the policymaking process—that is, why a particular proposal is enacted or defeated. Chapter 5 set forth several models for policy analysis. These can clarify how an issue is placed on the formal agenda for authoritative decision-making. Nurses who understand this process can better influence the system toward the development of sound health policies for their patients, their patients' families, and the profession of nursing.

This chapter will describe the path by which a bill becomes a federal or state law in the United States, with primary emphasis on federal processes. The legislative path differs only slightly between the federal and state levels and from state to state.

## INTRODUCTION OF A BILL

Only a member of the U.S. Congress (or of a state legislature) can introduce bills, though the idea for a bill can come from anyone, including constituents. A legislator can introduce any one of several types of bills and resolutions by simply giving their bill to the clerk of the house or, in Congress, placing the bill in a box called the *hopper* (Congressional

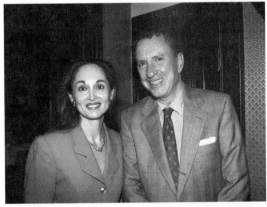

Yvonne Santa Anna, Director of Government Affairs, National Association for Home Care and Hospice and Senator Arlen Specter (R-PA).

Quarterly, 2000). In the U.S. Senate, a senator can postpone the introduction of another senator's bill by one day by voicing an objection. Legislation is often introduced simultaneously in the Senate and the House of Representatives as a pair of companion bills.

A member of Congress or state legislator who understands the legislative process in depth can contribute more to either the passage or defeat of a bill than one who is an expert only on its substance. However, the numerous players involved (the executive branch, the legislature, constituents, and special interest groups) and the complexity of the legislative process makes it far easier to defeat a bill than to pass one.

Of the thousands of bills introduced annually, relatively few rise to the formal decision-making agenda. For example, during the 108th Session of Congress (2003-2004), the House and Senate saw a total of 8468 bills introduced; 5432 in the House and 3036 in the Senate (Congressional Record, 2005). Of this number, 2394 were health care–related bills (1448 in the House and 946 in the Senate). Of the 8468 bills introduced, the President signed 498 bills into public law (U.S. Congress, 2005).

Every bill introduced in Congress faces a 2-year deadline; it must pass into law by then or die by default. Box 24-1 provides an overview of the various types of bills that can be introduced by members of Congress. Legislators introduce bills for a variety of reasons: to declare a position on an issue, as a favor to a constituent or a special interest group, to obtain publicity, or for political self-preservation. Some legislators, having introduced a bill, claim that they have acted to solve the problem that motivated it but do not continue to work toward enactment of the measure, blaming a committee or other members of the legislature if no further action is taken. Passage of a bill requires that at critical points in the policymaking process "a problem is recognized, a solution is available, the political climate makes the time right for a change, and the constraints do not prohibit action" (Kingdon, 1984, p. 93). Although meeting these conditions helps a bill to rise on the decision agenda, nothing can guarantee enactment.

---

**BOX 24-1** Types of Bills in the U.S. Congress

*Bill:* This is used for most legislation, whether general, public, or private (i.e., initiated by non-congressional sources). The bill number is prefixed with HR in the House, S in the Senate.

*Joint resolution:* This is subject to the same procedures as bills, with the exception of any joint resolution proposing an amendment to the Constitution. The latter must be approved by two thirds of both chambers, whereupon it is sent directly to the Administrator of General Services for submission to the states for ratification, rather than to the President. There is little difference between a bill and a joint resolution, and often the two forms are used interchangeably. One difference in form is that a joint resolution may include a preamble preceding the resolving clause. Statutes that have been initiated as bills have later been amended by a joint resolution and vice versa. The bill number is prefixed with HJ Res in the House and SJ Res in the Senate.

*Concurrent resolution:* This is used for matters affecting the operations of both houses. The bill number is prefixed with H Con Res in the House, S Con Res in the Senate.

*Resolution:* This is used when a matter concerns the operation of either chamber alone; adopted only by the chamber in which it originates. The bill number is prefixed with H Res in the House and S Res in the Senate.

From Congressional Quarterly. (2000). *Guide to current American government.* Washington, DC: Congressional Quarterly.

---

## INFLUENCING THE INTRODUCTION OF A BILL

Nurses can influence the introduction of bills as constituents and as members of professional associations that lobby Congress. They can call attention to problems in funding health care, such as the need for expanded services for uninsured children, the need for prescription drug coverage under Medicare, or the need to increase reimbursement for nursing services. Legislators like to work with organized groups that have strong positions on a bill, such as the American Nurses Association, American Association of Colleges of Nursing, American Association of

Nurse Anesthetists, American Nephrology Nurses' Association, or the state nurses associations.

Frequently, associations are asked to assist in drafting legislation and in lobbying members of the legislature. Coalitions of interested organizations are created to present a united front, a clear message, and a strong constituency to persuade legislators to support a particular bill (see Chapter 8). Enactment, if achieved at all, may take several legislative sessions.

Identifying the appropriate sponsor to introduce a bill is critical to its success. In selecting a primary bill sponsor, it is best to ask a member of a committee that has jurisdiction over the program or issue you wish to have addressed. For example, in the U.S. Senate, the Finance Committee has jurisdiction over the Medicare program and decides which Medicare-related legislation gets sent to the full Senate for a vote. Legislation that would address changes in direct reimbursement of nurse practitioners (NPs) or nurse anesthetists under Medicare would be less likely to be tabled (i.e., never acted upon) if a member of the Senate Finance Committee was a primary sponsor of the measure.

## COMMITTEE ACTION

Committees are centers of policymaking at both federal and state levels. It is in committee that conflicting points of view are discussed and legislation is often refined and amended. Successful committee consideration of bills requires organization, consensus building, and time; only about 15% of all bills referred to committees are reported out for House and Senate consideration.

The Senate and House have separate committees with distinct rules and procedures. Committee procedure provides the means for members of the legislature to sift through an otherwise overwhelming number of bills, proposals, and complex issues. Within the respective guidelines of each chamber, committees adopt their own rules to address their organizational and procedural issues. Generally, committees operate independently of each other and of their respective parent chambers (Schneider, 2001).

There are three types of committees at the federal level: standing, select, and joint. A *standing* committee has permanent jurisdiction over bills and issues in its content area. Some standing committees set *authorizing* funding levels and others set *appropriating* funding levels for proposed laws. This two-step authorizing-appropriating process is designed to concentrate the policymaking decisions within the authorizing committee and decisions about precise funding levels within the appropriations committees.

A *select* committee cannot report out a bill and is often created by the leadership to address a special problem or concern. A *joint* committee consists of members of both the House and Senate. One type of a joint committee is the *conference* committee, in which members of each chamber and party work together to address differences in their respective bills.

In congressional committees, leadership and authority is centered in the chair of the committee. The chair, always a member of the majority party, decides the committee's agenda, conducts its meetings, and controls the funds distributed by the chamber to the committee (Schneider, 2001). The senior minority party member of the committee is called the *ranking minority member* (or *ranking member*). The committee's subcommittees also have chairs and ranking members. Often, but not always, the ranking member assists the chair with some of the responsibilities of the committee or subcommittee. The committee chair usually refers a bill to the subcommittees for initial consideration, but only the full committee can report out a bill to the floor (Schneider, 2001). For example, the House Ways and Means Committee refer most Medicare bills to the House Ways and Means Subcommittee on Health. If the subcommittee wishes to take action on the bill, it usually will schedule at least one hearing to discuss the substance of the proposed legislation.

In very unusual circumstances, a few bills will bypass the committee process. This can only happen if the leadership of the majority consents. For example, according to a U.S. House Select Committee on Aging fact sheet, "Since the Roosevelt era, major pieces of social legislation, including civil rights reforms and labor reforms, such as the wage and hours bill, were forced to bypass committees of jurisdiction because the committees refused or delayed in allowing the House to consider them" (Pepper & Roybal, 1988, p. 1). In the end, however, committees and subcommittees usually select the bills they want to consider and ignore the rest. Committees thus perform a gatekeeping function by selecting from the thousands of measures introduced in each session those that meet their party's leadership priorities and that they consider to merit floor debate.

Consideration of bills whose content overlaps the jurisdictions of different committees falls to the leader of the chamber to decide. Health care issues, for example, can cut across the jurisdiction of more than one committee. When this occurs in the House, upon advice from the Parliamentarian, the Speaker of the House will base his or her referral decision on the chamber's rules and precedents for subject matter jurisdiction and identify the appropriate *primary* committee and other committees for the bill's referral (Schneider, 2001). The Parliamentarians in both chambers have a key role in advising the member of Congress presiding over a bill on the floor. While a member is free to take or ignore the Parliamentarian's advice, few have the knowledge of the chamber's procedures to preside on their own. The primary committee has primary responsibility for guiding the referred measure to final passage. Referrals to more than one committee can have a positive effect by providing opportunities for greater public discussion of the issue and multiple points of access for special interest groups, but this can also greatly slow down the legislative process (Davidson & Oleszek, 1996).

A committee can handle a bill in any of the following ways (Congressional Quarterly, 1993):

- Approve a bill with or without amendments.
- Rewrite or revise the bill and report it out to the full House or Senate.
- Report it unfavorably (i.e., allow it to be considered by the full House or Senate, but with a recommendation that the bill be rejected).
- Take no action, which kills the bill.

## AUTHORIZATION AND APPROPRIATION PROCESS

To understand the legislative process and to analyze individual pieces of legislation, it is important to know the distinction between *authorizing* legislation and *appropriating* legislation. Because a considerable amount of congressional activity is concerned with decisions related to spending money and because much of this activity has a direct effect on health care and nursing programs, it is especially important for nurses to be familiar with the authorization-appropriation process. Programs and agencies such as the Nurse Education Act, Scholarships for Disadvantaged Students, the National Health Service Corps, the National Institute of Nursing Research, the National Institutes of Health, and the Agency for Health Care Policy and Research are all subject to the authorization-appropriation process.

Before any of these programs can receive or spend money from the U.S. Treasury, a two-step process usually must occur. First, an authorization bill allowing an agency or program to come into being or to continue to exist must be passed. The authorization bill is the substantive bill that establishes the purpose of, and guidelines for, the program and usually sets limits on the amount that can be spent. It gives a federal agency or program the legal authority to operate. Authorizing legislation does not, however, provide the actual dollars for a program or enable an agency to spend funds in the future. Renewal or modification of existing authorization is called reauthorization (see Chapter 23).

Second, an appropriation bill must be passed. The appropriation bill enables an agency or program to make spending commitments and to actually spend money. In almost all cases, an appropriation bill for an activity is not supposed to be passed until the authorization for that activity is enacted. That is, no money can be spent on a program unless it first has been authorized to exist. Conversely, if a program has been authorized but no money is provided (appropriated) for its implementation, that program cannot be carried out (Collender, 1991).

The authorization-appropriation process is determined by congressional rules that, like most congressional rules, can be waived, circumvented, or ignored on occasion. For example, failure to enact an authorization does not necessarily prevent the appropriations committee from acting. If an expired program—for example, the Nursing Education

Act—is deemed likely to be reauthorized, it may receive funds. These must be spent in accordance with the expired authorizing language.

Today, much of the federal government is funded through the annual enactment of 13 general appropriations bills. Whether agencies receive all the money they request depends, in part, on the recommendations of the authorizing and appropriating committees. Each chamber has authorizing and appropriating committees, and these have differing responsibilities. For federal nursing education and research activities, the authorizing committees are the Senate Health, Education, Labor, and Pensions Committee and the House Energy and Commerce Committee. The appropriating committee for federal nursing education and research programs are the Senate and House appropriations committees and their subcommittees on Labor, Health and Human Services, Education and Related Agencies (Figure 24-1).

## COMMITTEE PROCEDURES

Committee consideration of a measure usually consists of three standard steps: hearings, markups, and reports.

**Hearings.** *Hearings* can be legislative, oversight, or investigative; each of these types of hearing may be either public or closed (Schneider, 2001). When the committee leadership decides to proceed with a measure, it will usually conduct hearings to receive testimony in support of a measure. From these hearings the committee will gather information and views, identify problems, gauge support for and opposition to the bill, and build a public record of committee action that addresses the measure (Schneider, 2001). Although most hearings are held in Washington, DC, field hearings in the members' respective states are also held.

Most witnesses are invited to testify before the committee by the chair, who is a member of the majority party and who sets the agenda for the hearing proceedings. The ranking minority member may have an opportunity to request a witness, but it is up to the discretion of the chair to agree to the selection of the witness. Written testimony can also be submitted to the committee by persons who do not have the opportunity to speak their position on a measure in person.

Nurses can influence the policymaking process by testifying at bill hearings. Frequently, committees prefer to deal with large, organized groups that have a position on an issue rather than with private individuals. Professional nursing organizations testify on behalf of their members. Congressional hearings are listed in the official House and Senate Websites at *www.house.gov* and *www.senate.gov*. C-SPAN provides live and recorded coverage of hearings *(www.c-span.org)*.

Constituents can influence the committee process by meeting with, and writing to, the members of the committee. Concerns expressed by constituents are given serious consideration.

Lobbyists often meet with all members of the committee to express their client's position on a measure. Professional associations often activate a grassroots network of members, asking them to contact the committee members to request co-sponsorship of, or opposition to, the measure.

The hearing process at the state level is similar, as is the importance of an organized approach to presenting testimony. When several representatives of nursing plan to testify on a bill, it is more efficient and effective for them to coordinate their testimony, raising different aspects of an issue rather than repeating the same points. It is also important for various nursing representatives to emphasize those issues where there is agreement; a unified message can strengthen the impression of a powerful coalition. And a hearing room packed with a supportive audience makes a powerful statement to legislators about support for an issue.

**Markups.** When legislative hearings are concluded, a subcommittee decides whether to attempt to report a measure. If the chair decides to proceed with the measure, she or he will generally choose to continue with the legislative process to "mark up" the bill. A *markup* is the committee meeting where a measure is modified through amendments to clean up problems or errors within the measure (Schneider, 2001). A quorum of one third of the committee is required in both chambers to hold a

# HOW A BILL BECOMES A LAW

### *The Federal Level*

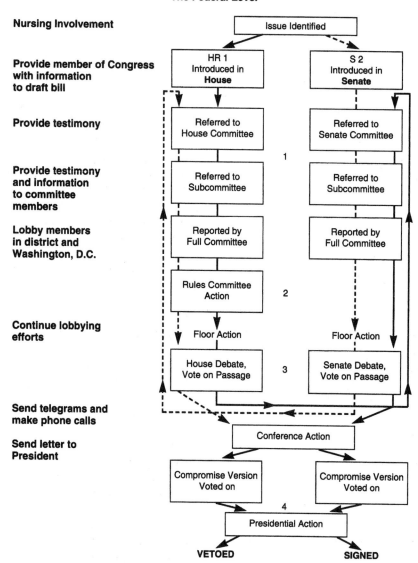

**Nursing Involvement**

**Provide member of Congress
with information
to draft bill**

**Provide testimony**

**Provide testimony
and information
to committee
members**

**Lobby members
in district and
Washington, D.C.**

**Continue lobbying
efforts**

**Send telegrams and
make phone calls**

**Send letter to
President**

[1] A bill goes to full committee first, then to special subcommittees for hearings, debate, revisions, and approval. The same process occurs when it goes to full committee. It either dies in committee or proceeds to the next step.

[2] Only the House has a Rules Committee to set the "rule" for floor action and conditions for debate and amendments. In the Senate, the leadership schedules action.

[3] The bill is debated, amended, and passed or defeated. If passed, it goes to other chamber and follows the same path. If each chamber passes a similar bill, both versions go to conference.

[4] The President may sign the bill into law, allow it to become law without his signature, or veto it and return it to Congress. To override the veto, both houses must approve the bill by a 2/3 majority vote.

**Figure 24-1** How a Bill becomes a law.

markup session (Schneider, 2001). A markup session can weaken or strengthen a measure. Pressure from outside interest groups is often intense at this stage. Under congressional "sunshine rules," markups are conducted in public, except on national-security or related issues.

After conducting hearings and markups, a subcommittee sends its recommendation to the full committee, which may conduct its own hearings and markups, ratify the subcommittee's decision, take no action, or return the bill to the subcommittee for further study.

**Reports.** The rules of both the Senate and the House dictate that a committee *report* accompany each bill to the floor. The report, written by committee staff, describes the intent of legislation (i.e., its purpose and scope). It explains any amendments to the bill, and any changes made to current law by the bill; estimates the cost of the bill to the government; sets out documentation for the bill's legislative intent; and often contains dissenting views on the measure from the minority-party committee members.

A committee's description of the legislative intent of the bill is extremely important, especially for the government agency that will implement and enforce the law. Sometimes the report contains explicit instructions on how the agency should interpret the law in regulations, or the report may be written without great detail. Sometimes an agency will interpret the law narrowly, particularly if it is written vaguely. For example, when certified nurse midwives received reimbursement authority under the Medicare program, the agency chose to reimburse them only for gynecologic services, not for all the services covered by Medicare, which they are legally able to provide. This was a narrow interpretation of the law and was not the intent of Congress.

The committee report is also important because it offers those interested in the bill an opportunity to promote or protect their interests. Committee staffs frequently include the report language suggested by special interest groups if it is congruent with the bill.

## FLOOR ACTION IN THE HOUSE AND SENATE

After a bill is reported out of committee, it can be placed on a calendar of chamber business and scheduled for floor action by the leadership of the majority party (Schneider, 2001). If the bill is not controversial, it may be dealt with expeditiously. Otherwise, it is placed on the chamber's calendar for future consideration. Both the rules governing the calendar on which a bill is placed and subsequent floor procedures differ between the House and Senate and among state chambers. Box 24-2 compares the House and Senate procedures for scheduling and raising measures.

The influence of the committee chair and ranking member of the committee that reports out a measure is maintained throughout the floor proceedings. They continue to manage the measure by "planning parliamentary strategy, controlling time for debate, responding to questions from colleagues, warding off unwanted amendments, and building coalitions in favor of their positions" (Schneider, 2001, p. 6). Box 24-3 compares House and Senate rules for floor consideration of a measure. In the House, the Committee on Rules governs proceedings on the floor; there is no such committee in the Senate.

When a bill moves to the floor, special interest groups continue to lobby its opponents, its proponents, and particularly undecided legislators, attempting to influence the outcome of the vote. This process is usually begun after the introduction of the bill, when lobbyists meet with the members of the referring committee to gather support for the measure, and continues until the bill is signed into law. When a bill moves to the floor, constituents are activated to contact the members of the legislature from their own districts. Members listen attentively to their constituents, and so lobbying should continue until the moment of the vote, especially lobbying of undecided members. Lobbyists are known to wait outside the cloakroom in the "lobby" to catch the attention of members as they move in and out of the chambers.

A vote on the bill is taken after the debate and amendment process is completed. There are three methods of voting: (1) *voice* vote, which calls for

**BOX 24-2** Scheduling and Raising Measures in the U.S. House and U.S. Senate

**HOUSE**

Four calendars (Union, House, Private, Discharge)

Special days for raising measures*

Scheduling by speaker and majority party leadership in consultation with selected representatives

No practice of "holds"

Powerful role for Rules Committee

Special rules (approved by majority vote) govern floor consideration of most major legislation

Non-controversial measures usually approved under *suspension of the rules* procedure

Difficult to circumvent committee consideration of measures

**SENATE**

Two calendars (Legislative and Executive)

No special days

Scheduling by majority party leadership in broad consultation with minority party leaders and interested senators

Individual senators can place "holds" on the raising measure, within limits

No committee with role equivalent to that of House Rules Committee

*Complex unanimous consent agreements* (approved by unanimous consent) govern floor consideration of major measures

Non-controversial measures approved by *unanimous consent* procedure

Easier to circumvent committee consideration of measures

Adapted from Schneider, J. (2005). *House and Senate rules of procedures: A comparison* (Congressional Research Service order code RL30945, CRS-6). Washington, DC: CRS.
*There are special days for calling up bills under the suspension of the rules and Calendar Wednesday procedures, for raising measures from the Private Calendar, and for bringing up legislation involving the District of Columbia.

**BOX 24-3** Floor Procedures of the U.S. House and the U.S. Senate

**HOUSE**

Presiding officer has considerable discretion in recognizing members

Rulings of presiding officer seldom challenged

Debate time always restricted

Debate ends by majority vote in the House and in the Committee of the Whole (i.e., the membership of the House)

Most major measures considered in Committee of the Whole

Number and type of amendments often limited by special rule; bills amended by section or title

Germaneness of amendments required (unless requirement is waived by special rule)

Quorum calls usually permitted only in connection with record votes

Votes recorded by electronic device; electronic vote can be requested only after voice or division vote is completed

House routinely adjourns at end of each legislative day

**SENATE**

Presiding officer has little discretion in recognizing senators

Rulings of presiding officer frequently challenged

Unlimited debate;* individual senators can filibuster

Super-majority vote required to invoke cloture; up to 30 hours of post-cloture debate allowed[†]

No Committee of the Whole

Unlimited amendments; bills generally open to amendment at any point

Germaneness of amendments not generally required

Quorum calls in order almost any time; often used for purposes of deliberate delay

No electronic voting system; roll call votes can be requested almost any time

Senate often recesses instead of adjourning; legislative days can continue for several calendar days

Adapted from Schneider, J. (2005). *House and Senate rules of procedures: A comparison* (Congressional research service order code RL30945, CRS-13). Washington, DC: CRS.
*Except when complex unanimous consent agreements or rule-making provisions in statutes impose time restrictions.
[†]Adoption of the motion to table by majority vote also ends Senate debate. Use of this motion, however, is generally reserved for cases when the Senate is prepared to reject the pending bill.

members to answer yea or nay (victory is judged by ear); (2) *division* vote, which requires a head count of those favoring and those opposing an amendment; and (3) *recorded* teller vote, which records each legislator's name and position taken on the vote.

Recorded votes are the most valuable to lobbyists and constituents because they document how the member voted—helpful information in determining whether to continue support for a legislator and as a predictor of a legislator's future stands on issues.

## CONFERENCE ACTION

Before a bill can be sent to the executive branch for consideration, identical bills must be passed in both chambers. Frequently, the bills originally considered by the House and Senate chambers are not identical, so members of each chamber must meet to resolve the differences. This is often where much of the hard bargaining and compromising takes place in the passage of legislation. The leaders of each chamber appoint *conferees*, usually senior members of the committees with jurisdiction over the bill, to meet with the conferees of the other chamber.

A joint conference offers another opportunity for groups and individuals to persuade members to support various positions on controversial aspects of the bill. Frequently, there is controversy over the amount of money allocated to a federal program. For example, House and Senate funding authorizations for nursing education programs can differ by tens of millions of dollars. Generally, supporters of a program would lobby for the version of the bill authorizing the largest amount of funding for it.

When agreement is reached on the controversial provisions of the measure, a conference report is written explaining the differences considered in resolving the issue. Both chambers must then approve the conference version of the bill for the bill to become law.

## SENATE ROLE IN THE CONFIRMATION PROCESS

The role of the Senate in the confirmation process is defined in the U.S. Constitution. Article II, Section 2 states that the President "shall nominate, and by and with the Advice and Consent of the Senate, shall appoint high government officials" (Tong, 2005). The Senate gives its advice and consent to presidential appointments, to Supreme Court nominees, and to other high-level positions in the cabinet departments and independent agencies of the government. The Senate also confirms

appointments of members of regulatory commissions, ambassadors, federal judges, U.S. attorneys, and U.S. marshals. Appointees named to be Supreme Court Justices and Cabinet secretaries receive close scrutiny by the full Senate and Senate committees.

There are several steps in the confirmation process. First, the President submits a nomination in writing and forwards it to the Senate. The nomination is read on the floor of the Senate and is given a number. Second, the Senate Parliamentarian, acting on behalf of the presiding officer, refers each nomination to the committee or committees of jurisdiction. Confirmation hearings, generally open to the public, can be held, but they are not held on all nominations. Supreme Court nominees and senior administration officials or controversial nominees are given the closest scrutiny in hearings. Senators can use the committee hearings as a forum to advance their own policy and political agenda, to determine or challenge the administration's positions on policy issues, and to receive commitments from a nominee. The committee has the option to report the nomination favorable, unfavorable, or without recommendation, or take no action at all. If the committee moves to report the nomination, it is filed with the Senate's executive clerk, who assigns a calendar number and places the nomination on the Executive Calendar.

The third step in the confirmation process involves floor consideration of the nomination. During this step, the Senate will meet in an executive session to consider the nomination. Nominations are subject to unlimited debate, subject to cloture being invoked (which requires 60 votes). The Senate has three options in its advice and consent role: confirm, reject, or take no action on the nomination. Confirmation requires a simple majority vote. Once the Senate has acted on a nomination, the Secretary of the Senate transmits the results of the nomination to the White House. In some instances, one or more senators can place a hold on a nomination, which can delay or prevent the nomination from reaching the floor for further action. Senate rules require any pending nominations to be returned to the President when the Senate is in recess for more than 30 days or adjourns between sessions. Presidents have made court appointments without the Senate's consent, when the Senate was in recess. These court "recess appointments" are temporary in nature, with the nominee's term expiring at the end of the Senate's next session.

## EXECUTIVE ACTION

After both chambers have passed identical versions of a bill, it is ready to go to the executive branch. The executive (President or Governor) has the power to sign a bill into law, veto it, or return it to the legislature with no signature and a message stating his or her objections. If no further action is taken, the bill dies; or, the legislature may decide to call for another floor vote to overturn the executive's veto. A two-thirds vote is required to override an executive veto in Congress and in many states. Under the U.S. Constitution, a bill becomes law if the President does not sign it within 10 days of the time she or he receives it, provided Congress is in session. Presidents occasionally permit enactment of legislation in this manner when they want to make a political statement of disapproval of the legislation but do not believe that their objections warrant a veto. If Congress adjourns before the 10-day period expires, the unsigned bill does not become law. In this case, the bill has been defeated by the *pocket* veto (Congressional Quarterly, 1993).

## REGULATORY PROCESS

As important as it is to become skilled at influencing the legislative process, it is equally important to influence the regulatory process (see Chapter 23). Regulations have a direct impact on a nurse's work and professional life. As changes in health care financing and delivery structures are driving changes in the current health care provider licensing system, many states are considering changes in the regulation of nursing, from amending the Nurse Practice Act to accomplishing a major overhaul of the entire licensing system. Many of these changes will take place in the regulatory arena within a nurse's state. Other health care–related regulations that can have an impact on nursing practice may also take place within the federal domain.

Though some regulations may be developed or amended without legislation, other regulations are created by the details of new or amended laws. The development of such regulations takes months and sometimes years. It is this important step—the development of regulations—that may be overlooked by organized groups and individuals working to influence policy and the political process (Figure 24-2).

One of the largest federal agencies having primary responsibility for health care programs is the Department of Health and Human Services (HHS). HHS is comprised of 12 major operating divisions with over 300 programs. It has responsibilities for public health, biomedical research, Medicare and Medicaid, welfare, and social services programs. Nurses interested in participating in the process of streamlining federal regulation of a specific HHS program should become familiar with the program's specifications, rules, and regulations. With this program knowledge, nurses will be in a position to provide informed feedback to regulators on the operation of the program. For example, nurses knowledgeable about the Medicare program, a federal insurance program primarily for people older than 65, younger disabled people, and those patients needing dialysis, can share their experience with policymakers as well as regulators. From their direct clinical experiences with these federal health insurance programs, nurses have much to share about the regulatory burdens and programmatic problems that impede efficient and quality patient care.

The Centers for Medicare and Medicaid Services (CMS) is the administrative agency that directs the Medicare and Medicaid programs. Under the leadership of the CMS administrator, Dr. Mark McClellan, the agency holds regular "Open Door Forums" for 14 individual health care provider groups *(www.cms.hhs.gov/opendoor)*. Although these forums are helpful to providers, because they often provide an avenue for discussing recently proposed regulations or draft guidance, they do not take the place of formal comment periods associated with the rulemaking process.

A major role of government regulation is to interpret the laws. The laws that Congress and state legislatures pass rarely contain enough explicit language

**THE REGULATORY PROCESS**

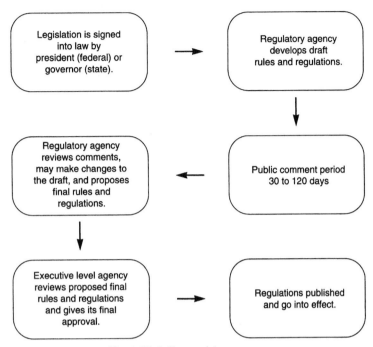

**Figure 24-2** The regulatory process.

to closely guide their implementation. It is the responsibility of the administrative agencies to promulgate the rules and regulations that fill in the details of those laws. The health policy positions of the executive or legislative branch of government will determine the laws that are passed, but once enacted, laws and their accompanying regulations will shape the way health policy is translated into programs and services.

Regulations specify definitions, authority, eligibility, benefits, and standards. Their development is shaped not only by the law but by the ongoing involvement and input of professional associations, providers, third-party payers, consumers, and other special interest groups (Box 24-4).

The administrative agencies, usually part of the executive branch of government, may enact, enforce, and adjudicate their own rules and regulations, thus assuming (in this context) the functions of all three branches of government (legislative, executive, and judicial). For example, some administrative

agencies can sit in judgment of previously enforced agency regulations that are now in dispute and judge whether to uphold or overturn them. Agencies are created through legislation that broadly defines their structure and function. They must develop their own regulations that set policy to govern the behavior of agency officials and regulated parties; spell out their procedural requirements, such as rules governing notices of intent, comment periods, and hearings; and develop enforcement procedures. For example, the Food and Drug Administration sets and monitors standards for foods and tests drugs for purity, safety, and effectiveness, while the Environmental Protection Agency, among other activities, controls health risks from water-borne microbes in drinking water through the development and implementation of regulations.

The promulgation of regulations is guided by certain rules. Key among these, at the federal level, is the requirement that the agency responsible for implementing a law publish a draft of any proposed

**BOX 24-3** How to Influence Legislative and Regulatory Processes

- Become informed about the public policy and health policy issues that are currently under consideration at the local, state, and federal levels of government.
- Become acquainted with the elected officials that represent you at the local, state, and federal levels of government. Communicate with them regularly to share your expertise and perspective on health care and nursing issues.
- Call, write, or send a fax or e-mail message to your legislator, stating briefly the position you wish him or her to take on a particular issue. Always remember to mention that you are a registered nurse and that you live and vote in the legislator's district.
- Request that legislation be introduced or a regulatory change made. Offer your expertise to assist in developing new legislation or in modifying existing legislation and rules.
- Become active in your professional association and work to activate a strong grassroots network of members who are prepared to contact their elected representatives on key health care issues.
- Attend a public hearing on a bill or regulation to show support for an issue, or actually testify yourself.
- Build your own political resume by becoming active in local politics in your area.
- Volunteer to work on the campaigns of candidates who are knowledgeable and supportive of nursing's perspective on health care issues.
- Seek appointment to a government task force or commission to have the opportunity to make legislative, regulatory, and public policy changes.
- Seek election to public office or employment in an administrative or executive agency.
- Explore opportunities to be involved with the policy and legislative process through internships, fellowships, and volunteer experiences at the local, state, and federal levels.

regulation or set of regulations in the *Federal Register*. The *Federal Register* is the official daily publication for administrative regulations, including rules, proposed rules, and notices of federal agencies and organizations, as well as executive orders and other presidential documents. The publication of proposed regulations offers an opportunity for interested parties to react to the draft before it becomes final. Commenting on draft regulations is one of the most important points of involvement in the entire legislative process (Longest, 1997). States follow similar procedures.

## A REGULATORY EXAMPLE: NATIONAL ASSOCIATION FOR HOME CARE AND THE OUTCOME AND ASSESSMENT INFORMATION SET

The following example is an illustration of the impact that home health nurses, home health agencies, professional associations, and consumers have had on the regulatory process as it relates to CMS' implementation of a Medicare home care patient assessment instrument—the Outcome and Assessment Information Set (OASIS). In the Omnibus Budget Reconciliation Act of 1987, Congress mandated that CMS (formerly known as the Health Care Financing Administration) develop a standardized patient assessment instrument to assist them in monitoring Medicare Home Health Agencies (HHAs). CMS used information from years of research and demonstrations in the development of OASIS, which contains 79 demographic, clinical, and functional data items for assessing patients and measuring outcomes.

In January 1999, CMS issued final rules requiring HHAs to conduct comprehensive patient assessments, incorporating the OASIS data elements, and electronically report the OASIS data collected. The rule stipulated that all Medicare-certified HHAs must collect OASIS data on both public and private pay patients, because section 1891(b) of the Social Security Act requires that the Secretary of Health and Human Services ensure that the conditions of participation and other requirements are adequate to protect all individuals under the care of the HHA.

Through the comment process and other means, home health agencies, advocacy groups, professional associations, and consumers expressed concerns regarding the privacy of OASIS information. According to a U.S. General Accounting Office (GAO) report:

Advocates commented that some of the OASIS questions were irrelevant and delved too deeply into the personal lives of patients. They cited the mental status questions, including one that asked about depressive feelings reported or observed in the patient, as well as a question regarding financial factors that could limit the patient's ability to meet his or her own basic health needs. They requested that patient identifiers be removed from the OASIS data before transmission to CMS or that CMS not require OASIS data to be reported on non-Medicare and non-Medicaid patients. (GAO, 2001)

In the spring of 1999, these privacy concerns led CMS to postpone the effective date of OASIS reporting, but not the collecting of OASIS data, for non-Medicare and non-Medicaid patients. In July of 1999, HHAs participating in Medicare had to comply with the new conditions of participation by (1) incorporating OASIS data items into the assessment process for Medicare, Medicaid, and private pay patients, (2) electronically transmitting accurate OASIS data to the state survey agency, and (3) maintaining the privacy of their OASIS data. CMS implemented several safeguards aimed at protecting the confidentiality of patient information collected (GAO, 2001). HHAs were directed to provide all patients with a written notice of their privacy rights. Even though HHAs were required to collect information on patients' financial condition, CMS eliminated the requirement for HHAs to transmit the information to data repositories. Additionally, CMS masked several OASIS patient identifiers for non-Medicare and non-Medicaid patients (Federal Register, 1999).

Since July of 1999, nurses and other advocates have continued to express their dissatisfaction to regulators and members of Congress with various aspects of the OASIS instrument. Testifying before the congressional committee with jurisdiction over the Medicare program and on behalf of the National Association for Home Care and Hospice (NAHC), one home health agency administrator testified that "while there are valid reasons to use a uniform patient assessment instrument, the extensive administrative responsibilities with OASIS must be streamlined to reduce costs, increase direct patient care time, and improve staff satisfaction and retention" (Wilson, 2001). NAHC continued to be actively engaged in working to influence CMS regulatory

policy by pursuing the streamlining and reduction of the OASIS instrument through their submission of testimony and recommendations to Congress, as well as working with the HHS Secretary Advisory Committee on Regulatory Reform and with the CMS administrator. Through these efforts, changes have been made to the OASIS instrument. One of the most recent changes occurred with the passage of HR 1, the Medicare Prescription Drug, Improvement, and Modernization Act of 2003 (Public Law 108-173). Congress directed CMS to suspend collection of OASIS information on non-Medicare and non-Medicaid patients until final regulations are published regarding use and collection of OASIS for non-Medicare and non-Medicaid patients. The provision also requires a study and report on the benefits and/or value and burden of collecting OASIS information from both large and small home health agencies. As of 2006, the suspension continues to be in effect, and CMS has not yet written the reports mandated by Congress.

## Key Points

- By participating in the legislative and regulatory processes of government, nurses can improve access to, and the delivery of, health care services.
- Nurses can also affect the practice of their profession in both state and federal programs.
- Understanding these processes is an important first step toward influencing them.

## Web Resources

**Environmental Protection Agency**
*www.epa.gov*
**The Federal Register**
*www.archives.gov/federal-register*
**House Energy and Commerce Committee**
*http://energycommerce.house.gov*
**Senate Appropriations Committee**
*http://appropriations.senate.gov*
**Senate Health, Education, Labor, and Pensions Committee**
*http://labor.senate.gov*

## REFERENCES

Collender, S. E. (1991). *The guide to the federal budget.* Washington, DC: Urban Institute Press.

Congressional Quarterly. (1993). *Congress and the legislative process.* Washington, DC: Congressional Quarterly.

Congressional Quarterly. (2000). *Guide to current American government.* Washington, DC: Congressional Quarterly.

Congressional Record. (2005). Daily Digest, February 15, 2005. Washington, DC: Government Printing Office.

Davidson, R. H., & Oleszek, W. J. (1996). *Congress and its members* (5th ed.). Washington, DC: Congressional Quarterly.

Federal Register. (1999, June 18). Part IV: Department of Health and Human Services. *Federal Register 64*(117), 32984-32991. Washington, DC: Government Printing Office.

GAO (U.S. General Accounting Office). (2001, January 30). *Medicare home health care: OASIS data use, cost, and privacy implications* (report no. GAO-01-205). Washington, DC: GAO.

Kingdon, J. (1984). *Agendas, alternatives, and public policy.* Boston: Little, Brown.

Longest, B. B., Jr. (1997). *Seeking strategic advantage through health policy analysis.* Chicago: Health Administration Press.

Pepper, C., & Roybal, E. (1988). *H.R. 3436 fact sheet: Financing and cost controls.* Washington, DC: U.S. House of Representatives Select Committee on Aging.

Schneider, J. (2001). *The committee system in the U.S. Congress* (Congressional Research Service order code RS20794). Washington, DC: Congressional Research Service.

Schneider, J. (2005). *House and Senate rules of procedure: A comparison* (Congressional Research Service order code RL30945, CRS-6). Washington, DC: CRS.

Tong, L. (2005). *Senate confirmation process: A brief overview* (Congressional Research Service order code RS20986). Washington, DC: Congressional Research Service.

U.S. Congress. (2005, February 15). Official resume of Congressional activity for the 108th Congress. Congressional Record, Daily Digest, pp. D96-D97.

Wilson, S. (2001, March 15). Testimony on bringing regulatory relief to beneficiaries and providers, made before the Committee on Ways and Means Subcommittee on Health, United States House of Representatives.

# *Vignette*  Mary L. Behrens

## From Sewage Problems to the Statehouse: My Life as an Elected Official

*"All politics is local."*

THOMAS P. "TIP" O'NEILL,
FORMER SPEAKER OF THE U.S. HOUSE OF REPRESENTATIVES

I have practiced as a family nurse practitioner, clinical specialist in pediatrics, and nurse educator. Running for political office had not been one of my early career goals. However, I did have a good political role model when I was young. My father was elected to our local school board and served for 12 years; for most of those 12 years, he served as chair.

He took my sisters and me to political rallies and speeches starting when I was about 10 years old. Because I was born, I came of age in the 1960s, I attended college during a period of student activism and protests and that experience influenced me.

### SEWAGE CHANGED MY LIFE

My first leap into the political arena came because of a call from an upset friend who lived on property along the river that ran through our community. She told me, "Mary, there is raw sewage on our lawn. I called the health department who told me to contact the state Department of Environmental Quality and when I called the DEQ, they said I should call the local health department. You should see what is floating up. It's totally disgusting and I am frustrated."

### Seeing is Believing

I drove out to my friend's neighborhood and saw firsthand the raw sewage that was being deposited on lawns. My friend told me it appeared like clockwork when everyone flushed their toilets and used their dishwashers in the morning and evening. Right then and there I decided to take action. I contacted the local day care centers and learned they had noticed an increase in diarrhea in the children. I then called the two local TV stations and three radio stations. I informed them of a serious problem on the river, and I gave them the time and location of a press conference I was planning.

At the press conference, I stated I was a nurse and was concerned about this sewage being a serious health threat to citizens in our town. I noted the increased diarrhea in children that was reported by the day care centers. The news media representatives who attended my press conference could see the raw sewage and captured images with their cameras. The train was moving down the track! The city, the health department, and the state Department of Environmental Quality had to deal with the calls from the press and the citizens. Our local city government and the state had to provide funds to connect this housing development to city water and sewer in order to stop the pollution.

### I CAN DO THIS!

As I took action on the sewage problem, I attended several city council meetings. When I observed the city council in action, I thought to myself, "I can do this and bring a perspective to the council as a nurse, mother, and concerned citizen." At the next election, I ran for city council in my ward along with 13 other candidates. I won, and since then, I have held three elected offices: city councilor and mayor, chair of the county commission, and representative in the state legislature. Also, I have recognized the importance of being involved in my professional associations. I have served as president of the Wyoming Nurses Association and second vice president of the American Nurses Association, and currently I serve as first vice president of the American Nurses Association, trustee of the American Nurses Foundation, and past chair and current treasurer of the American Nurses Association Political Action Committee (ANA-PAC).

### WHY DO NURSES MAKE GOOD ELECTED OFFICIALS?

Nursing education and experience provides us with many skills that are valuable in the political environment. The nursing process gives us a framework to solve problems through assessment, developing and implementing plans, and evaluating the outcomes. Executive director of the Minnesota Nurses Association, Erin Murphy (2004) wrote about nurses getting involved in politics:

Our minds, our hands and our voices are essential elements of our work. Each day we witness the miracles and the failings of today's modern health care. Because of what we know, we are obligated professionally, morally and ethically, to work to improve that which is failing.

I agree with Murphy and see the opportunities we have as elected officials to make a difference in addressing the failings.

### Nurses Listen

Nurses have expert communication skills and know how to listen. For example, one snowy night when I was mayor, I received a call from an angry resident who thought the city snowplow was making too much noise clearing his street. I thought most people would be grateful to have the plow cleaning up their street, but I said to the man, "I understand you are upset. Give me 20 minutes and I will have the plow off your street." The caller thanked me. My husband overheard the conversation and said, "That was quick thinking." I knew the plow would be long gone in 20 minutes anyway, and I did not have to call the city service department that night.

### Nurses Have Diverse Areas of Expertise

Nurses also know how to negotiate, partner with others, and resolve conflict. We understand culture, diversity, and teaching others. We know the importance of teamwork and consensus building. Nurses have experience with fiscal management and data management and are creative when resources are limited. When I served on the city council, I found the council had difficulty understanding the health department budget. I was able to help other council members grasp the importance of prevention programs, immunizations, maternal-child health, elder care, safe food preparation in restaurants, and safe drinking water.

### Nurses Are Seen as Credible, Trustworthy Professionals

According to a 2004 Gallup poll (2004), the profession of nursing is ranked number one in trust and respect—higher than physicians, teachers, and clergy. As a nurse, I was able to use my nursing knowledge and credibility effectively as a local leader.

## WHY RUN FOR OFFICE AT THE LOCAL LEVEL?

At the local level, you have the opportunity to help address problems that affect people's everyday lives. For example, a citizen came to a city council meeting one evening and said he wanted passing lanes on a street that was a major artery running north and south in the community. He had a persuasive personality and a reputation for getting what he wanted. His initial presentation was very convincing to other council members. I lived in this neighborhood and was concerned about the safety implications of this proposal. Part of this street abutted a park where children played sports after school. Parents parked along the street to watch or pick up their children. If passing lanes were established in this area, speeds would increase, and the potential risk of a serious accident would rise. I asked every councilperson to visit the area, particularly in the late afternoon. At the next meeting, I had 100% of the council behind me because of the safety issues. All of the members voted against establishing passing lanes on the street.

### Learn the Ropes

The local community is an excellent starting place if you want to run for higher office. You can gain experience, confidence, name recognition, and respect. I had the chance to testify before the Federal Energy Regulatory Commission in Washington, DC, about the high natural gas prices we were paying in our community. Because I was the only mayor to testify (the others providing testimony were senators, representatives, or governors), I was quoted and praised for bringing a refreshing perspective to the Commission.

### Network

As mayor, I worked with citizens, state legislators, and our state's congressional delegation in Washington, DC. Vice President Richard B. (Dick) Cheney was our lone U.S. Representative in Congress when I served as mayor of Casper, Wyoming. I formed an important connection with him because of my service. This type of connection was an important part of my network when I decided to run for the state legislature.

### Gain Expertise and Knowledge of Problems

Some of my efforts bridged both local- and state-level work. I had joined the "Seatbelt Coalition" in Wyoming before running for the legislature. The coalition's mission was to educate Wyoming citizens about the need for seatbelt legislation and develop a model law for the Wyoming legislature to enact. As a freshman legislator, I co-sponsored the first seatbelt legislation aimed at reducing fatalities on Wyoming highways. I also sponsored several pieces of legislation to help assist communities with high natural gas prices. My experience on the city council prepared me to hit the ground running with issues like this when I arrived at the Wyoming state house.

## DEVELOP AN ACTION PLAN TO GET INVOLVED IN POLITICS

### Join a Political Party

You don't have to agree with every part of a party's political platform, but joining a political party is an important step in learning the ropes of politics. Organized political parties provide support and guidance on how to get started with a political campaign. They can provide you with the opportunity to gain experience by working on someone's campaign before actually running yourself. You can learn the steps for running a grassroots campaign, for example, how much money you need to raise, what forms you need to fill out, how to organize a campaign committee, and how to access mailing lists, voter registration, and past precinct results. The parties also raise money, which is used to support the total slate of offices in that particular party. The party can help you get your message out and reach all voters, especially those who might "cross party lines."

### Connect with Other Nurses

Nursing colleagues and associations can be extremely helpful in any political campaign. A group of nurses can send a powerful message of support when they back a candidate. Many state nurses associations have political action committees to assist with endorsements and financial assistance.

### Learn from Others in Your Community

Another helpful activity is to join the League of Woman Voters. The name is derived from the woman's suffrage movement, but today membership is open to women and men. Local leagues will often hold public forums on various issues such as health care. It is a wonderful opportunity to contribute to the dialogue and make connections. The League of Women Voters is also concerned about getting the vote out and what motivates people to go to the polls. This is very important information for a prospective candidate.

### Develop Smart and Cost-Effective, Campaign Strategies

When you are a candidate, you cannot be afraid to ask for money, and you need to take advantage of free and low-cost opportunities to get your message out. Flyers, mailing labels (usually the party you have joined will provide this at a bulk price), newspaper and radio ads, yard signs, and billboards all cost money. Press releases, letters to the editor of newspapers, speaking at meetings and forums, neighborhood cafes, and news stories are free. My cheapest campaign was my first race for city

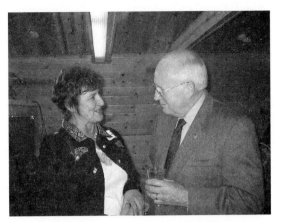

Mary Behrens and Vice President Dick Cheney.

council: We produced a one-page flyer and distributed it door to door. Whenever you choose a strategy like this, it is important to be aware of laws and regulations so you and your campaign staff don't run into problems. For example, you cannot leave flyers in a mailbox because it is a federal offense. If no one is at home, leaving a personal note stating "Sorry I missed you" can be an effective alternative.

### Get the Message Out

Getting out your message is critical to success. You must reach the voters. It does help to get some media training to help frame your messages. The press wants a good story and good "sound bites," so your words should be carefully selected. Don't say anything you would not want to see in print or on TV. The press may not fully understand an issue, and you can help frame the story with your nursing knowledge. If you give accurate information, members of the media will look forward to contacting you again. Experience with handling the media will help you be effective. I've learned from my experience. Don't be afraid to tell the TV crew that you want a "head and chest only" shot of you because you did not have time to change your clothes.

### SUMMARY

Nurses are often silent about political issues. Buresh and Gordon (2000) wrote about how nurses must communicate to the public what nursing does. Nurses bring important skills to the political environment. Now is the time for us to increase the number of nurses at the local level of government and make an important difference in people's lives. As the number of nurses increases, and nursing's contributions are more widely recognized, more nurses will seek and win elected office. As we develop more political leaders, we will be at more policy tables to influence change in the health of our cities, states, and nation. Serving as an elected official can be a very rewarding experience and a great opportunity for advocating for community health improvements.

We need nurses serving at all levels of government. We need nurses working for safe schools and safe drinking water at the local level, working for safe highways and seatbelt usage at the state level, and working for health care reform and funding for nursing education at the federal level. I know Florence Nightingale would be pleased with the progress nurses have made, but I think she would tell us there is a lot of work left to do.

## *Web Resources*

**Federal Energy Regulatory Commission**
*www.ferc.gov*
**How to Run for Local Office**
*www.ehow.com/how_135633_run-local-office.html*
**The League of Women Voters**
*www.lwv.org*
**Nursing's Legislative and Regulatory Initiatives for the 109th Congress**
*www.nursingworld.org/gova/federal/legis/109/initiatives.htm*

### REFERENCES

Buresh, B., & Gordon, S. (2000). *From silence to voice: What nurses know and must communicate to the public.* Ottawa, Ontario, Canada: Canadian Nurses Association.

Gallop Poll. (2004, December 7). Retrieved September 6, 2005, from *www.gallup.com'poll/content/default.aspx?ci=1654* (subscription needed).

Murphy, E. (2004, November/December). Nursing's leadership in American politics. The American nurse, 2004. Retrieved September 6, 2005, from *www.nursingworld.org/member/tan.*

---

## *Vignette*   Bethany Hall-Long

### *Farmgirl, Nurse, and Legislator: My Journey to the Delaware General Assembly*

*"I have come to the conclusion that politics are too serious a matter to be left to the politicians."*
GENERAL CHARLES DE GAULLE

### MY POLITICAL ROOTS

I am a nurse and I became the first health care professional elected into the Delaware General Assembly as well as the first registered nurse elected. The roots of my public involvement began in the farming community where I volunteered to help

others in my church and with neighborhood organizations. At the age of 12, I was a candy-striper in a local hospital and continued my civic work during my teen years. When I entered college, I joined a political party. Though my parents were not politically active, my great-grandfather was a member of the Delaware House of Representatives in the 1920s, and I am a descendent of Delaware's 16th governor.

My interest in politics began while working with underserved residents while completing my master's degree in community health nursing in the late 1980s. I used an earlier edition of this book in my graduate program and vividly recall reading the chapters about becoming involved in politics. I began working with my local city government, the League of Women Voters, and a federal health clinic that served the homeless. Before these experiences, I had thought that public policy was "remote" to nursing and somewhat "dry." These experiences changed my perspective.

## VOLUNTEERING AND CAMPAIGNING

I went on to volunteer with nonprofit and civic organizations, join professional associations, and complete my doctoral degree in nursing administration and public policy. During this time, I served as a U.S. Senate Fellow and as a U.S. Department of Health and Human Services policy analyst for the Secretary's Commission on Nursing. These experiences exposed me to national policy work, federal officials, leaders in the nation's health associations, and international researchers.

I became actively involved with veteran's organizations since my husband was active duty military. I also became a volunteer on political campaigns and with the Democrat Party. I had excellent mentors to assist me with both my nursing and my political career paths. All of these experiences helped me understand the policy process and the importance of building relationships.

I began my work in politics to make a difference in the lives of many citizens who lack life's necessary resources. As a public health nurse, I had an interest in improving the services available to vulnerable populations. I continue to work to advance issues important to the residents I represent; these issues include health care, the environment, land preservation, education, and economic development.

## THERE'S A REASON IT'S CALLED "RUNNING" FOR OFFICE

A number of factors contributed to my decision to run for public office in 2000, including my desire to make a significant contribution to the public's health. As a faculty member, I assigned students to various public health and health policy assignments. In these experiences, I witnessed the need for expert health knowledge in the Delaware General Assembly. The time was "ripe" within the political party and within my district to run for the Delaware legislature.

I ran for office for the first time in 2000 and lost by a mere 1%. I had run against a long-term, male incumbent and learned some important political lessons. In 2002, political redistricting left a vacant seat and I ran again. This time I won in a tough election against the president of the local school board.

## A DAY IN THE LIFE OF A NURSE-LEGISLATOR

One thing for certain in politics is that no two days are alike. Each elected official's experiences and perceptions are linked to his or her beliefs, the district's beliefs, the state's legislative rules, and any external economic or social pressures. In Delaware, serving as a legislator is a part-time job. Delaware's bicameral legislative session is a total of 45 days a year. Session convenes each January, and the legislature must pass the budget bill and recess by July 1. We meet three days a week—Tuesday, Wednesday, and Thursday. I spend the other days on constituent work, meetings, speeches, and continuing my other job as a nursing faculty member. Between July and January my days are filled with at least 8 to 12 hours of meetings, community work, and in election years, with campaign activities.

Much of a state legislator's time is spent on the capital and operating budgets of the state, as well as Senate confirmations. These central activities need to be completed by the end of the state's fiscal year, July 1. My most important role is to represent my constituents at committee meetings, public hearings, on task forces, and as a sponsor or co-sponsor of relevant bills. My district is both rural and suburban and has numerous policy needs: smart growth, transportation, education, health care, and economic development.

I juggle caring for my family, legislative work, and nursing education. I'm up at 5 AM to exercise, then I have breakfast meetings with constituents or campaign committee members. Then I usually put on my other "hat" and spend time with my nursing students. I return phone calls in my car as I head into the state capital.

When I arrive in my office, I'm greeted with phone messages, e-mail, and the pressing issues of the day. I share one staff member with two other officials. Session begins around 2 PM when we enter caucus for 30 to 45 minutes to discuss the legislative agenda and bills to be voted upon. One day a week there are committee hearings. In the afternoon, I squeeze in more phone calls, RSVPs, research with the lawyers, and head back to the House floor for votes.

After each legislative day, there are usually receptions sponsored by interest groups. These provide time for lobbyists and members to review issues and concerns and highlight state funding efforts or programs. Typically, I attend several civic or association meetings each evening after the session in my district. (I balance these with my son's sporting and school events.) These meetings are important for gathering community input, staying current on issues, and letting my constituents know that I am concerned about their issues. It all takes a lot of time, energy, and a few cups of coffee.

## WHAT I'VE BEEN ABLE TO ACCOMPLISH AS A NURSE-LEGISLATOR

I have co-sponsored a range of legislation as a member of the Health and Human Development, Agriculture, Natural Resources and the Environment, Homeland Security, and Education Committees. As the only health care professional in the Delaware General Assembly, I have been the prime sponsor of some important health bills and on task forces such as the Governor's Cancer Council and the Health Fund Advisory (Master Tobacco Settlement Committee).

I have worked on public health and environmental policies as a State Representative and as an appointed public member of blue ribbon commissions and legislative task forces. These policy issues have included occupational health, cancer, minority health, health professions, environmental justice, chronic illness, mercury removal form the environment, school health, early childhood education, prescription assistance, and end-of-life care decisions. I have found that having a nursing background is extremely valuable in influencing a wide variety of policy issues.

I have worked very closely with the farmers in my district—I was raised on a farm and know how vital farming is. I was pleased to sponsor, as my first piece of legislation, the farmland preservation license tag. I am working with community leaders to establish a non-profit land trust. The community I represent is experiencing rapid development pressures, so there is a need to mix private and public monies to assist farmers. In addition, I have sponsored land use legislation that helps with county, municipal, and state communication.

One percent of the U.S. population consumes more than 25% of all health care expenditures, and 5% of the population accounts for more than 50% of the total expenditure (U.S. Department of Health and Human Services, 2004). Chronic illness is a major issue for Delaware, as it is for the nation. I sponsored legislation to establish a blue ribbon task force to analyze the problem of chronic illness in Delaware and develop policy recommendations. The task force identified strategies including disease standards of care for health professions, improved communication between insurers and providers, outreach to the at-risk, and the use of a disease management approach with Medicaid patients and in the business community.

I was the prime House sponsor of legislation creating a cancer consortium for Delaware. This group has completed a comprehensive assessment and plans to tackle our high cancer mortality rates. I am pleased to say that the cancer incidence and cancer rates have dropped since the creation of this body. The state has implemented the consortium's many recommendations, including establishing a free treatment program for cancer patients who lack insurance, adding statewide caseworkers and creating screening programs. In addition, the Clean Indoor Air bill passed in 2002 and has eliminated smoking in public places in Delaware.

HIV infection rates in Delaware are among the highest in the nation. I co-sponsored needle exchange legislation. Unfortunately, given its ethical implications, this policy topic has not passed the House of Representatives. I co-sponsored the primary seatbelt law. For three years, I have tried to create a state Office of Health and Safety but have not been successful. This year, I am introducing a "scaled back" version of the bill to create a voluntary occupational health program.

## TIPS FOR INFLUENCING ELECTED OFFICIALS' HEALTH POLICY DECISIONS

What have I learned as a legislator that can help other nurses who are seeking to influence legislators? You must communicate well to influence policy, and nurses are naturally gifted communicators and problem solvers. In a study of nurse leaders in federal politics, I found that the political strategies used most frequently by nursing organizations are direct contacts, grassroots efforts, and coalition formation (Hall-Long, 1995).

Nurses should not be intimidated by needing to call, write, or visit their elected officials. It is important when meeting with elected officials that you are prepared, have a one-page fact sheet to leave behind (not a binder of information), and be prepared to summarize your issue and offer solutions in less than five minutes.

## IS IT WORTH IT?

If nurses don't speak on health care issues, who will? Physicians? Hospitals? Technicians? If nurses don't speak up, legislators will only hear from other groups. You've heard the expression, "It's not whether you win or lose but how you play the game." Well, in politics, how you play the game can determine whether you win or lose an issue. Increasing your influence by working in a group or coalition is an extremely effective strategy. Life as an elected official has been better than I could have imagined. Though it has taken some time away from my family and my scholarship, it has been worthwhile.

### REFERENCES

Hall-Long, B. (1995). Nursing education at political crossroads. *Journal of Professional Nursing, 11*(3), 139-146.

U.S. Department of Health and Human Services (DHHS). (2004). *The burden of chronic diseases and their risk factors: National and state perspectives 2004.* Washington, DC: DHHS.

---

# *Vignette* The Honorable Lois Capps

## A Nurse in Congress

*"Experience is not what happens to you; it's what you do with what happens to you."*

ALDOUS HUXLEY

If someone had told me on the day I earned my nursing degree from Pacific Lutheran University that I would become a member of Congress, I never would have believed it. But here I am today—a nurse, a mother, and a member of Congress. I didn't come to Congress under normal circumstances. My husband, Walter Capps, was elected to the U.S. House of Representatives in 1996 and I went with him to Washington, DC, where we were both excited about making a difference.

Tragically, our time together there was cut short when he died suddenly of a heart attack on October 28, 1997. Of course, my life changed forever. While grieving for the loss of my husband, I was also faced with questions about who would take his place in Congress. In the midst of the numbness and shock, I was approached about running to fill his seat. I was filled with so many questions. How could I run? What could I offer to the community? Was I qualified to be a member of Congress? To be true to myself, I had to be able to translate my life experiences into a tangible vision for how to improve the quality of life in California's central coast, the area I would represent. Although the campaign was hard, the answers to my questions were easy—I was and would always be a nurse.

While I never imagined running for office, I now know how relevant my nursing background is to my work in Congress. I spent most of my career as a public health nurse in schools, where, among other things, I helped teen mothers and fathers complete their education and learn to care for their children. Most of a school nurse's time is spent working for, and with, families whose children lack adequate resources for health care. Perhaps it is the child who fails a vision or hearing screening with no money for glasses or insurance for follow-up care. It may be the many children in our schools with gaping holes in their teeth who have never been to see a dentist. It may be those who experience abuse at home, who are depressed or even suicidal. Meeting these children and having countless other experiences during my nursing career have given me a unique perspective on the health care issues before Congress. Whether we're debating how to keep Medicare or Medicaid solvent or how to expand health care coverage to the uninsured, my years of training and experience give me firsthand knowledge not available to many of my colleagues. As I prepare to vote or speak on the floor of the U.S. House of Representatives, I often recall a particular student, young mom, or encounter that inspires me to work to improve the lives of people back home.

Nurses have a particular interest in how health care is delivered, how patients are cared for, and the continued advancement of health care delivery and services. We are advocates for our patients, and we aren't afraid to get our hands dirty. But we need to make sure our voices are heard. Special interest groups are everywhere, fighting for what's in their best interests, not in patients' best interests. At no time has this been more glaringly apparent than during the discussions on the Medicare prescription drug benefit—we could have used more nurses in Congress when that passed.

Practicing nursing for 30 years prepared me for service in Congress in many ways. First, both legislators and nurses must be good listeners. I believe that quality representation means taking the time to understand the views and problems of one's constituents. As a nurse, I was an advocate for my patients. Today as a Congresswoman, I'm an advocate for my constituents. Nurses learn to withhold premature judgment, to work as a team, to set goals and priorities, and to meet them. Also, nurses are taught to put the common good before their personal ambition and ahead of political interests. I developed these important skills during my nursing career, and they have served me well as a member of Congress.

Many of my legislative priorities come out of my experiences as a nurse. I worked hard to be appointed to the powerful House Committee on Energy and Commerce, which has jurisdiction over health issues. From this position, I have been able to play an active role in shaping health care policy in Congress. I'm proud of many of the things we have accomplished, including helping to pass the Breast and Cervical Cancer Treatment Act, increase funding for the National Institutes of Health, modernize the Food and Drug Administration, and improve children's health benefits. I've introduced my own legislation to help amyotrophic lateral sclerosis patients gain immediate Medicare coverage, to improve mental health care services, to recognize and help educate new mothers about postpartum depression, to eliminate youth drinking, and to teach cardiopulmonary resuscitation in schools—all of this legislation was enacted.

But there are still so many challenges before us, and we need your help to protect Medicaid from budget cuts, improve Medicare's coverage of prescription drugs, improve care for heart disease and stroke among women, and expand health care coverage to the uninsured. Another issue directly affects our profession: We are currently experiencing a shortage of nurses of crisis proportions, and we need to encourage more people to enter the nursing workforce. And who better to address the shortage than a nurse? In 2002, with the help of millions of nurses across the country, I was able to prod the Congress into passing the Nurse Reinvestment Act. This law establishes nurse education scholarships that would help pay for a nurse's education in exchange for a commitment to work for a period of time in a facility with a shortage of nurses. It also is designed to help current nurses afford more training and education so they can advance to the next level of nursing. The law also calls for greater efforts to help change the public's perception of nursing and for facilitating relationships between schools and health care facilities to help educate young people about the rewards of a nursing career.

In drafting this legislation, I called on my own experiences and sought the expertise of the people who know what needs to be done to fix the crisis—nurses. Furthermore, nurses around the country flexed their political muscle to help pass this important bill. Members of the American Nurses Association, the American Organization of Nurse Executives, the American Association of College Nurses, and many other nursing organizations lobbied members of Congress across the country—and the political spectrum—to support the bill. Since that time, we have been working hard to increase funding for these very programs, pass legislation that will improve working conditions in health care facilities, and provide assistance to schools of nursing so they can expand to meet our considerable needs. Because of the influence nurses can have when they get involved, I'm hopeful that we can get the federal government to more adequately address the nursing shortage. This is only one example of how nurses can significantly affect public policy.

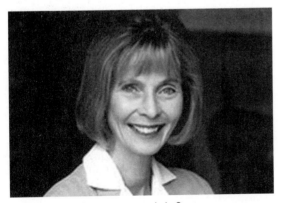

Congresswoman Lois Capps.

Nurses also can become part of the political process by volunteering on a campaign. Nurses in my district came out in droves to support my campaign. They organized phone banks, walked precincts, and made phone calls to support my candidacy. Having their support has been invaluable. I would not be in Congress today if it were not for the dedication and hard work of these nurses and other citizen groups, as well as the endorsement and support of the American Nurses Association's Political Action Committee.

Don't be afraid to put your own name on the ballot. As I've already pointed out, my nursing experience made me uniquely qualified to serve in Congress. The same is true for most nurses. Get out there and do it. Start serving on a local committee or run for city council or for the school board. Or if you're someone who feels less comfortable in the spotlight, volunteer on campaigns of candidates who share your ideals. It's never too late to get involved. I was 60 when I was first elected to Congress, my first elected office.

Nurses have credibility and respect. People trust us. Our professional knowledge enables us to advocate for safe, quality health care; promote education for children; and address other issues on patients' behalf. I am one of only three nurses in Congress. We need more nurses to become involved. When I first ran for office, my critics attacked me by saying, "What does a nurse know about politics or public policy?" But politics is everywhere—whether you're in a hospital, a school district, or in the halls of Congress. Nurses have unique experiences that distinguish us from traditional politicians. We have an important voice in the legislative process, and when we use it, there is no limit to what we can accomplish. As you move forward in your nursing career, I hope that you will consider becoming part of the political process as well. We need you—and your community will thank you.

# Vignette  The Honorable Carolyn McCarthy

## I Believed I Could Make a Difference

*"You gain strength, courage and confidence by every experience in which you really stop to look fear in the face. You are able to say to yourself, 'I lived through this horror. I can take the next thing that comes along.' You must do the thing you think you cannot do."*

ELEANOR ROOSEVELT

There are many routes to becoming a member of Congress. Few members' journeys to Capitol Hill, though, have gained the attention of the public—and the media—as Carolyn McCarthy's has. McCarthy was a suburban Long Island homemaker and licensed practical nurse most of her adult life. However, since 1996, she has had a movie of her life produced by Barbra Streisand, addressed the Democratic National Convention, appeared on Oprah, and had her story chronicled in a Lifetime Television "Intimate Portrait."

McCarthy's path to Congress has received great attention because it is like few others. She was thrust into the national media spotlight when the fabric of her family life was torn apart by violence. In 1993, McCarthy lived with her family in the same Long Island home in which she was reared. McCarthy's husband Dennis, a 56-year-old stockbroker, and her only child Kevin, then a 26-year-old employee of the same firm his father worked for, commuted together to and from New York City. On the evening of December 7, 1993, they were sitting together on a train on the Long Island Rail Road coming home. A lone gunman with a 9-mm semiautomatic pistol walked through two cars and shot 25 people. McCarthy's husband, Dennis, was one of 6 killed, and her son, Kevin, was one of 19 wounded. Kevin, shot in the head, was paralyzed and in a coma. He was given little chance of recovery. McCarthy devoted herself to his recovery and asked the question "Could this have been prevented?"

Was it the tragic shooting itself that motivated McCarthy to seek a seat in Congress? No—it was the action of her Congressional Representative on gun violence. A little over 2 years after the Long Island Rail Road shootings, Representative Daniel Frisa, the Republican Congressman representing her district, voted in March 1996 to repeal a ban on some types of assault weapons. McCarthy was outraged and sensed, correctly, that other citizens in her district were too.

After deciding to run against Frisa, she met many obstacles. Although she had been a lifelong Republican, the local Republican party would not back her, so she became a Democrat. Her opponent, incumbent Frisa, painted her as a "one-issue candidate" (Shapiro, 1996). She rejected that charge and demonstrated her commitment to many political issues. However, her gun control advocacy made her a target of the National Rifle Association. This served to harden her resolve.

Despite obstacles, McCarthy won a resounding victory and became the first woman to represent any part of Long Island in the House of Representatives.. She was sworn in on January 1, 1997, a few days before her 53rd birthday, and has been reelected four times.

My mother always said, "You can't go forward until you know where you've been." In that spirit, I have analyzed how my nursing background and other events in my life shaped my journey to Congress. When I was a teenager, I took care of a friend of mine who had been in a car accident. He and I were very close, and it hurt quite a bit to see him in pain, but I realized I could help, and I wanted to do that for the rest of my life. I find it ironic that the biggest challenge I faced as a young adult—losing someone—was the reason I became a nurse. The same event became the reason for my decision to enter politics.

December 7, 1993, is the date when havoc was wreaked in my family's life. Anticipation of the holiday season quickly turned to dread when my husband Dennis was killed and my son Kevin seriously injured as a result of the Long Island Rail Road incident. My family life changed dramatically in a span of mere minutes. Suddenly I was a wife without a husband, had a son without a father, and our extended family was without a brother, uncle, and nephew. Thankfully—but even more tragically—Dennis and Kevin had recently become closer than ever, commuting into the city together on the very train that tore them apart.

After Dennis' death and Kevin's recovery, I became committed to taking action on easy access to guns in our country. I asked my Congressman in Washington, DC, to vote against repealing the ban on assault weapons—but he voted to repeal the ban! I thought he was out of touch with his constituents on Long Island. A reporter caught me shortly afterward and asked if I was angry enough at my Congressman's vote to run against him. I said, "Sure, I'm Irish and I'm mad enough!" Well, the next day, the papers all said, "McCarthy to run against Frisa!" The phone started ringing, people started backing me, and the rest is history.

There are many days I wake up and still can't believe I serve in Congress. Since I've been here, I've used my nursing experience constantly. I've worked to educate the American people—and my colleagues—on gun violence and the costs of gun violence on our health care system. No one talks about those who survive gun violence and struggle for years to regain what they've lost, but I've lived that with my son Kevin and know the struggle all too well.

One of my top priorities in Congress is to alleviate the nursing shortage facing our country. The nursing shortage in America has reached dangerous levels: There are now over 120,000 job openings for registered nurses in hospitals nationwide. We are facing a national crisis; unfortunately, it will only get worse if we do not act now.

I am happy to report that in July of 2002, Congress took an important first step to alleviate the nursing shortage by passing the Nurse Reinvestment Act. This law, which President Bush signed on August 1, 2002, is designed to encourage people to enter and remain in nursing careers. Specifically, the law provides scholarships and loans to nursing students

---

## The Carolyn McCarthy Center for Gun Violence

### WHAT WE STAND FOR

- Ending the pattern of gun violence in America
- Renewing the Assault Weapons Ban
- Keeping guns out of the hands of criminals
- Instituting a national instant criminal background check system in conjunction with the no-fly list
- Restrictions on armor-piercing ammunition
- Closing gun show loopholes
- Child safety gun education
- Prohibiting cop-killer bullets
- Implementing tougher safety standards on gun makers
  - Child safety locks
  - Smart fingerprint technology

### WHAT WE DO

- Provide Americans with a voice to speak out against gun violence
- Provide candidates, both federal and local, with support to speak out on the issue without fear of being defeated by the National Rifle Association
- Act as a forum for victims of gun violence to tell their stories and meet others who have shared similar experiences
- Regularly update Americans on legislation and accomplishments in ending gun violence
- Establish and run a clearinghouse for gun-related resources

---

who agree to serve in a hospital with a critical shortage of nurses. The law also establishes outreach programs to encourage more individuals to enter the nursing profession.

After the Michigan school shooting when one 6-year-old killed another, I began looking into ways schools could use federal funding to pay for school nurses. Currently, only 14 states mandate a nurse in every school. I want to change that; there should be a nurse in every school.

In a single year, 2867 children and teens are killed by gunfire in the United States, according to the latest national data released in 2002 (Children's Defense Fund, 2005). That is 1 child every 3 hours, 8 children every day, and more than 50 children every week. If we are going to expel students from school for having guns, then we should educate children

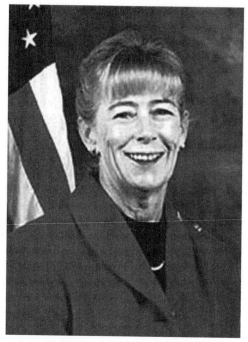

Congresswoman Carolyn McCarthy.

help more women come forward and ensure that more batterers and abusers get prosecuted for these vicious crimes.

On the grassroots level, nurses must face their legislators and ask them, "What are you doing to help me keep this country healthy?" You have to ask the questions because most politicians today are hoping nobody does. Demand an answer, and if you don't like the answer, tell them what you think and what you want them to do.

I often tell groups that one person can make a difference. However, even more can be done when one person is joined by two and three and four and then thousands. That's when a real difference is made! After 30 years of nursing, I learned to pray for patience and faith. I drew on that strength before I came to Congress. I often think being a member of Congress is not so different than the years I was a working in a hospital. Back then, I had a floor of patients to take care of; today, I have 435 patients! Nursing is a practice built on patience and education, and so is service in Congress.

and parents about the importance of using child safety locks. We should print brochures to send home to parents and guardians and educate children and adults about child safety locks. Only then will American school children have a fighting chance to learn their school lessons rather than the lesson that life is too short.

In 2005, I announced co-sponsorship of legislation reauthorizing the Violence Against Women Act (VAWA). Since 1994, VAWA has been a great success as many battered women now have places in their communities to turn to escape abusive relationships. But incidences of domestic violence still occur at a disturbing rate, and Congress must continue what we started in 1994. This legislation makes a good law even better. We have come far in eliminating the social stigma attached to being a victim of domestic violence; this legislation will

## *Web Resources*

**Brady Campaign to Prevent Gun Violence**
*www.bradycampaign.org*
**The Carolyn McCarthy Center on Gun Violence and Harm Reduction**
*www.cmccenter.org*
**Congresswoman Carolyn McCarthy**
*http://carolynmccarthy.house.gov*

### REFERENCES

Children's Defense Fund. (2005). Protect children, not guns. Retrieved March 14, 2006, from *www.childrensdefense.org/education/gunviolence/gunreport2005/gunreport2005.pdf*.

EMILY's List. (2000). EMILY's List honors Rep. Carolyn McCarthy and Sen. Dianne Feinstein for their leadership on gun-safety issues. Retrieved from *www.emilylist.org*.

Shapiro, B. (1996, November). Running against the gun: McCarthy on Long Island. *The Nation*.

## My Path to Congress

*"Each person must live their life as a model for others."*

ROSA PARKS

*Congresswoman Eddie Bernice Johnson (D-TX-30) has had a long career of service to others, beginning with a career as a nurse and leading to election as a member of Congress in 1992. Johnson was born and reared in Waco, Texas. Johnson's father insisted she attend college, and a high school counselor sparked her interest in nursing. In 1955, Johnson graduated with a diploma in nursing, completed a bachelor's degree in nursing in 1967, and a master's of public policy in 1976. She served as Chief Psychiatric Nurse at the Dallas, Texas, Veterans Administration Hospital for five years.*

*Johnson's political career began at the urging of friends in 1972. She waged a successful campaign for the Texas House of Representatives, becoming the first woman since 1935 to be elected to the Texas House from Dallas County. She chaired the Labor Committee, becoming the first woman in Texas history to lead a major Texas House committee. Her reputation as a hard-working negotiator earned her an appointment by President Jimmy Carter to become Regional Director of the Department of Health, Education and Welfare in 1977. In 1986, she was elected Texas State Senator. In 1992, she became the first black female to be elected to represent the Dallas area in the U.S. House of Representatives. Johnson was the chair of the Congressional Black Caucus during the 107th Congress, and in 2001 Ebony Magazine named Johnson one of the 10 most powerful black women in America.*

My parents instilled in me the value of a good education. They taught me to always be ethical and truthful. My father used to say, "You can be anything you want as long as you are law-abiding, self-supporting, and God-fearing," though I have rephrased that over the years to be "God-respecting." My mother has truly been an inspiration in my life. She remains one of the greatest volunteers I've ever known. It is due to her encouragement that I became a volunteer and learned to care for others and my community.

When I decided to become a nurse, I gave it my all. As a nursing student, I worked with children and eventually moved into psychiatric nursing. I spent five years serving at the Dallas Veterans Administration Hospital. During that time, I worked with hundreds of veterans who served our nation with grace and without question. I consider it an honor to have been able to care for them.

Fifteen years into my nursing career, due to the urging of my friends and community leaders,

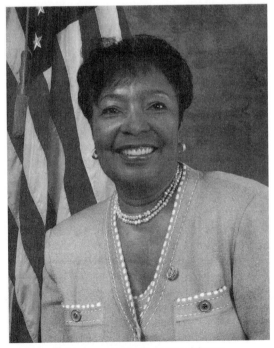

Congresswoman Eddie Bernice Johnson.

I decided to make a run for public office. It wasn't a decision reached without reservation. Like many women with a career, I had to balance family life, parenting, and my professional responsibilities while trying to be successful in the world of politics. My son, Kirk, was 11 years old at the time of my first campaign, and I knew the campaign would take me away from him. Kirk didn't think twice. He signed up for a home economics class at school and told me not to worry about the dishes or laundry. Kirk was determined to help me win, and he remains one of my strongest supporters. I knew running for office would not be easy.

I was able to transition to a career in public service successfully because of my experience as a nurse. Nursing taught me to be responsible, to pay attention to details, to work hard, and to get the job done. What I learned as a nurse has helped me tremendously in Congress.

I am now in my seventh term in Congress, representing the citizens of the 30th congressional district. I've been engaged in a wide variety of issues including science, technology, transportation, the environment, health care, election reform, and civil rights. I sit on the House Transportation and Infrastructure Committee, and I am the Ranking Democratic Member of the Subcommittee on Water Resources and the Environment.

During the 107th Congress, I sponsored legislation designed to reauthorize federal welfare programs and add stronger anti-discrimination provisions, remedy environmental injustice, and make the tax code fairer for workers whose primary tax is the payroll tax. I've sponsored bills to address HIV/ AIDS, to honor veterans, and to double funding for the National Science Foundation. I've spoken out about shortcomings in Medicare and have joined others in seeking increased funding for osteoporosis research funding.

I serve on the House Committee on Science and have spent many years advocating for a federal initiative program to encourage children to study science and math. I am very proud to have had the University of Texas at Dallas establish a lecture series in my name that is designed to encourage Dallas-area high school students to consider careers in science and engineering.

After the tragedy of 9/11, I began an initiative called A World of Women for World Peace. The program's mission is to encourage people to move beyond politics, race, class, and geography to work together to build a culture of peace in the world.

I believe once a nurse, always a nurse. I know now that my career in nursing not only paved the way for my career in public service but also prepared me in more ways than I ever thought possible. As a nurse I was able to care for others, and now as a member of Congress I am able to use my skills to serve my constituents with sensitivity.

## *Web Resources*

**Congresswoman Eddie Bernice Johnson**
*www.house.gov/ebjohnson*
**A World of Women for World Peace**
*www.house.gov/ebjohnson/wow_ebj/index.shtml*

## Hog-Housed: The Life and Death of Bachelor of Science in Nursing Entry to Practice in North Dakota

*"Sometimes I lie awake at night, and I ask, 'Where have I gone wrong?' Then a voice says to me, 'This is going to take more than one night.'"*

CHARLIE BROWN

Consensus about the type of education needed for entry into professional practice has long eluded the discipline of nursing. Other professions have consistently upgraded their educational standards without the noise, confusion, and protest that have accompanied nursing's attempts in this area. One state, North Dakota, was successful in establishing the baccalaureate degree as the educational criterion for entry into practice. Unfortunately, the citizens of North Dakota were unsuccessful in maintaining their accomplishment. This is the story of how and why such a novel attempt failed. It is a story of being "hog-housed."

### HISTORICAL BACKGROUND

In 1948, Esther Lucille Brown published *Nursing for the Future*. Brown's research led her to conclude that professional schools of nursing should be placed in degree-granting institutions. Her report received little attention, and there were few voices calling for significant change in nursing education.

The American Nurses Association (ANA) published its position paper on nursing education in 1965. Rapidly advancing technology, social changes, and the enactment of Medicare and Medicaid were changing the hospital business (ANA, 1965). Enrollment in diploma nursing programs was declining, and the number of associate degree programs in community colleges was increasing. This publication received much attention, and its recommendations about education divided the nursing community.

Although no deadline was established, the authors of the position paper envisioned an orderly transition to a time when the minimum preparation for beginning professional nursing practice would be baccalaureate degree education and preparation for technical nursing practice would be an associate degree in nursing. Unfortunately, the terms "technical nursing" and "professional nursing" were not defined. The graduates of diploma, associate degree, and baccalaureate degree programs took the same licensing exams and became registered nurses (RNs) subject to the same state laws and regulations.

Nurses in practice, as well as nurses in education, however, were very aware of the increasing responsibility nurses had in patient care and of the need to ensure an adequate grounding not only in psychomotor and comfort skills but also in the knowledge, abilities, and attitudes embedded in the liberal arts. In 1978, the ANA spoke out again on nursing education when its House of Delegates passed a resolution to require the baccalaureate degree as the minimum preparation for entry into professional nursing practice by 1985 (Donley & Flaherty, 2002).

Because entry into nursing practice is regulated by individual states, action to effect a change in requirements needs to be done through state legislation or regulation. Each state board of nursing is charged with protection of the public and has the authority and obligation to determine requirements for admission to practice in the particular state. Until 1984, all states deemed that graduates from associate degree, diploma, baccalaureate, or generic graduate programs were eligible to take the RN licensing exam. As the 1985 deadline approached, nurses in several states ratcheted up their efforts to require the baccalaureate degree in nursing for entry into practice. North Dakota was one such state.

## THE NORTH DAKOTA EXPERIENCE

In 1980, the North Dakota Nurses Association (NDNA) resolved to support the 1965 ANA recommendation and to work with the board of nursing to put bi-level entry requirements into place. Representatives of many interest groups (practical, associate degree, diploma, and baccalaureate nursing programs; the board of nursing, the state nurses association, the state licensed practical nurses association, the board of higher education, the state hospital association, and the vocational education association) met to identify risks and benefits and to develop strategies to implement the resolution. The majority of participants in these meetings were in favor of two levels of nursing. According to George and Young (1990), no action toward baccalaureate entry was likely in states where the number of associate degree in nursing programs was double or more than the number of bachelor of science in nursing (BSN) programs. In 1983, North Dakota had three diploma nursing programs, four baccalaureate programs, and three associate degree programs. The odds for success were favorable.

Eight of the ten nursing programs were in favor of the change. Opposition to the baccalaureate requirement came primarily from two of the diploma programs and other members of a small group calling themselves "concerned nurses."

Given the support for the resolution, NDNA in 1983 established a statewide coordinating committee on entry into practice. The committee determined that the associate degree should be established as entry level for licensed practical nurses (LPNs) and the baccalaureate degree as the entry level for licensed RNs.

The establishment of educational standards for nursing in North Dakota was a responsibility of the state board of nursing. Thus, changing entry into practice requirements was a regulatory process and not a legislative one. In the spring of 1984, the state board of nursing responded positively to the coordinating council's request to revise its administrative rules and regulations and to specify the associate degree as preparation for the LPN and the baccalaureate degree as required preparation for the RN as referred to in the Nurse Practices Act. The board of nursing formed an ad hoc committee to rewrite the rules for nursing education.

Even though support from nurses and from the public was strong, there were vocal opponents. Administrators of two of the hospitals that had diploma schools were adamant in their opposition. The "concerned nurses" and the administrators of the diploma programs had a bill introduced into the state legislature that would have prevented the North Dakota state board of nursing from setting new education standards. There was vigorous lobbying on both sides. More than 300 nurses attended the hearings. Proponents contended that the board of nursing was exceeding its statutory authority. Others felt strongly that the legislature was no place to settle internal professional issues. The bill was defeated by a substantial majority (personal communication with Betty Maher, former Executive Director of the North Dakota Nurses Association, March 2002).

In January of 1986, the state board of nursing adopted the rules for nursing education that required the baccalaureate degree for entry into professional nursing practice and the associate degree for licensure as a practical nurse. The revisions were filed with the North Dakota Legislative Council for publication and would have the effect of law upon publication.

In March of 1986, the board was served with a temporary restraining order in response to a lawsuit filed by two hospital diploma programs. The court decided, without dissent, in favor of the North Dakota Board of Nursing (*Trinity Medical Center v. North Dakota Board of Nursing*, 1987). The baccalaureate degree was established as the minimum academic requirement for entry into practice as a professional RN in North Dakota.

### Mission Accomplished—For a Short Time

How nurses in a state known for its political conservatism and not known for social innovation could have actualized the controversial 1965 ANA position paper is a study in effective political action. The following are reasons why it worked.

*Goal clarity.* The goal was simple, clear, attainable, and reflected the same central themes as were articulated in the original 1965 ANA position paper and in Brown's report:

■ Recognition of the importance of preparation for professional practice of a liberal education with its consequent impact on patient safety and other positive health care outcomes

■ Acknowledgment that nursing is a scholarly activity with scientific foundations

*Goal attainability.* The goal was attainable. All but one of the six non-BSN programs preparing for RN licensure were situated in a 4-year college or in a city where there was a 4-year college/university. This meant that there was little competition for students.

For reasons unrelated to entry-into-practice regulatory changes, a closing date had already been set for some of the LPN programs. Those that remained welcomed the opportunity to enrich their curricula and further invest in the community college structure.

The process of increasing educational requirements for a profession was not foreign to the state. Within the collective memory of North Dakota citizens was a time when elementary school teachers needed only a certificate earned in two or less years of postsecondary education. In 1987, a baccalaureate degree, as well as continuing education, was established as the minimum requirement for a teaching position. This supported baccalaureate entry for nursing, and the public response made it clear that it was reasonable to expect a registered nurse to have an education at least comparable to that of an elementary school teacher.

*Unity and collaboration.* Equally important, the nursing community was united. Yes, there were the "concerned nurses" who opposed the change, but this group constituted a small minority of the RN population. Most nursing leaders were vocal in their support of the proposed changes. The majority of nurses who were teaching in diploma, associate degree, and baccalaureate programs were solidly in favor of the revision. In addition, the change in entry-level requirements had the support of leaders in major clinical agencies who saw the upgrade of nursing education as a means to improve the quality of patient care.

The process used to bring about the change was an inclusive one. At every step, all stakeholders were invited to the table. LPNs; RNs in direct care, administrative, and educator roles; hospital and other health agency administrators; representatives of regulatory bodies; legislators; and consumers participated in committee work, the coordinating council, public hearings, and the ad hoc rule-writing committee.

*Protection of stakeholders.* There was attentiveness to do "no harm" to nurses or their employers. RNs and LPNs in practice at the time of the change in regulations were "grandfathered" into the process; that is, they could continue to renew their licenses with their original designation, no matter what their educational preparation had been. The new standards applied only to persons enrolling in a nursing program after January 1, 1987.

*Staying focused.* Finally, the message was kept on target. Once the outcome was determined—two levels of entry into nursing practice, technical (LPN) and professional (RN)—the focus was on achieving the regulatory changes in a timely manner. Other states had done preliminary work to institute the regulatory or legislative change. There was friendly competition to see who would be first to achieve the goal. North Dakota nurses were pleased to be the first (and only) state in the nation to attain the goal and expected that other states would soon have similar regulations.

## Demise of the Regulation

The finely knit entry-into-practice coalition began to unravel soon after the last knot was tied. During each legislative session after "entry" regulations had been instituted, bills were introduced to weaken or substantially change the educational requirements for the RN and by default for the LPN. In response to concerns about the shortage of nurses, a provision for temporary (later called transitional) licensure was inserted into the practices act in 1989. Under this provision, licensed nurses without the proper academic credential who moved into the state could receive a temporary license to practice for a period of time, provided they showed progress toward achieving the appropriate degree for the desired level of practice. The temporary license was touted as a way to secure adequate staffing, particularly in long-term care facilities where most nursing vacancies occurred.

### Strategies for Defeat

In 1995, legislation was again introduced to undo the changes of 1987. In an attempt to defeat that proposed legislation and to keep the issue from reappearing every legislative session, another bill was introduced to remove establishment of educational standards from the authority of the state board of nursing and to define educational levels in the Nurse Practices Act legislation. The bill passed, and educational requirements were moved outside the authority of the board of nursing.

*Loss of unity.* In 2003, a small group of nurses had a legislator introduce a bill to move oversight of nursing education from the jurisdiction of the board of nursing to the board of higher education. The bill's supporters were distressed that the board of nursing was vulnerable to outside pressures and lacked enthusiasm for the established educational standards. However, most nurses were not convinced it was wise to revoke the board's oversight of nursing education. The unity that had been the sustaining force of the movement toward baccalaureate entry in the 1980s was shattered.

*Co-Opting the message.* Lobbyists for health associations carefully orchestrated their opposition by blaming education requirements for the difficulty in recruiting nurses to rural long-term care facilities. The bill changed daily as nurses testified for and against the various versions, creating a picture of a profession divided. Legislators heard a muddled message and conflicting conclusions. On the other hand, the nursing home industry gave a very clear message. Representatives of long-term care facilities testified that it was too costly to have baccalaureate educated RNs. Although this seems counter to the general belief that a well-educated workforce is essential to economic development, legislators were getting tired and confused, and "economic benefit" sounded good.

Community college administrators began to realize that an associate degree program that prepared students for RN licensure would increase enrollment and state funding for their programs. In their

testimony, they questioned why North Dakota should be different from other states (American Association of Community Colleges, 1999).

### The Outcome

The original bill, which would have moved responsibility for nursing education from the state board of nursing to the state board of higher education, was eviscerated. A series of amendments were inserted. The bill that was finally signed into law by the governor bore resemblance neither to the original bill nor to anything else supported by the majority of nurses. In essence, the bill was hog-housed. *Hog-housed* is legislative jargon that means a bill is essentially rewritten to remove all language and substitute all new language. The intent is to decimate the original legislation. The requirements of the baccalaureate degree for entry into practice as a registered professional nurse and the associate degree for entry into practice as a licensed practical nurse were erased and the authority of the board of nursing diminished (Mooney, 2003).

## *Lessons Learned*

- Arguments for baccalaureate entry into nursing are consistent with positions supporting education for other professions.
- Nurses need to unite around an issue before it is taken to a public forum.
- The best policy can be hog-housed if supporters are not vigilant and mindful of maintaining unity.

### REFERENCES

American Association of Community Colleges. (1999). Position statement on associate degree nursing. Retrieved February 4, 2005, from *www.aacc.nche.edu.*

American Nurses Association (ANA). (1965). Education for nursing. *American Journal of Nursing, 65*(12), 106-111.

Brown, E. (1948). *Nursing for the future.* New York: Russell Sage Foundation.

Donley, R., & Flaherty, M. (2002). Revisiting the American Nurses Association's first position on education for nurses. *Online Journal of Issues in Nursing, 7*(2). Retrieved February 4, 2005, from *www.nursingworld.org/ojin/topic18/tpc18_1.htm.*

George, S., & Young, W. (1990). Baccalaureate entry into practice: An example of political innovation and diffusion. *Journal of Nursing Education, 29*(8), 341-345.

Joel, L. (2002, May 31). Education for entry into nursing practice: Revisited for the 21st century. *Online Journal of Issues in Nursing*, 7(2). Retrieved from *www.nursingworld.org/ojin/topic18/tpc18_4.htm*.

Mooney, M. (2003). Hog-housed. *Reflections on Nursing Leadership*, 29(4), 8-9.

*Trinity Medical Center v. North Dakota Board of Nursing.* (January 8, 1987). Retrieved February 5, 2005, from *http://court.state.nd.us/court/opinions/11257.htm*.

# **POLICY**SPOTLIGHT

# THE POLITICS OF NURSING REGULATION AND LICENSURE

Donna M. Dorsey

*"Although partially aware of the limitations of registration, nursing leaders believed...that legislation would transform their field by placing the power of the state behind their efforts."*

SUSAN REVERBY

Controversy and misunderstanding often surround professional regulation and licensure. Even the beginnings of nursing regulation caused controversy when the Royal British Nurses Association proposed that nurses be registered in order to practice nursing in England. Florence Nightingale was opposed to the movement because she felt "that the true qualities of a nurse could not be judged by registration" (Nightingale, 1893, p. 1). Despite the concern by Ms. Nightingale and others, regulation and licensure prevailed.

## HISTORY OF REGULATION OF THE NURSING PROFESSION

The New York State Nurses Association proposed the first registration act. At about the same time, the New Jersey, North Carolina, and Virginia Nurses Associations began the process of seeking legislation for regulation. North Carolina was the first state to put into place a nurse registration law in 1903, followed by New Jersey, New York, and Virginia later in the same year. The New York law was the strongest of the laws; it was passed in 1903. These states set the standard for other early registration acts (Kelly & Joel, 1999).

## WHY REGULATE?

How does regulation impact the nurse and nursing practice? What is the public benefit? Why is regulation or licensure needed? The purpose of nursing regulation is to provide for public protection by ensuring that safe, competent nurses are in practice. The regulatory scheme is based on what is known about the profession and the world in which the profession provides care. Licensure is the regulatory mechanism used to identify the individuals who meet the qualifications for practice. Regulation and licensure should not be designed as a barrier to practice. This requires that any regulatory decisions be made at the least restrictive level that will provide public protection. This is accomplished by creating a regulatory scheme that accomplishes the following:

1. Restricts who can practice by requiring licensure of the individual
2. Establishes qualifications for licensure
3. Limits use of the term *nurse*
4. Defines what constitutes practice
5. Provides grounds for loss of a license
6. Creates an agency (the board) to monitor and enforce the regulatory requirements

The regulation of nursing and other health professionals is a state, rather than a federal, responsibility. This is because it is the individual state's responsibility and right to protect the health and welfare of its citizens. Any differences in how nursing is regulated from state to state are a result of individual decisions made by state governments.

## LEGAL BASIS FOR LICENSURE AND PROFESSIONAL PRACTICE

Three elements define nursing regulation:
1. The Nurse Practice Act
2. Regulations
3. Policies, opinions, or declaratory rulings

### The Nurse Practice Act

The statute regulating nursing practice, commonly known as the Nurse Practice Act (NPA), is adopted by the state legislature and signed into law by the governor. It is the NPA that defines nursing or nursing practice, establishes a board, defines licensing requirements, protects the title of nurse, defines the powers and duties of the board, provides for staff and funding, details violations of the law and sanctions, and defines any other responsibilities of regulation, such as an alternative discipline program. Although there are differences among states, the basic components are similar.

The definitions of nursing or nursing practice are general in nature, thus allowing the board to interpret the boundaries. A more specific definition would be limiting. Nursing constantly changes, and with a specific definition, any change in practice would have to be approved by the legislature. The time alone to move new legislation through the legislative process could adversely impact the ability

of nurses to take advantage of new knowledge and skills for patient care.

The NPAs are more similar than different from state to state but do differ in some significant areas such as advanced practice nursing and prescriptive authority. It must be remembered that the NPAs are a product of state legislation. As with any legislation introduced in a legislature, it is subject to debate and compromise. It is the debate and compromise in state legislatures that explain the variation in the NPA from state to state. All changes in the NPA must move through the legislative process. Amendments to the NPA may be proposed by the board, professional association, legislator, nurse, or citizen. It is important that nurses take notice of any legislative proposals that may impact the NPA.

### Regulations

Regulations are written to interpret or better explain the law. For example, the NPA requires that an applicant pass a licensing examination approved by the board. It does not detail the examination required, the process for accessing the examination, or any costs. The regulations specifically name the approved examination(s) and define the requirements for accessing the examination. It is important to understand that regulations hold the force of law, but they cannot go beyond the law. A board cannot decide to exempt an applicant from the examination in regulation unless the NPA provided the authority to do so.

The precise regulatory process differs from state to state, but the general process is similar. The board itself may develop a regulation, an outside group may initiate it, or the board may establish a committee to develop a proposal. Often during the development phase, advice is sought from nurses, the public, and the health care community. Following consideration of the proposal, the board must vote to promulgate (move the regulation forward) the proposal as a regulation. The regulation is published by the state government and made available for public comment. Some states also have requirements for a public hearing on the regulation to gather comments. Following the prescribed public comment period, the board must address each of the comments and determine if it believes changes are required. In some states, a legislative committee can call a hearing on a regulation. The regulation cannot be changed by the legislature, but the regulation can be sent back to the board to address the issues identified at the hearing or to withdraw the regulation.

Once the regulation has passed through all the steps of the process, it is again published and, after a prescribed period, becomes effective. The time to adopt a regulation ranges from months to years. The process is deliberately slow to allow for comment and review by all interested parties. In the case of a regulation that is needed immediately, such as a fee change, an emergency process exists. The emergency regulations are time limited, and the board is required to move the regulation through the normal process while the emergency regulation is in place.

***Opportunities to influence regulations.*** There are a number of opportunities to influence a regulation. The first is during the development process. Boards often seek input from interested parties when developing a regulation. Both the comment period and the public hearing offer an opportunity to address any specific issues with the regulation. Enough public pressure may require that the board pull the regulation back from the promulgation process and reconsider the identified issues. The final decision regarding the regulation rests with the board and the governor. But if the regulation is extremely controversial, adoption becomes difficult.

### Policy, Opinion, or Declaratory Ruling

The ability of a board to issue a policy, opinion, or declaratory ruling (ruling) is dependent on state law. The process for issuing a ruling differs widely among boards. In general, these rulings are made by the board in response to a question for interpretation of the law. Most often, the questions are related to practice. Many boards use the opinion or policy to communicate a decision about practice or licensure. The declaratory ruling is a more formal process. Unlike the NPA or regulation, rulings do not hold the force of law, but they do set a legal precedent. The board is considered an expert in nursing regulation, and courts may use the rulings in decisions.

The rulings are based on research that includes the community standard, the current literature, legal review, and similar rulings from other state boards. Committees may also be established to study the question. The rulings can reject the question as outside the scope of practice or law or determine that it is within scope. Often a ruling, particularly one that addresses practice, is issued with conditions. Those conditions can be related to experience, education, specialized training, supervision, or worksite. Rulings reflect the best judgment of the board and impact all nurses. Nurses can impact rulings by offering expertise to inform the board about the issue under study.

### THE STATE BOARD OF NURSING

### State Board of Nursing Membership

The numbers of members of state boards range from 7 to 28. The majority of board members are nurses. Consumers are now represented on all but four state boards in the United States. Four boards have a physician member, and eight boards have other types of individuals represented (Crawford & White, 2002). Appointments are made by the governor though a process determined by the state. In 50% of the states, the governor appoints the members directly. Some states require confirmation of the appointment by the state senate or legislature. North Carolina is the only state where members are elected directly by the nurses in the state. The remaining states use other methods for appointment (Crawford & White, 2002).

Qualifications vary from state to state with requirements such as active practice, minimum years of practice, and residence in the state. Many boards require that the nurse members represent a specific area of practice. Most common are nursing education, nursing administration, and practice. Practical nurses are also represented on boards, with the exception of the four states with separate practical nurse boards. Some boards have specific positions for advanced practice nurses. Terms range from three years to an indefinite period (Crawford & White, 2002). The decisions made by the board directly impact the way nurses practice, and yet most nurses pay no attention to who is on the board. It is critical that nurses be actively involved in the recommendation and appointment process to ensure that the best individuals are appointed to the board.

### Role of the State Board

The role of the board is to carry out the provisions of the NPA to ensure public protection through safe, competent nursing care. This is accomplished through the development of regulations that detail the broad provisions of the NPA. The powers and duties detailed in the act create the framework for the board activities. Those powers include determining eligibility for licensure, issuing licenses, approving nursing education programs, investigating complaints, taking disciplinary actions for violations of the law, determining scope of practice, and licensing advanced nurses. A staff is employed to carry out the policies set by the board and the daily activities that support the work of the board.

*Complaint resolution.* A key role in public protection is complaint resolution. Boards are responsible for investigation of complaints, determining if there is adequate evidence to support charges against a nurse, and determining any actions to be taken. The NPA gives the board authority to reprimand or sanction a nurse, place a nurse on probation, revoke or suspend a license, or fine the nurse if found guilty of a violation. The board hears the case in accordance with the state's administrative law. The rights of the nurse must be preserved throughout the process. A board may negotiate a settlement and, if that fails, move the case to a full evidentiary hearing. If the decision is to revoke or suspend the license, the nurse may ask for reinstatement after the prescribed time set by the state, but it is the board that must determine the nurse's fitness to return to practice. For a nurse placed on probation, the board must monitor compliance and take action if the nurse fails to comply with the probationary order. Boards also provide alternative processes to deal with specific violations. Rehabilitation programs or alternative discipline processes are available for nurses with drug, alcohol, or mental health problems.

*Scope of practice.* Another responsibility of the state board of nursing is determining what safe nurse practice is, what constitutes the scope of practice, and what the basic standards of practice will be. This is accomplished through regulations, declaratory rulings, opinions, and decision trees. Committees are often used to provide the board expert input on the issue. Regulations are adopted that describe the standards of practice, delegation process, and various practice issues, such as IV therapy. The board also works with health care agencies, government agencies, and health professionals to interpret nursing practice.

*Crafting legislation.* The legislative role of the board varies widely among states. In some states, there is no role at all—another agency within the state government is responsible for communicating concerns of the board and for proposing any legislation related to the board. In other states, direct lobbying by the board is prohibited. Most states, however, have an active role in the legislative process. Boards develop legislation that is submitted either by the governor or by a legislator; they also provide testimony on bills that impact nursing and work with legislators to move legislation and legislative initiatives through the legislative process.

### Influencing the State Board of Nursing

To effectively influence a board, one must understand the board's decision-making processes. Board meetings are held at least quarterly and as often as monthly. Meetings are open to the public, and the general session agenda is available for public view. Boards use Websites to communicate information, including board meeting information.

It is the board meeting where decisions are made. A few boards have a public forum during the meeting to obtain input from the public on any issue of concern. It is not unusual for the board to request interested parties or experts to present information on an issue under consideration. Providing information at board meetings is an ideal opportunity to address an issue with the board.

Boards use committees to study issues and make recommendations for board action. It is at the committee level where one can have a great deal of influence. The opportunity to work directly with a committee and provide direct input into the decision-making process is invaluable. Committees do research, investigate the issue, prepare reports, and make recommendations to the board. Committees provide valuable information that may ultimately impact how nurses practice in the state.

## THE NATIONAL COUNCIL OF STATE BOARDS OF NURSING

The National Council of State Boards of Nursing (NCSBN) is composed of 60 boards representing the 50 state boards, four additional state boards with separate practical nurse boards, and the boards of the island territories. For many years, nurse regulators met as a committee of the American Nurses Association. In 1978, NCSBN was established as a separate organization. It was important to separate from the American Nurses Association in order to clarify the role of regulation in public protection versus the role of the professional organization in advancing the profession.

The mission of the organization is established to advance regulatory excellence. The NCSBN is a voluntary organization and, unlike its members (the state boards), has no authority rooted in federal or state law. It serves the member boards by providing an organization where boards can come together to act and counsel on issues of mutual concern that affect public health and welfare. Member boards conduct the work of the NCSBN through the Delegate Assembly and committees established to address identified issues. The Delegate Assembly is composed of two representatives of each member board, meets at least annually to discuss issues, elect officers, and conduct any other business as described in the bylaws.

### NCLEX Exams

NCSBN develops and administers the licensing examination, NCLEX-RN® and NCLEX-PN®. The NCSBN Board of Directors is responsible for setting the passing standard. An examination committee, composed of representatives of member boards, monitors the development process,

administers the examination, and develops any policies related to the examination. The Delegate Assembly approves the test plan for the examination, fees related to the examination, and any significant changes to the examination contract. Boards are responsible for determining candidate eligibility for the examination and licensing.

The research role of NCSBN is designed to assist member boards in making evidenced-based regulatory decisions. Understanding what elements are essential in regulation, what methodologies best provide for public protection, and how to best implement regulation are critical questions addressed by NCSBN research. Commitment to Ongoing Regulatory Excellence is an example of a project designed to identify best practices of member boards. Examples of other types of research include member board profiles, practice analyses, evaluation of regulation, and analysis of disciplinary actions.

In the practice and education arena, NCSBN examines issues related to regulation, such as discipline, assistive personnel, education, advanced practice, scope of practice, standards, and licensure qualifications. NCSBN uses committees, experts, and stakeholder meetings to gather input on issues. The outcomes of work are position papers, model regulations, and evaluations for member board use in decision-making.

NSCBN also analyzes federal and state legislation and policy. The organization does not lobby, but it does work to keep policymakers informed of regulatory issues and the impact of legislation on nursing regulation. Working with national and international nursing and regulatory organizations, NCSBN collaborates on issues of mutual interest.

### NURSYS

One of the most ambitious projects of NCSBN is NURSYS®, a national database of nurse licensure. Member boards submit to NSCBN licensure data that are entered into NURSYS®. The goal is to create a comprehensive national database of reliable and timely licensure information (Business Book, 2004).

## CURRENT ISSUES IN NURSING REGULATION

### The Nurse Licensure Compact

The state-based licensure model creates regulatory barriers. The population is mobile: Nurses who work as travel nurses usually hold multiple licenses, and disasters create the urgent need for nurses. More health care agencies cross state borders to provide care requiring that nurse maintain multiple state nursing licenses. Telehealth advances allow nurses to care for patients in multiple states, requiring multiple licenses. Therefore the question became, how can a system be created that preserves the state's authority and reduces the barrier to nurse mobility? The solution was the Nurse Licensure Compact (NLC), also known as the Multistate Licensure Compact.

*A regulatory milestone.* Between January 1 and July 1, 2000, the first major change in licensure in nearly 100 years was launched. Four states, Utah, Texas, Maryland, and Wisconsin, implemented the NLC, a state nursing license recognized nationally and enforced locally. Implemented through an interstate compact, the NLC allows nurses who reside in a compact state to work in any other compact state without obtaining another license. Passed by the state legislature, an interstate compact is defined as "an agreement between two or more states established for the purpose of remedying a particular problem of multi-state concern, in this case licensure" (Black, 1999, p. 274).

The NLC is similar to the driver's license model. The nurse must obtain a compact license in the state of the nurse's primary residence, giving the nurse a multistate privilege to practice in any other compact state without additional licensure. The nurse is expected to practice in accordance with the laws of the state where practicing. Should that nurse change the state of residence, he or she must obtain a license in the new state. Under the NLC, a nurse may hold a license only from his or her primary state of residence. Therefore, if the nurse holds a license in another compact state, that license must be made invalid. If the nurse is practicing in a non-compact state, the nurse must obtain a license in that state to practice. A nurse whose primary state of residence is in a non-compact state and practices

in a compact state must obtain a license in that compact state. The nurse does not receive a multistate privilege. The nurse's primary state of residence must be in a compact state in order to be entitled to multistate privilege.

*Barriers to joining the nurse licensure compact.* As of 2006, 21 states had joined the NLC. There are a number of issues that must be resolved before a board can make the decision to join the NLC. Most boards are not well funded and generally must rely on all, or a portion of, the revenues collected to fund their operations. Boards are concerned that once the board has joined the NLC, there will be revenue losses in the areas of endorsement, renewal, and verification that cannot be overcome through other sources of revenue. Experience has demonstrated that the losses in revenue are not nearly as dramatic as anticipated. States have been able to manage the revenue loss without adverse impact.

*Legislative issues.* All NLC language must be the identical to the NLC passed by the other states. Modifications to the NLC may result in a state being ineligible for participation in the NLC. The NLC administrators have agreed on a uniform set of core requirements, and all states in the NLC are moving toward meeting the requirements. The requirements include graduation from an approved nursing program, passage of the NCLEX, a criminal background check, and standards for international nurse evaluation. There also are concerns from nurses that the NLC will adversely affect collective bargaining. There is no evidence of any adverse impact on collective bargaining. Many states have clarified the issues related to labor by enacting enabling legislation that specifically states the NLC does not supercede any of the state's labor laws.

### The Advanced Practice Compact

The NCSBN passed the Advanced Practice Registered Nurse Compact (APRN Compact) in 2002. The APRN Compact supports increased mobility of advanced practice nurses (APNs), new technology and practice models, and a need to reduce barriers to practice across state lines for APNs. The current system of licensure is duplicative, with each state reviewing the same information. Finally, the APRN

Compact will move the requirements for certification or licensure toward uniformity, further providing for public protection.

The provisions of the APRN Compact are similar to those of the NLC. The APN's primary state of residence must be an APRN Compact state. The APN is granted a privilege to practice in any other APRN Compact state. The APN must comply with the laws of the state where practicing. In states where a collaborative agreement or other prerequisites are required, the APN also must comply with all additional requirements. Practice cannot commence until the additional practice requirements are approved. However, the time frame to complete the process is greatly reduced because of the APRN compact.

APNs also must comply with all requirements for prescriptive practice in the state. States vary greatly on prescriptive practice, so it is important that the APN understand the requirements of the state where the APN plans to work. In addition, the Federal Drug Administration requires that the APN with prescriptive authority obtain a separate Drug Enforcement Agency number in each state where practicing. The NCSBN believes this is an additional burden but has been unsuccessful in obtaining a change in the requirement.

Prior to introducing legislation to establish the APRN Compact, a state must enact the Nurse Licensure Compact. Both compacts could be passed at the same time, but most boards find it administratively efficient to pass the NLC first. In 2004, Utah became the first state to pass the APRN Compact. Iowa passed the APRN compact in 2005. It is expected that other states will move forward with the APRN Compact in the near future.

### Continued Competence

Competence is the foundation of public protection, making it a critical issue for boards. Clearly an unsafe or unethical nurse is a danger to public health, safety, and welfare. Mechanisms must be available to determine if a nurse cannot practice safely and provide whatever remediation is necessary for safe practice. Where a nurse cannot practice safely, board action may be the only option. With the practice of nursing continually evolving, the explosion of

knowledge, and rapid pace of changes in health care, the measuring competency is no easy matter; it is, however, a requirement.

In 1998, the Pew Commission recommended that all health care professionals be required to meet specific competency requirements throughout their careers (Finnocchio, Dower, Blick, & Grangnola, 1998). Two years later, the Citizen Advocacy Center convened a meeting on continuing competency, reinforcing that it is the responsibility of the professional licensing boards to ensure the competence of health care professionals throughout their career (LaBuhl & Swankin, 2001). However, little has been done to make the recommendations a reality. A first step is agreeing on a single definition of continued competence. In a literature review by Waddell (2001), no common definition of the term *continued competence* was found.

Cost and efficiency must be incorporated into any model of continued competence. Employers are hesitant to pay for mandated continued competence. Nurses will not pay for programs that are costly. Any legislative requirement for continuing education must carry reasonable fees. In the face of the nursing shortage, it is even more imperative that models be developed that do not take nurses away from patient care for long periods of time and do not adversely impose on nurses' personal time. Added to the dilemma is the diversity of nursing roles and practice settings. Developing a single approach becomes challenging. For these reasons, boards of nursing have yet to embrace a single methodology for assessing continued competence.

Continuing education has been the traditional mechanism for ensuring continued competence. Currently, 24 boards require some form of continuing education at the time of license renewal (Crawford & White, 2002, p. 178). The link between continuing education and continued competence has not been well established. Smith (2003) found there was no significant difference between nurses who received continuing education and nurses who had not in the perception of their professional growth. Boards have also found that some nurses tend to find whatever programs are available at the time of renewal to meet the renewal requirement, even when those programs are not germane to the competencies needed for the practice of the nurse. Smith (2003) found that nurses obtained about the same amount of continuing education whether mandated or not. The question raised is the value of mandating continuing education. Perhaps the easiest to regulate, it is still costly for boards to administer, and the outcomes are subject to question.

Another mechanism used by boards is an active practice requirement that mandates practice be verified at the time of renewal. Commonly, 950 to 1000 hours of practice are required in a five-year period for active licensure. Nurses not meeting the practice requirement must take an approved refresher course. The most frequent complaints about the course are the time it takes to complete the program and the focus of the content on care in the hospital.

*Re-entry to practice.* There are a few boards that require the NCLEX for nurses who have been away from nursing practice. The NCLEX was never designed to measure re-entry competence. There has been no study to determine if it is an effective measure for re-entry. In addition, some boards are faced with a dilemma. What if a nurse fails the examination? The cost to both the board and the nurse is high, with no clear evidence of public protection.

Regulations governing the practice of nursing address the concept of competence by creating the expectation that nurses will remain competent in their areas of practice. Regulations support the nurse's right to refuse assignment when the nurse does not have the requisite skills to act safely. By statute, boards have the authority to take disciplinary action on the license if a nurse has (a) failed to maintain generally accepted standards of practice, (b) failed to comply with the regulations, or (c) is incompetent.

The NCSBN established a committee to study the options for addressing continued competence. The committee is to review all options, including an examination. Many states are evaluating new models. North Carolina is using the reflective model that is a self-assessment and development of an individual learning plan (Continued Competence, 2005). Other boards are offering a variety of

options to demonstrate competency. Boards will continue to work on developing the best model for assessment of continued competence.

### Licensure and Certification of Advanced Practice Nurses

In the early 1970s, boards began to license advanced practice nurses (APNs). States approached the regulation of APNs differently, varying in interpretation and regulatory solutions. For example, some states used different terms to describe APN regulation, and some varied in the definition of APNs. Qualifications for licensure differed from state to state, and scopes of practice were not consistent. Even the term *APN* varied, with some states recognizing nurse practitioners, nurse midwives, nurse anesthetists, and clinical nurse specialists and others not including the clinical nurse specialists in regulation. These differences reflect the early development of advanced practice nursing and the political realities of the time. It is also these differences that have made the regulation of advanced practice nursing so challenging.

*Specialty certification.* One prominent issue is the use of specialty certification examinations developed and administered by professional organizations to grant licensure or certification. The use of specialty examination for the purposes of licensure must be beyond reproach. It must be legally defensible and psychometrically sound. This means that the examination must effectively measure entry-level competencies essential to the practice of the specialty. The examination must not be too broad or narrow in its scope of measurement when used for licensing decisions. It is expected that the examination will measure the competencies required to ensure that the practitioner has the ability to practice safely. Boards remain concerned that the specialty examination used for licensure is inappropriate. The current debate is whether there is a need for a new examination specifically for licensure. Certification bodies and advanced practice nurses are against such a proposal.

*Types of practitioners.* The growth in the types of nurse practitioners has created a number of concerns from a regulatory perspective. Boards want to ensure that there is a core set of competencies for all nurse practitioners and not just competencies within a narrow focus. Programs of study that focus on the narrow scope of practice raise questions for regulation as well, especially when the clinical experience is less than 500 hours of supervised experience in the specialty category and the didactic portion of the program is narrowly focused. An alternative would be to license APN at the broadest level while allowing specialization based on professional qualifications rather than licensure. The professional organizations, regulation, and education are working together to reach a consensus on how to best educate, examine, and regulate APNs.

## APRN Practice

APNs have been regulated for 30 years, and there has been little change in how they are regulated. Any activities that are perceived as an expansion of practice, any new practice arena, or any changes in laws or regulations are usually met with opposition from organized medicine.

*Tensions with medicine.* There is tremendous tension between medicine and nursing regarding scope and independence of practice. This resulted in compromises causing the variations in scope of practice and independence from state to state. Such compromises included limited prescriptive authority; joint regulation between the medical and nursing boards; physician supervision requirements; and requirements for collaborative agreements, practice agreements, and protocols. These processes create tensions with respect to the roles.

*Prescriptive practice.* Prescriptive practice is one of the hottest issues. States vary widely on how advanced practice nurses may prescribe. Some states have no limitations, other limit via a formulary, others by type of drugs such as narcotics, and a few do not grant prescriptive authority at all. There is no logic for these differences. If the advanced practice nurse has the requisite education, why should there be barriers to practice?

More than half of the states have a requirement for a practice agreement, collaborative agreement, or protocols, which must be approved prior to initiating practice (Crawford & White, 2002). The agreements outline the practice of the nurse and the role of the physician and must be approved either by the board or both the board and the medical board. Both the protocols and agreements can limit the scope of practice of APNs. Again, the requirements were enacted in response to political pressures and compromise. The rationale for the agreements is that APNs perform medical functions, and those functions must be reviewed and supervised by the physician. Attempts to pass legislation that would remove the requirement for agreements have met with resistance. Although a few states have been successful in changing the requirements, the majority of states have experienced little change.

## Use of Assistive Personnel

The growth in the use of assistive personnel has created new issues for boards. *Assistive personnel* is the umbrella term used for nursing assistants, home health aides, medication technicians, and any other unlicensed persons performing delegated nursing functions. There are a number of forces that have influenced the growth of assisted personnel. These include the nursing shortage, increase in non-traditional health care facilities such as assisted living facilities, the aging population, and costs of health care personnel. The major concern faced by boards is that unlicensed individuals will be used to substitute for nurses.

Boards receive a multitude of questions and concerns about delegation. Most often, the question is regarding the appropriateness of the delegation. If the nurse delegates, following the process for delegation, and an error occurs the nurse would not be held responsible as long as the delegation was appropriate. There is also misinformation regarding the role of the job description. The job description is a list of activities or tasks one may be asked to perform. The nurse retains the final authority to determine if it is appropriate for an unlicensed person to carry out particular tasks. Nurses need to understand the requirements related to delegation in the state where they are practicing. Such information helps to empower the nurse to authorize delegation or determine it is unsafe to delegate.

In 2002, 49 of 61 boards reported that delegation was either referenced in the NPA or in regulations.

Six of the boards reported the delegation was inferred in their laws or regulations (Crawford & White, 2002). These documents provide nurses with the information to delegate safely. A number of boards have created decision-making trees to assist the nurse in determining when to delegate and when not to delegate.

But the requirement for nursing delegation is viewed a burden by some. Boards have been faced with a great deal of pressure to permit assistive personnel, for example, to administer medications without nursing involvement. With more individuals being cared for in non-traditional care settings such as group homes, assisted living facilities, schools, and day care centers, lobbying is intense to allow others to administer medications. Cost is often cited as the barrier to hiring nurses. In addition, medication administration is viewed as a mechanical activity of simply removing the medication from the bottle. The dilemma is how to balance the needs of the patient for affordable health care in a setting of their choice and patient safety. There is continued pressure by employers to reduce the requirement for nurse delegation. Legislators may not adequately understand the risks when assistive personnel are permitted to perform tasks without nurse supervision.

### Certification of Assistive Personnel

The continued growth in the use of nursing assistants brings additional regulatory issues. For example, there are over 250 titles in use referring to assistants. There is no standardized training. Competency issues are difficult to address. There is no mechanism for identifying individuals who pose a danger to the public and for preventing them from working as nursing assistants. Employers are often unclear about the role of the nursing assistant.

By 2002, 13 boards were regulating nursing assistants of various types (Crawford & White, 2002). But the number and type of assistive personnel regulated varied from state to state. The obstacle for boards in moving forward with regulation is costs and human resources. In addition, there is often some industry pushback. Many people viewed regulation as a barrier because of the requirements for certification or licensing and other restrictions required by the regulation, such as active practice or limitation of the practice setting based on education.

In the 2003 NCSBN Delegate Assembly, the Kentucky Board of Nursing presented a resolution asking that NCSBN develop a position paper on the regulation of assistive personnel to include a model act and regulations. They felt strongly that as boards, it was time to move forward on the issue of regulation of assistive personnel. At 2005 Delegate Assembly, the members adopted the proposed Model Act and Rules for a Nursing Assistant Regulatory Model (Business Book, 2005, pp. 196-215). The model provides a blueprint for regulation of assistive personnel that will provide for public protection.

### U.S. Licensing of Non–U.S.-Resident Nurses

The migration of international nurses has increased because of the nursing shortage. The United States has always been an attractive destination for internationally educated nurses, but the nursing shortage stimulated more active recruitment of the nurses. The statistics from the Testing Department of the National Council of State Boards (C. Marks, personal communication, February 18, 2005) reveal that in 2001, 8612 internationally educated registered nurses took the NCLEX for the first time, and in 2004, 16,489 took the examination. In a survey of internationally educated nurses, Smith and Crawford (2004) found that the average number of days from licensure to the first assignment was 18.9 days in the hospital setting and 9.9 days in the nursing home or long-term care facility. They also found that the internationally educated nurse tended to carry a larger patient assignment.

*Language issues.* Language and communication are an issue. Even though a nurse may speak English as a second language adequately, medical terminology, abbreviations, medication names, and colloquial terms can create confusion and frustration. Physician orders may be difficult to interpret. Medications may have names different than those the nurse is familiar with, or there may be two medications with similar names, which causes further confusion. Nurses often use trade names for equipment, making difficult for the international nurse to understand what is needed. All of these examples may place patients at risk.

Boards require evidence in both oral and written English as part of the licensure procedure. The Test of Spoken English, International English Language Testing System, the Test of English as a Foreign Language, or similar examinations are used for evaluation. The issue with the examinations is that the tests are not specifically designed for health care providers. There is also some misunderstanding that if the nurse can pass the NCLEX, the nurse understands English health care terminology. The NCLEX is not an English test; rather, it is a test of nursing knowledge. The examination provides no measure of language competence, written or oral, and should not be relayed on any purpose other than determining competence.

A specialized orientation program for all international nurses seeking to work in the United States may be an approach in assisting international nurses. Currently, there is no organized program that assists the nurse to understand the professional practice of nursing in the United States, including its standards of practice, ethics, and the health care system. This has been left to the employers.

### SUMMARY

The issues faced by boards are continually evolving. The complexity of the issues will challenge boards, nurses, other health care providers, employers, and consumers. The nursing shortage, political forces, health care costs, advances in technology, and the explosion of knowledge are just some of the factors that will continue to influence issues. Emerging issues include the impact of globalization, alternate language licensure examinations, new categories of health care workers, scope of practice, nursing education, a new model of nursing practice to address the nursing shortage, and new testing modalities.

Boards alone cannot resolve all of the issues facing nursing. Many more groups and individuals are involved in the decisions related to regulation, and the stakes are high for all. It will require continued collaboration with nursing organizations, other professional associations, employers, other health care providers, and consumers. Regulation and licensure must not be barriers to practice, but rather the process designed for public protection. There is often a fine balance between regulation that creates barriers and public protection. It is the responsibility of boards, in collaboration with others, to find the right balance and enforce the requirements. Public protection must be the foundation for decisions made to address the issues of today and tomorrow.

## Key Points

■ The purpose of nursing regulation is to provide for public protection by ensuring that safe and competent nurses are in practice.
■ Amendments to the NPA may be proposed by the board, professional association, legislator, nurse, or citizen.
■ Competence is the foundation of public protection, making it a critical issue for boards.
■ State boards of nursing alone cannot resolve all of the issues facing nursing.

## Web Resources

**National Council of State Boards of Nursing**
*www.ncsbn.org/*
**National League for Nursing Test Products**
*www.nln.org/testprods/index.htm*
**Nurse Competence in Aging**
*www.nursingworld.org/nca/*
**NURSYS Licensure System**
*www.nursys.com/*

### REFERENCES
Black, H. C. (1999). *Black's law dictionary.* St Paul, MN: West Group.
The Business Book, Mission Possible. (2005). Chicago: National Council of State Boards of Nursing.
The Business Book, Shared Visions and New Pathways. (2004). Chicago: National Council of State Boards of Nursing.
Continued Competence. (2005). Retrieved from the North Carolina Board of Nursing Website: *www.ncbon.org/prac-contcomp.asp.*
Crawford, L., & White, E. (2002). *Profiles of member boards.* Chicago: National Council of State Boards of Nursing.

Finnocchio, L., Dower, C. M., Blick, N. T., & Grangnola, C. M. (1998). *Strengthening consumer protection. Priorities for health care workforce regulation.* San Francisco: Pew Health Professions Commission.

Kelly, L. Y., & Joel, L. A. (1999). *Dimensions of professional nursing.* New York: McGraw-Hill.

LaBuhn, R. A., & Swankin, D. A. (2001). Measuring continuing competence of health care providers: Where are we now—where are we headed? Proceedings of a Citizen Advocacy Center Conference, June 2000, Washington, DC.

Nightingale, F. (1893, June 19). Letter to Miss Luckes. Retrieved April 2, 2005, from the Clendening History of Medicine Library Website at *www.clendening.kunc.edu/dc/fn/luckes1.html.*

Smith, J. (2003). Exploring the value of continuing education mandates (NCSBN Research Brief, Vol. 6). Chicago: National Council of State Boards of Nursing.

Smith, J., & Crawford, L. (2004). Nurses educated outside the United States. Report of findings from the Practice and Professional Issues Survey (NCSBN Research Brief, Vol. 12). Chicago: National Council of State Boards of Nursing.

Waddell, D. L. (2001, May-June). Measurement issues in promoting continued competence. *Journal of Continuing Education Nursing, 32*(3), 102-106.

# chapter 25

# Lobbying Policymakers: Individual and Collective Strategies

Mary Foley*

*"The greater the obstacle, the more glory in overcoming it."*

MOLIÈRE

What does the word *lobbying* mean to you? The word has the effect of intimidating many people, who assume that lobbyists wield power and influence that regular citizens don't enjoy. Actually, the way the term came into usage was very simple and practical.

The word *lobbyist* comes from the early days of the U.S. government when constituents with interests in legislation or policy would wait outside the doors of the U.S. House or Senate chambers—in the lobby—to approach their legislators as they entered or exited. The idea of a citizen government may seem far removed from today's hectic political environment. Still, with the right combination of dedication, strategy, and persistence, individual citizens can and do have access to and accountability from elected officials—and you don't have to be a paid lobbyist to make a difference.

The number of paid lobbyists has increased over the last hundred years. Since 1920, we have seen the development of special interest groups and the relocation of many national headquarters to the Washington, DC, area. If an association does not have its headquarters in Washington, DC, it will often establish a satellite office there. Paid lobbyists must file with the Federal Election Commission (FEC) and comply with the regulations and guidelines set forth by the FEC in pursuing their lobbying efforts. What hasn't changed is that regular people have the most important power: the power of the voter. And you have even more power on your side: the power of the nurse.

Nearly everyone knows a nurse. Nurses are recognized as the most trusted group of professionals, ranking number 1 for trustworthiness in the Gallup Organization's most recent poll on honesty and ethics in professions (Gallup Organization, 2005) and in each Gallup poll ranking since nursing was added to the poll in 1999, except for one year: In 2001, firefighters were rated number 1 after their heroic acts during the September 11 terrorist attacks. Nursing is 2.7 million individuals strong, comprising the largest group of health care professionals in the United States. The combination of reputation

---

*This is an updated version of the chapter by Melinda Mercer Ray and Shelagh Roberts that appeared in the fourth edition of this book.

and presence is important to legislators. Think of the number of times people have said to you, "I could never do what you do." It is this profound respect that will assist you with your lobbying efforts.

Have you ever written a letter to a local, state, or federal legislator to express your opinion on a current issue? Have you ever come face to face with an elected official and asked why funding is being cut for a program you support? Have you ever presented administrators in your workplace information or resources to support or oppose a certain internal policy? If you answered yes to any of these questions, congratulations, you are already a lobbyist!

This chapter contains information to help you develop specific strategies to make the most of your expert knowledge and to communicate with legislators in ways most likely to bring success. Much of the chapter utilizes examples from the national experience in lobbying the U.S. Congress and Senate. Many of the principles will apply to lobbying efforts at a state or local level. Always check with state rules and regulations governing campaigns and lobbying to be fully compliant and successful.

## WHY LOBBY?

The most common reason people get involved with lobbying is because they see something that needs to be fixed. As a nurse, you may see circumstances on a daily basis in your practice that inspires passionate feelings about the way things should be. Perhaps you see patients and families struggling with insurance companies to get approval for medically necessary procedures. Like the founder of Mothers Against Drunk Driving and other activists who got involved after a personal event, each of us is just one personal or social injustice away from being involved in politics and each one of us can make a difference (Dodd, 2004).

Unless you represent your professional association as a paid staff person or you serve as an appointed or elected representative in local or state politics, you will take on the task of lobbying most likely for the sake of your personal and professional convictions. You will lobby because you feel strongly that certain policies should be enacted,

and your motivation will be strong enough to translate your concern into action. The elected officials you will most successfully influence are your own elected officials. That fact, and a few exceptions to that fact, will be reviewed in the steps that follow.

## PREPARE YOURSELF WITH KNOWLEDGE

The first step in the lobbying process is to find out as much as you can about your area of interest or the issue that concerns you. Aside from paying attention to what you see in your workplace, in the newspaper, the Internet, or on television, you should become a kind of detective. Discover the legislative history, dynamics of power, and policy particulars of bills related to your issue of interest. Your job is to learn as much as you can about the issue so that you can decide what your best lobbying approach will be.

Many professional nursing or other health care associations and think tanks regularly post position statements on controversial issues on their Websites. The American Nurses Association (ANA) and the Association of Women's Health, Obstetric and Neonatal Nurses (AWHONN) are two examples. Many such Websites have legislative affairs sections that display sample letters or issue briefs to help you frame your arguments in favor of, or in opposition to, a particular bill.

If you are a member of a professional organization, you can do some individual research using the Websites. For additional guidance, or if you have an expertise to offer, contact someone in the federal or state government affairs department.

Now that most government agencies and legislative branches make detailed documents, including bill texts and summaries, federal agency reports and studies, and countless sources of federal data available online, the Internet is a great place to search for information. The Library of Congress's Website, *www.thomas.loc.gov*, offers complete listings of bills that can be searched by subject, key word, co-sponsor, date of introduction, and bill title or number. In addition, every state has its own webpage with detailed information regarding elected officials and legislative activity. While the states' Websites vary in the degree of detail they provide, almost every state Website includes the names of, and contact information for, state senators and representatives, as well as a search function to identify your legislator according to zip code or city name. These searches will identify bills on your issue of interest in great detail and can help you gain thorough knowledge of the legislative histories behind a given subject. Tracking the bill is also very important, as the legislative process is, by design, one of compromise. Knowing where a bill is in the process, and what has changed or remained the same, will enable you to speak accurately about your support for, or opposition to, a bill at the right time. Obtain a copy of past voting charts and a list of bills introduced or co-sponsored by a legislator. Knowing the legislative history of an issue is vital if you are to make suggestions consistent with possible legislative remedies, identify allies who support your issue, and present yourself as a credible representative on the issue.

First, you must identify members of Congress or state legislatures who have been leaders on the particular issue. For example, if you search a legislative site using the key word *breastfeeding*, you can identify several legislators with a long history of introducing or co-sponsoring breastfeeding legislation. When approaching the legislator for support, you will be able to build on his or her previous knowledge and initiatives to craft a workable legislative strategy.

Once you identify the issue that you want to lobby on, and you have educated yourself as to its legislative history and the current status of bills related to it, the next step is to determine (1) whom you need to contact to bring about change and (2) the best mode of communication to accomplish that change.

## WHO TO LOBBY

At the federal level, your primary contacts are the congressional staff people in the offices of your representatives and senators. They work with other offices and outside interest groups to create and iron out detailed provisions in legislation. Your first step in building relationships at the federal level is to identify the person in your legislator's office who is responsible for your issue. Nursing and health related issues will likely be the staff liaison who works on health care policy. Sometimes, though, responsibility for health care issues can be divided among several staff people, particularly if the member of Congress serves on a committee that has jurisdiction over such issues; therefore, it is best to obtain specific information about who covers your particular issue of interest, not just who covers health care issues. Usually, the easiest way to identify the correct person on your issue is to telephone your member's Capitol Hill office and simply ask the person who answers the phone for the name of the individual who handles that issue. Once you have identified the proper staff member, you should address all correspondence or requests for meetings to that person.

At the federal level, there are two types of staff: those in the members' personal offices and those who work at the committee level. Some members of Congress are leaders on an issue because they have a personal or constituent-related connection to it, whereas others serve on committees that have jurisdiction over significant health care matters, such as the committees that oversee federal health programs or appropriations. Although there also are district offices for both representatives and senators in the members' home states, these offices generally handle constituent services rather than policymaking responsibilities, and they are not usually the place to turn to for policy issues except for those related to a specific constituent.

Political staff often experience high turnover rates, so you should always double-check that the contact information you have is current, particularly if you are relying on a published directory. Staff usually rely on experts in the field to help them understand the background of certain legislative issues. For example, the nursing shortage is an important issue in every district across the country. A staff member would need input from experts who actually work in nursing in order to get a firm grasp on what might be short-term and long-term strategies to recruit, and retain, nurses. Registered nurses and professional nursing organizations have the insight and the credibility to explain the complexities of the educational needs, overtime requirements, harried work environments, or the implications of an aging nursing workforce. Staff will rely on the firsthand professionals to help demonstrate why certain policies or practices are working or why they need to be changed.

Opportunities to build personal relationships are often easier at the local and state levels than at the federal level, for the simple reason that there are more occasions for networking and building informal personal relationships with policymakers where you both live. In your community, you can invite an official to meetings of your professional organization or provide him or her with an invitation to address the group at a meeting or luncheon. You should also regularly attend local and state meetings or committee hearings on issues in the home district. Additional opportunities for networking and visibility occur when you volunteer to serve on a task force in your community, take part in a political campaign, become involved in the political party structure, or run for office yourself. Through the informal exchanges with legislators and policymakers these activities provide, you can build the foundations for lasting relationships.

Staff members also enjoy tremendous responsibility and influence at the state and local levels. As at the federal level, at the state level it is important to identify the appropriate staff contact and to work with that individual to exert some influence on developing legislation. The chances are higher at the state or local level that a staffer or legislator will have some direct knowledge either of your place of work or of the specific issues you face in your town or city. Officials and staff at the state or local level will also likely be more concerned with issues that are particular to your geographic location than federal officials, simply because they have a smaller jurisdiction and constituency to serve. At both state and federal levels, it is very important to recognize the critical role that the staff plays in crafting legislation and helping to determine legislative priorities for the member of Congress he or she works for. You should always treat a personal office or committee staff representative with the same respect you reserve for the legislator. With the broad range of issues that members of Congress must address, they rely on staff to brief them on issues that are assigned to them. They also look to staff to craft legislation and make recommendations about what issues to champion. It is unrealistic to expect a meeting with a member of Congress in most circumstances. Although it may be more feasible to meet with a local or state representative, it takes careful planning and advanced notice to arrange meetings with all elected officials because of the demands on their time. Exceptions to the rule are if you have a personal relationship or connection with the member, although you should be careful not to exaggerate the relationship in order to get a meeting. Additional avenues of access may result from your participation in an association or coalition that has broad appeal to the member (Box 25-1).

## COMMUNICATING WITH POLICYMAKERS AND STAFF

### COMMUNICATING BY PHONE

Some pitfalls of communicating by phone are that there is no written record of a phone call, and you have no visual proof that you actually made the call. Additionally, when you communicate with staff via telephone, you have no way of guaranteeing that either your message or your personal information, such as your name, telephone number, or address, is recorded correctly. And even if they are recorded correctly, you have no assurance that they will be forwarded to the correct person. A telephone call may be worthwhile simply to express your support for, or opposition to, a legislative issue that is currently on the floor of the House or Senate for debate and will be coming up for a vote. Most congressional offices keep a running tally of yes or no votes from constituents who call the office during a contentious debate. Telephone calls can also be a good means of obtaining brief information or following up with someone with whom you have already established a relationship. Always follow up with a personal thank you note or e-mail acknowledging the call.

In general, telephone calls are not ideal for introducing yourself to a legislative assistant. It is better to write a letter or make a personal

---

**BOX 25-1**  Ten Tips for a Lobbying Visit to a Public Official

These are suggestions for visiting a public official or their staff on an issue of concern, whether you are alone or with a group.

1. Identify the best time and the purpose of the visit.
   a. Is it a "get acquainted" meeting?
   b. Is it to provide background about a particular topic?
   c. Is it to appeal for a specific action on a particular piece of legislation?
2. Do your homework.
   a. If you are meeting with the legislator, know as much as you can about his or her record on your issues and his or her general areas of interest.
   b. You may very likely meet with staff, even if you have an appointment with the legislator. Know who the staff is and be willing to meet with them. The staff member responsible for health will likely be the best match for your area of interest.
   c. Know the current status of legislation if you are speaking about a particular issue.
3. Be prepared to share an anecdote that illustrates the problem at hand and the need for a policy solution. But also come armed with key statistics and facts that can provide the data to demonstrate that the issue is more than one anecdote.
4. Provide a one- or two-page fact sheet to staff in advance of the meeting, and have it available to leave with whomever you meet. Also, if there are any key articles or reports that illustrate your position, bring a copy to leave behind.
5. Always bring several copies of your business card.
6. If you don't have an answer to a question at the time of the meeting, be sure to find that information later and provide it to the elected member of staff with whom you met.
7. Avoid getting into a rancorous argument with a public official or staff member. This may be the beginning of a long-term relationship and efforts to build the person's trust in your authority, expertise, and position on the issue.
8. Ask the legislator (or staff member) how he or she will vote on your issue if a bill is already before the legislature.
   a. If the legislator supports your position, thank him or her and ask what else you can do to build support for your position.
   b. If the legislator opposes your position, tell him or her that you will continue to provide information about the issue and hope that he or she will reconsider.
   c. If the legislator is reluctant to commit to a position, ask what information or other factor is needed for him or her to make a decision. Offer to provide what is needed, if you can do so.
9. Send a thank you note to whomever you met.
10. Make sure you follow up on commitments you make during the visit and share the legislator's position with your nursing organization and other interested parties.

---

introduction at an appropriate forum, such as a legislative briefing, to make the initial point of contact. After a letter has been received, it is perfectly acceptable to call the legislative assistant to whom you have written in order to confirm that the letter was received or to ask if he or she would like any further information. Telephone calls are, of course, expected if you are actively working with a legislative assistant or other staff member on a particular piece of legislation or if you have an ongoing relationship with that person. Placing numerous telephone calls to someone with whom you have no established relationship, however, can identify you as a nuisance. With written communication or e-mail,

the person can respond according to his or her own timetable, whereas a phone call is sometimes an interruption.

## THE THREE RIGHTS OF LETTER WRITING: SENDING THE RIGHT LETTER TO THE RIGHT ELECTED OFFICIAL AT THE RIGHT TIME

Most, if not all, members of Congress consider constituent mail services as essential elements in their constituents' perceptions of them. Members of Congress have been known to say that their constituents place a far greater value on their personal responses and experiences with their congressional offices than on familiarity with their voting records when it comes time for reelection. The two-way communication between legislator and constituent relies on the correct "mix of elected officials motivated to respond and capable citizens motivated to make demands, with an active two-way communications network between the two" (Frantzich, 1986, p. 116).

When you write a letter to a member of Congress or a state or local official, there are some general guidelines to follow. First, direct your letter according to the legislator's responsibility. Do not write a letter regarding problems with your state's practice act to a federal legislator, who has no authority on that issue. As an individual, your correspondence will be considered only if you write to the elected official who represents you. If you have a reputation as an expert or you have a personal relationship with an elected official, your letter may have impact. Personal letters still carry more weight than form letters, petitions, e-mails, or phone calls. If the elected official has a history of support of the issue, it is always important to start each communication with a thank you and an acknowledgement of their support

A further clarification of who to write pertains to an issue you may want to influence at the committee level, but your elected official is not on that committee. At the federal level, if your member of Congress is not on the committee, you can still communicate your opinion by addressing your letter to the chair of the committee at the committee address (not at the chair's congressional personal office address). Committee information, such as chair names, committee members, and committee address, is available on the Internet. State practices may vary, so again, check with your local guidelines.

As described by Catherine Dodd, RN and District Director for House Democratic Leader Nancy Pelosi (D-CA), politics is the art of the possible and the result of the compromise and strategy (Dodd, 2004). The best possible options may not be drafted in the initial version of a legislative proposal; through negotiation among elected officials and modifications made through amendments, the final proposal will not necessarily resemble the original ideas. This is an opportunity

to continue to communicate support, opposition, or proposals for improvements in the legislation. That first letter is no longer sufficient to address all of the permutations a legislative proposal may undergo. It is important for you to address the proposal as it appears at each phase of the legislation.

When possible, you should time your letter to give the staff or member plenty of time to address and work with you on the issue before any pressing legislation goes to the floor. Last-minute attempts to influence policy are rarely successful, and when they are, it is usually because a trusted colleague or expert, not a first-time constituent, has convinced the member to listen to his or her concerns (Frantzich, 1986).

In crafting the message of your letter, identify yourself as a nurse, particularly if the legislation has anything to do with health care. As a nurse, you are qualified to speak not only about health care issues but also about issues related to the environment, children's safety, seniors, and many other areas. Include hospital or other practice setting information as well as professional credentials, and make sure to include a return address, telephone number, and e-mail address if appropriate.

Identifying yourself as a nurse identifies you as an expert. Include information about how proposed legislation would influence your personal experiences, or provide personal anecdotes that demonstrate your firsthand knowledge of, and experience with, a certain issue. State clearly what your position is, what your major concern about the proposal is, and whether you want the official to support, or oppose, the proposal. Again, tracking the legislation throughout the process will require that you include relevant committee or hearing information and bill numbers in your correspondence. Keep your letter brief (no more than two pages) and to the point (Box 25-2).

## PERSONAL VISITS

Face-to-face lobbying is generally perceived by both staff and members of Congress as the most effective lobbying strategy. If you have arranged a personal visit with a legislative assistant or other staff member, or with a member of Congress or state or local official, you can apply many of the same guidelines

**BOX 25-2**   Lobbying by Letter

**WHO?**

**Elected Officials: President, Governors, and Legislators**

Call the Registrar of Voters in your county to find out which districts you live in and who represents you in the *State* House/Assembly and Senate. Access *www.thomas.loc.gov* to find our information on your federal officials.

**WHAT?**

**Legible Individual Letters**

Handwritten or typed, letters should express your support for, or opposition to, pending legislation (such as SB 255).

General "opinion" letters receive little attention. Avoid form letters and postcards or mass e-mails. They are given little attention.

THANK YOU letters are very impressive. They assure your elected representatives that you are monitoring their record.

**WHEN?**

**Immediately**

Letters should be sent as soon as the need for one arises. Letters must arrive before any hearing. Don't wait!

**WHY?**

**Influence**

Elected Representatives are GREATLY influenced by INDIVIDUAL letters.

**HOW?**

**Examples of Letters**

It is nice but not essential to include the room number; letters can be addressed this way:

> Legislator's Full Name
> California State Assembly or Senate
> State Capitol
> Sacramento, CA 95814

Address it properly.
> *Envelope:* The Honorable _____
> (first and last name)

> *Letter:* Use full name and address, as above
> Use personal or organization letterhead if you have it. Be sure to include your own name and address on the letter (not just on the envelope).

Use the following steps to write your letter:

- *Greeting.* Include formal title and last name (e.g., Dear Assemblywoman Smith, Dear Senator Jones).
- *Identify yourself.* Assert your credibility as a nurse, a member of a specialty or organization, a professional, a registered voter concerned about _____.
- *Identify the legislation you favor or oppose.* Show you understand the purpose of the legislation. Be specific with bill number, author and title. If you do not know the specifics, briefly describe the issue that concerns you. Write a separate letter for each bill/issue. **Never cover more than one bill in a letter**.
- *Explain your position.* Predict the impact of the legislation. Personalize; if you have expertise or experience, share it. Give pertinent facts. Be as concise as you can be. **Be accurate and honest**.
- *Urge support or opposition.* As legislation moves through the legislative process, it often changes. So, urge opposition to crippling amendments and support for strengthening ones.
- *Request a response.* Do not threaten or demand.
- *Sign it and mail it.*
- *Fax/mail copy to your association or interest group.*

*Continued*

**BOX 25-2** Lobbying by Letter—cont'd

**HINTS**

Be brief.
Be personal.
Be specific.
Be polite.
Be sure to sign your name and include your address.
Remember: Thank-you notes are IMPORTANT!

**SAMPLE LETTER**

Mary Breckenridge, RN
2500 Market Street, Suite 100
San Francisco, CA  94109

The Honorable Jackie Smith
California State Assembly
State Capitol
Sacramento, CA  95814

Dear Assemblywoman Smith:

I am a certified nurse-midwife and a member of the California Nurse-Midwives Association. I am writing to urge your support for Senator Jones' bill, SB 255, which will replace the word physician "supervision" in the language of our Nursing Practice Act with the more accurate word "collaboration," thereby defining the relationship between physician and nurse-midwife in accordance with the Joint Statement of Practice Relations Between Obstetricians and Gynecologists and Certified Nurse-Midwives. The bill will also allow hospitals to consider granting staff privileges to certified nurse-midwives, thereby expanding access to low cost, effective, safe care to women who wish to use our services.

I am a graduate of UCSF School of Nursing and practiced as a registered nurse in Maternal and Child Nursing prior to returning to school to become a certified nurse-midwife. I have practiced nurse-midwifery for the past 10 years and can vouch for the fact that the relationship I enjoy with my referring obstetricians is collaborative and supportive. In most instances, they never see my patients, nor are they required to do so, although under the current law they *are* required to sign off on the charts related to those patients. They, and I, see this as an unnecessary step which bears no relationship to patient care or safety. Barriers such as this supervisory requirement add additional expense and may delay access to care by requiring sign off of charts prior to initiation of essential care. ⑤ I urge you to support SB 255.

I would appreciate knowing your position on the bill.

Sincerely,
Mary Breckenridge, RN

Special thanks to Catherine Dodd, RN, for providing this sample letter.

for crafting your message that you would employ in letter writing on the issue. Know the current status of legislation; keep the visit brief, as time is usually short; keep your points succinct and germane to the topic; illustrate your expertise or concern with personal, firsthand examples; and identify your practice setting, particularly if you think the person you are meeting with is familiar with it. Finally, don't forget to ask for a specific action or request to close the meeting—for example, "We hope we can count on you to vote next Wednesday to increase funding for nursing education."

It is highly recommended that you provide a one- or two-page fact sheet to staff in advance of the meeting, and have a copy available to leave with whomever you meet as well. For example, if you are demonstrating the need for increased funding for nursing scholarships, you could provide a graphic representation—a chart or table—that illustrates the low rate of increase for nursing scholarships since they were initiated, particularly compared with grants or scholarships for other medical professions. Any resource that provides data or illustrates points in the form of easily digestible tidbits ("talking points") can be a useful resource to the staff member when he or she is briefing the elected official, writing speeches, or drafting a press release. You should always bring several copies of your business card.

If the person you are scheduled to meet with is unavailable for some reason, it is best to politely and enthusiastically accept an offer to meet with another staff member. You should then follow up with the person you met with as well as with the person you were originally scheduled to meet with. Do not be intimidated if you do not have the answer to a question during the meeting, but do make and keep the commitment to provide the information or supporting documentation in a timely manner. Always follow up a personal meeting with a note thanking the person for his or her time.

## E-MAIL CORRESPONDENCE

The rapid growth of e-mail correspondence and the sheer volume of e-mail communication account for the mixed review e-mail receives as a recommended tool for lobbying. For many members of Congress and their staffs, E-mail is the preferred mode of communication within and between staffs and with experts with whom they already have an established relationship. E-mail correspondence has many advantages:

- *Directness.* The information is sent directly to the person you identify.
- *Timeliness.* Correspondence is immediate, in most cases.
- *Flexibility.* Legislative staff can open e-mail in their own time frame, unlike phone calls, which are often unscheduled interruptions.
- *Attachments.* Important articles, reports, or other information that support your ideas can be attached with e-mail. (Note that if you do not have an established relationship with the person

you are e-mailing, he or she most likely will not open attachments for fear of computer viruses).

The very attributes of e-mail also account for the criticism levied at it. It is direct, and inboxes can be bombarded by e-mails that may not be relevant or from constituents. The concern about attachments is real, and in a climate of worms, viruses, and computer hacking, there are limits placed on what an unknown sender will be able to transmit.

If you do choose to send an e-mail at the time of a vote, it will be counted like a phone message. At that time, staff may be keeping a tally of constituent opinions, and a personal e-mail may be useful. When sending e-mail, always remember to include your name, address, phone number, and e-mail address so that your correspondence can be responded to or you can be contacted for further information. Observe the usual rules for written correspondence, as well as issue tips listed in the previous section on letter writing. With the development of e-mail lists from Websites, many organizations now have the capability to generate an immediate call to action for groups who share a common interest. Many organizations, associations, and interest groups keep legislative alert lists in house so they will have a list of parties who are interested in legislative affairs at their fingertips, but, just as with letter writing, it is important to personalize your e-mail. Some staff and members of Congress have indicated that group or "spam" e-mails have acquired the same status as other bulk postal mailings. One congressional staffer commented, "The e-mail address for the Congressman has to be one of the biggest wastes of taxpayers' dollars—the whole thing is a real headache for staff and of no value to the actual constituents" (Davis, 1999, p. 81). Simply signing onto a host Website, selecting a draft letter provided, and filling in your name will not have a significant effect; letters should be personalized whenever possible.

E-mail is clearly a valuable tool if you are actively working with other organizations or with congressional staff on documents that need to be shared, such as when you are drafting legislation. It is a wonderful tool for networking and for sharing ideas quickly among large numbers of people with diverse opinions. E-mail is probably most useful as a lobbying tool when it is used in conjunction with other lobbying strategies.

## THE INTERNET'S ROLE IN LOBBYING

The Internet has undeniably revolutionized both the content and the delivery of information. The Internet and its partner, e-mail, have come out of the 1990s as equal and complementary partners to more traditional modes of communication.

In terms of revolutionizing politics and lobbying, the most influential change has been an increase in the quantity and depth of information related to legislative affairs that is now accessible to all Americans, instantaneously. The Freedom of Information Act, coupled with the instant access of information from the Internet, has allowed Americans to view in great detail full bill texts, voting records, texts of committee hearings, government agency reports and recommendations, and campaign contributions as reported to the FEC. Many predicted that public interest groups, such as trade associations, membership organizations, and other traditional centers for like-minded people to come together, would be replaced by countless individuals who could find out everything and communicate to Congress instantaneously—during a speech on the floor of the House or Senate, for example—and assume control of lobbying at the grassroots level. After all, the Internet provides a low-cost mode of communication that can be a great equalizer, enabling individuals to compete with organized groups in ways they couldn't have imagined in the past.

What has happened, though, is that the large, traditional interest groups that have helped shape and generate grassroots interest in the past have utilized the Internet to expand membership, increase their public presence, and utilize their Websites to provide enhanced information and value-added services for their members. They are using their Websites to communicate with their respective constituencies and are "adapting their communication strategies to the presence of the Internet, rather than being left behind" (Davis, 1999, pp. 63-64). In addition to being the great equalizer, the Internet allows the opportunity for

traditional groups to communicate with an interested general public as well as with its membership. Organizations fill their Websites with information that highlights their accomplishments and instructions on how to become a member. They post position and policy statements, overall mission and goals of the organization, news releases, resource or publication information, and details about meetings or conventions (Davis, 1999).

In the 1996 presidential election, Republican candidate Bob Dole was the first presidential candidate to announce his World Wide Web homepage at the end of one of the debates. In 2004, Governor Howard Dean was an unsuccessful democratic candidate for president. Despite his loss, his campaign was acknowledged as breaking new ground in use of the Internet. As was described by many media and Internet watchers, the Dean campaign utilized some of the newer strategies, such as meet-ups and blogging (defined as a Web-based personal journal). In an article written for *Wireless,* the author wrote:

The biggest news of the political season has been the tale of this small-state governor who, with the help of Meetup.com and hundreds of bloggers, has elbowed his way into serious contention for his party's presidential nomination. As every alert citizen knows, Dean has used the Net to raise more money than any other Democratic candidate. He's also used it to organize thousands of volunteers who go door-to-door, write personal letters to likely voters, host meetings, and distribute flyers. (Wolf, 2004)

## TESTIMONY

Providing testimony for a political hearing is a prominent method used to go on record about an issue on behalf of an organization or as a constituent. Hearings are increasingly designed by the committee staff to highlight an issue, but they are not, in fact, where most of the key information is shared or decisions are made. As an individual, or on behalf of an association, you may request to testify on a particular issue. It is more likely that your coalition or organization will receive a call from a legislative office requesting that testimony be given from your group. Testimony is accepted in two forms for most committees: as oral remarks (those who are asked to testify) or as written testimony. Written testimony can be provided to the committee by the witness as a supplement to the oral remarks, or it can be provided by any association or individual choosing to submit it for the record. This testimony, including the transcript of the hearing, will eventually be compiled and published as a permanent record of the hearing.

Although very few nurses have the opportunity to testify at a hearing, it is important that you know how to prepare and conduct yourself in the event that you do testify. The principles of preparation are the same for these meetings as they are for a personal meeting: Be prepared, be pleasant, and be persuasive. Being asked to testify as a witness is very exciting, as it provides visibility for you and your organization. There are some things to keep in mind that will help make the experience positive for you.

**Know the Rules.** All committees and their subcommittees have a format they use to conduct the hearing; formats differ not only from state to federal committees but also from one committee to the next. Generally, there is a time limit placed on the length of an individual's remarks. As a guideline, the time limit usually falls between 3 and 10 minutes. You will use this time to present your position on the legislation or issue in an interesting and informative way. Some committees use a green-yellow-red light system to keep the witnesses on track. It is important that you follow the rules and conclude your comments when the red light comes on or your time has elapsed. Frequently, this is not your last word on the subject, as the committee will often engage in a question-and-answer period with a witness following the presentation of testimony.

A senior legislator chairs the committee hearing. The hearing is called to order, and the chair often begins with remarks. Following the chair's remarks, any other legislators on the committee that choose to provide opening remarks will be given the opportunity to do so. Do not be surprised if the elected officials come and go during the meeting. The staff is always present and, in fact, will be responsible for the key messages you bring, and they will also rely on the written materials. The hearing then turns to the panel(s) of witnesses for their comments on the legislation or issue being considered at the hearing.

**Know the Issue.** You do not need to be *the* expert on an issue to present coherent, strong testimony, but it is essential that you know the issue well enough to represent it to the committee and be able to answer questions. Witnesses are often selected based on their constituency and not necessarily on their expertise, although the best witness is a constituent who has expertise in the subject matter of the hearing.

If you are asked to testify, it is important that you learn all you can about the politics and the issue before your testimony. This is where association representatives are invaluable. Typically, they will be the ones who call and ask if you would be willing to testify. If you receive the call from them, rely on them for the drafting of remarks, briefing on the issue and the politics, rules of the hearing, and other matters. Request that they attend the hearing with you and support you through the process. If you receive a request directly from a legislator's office, you may choose to call your association representative to see if he or she is willing to provide support for your testimony. Frequently, associations are very willing to provide this support.

**Be Familiar with Your Prepared Remarks.** Very few of us are expert public speakers who can give a cogent speech under the scrutiny of a House or Senate panel. Therefore, unless you are one of these talented folks, take the time to prepare and practice your remarks before the hearing. Here are some tips that might help:

- Have your remarks printed in large, bold font. Everyone has a different preference for style, but the format may make a difference in your comfort level while giving your testimony.
- Practice, practice, practice. Review your remarks; practice them before friends, family, and colleagues—even your bathroom mirror. Make sure you personalize your testimony and use phrases that are comfortable for you.

- Identify some of the questions you might be asked and think through your responses. That way you won't be caught off guard or become discomfited by the questions.
- Prepare an appropriate response for occasions when you do not know the answer to the question. If you do *not* know the answer, do *not* make something up. Instead, state that you are not able to respond to that question but will try to find the answer and communicate it to the committee. Of course, if you commit to this kind of response, it is important that you follow up.

## POWER IN NUMBERS

Although the power of the individual nurse-constituent is great, the power base multiplies when nurses come together with a unified voice to advocate for change. There are a number of ways to add your voice to the collective voice for nursing leaders. Public interest, professional, or networking groups can begin at the local, or grassroots, level. Joining a local nursing organization or networking group is often a first step toward lending your voice to nursing concerns. Many local groups provide excellent resources for sharing information about public policy, networking with colleagues to discuss the state of nursing practice, or providing opportunities to advocate for health issues.

Nursing groups or organizations at the local level can be influential with policymakers at all levels of government—from a local board of supervisors to the U.S. Representative for their district. Elected officials often welcome opportunities to address the core constituencies in their districts to show that they care about the issues back home, and the possibility of good coverage in local newspapers can also be an incentive to those representatives with an eye toward reelection.

Local nursing groups can sponsor legislative luncheons or celebrate National Nursing Week by inviting a policymaker to either join them at a meeting or address the group. Groups can award legislators with annual "leadership" or "advocate" recognition. Such grassroots activities are excellent ways to increase awareness of nursing issues and to

make sure that nurses are represented when health care policy is being developed at any level.

The other model for grassroots action works in a reverse organizational pattern. Many national nursing organizations have local or statewide chapters. The headquarters of an association might be in Washington, DC, while the local chapters, sections, or branches can be spread out nationwide. This model is effective because the local or regional branch of the organization has the name recognition, resources, and prestige of the national association on their side as they pursue activities at the local level. In this way, local chapters enjoy the added strategic benefit of integrating their grassroots activities with the overall strategic lobbying goals of the national organization. The local group can then look to the national organization for position papers, copies of testimony, briefing documents, or other data on a given issue for use at the local level. Coordination of activities at the local and national levels of the same organizations is critical to ensure that all representatives of the umbrella organizations are spreading consistent messages and positions with policymakers and to avoid any conflicts that might undermine the overall lobbying strategy.

In terms of collective lobbying strategies, one of the most common, and increasingly most effective, options for bringing about change is to create or join a coalition. As the number of interest groups has increased, with almost every niche group having its own association or group, it has become more important to reach consensus and refine priorities with groups that share your interests before approaching federal policymakers with priorities or legislative remedies. Coalitions simplify the workload of legislators and their staff by saving them time: A meeting with one coalition representing 25 groups will take much less time than 25 separate meetings with individual representatives from each group. In fact, coalition expert Kevin Hula (1995) states that because of increasing demands on time, "groups are pressured to work out their differences before approaching Congress, rather than requiring Congress to sort out a seemingly infinite number of differences among groups" (p. 243).

## SUMMARY

You can make a difference. Whether you exercise your power as the power of one—the power of the nurse—or as part of the voice of nursing with collective lobbying strategies, you can make a difference. Nurses are experts in health care and enjoy the respect and trust of the American people, as well as the respect of policymakers who recognize that nurses are highly skilled professionals who work in stressful and life-threatening situations every day. The hardest part is getting started, and there are countless ways to begin to get involved at every level of decision-making to make a difference in the policies that affect the nursing profession and the health of all Americans.

## Key Points

- Lobbying public officials is essential for changing public policies.
- The public officials' staff can be key to persuading the official to adopt your position.
- The various routes to lobby public officials include personal visits, letters, e-mails, phone calls, and presenting testimony.
- Nurses need to be knowledgeable about the issues they are discussing with legislators; the Internet and nursing organizations can provide nurses with such information.
- Know your public official's positions, interests, committee roles, and record on issues related to yours.
- Lobbying as a collective action rather than as a single individual is likely to be more effective; however, never underestimate the power of one voice that speaks at the right time, to the right person, in the right way.

## Web Resources

Access a specialty nursing organization or professional association Website and look for information on legislative issues or government affairs.

**American Nurses Association, Government Affairs**

*http://nursingworld.org/gova/*

**American Women's Health, Obstetric and Neonatal Nurses**

*www.awhonn.org*

**GovSpot**—a non-partisan government information portal to access government information online; it provides a directory of state legislators.

*www.govspot.com/shortcuts/legislators.htm*

**The Library of Congress, Thomas**—a Website launched in January of 1995 to make federal legislative information freely available to the public.

*http://thomas.loc.gov/*

## REFERENCES

Davis, R. (1999). *The web of politics: The Internet's impact on the American political system*. New York: Oxford University Press.

Dodd, C. (2004). Making the political process work. In C. Harrington & C. Estes (Eds.), *Health policy: Crisis and reform in the U. S. health care delivery system* (4th ed.). Sudbury, MA: Jones and Bartlett.

Frantzich, S. E. (1986). *Write your congressman: Constituent communications and representation*. New York: Praeger.

Gallup Organization. (2005). *Annual honesty and ethics poll*. Princeton, NJ: Gallup Organization.

Hula, K. (1995). Rounding up the usual suspects: Forging interest group coalitions in Washington. In A. J. Cigler & B. A. Loomis (Eds.), *Interest group politics* (4th ed.). Washington, DC: Congressional Quarterly.

Wolf, G. (2004). How the Internet invented Howard Dean. Retrieved March 7, 2006, from *www.wired.com/wired/ archive/ 12.01/dean.html*.

# Vignette

Betty R. Dickson

## An Insider's View of Lobbying

*"There are two things you don't want to see being made—sausage and legislation."*

ATTRIBUTED TO OTTO VON BISMARK

I watch hundreds of school kids, parents, teachers, and single-issue citizens converge on the Mississippi state capitol every year during the annual January through March legislative session. I watch as they wander the halls of what is probably one of the most beautiful capitol buildings in the United States. They come to observe, take a stand on their issue, be recognized from the galleries reserved for visitors on the fourth floor, and/or tour the magnificent capitol building. Then they go home.

For 16 years, I have mentored nursing students as they come in groups to observe and be publicly recognized in the respective chambers by various legislators. A few have spent the entire day with me, following closely as I attend committee meetings, listen to testimony and debates, and conduct personal visits with legislators. Those who spend any time at all with me come away with a new respect for the role of a lobbyist and the importance of having someone represent nursing during the legislative session.

There's an old cliché—There are two things one ought not to watch: making sausage and observing the legislative process. Watching the lack of debate, the uninspiring debate, or the grandstanding by legislators can be strange to the novice observer. Most of those who look behind the scenes or witness the process in depth are fascinated. Some even become "hooked" and come back again and again.

With these one-day visits, visitors miss stories like the Bilbo statute, a bronze, life-size rendering of one of Mississippi's most notorious racist governors who also served in the U.S. Senate. It once stood in a prominent place in the capitol, and as more and more African Americans were elected to the legislature, the statue began to be moved around until today it has been relegated to one of the conference rooms, an insignificant place on the first floor of the capitol. Many of the older lobbyists know the significance of Bilbo's positioning today—a tribute to how far Mississippi has come and a testimony to the rise in power and the influence of African American legislators.

Visitors may miss the excitement of watching a plan for legislation come to fruition; they miss the interaction with the powerful legislative leaders and they miss the reality of what could happen if a profession, business, or organization does not understand the importance of having representation, in the form of a lobbyist, working on their behalf.

### GETTING STARTED

I started working as a lobbyist in 1989 when I began a long journey learning the ropes of lobbying in a small state, rich with tradition and history—some

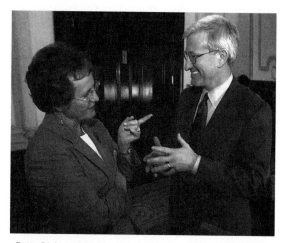

Betty Dickson lobbying former Governor Ronnie Musgrove.

760

bad, some notorious. In 1988, I became executive director of the Mississippi Nurses Association (MNA) and, soon thereafter, began a 16-year lobbying stint for nurses.

During those years, MNA had 95% of its legislation passed, including the following:

- Securing significant annual funding for nursing education
- Creating a $12,000 per year stipend for nurses to obtain a master's or doctoral degree if they teach in a school of nursing
- Securing inclusion of nurse practitioners in most health care networks in the state, including Blue Cross–Blue Shield, who paid nurse practitioners at the same rate as physicians
- Obtaining controlled substance authority for nurse practitioners
- Establishing the Office of Nursing Workforce

I worked for a group of nursing leaders at the MNA who understood the value of using the political arena to protect and advance the profession.

## POLITICAL STRATEGIES

### Getting Nurses on Every Health-Related State Agency

My lobbying career got off to a big start. Innocently, I took the MNA leadership seriously when they told me their major objective was to have nurses at the seat of every table where health care decisions were made. During my first year at MNA, our lobbyist was a nurse-attorney. During Desert Storm, the nurse/lobbyist went to work full-time for a law firm to fill a vacancy created by an attorney/guardsman who was called to active duty. I became MNA's only lobbyist.

During that first year, the lobbyist and I developed a strategy to access every code section in the law for every health care agency. We planned to try and amend the law to mandate that a nurse be on every governing board of any health-related agency, including the department of education. Although the legislation would define my career and reputation, I was totally unaware, at the time, of the enormous opposition to "touching" any board's composition. That legislative session turned out to be one of getting acquainted with division and department heads, getting a great education about

government agencies, and getting a ton of teasing from other lobbyists who thought this was a pretty gutsy move for a newcomer.

Of course, the bill had little chance of passage, but once we searched the Mississippi code, drafted the bill's language, asked a legislator to introduce the bill, and attempted to get a committee hearing on the bill, I learned the legislative process from the bottom up. To this day, those agency heads who are still around ask me at the beginning of each session if I have any surprises up my sleeve. It's good to keep them guessing.

Interestingly enough, as a result of that initiative and even without passage of the bill, the mental health division and the state board of health, to this day, keep a registered nurse (RN) on the board, including one who served as chair. Today, there are three RNs on the Mississippi State Board of Health, proof that you don't have to get a law passed to accomplish your goal, or, there's more than one way to skin a cat.

### Numbers Connote Strength

Lobbying is also about counting. I could count, nursing leadership could count, and legislators especially know the value of numbers. We used the strength of numbers to influence legislators. In 1994, there were over 40,000 RNs and licensed practical nurses (LPNs) practicing in Mississippi, and we had to establish a mechanism to bring representatives from all those nurses together.

Through the Nursing Organizations Liaison Committee of MNA, we brought 25 nursing organizations together and worked to plan and agree on a legislative agenda. There were representatives from each group who worked collaboratively on a statewide nursing summit where 700 to 800 RNs and students attended annually. We invited key legislators to join us, and they could count the numbers for themselves. It was through this coalition that nursing began to be recognized as a significant force at the state capitol.

### INGREDIENTS OF A GOOD LOBBYING RECIPE

There are no secret ingredients to lobbying. Legislators really do depend on lobbyists to provide information about issues, to muster support for pet projects, to help with constituents' problems, and to help with their campaigns.

## Call in the Nurses

It helps to have a successful political action committee behind you, and it helps to have a plan to "call in the nurses" when the need arises. I know that legislators really fear having large droves of citizens come to the capitol—whether it's truckers, physicians, loggers, hair braiders...or nurses.

I think back to one issue in the early 1990s when an attempt was made to establish medication technicians in nursing homes. Nurses were strongly opposed to this new provider whose only requirement was a high school education and a few weeks of training. The vice chair of the House of Representatives Public Health and Welfare Committee was assigned the bill and scheduled a public hearing. MNA arranged for over 100 nurses, in uniform, to attend the hearing. When the committee chair couldn't get everyone in the regular conference room on the first floor, he moved us to the second floor to a larger room. It became apparent that the second room was too small, so he moved us to an even larger room back again on the first floor. Imagine 100 nurses marching to a room on the first floor, then marching upstairs to another room, then down the stairs and to the room on the opposite end of the hall. It created a lot of excitement, lots of stares, and lots of curiosity. It also established several points about the nursing community: We are well organized, there are a lot of us, and we will make plenty of calls to our legislators.

When the chair finally got the hearing under way, the nurses were already breathing pretty heavily. When testimony began, the breathing became a little more pronounced. And when one of the opponents, during testimony, said something disparaging about nurses, all 100 gasped in unison. It even scared me, and I was on their side. Needless to say, he ended the hearing without a vote on the bill. Mississippi still does not have medication technicians.

## Be in the Right Place at the Right Time

Successful lobbying sometimes depends on being in the right place at the right time. Once a state senator called me to review an immunization bill he wanted to introduce. After reading through the bill, I told him that I thought we were already doing what he wanted to do with the legislation. His reply was that he wanted an immunization bill! I told him I would get back with him with a suggestion. I was MNA's representative on the Mississippi State Health Department's Immunization Task Force, so I called the chief of staff at the health department, a nurse. She suggested that we convince him to introduce a bill for a statewide immunization registry, one of the goals of the task force. I did. He loved the idea. He introduced a bill, and we worked very hard for passage. Today there is a statewide registry for tracking immunization. Mississippi also has one of the highest immunization rates in this country.

That same nurse and I were in the capitol during a legislative session when we were called by the chair of Public Health and Welfare committee who wanted to implement a school-based clinic pilot for the state. We were given the assignment to come up with language for an amendment to an education bill. She grabbed an envelope, and we crafted the language on the back. Reading it over carefully, we went back into the meeting where she handed the chair the envelope, and he passed it to the bill writer. It became law.

## Putting Frogs in a Wheelbarrow: Use Humor as a Tool

Sometimes humor can disarm even the most stoic adversary. After we were successful in getting the bill to create the Office of Nursing Workforce (ONW) passed through the House and the Senate and then back to the House for final approval, a community college president appeared at the weekly committee meeting and told the chair that the community colleges were opposed to our bill. We were completely blown away at this final hour. The chair gave us one day to work out the problem. Luckily, the community college presidents were meeting the next day, so I arranged an audience with them by convincing an old friend, who was a president, to get a group of us on the agenda. Several of us appeared the next day but were getting nowhere. The head of the community college board kept saying we didn't need ONW. We tried to reason with him: "We have no accurate data on nursing in Mississippi; we need better communication between the schools of nursing and nursing administration; we need to develop workforce strategies." Nothing was working with the all-male audience. Finally I placed both hands on the table and asked: "Mr. Chairman, have you ever tried to put frogs in a wheelbarrow?" A slight smile appeared on his face. "Where are you going with this?" he asked. I explained, "We have been trying to get these folks working together. First, we get the community college nursing programs in the wheelbarrow. Then we turn around and try to pick up the bachelor of science in nursing (BSN) or higher programs and put them in the wheelbarrow. Then we try to get hospital administration in the wheelbarrow. Then we turn around and the other two have jumped out. We need a way to get them all in the wheelbarrow at the same time." They all laughed and, with further discussion, agreed to support our bill.

### Use Your Best Assets

When Mississippi's first Republican governor since reconstruction, Kirk Fordice, created the state's Health Care Commission, I was appointed to represent nursing. When it came time for nursing to make a presentation on nursing's role in health care and how we could improve the status of health care in Mississippi, MNA chose three outstanding leaders to make our case. The first was a diminutive, perky nurse president of MNA who could spit out data in rapid fire delivery; the second was our impressive board of nursing executive director, whose ability to think on her feet and whose sense of humor was incredible; and finally, a tall blond dean of a school of nursing and former Alabama Maid of Cotton, whose intelligence was only exceeded by her good looks.

When the nurses finished their presentation and as we walked back to our chairs, the president of the hospital association whispered to me, "You don't play fair." As a result of our unfair play, the commission recommended, and the legislature passed, legislation to increase funding to three existing nurse practitioner programs and to add two new programs—all to increase the numbers of NPs so that rural Mississippi could experience better health care coverage. That led to a need for further legislation.

### Use Proven Strategies

Learning from past experiences was helpful as nurse practitioners called upon MNA to help with the issues of signing forms that, by law, required a physician signature. Once again, we did a code search and found every law requiring a physician signature and drafted a bill to change the language to say "or nurse practitioner". It included numerous forms, one of which was an authorization for handicapped parking. The bill was huge and affected many agencies, thus creating a lot of attention. We explained that the NP was the provider and the physician was not always on site. In order to get a physician signature, the patient had to schedule an appointment with the physician, thus creating additional cost and additional paper work. The bill passed and the result was that the State Department of Health changed all their forms to include NP signatures.

### Be Prepared for a Big Fight

Because of these legislative successes and other efforts through MNA, NP numbers grew and began spreading out across the state; eventually, some NPs opened their own practices. This was perceived as a threat by the Mississippi State Board of Medical Licensure (MSBML) and the Mississippi Medical Association.

To set the stage for the fight, it must be understood that under state law enacted in the Nurse Practice Act, NPs must work with a collaborating physician who does not always have to be in the same setting. Existing law also requires the Mississippi State Board of Nursing (MSBN) to jointly promulgate any NP regulatory change with MSBML. This language was agreed upon in the early 1980s when the NP practice was established. MSBML regulations passed in the early 1990s use the term "supervising" rather than "collaborating physician" and require that any physician supervising an NP in a "freestanding" clinic must appear before the MSBML before receiving permission to supervise. "Freestanding" is defined as being 15 miles or 15 minutes away from the physician. For this arrangement, the physicians had to take a day away from their practice and come to Jackson, the capitol, to be interviewed by the board. This, in effect, created a barrier to the NP practice in a freestanding clinic. We began to take steps to remove the barrier.

The fight that ensued lasted through several legislative sessions but taught me a lesson in electoral politics. The lesson was that if one loses power in one chamber but gains it in another, one must still work to maintain strength in both.

The story began in the early 1990s when the MSBML, through their regulatory process, began adopting regulations supposedly aimed at physicians who were supervising NPs. What the regulation actually did was place severe restrictions on the practice of NPs. The first regulations were adopted in 1990; several years later, an attempt was made to make those regulations even more restrictive.

MNA countered by asking for help from the Mississippi legislature. A bill was introduced by a great friend of nursing, a woman who had introduced NPs back in her small hometown where she served as mayor prior to running for the legislature. She was chair of the House Insurance Committee and helped us find a pretty obscure insurance statute related to NP reimbursement. Her bill amended that law to state simply that "any regulation that impacts the practice of nurse practitioners must be jointly promulgated with the Board of Nursing." The bill passed the State House of Representatives where nursing had much more influence because of friends like the chair and vice chair of the Public Health and Welfare Committee. Because the bill was in the House Insurance Committee, it was passed without much scrutiny from the medical community—what we call "flying below the radar screen." The House bill was referred to the Senate Public Health and Welfare Committee instead of the Insurance Committee. It was the best thing that could have happened because the chair of the Senate Public Health and Welfare Committee had a daughter who was a pediatric nurse practitioner. Utilizing her, along with other NPs from his district, we convinced him that the MSBML was stepping outside their boundaries by passing restrictive regulations that affected nursing.

When the bill reached the Senate, the chair took up the House bill and guided it to passage in spite of the late efforts by the medical community. Round one, advantage nurses.

### Be Aware That Elections Can Change Everything

State elections are held every four years. When our Senate chair decided not to seek reelection, nursing lost some powerful support. But we maintained strong support in the House where the chair of Public Health and Welfare was a great friend.

In an attempt to abolish the deadlock created by joint promulgation and to fly something out there to see where our opposition was, we had a very controversial bill introduced in the House that would remove all joint promulgation language. The medical community perceived this as an opening for independent practice by NPs. We knew it would create quite a stir and watched with interest at the havoc it created. Of course, neither chamber passed the legislation, but it did get a hearing in the House where we were able to get the issues on the table. The lesson: We used our friends in the House when we lost our Senate support.

The following year, NPs convinced MNA that they should be allowed to write prescriptions for controlled substances. My own NP told me that I could go to the pharmacy, ask for codeine in my cough syrup, and sign for it but that she could not prescribe it for me. That made no sense. So I went to the pharmacy, requested cough syrup with codeine, and signed for it. I would use that experience later to argue for NPs' right to prescribe.

### Understand That Sometimes the Regulatory Process Is the Best Strategy

MNA talked with the executive director of the MSBN and determined that controlled substance authority could be granted through the regulatory process. It would require joint promulgation, but that was a chance we would take. The board of nursing was extremely cooperative, and together, we took the regulatory language used by the MSBML for physicians and constructed language to apply to NPs. At the time, the MSBML staff was being cooperative.

They discovered an existing law that would have to be amended before we could go forward with joint promulgation. A Bureau of Narcotics law stated that the MSBML would have jurisdiction over the legal distribution of narcotics by physicians, *nurses*, podiatrists, and veterinarians. It was the MSBML staff who told us the law would have to be changed because they did not want to deal with the NPs.

Our first stop was with the Mississippi State Medical Association to communicate our plan of action. An old circuit judge told me years ago that he did not like surprises, so my plan was to completely apprise the medical community of our intentions. My offer: Support us in changing the language in the Bureau of Narcotics bill and controlled substance authority through the regulatory process and we will not pursue legislation to remove joint promulgation during this term. They declined our offer...and the game began. We had the bill introduced to remove all joint promulgation and allow only the board of nursing to control the NP practice as well as the bill to change the Bureau of Narcotics legislation.

### Make Real Friends in the Legislature

To get physicians worked up, the Mississippi State Medical Association began faxing physicians with information that NPs would be allowed to do surgery under this bill. They conducted a survey that reportedly indicated that patients preferred physicians to write their prescriptions. They held a press conference touting physician education, their survey, and numerous other silly admonitions—all to disparage NPs and imply that NPs were taking over medicine.

We countered the next day with a press conference, citing research documenting that nurse practitioners have the same or better outcomes as physicians and citing the number of NPs practicing in rural areas where no physician would go. We also used my example of how patients could sign for their own codeine if they wished.

There was one key legislator who was not happy with the medical community because physicians in his area were refusing to sign a contract with Blue Cross–Blue Shield to provide coverage to patients. He was also not too happy with the number of physicians in Mississippi refusing to see Medicaid patients.

As a result, this legislator was very supportive of the NP practice because the only health care provider in his community was an NP. Despite the extreme opposition by the physicians, the bill to amend the Bureau of Narcotics law passed after we agreed to withdraw the joint promulgation bill. We worked with the Mississippi State Medical Association, through an informal committee, to agree on regulatory language allowing NPs to write prescriptions for controlled substances, including Schedules II through IV.

Later, that same legislator was elevated to chair of the House Public Health and Human Services, and with that came his continued support to keep the MSBML in check. For instance, he requested that both the MBON and the MSBML address the lack of collaborating physicians in rural Mississippi—all a result of restrictive regulations from the MSBML. Because of his efforts, new regulations have been passed, and now the MSBML regulations identify the physician as "collaborating" rather than "supervising," corresponding with MSBN regulations.

### THERE REALLY IS A NEED FOR LOBBYISTS

There is so much health care legislation today affecting the nursing community. From Medicaid to the State Department of Health, from school nurses to nursing education, from the nursing shortage to mandatory overtime, all of these areas can benefit from nursing representation in state and federal legislative arenas. Someone who knows the ins and outs of the legislative process and is respected can make a significant difference for the practice of nursing.

Lobbyists keep their fingers on the pulse of health care legislation and regulations. They are skilled communicators, some with a sense of humor, who know when to call out the nurses. They have the expertise to help with political campaigns. Lobbyists know how to assist legislators with constituent problems and can be in the right place at the right time. Organizational success in policy arenas is often directly related to the effectiveness of the lobbying effort. Unless nurses do this as a full-time job, they rarely have the time to assume the lobbying function. My advice to nursing: Don't be caught without one.

# Interest Groups: Powerful Political Catalysts in Health Care

Patrick S. Malone & Mary W. Chaffee*

*"There are two things you need for success in politics. Money...and I can't think of the other."*
SENATOR MARK HANNAH

As thousands were responding to the devastation left in the wake of hurricane Katrina along the Gulf Coast of the United States in September of 2005, another flurry of activity was occurring in Washington, DC: Congress was considering $200 billion worth of hurricane aid packages. Like sharks drawn to blood, lobbyists acting on behalf of special interest groups moved in to take advantage of a rare opportunity. Special interests including the oil lobby, the American Institute of Architects, the Air Transport Association, the American Farm Bureau, and the Federation of American Hospitals (representing for-profit hospitals) were elbowing one another out of the way in an attempt to capitalize on the abrupt change in the nation's policy agenda (Birnbaum, 2005). The hurricane's damage opened the door to lucrative policy changes that interest groups had sought for years.

In his earliest writings on life in the United States, Alexis de Tocqueville presented a thought-provoking opinion as to the explanation for America's successful democratic system. One reason for success, he wrote, was the propensity for Americans to participate in voluntary associations or interest groups. Today, de Tocqueville would be proud. Interest groups in the United States number in the thousands, representing every conceivable interest from business to education to wildlife conservation. During the 2004 presidential election the prominence of interest groups was staggering, with Senator John Kerry and President George W. Bush both claiming the other's link to powerful interest groups (Tichenour, 2006).

Are interest groups good or bad? A simple yes or no cannot fully answer the question. Indeed, interest groups represent everything good about our system: organizations looking after their constituents and advocating for preferred policy choices. But interest

*The authors wish to acknowledge the contribution of Mary Wachter to the original version of this chapter.

groups can also wield untoward power. Regardless, through their use of professional expertise, lobbying tactics, coalition development, and political action committees (PACs), there is little argument that interest groups exert significant influence on policy, on politics, and ultimately on society. However, interest groups are also seen as devoted to private interests rather than the public good. They are even called "pressure groups" when they demonstrate particularly aggressive advocacy tactics. In this chapter we take a comprehensive look at interest groups, their origins and development, their strategies, and their impact on health care and health care systems.

## A BRIEF HISTORY OF INTEREST GROUPS

Occupational and professional organizations gave birth to the first interest groups. Early development was influenced by the rapidly budding industrial era in the late nineteenth century. The subsequent expansion and professionalization of the economy led to the growth of many types of organizations; the development of one group would often lead to the appearance of an opposing body. Nonprofit associations such as the American Cancer Society would be countered by profit-based associations such as the Tobacco Research Council. Large corporations tended to sponsor for-profit–sector interest groups, whereas the government and nonprofit organizations would support nonprofit groups.

### IRON TRIANGLES

In the 1940s and 1950s, "iron triangles" developed. These were networks of private interests, bureaucrats, and government officials linked in mutually beneficial relationships, and they are powerful fixtures in American politics even today. In typical cases an iron triangle would be composed of a congressional committee or subcommittee, interest groups (trade or industry associations), and a federal agency. For instance, in the timber industry, an iron triangle may include the Agriculture Committee's Subcommittee on Forests, the U.S. Forest Service as the federal agency, and an interest group representing the timber industry. These groups all support and benefit from one another.

### LIBERAL FOUNDATIONS

In the 1960s, interest groups with more ideologic and liberal foundations emerged. Fueled by the tumultuous social climate of the Vietnam era and the fight for civil rights, Americans began questioning their democratic system of government and raising their voices about race relations, economic policy, and foreign involvement. Sit-ins, boycotts, and protests punctuated the decade.

### RIGHT-WING INFLUENCE

In the 1970s and 1980s the United States witnessed a rebound response to the liberalism of the 1960s. There was a proliferation of right-wing conservative interest groups such as the New Christian Right. Interest groups also began to take center stage in American politics. For example, President Jimmy Carter battled with the American Medical Association (AMA) over health care spending controls. Ultimately, as a result of the Federal Election Campaign Act amendments of 1974, revisions in campaign finance laws led to a more prominent role for interest groups in the electoral process. This legislation laid the foundation for future debates about interest groups, their influence, and the integrity of the political process (Berry, 1997).

### A DOMINANT ROLE

In recent years, interest groups have come under increasing scrutiny for their powerful political influence. This comes as no surprise, given the expansion of the funds, staff, and expertise of interest groups. Furthermore, the changing demographic and religious makeup of the country has introduced many groups, some previously disenfranchised, to the political scene, and many minorities find themselves better represented than ever before. As more players arrive on the political stage, the mix of power, influence, and policy alternatives grows more enigmatic—and outcomes more difficult to predict.

## WHY DO INTEREST GROUPS EXIST?

Interest groups have long been a part of the American political landscape. Although they have not always met with favor, they tend to be an accepted fact of political reality. James Madison considered interest groups to be simply an extension of human desire, based on the propensity of the citizenry to have different opinions concerning religion and government. He also believed the causes of factions to be "sown in the nature of man" (1961, p. 79). From a policy perspective, Lindbloom considered the interest group's role in the policy process to be "indispensable" (Lindbloom, 1980).

With Madison's views as background, it is important to note that interest groups have not always been met with open arms. Some question their value as agents of mobilization. Indeed, one of the more interesting dilemmas regarding interest groups centers on their role in political mobilization, versus that of political parties. Political scientists have traditionally taken the position that parties were more beneficial than interest groups as mechanisms for mobilization (Walker, 1997). In truth, there is room for both. By serving as a check on majoritarianism, interest groups ensure there is a political voice for special, often minority, interests. Parties, conversely, fight for the majority interest (Dye, 1998). Still, others argue that interest groups are elitist and nonrepresentative in nature. Schattschneider's (1960) description of the flaw in the pluralist heaven is often quoted: "The heavenly chorus sings with a strong upper class accent."

This leads to a crucial distinction between interests and interest groups. Although it may seem trite, the distinction is an important one. To borrow an example from Berry (1997), farmers are not an interest group, but the American Farm Bureau Federation (AFBF) is. The difference lies in one thing— organization. Although not all farmers belong to the AFBF, the AFBF represents the interests of all farmers. Therein lies an indicator of the political power of the interest group. Their influence lies not only in their membership, but also in their ability to represent the interests of a much larger body.

## FORMING AND JOINING

Political scientists have long struggled with the reasons that make people join interest groups and why interest groups form. Truman (1951) considered interest groups to be a group of people with shared values who join together to influence other groups in society. In essence, he felt that their creation is a result of natural interaction and societal disturbances. Mancur Olson (1965) argued that people join groups for selective benefits or as a result of coercion. In his view, group development is problematic. Salisbury's (1969) answer to the formation problem lay in the role of the entrepreneur. As part of his Exchange Theory, Salisbury argued that it takes the work of individual catalysts to ensure group formation. These entrepreneurs seek to assume the early organizational costs in return for a staff job with the group. Scholars since Salisbury have suggested that politics may play a greater role in that there may be more incentive involved in contributing to the collective political benefits than originally thought.

Quite simply, people join interest groups to realize one of three types of benefits: material, solidary, and purposive (Clark & Wilson, 1961).

- Material benefits involve tangible rewards.
- Solidary benefits designate social rewards that occur from association with the group.
- Purposive benefits tend to be ideologically based or issue-oriented goals, not tangible in nature.

Olson (1965) later added selective benefits (benefits available only to members of the organization) and collective benefits (those that accrue to both members and nonmembers) to this list.

## CLASSIFICATION OF INTEREST GROUPS

Interest groups have a number of forms, structures, missions, and types (Dye, 1998). Some of the more common differentiations follow:

- *Organizational structure.* Interest groups may be national, regional, state, or local. They may have centralized or decentralized structures. They may cater to groups or individual members, organizations (e.g., trade associations), or even governments (e.g., National League of Cities). Finally, they may have large or small staffs, be mail based, or even be Internet based.
- *Economic focus.* Economic interest groups, such as the Business Roundtable, base their mission in the economic interests of their members. People

for the American Way and other noneconomic interest groups have goals that are more ideologic in nature. Interest groups may even bridge the gap between economic and noneconomic goals depending on their ideologic, informational, and instrumental functions.

- *Type of benefit.* Interest groups vary widely in the types of benefits they seek to obtain for their members (Box 26-1). Groups such as Greenpeace and the Christian Coalition offer mainly ideologic benefits that are more purposive in nature. Members of the United Auto Workers enjoy material benefits from their membership such as higher pay and health benefits. Members of the National Organization for Women gain a feeling of solidarity in their relationship with others in the organization. Finally, some organizations, such as AARP, offer a combination of all these types of rewards for their members.
- *Goals and mission.* Interest groups pursue unique goals. Business groups and trade associations seek to influence lawmakers to enhance their business interests. Professional associations and labor groups attempt to further the specialized status and interests of their fields. The goal of a group may involve the public interest, seeking a collective good on behalf of the general public, or a group may exist to pursue a single agenda, focusing its energy on one cause. An example of a single-issue group is the AMA.

## INTEREST GROUP ACTIVITY

Lobbying legislators is considered the primary tool of interest groups to further their causes. This is not surprising. Indeed, interest groups are expert at using lobbying to influence agendas, legislation, and policymaker actions. The way that interest groups exert influence, however, is more complex than lobbying alone. The strength—indeed, the currency—of the interest group is information. The data and expertise of the staff and membership of interest groups represent a tremendous force. Because information is power, this places interest groups in an excellent position to be creative in determining strategic approaches to electoral influence or political mobilization.

---

**BOX 26-1**  Examples of Interest Groups (by Type)

**BUSINESS**
Business Roundtable
National Small Business Association
U.S. Chamber of Commerce

**TRADE**
American Petroleum Institute
Home Builders Association
Motion Picture Association of America

**PROFESSIONAL**
American Medical Association
American Nurses Association
National Education Association

**UNION**
American Federation of Labor and Congress of Industrial Organizations
American Federation of Teachers
United Steel Workers

**AGRICULTURE**
National Cattlemen's Association
National Grange
The Tobacco Institute

**WOMEN**
League of Women Voters
National Organization for Women

**PUBLIC INTEREST**
Common Cause
Public Citizen

**IDEOLOGIC**
American Conservative Union
Americans for Democratic Action
People for the American Way

**SINGLE ISSUE**
National Rifle Association
National Right to Life Committee
National Taxpayers Union

**ENVIRONMENT**
Environmental Defense Fund
Nature Conservancy
Sierra Club

*Continued*

**BOX 26-1** Examples of Interest Groups (by Type)—cont'd

**RELIGIOUS**

American-Israeli Public Affairs Committee
Catholics for Choice

**CIVIL RIGHTS**

American Indian Movement
National Urban League
Rainbow Coalition

**AGE RELATED**

American Association of Retired Persons
Children's Defense Fund

**MILITARY VETERANS**

American Legion
Veterans of Foreign Wars
Retired Officers Association

**GOVERNMENT**

National Association of Counties
National Conference of State Legislators
National League of Cities

## INTEREST GROUP STRATEGY

Interest groups use a variety of tactics to persuade lawmakers or sway public opinion. Most can be defined as one of two types: inside strategies or outside strategies (Walker, 1997). *Inside* strategies are direct and focused in nature. These include tactics such as direct lobbying or PAC contributions. Interest groups using inside strategies often depend on the use of financial resources and subject matter expertise to influence public officials. Conversely, *outside* strategies are more broadly focused. Although they may be used in concert with inside schemes, outside strategies are generally used to influence the general public or a segment of the population. Outside strategies may simply plant the seed for future political support—months or even years down the road.

Aside from direct and more informal contacts with legislators and government officials, interest groups may exert their influence on legislation in the form of lawsuits or the filing of *amicus curiae* (friend of the court) briefs. They may organize coalitions or protests to pressure legislative decision-makers. Interest groups will often target constituents directly through letter writing, telegrams, e-mail, or telephone calls to mobilize support. They may enlist the media to mobilize the public around a specific policy issue, a strategy known as *media advocacy*. Groups may also attempt to influence elections through campaign contributions, candidate endorsements, or volunteer campaign work. Finally, using their subject matter expertise, interest groups play an important role in drafting legislation and regulations. By assisting congressional staffs through this type of inside strategy, interest groups wield tremendous power in shaping policy and law.

Which strategy is the best? Given the number of approaches available to interest groups, one may wonder when an interest group will choose a particular tactic. Unfortunately, interest group scholars find themselves at a loss to explain the strategy choices interest groups make. Baumgartner and Leech (1998) note that interest group behavior is unpredictable. First, most groups use a variety of strategies as opposed to a single tactic. Second, the choice of strategy depends on the contextual nature of the situation as well as the unique characteristics of the group.

## POLITICAL ACTION COMMITTEES

PACs are the campaign funding arm of special interest groups. They are money-making machines that raise funds to contribute to candidates' legislative, gubernatorial, congressional, and presidential campaigns. The term *political action committee* usually refers to one of two types of political committees registered with the Federal Election Commission (FEC):

- Separate segregated funds (SSFs) and nonconnected committees. SSFs are political committees established and managed by corporations, labor unions, membership organizations, or trade associations. SSFs are limited in their ability to solicit contributions. They may seek donations only from individuals associated with connected or sponsoring organizations.
- Nonconnected committees, in contrast, are not connected to corporations and so on, and they may solicit contributions from the general public (FEC, 2005).

Political incumbents receive the majority of PAC contributions. PAC contributions, however, do not buy votes. In fact, there is very little evidence that PAC funding directly affects a legislator's vote on a given bill (Weissert & Weissert, 2002). What PAC contributions buy is *access*.

## POLITICAL ACTION COMMITTEE FUNCTIONS

The PACs are one part of a three-pronged approach—direct lobbying, grassroots lobbying, and PAC contributions—used by special interest groups to influence policy decisions (Weissert & Weissert, 2002). The influence exerted by PACs is directly related to the amount and timing of contributions made to candidates. Candidates who receive PAC dollars, particularly when this support is rendered early (e.g., before primary elections), are more likely to meet with those groups and listen to their positions on issues. Thus PAC contributions gain access to decision-makers at critical times (Heineman, Peterson, & Rasmussen, 1995).

There are other functions of PACs that can influence policymakers besides direct monetary contributions. Organizations with large memberships are impressive voting blocks that candidates and elected officials pay close attention to—especially if their race is hotly contested. The endorsement of a candidate by the PAC of a large group can be leveraged into votes. Endorsements by PACs are publicized to the membership of the interest group. The endorsement is the group's seal of approval and indicates that the candidate being endorsed has met a number of criteria. Possible reasons for endorsement include:

- Alignment of the candidate's position on issues with that of the group
- Sponsorship of legislation supported by the group
- The electability of the candidate (Heineman et al., 1995)

In the case of incumbents, a voting record that is favorable to the group and the candidate's holding of a key leadership position may also be conditions for endorsement (Weissert & Weissert, 2002). Decisions about contributions and candidate endorsements are generally made by the governing body of the PAC. This usually consists of members of the interest group who are either appointed or elected by the membership.

## HOPPING DOWN THE CAMPAIGN MONEY TRAIL

There are ethical implications of a political process in which interest groups give money to elected officials who are then supposed to make unbiased policy decisions in the best interests of their constituents. For this reason, PACs are heavily regulated political entities. There are federal, state, and local PACs, and each is subject to specific designated regulations. State and local PAC regulations vary widely throughout the United States. The regulations set forth by the FEC, the government agency with regulatory oversight of federal PACs, are discussed here.

The PACs raise money primarily through contributions by special interest group members. Individuals may contribute up to $5000 per calendar year to a PAC. There are limits on the amount that a PAC can contribute to a candidate's campaign. This amount may range from $1000 to $5000 per candidate per election depending on whether the PAC has been approved by the FEC as a one-candidate or multi-candidate PAC. Candidates use PAC money to pay the ever-increasing costs of running a campaign, especially the cost of advertising. In the 2000 campaign cycle, candidates, parties, and interest groups spent $3 billion to secure elected positions. This represents a 50% increase in expenditures from the 1996 election cycle (Dwyer, 2000).

Historically, PACs are well-known for their contributions to political parties, especially the National Democratic and Republican Committees. The parties then spend this money on activities that benefit the candidates. The FEC limit on contributions from a PAC to a political party is $20,000 per calendar year. All contributions must be reported quarterly to the FEC and represent public information (FEC, 2005).

## AMERICAN NURSES ASSOCIATION POLITICAL ACTION COMMITTEE

The American Nurses Association Political Action Committee (ANA-PAC) is the campaign funding arm of the American Nurses Association (ANA), the most prominent nursing special interest group, which speaks for all 2.7 million registered nurses (RNs) in the United States. ANA-PAC was established in 1974 to strengthen ANA's voice in the nation's capitol. Since that time ANA-PAC has grown to become one of the top health care PACs in the United States. For the third consecutive election cycle, ANA-PAC has raised more than $1 million from nurses throughout the country. There are many nurses who are high donors, but the average contribution is about $42 per year per nurse.

The purpose of ANA-PAC is to assist candidates who are friends of nursing win elections for federal office, thus increasing the number of federally elected officials who understand and support the ANA's policy agenda. ANA-PAC is committed to increasing the number of RNs in public office at every level of government. During the 2000 election cycle, ANA-PAC was successful in helping to reelect three nurses to the U.S. House of Representatives. ANA-PAC also endorses candidates for office (ANA, 2005b).

## FOLLOW THE MONEY

### MONEY AS INFLUENCE

Money plays a prominent role in the ability of interest groups to achieve their goals. Money reflects the power of the group, buys access to policymakers, and ensures the visibility of the interest group. Money is important to incumbents and even more important to challengers (Berry, 1997; Jacobson, 1990). Along with information, it is the lifeblood of interest groups.

### HARD AND SOFT MONEY

Political contributions are described as *hard* or *soft*. Hard-money donations are those made directly to candidates. Soft-money donations are earmarked for party-building activities (e.g., registration voting drives) but have often been used for advertising candidates, an activity now regulated by new campaign finance laws. In the 1999-2000 election cycle, Republicans raised $447 million in hard money and $244 million in soft money. Democrats

raised $270 million in hard money and $243 million in soft money (Dwyer, Cohn, McNamee, & Palmer, 2001).

Let there be no mistake: Interest groups do not hesitate to use money to influence elections. Interest groups spent tens of millions of dollars in the U.S. House and Senate races in fall 2000. One study by the Center for the Study of Elections and Democracy at Brigham Young University (BYU) suggests that some of the closest races of the recent election cycle may have been strongly influenced by interest groups (Allen, 2001). The study found that interest groups spent over $95 million for radio and television advertisements alone. Other interest group–funded activities included phone calls, direct mailings, and billboard advertisements.

## CAMPAIGN FINANCE REFORM

Campaign finance reform has threatened to curb the influence of money on the political system. The 1974 campaign finance reforms, well intended as they were, provided legitimacy to fund-raising. Post-Watergate efforts to reform campaign finance laws have proven relatively ineffective because of the fund-raising prowess of clever campaign managers. Indeed, campaign officials have historically met with great success in securing large donations to political parties that subsequently end up in the hands of the candidates.

By far the most significant attempt at reform has been the Bipartisan Campaign Reform Act—Public Law 107-155 (also known as the *McCain-Feingold Bill*), sponsored by Senator John McCain (R-AZ) and Senator Russ Feingold (D-WI). The final version of the bill, sponsored by Representative Christopher Shays (R-CT) and Representative Martin T. Meehan (D-MA) was signed into law by President George W. Bush on March 27, 2002. The bill bans corporations, individuals, and unions from giving unregulated soft money to national parties, an amount that totaled nearly $500 million in 2000. It also limits soft-money contributions to state and local parties, capping them at $10,000 and barring their use in federal campaigns. The campaign finance reform also increases contribution limits for candidates running against wealthy candidates who finance their own campaigns; creates stricter disclosure requirements; and prohibits fund-raising on federal property and from foreign sources (Brookings Institution, 2002; Center for Responsive Politics, 2005a).

The bill also raises hard-money contribution limits by individuals to $2000 for House, Senate, and presidential candidates and to $25,000 for parties. Most significantly for interest groups, the McCain-Feingold Bill limits the ability of unions, nonprofit organizations, and corporations to broadcast political advertisements (issue advertisements) targeting specific federal candidates for the 60 days before a general election and for the 30 days before a primary election (Dewar, 2002).

Despite the passage of the Bipartisan Campaign Reform Act, campaign finance reform will remain on the national agenda, and deliberations on both sides of the issue continue. Some interest groups have raised concern that the portions of the bill restricting issue advertisements in the final phases of a campaign may tread on rights of free speech. Others believe reform efforts are imperative in rescuing a political system controlled by big money and large corporations. Democrats and organized labor groups will continue to express concern about the fairness of the legislation. Republicans, meanwhile, appear poised to benefit early from reform efforts as a result of their prowess at securing hard-money donations. Representative Albert Wynn (D-MD) stated, "A Republican passing a hat in a country club can make a lot more hard money than a Democrat talking to regular people" (Squitirei, 2001). Whatever the ultimate outcome, the implications of reform are significant. Kuttner (2001) writes, "How societies' richest and most powerful interests are permitted to undermine democracy by substituting a large check for a democratic mobilization of voters has its most profound implications for substantive politics" (p. 4).

## EVOLVING ROLE OF POLITICAL PARTIES

Political scientists have come to question the viability of the American political party in the face of the growing power of interest groups. Are the two alike?

Do they serve similar functions? Are they compatible, or in conflict with each other?

Early political party structure was heavily influenced by religious, geographic, and ethnic loyalties. Immigrants to the United States found connections and jobs through the patronage system by affiliating with a local political boss. The resulting strength and allegiance of these relationships were solid. As the U.S. political system matured, other mechanisms evolved to mobilize the public. Foremost among these were interest groups.

Political scientists have debated the compatibility of the interest group and the political party system. Some contend that the rise in interest groups splinters party influence, and when parties have control of the national agenda, the influence of interest groups is lessened (Schattschneider, 1960). Others suggest that parties and interest groups have unique roles in different circumstances (Walker, 1997). As noted earlier, interest groups ensure that there is a political voice for special, often minority, interests, whereas parties fight for the majority interest (Dye, 1998). During election cycles, political parties tend to be more active. Between cycles, interest groups are extremely active.

## HEALTH CARE INTEREST GROUPS

### INTEREST GROUP POWER

Health care interest groups compete no differently than others do in their quest for influence on the political stage. In the 1960s the AMA reigned as the heavyweight of health care lobbies. By 1994, the year of President Clinton's intense efforts at health care reform, the AMA's preeminent status had changed. The AMA was still a force to be reckoned with, but it was competing with many other groups that had emerged or strengthened their political footing—including nurses. Broder (1994) writes that more than 1100 interest groups weighed in on the 1994 health care reform initiative. The BYU research makes specific note of the influence of Citizens for Better Medicare (underwritten by the pharmaceutical industry) on the fall 2000 federal elections, and the 2004 election cycle proved to be no different.

Health care interest groups were a potent force in the 2004 election cycle (Center for Responsive Politics, 2005b). The health industry, led by the AMA, contributed over $123 million, 61% of which went to Republicans and 39% to Democrats (Box 26-2). Presidential candidate George W. Bush topped all candidates, with $10.8 million in donations from health care interest groups. Rounding out the top five recipients of health care largesse were presidential candidate John Kerry ($6.9 million), presidential candidate Howard Dean ($1.4 million), Senator Arlen Specter (R-PA) ($1.3 million), and Senator Richard Burr (R-NC) ($1.1 million).

Physicians, nurses, and other health professional associations are generally the largest campaign contributors in the health care industry, but the pharmaceutical industry, health maintenance organizations, and other health service companies continue to grow in importance. Undoubtedly the

Medicare legislation signed in November 2003 by President Bush is evidence of the growing influence of these health care interests (Center for Responsive Politics, 2005b).

## INTEREST GROUPS AND THE FAILURE OF HEALTH CARE REFORM

To see evidence of the power of health care interest groups, one need look no farther than the health care reform attempts of the first Clinton administration. The historic role of interest group activity in health care reform is nothing new. Blue Cross successfully stopped post–World War II reform efforts by developing extraordinary advertising campaigns asserting that private mechanisms were superior to government programs in meeting the health care needs of the citizenry. In 1948, the AMA mobilized physicians in grassroots efforts to defeat President Truman's plan for a national health insurance program. The AMA also played a critical role in the passage of the 1966 law creating Medicare and Medicaid. In the most recent health reform attempt, the role of interest groups was prominent as well.

The attempt toward reform of the U.S. health system in the early 1990s was a significant one. In fact, the Center for Public Integrity found that the 1993-1994 health care reform effort was the most heavily lobbied initiative in U.S. history, with expenditures exceeding $100 million. Although President Clinton's initial proposal was strong, symbolic, and persuasive, neither he nor his staff were prepared for the opposition that would follow, opposition orchestrated largely by interest groups.

President Clinton's inability to effectively communicate his vision caused problems from the beginning, and the lack of support from major interest groups was a fatal blow. In his attempt to build a cadre of experts to guide national health care reform, President Clinton depended on alliances of hospitals, physicians, labor, and the elderly (Morone, 1994; Skocpol, 1994, 1996; Waldman, Cohn, & Clift, 1994; Yankelovich, 1995). Although these parties agreed on the need for universal coverage, they differed significantly on how to finance it. One of the most serious blows to

---

**BOX 26-2**　Top Ten Health Care Contributors to Federal Candidates and Parties: 2004 Election Cycle (Total of All Contributions, $123,185,922)

1. American Medical Association ($2,326,060)
2. American Hospital Association ($2,169,152)
3. American Dental Association ($1,735,069)
4. Pfizer Inc. ($1,630,556)
5. GlaxoSmithKline ($1,086,567)
6. American Health Care Association ($978,481)
7. American Optometric Association ($951,775)
8. American Academy of Ophthalmology ($940,250)
9. American Physical Therapy Association ($912,056)
10. Eli Lilly & Co. ($885,252)

Note: numbers are based on contributions from PACs, soft-money donors, and individuals giving $200 or more. In some cases, money comes from the organization's PAC, its individual members or employees or owners, and those individuals' immediate families. Organization totals include subsidiaries and affiliates.

From Center for Responsive Politics. (2005). *Who gives.* Washington, DC. Retrieved October 1, 2005, from *www.opensecrets.org.*

the Clinton plan was the lack of supportive major business groups and trade associations (though some initially supported it). The Business Roundtable, the Chamber of Commerce, the National Association of Manufacturers, and the AMA all refused to support the Clinton proposal (Shick, 1995).

Many groups played a role in the opposition effort. The AMA led all PACs by spending $1.3 million to lobby physicians to fight a reform plan that could limit physicians' personal earnings (Birenbaum, 1995; Glied, 1997; Laham, 1996). The American Hospital Association (AHA) sent information packets to each of its 4900 member hospitals containing advice on how to mobilize 4 million health care employees and thousands of volunteers (Center for Public Integrity, 1994). The Federation of American Health Systems, representing a membership of 1400 for-profit hospitals, formed the Health Leadership Council, composed of the chief executives of the 50 largest health care companies. Their efforts included convincing politicians, journalists, and citizens of the dangers of Clinton's reform proposal. Meanwhile, the National Association of Health Underwriters embarked on a campaign to support their interests.

Opponents of the Clinton plan capitalized on the fear of the unknown, convincing Americans to mistrust changes to the health care system they did not understand (Birenbaum, 1995). An effective combination of advertising, mailings, television ads, lobbying, and grassroots activity was enough to destroy any hope of significant health care reform.

Particularly noteworthy were the efforts of the Health Insurance Association of America (HIAA), a coalition of midsized and small insurance companies that would have been negatively affected by the success of Clinton's proposal (Jacobs, 1994; Jacobs & Shapiro, 1995; Laham, 1996; Skocpol, 1994). The HIAA, using its established infrastructure, used print and television advertisements in their "Campaign to Insure All Americans." Directing their message at insurance company employees, small business, veteran's organizations, and the elderly, the HIAA and its members contended that the Clinton plan would "cost jobs and would mean bureaucratic controls" (Kosterlitz, 1992). In addition to hiring former Ohio Republican Congressman

Willis Gradison as its chief strategist, the HIAA spent almost $15 million on the infamous "Harry and Louise" advertisements, featuring a middle-class couple who bemoaned the risks of the Clinton plan (Kosterlitz, 1994).

The Clinton plan for health reform was doomed. Opposition by interest groups and multiple stakeholders, coupled with a divide in the Democratic party over the best method for achieving reform, dealt the Clinton reform effort its fatal blow (Gergen, 1996; Laham, 1996; Patel & Rushefsky, 1995).

## NURSING AS A SPECIAL INTEREST GROUP

### EARLY SUCCESS AS AN INTEREST GROUP

One of nursing's greatest successes as an interest group working to influence public policy occurred in the early years of the twentieth century. Nurses sought to control their profession by developing standards of practice and educational requirements, but the profession had no means to do so because it was unregulated. Not only was nursing unregulated, but nurses were women. Women had no political voice—because they had no vote—in the United States at the turn of twentieth century.

The key to obtaining professional control lay in passing state practice acts, but a profession without the right to vote was at a huge disadvantage. Acquiring the vote would increase the chance of success in passing state laws regulating nursing. Nursing therefore actively supported the women's suffrage movement. In another act of collaboration that would contribute to success, the four active nursing organizations built a strong coalition. These organizations included the Nurses Associated Alumnae of the United States and Canada, later the ANA; the American Society of Superintendents of Training Schools for Nurses (later the National League for Nursing [NLN]); the National Association of Colored Graduate Nurses (later absorbed into the ANA); and the National Organization for Public Health Nursing (which later joined the NLN) (Lewenson, 1996).

The collaborative work toward a common goal paid off. The first nurse practice acts were passed by state legislatures in 1903, 17 long years before women would achieve the right to vote. This was an extraordinary political achievement that set the standard for what nurses could achieve through focused political efforts. Other legislative victories have occurred as well, such as the passage of the Needlestick Safety and Prevention Act in October of 2000, a federal law designed to protect nurses and other health care workers from needlesticks in the workplace. Finally, the ANA-PAC and other nursing-related PACs made significant contributions to candidates and parties (Box 26-3) in the 2004 election cycle (ANA, 2005b; Center for Responsive Politics, 2005b).

## BARRIERS TO NURSING'S POLITICAL INFLUENCE

Despite a three-pronged strategy, nursing's success as an interest group has not been steady. Nursing's influence has suffered because of two weaknesses: a lack of focus on core issues and the "free rider" problem.

**Lack of Focus on Core Issues.** Feldstein (1996) writes that when members of a group have similar interests, the costs of organizing are less. Large differences in position may be viewed as political weakness and may cause members to defect. Feldstein further notes that legislators may be confused about who speaks for members' interests

if there are multiple voices supporting different positions. Another reason for the lack of focus on core issues is the great range of levels of nursing education, practice settings, and specialties. The ongoing specialization of nursing has led to the growth of over 100 nursing specialty groups, each with its own agenda and political goals. Although membership in a specialty association may meet the educational and networking needs of nurses, it also may be contributing to the overall fragmentation of nursing's image, message, and political influence.

**"Free Rider" Problem.** When individuals with a common interest organize to achieve favorable legislation, all individuals with that common interest gain, whether or not they are members of the organization (Feldstein, 1996). The individuals who do not participate as members yet still benefit from the activities of the group get a "free ride." Every nurse in the United States benefits from the political activity that the ANA conducts on behalf of all 2.7 million American nurses—yet less than 10% of American nurses are members of state nurses associations and the ANA. Feldstein (1996) points out a critical issue for nurses: Unless a group overcomes the "free rider" problem, they may be unable to raise sufficient funds to lobby for desirable policies.

To overcome these two barriers to political influence, as well as to maintain the organization's viability, the ANA created the Futures Task Force in 2000 to define its future direction and organizational focus. Five core issues have been identified that will drive the ANA's work in the future: appropriate staffing, workplace health and safety, workplace rights, patient safety and advocacy, and continued competency (Foley, 2000).

Interest groups competing with others may attempt to carve out a political niche or policy domain that is recognized as theirs alone (Weissert & Weissert, 2002). A group does this by defining specific issues for itself. The ANA's identification of five core issues that will define its policy agenda clearly stakes out the organization's territory, and ANA continues to focus on these core issues today (ANA, 2005a).

---

**BOX 26-3**   **Top Nursing Association Political Action Committee Contributors to Federal Candidates and Parties: 2004 Election Cycle (Total of All Contributions, $1,176,841)**

1. American Association of Nurse Anesthetists ($542,135)
2. American Nurses Association ($496,846)
3. American College of Nurse-Midwives ($66,860)
4. American Academy of Nurse Practitioners ($62,500)

From Center for Responsive Politics. (2005). *Who gives.* Washington, DC. Retrieved October 1, 2005, from *www.opensecrets.org.*

## SUMMARY

From their earliest days, interest groups have met with equal amounts of disdain and admiration. Some view them with skepticism as elite influences on the political system, restricting the access of average citizens to legislators. Others perceive interest groups to be of great value, providing expertise to legislators and a political voice to millions of Americans. Whatever one's view, the place of interest groups is firmly woven into the fabric of American political life. Furthermore, despite recent reform efforts, it is unlikely that their influence will unravel anytime soon.

## *Key Points*

- Special interest groups play an influential role in shaping legislative outcomes in the American policy environment.
- Health care interest groups were a potent force in the 2004 election cycle, contributing over $123 million to political candidates.
- Nursing's influence as a special interest has suffered because of two weaknesses: a lack of focus on core issues and the "free rider" problem.

## *Web Resources*

**Center for Public Integrity—LobbyWatch**
*www.publicintegrity.org/lobby*
**Federal Election Commission (FEC)**
*www.fec.gov*
**Guide to the Lobbying Disclosure Act**
*http://clerk.house.gov/pd/guideAct.html*
**OpenSecrets.org**
*www.opensecrets.org*

## REFERENCES

Allen, M. (2001, February 5). Interest groups a force in congressional elections. *Washington Post*, A5.

American Nurses Association (ANA). (2005a). American Nurses Association annual stakeholders report—2004. Retrieved October 1, 2005, from *http://nursingworld.org/about/lately/ceohome.htm*.

American Nurses Association (ANA). (2005b). American Nurses Association Political Action Committee (ANA-PAC).

Retrieved October 1, 2005, from *www.nursingworld.org/gova/federal/anapac*.

Baumgartner, F. R., & Leech, B. L. (1998). *The importance of groups in politics and political science*. Princeton, NJ: Princeton University Press.

Berry, J. M. (1997). *The interest group society*. New York: Longman.

Birenbaum, A. (1995). *Putting health care on the national agenda*. Westport, CT: Praeger.

Birnbaum, J. H. (2005, September 28). Lobbies line up for relief riches: Groups portray projects as storm aid. *Washington Post*, D1.

Broder, D. (1994, January 31-February 6). Can we govern? *Washington Post National Weekly Edition*, 23.

Brookings Institution. (2002). *Governmental studies*. Washington, DC: Brookings Institution. Retrieved October 1, 2005, from *www.brook.edu*.

Center for Public Integrity. (1994). *Well-healed: Inside lobbying for health care reform*. Washington, DC: Center for Public Integrity.

Center for Responsive Politics. (2005a). *Elections: Campaign finance reform*. Washington, DC. Retrieved from *www.opensecrets.org*.

Center for Responsive Politics. (2005b). *Who gives*. Washington, DC. Retrieved October 1 from *www.opensecrets.org*.

Clark, P., & Wilson, J. (1961). Incentive systems: A theory of organizations. *Administrative Science Quarterly, 6*, 129-166.

Dewar, H. (2002, March 21). Campaign reform wins final approval: Senate votes 60-40; Bush says he will sign "flawed" bill. *Washington Post*, A1.

Dwyer, P. (2000, December 4). The candidate as a campaign spectator. *Business Week*, 38.

Dwyer, P., Cohn, L., McNamee, M., & Palmer, A. (2001, April 16). Campaign reform: Where do we go from here? *Business Week*, 42.

Dye, T. R. (1998). *Politics in America*. Upper Saddle River, NJ: Simon & Schuster.

Federal Election Commission (FEC). (2005). *Quick answers*. Retrieved October 1, 2005, from *www.fec.gov*.

Feldstein, P. (1996). *The politics of health legislation: An economic perspective* (2nd ed.). Chicago: Health Administration Press.

Foley, M. (2000, June 23). President's opening address, American Nurses Association Biennial Convention, Indianapolis. Retrieved October 1, 2005, from *www.nursingworld.org*.

Gergen, D. (1996). And now, the fifth estate? *U.S. News and World Report, 120*(17), 84.

Glied, S. (1997). *Chronic condition: Why health reform fails*. Cambridge, MA: Harvard University Press.

Heineman, R. A., Peterson, S. A., & Rasmussen, T. H. (1995). *American government* (2nd ed.). New York: McGraw-Hill.

Jacobs, L. R. (1994). The politics of American ambivalence toward government. In J. A. Morone & G. S. Belkin (Eds.), *The politics of health care reform: Lessons from the past, prospects for the future*. Durham, NC: Duke University Press.

Jacobs, L. R., & Shapiro, R. Y. (1995). Don't blame the public for failed health care reform. *Journal of Health Politics, Policy, and Law, 20*(2), 411-423.

Jacobson, G. C. (1990). The effects of campaign spending in House elections: New evidence for old arguments. *American Journal of Political Science, 34*, 334-362.

Kosterlitz, J. (1992, March 25). Insurers are gearing up. *National Journal*, 706-707.

Kosterlitz, J. (1994, June 25). Harry, Louise, and doublespeak. *National Journal*, 1542.

Kuttner, R., (2001). The McCain mutiny. *American Prospect, 12*(7), 4.

Laham, N. (1996). A lost cause: Bill Clinton's campaign for national health insurance. Westport, CT: Praeger.

Lewenson, S. B. (1996). *Taking charge: Nursing, suffrage, and feminism in America, 1873-1920.* New York: National League for Nursing Press.

Lindbloom, C. (1980). *The Policy Making Process.* Englewood Cliffs, NJ: Prentice-Hall.

Madison, J. (1961; original 1788). *Federalist papers.* New York: New American Library.

Morone, J. A. (1994). Introduction. In J. A. Morone & G. S. Belkin (Eds.), *The politics of health care reform: Lessons from the past, prospects for the future.* Durham, NC: Duke University Press.

Olson, M., Jr. (1965). *The logic of collective action.* New York: Schocken.

Patel, K., & Rushefsky, M. E. (1995). *Health care politics and policy in America.* New York: M.E. Sharpe.

Salisbury, R. H. (1969). An exchange theory of interest groups. *Midwest Journal of Political Science, 13*(1), 1-32.

Schattschneider, E. E. (1960). *The semi-sovereign people.* New York: Holt, Rhinehart and Winston.

Shick, A. (1995). How a bill did not become law. In T. E. Mann & N. J. Ornstein (Eds.), *Intensive care: How Congress shapes health policy.* Washington, DC: Brookings Institution.

Skocpol, T. (1994). Is the time finally ripe? In J. A. Morone & G. S. Belkin (Eds.), *The politics of health care reform: Lessons from the past, prospects for the future.* Durham, NC: Duke University Press.

Skocpol, T. (1996). Boomerang: Clinton's health security effort and the turn against government in U.S. politics. New York: W.W. Norton.

Squitieri, T. (2001, May 8). Campaign reform in jeopardy: Congressional Black Caucus may oppose finance overhaul. *USA Today,* A-1.

Tichenour, D. J. (2006). Allies, adversaries, and policy leadership. In M. Nelson (Ed.), *The presidency and the political system.* Washington, DC: CQ Press.

Truman, D. B. (1951). *The governmental process: Political interests and public opinion.* New York: Knopf.

Waldman, S., Cohn, B., & Clift, E. (1994). How Clinton blew it. *Newsweek, 123*(26), 28.

Walker, J. L. (1997). *Mobilizing interest groups in America.* Ann Arbor, MI: University of Michigan Press.

Weissert, C. S., & Weissert, W. G. (2002). *Governing health: The politics of health policy.* Baltimore: Johns Hopkins University Press.

Yankelovich, D. (1995). The debate that wasn't: The public and the Clinton health care plan. *Brookings Review, 13*(3), 6.

# *Vignette*　　Joanne Disch

## Extending Your Influence: Serving on the AARP Board

*"To have courage for whatever comes in life— everything lies in that."*

MOTHER TERESA

Several years ago as I was approaching 50, some of my friends began saying to me, "You should run for the board of AARP." We'd have a good laugh, and the subject would be dropped. But one friend persisted and sent me to the Website address a few years later to view the board application process. I read the criteria and reviewed the application. Surprisingly, I had relevant experience in four of the five categories in which they were interested.

The one category—prior experience in AARP— was a *big* gap, but surely there would be a way to address that. Furthermore, thinking of the country's demographic shifts, and anticipating the kind of member they might be seeking, I thought my qualifications were strong: a nurse, a woman, a "baby boomer." I decided to give it a try.

### THE APPLICATION PROCESS

I spent a great deal of time gathering information about AARP and talking with leaders in gerontology and public policy. I spoke with a former chairman of the AARP Board from Minnesota and contacted national leaders I knew who had had experiences with AARP—all with an eye toward gaining an appreciation for the organization's priorities and strategic direction. Naturally, I read the Website and other materials, including a book that had been written, albeit in a very negative light, by Alan Simpson. A former senator, he had coined the term "greedy geezers" to reflect his view of the mindset of most AARP members.

The application form requested that respondents provide information on their experiences in five areas: leadership, governance, interpersonal relationships, public speaking, and experience with AARP. Given my career experiences as an administrator and perennial volunteer in professional nursing and health care organizations, I was able to cite a number of concrete examples that addressed the first four categories. Each area was limited to 150 words. I developed several drafts and circulated them to colleagues.

For the fifth area, I decided that my only hope was to frame a major vulnerability as a strength. I've always believed that "framing is everything." This would be the ultimate test: I wrote about the benefits of boards being composed of a combination of seasoned veterans who knew the organization thoroughly and a few members who could offer a new perspective and a fresh approach. That would be me. I also indicated that I had been a member since turning 50, had read their periodicals, and used the website frequently.

And then I waited.

## THE INTERVIEW

That year, approximately 600 people applied to be on the board. The National Nominating Committee, of which I am currently the chair, uses a very effective, thoughtful process for winnowing the number of applications down to approximately 18, who are then invited to Washington, DC for a 1-hour interview.

In preparation for that interview, I again sought out individuals for consultation who knew the organization and key issues facing elders. Colleagues from the Center for Gerontological Nursing at the University of Minnesota were particularly helpful in assisting me in outlining issues and proposing solutions that could help shape AARP's policy agenda. A mentor, Claire Fagin, helped me anticipate questions and possible answers for the interview.

At this point in the process, three letters of reference were requested. I asked three individuals who are nationally known and/or whose work relates to AARP's mission, and who could reflect different dimensions of how I could contribute to AARP: the CEO of Minnesota's quality improvement organization; a former U.S. senator from Minnesota; and a nursing colleague who is dean of a leading school of nursing.

Also during this time, staff at AARP were formally and informally conducting a background check, as had been disclosed on the application form. My philosophy of "Information is power, but relationships are the key" was being tested here.

AARP's interview process is set up so that the nominating committee of 10 people is present (three board members and seven national AARP volunteers), and three of them ask the majority of questions while the other seven observe and take notes. It was a very cordial process, held in a hotel suite. Questions included the following: *What should AARP do to be more relevant? What experiences have you had speaking to a large audience? How would you arrange your schedule to accommodate AARP's heavy time commitments?* (at a minimum, 30 days a year are required). At the end of the day, there was a reception for the individuals who had interviewed that day, along with the nominating committee and support staff. At that point, I truly felt that I would *not* be selected, because one committee member believed that the minimum time commitment was closer to 60 days, and I clearly could not commit to that.

## THE INVITATION

Within several weeks, I received a phone call from the chairman of the nominating committee, indicating that I had been selected as one of six new board members, the class of 2008. This was not formalized until the board voted on the slate in February of 2002, so I was asked to not share the good news until then. Formal installation occurred during the Leadership Conference in April.

## RECOMMENDATIONS FOR GETTING APPOINTED

Through my experiences applying for a position on the board and serving on the National Nominating

Committee, for 2 years as a member and now as chairperson, I offer several recommendations on maximizing one's chances to be selected for a board position:

- Read the application carefully, and answer every question asked; leave no blanks. If you are weak in one area, determine whether you can shift an experience from one category to another.
- Follow the directions to the letter. If it says, as the current AARP Board application form does, "No additional documentation will be accepted," don't attach a CV or resume. If the form says, "Use the form provided," use it—even though it means transferring information from your CV. This year, there are 850 applications, and we definitely do not want to pore through someone's CV to see if he or she meets the minimum criteria to advance in the process.
- Provide detailed information that's requested. Don't answer, "Lots!" as one current applicant did when asked to provide examples of volunteer experience.
- Offer concrete examples. For example, in addressing leadership ability, avoid answers such as "Everyone says I'm a leader" or "My leadership ability speaks for itself." Instead, cite examples in which you were a leader and be explicit in what you did and what resulted.
- Gather as much information as you can about the organization; talk with current and former members and officers; read the website and publications; and examine financial statements and stockholder documents, if applicable.
- Practice being interviewed by individuals who know the organization and/or the industry, and develop recommendations for how the organization could better position itself and meet constituents' needs.
- If you know individuals currently on the board, do not ask for their support. Often they have nothing to do with the selection, and even if they do, it could put them in an awkward situation. You could, however, ask if there are any suggestions that they would have as you progress through the process.
- Avoid lobbying for a particular issue or agenda and being viewed as a single-issue candidate.

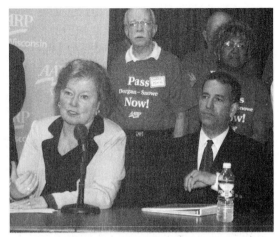

AARP board member Joanne Disch joined U.S. Senators Russ Feingold (on the right) and Herb Kohl (not shown) at a press conference in Milwaukee in July 2004 in support of efforts to legalize the safe importation of prescription drugs from licensed and registered pharmacies in Canada. Behind them are members of the Washington Park Senior Center in Milwaukee. The bipartisan bill, known as the Dorgan-Snowe Bill, counts both Feingold and Kohl among its cosponsors.

It's one thing to have a perspective or a lens, such as nursing, which is often very desirable. It's another to frame every discussion in terms of your singular viewpoint.
- Identify the specific information that you want to ask the members present during the interview.

## Lessons Learned

Observing firsthand the contributions that nurses make to the work of nonprofit boards makes me want to encourage every nurse to get involved. *They need us*—to view issues broadly, to consider the human impact, to appreciate the logistics of creating change, to interact effectively with a wide array of constituencies, to get things done. However, just being a nurse is not enough. Over the years my mentors in nursing, health care, and the voluntary sector have taught me much about serving as an effective board member. Some of these tips are unbelievably simple but often overlooked:
- Be on time, and be prepared. Read the materials, understand the issues, and develop questions

to ask. Avoid asking for something to be explained when it's clearly covered in the minutes or supporting materials.

■ Turn your beeper off. It impresses no one when you are called out of meetings. If something at home or work is critically important, make arrangements to be contacted during a break or lunch.

■ Get to know your fellow board members at board-related social events or at breaks or meals during board meetings. You will certainly enjoy some people more than others, but you do not want to be perceived as being part of a clique that always hangs out together.

■ Frame issues and questions in terms of what's good for the organization and is consistent with its strategic plan and objectives. Although each of us has particular agendas or viewpoints, such as making nursing more visible, exercise extreme caution to not be the "nurse board member" who brings every issue back to nursing. Not surprisingly, nurses are not the only ones who do this. Regardless, the end result is eventual marginalization of anything the person says. Claire Fagin suggests that, in any interprofessional or business group, you should first make at least two or three comments from a broad perspective before making one even remotely related to nursing.

■ Listen to what others are saying in discussions, and seek to understand their points of view. "Credit" doesn't go to the person who talks the most but to the individual who adds a new dimension to the discussion or suggests a strategy for reconciling different points of view... which means you have heard the different points of view.

■ If you have made your point, you have made your point. Think through what you want to say before you say it, and then say it... once. Board members who bring up the same points, time after time, on the same agenda item risk aggravating their colleagues and gaining a reputation for being more interested in advancing their own points of view rather than the group's collective intent.

■ Enjoy your experience. Being exposed to different ways of thinking and new colleagues offers an extraordinary opportunity to influence and be influenced.

Serving on a national board such as that of AARP is a professional honor and an opportunity for the individual, yet what has been reaffirming to me is to see the benefits that accrue to a large national or international organization when individuals with a nursing background sit on the board. Currently, there are two nurses on the AARP Board, and we contribute in a number of ways through knowledge and skills that nurses routinely possess: a systems orientation; an ability to see the big picture and yet be aware of the "devil in the details"; management skills; interpersonal skills that are especially useful when reconciling differing points of view; and knowledge of the health care system and the human condition.

Many people ask what it's like to be on the AARP Board. At this point in my career, it's a perfect fit. AARP's vision is for "a society in which everyone ages with dignity and purpose and in which AARP helps people fulfill their goals and dreams." Can't we all support that?

## *Web Resources*

**American Association of Retired Persons**
*www.aarp.org*

# chapter 27

# The American Voter and Electoral Politics

Candy Dato

*"It is the duty of every citizen according to his best capacities to give validity to his convictions in political affairs."*

ALBERT EINSTEIN

The most political act that every nurse—indeed, every citizen—can perform is to vote. Voting, the very symbol of democracy, has been shown to be both flawed and forgotten in the United States in modern times. It is forgotten in the sense that voter turnout among Americans still remains very low despite some improvement in recent elections. It is flawed with regard to the actual process of determining who can vote and how votes are counted, as was demonstrated in the hotly contested and problematic 2000 and 2004 presidential elections.

American voters continue to be courted relentlessly by a stream of media reports, phone calls, e-mail campaigns, and old-fashioned paper messages throughout what often feels like an endless campaign season. Their turnout is low, and the cynicism of the past several years is now accompanied by anger and suspicion. Yet the process continues—and nurses continue to be involved in political campaigns.

Nurses can make certain that family, friends, colleagues, and students vote. Nurses and other health care workers can have considerable influence on those with whom they come into contact by explaining the importance of voting and its effect on their daily lives. Nurses affect the political process through their individual and collective support of candidates. Health care issues are tied to

public policy and are thus dependent on the votes of elected officials. Pushing for the passage of health care legislation is one way nurses can show the public that patient advocacy does not stop at the health facility door. Imagine 2.2 million nurses with buttons saying, "I am a nurse. I vote—do you?"

Nurses must take part in the discussion of the complex issues surrounding campaigning and electioneering. We must understand the issues related to electioneering and campaigning in addition to developing the knowledge and skills to participate effectively in these processes.

## CURRENT ISSUES AND TRENDS

For many years, government relations professionals and political scientists have sounded the alarm about national trends of declining participation in electoral politics in the United States. The controversial presidential elections of 2000 and 2004 raised the public awareness of flaws in the election process as well. Proud Americans had their sense of security with the election process, the solid foundation of democracy, shaken. The long history of corruption (Gumbel, 2005) had been seen as part of a colorful past, and incidents of corruption in elections were viewed as atypical, isolated events. The long-standing problems with the entire election process came to the awareness of the general public with the chaotic 2000 presidential election. The disputed outcome involving the Supreme Court led to demands for election reform, heightened voter mobilization, and greatly increased voter turnout in 2004. But the 2004 election was also flawed—absentee and other provisional ballots were not counted in a consistent manner, voters found themselves removed from registration lists, use of irregular felon purge lists continued, the actual machines were still a problem, and there were many very long lines. These issues continue to warrant our nation's focused attention if our democracy is to thrive and be the model for other nations.

## VOTING PATTERNS

The highest level of voter participation was in the 1964 presidential election, when 69% of the voting-age population actually voted. Between 1976 and 1988 the levels did not exceed 60% in any presidential election year. There was an increase during the 1992 election, when numbers reached 61% and caused many to question whether this was a sign of a shift in behavior. The 1996 elections demonstrated that there had not been a sea change. The 54% turnout represented a decline in both the percentage and the actual number of voters from 1992. The 1996 election witnessed the lowest voter turnout for a presidential election since 1924, when women were first enfranchised and still unfamiliar with voting, and when laws discriminated against the registration of immigrants. The turnout in 2000 went up only slightly, to 55% (U.S. Census Bureau, 2005).

Following the vehemently contested and chaotic election of 2000, there were unparalleled, dynamic, forceful, and expensive voter mobilization drives by the Democratic and Republican parties, with a resultant increase in voter turnout in 2004. The 58% turnout was the highest since 1984, although still lower than the elections of the 1960s and 1970s (U.S. Census Bureau, 2005). Midterm elections fare worse, with one third of the electorate voting, and local elections may only draw one fourth of the electorate. The U.S. government gives legitimacy to countries that have elected governments, but the United States itself rates low: 20, out of 21 counties with established democracies, most having voting rates of 80% and higher (Center for Voting and Democracy, n.d.). There has been concern with declining voter turnout worldwide since 1990. Still, when comparing the voter turnout rates from 1945 to 1998, the United States ranks

139 out of 172 countries (International Institute for Democracy and Election Assistance, 2005). Countries such as South Africa, Tajikistan, and Kazakhstan, which have only recently won the right to vote for their leaders, see huge turnouts (U.S. Election Assistance Commission [EAC], n.d., b). It is ironic that in 2004 the United States was fighting a war to win the right for people in the Middle East to vote when voting turnout was so low at home.

Another cause for concern is the demographics of those who do vote. Nonvoting has been disproportionately more common among those of lower socioeconomic status, people of color, and the young. The very low rate of 32% of the 18- to 24-year-olds voting in 2000 has been eased somewhat by the dramatic increase in 2004 to 42%; however, the entire electorate is older, with the highest turnout being among those 45 and older. Turnout among Black voters has been rising gradually, closing the gap with white voters, although it remains low among Hispanic and Asian and Pacific Islander voters (Table 27-1) (U.S. Census Bureau, 2005).

Reasons for nonvoting among all groups have been attributed to personal reactions such as cynicism, alienation, social disconnection, boredom, satisfaction with the status quo, and a lack of a sense of political responsibility. Structural problems in the voting process such as political action committees (PACs), negative campaigns, lackluster candidates, political media, television, the educational system, and a lack of interest by the so-called "me generation" are also blamed.

A survey taken by the U.S. Census Bureau (1998) shortly after the 1996 presidential election found 22% of the sample said they were "too busy to vote," and 17% said they had "no interest" or they "did not care." Of note is that these numbers were up from 8% and 11% in 1980. The League of Women Voters (1996) found in a survey that nonvoters are less likely to grasp the impact of elections on issues that concern them, discuss political issues less often than voters, believe that they lack sufficient information on which to base their votes, and find the voting process difficult and cumbersome. In addition, they are less likely to be contacted by organizations that encourage voting, and they attach less importance to voting than to other,

**TABLE 27-1**  Percentage of Voter Turnout of Voting Age Population in Presidential Elections by Race or Ethnicity, Gender, and Age

|  | 1988 | 1992 | 1996 | 2000 | 2004 | 2004* |
|---|---|---|---|---|---|---|
| Total U.S. | 57 | 61 | 54 | 55 | 58 | 64 |
| Men | 56 | 60 | 53 | 53 | 56 | 62 |
| Women | 58 | 62 | 56 | 56 | 60 | 65 |
| **RACE** | | | | | | |
| White[†] | 62 | 67 | 60 | 60 | 60 | 65 |
| Black | 52 | 54 | 51 | 54 | 56 | 60 |
| Hispanic[‡] | 29 | 29 | 27 | 28 | 28 | 47 |
| Asian or Pacific Islander | N/A** | 27 | 26 | 25 | 30 | 44 |
| **AGE** | | | | | | |
| 18 to 24 years | 36 | 43 | 32 | 32 | 42 | |
| 25 to 44 years | 54 | 58 | 49 | 50 | 52 | |
| 45 to 64 years | 68 | 70 | 64 | 64 | 67 | |
| 65 years and over | 69 | 70 | 67 | 68 | 69 | |

From U.S. Census Bureau. (2005). Statistical abstract of the United States. Retrieved September 1, 2005, from *www.census.gov/population/www/socdemo/voting.html*.
*Percentage of citizen population.
[†]White alone (non-Hispanic).
[‡]Any race.
**Statistics not available until 1996.

daily activities. The researchers also found that forms of personal contact such as encouragement by family and friends were instrumental in changing voting behavior.

One group of Americans—African Americans—has shown some contrary patterns. A U.S. Census Bureau study (2005) showed that voter turnout was down from 1994 to 1998 for Caucasians and Asians and Pacific Islanders, as well as all ages and genders; turnout among Hispanics remained the same. However, African-American turnout percentages increased during this time. On the other hand, African Americans felt more strongly about the contested presidential election of 2000, which divided the country along both party and racial lines. African Americans felt more "cheated," "bitter," and "angry" than white Americans about the election. Indeed, there are many allegations that the black vote was suppressed in the 2000 election. This negative perception extends beyond the election, with 76% of African Americans saying that the election system in the United States is discriminatory, versus 62% of

white Americans (Simmons, 2000). A Democratic National Committee (DNC) study asserts that one in four Ohio voters had difficulties voting in the 2004 election such as excessively long lines, with African-American voters having twice as many problems, and five times as many voters being questioned about identification than would have been predicted based on registration statistics (McFeatters, 2005; U.S. House of Representatives, 2005).

The Center for Information and Research on Civic Learning and Engagement (Lopez & Kirby, 2005) reports study findings that white youth are the most likely to view voting as important (57%, versus 44% of African-American and 40% of Latino youth). Voting behavior is related to feelings of efficacy, and a majority of youth ages 15 to 25 feel they can "make little difference in solving the problems of their communities," with African-American (63%) and Latino (61%) youth feeling even less efficacious than white youth (51%). The study also reveals that discussing politics with parents is positively correlated with voting behaviors: 63% of white youth reported talking with their parents often about politics, versus 52% of African-American and 47% of Latino youth.

Some concerns and myths about indifference among college students were crushed by the results of a survey of college students who were registered to vote in the 2004 election (Eagleton Institute of Politics, 2005). It found that college students who registered did actually vote (87%); they did not find tremendous obstacles to registering and voting, including the use of absentee ballots; a majority favored traditional voting; they were influenced more by family than by other influences; and they believed that college students' votes mattered in the election. A Harvard University Institute of Politics (2005) study revealed that the deep-rooted distrust that college students held for the political system had changed over a 5-year period. The 2004 election "galvanized college students," who voted, spent time and money, and expressed a strong commitment to being heard.

Another divergence in voting—the gender gap—is the percentage difference between men and women related to their support of a candidate. The gender gap has been present in every presidential election since 1980. In the 2000 election, women were more likely to vote for Gore than Bush by 12 percentage points (54% versus 42%), and men were more likely to vote for Bush than Gore by 10 percentage points (53% versus 43%) (Center for the American Woman and Politics, 2005b). This gender gap was again seen in 2004 when 55% of men versus 48% of women supported Bush and 51% of women versus 41% of men supported Kerry. Bush increased his percentage of women's votes from 43% to 48%, "a major reason why he took the popular vote this time around" (Center for the American Woman and Politics, 2004).

In addition to their voting patterns, women affect elections through their numbers, influence, and different concerns. More women register to vote and more women vote than men. The percentages of women voting have been greater than men in every election since 1980, and the actual numbers of women voting have been greater than the numbers of men voting since 1964 (U.S. EAC, n.d., c). There are 41 PACs and donor networks that

either give money primarily to women candidates or have a predominantly female donor base (Center for the American Woman and Politics, 2005d). There are also differences in women's identification with political parties and their ratings of presidential performance (Center for the American Woman and Politics, 2005c). One area in which there is a sizeable gender gap is in the perceived importance of women's equity and equality under the law: 10% for equal pay; 13% for equality under the law; and 14% for appointment of women to government leadership positions. Of note, women also place more importance on the abortion issue than men (9% gap) (Lake et al., 2004). In 2004, preelection polls showed that both men and women viewed terrorism and the war in Iraq as very important, along with the economy and jobs. Women differed in that they believed that the United States was less safe from terrorism than men did, they had stronger concerns about Iraq, and they were more likely to say that the United States was moving in the wrong direction. Women also had strong concerns about health care and retirement security (Carroll, 2005).

## NATIONAL VOTER REGISTRATION ACT

Another view of low voter turnout is that it is reflective of a structural problem—access to the voting process. Starting in the 1980s, several national groups (e.g., Project VOTE, Human SERVE, the National Coalition of Black Voter Registration) were mobilizing local groups to change the power structure. Grassroots efforts for inclusion were begun to challenge the prevailing political system, which was seen as victimizing the poor and disadvantaged. Past movements had successfully led to legalization of the right to vote for many people. Later, voting rights were extended to women (1920) and youth (1971). However, barriers to voting persisted for a while; poll taxes were not eliminated until 1964 and literacy tests not until 1965 with the passage of the Voting Rights Act.

Local barriers were initially targeted until it became evident that it was more efficient to join together to work on the problem nationally in order to bring sweeping reforms of voter registration to the struggle for the disenfranchised. The League of Women Voters was a major leader in the coalition to support the passage of legislation designed to reform the current system and encourage voter participation by making it easier to register.

In the late 1980s, voter registration reform was seen as a partisan issue that the Democrats supported and the Republicans did not. President Clinton came into office with the expansion of voter registration as part of his platform. The goal was to empower those without money to have access to government. He signed the National Voter Registration Act (NVRA) into law on May 20, 1993, and it went into effect January 1, 1995. Clinton's success is the success of a broad and influential political struggle and social movement and an appealing attempt to engage the masses. It was hoped that through the expansion of the population registered to vote, the NVRA would expand the numbers of citizens voting and therefore lead to a reconfiguration of power relations.

The NVRA, also known as the "Motor Voter Act," provides for the establishment of several mechanisms to increase voter registration, the key one being "motor voter" registration. Any application, renewal, or change of address for a driver's license or nondriver's identification card triggers an application for voter registration. Agency registration established distribution of voter registration application forms and assistance at a variety of governmental and nongovernmental agencies, including unemployment, public assistance, vocational rehabilitation, and Social Security agencies, as well as libraries. Mail-in registration was also established in those states where it did not already exist. The NVRA also eliminated the purging of nonvoting registrants from voter registration lists and required election officials to send all applicants a notice informing them of their voter registration status.

Human SERVE (1996) and the League of Women Voters (Duskin, 1997a) reported that the NVRA brought about the largest expansion of voter registration in a 2-year period in the history of the United States, an estimated 12 million new voters. Some states such as Georgia had phenomenal increases (from 85,000 registering in 1994 to 181,000 in the

first 3 months of 1995). Although it had been projected that nearly half of the added registrants would actually vote, the numbers were much lower in the 1996 presidential election, suggesting that structural issues are not the only reasons for low voter turnout. The trend toward increased voter registration continued in the second 2 years after the NVRA; however, the number of Americans actually voting declined from 1994 to 1998 (Federal Election Commission, 2001). In its first report to Congress, the U.S. EAC, the government agency that began administering Federal Elections in 2002 (see the discussion of the Help America Vote Act [HAVA] later in this chapter), noted that voter registration increased in terms of numbers in the 2004 general election compared with the 2000 election by at least 12 million people based on their information (which they note is incomplete). Yet the rate of growth declined from 78.9% of the voting age population being registered in 2000 to 78.5% in 2004 in the 48 states that reported data to EAC (U.S. EAC, 2004).

## THE 2000 PRESIDENTIAL ELECTION

The electoral college; butterfly ballots; dimpled, pregnant, and hanging chads—American voters dusted off their memories of high school civics class and sprinkled their conversations with previously unfamiliar terms after the disputed 2000 presidential election. The media made critical errors in their declarations of winners on election night, and American voters—indeed the whole world—waited 5 weeks for a definitive answer to the question of who had won the presidential election. The impact of this hotly contested election on the American voter will not be fully known for years to come.

The Florida recall battle ended up with the 2000 presidential election being sent to the Supreme Court for a decision. The aftermath of this muddled and controversial election continues to drive legislative actions. Florida was not the only state or locality found to have serious flaws in its voter registration process and methods of counting votes. Thousands of qualified voters around the country lost their voting rights because of administrative errors and faulty equipment, and others were sent home feeling disenfranchised. The Democratic Investigative Staff of the House Judiciary Committee (U.S. House of Representatives, 2001) found a "national epidemic of disappearing votes" (p. 4) related to the many problems with voting machines, confusing ballots, registration, inaccessible polling places, voter intimidation, and improper recounts. Their data showed that in 31 states the votes of a minimum of 1,276,916 citizens were discarded without a presidential vote. They note that this is larger than the margin of the popular vote between Gore and Bush. The 2000 election was a wake-up call for Americans.

## HELP AMERICA VOTE ACT

HAVA was enacted by Congress in 2002 to improve voting systems across the nation and ensure the integrity of elections in the United States. HAVA established the EAC to assist in the administration of Federal elections, act as a national clearinghouse, provide funds and guidance to improve states' voting systems (including replacing punch card voting, mandating centralized voter registration lists), and establish minimum election administration standards. HAVA also established mandatory provisional ballots for voters when their voter registration was in dispute (U.S. EAC, n.d., b). The adoption of HAVA by Congress was marked by division, and the response to HAVA's provisional voting rules has also been divided. It is the first time that there has been a federal role in the administration of elections of federal offices, rather than the historical precedent of local and state government control.

## THE 2004 PRESIDENTIAL ELECTION

Voter turnout rose dramatically in the 2004 election. There was a lot of interest in the presidential election by voters who remembered the faulty process in 2000. Voters were also polarized in their strong views of the president himself, and they had been courted endlessly by the campaigns, which recognized that the elections would be close.

The campaigns involved forceful and expensive voter mobilization of the parties' voter bases and convincing a relatively small number of undecided voters. The Republicans used centralized professionals, targeting their base and working on getting out the vote, whereas the Democrats' vigorous efforts were more decentralized.

Citizens had different reasons for voting. Senior citizens continued to have the highest voter turnout rates. As the American electorate ages, the importance of issues of concern to senior citizens, such as Social Security and Medicare, will increase. At the other end of the age spectrum, the percentage of young people aged 18 to 24 had an increase in their turnout. Young adults were one group that was courted and mobilized in preparation for the 2004 election. The Vanishing Voter Project (Patterson, 2004), a large study of young voters, found that young voters believed that the election results would significantly affect the future of the country. Their interest in the election continued throughout the campaign, spurred on by outside events like the 9/11 hearings. They were more interested in the war in Iraq and less interested in the economy than older adults. They were also strongly motivated to vote by their dislike of one of the candidates. The issues that were most important to women in the 2004 election included jobs and the economy, homeland security and terrorism, Iraq, moral values, health care and prescription drugs, Social Security, and Medicare (Lake et al., 2004).

Many viewed the 2004 election as more problematic than the 2000 election, beginning with voter registration irregularities such as multiple registrations (duplicate registration in more than one state); multiple errors in the lists of voters, eligibility documents, and information given to voters about the location of their polling place; overly complex or outdated voter registration forms; conflict of interest for administrators; voting roll purges (especially because of incorrect information about felony convictions); and voters' uncertainty about their registration status or finding that they were not registered because of registration errors. There were also new concerns about possible identity theft with voter registration information (Electronic Privacy Information Center, 2005).

The concerns about fraud did not center on paper ballot technology but on concerns about security and the possibility of electronic fraud. In additions to fears of hackers breaking into the system, lack of a paper trail, vote buying, absentee ballot fraud, and possible conflict of interest, there was also the fact that one of the executives of a touch-screen voting machine had promised to "deliver" votes to Bush (Campbell, 2004; Corn, 2004).

Voting in the 2004 election was done by optical scan (39%), electronic systems (22.6%), mechanical lever (12.2%), punch cards (8.9%), paper ballot (1.7%, largely for absentee ballots), mixed (7.3%), and unknown (8.2%) (U.S. EAC, 2005). Problems were cited with the technology as well as the lack of it in areas where there were insufficient numbers of voting machines, which resulted in excessively long lines of 5 or 6 or even 10 hours. The 2004 election "lacked the drama" of the 2000 election—not because all the votes cast were counted in a way that satisfied the voters, but because the Bush margin of winning was large enough that resolved voting issues would not have made a difference. "And while the margin of victory exceeded the margin of litigation, it did not exceed the margin of concern" (Election Reform Information Project, 2004, p. 2).

The HAVA federal mandate for states to provide for provisional ballots was carried out by different states in vastly different ways such as which were counted and which were not. The Election Reform Information Project (2005) reports progress was made in that 1.6 million provisional ballots were cast and problems in that only 1.1 million were counted. Some alleged that there was a heightened level of manipulation related to the highly charged race. A study of the election, commissioned by the DNC (McFeatters, 2005), does not allege that votes were stolen but rather suppressed through long lines, inadequate numbers of machines, particularly in areas likely to see Democratic votes, and unnecessarily forcing voters to use provisional ballots, many of which were rejected. The DNC report showed failures in Ohio, particularly for African-American voters, younger voters, and those using touch-screen machines. Bush needed Ohio's 20 votes.

Identification requirements especially disenfranchised poor, minority, and young citizens, who are less likely to have drivers' licenses or other forms of identification. Some states called for identification to be brought to the poll by the end of Election Day (contrary to HAVA guidelines). The League of Women Voters took this to court and lost. Concerns for the future include identification requirements as a continued barrier to voting rights. The American Civil Liberties Union (2005) and other groups have also expressed concerns about the 2007 expiration of sections of the 1965 Voting Rights Act, noting that racial discrimination in voting still continues.

Andrew Gumbel, in his book "Steal This Vote" (2005, p. 1) quotes Jimmy Carter, speaking about why he saw the U.S. voting system as a failure that his international election-monitoring team would not observe: "We wouldn't think of it … the American political system wouldn't measure up to any sort of international standards…" International poll watchers who did observe U.S. elections in three states found that the administration of the U.S. electoral system was compromised (Election Reform Information Project, 2004).

More HAVA mandates are going into effect in coming years. HAVA will be making funding available to states to improve both technology and accessibility of voting machines, as well as the overall administration of elections. In response to proposed federal guidance on state voter registration, the League of Women Voters (2005) reported that election management is inadequate and that states need clearer lines of responsibility, stronger security measures, and "protection against erroneous purges of voters." Concerns about the integrity of the voting system have prompted responses such as Caltech-MIT Voting Technology Project's guidelines for voters to safeguard their votes (Caltech-MIT/ Voting Technology Project, n.d.).

# CANDIDATES

## WOMEN AS CANDIDATES

Elected officials at all levels of government do not reflect the gender composition of the United States. Women have largely been restricted in their journey to the heart of political power in this country.

In 1992, the "Year of the Woman," that pattern was altered somewhat when women moved into national and statewide elected offices in greater numbers than ever before. The number of female candidates for Congress, statewide elective executive offices, and state legislatures has been climbing steadily for the past 20 years. In 1976 there was one woman candidate for the U.S. Senate and there were 54 for the House of Representatives, two for governorships, and 1258 for state legislatures. Records were set in 1992, with 11 for the U.S. Senate; in 1994, with 10 for governorships and 2285 for state legislatures; and in 2000, with 124 for the House of Representatives. The number of female candidates declined for some offices in 1996, with nine candidates for the senate, six for governorships, and 2274 for state legislatures (Center for the American Woman and Politics, 2005a).

Record numbers of women were serving in the senate (14) and the House (81) in 2005. The number of women in statewide elective executive posts, such as governor or comptroller, dropped from the 1995 record of 85 to 81 in 2005, representing 25.7% of available positions (down from the 27.6% high in 1999 and 2001). The number of women of color remains a particular concern; for example, only 30 have ever served in the U.S. House of Representatives. The first and only woman of color to serve in the senate was Carol Moseley Braun, an African American, who was elected in 1992 and served from 1993 to 1999. Women of color comprised 3.5% of the members of Congress and 1.6% of the total statewide elective executives in 2005 (Center for the American Woman and Politics, 2005a).

Congresswoman Carolyn McCarthy (D-NY), a nurse, embodies many of the characteristics of a female candidate coming up against a male incumbent. She overcame numerous obstacles and is viewed as a hero to many. Like many other women, she was not considered to be a serious contender and was thought of as a one-issue candidate because of her strong stance on gun control after her husband's death in the much-publicized Long Island Railroad Massacre. What mobilized people to support her were her media exposure and her commonsense approach to a variety of issues.

The well-publicized and well-financed 2000 race for the senate seat from New York tells another story. Hillary Clinton (D-NY) ought to have had a natural base among women voters; however, her campaign staff was concerned about the very mixed reactions of women to candidate Clinton. These concerns proved unfounded, and she won the election with an unexpectedly strong 12-point lead. Exit polls found that 60% of women voters supported her (Bumiller & Murphy, 2000), and she became the first female U.S. senator from New York—and what's more, the first First Lady to hold national office. A May 2005 Marist poll shows that she is a polarizing figure; however, women continue to show more support for her than men, with 54% of women versus 44% of men saying they want her to run for president in 2008 (Marist College Institute for Public Opinion, 2005).

Male candidates still outnumber female candidates. Many female candidates belong to or receive formal and informal campaign support from women's organizations, women's PACs, and professional associations such as the American Nurses Association (ANA), whose members are mostly women. Incumbents, who are largely men, win elections more easily and consistently. The current campaign finance laws favor incumbents. Women candidates have the same problems as challengers in general: they are lacking in money, name recognition, and the built-in advantages that incumbency offers. The dual, and often related, concerns about the power of the media and the exorbitant cost of campaigns geared to short television spots without substantive discussions of issues plague American voters.

The 109th Congress had more women than any other. A December 2000 Gallup poll (Simmons, 2001) reported that 57% of Americans say the United States would be governed better if more women were in office (only 28% thought so in 1984). Further optimism for women in U.S. politics can be found in a 2005 Gallup report (Jones, 2005) that 86% of Americans would personally vote for a woman for president and, more conservatively, 47% thought their neighbor would. Just under half of the people polled thought the United States would have a female president within the next

10 years; most thinking it will be within 2.5 years. A substantial proportion of those polled felt that there would be no difference in how a man or woman would handle national security and domestic policy.

## DIVERSITY AND REDISTRICTING

Nurses have been concerned about the lack of balanced ethnic representation by candidates for public office. The power of incumbency is a major obstacle to increasing diversity—ethnically and racially, as well as by gender. Ethnicity, race, or gender alone is not sufficient for a candidate to win. Candidates must have a broad understanding of the issues and must form alliances with groups other than their own.

In 1965 the Voting Rights Act required equality of opportunity for racial minorities to vote. That major piece of civil rights legislation gave the U.S. Department of Justice authority to ensure that redistricting plans reflected racial balance. Redistricting is designed to equalize the population among congressional and state legislative districts, and it is a highly political process. On the one hand, it has enabled more minority candidates to seek elected office (Duskin, 1997b). It is, however, a limited strategy for increasing minority representation in state legislatures and in Congress. It has often been used to protect incumbents through gerrymandering (manipulation of district boundaries to favor one party over another). Legislators thought that the creation of *majority minority districts* (in which a minority group represents the majority in the district) through redistricting would increase voter turnout in those areas. Preliminary studies have not upheld this belief. "Empowerment, in the sense of having a much greater chance of electing a legislative candidate of one's choice (frequently equated with 'of one's own group'), does not invariably lead to greater participation" (Brace, Handley, Niemi, & Stanley, 1995, p. 201).

Gumbel (2005) discusses the long history of suppression of the African-American vote in the United States through gerrymandering, instituting obstacles to voting, intimidation, and felony voting restrictions (especially from 1980 on, when there were rising incarceration rates among African Americans). In the south, districts were gerrymandered so that African Americans were either limited to a small number of districts or spread so thin that they could not have any control. For example, Arkansas, a state with just under 50% African-American citizens, didn't send an African American to Congress for several decades.

The 2000 census and the redistricting that followed had a major impact on the composition of Congress and state legislatures. The U.S. Constitution requires that every state's representatives must be elected from districts of equal population. The total number of congressional districts must be 435. Each state is entitled to at least one representative, and the remaining members are apportioned among the states by population. It is primarily the responsibility of state legislatures to redraw congressional districts, after the decennial census, with the majority party clearly having an opportunity to redraw districts to its own advantage. In the 2000 census, some states lost members and others increased their representation. The congressional elections in 2002 reflected redrawn districts, the result of partisan battles.

Pennsylvania and New York are protecting incumbents through restrictive measures that require candidates to get thousands of signatures within a short period in order to have their name placed on the ballot. In one election district in Brooklyn, New York, 21.3% of registered voters in 1996 and only 13.3% in 1998 voted. This particular district had been redrawn in the last round of redistricting. It seems to have no sense of community, a lack of cohesiveness, and a sense of alienation (Barnes, 2000).

Gerrymandering is truly bipartisan, with both parties shifting boundaries in their favor when they can. In 2000, a New York state Republican senator and a Democratic assemblyman had very tight races. Two years later, during redistricting, the homes of the two close opponents were drawn out of the districts. One of the opponents described her district, "Think of a balloon, and how when you put your finger in a balloon, it changes shape. That was the district, and that part of the balloon where your finger would be was my house" (Cooper, 2005).

Redistricting came into the national public limelight with Majority Leader Tom DeLay's 2003 bold extra round of Republican-controlled gerrymandering designed to shift districts from Democrat to Republican, which it did, sending four new Republicans to Congress. Outcomes include a disillusioned electorate with low motivation to vote and loss of confidence in democracy, a decline in centrists in both parties, and weakened political influence for minorities (*Business Week*, 2005). A specific effect of the 2004 election is a distinct Republican press forward, which some say may take a long time to be equalized.

One analysis (Center for Voting and Democracy, 2005) of the state of democracy in U.S. elections found "sky-high incumbency rates" and alarmingly low degrees of voter choice, with the 2000 and 2004 elections being the least competitive elections in U.S. history. In 2004 House races, only five incumbents lost, 83% of the races were won by margins of at least 20%, and the average victory margin was 40%. A predictable result of this unhealthy lack of voter choice is voter apathy and alienation. Even with a surge of voter turnout for the presidential election, more than 62% of voters skipped over their House races.

Gerrymandering, with its long history, has been heightened by the use of computers, enabling politicians to create designer districts with surgical precision. Political parties, not voters, are choosing elected officials. Numerous states and groups are working diligently on effecting redistricting reform so it would be enacted in the public interest

Another reform measure against incumbency, term limits, was implemented in many states and localities. In state legislatures there has been an increase in attempts to reverse the term-limit legislation from the late 1980s. Lawmakers mourn the loss of experience, but voters' responses are harder to predict with regard to repealing term limits (Verhovek, 2001). The future of federal term limits will require action by Congress. Many believe that its members will refuse to support term limits out of self-interest. But in 2005, Elliot Spitzer, Democratic candidate for the 2006 New York gubernatorial race, announced that he was committed to making redistricting a nonpartisan activity.

Others may follow suit as the American public becomes increasingly disturbed at the bias built into the nation's electoral politics.

## ROLE OF POLITICAL PARTIES IN CAMPAIGNING AND ELECTIONEERING

Political parties, activists, and interest groups recruit candidates to run for office. Incumbents leaving political life often endorse a successor. The political parties promote candidates from within their ranks, support them, and get them elected.

There has been increasing interest in "third parties" by those Americans who do not feel well represented by our predominantly two-party system. The basic difficulty lies in the inability of third parties to deliver enough resources and votes to get their candidates elected. Some wind up aligning themselves with one of the major parties in the end, whereas others are viewed as losing the election for one of the major parties. In the 2000 presidential elections, Ralph Nader and the Green Party failed to garner the minimum of 5% of the popular vote to qualify the party for public campaign financing in the 2004 elections (Federal Election Commission, 2001); however, the closeness of the Bush-Gore race suggests that had Nader withdrawn from the race and supported the Gore ticket, Gore would likely have won.

### ELECTRONIC DEMOCRACY

There has been a growing trend toward "electronic democracy" through the use of computer-mediated political communication, the systematic use of the Internet to reach large numbers of citizens with a potentially interactive approach to communication. In the political arena the Internet has been used to inform constituents, to raise money, and to gather support via petitions and requests for e-mail messages. There has also been an exponential increase in electronic access to federal, state, and local elected officials. There has been an expansion of the number of computers available to citizens in their own homes, schools, libraries, commercial sites, and government offices. The Internet also provides a means of communication for all candidates, regardless of their relative campaign budgets, thus giving more access to candidates of all political parties. There was a tremendous growth in the use of the Internet in the 2004 election (see Glazer chapter); however, one study found that 46% of college students surveyed did not obtain information about voting from any Websites (Eagleton Institute of Politics, 2005). "A majority of students (56%) said they would rather vote in a booth on Election Day than on-line or through the mail, a sign that traditional election rituals may be more appealing to students than the convenience of Internet voting" (Eagleton Institute of Politics, 2005). The Internet will continue to influence political campaigns and possibly the actual process of voting.

## INVOLVEMENT IN CAMPAIGNS

Political campaigns are often paradoxic scenes of chaos and organization. Nurses are highly sought as campaign volunteers or as staff because of their experience in creating order out of chaos.

### NURSES AND CAMPAIGNS

Nurses have been expanding their collective experience in political campaigns since the early 1980s. Nurses were encouraged to take advantage of a variety of political training workshops offered by the National Women's Political Caucus, the Women's Campaign Fund, the political parties, the ANA, and others. Nurse campaigners are now a part of the cadre of experienced volunteers and paid staff available to candidates and campaigns of both political parties. Elected officials regularly recommend nurse campaigners to their colleagues.

Campaign experiences have provided nurses with the knowledge and skills needed to become candidates themselves. The number of nurse candidates running for and winning state legislative and county races is increasing. In 1997, approximately 80 nurses held seats in state legislatures. Nurses continue to be seen running for mayor, city council, school board, and other state and local offices throughout the United States.

In 1992, Eddie Bernice Johnson of Texas became the first nurse elected to Congress, followed by Carolyn McCarthy in 1996 and Lois Capps from California in 1998. Voters are looking for candidates who offer a credible and fresh approach to problem solving. Nurse candidates fill that vacuum.

Nurses must make sure that the campaign staff knows they are nurses. Being a nurse is a professional identity and can add to political identity. Nurses should introduce themselves as nurses, sign their checks with RN after their names, let staff know about their ability to bring other nurses into the campaign, and always look for opportunities to let staff and others know they are nurses and are part of a very large group of women voters.

Nurses have numerous skills that are invaluable in a campaign, so they should make their talents known. As volunteers, nurses must take the initiative to make sure their worth is recognized. Nurses considering volunteering for a political campaign should assess campaign needs and their own availability, interests, talents, and experiences. After identifying the leadership of a campaign, nurses can introduce themselves, explain how much their time is worth, and tell about what they are doing or would like to do in the campaign. To get what they want, nurses have to use their communication and negotiation skills to make a place for themselves in areas of responsibility, such as scheduling and coordinating other volunteers or even running the overall campaign. High visibility in a campaign can earn nurses enormous political credit.

### RECRUITING CANDIDATES

Politically active nurses recruit candidates. These candidates include both nurses and non-nurses who support important issues in nursing. There are responsibilities associated with the recruitment of candidates. Some candidates will need education and support as they run for office at various levels. Nurses have taken advantage of political training programs for women candidates.

Campaigns need time, money, and volunteers. Nurses encouraging someone to run for office must deliver each of these commodities. If the recruited candidate wins, nurses will have influence with this new member of a particular political body. They may also have accomplished the additional goal of delivering a clear message to the opposition, who may, in fact, have been one of nursing's opponents. If nurses can affect just one election, they will already have political power, and for politicians, whose main goal is getting elected and reelected, the political power of nurses will be not only acknowledged but sought.

Nurses have developed long-range plans for grooming nurse leaders who will take on increasingly advanced leadership roles in electoral politics, including running for office. This type of visionary planning will ensure nursing's rightful place at the policymaking levels of health care. It will also help increase the number of women and minority-group members in public office. Nurses are challenged by the power of incumbency and the barriers it presents to having greater diversity among elected officials.

Voter registration drives provide an excellent opportunity for nursing students or nurses new to political action to get involved. In university settings they are an opportunity to reach the younger population who are eligible to vote but may not have been exercising that right. Such drives can also provide a public relations opportunity by enabling nurses to become visible in large educational, health care, and other facilities, thereby gaining credit for promoting community involvement. Increasingly, nursing has built stronger ties with consumers in order to generate support for its health care agenda. Nurses can get specific details about organizing and conducting a voter registration drive from organizations such as the National Women's Political Caucus, the Women's Campaign Fund, and the League of Women Voters.

Voter registration efforts have targeted both the general public and, more specifically, nurses. The ANA and state nurses associations (SNAs) increased efforts to register nurses in 1996 in their "Registered Nurse/Registered Voter" campaign, which was launched during the ANA's centennial and reached almost 200,000 nurses. The ANA and SNAs sent out colorful posters featuring a photo of Isabel Hampton Robb with the caption, "This nurse couldn't vote" (ANA, 1996).

Think of the effect on an election if the more than 2 million nurses in this nation voted! As the 2000 presidential elections illustrated, every vote does count.

## CHOOSING A CANDIDATE TO SUPPORT

Nurses often work on campaigns through their affiliation with organized nursing efforts such as ANA-PAC, the PAC of the ANA. Through PACs, nurses are able to pool their financial resources for a candidate endorsed by their nursing organization. (Although either the organization or its PAC can endorse a candidate, only the PAC can make a financial contribution to the candidate's campaign fund.) Endorsement decisions are made based on knowledge of the candidate, the organization's priorities, and the political landscape. The organization or PAC usually conducts interviews with candidates or sends them questionnaires to complete, to ascertain their positions on nursing and health issues. Sometimes organizations will decide to make endorsements based on a single issue. At other times there is a broad agenda to consider, and other political factors become important. For example, an organization may be displeased with an incumbent who has not been fully supportive of its legislative priorities, but the incumbent is the chair of the health committee and is unlikely to be unseated by the challenger.

Nurses also join local groups working with a particular candidate or groups of nurse colleagues. Many work on campaigns of candidates they support as individual citizens, nurses, or members of other organizations. Whatever the situation, choosing the right candidate is important, because nurses have a positive public image to uphold and want to use their time wisely and effectively.

Nurses choose candidates whose values, beliefs, and priorities are closely aligned with their own and those of the profession. Candidates may be evaluated based on their previous legislative work. Nurses may know candidates as a result of their political party activities, because of their participation in community organizations, or from the neighborhood. Candidates are evaluated on their positions on issues, voting records, qualifications, and electability. Many factors that have an impact on a candidate are taken into account (Box 27-1).

## EXPLORATORY COMMITTEES

Exploratory committees enable candidates to test the political waters. Before a campaign begins, they

---

**BOX 27-1**   Questions to Ask When Considering Support of a Candidate

**CANDIDATE**

- What kinds of experiences would the candidate bring to the office?
- Are the candidate's political knowledge and skill respected by his or her peers?
- What is the candidate's voting record in the office for which he or she is running or in a previous office?
- What is the candidate's position on issues of concern to nursing and health care?
- In what committees and positions of leadership has the candidate served while in office?

**CAMPAIGN STAFF AND PLAN**

- Does the campaign have an overall plan and component parts?
- Has the staff researched the political unit and obtained an up-to-date profile of the district where the candidate is running?
- Is the campaign plan realistic?
- What is the budget, and are the plans for raising funds realistic? Is the candidate prepared for his or her fund-raising role?
- Is the campaign managed in a professional manner?
- Are schedules adhered to and tasks completed on time?
- Do the candidate, campaign manager, and team work well together?
- Do they recognize that in areas such as polling, public relations, and fund-raising, hiring political professionals may be well worth the cost?
- Are there creative plans to combine professional and volunteer help?
- Is the volunteer coordinator personable and capable of planning and staffing key events?
- Is there a "get out the vote" plan?

**ELECTABILITY**

- What is the likelihood of the candidate's being elected?
- Do polls show a high positive or negative rating for the incumbent?
- Does the voting public recognize the challenger's name?
- Does the candidate have the party's backing? If not, why not?
- Is the candidate a good public speaker, and does he or she appear to enjoy campaigning?
- How much does the candidate want to win?

- What are some of the factors that will influence electability, including the political, economic, and ethnic makeup of the district and the financial base of all candidates?
- What is the percentage of voters who voted in the last election? Is this a presidential election year, in which one can expect a higher voter turnout?
- Is this candidate challenging an incumbent? What was the incumbent's margin of victory in the previous election? Is this an open seat because of the incumbent's retirement, or is it a new seat created as a result of redistricting? Are there any particular or new issues that would affect the incumbent's race?
- What are the major media sources?

**OVERALL ASSESSMENT**

- What is the risk/benefit ratio?
- What is the potential damage to the nursing organization supporting a candidate if the candidate loses?
- What is the candidates relationship with the political parties (considering members' responses, organization's public image, relationships with other organizations and coalitions)?
- Does this potential damage outweigh the benefits of supporting the candidate?

---

must determine which of the people encouraging them to run for office are ready to commit time and money. It is a time for candidates to assess their relationship with the political party and gauge the amount of support, financial and otherwise, available for a campaign. Candidates use this period to determine what segments of the registered voter population will be in their corner and how to reach those who are swing voters or independents. It is a time to develop relationships with both individuals and groups and is invaluable to a campaign.

Exploratory committees may be formal, with a long list of prominent names on a raised letterhead, or informal and small. Seats on these committees are often prestigious, with membership a sign of having "arrived" as a valued political participant. The significance of these committees increases with the level of office sought. The legalities surrounding the formation of exploratory committees for fund-raising purposes are regulated by the Federal Election Commission or by state election commissions.

## CAMPAIGN MANAGERS

An important early step for candidates is choosing a campaign manager. This critical decision may be influenced by the political party, as well as by the candidate and those working closely with him or her. The political network of former candidates and current activists will supply a candidate with suggestions for a manager. Politics involves finding out who knows what and whom and keeping in touch with them.

Experience, especially in successful campaigns, is important. Campaigns for higher public office often require an experienced campaign manager. Nevertheless, enthusiastic, energetic, and talented organizers can manage their first campaigns successfully.

From the beginning, the candidate and the manager must understand each other's roles. A campaign can begin to fall apart if the candidate is managing the campaign instead of the person hired to do so. A trusting relationship is essential.

## CAMPAIGN CALENDAR

A campaign calendar is a critical part of campaign planning. It is a tool used to divide the numerous campaign activities into manageable pieces. A good campaign will have carefully thought-out goals, priorities, and phases that are meticulously scheduled throughout the campaign period.

The calendar outlines a schedule for the campaign, supports the staff's focus on details, and helps to prevent internal crises. For example, planning "get out the vote" telephone banking before Election Day involves knowing that the telephone company needs 3 weeks' notice to install additional lines, and that a friendly union will be scheduling its phones for several candidates. Building this requirement into the plan ensures that the telephones will be in place on schedule. Without such planning, the campaign might have no telephones, but it would have many angry and frustrated volunteers as well as additional expenses as a result of the effort to obtain telephones on short notice.

## CAMPAIGN VOLUNTEERS

Volunteers are the core of any political campaign. In a low-budget campaign, they can be the campaign themselves. First, volunteers must be recruited. Active, enthusiastic nurses can be drawn from all health-related areas: hospitals, clinics, doctors' offices, temporary agencies, community health agencies, schools of nursing, and others. If enough volunteers are recruited, no one will be overburdened.

One way to recruit volunteers is through a "candidates' night," to which all candidates for a particular office are invited by a nursing organization. Nursing organizations can also seek out other organizations, such as other health care professional groups, to co-sponsor "candidates' nights." Once the slate of candidates is determined, ask all of the candidates for their schedules (well in advance), and select a date when all will be available. Advertise the event as a special reception for nurses. Work backward from the date of the event, and plan every detail. Create a flyer and distribute copies to area nurses; arrange other publicity; contract for a meeting place; order refreshments; and decide who will introduce the candidates and determine the format, including how long each is to speak and whether there is to be a question-and-answer period. Then delegate the tasks to get the job done. At the event itself, have an attendance sheet at the entrance, requesting name, address, and telephone number. If it is feasible, spend time with each guest and ask if he or she is interested in volunteering for upcoming political activities. Take notes (name, address, telephone number, and e-mail address), and follow up later with a telephone call to confirm the volunteer's commitment. For larger crowds, distribute volunteer cards and make a strong pitch for volunteers (Box 27-2).

Local community issue groups can provide additional information on volunteer recruitment. Handbooks are developed on a regular basis by a broad range of organizations such as AARP and the League of Women Voters. Nursing organizations and student nurses are natural sources for volunteers.

Volunteers should be carefully cultivated, cared for, trained, appreciated, and treated with respect; their time should be well used, accounted for, and recognized. Volunteers can enjoy the time they

---

**BOX 27-2** Recruiting Volunteers

- Schedule an event that will involve one or more candidates—perhaps a coffee hour in someone's home or at a public meeting place. Candidates should make opening remarks, respond to questions, and ask for the support of nurses.
- Host a social event with a political theme for area nurses. Make it festive and fun. Invite several local political personalities to attend.
- Co-sponsor an all-day political skills seminar in conjunction with local political parties. At the conclusion, sign people up for jobs that appeal to them.
- Call a meeting to discuss upcoming political projects. Encourage each member of the core group to bring two friends. Then involve the guests in the conversation, planning, and strategy. By evening's end, they will be ready to help.
- Organize informal get-togethers ("brown bag lunches") at or near nurses' workplaces. Invite a local campaign manager or politically active nurse to speak, then sign up volunteers.

---

**BOX 27-3** Effective Use of Volunteers

- Plan work for volunteers in advance of their scheduled time to volunteer.
- Give volunteers information about the type of work they will be involved in ahead of time.
- Keep to a realistic and accurate work schedule.
- Have the work ready for the volunteer's arrival, including any necessary equipment and supplies.
- Provide clear, detailed instructions.
- Have an experienced staff member or volunteer available for questions.
- Enlist the volunteers' help in making the most appropriate assignments, based on their strengths and weaknesses and the campaign needs.
- Maintain a comfortable and pleasant work atmosphere.
- Arrange for volunteers to work with friends or colleagues when possible.
- Provide appropriate snacks and cold drinks.
- Keep records of jobs that volunteers have done so that they may be called on again.
- Ask volunteers for feedback on the work assignments.
- Invite all volunteers to the election night celebration.
- Remember that not enough can be said about voicing appreciation. Whether the campaign is successful or not, people who gave their time to the campaign should be recognized and appropriately thanked.

---

spend working together. The team of volunteers in a campaign should feel as though they are an integral part of that effort, and they should be thanked and thanked—and thanked again (Box 27-3).

## FUND-RAISING

Candidates' war chests and their ability to raise money demonstrate their seriousness. One must raise money to get money. Major contributors who give large donations to a campaign want to know how much money a candidate has raised before they will contribute. It is also the first question asked by PAC directors. A volunteer or group that successfully raises money will definitely be appreciated.

Fund-raising is both an art and a skill. Most organizations recognize the value of contracting with professional fund-raisers and find that it is worth the initial outlay. The manner in which a fund-raising appeal is conducted is vital. An error-free, attractive, and creative appeal for donations is worth the effort. An expert fund-raiser knows how to do it and how to get the best price.

Candidates or volunteer fund-raisers should start with family, friends, and colleagues. If time and money permit, messages should be targeted at specific groups in order to get the most from the appeal.

Much can and should be explored with respect to fund-raising. Additional tips are provided in Box 27-4.

## INDIVIDUAL VOTER CONTACT

Everyone involved in a campaign—the candidate, staff, and volunteers—is in the campaign to win, which means garnering more support than the opponent does. This is accomplished with a plan that is based on knowledge of the district voters—that is, who will support the candidate, who will not support the candidate, and who is undecided. Once voters have been identified, they must be contacted personally. One important fact here that often surprises those new to politics is that campaigners do not want to contact all voters—just those who will or might vote for their candidate.

**BOX 27-4** Fund-Raising Tips

- Determine the amount of money the campaign wants to raise, and state it publicly.
- Remember that the most effective method of fund-raising is one-on-one, direct, personal contact with a potential donor. (It is much harder for people to say no in a face-to-face situation.)
- Know that the most effective fund-raiser is often the candidate. The candidate's time should be used wisely for the expected high-level donors.
- Remember that people expect to be asked to give money, and most people don't give unless asked. Fund-raisers cannot be shy. If you believe in your cause and organization, you should be asking for support and contributions of money.
- Always ask individual donors for more than they might be expected to contribute. (People never give more than what is asked of them.)
- When planning a fund-raising event, keep in mind that expenses should not exceed one third of the price of the ticket; otherwise the effort cannot be justified.
- Remember that people like raffles and 50/50 drawings, which produce many small individual contributions. They can be included in any fund-raising event, meeting, or gathering.
- Keep asking. The techniques of fund-raising (mail solicitation, phone calls, personal contact) can be varied, but ask repeatedly.
- Keep records of those who contribute. Never give the list of donors away; lists are power. (If some other group asks for money, the people on your list may give to them and not to you the next time.)
- Thank people in person if possible. Send a thank-you note immediately. If the fund raiser is for a candidate, the campaign staff should send a thank-you note from the candidate.

An effective campaign gets the voters' attention. Voters are bombarded by information during a campaign. The goal is to get voters to notice the candidate, think about his or her commercial, and open mailed advertising pieces. Candidates are noticed when their messages are presented clearly and creatively and repeated over and over. Repetitive contact and following up that contact are essential to persuading voters.

The three most traditional ways to contact individual voters are through telephone banks, canvassing (direct face-to-face contact, often with written material being distributed), and direct mail. Telephone banks and door-to-door canvassing are labor intensive, so a large number of volunteers must be recruited. They will also be needed to make follow-up contacts. Telephone banks, if well organized, can reach more voters in a shorter amount of time than canvassing. For telephone banks, a well-prepared script for volunteers is necessary. The numerous details involved in these efforts necessitate good planning. For example, 2 or 3 hours of telephoning per night is all a volunteer can usually do, so you must consider a number of variables when planning a telephone bank project: the hours, the number of telephones, the number of calls to be made, and so on. Telephone lists must be obtained, or numbers will have to be looked up before the telephoning can be done. In some areas, electronic dialing is available, using names or numbers of members of political parties or organizations. Nurses and other volunteers new to phone banking may prefer coming in as a small group. Organizing groups of nurses from a particular hospital or students and faculty from a school of nursing may be a way to bring in new volunteers.

A campaign kit is essential for canvassing. This kit can include information about the candidate, his or her position on issues of interest to the target group, volunteer cards for interested individuals to complete, campaign buttons, maps of the area, and sample outlines of what to say to the voters. It is necessary to avoid planning telephone or canvassing events that conflict with popular events such as the World Series.

Direct mail should be well designed, attractive, and personalized. If possible, a specific message should be directed to the concerns of particular voters, such as nurses, senior citizens, parents, or teachers. Such targeted messages are known to be among the most effective. Many campaign managers believe it is worth the expense to obtain professional help in writing direct-mail pieces.

New approaches to voter contact include organized efforts through churches and social organizations. Technology is expanding the horizon as well, with Internet pages and e-mail messages abounding. The increase in voter turnout in 2004 was a result of heightened party efforts to strengthen their bases, much of which was done through Internet communications such as newsletters, blogs, and online fundraising.

## MEDIA

Successful campaigns combine a well-funded and strategic media plan with a well-funded and carefully targeted voter contact program and field operation. The media plan should complement efforts to contact the individuals. Next to personal contact, television and radio are the most persuasive methods. Advertisements or articles that appear in local newspapers are often useful in local races, especially when money is tight. Television time is expensive, although creative campaigners can get free coverage through innovative campaign techniques. For example, a candidate can schedule "work days," such as spending a day in a clinic with a nurse or in an elementary school with a teacher, and obtain coverage for the experience. (See Chapter 9 for a discussion of gaining access to and using media.)

## GETTING OUT THE VOTE ON ELECTION DAY

The final campaign step is getting people to vote on Election Day. Volunteers will be needed to telephone people, reminding them to vote. The intensity of the campaign heightens in the last few days. Voters may need babysitters or a ride to the polls. It is important to assist voters in many ways. Besides poll watchers, volunteers are needed to circulate near the voting place to persuade voters who are as yet undecided.

## AFTER YOUR CANDIDATE WINS

After the glow of the victory celebration has worn off, it is important to build on one's relationship with the candidate, who is now an elected official. Most elected officials take their role in representing their constituencies seriously and need to hear from a broad range of voters. Nurses can continue to offer these officials a wealth of information about issues affecting the health and welfare of the community. Nurses interested in paid or appointed positions can then campaign for themselves, using the same skills that were successful in electing their candidate. Nurses frequently take on volunteer advisory roles on health issues. Those seeking staff positions may have assumed considerable responsibility during the campaign. They may continue to do so by, for example, creating events that help the newly elected official have access to a greater number of constituents. They may ask other supporters to recommend them to the elected official.

*Key Points*

- Nurses have a potentially important voice and role in all aspects of the political and electoral process.
- Decades of low voter turnout took an upward turn after the contentious 2000 presidential election, with some promising increases among young voters. Women voters continue to vote more regularly than men, with differences in whom they tend to support, as well.
- The U.S. electoral process is under scrutiny. The full effects of election reform are yet to be seen as the debate continues about the actual mechanisms for voting and the regulation of the system. Recent elections have been fraught with problems and fraud, fueling the call for reform.
- Concerns for voting technology and preventions of election fraud will continue to be of prime interest over the next several elections.
- Nurses bring important skills to public office and campaigns for these offices.

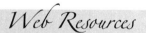

*Web Resources*

**Center for the American Woman and Politics**
*www.cawp.rutgers.edu*
**Eagleton Institute of Politics**
*www.eagleton.rutgers.edu*
**International Institute for Democracy and Electoral Assistance**
*www.idea.int*
**League of Women Voters**
*www.lww.org*

## REFERENCES

American Civil Liberties Union. (2005). ACLU voting rights: About the VRA. Retrieved October 1, 2005, from *www.votingrights.org/more.php#sect5.*

American Nurses Association (ANA). (1996). *Help make nursing count in election '96.* Retrieved October 1, 2005, from *www.nursingworld.org/gova/voteintr.htm.*

Barnes, J. E. (2000, October 1). The empty booth. *New York Times,* CY1, 15.

Brace, K., Handley, L., Niemi, R. G., & Stanley, H. W. (1995). Minority turnout and the creation of majority-minority districts. *American Politics Quarterly, 23*(2), 190-202.

Bumiller, E., & Murphy, D. (2000, November 9). First Lady emerges from shadow and is beginning to cast her own. *New York Times,* A1, B18.

*Business Week.* (2005, June 13). Gerrymandering: A partisan game of gotcha! (electronic version). Retrieved March 21, 2006, from *www.keepmedia.com/pubs/BusinessWeek/2004/06/14/481695?ba=a&bi=0&bp=7.*

Caltech-MIT/Voting Technology Project.. (n.d.). Seven steps to make sure your vote is counted. Retrieved March 21, 2006, from *www.vote.caltech.edu/sevensteps.htm.*

Campbell, T. (2004). Motherhood, apple pie, and election fraud (electronic version). *Chronicle of Higher Education, 51*(16), 11.

Carroll, S. (2005). Women voters and the gender gap. American Political Science Association Website. Retrieved March 17, 2005, from *www.apsanet.org/print/printer_content_5270.cfm.*

Center for the American Woman and Politics. (2004). *Gender gap persists in the 2004 election.* Eagleton Institute of Politics, Rutgers—the State University of New Jersey. Retrieved March 21, 2006, from *www.cawp.rutgers.edu/Facts/Elections/GG2004Facts.pdf.*

Center for the American Woman and Politics. (2005a). *Facts and findings.* Eagleton Institute of Politics, Rutgers—the State University of New Jersey. Retrieved October 1, 2005, from *www.cawp.rutgers.edu/Facts2.html.*

Center for the American Woman and Politics. (2005b). The gender gap: Voting choices in presidential elections. Eagleton Institute of Politics, Rutgers—the State University of New Jersey. Retrieved September 1, 2005, from *www.cawp.rutgers.edu/Facts/Elections/GGPresVote.pdf.*

Center for the American Woman and Politics. (2005c). The gender gap: Party identification and presidential performance. Eagleton Institute of Politics, Rutgers—the State University of New Jersey. Retrieved September 1, 2005, from *www.cawp.rutgers.edu/Facts/Elections/GGPrtyID.pdf.*

Center for the American Woman and Politics. (2005d). Women's PACs and donor networks: A contact list. Eagleton Institute of Politics, Rutgers—the State University of New Jersey. Retrieved September 1, 2005, from *www.cawp.rutgers.edu/facts/pacs.pdf.*

Center for Voting and Democracy. (2005). Dubious democracy 2005. Retrieved October 3, 2005, from *www.fairvote.org/?page=543.*

Center for Voting and Democracy. (n.d.). Voter turnout. Retrieved September 1, 2005, from *www.fairvote.org/?page=262.*

Cooper, M. (2005, March 11). Civic groups back a bill to stop gerrymandering. *New York Times,* late edition, section B, p. 4.

Corn, D. (2004). A stolen election? *The Nation, 279*(18), 5-6.

Duskin, M. S. (1997a). League reaches out to push participation. *National Voter, 46*(2), 4-7.

Duskin, M. S. (1997b). Number of women officeholders edges upward. *National Voter, 46*(2), 11-12.

Eagleton Institute of Politics. (2005). Four myths of collegiate cynicism exploded. Retrieved September 20, 2005, from *www.eagleton.rutgers.edu/news-research/press_studentsurvey.html.*

Election Reform Information Project. (2004). Election reform briefing: The 2004 election. Retrieved September 1, 2005, from *http://electionline.org/portals/1/publications/election%20reform%20briefing%209.pdf.*

Election Reform Information Project. (2005). Briefing—Solution or problem? Provisional ballots in 2004. Retrieved September 2, 2005, from *http://electionline.org/Portals/1/Publications/ERIP10Apr05.pdf.*

Electronic Privacy Information Center. (2005). Statewide centralized voter registration databases. Retrieved September 20, 2005, from *www.epic.org/privacy/voting/register.*

Federal Election Commission. (1997). The impact of the National Voter Registration Act of 1993 on the administration of elections for federal office 1997-1998. Retrieved March 22, 2006, from *www.fec.gov/votregis/nvrasum.htm.*

Federal Election Commission. (2001). 2000 Presidential popular vote summary. Retrieved March 21, 2006, from *www.fec.gov/pubrec/fe2000/prespop.htm.*

Gumbel, A. (2005). *Steal this vote.* New York: Nation Books.

Harvard University Institute of Politics. (2005). Harvard Institute of Politics survey of student attitudes: The Global generation. Retrieved March 22, 2006, from *www.iop.harvard.edu/pdfs/survey/spring_poll_2005_execsumm.pdf.*

Human SERVE. (1996). *The impact of the National Voter Registration Act (NVRA) January 1995-June 1996: The first eighteen months.* New York: National Motor Voter Coalition.

International Institute for Democracy and Election Assistance. (2005). Retrieved September 22, 2005, from *www.idea.int/vt/survey/voter_turnout_pop2.cfm.*

Jones, J. M. (2005). Nearly half of Americans think U.S. will soon have a woman president. Retrieved October 5, 2005, from *http://poll.gallup.com/content/default.aspx?ci=18937.*

Lake, C. C., Snell, A. R., Perry, M. J., Mermin, D., Gotoff, D. R., & Kannel, S. (2004). The gender gap and women's agenda for moving forward. Retrieved September 20, 2005, from *www.votesforwomen2004.org.*

League of Women Voters. (1996). League of Women Voters. Retrieved March 6, 2006, from *www.lwv.org.*

League of Women Voters. (2005). Helping America vote: Safeguarding the vote. Retrieved March 22, 2006, from *www.lwv.org.*

Lopez, M. H., & Kirby, E. (2005). Electoral engagement among minority youth. Retrieved September 20, 2005, from *www.civicyouth.org/PopUps/FactSheets/FS_04_Minority_vote.pdf.*

Marist College Institute for Public Opinion. (2005). National poll: Campaign 2008. Retrieved September 1, 2005, from *www.maristpoll.marist.edu/usapolls/PZ050506.htm.*

McFeatters, A. (2005, June 23). Democrats fault voting process in Ohio. *Toledo Blade.* Retrieved September 20, 2005, from *http://toledoblade.com/apps/pbcs.dll/article?AID=/20050623/NEWS09/506230466&SearchID=73223283474434.*

Patterson, T. E. (2004). Young voters and the 2004 election. Retrieved September 1, 2005, from *www.ksg.harvard.edu/presspol/vanishvoter/Releases/Vanishing_Voter_Final.*

Simmons, W. (2000). Black Americans feel "cheated" by election 2000. Gallup News Service. Retrieved March 22, 2006, from *http://poll.gallup.com/content/default.aspx?ci=2188&pg=1.*

Simmons, W. (2001). Majority of Americans say more women in political office would be positive for the country. Gallup News Service. Retrieved March 22, 2006, from *http://poll.gallup.com/content/default.aspx2ci=21438pg=1.*

U.S. Census Bureau. (1998). Census brief: Too busy to vote. Retrieved March 22, 2006, from *www.census.gov/prod/3/98pubs/cenbr984.pdf.*

U.S. Census Bureau. (2005). Statistical abstract of the United States. Retrieved September 1, 2005, from *www.census.gov/population/www/socdemo/voting.html.*

U.S. Election Assistance Commission (EAC). (2004). The impact of the National Voter Registration Act of 1993 on the administration of elections for federal office. Retrieved September 20, 2005, from *www.eac.gov/election_resources/Nvra2004-SURVEY.pdf.*

U.S. Election Assistance Commission (EAC). (2005). Election day survey. Retrieved September 27, 2005, from *www.eac.gov/election_survey_2004/pdf/EDS%20exec.%20summary.pdf.*

U.S. Election Assistance Commission (EAC). (n.d., a). About the EAC: Mission statement. Retrieved September 20, 2005, from *www.eac.gov/mission_statement.asp?format=none#hava.*

U.S. Election Assistance Commission (EAC). (n.d., b). International voter turnout statistics. Retrieved September 20, 2005, from *www.eac.gov/election_resources/internatto.htm.*

U.S. Election Assistance Commission (EAC). (n.d., c). Voter registration and turnout in federal elections by gender 1972-1996. Retrieved September 1, 2005, from *www.eac.gov/election_resources/genderto.htm.*

U.S. House of Representatives. (2001). How to make over one million votes disappear: Electoral sleight of hand in the 2000 presidential election. Democratic Investigative Staff, House Committee on the Judiciary. Retrieved September 20, 2005, from *www.house.gov/judiciary_democrats/electionreport.pdf.*

U.S. House of Representatives. (2005). Status report of the House Judiciary Committee Democratic Staff. Preserving democracy: What went wrong in Ohio. Retrieved September 20, 2005, from *www.house.gov/judiciary_democrats/ohiostatusrept 1505.pdf.*

Verhovek, S. H. (2001, May 21). In state legislatures, 2nd thoughts on term limits. *New York Times.* Retrieved August 23, 2001, from *www.nytimes.com.*

# POLICYSPOTLIGHT

## POLITICAL ACTIVITY: DIFFERENT RULES FOR GOVERNMENT-EMPLOYED NURSES

Tracy A. Malone & Mary W. Chaffee

*"Government of the people, by the people, for the people, shall not perish from the Earth."*

ABRAHAM LINCOLN

■ Donald Thompson, a member of the U.S. Air Force, forwarded what he thought was a humorous e-mail to about 70 friends. The e-mail made fun of the U.S. President. Thompson faced charges of violating the Hatch Act and could be suspended or fired from his job (Robb, 2004).

■ Mike McEntee, a Federal Aviation Administration air traffic controller, ran for mayor of Albuquerque, New Mexico in 2001. Because he identified his political party affiliation, he was charged with violating the Hatch Act, served a

4-month suspension, and spent over $100,000 on attorney's fees (Robb, 2004).

Citizens of the United States celebrate many freedoms—speaking out on radio call-in shows, conducting public demonstrations when a political issue lights a personal fire, and campaigning for political candidates. It seems to be a paradox, then, that the U.S. government restricts the type of political activity in which government-employed nurses, as well as other employees, may participate. This policy may appear to be a restriction of political freedom and the right to free speech, but the limits serve as a means of protecting government employees from coercion. Nearly 60,000 nurses nationwide are subject to these restrictions.

Two major regulations affect the political behavior of government-employed nurses. First, the Hatch Act limits the political activity of civilian nurses serving in a variety of government agencies, including the Veterans Administration, the Department of State, the U.S. Public Health Service, and the civil service system. Second, a Department of Defense regulation limits the political activity of nurses who serve on active duty in the Army, Navy, or Air Force.

## THE HATCH ACT

The Act to Prevent Pernicious Political Activities, more commonly known as the *Hatch Act*, was passed in 1939. The Hatch Act restricts the political activity of executive branch employees of the federal government, the District of Columbia (DC) government, and certain state and local agencies. Because the original Hatch Act was extremely restrictive, multiple attempts have been made to amend the legislation and loosen restrictions. In 1993, Congress passed legislation that substantially amended the Hatch Act, allowing most federal and DC employees to engage in many types of political activity. Although these amendments did not change the provisions applying to state and local employees, they do allow most federal and DC government employees to take an active part in political management or in political campaigns. The Office of Personnel Management (OPM) published the translation of the amendment into specific regulations in the *Federal Register* on July 5, 1996.

Nurses employed by the federal government in any status (i.e., full-time, part-time, permanent, temporary) are subject to restrictions on political activity. Nurses covered by the Hatch Act include the following (American Nurses Association [ANA], 1992):

- Federal employees
- DC employees
- Employees of state or local agencies in programs funded by the federal government
- Commissioned officers in the U.S. Public Health Service

The political activity of government employees is restricted to protect employees from coercion by corrupt politicians and political organizations. In the 1930s a Senate panel discovered that certain federal employees had been coerced to support specific political candidates in order to keep their jobs. Senator Carl Hatch of New Mexico introduced legislation that was enacted in 1939 to end this practice. Senator Hatch also feared the development of a national political machine made up of federal employees following the directions of their employers. In addition, the Hatch Act maintains the political neutrality of government offices.

## THE LURE OF THE INTERNET

Using the Internet for partisan political communication has caused some government employees to wind up in trouble. Scott Bloch of the Office of Special Counsel (OSC) has cautioned federal employees about using the Internet for what might be considered political banter. Bloch reminded federal employees to be "vigilant about following the Hatch Act, because we [the Office of Special Counsel] will consider this activity a form of electronic leafleting, and thus a violation of the prohibition on partisan political activity in the workplace" (*About.com*, 2004).

## HOW IS "POLITICAL ACTIVITY" DEFINED?

*Political activity* is defined as any activity that is directed toward the success or failure of a political party, candidate for partisan political office, or partisan political group. For nurses covered by the Hatch Act, a wider range of political activities is now possible because of Hatch Act reform, with some specific restrictions.

---

### How to Contact the U.S. Office of Special Counsel with Hatch Act Questions

The U. S. Office of Special Counsel (OSC) provides advisory opinions to anyone seeking advice about political activity and the Hatch Act. Advice may be requested in writing or by calling the OSC using the following contact information: Hatch Act Unit, U.S. Office of Special Counsel, 1730 M Street, NW, Suite 300, Washington, DC 20036-4505; phone: (800) 854-2824 or (202) 653-7143; *www.access.gpo.gov/osc.*

Nurses covered by the Hatch Act *may:*

- Register and vote as they choose
- Assist in voter registration drives
- Express opinions about candidates and issues
- Participate in campaigns where none of the candidates represent a political party
- Contribute money to political organizations
- Attend political fund-raising functions
- Attend and be active at political rallies and meetings
- Join and be active members of a political party or club
- Sign nominating petitions
- Campaign for or against referendum questions, constitutional amendments, or municipal ordinances
- Campaign for or against candidates in partisan (political party–affiliated) elections
- Be candidates for public office in nonpartisan elections
- Make campaign speeches for candidates in partisan elections, as long as the speech does not contain an appeal for political contributions
- Distribute campaign literature in partisan elections
- Help organize a fund-raising event, as long as they do not solicit or accept political contributions
- Display a partisan bumper sticker on a private automobile used occasionally for official business
- Contribute to a political action committee through a payroll deduction plan

  Nurses covered by the Hatch Act *may not:*

- Solicit or receive political contributions from the general public
- Coerce other employees into making a political contribution
- Become personally identified with a fund-raising activity
- Participate, even anonymously, in phone-bank solicitations for political contributions
- Solicit political contributions in campaign speeches
- Display partisan buttons, posters, or similar items on federal premises, on duty, or in uniform
- Participate in partisan political activity while:
  On duty
  Wearing an official uniform
  Using a government vehicle
  In a government office

- Sign a campaign letter that solicits political contributions
- Use official authority or influence to interfere with an election
- Solicit or discourage political activity of anyone with business before their agency
- Be candidates for public office in a partisan election
- Wear political buttons on duty

Although Hatch Act reform has resulted in greater opportunity for political participation, handling political contributions remains off limits. Personally accepting, soliciting, or receiving political contributions is not permitted under current regulations.

## ENFORCEMENT OF THE HATCH ACT

The OSC is an independent federal agency charged with enforcing the Hatch Act and several other federal laws. Headquartered in Washington, DC, the OSC investigates and, when warranted, prosecutes violations before the Merit Systems Protection Board. The OSC serves a dual role under the Hatch Act. Its mission includes preventing Hatch Act violations through the use of advisory opinions, and enforcing and prosecuting violations of the act when they do occur. Each year the OSC issues approximately 2000 advisory opinions, enabling individuals to determine whether and how they are covered by the act and whether their contemplated activities are permitted under the act. The OSC also enforces compliance with the act, receiving and investigating complaints alleging Hatch Act violations (OSC, 2004).

The OSC reports increased requests for advisory opinions on political activity during presidential election periods. During the 2004 election period the OSC received and is investigating a record number of Hatch Act violations—more than 60% of what was expected going into the 2004 election period. The OSC credits the surge to more political activism by government employees taking advantage of the freedoms to be politically active that were granted in 1993 when Congress loosened some Hatch Act restrictions. With a rise in political advocacy by federal employees, there are more possibilities for violations. Today the most common way federal employees run afoul of the Hatch Act is through misuse of e-mail. When a federal employee sends an e-mail that advocates support or opposition of a partisan candidate running for office and does so from a government computer, in a government building, or while on duty in a federal job, he or she violates the Hatch Act. Most of the state government employee violations involve members who were unclear as to their ability to run for public office while serving in state government.

With the wave of new political appointees that entered government service as a result of the 2004 presidential election, the OSC stepped up efforts to get the message out that federal employees, political and career, must use the many opportunities available to them to learn about the Hatch Act's requirements. Although the OSC will prosecute violations of the Hatch Act, it views its primary role as helping federal employees avoid such violations in the first place.

## PENALTIES FOR VIOLATING THE HATCH ACT

Federal employees who violate the Hatch Act may be punished by removal or by a minimum 30-day suspension without pay. Violations of the Hatch Act applicable to state and local employees are punishable by removal or by forfeiture, by the employer, of an amount equal to up to 2 years of the charged employee's salary. In matters not sufficiently serious to warrant prosecution, the OSC will issue a warning letter to the employee.

## DEPARTMENT OF DEFENSE REGULATIONS

Restrictions similar to those in the Hatch Act regulate the political behavior of the nurses on active duty in the U.S. Army, Navy, and Air Force. The "spirit and intent" of Department of Defense Directive 1344.10 (Department of Defense, 2004) prohibits any activity that may be viewed as associating the Defense Department with a partisan political cause or candidate.

Nurses in the U.S. Army, Navy, or Air Force *may:*
- Register, vote, and express their personal opinions on political candidates and issues, but not as representatives of the uniformed services

- Encourage other military members to vote, without attempting to influence or interfere with the outcome of an election
- Contribute money to political organizations, parties, or committees favoring a particular candidate
- Attend partisan and nonpartisan political meetings or rallies as spectators when not in uniform or on duty
- Join a political club and attend meetings when not in uniform
- Serve as nonpartisan election officials, if:
  They are not in uniform
  It does not interfere with military duties
  Approval is provided by the commanding officer
- Sign a petition for legislative action or for placing a candidate's name on a ballot, but in the service member's personal capacity
- Make personal visits to legislators, but not in uniform or as official representatives of their branch of service
- Write a letter to the editor of a newspaper or other periodical expressing personal views on public issues or political candidates
- Display a political bumper sticker on a private vehicle
- If an officer, seek and hold nonpartisan civil office on an independent school board that is located on a military reservation

Nurses in the Army, Navy, or Air Force *may not:*
- Use their official authority to influence or interfere with an election
- Solicit votes for a particular candidate or issue
- Require or solicit political contributions from others
- Participate in partisan political management, campaigns, or conventions
- Write or publish partisan articles that solicit votes for or against a party or candidate
- Participate in partisan radio or television shows
- Distribute partisan political literature
- Participate in partisan political parades
- Display large political signs, banners, or posters on a private vehicle
- Use contemptuous words against the president; the vice president; Congress; the secretaries of defense or transportation or the military

departments; or the governors or legislators of any state or territory where the service member is on duty

- Engage in fund-raising activities for partisan political causes on military property or in federal offices
- Attend partisan political events as official representatives of the uniformed services
- Campaign for or hold elective civil office in the federal government, or the government of a state, a territory, DC, or any political division in those areas

Nurses serving in the military are encouraged to obtain an official opinion from a military lawyer if they are unsure about participating in a specific political activity.

American nurses have created new horizons in policy and politics by becoming increasingly sophisticated in their political knowledge and by becoming actively involved in influencing health care in many environments. Many have translated professional nursing skills into effective political skills. Government-employed nurses should have their voices heard, as all other nurses have the opportunity to do, and participate actively in the political process. However, it is critical that they be aware of and abide by the laws and regulations designed to offer them a nonpartisan workplace and protection from coercion. Although the availability of information and educational materials on political activity and government employment is abundant, it is the nurse's responsibility to review and understand the provisions of the Hatch Act and Department of Defense regulations to avoid any unnecessary violations or misuse of their key positions in the U.S. government.

## Key Points

- Although government-employed nurses should actively participate in the political process, they need to be aware of regulations limiting their political activity.

- Two major regulations affect the political behavior of government-employed nurses. The Hatch Act limits the political activity of civilian nurses serving in government agencies, and a Department of Defense regulation limits the political activity of nurses who serve on active duty in the Army, Navy, or Air Force.
- It is the responsibility of nurses working in government service to review and understand the provisions of these regulations to avoid any unnecessary violations or misuse of their key positions in the U.S. government.

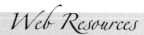

Web Resources

> **U.S. Office of Special Counsel (OSC)**
> *www.osc.gov/hatchact.htm*
> **U.S. Department of Defense Directive—**
> **Political Activities by Members of the**
> **Armed Forces on Active Duty**
> *www.dtic.mil/whs/directives/corres/html2/d1344*
> *10x.htm*

## REFERENCES

About.com. (2004). Federal employees accused of Hatch Act violations: Pair busted for sending politically-charged email while on duty. Retrieved October 6, 2005, from *http://usgovinfo.about.com/od/thepoliticalsystem/a/ hatchbadboys.htm.*

American Nurses Association (ANA). (1992). The political nurse: Your rights under the Hatch Act. *Capital Update, 10*(1), 4-5.

Department of Defense. (2004). DoD Directive 1344.10, Political activities by members of the armed forces on active duty. Retrieved October 6, 2005, from *www.dtic.mil/ whs/directives/corres/html2/d134410x.htm.*

Robb, K. (2004, October 4). Hatch Act minefield: As political activism rises, so do violations, prosecutions. *Federal Times.* Retrieved October 6, 2005, from *www.federaltimes.com.*

U.S. Office of Special Counsel (OSC). (2004). *U.S. Office of Special Counsel fiscal year 2003 report to Congress.* Washington DC: OSC.

# *Taking Action*   Colleen Conway-Welch

## *The Power of Political Contributions*

*"You're more likely to see Elvis again than to see McCain-Feingold Bill pass the Senate."*

SENATOR MITCH MCCONNELL

Political fundraising is both an art and a science and some would say unfortunately, the lifeblood of the political process. Funding campaign costs associated with a candidate's efforts to win elected office is an essential first step to a successful election. The sources of political contributions are varied and include individuals, business trade unions, political organizations, and registered political parties.

## THE IMPORTANCE OF POLITICAL DONATIONS

In order to secure the attention of politicians, some believe that the *amount* of political contributions carries more impact than the *source*. In fact, Mueller (1989) suggested that the likelihood of winning an election is positively related to the amount. However, "signaling" literature (Ball, 1995; Lohmann, 1995) suggests that contributions serve the main purpose of signaling support of a policy position and that impact is not necessarily related to amount. For example, a good case can be made for the importance of a grassroots "groundswell" of small donations as opposed to a few large donations. Regardless, political contributions also signal the candidate's ability to raise funds.

Bennedsen and Feldmann (2006) suggest candidly that, ultimately, providing financial support is a better way to sway a decision in a particular direction than providing relevant information to influence the political process. However, they also suggest that there is more than an occasional connection between donating to a campaign and providing information, which the literature has historically treated as separate issues. They suggest that the two activities are often strategic trade-offs, because

information can raise the interest and therefore the financial commitment of contributors. In fact, their research lends support to a rather cynical view that interest groups with intense preferences and high stakes in their preferred policy issues tend to prefer the use of contributions in contrast to the acquisition and provision of useful information!

Politicians are aware that interest groups generally gather and transmit only information that serves their own interest; rarely are both sides of an issue well represented by one interest group. In fact, collecting information and deciding *not* to provide it to the politician is strategic in and of itself, and a donor interested in influencing policy will frequently make use of this strategy (Bennedsen & Feldmann, 2006). For example, in attempting to restrict the scope of practice of non-physician providers in one state, a lobbyist for the state medical association may give an example to a Senate or House member of a state that has an equally restrictive scope and not the states that have broader scopes. Or, a candidate running for office may want information on gun control issues that have been "hot" buttons in his area. Her aide calls the National Rifle Association (NRA) lobbyist and asks for data. The lobbyist does an extensive search and finds several issues that have drawn much publicity. The lobbyist also finds data that could be considered detrimental to the NRA. The lobbyist decides to discard the detrimental data and not share it with the candidate.

## STEREOTYPES OF WOMEN DONORS

Many of us have seen a politician's ignorance or unfamiliarity with an issue result in him/her being persuaded to choose a position that is coincidentally consistent with that of a constituent who has made a campaign contribution. Because most nurses are women, what are some of the dynamics involved in being female and being a political donor? Stereotypes

**805**

of women donors have evolved from a time when we still had laws prohibiting women from possessing and controlling money they had earned or inherited.

Political parties are particularly interested in finding the key to maximizing donations by women because women make up 53% of the work force, start new businesses at three times the rate of men, control more than half of the personal wealth in the United States, and are key players in the trillion-dollar intergenerational transfer of wealth in the United States. In philanthropy, women actually give away a larger portion of their income, even though they earn about 70% of what men earn (Mueller, 1989). Issues that interest women relative to philanthropy easily translate into political issues, such as quality of life, peace, and justice. It is also important to women to be engaged in the cause, so getting women involved politically at the local level is usually an important first step in convincing them to be involved financially. Once women give to an organization, they are more likely than men to have a long-term relationship with that cause or candidate. Although some men say that "who does the asking" is important, women are usually more interested in "why" someone asks for money and are more likely to have a long-term relationship with the organization if the "why" or the value of the gift is clear and tangible. This dynamic also suggests that women

**TABLE 27-2** Federal Election Commission Campaign Contribution Limits: 2005-2006

| | TO EACH CANDIDATE OR CANDIDATE COMMITTEE PER ELECTION[6] | TO NATIONAL PARTY COMMITTEE PER CALENDAR YEAR(FEDERAL ACCOUNT) | TO STATE, DISTRICT, AND/OR LOCAL PARTY COMMITTEE PER CALENDAR YEAR | TO ANY OTHER POLITICAL ACTION COMMITTEE (PAC) PER CALENDAR YEAR[1] | SPECIAL LIMITS |
|---|---|---|---|---|---|
| Individual may give | $2100[2] | $26,700[2] | $10,000 (combined limit) | $5000 | $101,400[2] overall biennial limit: $40,000[2] to all candidates, $61,400[2] to all PACs and parties[3] |
| National party committee may give | $5000 | No limit | No limit | $5000 | $37,300[2] to senate candidate per campaign[4] |
| State, district, and local party committee may give | $5000 (combined limit) | No limit | No limit | $5000 (combined limit) | No limit |
| PAC (multicandidate)[5] may give | $5000 | $15,000 | $5000 (combined limit) | $5000 | No limit |
| PAC (not multicandidate) may give | $2100[2] | $26,700[2] | $10,000 (combined limit) | $5000 | No limit |

From Federal Election Commission, 2005. Available online at *www.fec.gov/pages/brochures/fecfeca.shtml#Contribution _Limits.*

[1] A contribution earmarked for a candidate through a political committee counts against the original contributor's limit for that candidate. In certain circumstances the contribution may also count against the contributor's limit to the PAC.

[2] These contribution limits are increased for inflation in odd-numbered years.

[3] No more than $40,000 of this amount may be contributed to state and local party committees and PACs.

[4] This limit is shared by the national committee and the Senate campaign committee.

[5] A multi candidate committee is a political committee with more than 50 contributors that has been registered for at least 6 months and, with the exception of state party committees, has made contributions to five or more candidates for federal office.

[6] A federal candidate's authorized committee(s) may contribute no more than $2000 per election to another federal candidate's authorized committee(s). An individual may give $2100 in the primary *and* $2100 in the general election. No matter how an individual splits her donations, they cannot exceed $101,400 every 2-year cycle.

are more likely to volunteer, want an emotional connection with the cause and/or candidate, want to be kept informed about progress and/or problems, and want to be acknowledged and thanked accurately and precisely, using the name (e.g., Jane Doe, Dr. Jane Doe, Mrs. John Doe) they have requested.

Women also like to be part of a new initiative and sometimes will take a risk on an unknown candidate if they feel she or he represents their own values. Women generally agree that they give to change, to create, to connect, to commit, and to collaborate.

## HARD MONEY AND SOFT MONEY

Campaign laws are complicated. You will hear reference to "hard" money and "soft" money. In the past, hard money was money given by an individual and soft money was money given by corporations or political action committees (PACS), created by groups who pool their money to be more influential.

Today, hard money is a personal, individual contribution given to a candidate and soft money is money that exceeds the limits an individual can give to an individual candidate (Table 27-2). It may also be a "527" account, which may take corporate money (Federal Election Commission, 2005).

## WHAT DOES THIS MEAN FOR NURSING?

What does this all mean for nursing? Many nursing organizations have started PACS. PACs seek monetary contributions to endorse local, state, or national candidates who reflect their particular political persuasion. However, although PAC contributions are influential, individual contributors are very important, too (Box 27-5).

The bottom line is that without money there is no campaign. Without money there is only a candidate who has a dream.

## EMILY'S LIST

"Early Money Is Like Yeast" (EMILY's List). "EMILY's List" fund is an important vehicle for political fund-raising among Democrats, and the fund is aptly named. Early money will give a candidate a strong start, scare other competitors away from the race (even the primary), and put a face on the individual

---

**BOX 27-5   Why Political Contributions by Nurses Are Powerful**

- Poll after poll shows that nurses are among the most trusted professionals in the country. Our support sends an important message about the reputation and values of a candidate that is useful to him or her from an advertising and fund-raising perspective.
- Nurses can and should *combine* the amount given with "face time." In other words, get involved with your candidate's office, staff, and efforts. Be sure they know your name, where you work (if you do), where you volunteer, and that you are a nurse.
- Contributions on either side support our two-party system. Passionate Republicans and Democrats have more in common with each other than lukewarm members of each party have with one another.
- No matter the amount, contributing makes you a player rather than an observer. As you get more involved with players, a sense of community and camaraderie builds and networking begins; this networking can open important career opportunities and give you greater access to the candidate.
- Your beliefs and persuasions have a platform where they have the opportunity for equal consideration.
- If you don't financially support a candidate or a political action committee (PAC) even minimally, you should not complain about the results. The ultimate success of our government is directly related to the number of people who participate in the process, and political contributions are an important part of that participation.
- If you give money, you are more likely to vote, even if it turns out to be an inconvenience.

---

or group who took a risk to "step up" with early money. EMILY's List is an example of an organization that recognizes the critical influence of early money and has developed effective political strategies to capitalize on that knowledge (Box 27-6).

Nurses and nursing groups are not known as early or substantial givers. One reason is that we are not generally a profession of wealthy individuals. Another reason is that nurses sometimes feel that their work is their contribution to the community, and political contributions should not be necessary

---

**BOX 27-6** What Is EMILY's List?

EMILY's List *(www. Emilyslist.org)* is the largest grassroots political network in the United States—a network of over 100,000 Americans committed to recruiting and supporting viable female political candidates. EMILY's List was established in 1985 and is partisan, focused on electing Democratic women. The name is an acronym derived from the phrase, "Early money is like yeast."

---

*Web Resources*

Federal Election Commission
*www.fec.gov*
U.S. House and Senate Disclosures
*www.fecinfo.com*
Voter Research Hotline
*www.vote-smart.org*

---

to improve health and health policy. Nothing could be further from the truth.

*Key Points*

- Political contributions are the lifeblood of politics.
- Early giving in a primary brings the donor to the attention of the candidate.
- Women give political contributions for different reasons than men do.

**REFERENCES**

Ball, R. (1995). Interest groups, influence and welfare. *Economics & Politics, 7*(2), 119-146.

Bennedsen, M., & Feldmann, S. E. (2006). Informational lobbying and political contributions (with Anthony Bertelli), *Journal of Public Economics, 90*(4-5), 631-656.

Federal Election Commission. (2005). Quick answers to common questions. Retrieved September 26, 2005, from *www.fec.gov/ans/answers.shtml.*

Lohmann, S. (1995). Information, access, and contributions: A signaling model for lobbying. *Public Choice 85,* 267-284.

Mueller, D. C. (1989). *Public Choice II.* Cambridge: Cambridge University Press.

---

*Taking Action*   Greer Glazer, Shari Dexter, & Michele Artz

## *Anatomy of a Political Campaign*

*"The hardest thing about any political campaign is how to win without proving that you are unworthy of winning."*

ADLAI E. STEVENSON

Is it hard to imagine why anyone would stand in the rain or snow from 6:00 AM to 6:00 PM on Election Day handing out information about a political candidate? How about someone driving a candidate to eight events in one long 14-hour day covering 250 miles? People work on political campaigns for a variety of reasons, and understanding their motivation is critical to building a strong volunteer program.

### WHY PEOPLE WORK ON CAMPAIGNS

People's motivations for working on campaigns fall into four general categories:
- Belief in an issue or a candidate
- Network building
- Party loyalty
- Personal payback

## Belief in an Issue or a Candidate

Some people work for a candidate because they feel strongly about issues they support and champion or conversely want to defeat the opponent because of where he or she stands on the issues. Volunteers are usually passionate about their issues, and if focused on a single issue will often try to keep their issue at the forefront of the campaign. Nurses bring the health focus. In the 2004 elections, when the war in Iraq and homeland security were top issues, nurses working on campaigns helped maintain a focus on health issues. Carol Roe, RN, MSN, JD, a nurse activist, represents people who work on campaigns to effect policy. She volunteered for Gerald Ford's presidential campaign in Cincinnati, Ohio. She was drawn to the campaign because of what his wife, Betty Ford, was saying about the role of women and support for the Equal Rights Amendment and "the way she used her breast cancer experience to promote discussion about a subject that, at the time, few discussed" (Carol Roe, personal communication, April, 15, 2005).

## Network Building

Some people are drawn to campaigns to build their own social network. They may be high school or college students or retired adults who are looking for fun and opportunities to socialize. Getting these volunteers involved in social activities will keep them involved in campaign activities.

## Party Loyalty

Some people work for the candidate because they are loyal to the political party. Although they may be very supportive of a particular candidate, their reason for involvement is the knowledge that the campaign needs workers. The Democrats and Republicans target close races in which they believe an infusion of financial and human resources can change the outcome of the election. Party loyalists will travel to different states to work on campaigns in which they can make a difference in the election. In 2004, nurses traveled to a variety of states to attend rallies and events to support presidential candidates and help them gain visibility to garner press coverage.

## Payback

Tangible paybacks include paid work for the campaign, course credit for students, and if the candidate is elected, appointment to the staff, appointment to key commissions or boards or other political appointments, and support for specific legislation. Greer Glazer worked on former Ohio Congressman Eric Fingerhut's campaign by coordinating house parties in one city in his district and was appointed to his 19th Congressional District Healthcare Advisory Committee. People also work on campaigns for intangible benefits, which may include recognition for their work and a desire to contribute to the democratic process.

Understanding the reasons why people work on campaigns enables the campaign to successfully plan and recruit volunteers. It does not necessarily help to retain them. You must be aware of the reasons why people stop working on campaigns.

## WHY PEOPLE STOP WORKING ON CAMPAIGNS

The major reason why people stop working on campaigns is that their roles and campaign activities are not aligned with their motivation for working on the campaign. It would not make sense to ask someone who is pro-choice to work on the campaign of a candidate who is not pro-choice. It would also be counterproductive to ask someone who just moved to town and wants to meet people to spend hours alone stuffing envelops. Even if the activities match the campaign worker's motivation, people leave campaigns because they lose interest, aren't given enough positive feedback and recognition, don't feel a part of the larger whole, lose faith that the candidate can win the election, feel that they are only doing boring work, have competing outside interests such as family and work obligations, and aren't enjoying themselves. What are campaign activities that either engage or disengage campaign workers?

## THE INTERNET AND THE 2004 ELECTION

The Internet became an essential part of American politics in 2004 (Pew Research Center, 2004), as 75 million Americans (37% of the adult U.S. population) used the Internet to get campaign information and news, discuss and debate issues, and participate in the campaign by donating to candidates or volunteering to work on their campaigns. Convio created a free handbook, *Using the Internet for Effective Grassroots Advocacy: Strategies, Tools and Approaches for Inspiring Constituents to Take Action*, about the fundamentals of online advocacy (Convio, 2005a). Specific online activities grew from 2000 to 2004 and included the following (Pew Research Center, 2004):

- Voting information: The number who got information on where to vote grew more than 150% to nearly 14 million people.
- Donations: The number who gave campaign contributions online grew 80% to about 4 million people.
- Discussion and chat: The number who participated in online political discussions or chat groups grew 57% to about 4.5 million people.
- Candidates' voting records: The number who got information about candidates' voting records grew 38% to nearly 16 million people.
- Surveys: The number who participated in online surveys about politics grew 15% to just under 14 million people.
- Candidates' positions: The number who researched candidates' positions online grew 14% to more than 27 million people.
- 32 million people traded e-mails with jokes in them about the candidates.
- 31 million went online to find out how candidates were doing in opinion polls.
- 25 million used the Internet to check the accuracy of claims made by or about the candidates.
- 19 million watched video clips about the candidates or the election.
- 17 million sent e-mails about the campaign to groups of family members or friends as part of listserves or discussion groups.
- 16 million people checked out endorsements or candidate ratings on the Web sites of political organizations.
- 14 million signed up for e-mail newsletters or other online alerts to get the latest news about politics.
- 7 million signed up to receive e-mail from the presidential campaigns.

- 4 million signed up online for campaign volunteer activities such as helping to organize a rally, getting people to register to voters, or getting people to the polls on Election Day.

Sixty-three million online political news consumers (52% of Internet users) said the Internet was an important source of information that contributed to their voting decision, and 27% said that this online information made them vote for or against a specific candidate. They used the Internet for its convenience as well as to supplement information obtained through television and other print media. Campaigns met this information need by using the Internet to communicate targeted messages to specific constituencies and were able to track responses to these messages.

## CAMPAIGN ACTIVITIES

Campaign activities can be divided into basic-level campaign activities and advanced-level campaign activities. The activities in which one participates are largely determined by the amount of time one has to give to the campaign, the motivation for participation, and the needs of the campaign (Robinson, 1995a). Of all Americans, 26% participated directly in at least one campaign activity in 2004. About 4 million people signed up online for activities that included registering voters, getting people to polls on Election Day, and organizing a rally (Pew Research Center, 2004). Many nurses have worked on basic-level campaign activities. These include organizing phone banks and literature drops, office work, poll watching, organizing house parties, driving candidates, fund-raising, serving as health policy advisors, organizing voter registration, and providing Internet communication about a candidate. Advanced-level campaign activities and roles usually require full-time involvement and include campaign manager, finance director, political director, communications director, and operations director.

### Basic-Level Campaign Activities

Basic-level campaign activities are easily undertaken by nurses because we are used to working on teams and in groups, have good communication skills, and are well organized. There are some issues you need to think about before volunteering. First, are you doing this for your personal benefit or for an organization's benefit?

Although there are no limitations on your involvement in a campaign as a private individual, it is important to note that in some cases it may be inappropriate for you to work on a political campaign as a representative of a particular organization. Some organizations are actually prohibited from engaging in political activity or candidate endorsements based on federal election law and their tax status (see *Political Activity: Different Rules for Government-Employed Nurses*, which precedes this section). Political involvement on behalf of that organization could cause problems for the organization as well as the campaign. Check to be sure that your participation in a campaign is approved by the organization that you represent. Many organizations have detailed processes and procedures for official endorsement. It is best to check before engaging in campaign work as an organizational representative.

Once you have the green light, don't be shy about making sure the campaign is aware of your affiliation. If you want an organization to get credit for your participation, you need to identify yourself as a representative of that organization. It would be best to have a group of individuals from your organization take responsibility for a specific campaign activity or project. The American Nurses Association organizes Campaign Activity Night (CAN) in the fall of each national election year. That night nurses nationwide are asked to work on campaigns. It is much more powerful to report to a campaign manager that 10 nurses worked 4 hours each telephoning 1200 constituents at campaign headquarters than to report that one nurse worked for 4 hours and called 120 constituents.

The second issue to consider is how much time you have to volunteer. Campaigns count on their volunteers, and if you sign up to do something, it is important that you follow through. If you have time to volunteer only once, a little help is better than no help. Obviously the more time and involvement you have, the greater will be the payback. For those who have more time, decide whether you want to be involved in many activities or stay focused on one activity. Keep in mind that it is easier to quantify one's contribution and get credit for the work when you can be identified as filling a specific role such as driver, house party coordinator, or health policy advisor, rather than filling many nonspecific roles.

The last issue to consider is when to get involved in the campaign. If possible, it is best to get involved early in the campaign. Candidates remember their early supporters. It is easier to carve out your niche when there are fewer people involved in the early stages of the campaign.

### Types of Campaign Activities

*Phone banks.* Phone banks are frequently used to contact voters for voter identification, to communicate the candidate's message, to determine support or nonsupport of a specific candidate or issue, and to ensure turnout on Election Day. They are also used to recruit volunteers, raise money, and ensure turnout at campaign events. You will be given a list of names and phone numbers and asked to read a script created by the campaign. There are usually written directions about how to deal with answering machines, wrong numbers, voter comments, and busy signals. Most campaigns provide a short training session before calls are made. Nurses are usually skilled at phone banking because of their excellent communication skills.

*Literature drops.* Volunteers often go door to door to drop off campaign literature. Usually there is a short training session about where to place the literature and legal limitations such as avoiding placement in mailboxes. You will need a name tag, written instructions, map, directions to the area, and a telephone number to call if problems are encountered. Leafleting is a form of literature distribution that is limited to public places.

Literature drops and leafleting are low-impact voter contacts with low cost and little ability to target voters. Other low-impact voter activities include buttons and bumper stickers, lawn signs, billboards, and human billboards. High-impact voter contact activities include: door-to-door canvassing, house parties, special events, and get out the vote (GOTV) activities. The latter include door-to-door canvassing, acting as poll workers, phoning to remind people to vote, and providing rides to the polls.

*Door-to-door canvassing.* Door-to-door canvassing is a traditional type of voter contact in which the volunteer knocks on the door and speaks with the voter. In your training you will receive a script to follow. You will leave literature about the candidate with the voter. Your goal may be to share the candidate's message or to determine the voting preference of the voting inhabitants of the house. You will receive a kit with names; addresses; the order in which houses are to be visited; the script; a number to call if problems are encountered; written candidate information; supporter items such as buttons or bumper stickers; volunteer cards; a form to report voting preferences, questions, or requests for more information; and a thank-you card.

*House parties.* House parties are given by a volunteer in a targeted area where neighbors, friends, and colleagues or acquaintances are invited to the volunteer's house to meet the candidate. The candidate usually makes a brief presentation (10 to 20 minutes) followed by a question-and-answer period. The campaign usually provides the host with written instructions including a sample invitation and thank-you cards. The host is responsible for distribution of invitations, follow-up calls, purchase of food and drinks, physical setup of the house space, managing the event, collection of funds, and sending thank-you notes to attendees. House parties can be fun to host or attend. Greer Glazer served as house party coordinator in University Heights for Lee Fisher during his campaign for Ohio State Senate. Most of the house parties gathered between 10 and 30 people, eager to meet the candidate. Some parties had lavish food; others were limited to coffee, tea, and cookies. The events were casual, were relaxed, and provided everyone with the opportunity to have one-on-one contact with the candidate. When Lee Fisher was elected State Senator, Greer served in an advisory capacity on nursing and health issues. He subsequently ran for the office of Ohio's Attorney General and was elected. The relationship that had been developed by working on all of his campaigns was very helpful when Greer was able to have access to discuss Medicaid payments for advanced practice nurses.

*Created events.* Created events are the best way to create the environment for the candidate's message and to target it to a specific group. Congressman Sherrod Brown of Ohio (D-OH) routinely holds such events. These include meetings with nurses to discuss health care issues, meetings with senior citizens to discuss prescription drug coverage, or town hall meetings to discuss larger policy issues such as social security. These events are likely to get media coverage. Every detail is planned in advance. The campaign uses these events to elaborate on a candidate's position and to provide visual images that enhance public support.

Timing for media events can be created by the campaign or dictated by opportunities that arise to highlight a candidate's position. Examples of events created by the campaign might include staging a worker rally, holding a press conference in front of a hospital to discuss the need for enhanced medical insurance for children, or interviewing senior citizens about Medicare. For added exposure, clips from rallies or interviews might also be posted as a flash video on the candidate's Website.

Unplanned media opportunities use news events to highlight a candidate's position with regard to a current event. It can provide an opportunity to differentiate the candidate from the opposition

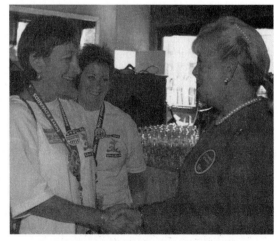

Greer Glazer (left) and Erin Murphy with Congresswoman Carolyn McCarthy at an American Nurses Association Political Action Committee (ANA-PAC) event.

candidate or to highlight one's leadership on the topic. For example, a few days after 9/11 President Bush was able to show his respect and sorrow for his fellow Americans at Ground Zero by standing arm in arm with firefighters helping with the recovery effort. Such media events create powerful messages (see Chapter 9).

In addition to candidate media events, supportive organizations and individuals may use their own resources to generate media coverage for a particular issue. For example, ANA's political action committee, ANA-PAC, has actively taken out newspaper ads, made radio spots, and purchased political paraphernalia to advocate for nurse-friendly candidates.

***Get out the vote activities.*** The candidate can have the most campaign funds, best message, and most efficient operation, but if the campaign is unable to get supporters out to vote on Election Day, the candidate will not win. Phone banks are used to get out the vote using scripts that provide a sense of urgency about the race and election. The voter may be offered a ride to the polls if needed. The same messages can be e-mailed to listserves of supporters. Door-to-door canvassing is also effective in getting out the vote. Campaigns also have poll workers who distribute information and sample ballots and poll watchers who track supporters voting and report back to the campaign so that nonvoters can be contacted (Robinson, 1995b).

### Advanced-Level Campaign Activities

The *campaign manager* has overall responsibility for the strategic and technical decisions of the entire campaign and creates the campaign and business plans. The campaign manager sets the tone to motivate staff and volunteers who work long hours for little or no payment. For example, the 2004 election illustrates that an Internet strategy should be an integral part of any campaign (Convio, 2005b).

The *finance director* has overall responsibility for finances. This individual manages fund-raising and oversees a finance committee and fund-raising events, as well as how money is spent. This is the person who determines with the political director and the communications director how much to spend on media, special events, travel, staff, and so on. The 2004 election proved that fund-raising via the Internet should be a critical component of any campaign. Fund-raising through the Internet raised $82 million (33%) of Senator John Kerry's $249 million, $14 million (5%) of President George Bush's $273 million, and $20 million for Dr. Howard Dean, which represented 40% of his total fund-raising (Pew Research Center, 2004). Dean's campaign enlisted grassroots volunteer fund-raisers to be "Dean Team" leaders. The campaign supplied Internet tools so that these "Dean Team" members could recruit and raise money from those they contacted. They created personal Webpages telling their stories about why they were campaigning for Dr. Dean, had a personal Internet-based fund-raising center, could check responses, and could thank the contributors, all through the personalized Website. The majority of online donations were under $200 (Convio, 2003).

The *political director* has overall responsibility for campaign strategy to determine how to position the candidate as the person to win. The director oversees a field director, outreach director, recruitment director, and Web director. A major responsibility is developing opposition strategy. In the 2004 election the Internet not only became an effective medium for fund-raising, but it also provided extensive constituent outreach that resulted in an online constituency. Governor Dean's campaign did an outstanding job of recruiting and developing online constituency by having people register on the campaign's Website; sending routine e-mail messages with consistent and compelling messages; creating online polls, surveys, and discussions (weblogs, or blogs); asking those visiting the Website to forward messages to friends and relatives ("viral marketing"); and creating urgency. Dean's Webpages were updated so that new fund-raising results were displayed every 45 minutes, and messages were created to ask for a specific contribution to meet a goal by a deadline.

The *communications director* has overall responsibility for theme and message and oversees a scheduler, research director, and press secretary. A campaign message is the basis of communications. Paul Tully, former Political Director of the Democratic National Committee, defined the message as "a limited body of truthful information which is consistently conveyed by a candidate and an organization in order to provide the persuasive reasons for an audience to choose and act on behalf of their choice of our candidate" (Robinson, 1995c, p. 8). The message should be simple, clear, concise, constructive, and convincing. Paul Tully developed a message box as a practical tool for planning and action. It looks like this:

> What the candidate says about himself
> What the opponent says about himself
> What the candidate says about his opponent
> What the opponent says about the candidate

Throughout a campaign, candidates seek as much control as possible over how they and their opponents are perceived by the media and the electorate. Communications directors carefully craft messages about their candidate as well as about the opponent, often based on research and polling. The goal is to ensure that their campaign defines the candidate and, to the greatest extent possible, the opponent on their own terms.

The tug of war for achieving the upper hand in crafting this definition was evident in the 2004 presidential race. The Bush campaign successfully defined Senator Kerry for the public, making it extremely difficult for the Kerry camp to conduct the campaign on its own terms. Through consistency of message and with the help of outside efforts such as the "Swift Boat Veterans for Truth," the Bush Campaign tapped into the public's core concerns about Senator Kerry's background and qualifications as a leader and often controlled the electorate's perceptions of Kerry more effectively than the Kerry campaign itself.

The last part of planning the message involves research about the voters: Who are the voters most and least likely to vote for your candidate, and who are most persuadable? What are the issues that are important to them, and what positions taken by a candidate would influence them to vote for or not for the candidate? When will the voter likely make a decision about who he or she will vote for? Where do the voters live? Why do they support, do not support, or are undecided about the candidate?

The Internet proved to be an effective communication tool for developing and executing candidates' messages in the 2004 campaign. Fourteen million people participated in online surveys; 27 million people researched candidates' positions online, and 17 million people sent e-mails about the campaign to friends and family (Pew Research Center, 2004).

The *operations director* has overall responsibility for the administrative activities and provides oversight for an office manager and staff, treasurer, and volunteer coordinator.

Involvement in political campaigns provides a wonderful opportunity for influencing candidates about health issues, for meeting people, and for bringing a nursing perspective to the political process.

## Lessons Learned

- The Internet became an essential part of American politics in 2004.
- The basic or advanced campaign activities are largely determined by the amount of time you have to give the campaign, your motivation for participation, and the needs of the campaign.
- Nurses' education and experience have prepared them to effectively participate as a candidate or campaign worker.

## Web Resources

**Democratic Congressional Campaign Committee**
www.dccc.org
**Democratic Senatorial Campaign Committee**
www.dscc.org
**Green Party of the United States**
www.gp.org
**Independent American Party**
www.usiap.org
**MoveOn.org**
www.moveon.org
**National Republican Senatorial Committee**
www.nrsc.org
**Republican National Committee**
www.rnc.org

## REFERENCES

Convio. (2005a). Using the Internet for effective grassroots advocacy: Strategies, tools, and approaches for inspiring constituents to take action. Retrieved on March 29, 2006, from *www.convio.com/advocacyguide1*.

Convio. (2005b). The basics of email marketing for nonprofits. Retrieved August 2, 2004, from *www.convio.com/emailbasics*.

Convio. (2003). Using the Internet to raise funds and mobilize supporters: Lessons nonprofits can learn from the Dean for America Campaign. Retrieved on March 29, 2006, from *www.convio.com/downloads/Dean_whitepaper_121703.pdf*.

Pew Research Center. (2004). The Internet and campaign. Internet and the American Life Project. Retrieved March 26,

2005, from *www.pewinternet.org/ pdfs/pip_2004_campaign.pdf*.

Robinson, W. C. (1995a). Campaign planning. In S. Snider (Ed.), *Democratic National Committee campaign training manual*. Washington, DC: Democratic National Committee.

Robinson, W. C. (1995b). Voter contact. In S. Snider (Ed.), *Democratic National Committee campaign training manual*. Washington, DC: Democratic National Committee.

Robinson, W. C. (1995c). Message. In S. Snider (Ed.), *Democratic National Committee campaign training manual*. Washington, DC: Democratic National Committee.

# *Vignette*   Barbara B. Hatfield

## Truth or Dare: One Nurse's Political Campaign

*"All serious daring starts from within."*

HARRIET BEECHER STOWE

My dream had always been that of being a wife, mother, and nurse. Never in my wildest dreams did I envision a career in politics. Having graduated from a hospital-based diploma program, I was content to raise my family and work as a staff nurse in Charleston, West Virginia. As I became more experienced in my career, I began to become increasingly frustrated by the lack of power that nurses have in health care decisions. My colleagues and I saw the problems on a daily basis but felt powerless to make needed changes. Living and working in the capital city, we constantly heard about the activities of the West Virginia legislature. The legislative meeting schedules were printed daily in the local newspapers.

After one particularly discouraging day, some of the nurses on my unit suggested that we sit in on a Health Committee meeting at the House of Delegates. Working full time and raising our families didn't leave much time for outside activities,

but one day after work we decided to go and listen for ourselves. In the 1980s, nurses still wore white uniforms. Because we hadn't had time to change, we were immediately recognized as nurses. To our amazement no one serving on the Health Committee had any health care experience. In a moment of levity I commented to my friends that if these guys could get elected, I probably could, too. At least I would understand what they were discussing. We all laughed because, of course, I had no intention of ever running for office.

My offhand comments, intended to be funny, were taken quite seriously by two of my colleagues. They decided that one of them would be my campaign manager and the other my public relations chairperson. I still had no intention of actually running but agreed to go with them to a workshop entitled "How to Get Women and Minorities Elected to Office," which was sponsored by the National Organization for Women. After attending the workshop and reading the book that they provided, I was more convinced than ever that my running for office was a futile cause. I promptly forgot about my threat.

My friends, however, didn't forget and began to spread the word. Before I knew it, I was being contacted by other nurses who wanted to help with my campaign for the House of Delegates. To pay the filing fee, they had collected $33.00 by asking 33 nurses for a dollar each. I called a meeting at my house, and 15 nurses showed up, excited and ready to go. All of us realized that the power that we wanted and needed was in the political arena. Suddenly, I found myself on a roller coaster, and I couldn't get off.

In my House of Delegates district at this time there were 12 vacant seats. The 12 top vote getters from the Democratic party ran against the 12 from the Republican party in the general election. Our first challenge was to make it through the primary. Thirty-four other candidates were running, many of whom were seasoned politicians. Our first big obstacle was money, or the lack of it. None of my backers had money, and I certainly had no personal wealth. We began by collecting small donations of $15 to $25 from individual nurses. The nurses that donated were charged to collect from other nurses. The campaign manual suggested going after endorsements from groups and organizations. I received support from the West Virginia Nurses Association and the West Virginia Association of School Nurses, which were small but very politically active, the teachers' associations, the Hospital Association, and the Medical Association. The last two groups endorsed me because I was a nurse but never expected me to win and dropped their support after my first election. They never quite understood that my first loyalty was, and still is, with nurses and their patients rather than with doctors and hospital administrators.

My campaign "staff" consisted of volunteer nurses who took pictures, researched key issues, designed brochures and flyers, and formed phone banks. We found out that if you aren't one of the "good ole boys," you get very little help or advice from the party. There was no money to buy mailing lists, so we had to be creative. For 2 months we went to the Voter's Registration Office every night after work, looked at every voter's card in the targeted precincts of my district and got the names and addresses of the voters who had voted in the last three elections. From these we developed mailing and walking lists.

The guide instructed us to do three mail-outs. We had the money to do one. There was only one way to get our literature out. The volunteer nurses formed teams and walked from house to house, knocking on doors and leaving brochures. To our delight, we discovered that everybody loves nurses and enjoys talking to them. Two weeks later, I covered those same precincts to introduce myself.

Through all of these efforts, I became known as the "nurse" candidate. This helped to pull me out of the pack of 35 candidates. To get free publicity, we stood on street corners and along the highways, often in uniform, holding signs with slogans like "Elect a Nurse" and "Every House and Senate needs a Nurse." By now, my volunteer nurses and their friends were so excited and encouraged that my biggest fear was letting them down, so I never stopped. Although I tried not to think about it, deep down I still didn't think we stood a chance of winning.

The night of the primary election, I didn't plan a party because I couldn't face the nurses if I lost. My close friends, who had worked so hard, sat with me as the first returns came in. In disbelief, we listened as my name began to be mentioned in the top 12. At the end of the evening, I was not only one of the 12 winners but had come in third. The nurses had won a big one! Suddenly reality set in. We looked at each other and exclaimed, "We have to do this all over again for the general election," which was less than 6 months away.

After a month's rest, we did it all over again, and once again were victorious in the general election. When the elation faded, I realized that I didn't have a clue what to do next. The campaign manual had instructed you how to win but didn't say anything about how to be a good legislator. I quickly discovered that my past training had prepared me well. As a nurse, I had been playing politics throughout my hospital career.

With name recognition and a positive voting record, I have continued to win elections. We still struggle to raise money, and I still depend heavily on the dedicated nurses and other friends who volunteer to help me. The grassroots campaign is still an effective way to win, although, with the growing importance of the media, candidates must raise more money than ever. Those of us without large corporate donations have to rely on small donations from a lot of people. Fortunately, over the years we have broadened our base to include social workers, teachers, labor unions, and others who fight for the "little guys." The nurses, however, are always my mainstay.

During each campaign, I have, in addition to the volunteers, a few nurses who stay close to me. They are always there to provide support when I get discouraged and give me strength when I want to quit. As the battles get tough, they keep me focused on our real objective—making life better for the people of West Virginia.

I am currently serving my fourteenth year in the West Virginia House of Delegates. I am very proud to be known as the nurse in the House. My office is often full of nurses and other health care workers. They are such an inspiration to me. I never tire of seeing the glee on their faces when we win a battle and the determination when we lose one. Being in the legislature has opened other doors for me, giving me new ways to serve as a nurse.

I use my experience to inspire other nurses to step up to the plate and get into politics. We need

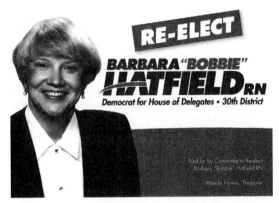

Barbara Hatfield, RN: Campaign postcard for 2004 election.

nurses to run and serve on school boards, commissions, and city councils. They must be a part of state legislatures and run for seats in the United States Congress to join the three nurses who are currently serving there. Nurses are respected for their knowledge and dedication. They can have a tremendous influence on health care policy. I will continue my service in the West Virginia legislature until I can convince another nurse to run in my place. Then I will gladly step aside for the next generation of nurses.

# Vignette — Christine W. Saltzberg

## There's Nothing Quite Like Campaigning for Office

*"A hero is an ordinary individual who finds the strength to persevere and endure in spite of overwhelming obstacles."*

CHRISTOPHER REEVE

Without a doubt I count campaigning for public office as one of the most phenomenal experiences of my lifetime. Running for office is exciting, intense, and time limited.

My first campaign for an open seat in the New York State legislature took place over 5 very intense months and cost about $400,000. Besides putting together a campaign committee and raising a lot of money in a short amount of time, each and every day was filled with phone calls, meetings, interviews, events, and writing and editing materials. I met thousands while walking door to door for about 2 hours a day in the beginning weeks of the campaign and then as much as 8 hours a day toward the end. Some nights I had to soak my feet they were so sore, and eventually I wore out at least two pairs of shoes. With all the activity, fresh air, and exercise from walking I had tremendous energy and rarely slept more than 4 hours a night. I would answer e-mail and read well after midnight, because I could do those things when the rest of the world was sleeping. Of course, no one would want me to call asking for money at that time anyway, plus my mind was racing, still busy reviewing the day and making plans for the next.

It is very important to understand that a campaign demands a lot of attention from everyone, especially the candidate. Campaigning for office can be at least as demanding and requires as much involvement as full-time employment and some-times even more so depending on the office one seeks and the attention one focuses on it. In addition, there are associated costs and benefits to campaigning. First of all the candidate does not earn a salary for pursuing elected office, and so will need to determine how much time and personal resources, including finances, can be devoted to the effort. There are constant interruptions by the phone and fax, and everything seems to be urgent and needs to be done immediately—or better yet, yesterday. One learns very quickly that interpersonal skills, flexibility, and spontaneity can be important assets. One also learns a great deal in a very short time, including, for exam-ple, that campaigning for state office and writing a dissertation are incompatible with each other. A registered nurse since 1971, I had practiced across the continuum of care, held a masters degree in community and public health nursing, and most recently had served on the faculty in a school of nurs-ing where I taught at the undergraduate and gradu-ate levels. When I decided to throw my hat into the political arena the first time, I was in the midst of writing my dissertation to complete the PhD in education at Cornell University.

Relatively unknown before the first race, I successfully garnered 48% of the vote in a legislative district that, although not as geographically chal-lenging as some districts are, covered major portions of three counties and included both suburban and rural towns and communities. I began my second campaign a little earlier in the year and raised more money than before, which was helpful in many ways. Both campaigns were for the same seat and against the same person. I was not elected either time, and believe that each time the public missed an excellent opportunity to elect someone who understands systems, is open to and knows how to effect change, and has the educational and experi-ential background to develop policy and address myriad concerns including public health issues, the nursing shortage, and education.

## PREPARING FOR CANDIDACY

Not all nurses will choose to seek public office, nor should they, any more than every person should become a nurse, as nurses can all attest. Yet nurses are better prepared to become candidates and to hold public office than they may realize. I recall entertaining thoughts about the possibility of running for public office the first time, as I watched Congress impeach President Clinton. During these proceedings and what could be viewed as historic moments, I was conducting research for my doctoral dissertation on nursing students' episte-mological perspectives, because I was interested in how people think about the world and knowledge, how they construct their experiences, and how they go about making judgments when faced with uncertainty (Saltzberg, 2002). I was struck by the reasoning abilities and arguments displayed by various elected officials, many of whom had been in office for years. I remember wondering how some of them ever got elected and concluding that we need better thinkers in the legislature.

I believe that the kinds of issues, problems, and concerns with which legislators grapple require people with diverse life experiences who are open to hearing and considering others' perspectives while constructing their own, and who are wise decision-makers even in the face of uncertainty. Most legislators in New York State are attorneys or have major connections with businesses, and what-ever their background, most are men. Nowhere in the state or U.S. Constitution does it say that only attorneys or business owners should be elected to the state legislature or Congress. There are other views of the world and experiences worth know-ing and considering when making laws and developing policy. People from diverse backgrounds can make important contributions to the directions our states and country take.

## MAKING THE DECISION TO RUN

I believe that there are several crucial questions to ask oneself when considering the possibility of running for public office. I asked myself these same questions before agreeing to become a candidate for the state legislature the first time:

- How do I feel about privacy?
- How do I feel about raising money?
- How does my family feel about my running for office?

Mounting a successful campaign depends on serious and realistic appraisal of each area before making the decision to take up the challenge.

### Privacy

Privacy has always been very important to me, so it was one of the first things I considered when making the decision to run. I knew that once I announced my candidacy privacy would become much more difficult to achieve. Computers make it very easy to conduct electronic searches and gather information about people on everything from their charitable contributions to statements given to the media, and anything from where children attend school to parking tickets. Even when one has never had a parking ticket or a traffic violation, such searches will often be made and are intended to uncover all kinds of information that may prove useful during a campaign. This is why it is so important to take whatever time is necessary to honestly reflect on your own life before making the choice to become a candidate. Such reflection can help prevent future possible heartache and anguish and help prepare you to address an issue that becomes public knowledge during a campaign. Being open to the world and the experiences that follow candidacy involves taking risks and yet can be very positive. I knew that my life and background could withstand the scrutiny and curiosity that come with candidacy, and because of that I also knew it would serve me well on the road to public office.

Initially when you become a candidate, the phone never seems to stop ringing, mail and e-mail increase significantly, and, as you become more known, people want to talk with you every place you go. During my first campaign for the New York State legislature, I ended up with three phones. One phone line was set up with a fax machine, was solely devoted to the campaign, and came in very handy for sharing information and meeting various deadlines. I also carried a cell phone everywhere. Another phone with a private number eventually became necessary because the others were always so busy my family members and I needed a way to communicate in an emergency. I strongly recommend that all phones have caller identification, call waiting, and message capability. It is great to know that the press is calling before you pick up the phone, because it gives you a chance to decide if you want to speak with a reporter at that particular time and gives you a moment or two to prepare before doing so.

### Fund-Raising

Raising money is necessary to running for office, but especially in contested local races and those at the state and federal levels, where campaigns can become very expensive. No matter what office one seeks the person most responsible for raising money is the candidate. Once these basic things are understood and once the decision is made to become a candidate, a variety of fund-raising strategies need to be employed as early and continuously as possible throughout the campaign. What happens with the money? This of course depends on what the particular campaign requires to get the message out about the candidate, the candidate's positions on issues, and the geography involved. For example, in a campaign for a state office, campaign staff may be printing and mailing literature to well over 100,000 people and doing so multiple times. The needed media exposure through television and radio will probably be the most costly campaign expenditures whatever the office level, and especially if one has to purchase time in multiple media markets.

Effective campaign finance reform could help make raising money easier for candidates who are not independently wealthy and could lower contribution limits, possibly decreasing the total amounts spent on campaigns. I believe that if campaigns become publicly financed, then more people including nurses will consider running for office and more races will be contested at all levels of government. Furthermore, I believe that candidates should not have to go into major debt or mortgage their homes, thus potentially jeopardizing their families' futures, in order to campaign for office and enter public service. Entering public service should not be a privilege determined by wealth or gender.

I will discuss some actual strategies for fundraising in a later section.

### Family Support

Most of us have a family in some form or another, and I believe that family support is paramount to campaigning for public office, because their lives will be affected in a variety of major ways. My family has always supported my interests and pursuits, and yet I still recommend asking for family support before becoming a candidate. My family believes in me and wants to be helpful; as wonderful as that is, decisions may have to be made about their roles. For example, a candidate needs to decide if any family members or others will be surrogate speakers at events, at gatherings, or with the media. Still other involvement may need to be negotiated.

My oldest son was willing to move back to New York and home to work full time as my primary assistant on my first campaign. On any given day he might research a piece of legislation or an organization's views, take phone calls and schedule appointments, write a press release, coordinate a mailing to reach thousands of district voters, represent me at a campaign staff meeting, or accompany me to meet with government officials or to attend a fundraiser. Toward the end of the campaign my son found himself doing some slightly more mundane yet equally important things like shopping for shoes and makeup for me, picking up groceries for the family, making a sandwich for me, or doing my laundry, because I had no time to do any of it myself. He also drove me to events so I could focus on making phone calls, reviewing information, and preparing along the way. Every minute can be filled with campaign-related activities, so how the

candidate spends every minute is important. The experiences on my campaign were eye openers for my son; currently in his final year of law school, he has no plans at this time to pursue elected office.

My husband took 7 weeks' vacation to work on my first campaign. He too was involved in multiple ways—taking pictures, accompanying me to events, marching with me in parades, preparing mailings, putting up signs, organizing and staffing phone banks, contributing campaign funds, and so much more. The second time I ran, he devoted another 3 months' vacation to working on the campaign. During each campaign he was my confidante and most loyal supporter. Family members from all over the country made financial contributions to my campaigns. In fact, I could not have run for office without their help and that of my many friends, neighbors, and nurse colleagues.

For me, having the ability to run a credible campaign and to accomplish the work once elected was never an issue. So, once satisfied with the answers to these three questions, I knew I was ready to accept the challenges that come with candidacy.

### BUILDING A CAMPAIGN

The most important thing to remember about choosing an advisory committee and campaign staff is that you have to be able to trust them. The candidate needs to be able to rely on each and every one not to divulge the campaign plan or strategies to others outside the campaign, especially to the opposition and the media, unless, of course, divulging specific information is one of the strategies. Staff members, including volunteers, need to be able to question your positions on issues and the decisions that are made in the campaign. They need to know that you will listen to them and to their ideas and suggestions even if after consideration you choose a different path. You need them to be able to openly and accurately support you to the public, even if confidentially a volunteer or staff member disagrees with you on some point. You are asking them all for a commitment and assistance to get elected, and you need to reciprocate by making a commitment to taking the campaign seriously, working hard to get elected, and being worthy of their respect and support.

In the beginning of a campaign my recommendation is to fill only the major staff positions such as coordinator or manager, treasurer, and volunteer coordinator. Then together develop the basic campaign plan and budget and grow from there. As the campaign and plan begin to take shape, you get a sense of what roles are still essential and when to fill them. As you spread the word about your candidacy, be open to considering everyone you meet as a potential supporter and volunteer. Take notes and pass that information along to your staff members to pursue. Building toward Election Day, more and more volunteers will be needed for certain activities, and people need to be matched with the right roles or activities. Not everyone is comfortable making cold phone calls to strangers to encourage them to vote for a particular candidate; however, the same volunteers might be more than willing to go door to door and drop off literature or put up lawn signs in their election districts. Without a doubt staff members, volunteers, family members, colleagues, and friends need to know that you appreciate everything they do to help get you elected. Everything, no matter how small, is a contribution and a vote of confidence in the candidate.

My campaigns depended heavily on volunteers from different political parties and included some nurse colleagues and staff members with no campaign experience whatsoever, so initially I had to help them learn their jobs while doing my own. I had previously worked on federal- and state-level campaigns and had attended the Institute for Public Leadership sponsored by the YWCA. The institute prepares women to be candidates and to manage campaigns.

I was adamant that the makeup of my campaign staff would represent my beliefs about the world and what I believe is important. During each of my campaigns I mentored others, including nurses, in their new roles as campaign coordinator, treasurer, volunteer coordinator, and more. In every campaign you will want to remember your base of support, as they will help you get elected.

## Fund-Raising and Endorsements

*Fund-raising strategies.* As I have stated previously, campaigns can be very expensive. To get your message out effectively requires setting a realistic budget for the kind of campaign you plan to wage and accepting that this may necessitate continuous fund-raising throughout the course of the campaign. Initially fund-raising may seem daunting to an inexperienced candidate, because it requires asking for support and possibly not getting it. Every dollar people contribute, however, helps the candidate raise more, and every time a candidate asks for contributions she gains more fund-raising experience in the process. In the beginning a candidate may need to spend time making phone calls to family members and friends to raise small amounts of money and gain confidence. As the campaign begins to take shape, the plan helps guide requests, and the candidate can mention specific purposes for the funds, such as printing and mailing costs or a media buy. Knowing the laws limiting campaign contributions is essential for the candidate and the staff. As the campaign accelerates and Election Day approaches, there will be less time available for fund-raising, so decisions will need to be made about how best to spend one's time.

*Endorsements.* Whether to seek political action committee (PAC) endorsements is one area each candidate will need to decide how to address. The endorsement process itself can be a competitive one. Often the process involves responding to written questionnaires and group interviews about one's views or positions on a whole variety of issues important to members of the PAC and the parent organization. Such questions are not limited to one issue, even if a candidate has decided to enter a race and focus the agenda on one issue, such as the nursing shortage or violent crime. The groups will seek to learn the candidate's views on a whole host of issues, what she will do while in office, and how accessible she will be once elected. The endorsement process can be time consuming, yet the process helps the candidate learn about issues from others' perspectives and helps the candidate garner support, whether financial or otherwise.

## Getting the Message Out

*The message.* "A lifetime of experience" was my first campaign theme. Ultimately, whatever theme is chosen, it should be the most appropriate for the

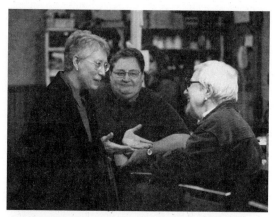

During her first campaign for the New York State Assembly, Christine W. Saltzberg, PhD, MS, APRN, BC (left) stops at a local diner to great seniors and to discuss health care issues such as the high cost of prescription medications, with them.

particular campaign and candidate. The candidate and campaign staff should adopt a theme and craft the message so that every statement reflects that theme and is consistent across time and media. What is at the core of the theme is the message you will strive to convey to voters every day of the campaign.

***The media.*** If you are willing to do the research for them, I have learned that reporters will gladly accept the information you provide. Some reporters will even rehash old news rather than seek out the new, and some are simply better writers than others. Reporters sometimes ask particular questions in order to get a reaction, and they may even inadvertently provide information about the opposition's views on an issue. Therefore it is very important to listen to the questions that are asked, even if you choose not to answer, and it is important to pay attention to any slips of the tongue reporters may make, as you may be able to use that information. A candidate does not have to accept the premise of a reporter's questions, and if an interview is being taped, the candidate can respond to questions any way she chooses, because what will be made public will be your responses, not what the reporter asks. It is always a good idea to consider what you say before speaking and take every opportunity to present your message clearly.

Stick to the campaign message. Remember, reporters are not interviewing you because they are your friends; it is their job, and nothing is off the record, although some reporters will try to be fair about what they write or report. I have met at least one reporter who tries to be as fair and as unbiased as possible; unfortunately he is no longer covering the political news in major races, although I am not sure why that is. He is a much better writer than many reporters I have met over the years. It is important to be cautious with what reporters tell you, as some are willing to pass along misinformation, such as telling a candidate where an opponent plans to hold a rally, or may agree to meet a candidate for an interview, then do not show up and refuse to take a phone call for clarification. Some will even misinform the public, whether intentionally or not, which may help the opposition.

It is the sensational, however, that gets media attention, sells newspapers, and holds an audience's interest even when a story is not true. For example toward the end of my second campaign I was doing so well that, fearing he would lose and at the behest of his handlers, my opponent went on television during an early morning news program and made accusations about me that were not true. Here was a great opportunity for free publicity and to repeat his campaign message, but instead he could not stop talking about me. The reporter finally had to interrupt and suggest that my opponent might want to tell the audience about his campaign. Nurses know from repeated national surveys that the public trusts us more than any other group, and so when nothing else was working and in an effort to derail what my opposition knew was a speeding train—me, heading toward election—it was the basis for that trust that got called into question by my opponent and those whose philosophy it was to win at any cost. The media loved it, because by then the race was being talked about across the state. The truth did not seem to matter to the media, and they would not report it even when it was provided to them. Making headlines and helping to manipulate the public's perceptions during a hotly contested race was what seemed all important to reporters. One has to wonder, though—if an elected official is willing to make untrue accusations to get reelected, how far is that person really willing to go to stay in office, especially if it's believed that the public will never know the truth?

## HIGHS AND LOWS

Being a candidate in one of the state's most highly publicized campaigns and one of the most organized campaigns the community has seen is certainly exciting and definitely leaves one feeling successful and truly proud of the accomplishments one has achieved, whatever the outcome. Not being elected afterward can be a surprise. It is, however, not the worst thing that has ever happened in my life. After the first campaign, person after person, including many former and current public officials from the opposing party, congratulated me on my campaign prowess. I can truly say that there is no other experience quite like it.

## LESSONS LEARNED AND OTHER PEARLS OF WISDOM

### Integrity

Whatever major decisions are made in a campaign, whatever positions are taken on issues, and whatever strategies are implemented, I believe a candidate has to consider the potential ramifications and consequences of each, because ultimately it is the candidate who has to live with them. Others may question this stance, and perhaps even label it "micromanaging," but I strongly disagree. It is the candidate who is the most visible during a campaign, and therefore her honor and integrity are tested in public throughout every day. Moreover, if one is not careful, a campaign can seem to take on a life of its own and carry the candidate along. To avoid this, the candidate must ask questions and be involved in major decisions. On a related issue, I chose not to use any surrogates during my campaigns, because I believe I am the one who best knows my views on issues and how they have developed and can articulate those most appropriately and emphatically.

### Stick to the Message

It bears repeating: Stick to the campaign message, even if you abhor repetition. This can be particularly difficult for someone who finds repetition

## Best Resources For Campaign Education

Over the past 6 years I have participated in various political training programs. Most tend to focus on three topics—the candidacy, campaign management, and fund-raising—and do so with varying emphasis on each. From my experience the best three programs are the Institute for Public Leadership, which is sponsored by the YWCA and involves an intensive 2 days of interactive sessions in which presenters attempt to be nonpartisan; the Political Opportunity Program presented by EMILY's List, a national organization dedicated to electing pro-choice Democratic women candidates; and the Campaign School, sponsored by the Eleanor Roosevelt Legacy Foundation of the New York State Democratic Committee. All three programs are excellent, invigorating, and interesting. Besides providing important and useful educational materials to take home, they bring candidates into contact with women who hold public office at the local, state, and federal levels of government and those who help them get there. One major particular feature that stands out among all the programs was that the Institute for Public Leadership actually has participants work in small groups to develop a campaign theme, a plan, and a budget for those interested in managing a campaign, while potential candidates are involved in developing a platform, presenting it to the entire audience, and videotaping it for future review and analysis.

Another program to consider is offered at Yale University law school in New Haven, Connecticut. Its Website *(www.wcsyale.org)* describes the program as nonpartisan, nonadvocacy political campaign training for women who want to manage campaigns or run for office. Unfortunately, critical points in my own campaigns have kept me from attending this particular program.

Registration is required to attend these programs, and depending on the program there may be fees and other associated costs. These may include travel, accommodations, and food; however, scholarships or sponsorships may be available and are definitely worth looking into if cost is a determining factor. Each organization has a Website offering additional details about training programs and contact information. The web addresses can be found at the end of this chapter.

boring; however, it is an important lesson to learn and in actuality simplifies things. The candidate does not have to create some new way of saying something each and every encounter with either the public or the media. It is also much easier to remember what you say and to be consistent over time when the message is essentially the same over and over.

### Educating the Public and Influencing Policy

I have long been a proponent of nurses' involvement in political action and public policy development (Pineiro-Zucker, 2004). Each political campaign affords nurse candidates and their colleagues great opportunities to keep professional nursing and public health issues in the media and in the forefront of people's minds for the duration of every campaign and thereafter. The more successful a nurse candidate is in doing so during a campaign, the more likely she will continue to influence the public debate and political agenda long after Election Day. I frequently see evidence of my influence.

*Web Resources*

---

**Eleanor Roosevelt Legacy Foundation**
*www.eleanorslegacy.org*
**EMILY's List**
*www.emilyslist.org*
**Women's Campaign School**
*www.wcsyale.org*
**YWCA**
*www.ywca.org*

---

## REFERENCES

Pineiro-Zucker, D. (2004, July/August). Christine Saltzberg: An advocate for public policy development. *New York State Nurses Association Report, 35*(7), 7.

Saltzberg, C. W. (2002). Nursing students' uncertainty experiences and epistemological perspectives. (Doctoral dissertation. Cornell University, 2002). *Dissertation Abstracts International, 62*(12), 4090.

*chapter*

28

# Nursing and the Courts

Virginia Trotter Betts, David Keepnews, & Jill Gentry

*"Social advance depends as much upon the process through which it is secured as upon the result itself."*

JANE ADDAMS

The courts are an important forum for nurses to advocate for their patients and themselves. The legal and judicial system is a major arena in which the American people have traditionally sought vindication of their rights. Legislative initiatives and administrative regulations are often tested, affirmed, or invalidated through the courts. The circumstances under which employees can bargain collectively have often been matters of court rulings. Professional licensing laws, scope of practice, and antitrust laws are statutes that reflect existing rights that are enforceable through the courts.

Nurses, like most nonlawyers, often think of legal and judicial processes as arcane, mystical, frightening, and/or highly technical and better left to legal experts to address and understand. However, just as nurses have learned that they can shape legislation and regulations that affect the profession, they need to understand how judicial decisions also affect nursing practice and how (especially through their professional associations) nurses can have a positive impact on the outcome of legal decisions. Nurses should not regard the legal system as the exclusive domain of lawyers and judges any more than they regard the legislative process as the exclusive domain of lobbyists and legislators.

As activists interested in achieving particular policy outcomes, nurses always need to consider their broadest set of alternatives in developing a plan for success in policy development and implementation. Policy analysts, social activists, and legal scholars have differing opinions as to the effectiveness of using the judicial branch of government and its action instrument, the courts, to bring about social change. Nevertheless, the courts can be an important arena for policy action by organized nursing and should be more widely and proactively used.

This chapter provides an overview of the legal and judicial system and the role of the courts in shaping policy by drawing on relevant examples from nursing and health policy. It is not a comprehensive overview; rather, it aims to provide the reader with a general understanding of this area and its critical importance for nursing.

## ROLE OF THE COURTS IN SHAPING POLICY

### THE JUDICIAL SYSTEM: A BRIEF OVERVIEW

The United States has two major, parallel court systems: federal and state. The federal courts have jurisdiction over matters that involve the U.S. Constitution and federal laws and regulations. Federal courts can also hear complaints that arise between parties in different states if a sufficient monetary amount (current minimum $75,000) is in dispute. The trial courts for the federal system, the entry point for most federal cases, are district courts; there are 94 federal district courts located throughout the United States and its territories. Federal courts of appeals are organized into 11 geographic circuits plus the District of Columbia Circuit Court and the Federal Circuit Court (Want, 1997). The U.S. Supreme Court is the federal court of last resort.

Each state has its own court system, which generally interprets its state's constitution and laws. State courts may also hear some claims that arise under federal law or the U.S. Constitution. Generally, the state court system includes trial-level and appellate courts, with a high court (usually known as the *state Supreme Court*) as the court of last resort. Often, trial courts are further subdivided on the basis of subject matter, an amount or a remedy in dispute, or another specific legal issue. (For instance, various states may have family court, probate court, municipal court, mental health court, and so on.) On certain matters, decisions of a state Supreme Court may be appealed directly to the U.S. Supreme Court, whose decisions become the law of the land.

## EVOLUTION OF THE COURTS

As the U.S. court system has evolved, there have been varied periods of judicial activity in shaping social policy for the nation. In *Marbury v. Madison* (1803), the U.S. Supreme Court first asserted its power to declare an act of the legislative or executive branch null and void if the act exceeded, by the Court's interpretation, the powers granted to that branch by the Constitution. This fundamental concept of *judicial review* has evolved into one of the most important powers belonging to the courts because it grants courts significant influence over governmental activities.

Another doctrine that has emphasized the role of the courts as a force in social policy is expressed in the legal maxim of *stare decisis*. *Stare decisis*, or "let the decision stand," sets the course for judicial precedents by adhering to previous findings in cases with substantially comparable facts and situations. Thus, courts grant deference to their own prior rulings. They are not completely bound by precedent, and it is of course not unheard of for courts to overrule prior decisions, but generally they depart from precedent based on compelling and clearly articulated reasons.

The scope of the Supreme Court's influence on American life expanded greatly in the years after the Civil War, when the Fourteenth Amendment to the Constitution, ratified in 1868, limited the states' abilities to restrict the rights of their citizens, including the right to due process and the equal protection of the law. This amendment made many state laws susceptible to being challenged in the federal courts, particularly as the Supreme Court ruled that the Fourteenth Amendment had the effect of making many aspects of the Bill of Rights (e.g., the right of free speech under the First Amendment) applicable to the states.

From the mid 1950s to the mid 1980s the Supreme Court, in part reflecting changing social values and public debate on social reform, extended concepts of individual liberties and civil rights. With the appointment of the late William Rehnquist as Chief Justice in 1986, the Court came to be seen as more conservative in its ideology, narrowing its views of individuals' rights in some regards and restricting the federal government's power over the states. President Bush's recent appointments of Chief Justice Roberts and Associate Justice Alito are likely to have a significant impact on future decisions of the court.

## IMPACT LITIGATION: ESTABLISHING RIGHTS

Over the decades, advocates have had a strong tradition of using the courts strategically to establish, affirm, or clarify rights at the federal or state level. Litigation with a potentially broad effect beyond the specific parties involved is often referred to as "impact" litigation. The goal of such litigation has been described as "win[ning] cases to establish good precedent for future cases" (Johnson, 1999; Parmet, 1999). A particularly prominent example of impact litigation is *Brown v. Board of Education*, the 1954 case in which the U.S. Supreme Court struck down school segregation and mandated that states begin a process of desegregating their public schools. The Court found that segregated public school education constituted a state policy of inferior education for African-American children and that it thus violated the Equal Protection Clause of the Fourteenth Amendment to the U.S. Constitution.

Another prominent example of using the courts to establish social policy is *Roe v. Wade* (1973), in which the U.S. Supreme Court found that women had a right to choose the medical procedure of abortion free of unreasonable state restrictions. The Court made this ruling on the basis of its interpretation of various amendments to the Constitution that, it found, together conferred a right of privacy that included self-determination in seeking a medical procedure to terminate pregnancy. Although *Roe v. Wade* has been modified and narrowed in some respects by subsequent Supreme Court decisions, the basic right of a woman to choose abortion to terminate an unwanted pregnancy as established by the Court in 1973 has remained intact and continues as current reproductive health policy.

The right to die is another important area in which litigation has been used to establish health-oriented rights. In *Cruzan v. Missouri Dept. of Health* (1990), the U.S. Supreme Court established the right of individuals to refuse life-sustaining treatment. This right is now reflected in measures such as the Patient Self-Determination Act (PSDA) (Public Law [PL] 101-508, 1990).

Despite cases such as *Cruzan* and the PSDA's provisions for individuals to make their end-of-life treatment choices known through written advance directives, most Americans have not completed such directives (Collins, 1999). In *Schiavo ex rel. Schindler v. Schiavo* (2005), one of the most litigated cases related to end-of-life decision-making, Theresa (Terri) Schiavo lay in a persistent vegetative state for 15 years after sustaining severe brain damage following cardiac arrest. Terri Schiavo's life was sustained by a feeding tube for 15 years. She had left no written directives about her care. Her husband stated that, based on conversations he had held with her, she would not wish to live in a vegetative state—a contention that Ms. Schiavo's parents vigorously disputed. His direction to remove her feeding tube was strongly opposed by her parents and by others who characterized removing the tube not simply as removing life-sustaining treatment, but as an act of euthanasia—that is, that this move would kill her by starving and dehydrating her. This question became a matter of immense public controversy. Not only was the decision to remove Terri Schiavo's feeding tube highly litigated (it was contested in at least 10 actions in federal court and 30 in Florida courts), it became highly politicized

as well, particularly after her feeding tube was removed and her parents sought to have it reinserted. Several lawmakers (including Florida Governor Bush and President Bush) publicly assailed attempts to remove the feeding tube. Congress even enacted legislation granting the federal courts jurisdiction to hear the case.

Terri Schiavo died almost 2 weeks after her feeding tube was removed. Ultimately, this case's most valuable precedent may lie in demonstrating the high level of drama and controversy that can be generated around conflicts over end-of-life decision-making. Anticipating and addressing such conflicts through legislation is likely to prove a more satisfactory (and certainly more dignified) mechanism than hotly contested legal and political battles over individual family tragedies.

Some groups have sought to establish physician-assisted suicide for terminally ill patients as a legal right. These advocates have challenged existing state enforcement actions against physician-assisted suicide or pushed state-level initiatives to establish such a right, as in Oregon. In 1997, the U.S. Supreme Court ruled for the first time on the issue of physician-assisted suicide. It rendered a unanimous decision, finding that there is no constitutional right to assisted suicide (*Vacco v. Quill*, 1997; *Washington v. Glucksberg*, 1997). However, the justices offered three different opinions, signaling a recognition that both the specific issue of assisted suicide and the broader issues of end-of-life decisions and care of the terminally ill will continue to be the subject of debate and reflection throughout American society. The Court basically determined that the states retain the authority to determine policy on assisted suicide and reaffirmed the distinction between withdrawing life-sustaining treatment and providing active assistance in committing suicide. Justice Stephen Breyer, in a concurring opinion, suggested an approach to the question of assisted suicide that "would use words roughly like 'a right to die with dignity.' [A]t its core would lie personal control over the manner of death, professional medical assistance, and the avoidance of severe physical suffering—combined" (*Vacco v. Quill*, 1997).

In contrast to Oregon, other state courts, such as the Michigan circuit court in *People v. Jack Kevorkian*

(2001), have decided that assisted suicide is not an action that will be afforded federal or state constitutional protections, finding that the state's interest in the preservation of life and the prevention of suicide are substantially greater than one's personal beliefs or self-determination decisions.

## COURTS AS ENFORCERS OF EXISTING LEGISLATION

The courts are commonly used as a means to enforce existing rights and legislative and regulatory requirements and processes. For nurses, this means that the courts can be a source through which nurse practice acts or other relevant laws are enforced.

For example, in 1992, the Alabama State Nurses Association and the Alabama Board of Nursing, with the support of the American Nurses Association (ANA) and the Emergency Nurses Association, sued local hospitals that sought to place emergency medical technicians in the emergency department to provide nursing care. The nurses alleged that such assignment violated the Alabama Nurse Practice Act by allowing individuals to practice nursing without being appropriately educated and licensed. The nurse plaintiffs prevailed in the suit, and the hospitals were forced to end this practice (*Alabama Nurses Association, Alabama State Board of Nursing, et al. v. Samuelson and the Alabama State Department of Public Health*, 1992).

In Oklahoma the state board of nursing, supported by the Oklahoma Nurses Association, sued a hospital over its practice of using unlicensed assistive personnel (UAPs) to provide some technical aspects of nursing care. This private hospital had sought to use an exception to the state's nurse practice act that permitted UAPs, in some circumstances, to provide care within public health programs. The hospital argued that because it served indigent patients, including Medicaid recipients, it should fall within this exception. The board of nursing challenged the hospital. The board lost at trial, and the case went to appeal. The ANA submitted an *amicus curiae* brief in support of the board of nursing's position. The appellate court judge concluded that the hospital was skirting the mandates of the Nurse Practice Act and remanded the case back to the

lower court for further review. At that point the matter was settled before going to trial again. Therefore, although this out-of-court–settled case produced a less definitive and less generalizable legal result than the Alabama case discussed previously, it does represent an example of the use of the courts to seek enforcement of the state nurse practice act. It is an effective method to protect the professional nurse's scope of practice.

## ANTITRUST LAWS

Federal and state antitrust laws are designed to protect consumers by prohibiting anticompetitive business practices. These laws have their roots in the end of the nineteenth century, when large and powerful businesses combined into alliances and colluded on prices, distribution, and other practices. Such collusion effectively eliminated competition among them and blocked newer companies from entering the market, which operated to the detriment of the consumer. Antitrust protections have been an area to which nurses and others have sometimes looked for relief from practices that block their full participation in the health care marketplace. Federal antitrust laws are enforced through two federal agencies, the Federal Trade Commission (FTC) and the Antitrust Division of the Department of Justice (DoJ). Individuals can also bring antitrust suits in federal court, although the cost of a private antitrust action can be extremely high. Several states have their own antitrust laws, which are generally enforced through the offices of the state attorney general and through private lawsuits in state court.

Traditionally, health professionals were largely free from antitrust scrutiny under an exemption for "learned professions." In 1975 the U.S. Supreme Court essentially eliminated that exemption (*Goldfarb v. Virginia State Bar*, 1975). Over the past three decades, antitrust laws have become significant to the health care industry. Merger activity among hospitals, insurance companies, and health systems has brought attention from antitrust enforcement agencies. In recent years, the DoJ and FTC have issued joint guidelines for antitrust enforcement in the health care industry, intended to offer general guidance on which practices are and are not likely to trigger action by these enforcement agencies

(U.S. DoJ and FTC Statement of Antitrust Enforcement Policy in Healthcare, 1996).

One case in which nurses brought an antitrust action to confront anticompetitive business practices involved a group of certified nurse midwives in Tennessee. In 1980 these nurse midwives were forced to close their newly opened family-centered nursing practice and midwifery service after meeting the concerted resistance of several Tennessee physicians, hospitals, and a prominent physician liability insurance company. Through the actions of these parties, the nurse midwives were barred from receiving hospital privileges, physician supervision, and an opportunity for collaborative practice. Nearly 9 years after closure of their practice, and following extensive litigation, the nurse midwives won settlements against some of the defendants (*Nurse Midwifery Associates v. Hibbett et al.*, 1990). In the end the Court found that several of the defendants had indeed violated antitrust laws.

On the other hand, the Minnesota Association of Nurse Anesthetists brought an antitrust action against Unity Hospital for firing its certified registered nurse anesthetists (CRNAs) after contracting with two groups of anesthesiologists. The court held that their dismissal from the hospital did not constitute a violation of the antitrust laws because an increase in competition for the same services did not prevent nurses from providing services to other hospitals (*Minnesota Association of Nurse Anesthetists v. Unity Hospital*, 1999).

Some physician groups have made "reform" of antitrust laws a policy priority and have sought at least a limited exemption for some activities by physicians that would otherwise violate antitrust laws. For instance, the American Medical Association (AMA), which has long championed antitrust exemptions for physicians, has supported congressional proposals to allow for joint negotiations by physicians with managed care organizations and other payers. The AMA has characterized "antitrust relief for self-employed physicians" as one of its "top priorities" (AMA, 2001). Such proposals pose significant concerns for nurses and other nonphysician health care providers, because they would remove an important means through which such providers can challenge anticompetitive activities by physicians.

Professional associations can also be subject to antitrust scrutiny. For example, courts have invalidated such practices as agreement by a county medical society to set fees for medical procedures (*Arizona v. Maricopa County Medical Society*, 1982). In *Wilk v. American Medical Association* (1990), the AMA was found to have violated antitrust laws for anticompetitive activities aimed toward chiropractors. The AMA had advised that physicians were guilty of unethical conduct if they referred patients to chiropractors or accepted referrals from them, since one of the AMA's ethical principles barred cooperation with "unscientific practitioners." A group of chiropractors filed suit against the AMA and prevailed in the Seventh Circuit Court of Appeals, which found that this was part of an attempt to boycott and ultimately eliminate the chiropractic profession.

## LIABILITY (TORTS, PRODUCT LIABILITY) AS A MEANS TO EFFECT SOCIAL CHANGE

Another area of the law that presents nurses with a means to effect change is the tort system. Tort law (laws through which individuals and corporations are held accountable for acts or omissions that cause injury to others) is often what nurses think of first when the subject of legal issues in nursing is raised, because professional malpractice is a particularly visible aspect of tort law. Nurses are indeed held legally accountable for their professional care and judgment (Smith-Pittman, 1998). Nurses should be aware of the provisions of their employers' malpractice insurance policies and the circumstances under which they are and are not covered. In our opinion, nurses are almost always well advised to carry their own personal liability insurance.

On a proactive note, nurses can use tort law to address problems and issues that affect them and their practice. Health care workers have, at times, successfully sued their employers for failure to take reasonable measures to protect employee health and safety. Some such suits have been for failure to provide reasonable security measures, which resulted in injury to health care workers, or failure to switch to needleless systems, resulting in nurses becoming exposed to human immunodeficiency virus or hepatitis B virus from needlesticks. The impact of such legal actions has broad implications, especially because other employers may be influenced to take measures to provide protection for employees to avoid potential future liability (General Accounting Office, 2000). The experiences of nurses and other health care workers infected with bloodborne pathogens as a result of needlesticks has also led to federal legislation addressing the issue, the Needlestick Safety and Prevention Act of 2000 (see *Needlestick Injures in the Workplace: Implications for Public Policy* following Chapter 17). This federal act directed modifications to the bloodborne pathogen standard of the Occupational Safety and Health Administration (OSHA). Since the act was signed into law, several states introduced and enacted legislation setting standards beyond what is required by the federal needlestick law.

Anti-tobacco advocates have also made much use of tort and product liability law. Through both individual lawsuits and class actions, advocates have sought to hold that industry accountable for illnesses and deaths caused by tobacco use. These legal efforts have also helped publicize important, previously undisclosed information about the tobacco industry and its practices and about the serious health effects of tobacco use, adding ammunition to both legal and political efforts to limit access to and use of tobacco. After years of important but generally unsuccessful litigation, 46 states settled a lawsuit against U.S. tobacco manufacturers, agreeing on payments to states of over $250 billion, as well as restrictions on advertising and marketing of tobacco products (Wilson, 1999; Levin & Weinstein, 1998). (See also the second Vignette in Chapter 25.)

Fast-food restaurants have become the target of lawsuits alleging their responsibility for contributing to obesity and obesity-related illness. The legal strategy behind these suits, which thus far have met with mixed success, is modeled on the approach used in suing tobacco companies—that is, that the industry has marketed products it knows cause illness and death (Heller, 2002).

## CLASS ACTION SUITS

Class action suits are another means through which advocates have sought to have an impact on health, safety, and social justice issues. Such suits seek to vindicate the rights of an entire class of individuals who share a common interest giving rise to the suit and who seek a common outcome. Such suits are brought on behalf of a large group by a smaller number of class representatives. Class action suits have been brought on behalf of recipients of silicone breast implants, of citizens of a geographic area who have suffered ill effects from the dumping of toxic wastes, of female employees of a public university system who have encountered wage discrimination, and of airline flight attendants who have been injured by second-hand smoke.

In 2005, President Bush signed into law the Class Action Fairness Act, which will move many class action suits into federal court that previously would have been heard in state courts (Wilson, 2005). This law was supported by defense attorneys and opposed by plaintiff's attorneys because federal requirements for class-action suits are often more stringent than those of state courts.

## CHALLENGING INAPPROPRIATE GOVERNMENT ACTION

The U.S. Constitution and state constitutions offer citizens and residents a number of protections, including protection from unreasonable government action in a number of areas. For instance, the government cannot take an individual's property or liberty without due process. Individuals are free from unreasonable searches and seizures. All individuals are guaranteed equal protection under the law. These guarantees have been made more specific as they apply to the actions of government agencies through a federal Administrative Procedures Act and similar acts at the state level that define the processes for and restrictions on administrative action. In addition, administrative agencies are generally limited to acting within the parameters set for them by legislation. Once an individual is granted a license to practice a profession such as nursing, she is considered to hold a property interest in that license, which therefore cannot be taken away without due process following established legal procedures.

Together, these protections provide a basis for challenging action by a government agency that an individual or group believes or alleges to be inappropriate or unreasonable. In 2005, California's Department of Health Services sought to delay implementation of a regulatory requirement that hospitals in medical-surgical units ensure that each nurse care for no more than five patients at a time. This requirement was part of a package of regulations that had been adopted by the Department under the state's previous administration; those regulations provided for an initial staffing ratio in medical-surgical units of 1:6, and set a date of January 1, 2005, to move to a more stringent 1:5 requirement (see *California Nurse Staffing Ratios* following Chapter 18). Under new leadership, the Department issued an emergency regulation to delay implementation until January 1, 2008. California law allows a state agency to issue emergency regulations (which go into effect without a public hearing) when necessary for the immediate preservation of public health and safety. A nurses' union sued to stop the delay. A Superior Court judge granted their request, finding that the Department had failed to follow required procedures for changing state regulations and that it had not demonstrated that the delay was needed for the immediate preservation of public health and safety (*California Nurses Association v. Schwarzenegger et al.,* 2005).

## ACTING "DEFENSIVELY"

Although court decisions can have a positive effect on issues that concern nurses and other health care advocates, they can also have an adverse impact. Nursing is sometimes faced with trying to react to, address, and mitigate the impact of a negative court decision. A recent example of this is action by the U.S. Supreme Court regarding the applicability of the National Labor Relations Act to nurses. That act provides employees, including nurses, with a number of protections, including the right to engage in concerted action regarding wages, hours, and working conditions, to organize unions, and to bargain collectively with their employers. Some employers have argued that nurses, because they direct the work of other employees, are "supervisors" and are therefore not covered by the act. In *NLRB v. Health Care and Retirement Corp.* (1994), the Supreme Court invalidated the rationale that the National Labor Relations Board (NLRB) had previously been using to find that nurses were not "supervisors." (The NLRB had argued that nurses direct the work of

other staff, such as licensed practical nurses and nursing assistants, in the interests of patient care, and not "in the interests of the employer.")

The decision understandably caused a great deal of concern among nurses because it eliminated the reasoning by which the NLRB had found most nurses to be eligible for collective bargaining. Because supervisors (as defined by the National Labor Relations Act) do not have the right to bargain collectively, the potential implications of the decision jeopardized the collective bargaining rights of many, if not most, registered nurses (RNs).

Following that decision, however, the ANA and nurses' unions worked to mitigate its impact. For example, ANA challenged employers' efforts to claim that large numbers of nurses are ineligible for collective bargaining and has supported the NLRB in its decision to find alternative approaches to ruling that directing the work of others in providing patient care does not make RNs ineligible for collective bargaining. In 2001 the U.S. Supreme Court revisited the issue of nurses as supervisors as presented in *NLRB v. Kentucky River Community Care.* This decision rejected the NLRB's argument that, in directing the work of others, nurses do not exercise "independent judgment" as used in the National Labor Relations Act to (in part) define "supervisors" (see Chapter 20). The issue remains a source of concern for nursing unions and professional associations.

## ROLE OF *AMICUS CURIAE*

*Amicus curiae,* or "friend of the court," briefs provide an important tool for advocacy groups to make their views known on a case with broad implications even when they are not parties to that case. An *amicus curiae* brief is filed (with the court's permission) by a group with an interest in the case in order to advise the court on how it should rule. Generally, the brief offers the court a group's unique knowledge of and perspective on the issue brought before it.

Nursing has used this avenue to make its perspectives heard in appellate-level federal and state cases throughout the country. In *NLRB v. Health and Retirement Corp.* and *NLRB v. Kentucky River,* discussed previously, the ANA filed *amicus* briefs with the U.S. Supreme Court in order to offer its unique perspective as the nation's largest professional and labor organization for RNs in explaining why direction and oversight of ancillary personnel is an integral aspect of nursing practice and not a "supervisory" function. The ANA joined with the AMA and other nursing and physician groups to offer the perspective of health care providers regarding physician-assisted suicide by filing joint *amicus curiae* briefs in *Washington v. Glucksberg* and *Vacco v. Quill*. The ANA has also made its voice heard in cases regarding appropriate bargaining units for hospital employees; the right of publicly employed nurses to speak out on the job regarding safe patient care; and the right of Medicare recipients enrolled in health maintenance organizations (HMOs) to receive adequate services and procedural protections (*Grijalva et al. v. Shalala*, 1996). The ANA has also addressed criminal prosecution of pregnant women for drug or alcohol abuse (*Whitner v. South Carolina*, 1996) and the issue of what constitutes a "serious health condition" under the Family and Medical Leave Act (FMLA) (*Victorelli v. Shadyside Hospital*, 1997). The *amicus curiae* brief is a particularly useful and attractive option for nurses to use in speaking out on important legal issues that affect the profession or policy issues for which the profession has important substantive concerns, but where nurses are not party to the action itself.

## ADVOCATING EXPANSION OF LEGAL RIGHTS THROUGH LEGISLATION

Because Congress and the state legislatures are sources of federal and state law, respectively, legislative authority provides the foundation for future legal action. In other words, laws passed at the federal or state level often create legally enforceable rights or remedies that can be legally enforced through the courts. The Americans with Disabilities Act (ADA) provides for equal treatment for disabled Americans and bars discrimination in a number of areas, including employment and public accommodations. For example, a person with a disability who is able to perform the essential aspects of a job with reasonable accommodation cannot be fired or denied a promotion on the basis of her or his disability.

Although many would argue that the ADA merely applies principles of equality and fair play that are basic to American law and public life, it also creates specific enforceable rights. Similarly, the FMLA grants specific rights for employees to take unpaid leave under certain circumstances in order to receive or provide care to a family member. The FMLA, signed into law by President Clinton after previously being vetoed by the first President Bush, was strongly supported by the ANA. The act defines a number of new and important parameters for families' rights.

In 1996, New York nurses developed and supported state legislation to grant professional licensing boards the power to seek judicial interventions to prevent the unauthorized practice of a profession. Under this proposed legislation, the board of nursing would have been able to seek to stop the use of UAPs to perform functions reserved to RNs, because this could constitute practicing nursing without a license. This legislation would have given nurses a significant tool to use in preventing the dangerous, inappropriate use of UAPs by health care institutions. Unfortunately, New York governor George Pataki vetoed the bill passed by the state legislature.

In 1996, the Health Insurance Portability and Accountability Act (HIPAA) was enacted. HIPAA is federal legislation that addressed two major issues. It created requirements and standards under which employees may be able to change jobs without losing health care coverage. In addition, HIPAA called for national protections for the privacy of individual health information, especially electronic records. The Centers for Medicare and Medicaid Services (CMS) approved regulations implementing this aspect of HIPAA in 2002. They provide basic standards for all individuals who seek and receive health care and provide a legal remedy to the individual when his or her private health information is not appropriately safeguarded. HIPAA violations may result in consequences that include fines and prison terms. Certainly HIPAA implementation has dramatically altered the collection, storage, transfer, and use of all patient health information, with both intended and unintended consequences in the health care arena.

# PROMOTING NURSING'S POLICY AGENDA

Health care is experiencing rapid and chaotic change in which the rules of the game are being developed more in closed corporate board rooms than in the halls and auditoriums of public policy assemblies. Therefore nursing needs a greater range of effective strategies to achieve its preferred outcomes. Organized nursing must become comfortable, proficient, and well prepared to be successful in all policy arenas and at all levels of government.

## *Key Points*

■ Understanding litigation as an effective strategic option, enhanced risk-taking skills, and sufficient resource building for litigation must be developed by organized nursing on a proactive basis.

■ This is particularly important at the state level, where significant issues arise that often have far-reaching implications for nursing and health care consumers.

■ Organized nursing, at the national, state, and local levels, must prepare nurses to evaluate issues and opportunities to promote health and social policy though the judicial system.

## *Web Resources*

**American Association of Nurse Attorneys**
*www.taana.org*
**American Bar Association, Section on Health Law**
*www.abanet.org/health/home.html*
**American Health Lawyers Association**
*www.healthlawyers.org*
**American Society of Law, Medicine and Ethics**
*www.aslme.org*
**FindLaw**
*www.findlaw.com*
**National Health Law Program**
*www.healthlaw.org*

## REFERENCES

*Alabama Nurses Association, Alabama State Board of Nursing, et al. v. Samuelson and the Alabama State Department of Public Health,* Case Nos. CV-92-2275 and CV-92-2477 (1992). 20 Am. Jur. 2d Courts § 147, 2004.

American Medical Association (AMA). (2001). Antitrust relief needed for physicians. Retrieved July 7, 2005, from *www. ama-assn.org/ama/pub/article/4030-3979.html.*

Americans with Disabilities Act of 1990, P.L. 101-336, 42 U.S.C.. § 12101 et. seq.

*Arizona v. Maricopa County Medical Society.* 457 U.S. 332 (1982).

Breyer, S. Concurring opinion in *Washington v. Glucksberg,* 521 U.S. 793 (1997).

*Brown v. Board of Education,* 347 U.S. 483 (1954).

*California Nurses Association v. Schwarzenegger et al.,* Case No. 04CS01725 (2005).

Class Action Fairness Act of 2005, Pub. L. No. 109-2, 119 Stat. 4, Sec. 2(a)(2)(A).

Collins, S. (1999). Rethinking the Patient Self Determination Act: Implementation without effectiveness. *Journal of Nursing Law,* 6(3), 29-46.

*Cruzan v. Missouri Department of Health,* 497 U.S. 261 (1990).

General Accounting Office. (2000). *Occupational safety: Selected cost and benefit implications of needlestick devices for hospitals.* GAO-01-60R. Accessed July 7, 2005, at *www.gao.gov/new.items/ d0160r.pdf.*

*Goldfarb v. Virginia State Bar,* 420 U.S. 905 (1975).

*Grijalva et al. v. Shalala,* 966 F. Supp. 747 (D. Ariz. 1996).

Heller, E. (2002, November 11). 'Fat suit' weighs in. *National Law Journal.* Retrieved July 7, 2005, from *www.law.com/servlet/ ContentServer?pagename=OpenMarket/Xcelerate/View&c=Law Article&cid=1039054412904&live=true&cst=1&pc=0&pa=0).*

Johnson, K. R. (1999). Lawyering for social change: What's a lawyer to do? *Michigan Journal of Race & Law,* 5, 201.

Levin, M., & Weinstein, H. (1998, November 28). Last of 46 state officials sign tobacco accord. *Los Angeles Times,* A1.

*Marbury v. Madison,* 5 U.S. 137 (1803).

*Minnesota Association of Nurse Anesthetists v. Unity Hospital.* 208 F. 3d 655 (8th Cir. 1999).

*NLRB v. Health Care and Retirement Corp,* 511 U.S. 571 (1994).

*NLRB v. Kentucky River Community Care,* 532 U.S. 706 (2001).

*Nurse Midwifery Associates v. Hibbett et al.,* 918 F. 2d 605 (6th Cir. 1990).

Parmet, W. (1999). Tobacco, HIV and the courts: The role of affirmative litigation in the formation of health policy. *Houston Law Review,* 36, 1663.

Patient Self-Determination Act of 1990, P.L. 101-508, §§ 4206 and 4571, 42 USC § 1395 et seq.

*People v. Jack Kevorkian,* 248 Mich. App. 373, 639 NW2d 291 (2001).

*Roe v. Wade,* 410 U.S. 113 (1973).

*Schiavo ex rel. Schindler v. Schiavo,* 403 F.3d 1223 (11th Cir. 2005).

Smith-Pittman, M. (1998) Nurses and litigation: 1990-1997. *Journal of Nursing Law,* 5(2), 7-20.

U.S. Department of Justice (DoJ) and Federal Trade Commission (FTC). (1996). Statement of antitrust enforcement policy in healthcare. Retrieved July 7, 2005, from *www.usdoj.gov/atr/ public/guidelines/0000.htm.*

*Vacco v. Quill.* 521 U.S. 702 (1997).

*Victorelli v. Shadyside Hospital,* 128 F. 3d 184 (3rd Cir. 1997).

Want, R. (Ed.). (1997). *Federal-state court directory*. New York: Want Publishing.

Washington v. Glucksberg, 521 U.S. 793 (1997).

*Whitner v. South Carolina*, 492 SE 2d 777 (SC 1997).

*Wilk v. American Medical Association*, F. 2d 352 (7th Cir. 1990; *cert. denied*, 498 US 982) (1990).

Wilson, H. (2005). Will tort reform cure the courts? *MarketWatch*. Retrieved July 7, 2005, from *www.cbs.marketwatch.com*.

Wilson, J. J. (1999). Summary of the Attorneys General Tobacco Settlement Agreement. Retrieved June 1, 2006, from *http://academic.udayton.edu/health/syllabi/tobacco/summary.htm*.

# chapter 29

# Contemporary Issues in Nursing Organizations

Katherine Kany

*"Turning and turning in the widening gyre, the falcon cannot hear the falconer; things fall apart; the center cannot hold…"*

WILLIAM BUTLER YEATS

An e-mail composed by the nurse after a long and arduous shift outlines a range of problems and an air of hopelessness about the work environment and practice issues she faces. She wants to take care of patients, but she can barely manage another shift. She wants to know what you—representing the professional organization—can do to help her now.

*An e-mail from another nurse arrives, full of anger about the issues facing health care consumers and health care providers, followed by finger pointing and harsh criticism toward organizations, such as yours, that haven't alleviated the problems.*

*A frightened nurse calls to tell you of the horrific staffing and overtime issues in her hospital. She tells you that patients have unmet needs, or worse, and that the facility needs to be reported to the appropriate regulatory agency. Can you explain how this gets accomplished? Will she be identified as the "whistleblower"? Can your organization do the reporting, or come in and investigate?*

*A letter from a longtime member questions the organization about what it is doing about the uninsured in the state, noting that there is no nurse on the new commission appointed by the governor to make recommendations for remedying the problem.*

For 17 years I have worked on behalf of fellow nurses and their workplace and professional priorities. Seven of those years were spent in the health care division of the American Federation of Teachers (AFT), and the ten remaining years at the American Nurses Association (ANA), split between the Departments of Labor Relations and Workplace Advocacy and the Department of Nursing Practice and Research.

Anyone who has ever worked for a membership organization will tell you that there are some people who will never be satisfied with the efforts made on their behalf, others who will always question what they are receiving in return for what they give in annual membership dues, and still others who are unaware of the organization's work. Holding organizations accountable to members is reasonable and appropriate. Misrepresenting what an organization can or does provide for a member is not.

National nursing organizations (and their state affiliates) vary in size and resources—factors that can significantly affect how they are perceived and whether or not they are invited to participate in meetings and committees convened to discuss issues and propose changes in local, state, and national policies. Presence in these other public and private sector arenas is critical if nursing wants to influence decisions and shape public policies that will improve the environment for care and increase reporting and accountability for the safety and quality of care delivered.

Generally, seats at these tables are limited, and competition for which organization, union, or specialty group representing nurses is invited to participate or testify can be stiff. The lack of unity within the profession, and the disparity of resources and expertise among the various organizations and affiliates, have resulted in a spotty presence at policy discussions and a fragmented approach to addressing problems facing the profession and nursing practice—a fact that is particularly important at this time.

A term currently used to describe the state of affairs for the nursing profession is "crisis." We see that idiom in the titles and bodies of reports and read it in newspapers. What do nurses, or people, do in times of crisis? Generally people seek out individuals or organizations that seem most appropriate to resolve their dilemmas, whether or not they would normally use those resources or support organizations that provide them. The needs of the nursing workforce at this point in the profession's existence require strong, collaborative, proactive, politically savvy nursing organizations to provide the venue for collective vision and action on a variety of issues. But are nursing organizations meeting this mandate?

## THE CRISIS IN NURSING

For the past 10 years in particular, a range of professional and workplace issues have driven nurses to the doors of professional associations begging for solutions. At first, early in the 1990s, the drive within the health care industry to redesign, reorganize, and restructure care delivery in an effort to contain health care costs prompted an enormous reaction and response from nurses. Calls to nursing organizations came from staff nurses and unit managers, and sometimes from nurse executives, extremely concerned about patient safety. With the calls came requests for any minimum safe staffing guidelines, position statements, or research that could be used to oppose reducing the use of RNs and replacing them with unlicensed and minimally trained assistive personnel.

As RN staffing reductions (under the euphemisms of "downsizing" and "reengineering") were implemented essentially unimpeded, fears about patient safety were realized and later captured in the 1999 seminal report of the Institute of Medicine (IOM), *To Err Is Human: Building a Safer Health System.* Shortly thereafter, nursing was placed under the microscope as the cause of the majority of errors in the three-part series in the *Chicago Tribune* in September 2000 that led with the first article, "Nursing Mistakes Kill, Injure Thousands: Cost-Cutting Exacts Toll On Patients, Hospital Staffs." Nurses were again asking for help in identifying appropriate numbers and mix of direct care staff. Others sought advice for reporting facilities for unsafe practices.

As the century turned and RN vacancies in hospitals went unfilled, hospitals moved to extended hours of work and the use of mandatory overtime to fill the staffing gaps. Nurses were overwhelmed and incredulous that what was being asked or required of them essentially further compromised the safety of patients and their own safety. Equally frustrating for them was the realization that, unlike other industries and professions, no limits existed on hours of work for health care providers (except for interns and residents). As nurses opposed these strategies for filling staffing gaps, the final insult came. Managers threatened to report RNs who refused to stay—or even to come to work—with patient abandonment, exacerbating the gulf and animosity between staff nurses and nurse managers.

Some of these issues are so critical that nurses said they would leave acute care environments because of professional frustration and despair over the safety and quality of care delivered and threats to their own safety and well-being (Cornerstone Communications Group, 2001). Nurses also said they would leave the profession prematurely because of burnout and difficult working conditions (Aiken, 2002).

Given the mounting severity of both the future shortage of nurses and the burnout and dissatisfaction among today's working nurses, one would expect professional associations to be thriving and flourishing, harnessing and channeling nurses' anxiety into a major political force. Have nurses' requests for help been answered? Are professional associations thriving? Can professional associations meet the needs of the profession in general or the professionals in particular? Or should nurses look elsewhere to resolve the surplus of problems that threaten their physical and emotional well-being, their livelihood, and their future?

## A TIME FOR COLLECTIVE ACTION

Committees and task forces have been convened within and among nursing and other organizations to study practice and workplace concerns confronting the profession that are contributing to the shortage. Chief among those assembling groups to study the issues and find solutions are the American Hospital Association (AHA), the ANA, the IOM, and the Joint Commission on Accreditation of Healthcare Organizations (JCAHO). Also included in this group is a report developed for the Robert Wood Johnson Foundation by Bobbi Kimball, RN, MBA, and Edward O'Neil, PhD, MPA, entitled *Health Care's Human Crisis: The American Nursing Shortage.*

Contained in and across these reports is consensus that many complex and interrelated issues need to be addressed in order to stem the nurse staffing crisis and to meet the exponential growth of consumer need and demand for nursing care. Uppermost among the issues identified are the following:

- Insufficient and/or inappropriate staffing
- Overtime and extended hours of work and implications for patient safety
- Occupational safety and health
- Limited professional autonomy
- Exclusion from essential decision-making affecting nursing practice and outcomes of care

Associations can and do work to shape public policies that affect these issues, as well as the safety and quality of care, accessibility and affordability of health care, RN scope of practice concerns, reimbursement for advanced practice nurses (APNs), and funding streams to support nursing education. With the nursing shortage on the national agenda, now is the time for nursing organizations to act. There is now public acknowledgement of the policies and practices that exclude nursing from its appropriate place in decision-making arenas and diminish its value (AHA, 2002; ANA, 2002; JCAHO, 2002; Kimball & O'Neil, 2002; Page, 2003).

These acknowledgments get to the heart of the value, power, and image issues that have beleaguered the profession. Included among the recommendations from the many reports on the nursing shortage are proposals that would increase the autonomy and authority of the profession. For example, the AHA (2002) report organizes its recommendations into five strategic actions. Two in particular hold great potential for positive changes for nurses from the bedsides to the boardrooms if used by nursing associations and unions:

- *Foster meaningful work* by transforming hospitals into modern organizations in which all aspects of the work are designed around patients and the needs of staff to care for and support them. Workers must find meaning in their work and be supported in their efforts to provide high-quality care.
- *Improve the workplace partnership* by creating a culture in which hospital staff—including clinical, support, and managerial staff—are valued, have a sustained voice in shaping institutional policies, and receive appropriate rewards ad recognition for their efforts.

With this public recognition of the need for action, the issue becomes whether nursing organizations have the will, resources, and expertise to act.

## ASSOCIATION STABILITY AND ABILITY TO MEET MEMBER NEEDS

There are over 100 discrete nursing and nursing specialty organizations or nursing divisions within broader-based associations such as the American Heart Association's Council on Cardiovascular Nursing and the American Public Health Association's Public Health Nursing Section. Only about 20% of the nation's 2.5 million registered nurses belong to one or more of these professional organizations.

The viability of so many niche organizations suggests they do meet special needs, or that at least members perceive that their distinctive issues are being addressed. No matter the similarities, nurses often distinguish what makes their situation unique and appreciate customized solutions—preferably those developed in similar units, settings, and specialties. Despite that, would it be better to have one or two large, multispecialty or umbrella nursing organizations so that they can use their cumulative power to meet member priorities and fight the large battles? Can ANA or any umbrella organization meet the needs and expectations of nurses? Perhaps the most telling measure of customer satisfaction can be found by looking at membership trends.

## EXAMPLE OF A NEW NURSING ORGANIZATION

As a relatively new organization, the Hospice and Palliative Nurses Association (HPNA) grew by 285%, with membership at 2800 in 2000 and 8000 in July 2005 (D. Butcher, personal communication, 1 August 2005). According to Deena Butcher, Director of Membership for HPNA, this phenomenal growth is attributed to the association's commitment to identifying and meeting member needs and providing opportunities for members' involvement. HPNA is somewhat unique in that it has opened its membership to include Licensed Practical and Vocational Nurses (LPNs), as well as Nursing Assistants (NAs), in addition to the RN and APN members. LPN and NA membership within HPNA totals 500 and 1000, respectively. Ms. Butcher also points out that HPNA's sister organization, the National Board for Certification of Hospice and Palliative Nurses (NBCHPN), is the only nursing specialty group to offer certification to all categories of nursing care providers.

## THE OLDEST NURSING ORGANIZATION

Over the same time period, membership in the ANA has dropped by close to 8000 nurses from almost 158,000 in 2000 to slightly over 150,000, or 6% of the nation's registered nurses, in 2005. The ANA has a broad mandate to advocate for the profession and nurses, regardless of their specialty, and sells itself on its size and ability to represent the diverse perspectives of all areas of nursing practice; its ability to provide considerable resources because of a large member and revenue base; and a voice that speaks for the profession. And yet, it has sustained an overall loss of over 54,000 nurses since its peak in 1994 when its membership was approaching 206,000.

Who has left the organization? The vast majority of ANA's loss consists of organized staff nurses. Included in the lost members are the collective bargaining arms of the California Nurses Association (CAN), the Massachusetts Nurses Association, the Pennsylvania Nurses Association, and the Maine Nurses Association. These nurses wanted a more radical advocate with stronger positions and actions against untested, cost-driven changes that compromised care. Those demands, however, tested the intentions of state associations and a national organization attempting to meet the divergent needs of staff nurses versus administrators, faculty, and APNs. And the responses were reflective of elected leadership not comfortable with aggressive policies that felt more like a union and less like a professional association.

A range of realities within the ANA has resulted in ongoing tensions and distrust among its nurse members. Disparities among member interests and priorities led to the collective bargaining membership's being contained within the United American Nurses (UAN), a separate but affiliated entity with its own budget, its own legislative agenda, and an AFL-CIO affiliation. ANA's union members voted in 1999 to form the UAN in order to gain more control over the resources that result from their dues dollars; ensure insulation of collective bargaining from management representatives who may sit on the ANA board and oversee budget and finances of the organization; and provide the autonomy to shape federal legislation that addresses staff nurse priorities and labor issues. For some nurses, collective bargaining is a "blue-collar" approach to resolving workplace concerns—it's "unprofessional." To others, it's the only recourse for protected collective work to make the changes that many workplaces desperately need in order to create nurse-friendly, safe environments.

Among the primary struggles between the collective bargaining and noncollective bargaining sectors of ANA have been the allocation of resources to labor relations programs within ANA and the need to maintain confidentiality (or insulation) regarding the specific use of these monies for organizing activities, particularly when some of the campaigns would occur in the facilities employing members of the ANA board of directors.

Membership makeup on the national and state boards of directors within ANA is another sore point among members. Traditionally the boards of directors have been largely composed of educators and administrators—constituent groups that do not represent the majority of ANA members, but who determine policy priorities and resource allocation that very much affect the staff nurses who are the majority of the association. Except for one seat allocated to a staff nurse representative, board seats are not tied to state associations or specific constituencies within ANA—a factor that potentially limits representation of any category of member and may reduce accountability on the part of board members.

Another major problem among the membership is the rivalry about who is getting more resources from the parent organization—collective bargaining, represented by the UAN, or workplace advocacy, represented by the Center for American Nurses (CAN), a coalition of ANA's state nurses associations that do not participate in collective bargaining. Fueling this fire are confused or incorrect notions about how the work, products, and resources of ANA are attributed to these two entities. As a result, several ANA products have had to be duplicated and customized for collective bargaining and non-collective bargaining members so that words such as "collective bargaining," "contract," and "organized nurses" do not appear universally. Also of political importance is the fact that ANA has been compelled to provide both groups with equal time in ANA publications and communications. Although the UAN and collective bargaining strategies are geared to nurses working as a group to accomplish changes in the workplace, the CAN philosophy is to provide "tools, services and strategies designed to make nurses their own best advocates in their practice environments" *(www.nursingworld.org/can)*. But sometimes the distinctions between the two entities override their common goal of serving the needs of nurses, the profession, and patients.

Perhaps the most significant blow to ANA's viability began with the 1995 disaffiliation of the collective bargaining members in CNA. CNA has worked across the continental United States and in Hawaii to fracture ANA's constituent member associations and fuel the frustration and dissatisfaction sometimes felt among the members. CNA actively supported the disaffiliation of the collective bargaining members in Massachusetts and Maine in 2001 but lost in Hawaii in 2004. CNA successfully preyed on the large and vulnerable Cook County Hospital bargaining unit in Illinois. The organization travels around, setting up workshops to convince organized nurses to disaffiliate from the UAN and join CNA—activity that further weakens the ANA and UAN state affiliates and siphons CNA member money and resources that could be applied to new organizing activities rather than destroying what currently exists. Not only does the work of CNA undermine existing UAN bargaining units, it makes those units more vulnerable to union-busting actions on the part of employers. All in all, there are many factors inside and outside the organization which continue to destabilize membership and further weaken the voice of the one organization that could potentially represent the overarching priorities of the nursing profession.

Why are niche organizations maintaining and increasing membership while the largest nursing organization withers on the vine? One could speculate that a primary difference is that specialty organizations do not provide services related to collective bargaining. Their focus is to set standards and provide support for professional practice. ANA has tried to do both. But the political reality is that ANA is unable to fully embrace the priorities and needs of collective bargaining nurses without offending the sensibilities of those members in management, academia, and entrepreneurial ventures and those staff nurses who do not see the role collective bargaining can play in enhancing professional practice.

The philosophical differences and ethical dilemmas nurses experience with regard to collective bargaining are enormous (Williams, 2004). Not only do these political differences play out within the organization, they often affect ANA's ability to relate to the other nursing associations as well. For instance, in planning for Nursing's Agenda for the Future (NAF), a national initiative to bring nursing together to develop a unified plan to address nurse staffing and patient safety issues, several of the nursing organizations argued to exclude all unions from the invitation list. ANA prevailed in this situation, but concerns about the strategies that might be forthcoming from these nurses during the meeting kept many of those managing small group sessions on guard.

Can professional nursing associations work effectively to address the myriad needs of the profession? Yes and no. If the needs relate specifically to nursing practice, then specialty organizations are well equipped to provide the expert tools and resources that their members desire. If the needs go beyond that to include effecting dramatic changes in policies and practices that affect care delivery, the likelihood diminishes significantly because that involves a true collective voice for the profession in order to be taken seriously in legislative arenas.

## POLITICS AND PROFESSIONAL INITIATIVES

In the past, there have been issues bigger than specialty or setting that have drawn nurses together for swift and effective action. Most successful of all was the nursing community's' rapid and effective quashing of the very short-lived 1987 proposal of the American Medical Association (AMA) to create a new health care provider called the *Registered Care Technologist* (RCT), who would function under the physician's license to supplement the insufficient supply of registered nurses. Nursing organizations swiftly pulled together to educate the public and policymakers that this plan would further burden the RNs working in direct care settings by making them responsible to oversee the work of minimally trained providers (RCTs) without the authority for such oversight, increasing their workload and jeopardizing safe, coordinated patient care. As a result, plans to move forward with this proposal were dropped.

Nursing organizations also strongly united around priorities for cost-effective, accessible, high-quality health care in the tumultuous days of health care reform activities during the first Clinton administration. Convened by ANA, nursing associations met and developed and signed onto a plan to address the profession's concerns, a plan that still

exists today: Nursing's Agenda for Healthcare Reform (ANA, 1992). Although Clinton's attempt to reform health care through the Health Security Act failed, nursing organizations worked together then, and still, around the principles developed over a decade ago.

## NURSING'S AGENDA FOR THE FUTURE

In late 2000, keenly aware of the crisis confronting nursing, the ANA began work on a plan to convene the profession to craft its own plan to address nurse staffing and quality of care issues. By early 2001, ANA secured funding to underwrite a major portion of the cost of bringing the nursing community under one roof to deliberate on a course of action that would come from nursing's own vision for itself and its future and that would preempt others who would attempt to determine their own plan for nursing.

The September 2001 "Call to the Nursing Profession" summit was a meeting attended by representatives of 60 of the 100 national specialty nursing organizations and unions invited. The summary report of the summit identified nursing's priorities and a complex plan and implementation strategy to accomplish its vision for the profession: *Nursing's Agenda for the Future: A Call to the Nation* (ANA, 2002). The anticipation at the close of the nursing summit meeting was that in the year 2020, when interviewed about its current state, nursing could say the following about the profession:

- Nursing is the pivotal health care profession, highly valued for its specialized knowledge, skill, and caring in improving the health status of the public and ensuring safe, effective, high-quality care.
- The profession mirrors the diverse population it serves and provides leadership to create positive changes in health policy and delivery systems. Individuals choose nursing as a career, and remain in the profession, because of the opportunities for personal and professional growth, supportive work environments, and compensation commensurate with roles and responsibilities (ANA, 2002).

Although the final plan is admirable, the struggles to move from initial concept to steering committee to summit meeting were *enormous* and revolved around political turmoil between and among some of the organizations on the steering committee and lack of consensus about the real issues confronting nurses in the trenches; a reluctance to call the nursing situation a "crisis"; and an initial reluctance by some of the steering committee organizations to include nurses representing unions in the deliberations. Rather than publicize the meeting and the discussions that took place during the 5-day summit, several nursing organizations insisted that any and all observers be banned for fear that some might see the nursing factions within the community and report that nursing "did not have its act together."

In the end, although many organizations signed on to accomplish work to move the profession forward to accomplish its agenda, the realities became clear. The majority of those interested in participating in the implementation process lacked human and financial resources to accomplish the work outlined. The work to develop and fund a proposal that would provide the participating nursing organizations with grant monies became bogged down in a mind-numbing bureaucratic process that couldn't even finalize a concept paper as of late 2004. And the momentum that began in 2001 had essentially died on the vine at a time when the other national reports from JCAHO, AHA, IOM, and others could have been used to further support the priorities that nursing had identified in its own report, *Nursing's Agenda for the Future*.

## A COALITION OF NATIONAL NURSING ORGANIZATIONS

In late 2001, two coalitions of national nursing organizations merged: the National Federation of Specialty Nursing Organizations (NFSNO), a coalition of nursing organizations founded in 1973, and the Nursing Organizations Liaison Forum (NOLF), a corresponding coalition of specialty organizations established by ANA in 1982. Called the "Nursing Organizations Alliance," or more simply "the Alliance," the group encompasses over 65 organizational members representing 305,000 registered nurses working in administration, research, education, and clinical practice. The Alliance describes its mission as follows: "to increase nursing's visibility and impact on health through communication, collaboration and advocacy." When the Alliance

was formed, Ann Manton, RN, PhD, the immediate past co-chair of NOLF, said "Nursing leaders believe there's strength in numbers, and the Alliance will be able to use the power of the collective membership of its member organizations to make a difference in the lives of nurses and their patients across the nation" (Nursing Organization Alliance, 2001).

As the first coordinator to lead the brand new Alliance, Patricia Seifert, RN, MSN, CRNFA, FAAN, espoused that its mission would be "to increase nursing's visibility through communication, collaboration, and advocacy by supporting and strengthening the individual organizations." Would that collaboration and advocacy include addressing the needs of a profession in crisis through joint legislative priorities or initiatives? According to Seifert, the Alliance believed that the ANA was the "leader in legislative activity." Instead, the Alliance members wanted to focus on building the current and future potential of their member associations. Among the challenges Seifert identified was "identifying the role of the professional organization as it relates to attracting new members, increasing or redesigning the 'value' of membership, and offering services that would benefit members—organizations and individuals" (P. Seifert, personal communication, June 27, 2005).

Will the Alliance use its collective size and voice to eventually tackle the issues that make for the current crisis? Seifert believes that it "would be a logical progression or evolutionary drive to consider issues such as staffing, overtime, etc.," but believes that "Alliance organizations increasingly will address these issues as they relate to individual members' satisfaction with their professional organization." In the meantime, nurses await signs of leadership from the profession's myriad nursing organizations in providing a collective voice and action to ensure the future of nursing.

## ROLE OF COLLECTIVE BARGAINING

Nursing associations struggle alone or in coalitions to craft legislative language and then lobby for years to promote passage of bills that would address nursing priorities such as safe staffing levels, elimination of mandatory overtime, protections involving health and safety issues, and patient safety priorities.

At the same time, nurses in collective bargaining units are negotiating, implementing, and enforcing contracts to address those same issues, in addition to working on state and federal bills to do the same. Although some nurses fear that pressing for legislative and regulatory approaches to maintaining minimal staffing levels means locking in numbers that may need to change down the road and are afraid to move forward, organized nurses believe they can work to finetune or improve laws and regulations through their contract.

Nurses have effectively used collective bargaining agreements to improve and protect the safety and quality of care they provide (Budd, Warino, & Patton, 2004). Nurses have made incredibly difficult decisions to go on strike over these issues. Whereas some see this as the ultimate unprofessional act, the nurses who vote to do so are risking employment, income, and benefits to make certain they can provide safe, high-quality care for their patients. To many, this is the ultimate in professionalism—putting personal needs aside in order to care for patients.

Nurses working under collective bargaining agreements have negotiated powerful language that addresses the professional concerns outlined at the beginning of this discussion. For example, nurses have:

- Developed contract provisions that allow them to close care units when staffing is insufficient
- Negotiated the right to include review of nursing-sensitive patient outcome data in comparison with the number and mix of nursing staff, as part of the work undertaken in joint labor and management committees that review safety, quality, and staffing issues
- Been successful in negotiating the right to participate in the selection of a patient classification system that will be the determining factor for nurse staffing levels
- Won contract language that allows them the right to refuse overtime work or "floating" to other units to which they have not been oriented
- Bargained language that provides them—and all staff—with safe needle devices, appropriate gloves and masks, and equipment and training to address ergonomic issues

The collective bargaining agreement struck between nurses and their employers is a legally enforceable document that gives nurses both a voice for professional priorities and recourse when the contract is violated. Contracts are often unique to the nurses, the patient population, and the facilities where they are negotiated. Because of the nature of these agreements, nurses also have an opportunity to renegotiate and strengthen these agreements every 3 to 5 years (or whenever the contracts expire)—an option not usually available through legislative approaches. As a result, nurses and other health professionals are turning to unions to meet their professional needs and to maintain more control over their workplace issues. Can any professional organization provide this level of control to its members?

## REALITY CHECK

Can and do professional associations accomplish what nursing needs to survive? It seems as though nurses are finding some or much of what they need from their specialty associations. However, the need for major changes within the health care industry and powerful legislation that addresses issues related to the safety of patients, for example, is largely not being met—with a few exceptions, such as vigorous opposition to any use of mandatory overtime except in times of crisis. Specialty organizations have been successful in legislative initiatives specific to their area of interest. Chapter 31 provides rich examples of how some of these organizations have influenced public policies through politically astute action.

Although the efforts for changes in national, state, and local policies must continue, nursing is not speaking with one voice about what the changes should be. The more diverse the membership within an organization, or the larger the coalition organized around an issue, the less likely consensus can be achieved and progress can be made. A better approach may be for nursing to work hard on building consensus on major issues but agree to go in separate directions on issues on which there is significant disagreement or to shift attention to resolving an issue to the local or organizational level.

Clearly, specialty groups are sustaining, and in some cases increasing, membership. The profession needs organizations that will develop practice standards; develop and promote research priorities; and translate research into practice. Organizations promising to meet the needs of all nurses and to be a powerful voice for all of nursing have misunderstood or misrepresented what can realistically be accomplished. As long as nursing remains fractured about what it means to be a professional nurse as well as what is right for nurses and for public policy, nursing organizations will better serve their members by providing services that meet very specific practice needs, allowing nurses to decide the best course of action for the delivery of safe, high-quality care, and acting locally through grassroots coalitions or collective bargaining agreements to see that those priorities are accomplished.

One wonders what the future holds for associations like ANA that have lost 26% of their membership during the critical years when nurses are desperately seeking help. Should nursing associations remain specialized and narrow their scope? Should nurses rethink the value of collective bargaining and what they can accomplish with powerful and cutting-edge contract language? What will stimulate nurses to join nursing organizations? The answers to these questions are difficult to know, but we all need to contemplate them forthrightly if our profession is to survive, let alone thrive.

## Key Points

- Professional associations and organizations have met member needs on many issues and in many ways, including development and maintenance of professional practice standards; development of policies and positions that advocate for safety and quality of care; performance of advocacy work on behalf of professional priorities; and development of tools and resources to enhance professional practice.
- Where these organizations have come up short is in aggressively pursuing a unified approach to implementing strategies and tactics they have developed for themselves—and that others

have echoed in their own reports and recommendations—to stem the nursing shortage, improve the safety of care delivery, and enhance the image of the profession and the value of nursing.

- Despite all the positions and policies proposed, little is changing at the point of care delivery, except where contract language establishes a level of control for the professional nurse and allows professional judgment to dictate the decisions that take place with regard to safety and quality of care.
- Improving the work environment provides the focus and opportunity for a partnership or coalition of professional nursing associations and unions. However, lessons learned from the ANA show that this is not a feasible option.
- The Alliance of Nursing Organizations has the potential to bring nursing organizations together for concerted action around the crucial issues confronting the profession.
- Specialty nursing organizations fill a niche for specialty-focused concerns of nurses and related public policy matters.

## Web Resources

**Center for American Nurses (CAN)**
*www.nursingworld.org/can*
**Nursing Organizations Alliance**
*www.nursing-alliance.org*
**Nursing's Agenda for Healthcare Reform**
*www.nursingworld.org/readroom/rnagenda.htm*
**Specialty Nursing Practice Organizations**
*http://nursingworld.org/rnindex/snp.htm*
**United American Nurses (UAN)**
*http://nursingworld.org/uan*

### REFERENCES

Aiken, L. (2002). Hospital nurse staffing and patient mortality, nurse burnout and job dissatisfaction. *JAMA, 288,* 1987-1993.
American Hospital Association (AHA). (2002). In our hands: How hospital leaders can build a thriving workforce. Retrieved July 10, 2005, from *www.hospitalconnect.com/aha/key_issues/workforce/commission/InOurHands.html*.

American Nurses Association (ANA). (1992). *Nursing's agenda for health care reform.* Washington, DC: American Nurses Publishing.

American Nurses Association (ANA). (2002). Nursing's agenda for the future: A call to the nation. Retrieved July 10, 1995, from *www.nursingworld.org/naf.*

Budd, K., Warino, L., & Patton, M. (2004). Traditional and non-traditional collective bargaining: Strategies to improve the patient care environment. *Online Journal of Issues in Nursing, 9*(1), Manuscript 5. Retrieved July 10, 2005, from *www.nursingworld.org/ojin/topic23/tpc23_5.htm.*

Butcher, D. (2005). Personal communication, August 1, 2005.

Cornerstone Communications Group. (2001). Analysis of American Nurses Association staffing survey. Retrieved July 10, 2005, from *www.nursingworld.org/staffing/ana_pdf.pdf.*

Joint Commission on Accreditation of Healthcare Organizations (JCAHO). (2002). *Health care at the crossroads: Strategies for addressing the evolving nursing crisis.* Oak Brook, IL: Joint Commission Resources. Retrieved June 18, 2005, from *www.jcaho.org/about+us/public+policy+initiatives/health+care +at+the+crossroads.pdf.*

Kimball, B., & O'Neil, E. (2002). *Health care's human crisis: The American nursing shortage.* Princeton, NJ: Robert Wood Johnson Foundation. Retrieved May 23, 2005, from *www.rwjf. org/news/special/nursing_report.pdf.*

Nursing Organization Alliance. (2001, December 17). Coalitions of nursing specialty organizations unite (press release). Retrieved June 23, 2005, from *www.nursingworld.org/pressrel/ 2001/pr1217.htm.*

Page, A. (Ed.). (2003). *Keeping patients safe: Transforming the work environment of nurses.* Washington, DC: Committee on the Work Environment for Nurses and Patient Safety, Institute of Medicine. Retrieved May 23, 2005, from *http://books.nap. edu/catalog/10851.*

Seifert, P. Personal communication, June 27, 2005.

Williams, K. (2004). Ethics column. Ethics and collective bargaining: Calls to action. *Online Journal of Issues in Nursing.* Retrieved March 19, 2006, from *http://nursingworld.org/ ojin/ethicol/ethics_15.htm.*

# chapter 30

# You and Your Professional Nursing Organization

Pamela J. Haylock

*"It is rewarding, in the sense of having shared the results of your work and efforts with colleagues, of having contributed in some small way to the nursing profession, and of having learned much about yourself in the process."*

MARY JANE MORROW WARD

Organizations are described as "alive and screaming political arenas that host a complex web of individual and group interests" (Bolman & Deal, 1997). This perspective, reflecting the underlying assumptions for the information presented in this chapter, is summarized in five central propositions:

1. Organizations are coalitions of individuals and interest groups.
2. Enduring differences in values, beliefs, information, interests, and perceptions of reality exist among members.
3. Most important decisions involve the allocation of the organization's resources.
4. Scarce resources and enduring differences make conflict a central feature in organizational dynamics, and power the most important resource.
5. Organizational goals and decisions emerge from bargaining, negotiation, and jockeying for position among different stakeholders.

It has been reported that fewer than 7% of the nation's registered nurses are members of professional nursing organizations (Beauregard et al., 2003). Yet, political involvement is a professional imperative for nurses, who must be knowledgeable about issues, laws, and health policy and must possess political competencies, including communication and leadership skills. The internal politics of professional organizations provide a relatively safe practice arena in which nurses can observe, learn, prepare, and perfect the skills needed to be influential within and outside of professional nursing and health care organizations. This experience can be parlayed into added influence in work settings, community-based activities, and the broader health policy arena. Understanding organizational processes and acknowledging political influences can augment members' organizational experiences and, ultimately, enhance the political impact of nursing. The processes through which members can be actively and successfully involved in professional nursing organizations are the foci for this chapter.

## JOINING A PROFESSIONAL ORGANIZATION

Most nurses join professional organizations for continuing education, to be updated on professional issues, and for networking opportunities. When a nurse joins an organization, it is with the expectation that there will be a reasonable return on the member's investment of dues and commitment of time and energy. New knowledge is essential to competent nursing practice, and professional specialty organizations play vital roles in providing members with continuing education opportunities (Murphy et al., 2005). Tangible membership benefits include such things as professional journals, newsletters, discounted purchases of the organization's publications and subsequent access to state-of-the-art information, discounted conference and certification fees, and other forms of professional education. Perhaps more significant are the intangible benefits of membership, including the ability to network with colleagues in similar work settings, the chance to contribute to the development of standards and materials useful in nursing practice, and opportunities to mentor and to be mentored. Finally, and perhaps most important, professional organizations generally provide members opportunities to develop and fine-tune leadership skills that are critical for nurses who aspire to any level of influence within and outside of their professional organizations.

Being a member of a professional nursing organization is a voluntary endeavor. One's voluntary membership can be compared to the evolution of a long-term relationship—one in which the individual member *and* the organization benefit from the affiliation. For the relationship to work for both parties, short-term and long-term goals must be complementary. The prospective member's and the organization's major priorities should match. For example, a member who seeks involvement in health policy should assess the organization's commitment to health policy, its political action in general, and its likelihood of addressing the prospective member's health-related concerns.

Nurses who aspire to influential roles within the organization should get a complete understanding of its mission, goals, priorities, and political agenda, as well as an individual member's potential to be heard within it. After joining, a member can work toward achieving his or her desired level of influence. Choosing carefully and wisely among the many nursing organizations can make the difference between an exercise in frustration and a truly enriching volunteer experience.

## WHICH ORGANIZATION TO JOIN?

There are many nursing organizations, each with a unique mission or reason for existence and varying degrees of compatibility between the interests of potential members and the organization's purposes. Some organizations outside of the United States focus on international issues of relevance to American nurses. The American Nurses Association (ANA) is the professional organization that advocates positions of relevance to all professional nurses. In addition, some 70 national specialty or ethnic nursing organizations offer members specific educational opportunities and collegial support through which members can address shared professional practice issues.

Sixty-six U.S.-based nursing organizations are represented in the Nursing Organizations Alliance, a coalition created in 2001, merging the National Federation for Specialty Nursing Organizations and the ANA's Nursing Organization Liaison Forum. Membership in the Alliance is open to any nursing organization and nursing components of multidisciplinary organizations whose focus is to address current and emerging nursing and health care issues. The mission of the Alliance is "to increase nursing's visibility and impact on health through communication, collaboration and advocacy" (Nursing Organizations Alliance, 2005). The Alliance focuses on member organizations' needs by identifying mutual concerns that can be best addressed collectively. In 2004, Alliance members agreed to focus on the nurses' working environment by advocating efforts to identify and promote healthy and supportive work settings (Mason, 2004).

The Alliance, or similar coalitions, has significant potential to affect human health and well-being. As globalization continues to evolve, health issues and health care delivery challenges will likely blur practice boundaries that have been created and reinforced by specialty organizations. For example, health care system response and readiness impose challenges for the nursing profession. The concept of health surge capacity, that is, the health care system's capacity to "rapidly expand beyond normal services" to meet the needs imposed by a large-scale public health emergency or disaster, highlights the necessity for nurses' collaboration and coordination with regard to education and training in preparation for such events (Phillips & Lavin, 2004, p. 279). Infectious disease outbreaks such as severe acute

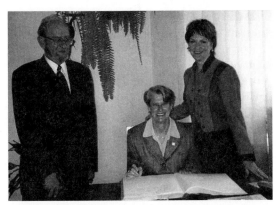

In 1998, Linda U. Krebs (seated) and Pamela J. Haylock, then President and Immediate Past President respectively, of the Oncology Nursing Society, were given the opportunity to travel to Lublin, Warsaw, and Krackow, Poland, offering organizational guidance to nurse-leaders of the newly established Polish Oncology Nursing Society. Here, Krebs and Haylock signed the guest register while meeting with the Medical School President at the University in Lublin, Poland.

respiratory syndrome (SARS), HIV/AIDS, and Human Papilloma Virus (HPV), the virus responsible for cervical cancer, are rarely limited to one geographic area, one nation, or even one continent. Tobacco use is a leading cause of preventable death worldwide, and the world's nursing organizations have the potential to promote health and reduce health risks by focusing on and promoting tobacco control policies and practices (Sarna & Bialous, 2004). Nurses and nursing organizations cannot afford to be uninvolved in women's health issues in general, or more specifically, deviations in health that increase risks of preterm births, a major public health concern with huge financial and emotional costs to families and communities (Sharts-Hopko, 2005).

Awareness of patient safety issues has increased over the past few years (Hughes, 2004). These realities diminish quality of care and rightfully undermine public confidence in health care delivery systems and health care professionals. Nurses, as the largest group of health care professionals and the health care professionals with the most direct and intimate contact with patients and families, should be in the forefront of developing policies and procedures to promote safety in all settings and for all individuals whose well-being is our primary concern (Burke, Mason, Alexander, Barnsteiner, & Rich, 2005; Hughes, 2004). The aforementioned issues are just a few of the health-related challenges that can be addressed through a coalition representative of professional nursing, interdisciplinary, and multi-disciplinary organizations that collaborate instead of compete (Whalen, 2003).

An essential element of any successful cooperative initiative to address these and other challenges is effective leadership. Kitson (2004) defined leadership as "having that ability to see into the future and to transform individuals, teams, systems and whole organizations (indeed, social systems) in ways that enable them to tackle the challenges that lie ahead" (p. 211). Traditionally, individual nursing organizations used informal leadership grooming methods (e.g., committee membership and ascendancy to committee leadership, elected board positions, and other specific appointments) and, more recently, proprietary or "members-only" leadership development programs. The value and cost-effectiveness of these programs have yet to be documented. Discipline-wide leadership development programs such as the Royal College of Nursing's Clinical Leadership Programme (Cunningham & Kitson, 2000) and the Nursing Alliance Leadership Academy (Nursing Organizations Alliance, 2005) can promote a discipline-wide vision focused on patients and contexts of care and collectively craft political strategies that promote nursing's policy initiatives. At the same time, these programs enhance the personal and professional development of nurses for more effective advocacy on behalf of the profession (Shaver, 2004; Sherman, 2005).

## ASSESSING COMPATIBILITY: MEMBER NEEDS AND THE ORGANIZATION

It is unlikely that any one organization will address members' array of professional needs and interests. Nurses are encouraged to join both the ANA, through which generic professional issues are addressed, and a specialty organization focusing on issues within a nurse's particular practice arena. Belonging to an organization with an intent to promote interdisciplinary collaboration such as that intended by the

Nursing Organizations Alliance, can be an added benefit of organizational membership. Organizations whose members represent the various disciplines connected to a specialty area—for example, organizations that include nurses, physicians, social workers, and administrators—expand the context of the issues being considered. The missions of social organizations, such as "gender equality in education and health," promoted by the American Association of University Women, may provide additional support and resources in addressing particular health policy–related concerns.

## ORGANIZATIONAL STRUCTURE AND PROCESSES

If a member hopes to find rewarding professional experiences through influence and power within an organization, it is important to have a thorough understanding of the organization's formal structure and processes—why it exists, what it purports to do, how it runs, and who runs it—as well as informal norms and expectations. Formal structure is determined by the organization's mission statement and bylaws, which are, in turn, operationalized by governing policies and processes. The mission statement, bylaws, and policies are published documents that are accessible not only to potential and current members but also to the general public. Processes, including step-by-step procedural directions, are generally made available to members on request. The subtle, implied, yet important, norms and expectations are discernible through formal and informal networking, collegial discussion, and astute observation.

### MISSION STATEMENTS

Mission statements define organizational purpose (Nanus, 1992). For example, the long-term mission of the ANA is to work to improve health standards and availability of health care services for all people, foster high standards for nursing, promote the professional development of nurses, and advance their economic and general welfare (ANA, 2006). Priorities addressed by the ANA include labor, wages and benefits, workplace safety, and nurse staffing. The missions of the following organizations allow

them the flexibility to address issues of concern to the majority of members through appropriate means: American Society for Pain Management Nursing (2005), to advance and promote optimal nursing care for people affected by pain; the Oncology Nursing Society (2005), to promote excellence in oncology nursing practice and quality cancer care; and the Association of Rehabilitation Nurses (2005), to promote and advance professional rehabilitation nursing practice through education, advocacy, collaboration, and research to enhance the quality of life for those affected by disability and chronic illness. As organizations evolve, stated missions are likely to change accordingly. Current mission statements, and organizational visions and goals, are usually offered on home or "about us" pages of organizational Websites.

### BYLAWS

Bylaws, the organizational "rule book," govern internal affairs and identify who has power and how that power works. They outline the purpose of the organization; membership criteria; financial and legal procedures; the number of board meetings; how the governing board operates; and the size, number, selection, and tenure of board members (Hummel, 1996). Most important, bylaws outline provisions for changes—amendments to the bylaws—defining who can bring suggested changes forward, and how the amendment process works. The significance of bylaw changes is reflected in the formality of the process. Most organizations require that proposed changes come forward in a specific format and within a designated time frame. It is often important that proposed bylaw changes be reviewed by legal counsel and a parliamentarian before being submitted to the governing board. The board then reviews proposed changes and may offer an opinion as to the value and consequence(s) of the changes. Rationale and arguments for and against the proposed changes are often required components of the proposal, and sponsors are usually identified when the change is submitted to the organization's voting body.

A look at just a few bylaw changes approved by nursing organizations demonstrates how profoundly these member-generated changes can affect an organization. A 1992 bylaw amendment allowed the International Association of Enterostomal Therapy (IAET) to change its name to the Wound, Ostomy, and Continence Nurses Society, reflecting recognition of the expanded focus of the specialty and the organization. A bylaw change proposed by members of the Oncology Nursing Society (ONS), voted down several times but finally approved in 1997, established provisions for "associate membership" offering non-registered nurse health care professionals and other interested persons (such as pharmaceutical company representatives) limited membership benefits. Another ONS bylaw change, approved by members in 1997, changed its mission statement from one that focused primarily on nursing education to a broader quality cancer care agenda. Clearly, changes in an organization's bylaws can have a lasting effect on leadership roles and the focus of the organization.

## GOVERNANCE POLICIES

The organization's values and perspectives are blended into policy that codifies what staff can or cannot do and also the governing board's process and relationships (Carver, 1997). John Carver, a theorist and consultant on governance design, suggests that organizational effectiveness is supported by board policies that fall into four groups: (1) the desired "ends"—the reason the organization exists; (2) the executive limitations, or the unacceptable means of achieving the ends; (3) governance process; and (4) the board-staff linkages (Carver & Carver, 2006).

## PROCESSES AND PROCEDURES

Step-by-step "how-to" directions are offered in organizational policy and procedure manuals. The most common processes available to general members who wish to influence organizational direction or agendas, aside from bylaw amendments, include

- Drafting and presenting organizational resolutions and position statements
- Suggesting organizationally branded projects, products, and services
- Introducing issues for consideration by the governing board

- Presenting issues for discussion in forums offered during general business meeting agendas

*Resolutions* are statements that reflect the organizational mission and goals and are proposed to the organization for endorsement and action by members. Resolutions are used to inform members or other designated constituencies about an issue and to show support (or lack of support) for programs or legislative initiatives. Many organizations use commemorative resolutions to recognize contributions of members, individuals, or organizations. Members who submit resolutions are usually required to follow a formalized process that includes meeting established deadlines and using a designated format. The procedure likely requires submission of the resolution itself, supporting data and information, recommendations for how the intent of the resolution is to be operationalized and its potential financial impact, and identification of supporting members. Resolutions that meet established criteria are then put before the organization's voting body. The actual procedure varies from one organization to another; meeting established and organization-specific criteria is essential for members to give thoughtful consideration to the implications of resolutions and their passage by voting members.

*Position statements* are documents, issued under the auspices of the governing board, that articulate the organization's official stance on issues relevant to its mission. They are intended as instruments of change, increasingly reflecting a theoretical and research foundation. Position statements promote a common understanding of and a collective response to issues of importance to organizational constituencies. The need for an organizational stance may be identified and suggested by general members as well as members in formal leadership roles. General members would communicate this need via formal and informal member-leadership channels. The board may choose to craft a position statement on its own or may appoint members with acknowledged expertise to the task. Position statements are released only after the governing board gives its final approval. Most nursing organizations post position statements on their Websites so that their perspective is accessible to a wide audience.

*Projects, products, and services* that are consistent with an organizational mission offer important and exciting opportunities for involvement and participation of members. Quite often, this is where the "Wow!" factor—described by Tom Peters (1994) as the excitement members get from being part of something important and meaningful—comes into play and is a critical factor in promoting members' commitment to the organization. Shepherding an idea from conception to completion and successful dissemination is probably one of the most rewarding aspects of organizational membership. Projects, products, and services come to be because they are identified as things that members need and are therefore critical benefits of membership. When they are perceived as valuable, these things reflect well on the organization. This level of work is generally assigned to committees, working groups or teams, and task forces composed of appointed expert members. Through such involvement, nurses get to exercise creativity while being part of a collaborative effort that also affords opportunities to be mentored or to mentor others, to be exposed to new ideas and new ways of doing things, and to achieve success in a potentially complex process. Volunteering to be part of a working group whose charge reflects a member's interests and expertise is a common route to gaining exposure and the credibility necessary to be influential enough to effect change. Most projects, products, and services mirror the creators, thus providing members with the ability to influence policy in subtle ways. For example, work on a patient education tool provides the nurse member with the opportunity to convey ideas she or he believes are important directly to the patient population and, ultimately, to effect changes in nursing practice. Organizational publications, generally an important benefit of membership, provide numerous ways to affect organizational direction. Serving as a manuscript reviewer, a contributing editor, or as an editorial board member for publications allows members to participate in shaping organizational publications, another avenue for influence within and outside of the organization.

*Application and selection processes* for these working groups vary widely among nursing organizations, but this procedural information should be easy to find. Authored submissions, "letters to the editor" in organizational publications, and other organizational endeavors provide ways to attract the attention of those responsible for making appointments. Performing successfully in these groups, once an appointment occurs, is essential. Group members need to understand group norms that will help establish a new member's standing as a valued colleague. By way of introduction to a new group, it is helpful to briefly identify the basis of one's interest in this group's work and describe the attributes one brings as a group member. Team leaders or committee chairpersons value knowledge of members' areas of interest, expertise, and skills and areas in which members would welcome mentoring or would be able to serve as a mentor. Public speaking and writing skills are especially valued.

*Board agendas* outline the work of the governing board. Most organizations offer members the chance to have issues placed on meeting agendas. Bylaws stipulate how and when board meetings occur and identify the means through which general members can contribute to board deliberations. Most often, informal communications with board members are enough to have an issue of concern placed on an agenda, but informal mechanisms will not guarantee that the issue is discussed. Formal communication, written letters, and/or electronic mail generally assure the member that a response of some sort will be forthcoming from the board. Of course, the response may not be the one the member hopes to receive, and as a result the member may seek alternative means—a resolution, a bylaw change, a position statement, or a discussion forum—to have the issue addressed.

*General business meeting agendas* offer another way members can bring issues and concerns to the attention of the governing board, other members, and colleagues. General business meetings are conducted according to some form of parliamentary procedure, often a variant of the tried and true *Robert's Rules of Order* (Robert, Evans, Honemann, Balch, & Robert, 2000). Members who wish to use the business meeting as a mechanism for addressing issues need to be fully informed about the procedure that allows this to occur. One or maybe two procedural blunders might be tolerated, but a number of them cast the member in a negative light that can be difficult to shed. Being knowledgeable of parliamentary procedure ensures that a member's concerns cannot be dismissed because of violations of that procedure.

Proficiency with the rules of order conveys the member's commitment to effectively presenting an issue to colleagues who may share the concern.

## TAX-EXEMPT STATUS

Tax-exempt status is allocated based on the mission, bylaws, and governance of the organization and is essential to understanding the degree to which advocacy efforts are allowed. Most voluntary nursing organizations are established as nonprofit organizations. Nonprofit status can lead to confusion because some board members, staff, and general members view political action as unseemly, irrelevant to an organization's mission, illegal, or having the potential to alienate existing and prospective members (Sparks, 1997). In fact, nonprofit advocacy and lobbying are both legal and necessary to promote organizations' missions (Sparks, 1997). Most nursing organizations are established around a variety of advocacy issues, such as improved nurse wages and work conditions, patients' needs for access to care, and evolution of a nursing specialty. Nonprofit status is granted under individual states' jurisdiction, but the classification for federal tax law directly affects what the organization can and cannot do (Yale, 1997). For example, organizations granted nonprofit status under Section 501(c)(3) of the Internal Revenue Code can accept tax-deductible contributions but are subject to severe restrictions on lobbying activities. Those classified as social welfare organizations under Section 501(c)(4) or as business leagues under Section 501(c)(6) may lobby (Hummel, 1996). Most nursing organizations operate under Section 501(c)(6) nonprofit status, in which there is no limit on lobbying. Support of specific candidates and any direct financial support to candidates, however, must be managed through separate political action committees (G. A. Yale, personal communication, August 6, 2002).

## NURSING ORGANIZATION LIFE CYCLE

Organizations go through life cycle stages from "conception" and "infancy" to "adulthood" and finally "old age" (Tecker & Fidler, 1993). For an organization to flourish and succeed in achieving goals, its leaders must adjust to changes in its environment and the resulting needs of members. An organization that is in its conception or infancy stage, characterized by struggles to survive, is unlikely to have either the resources or expertise to affect issues beyond its immediate survival. In the "young adulthood" stage, organizations formalize policies, and internal politics become evident. By "adulthood," an organization and its management are peaking, have mastered the environment, and serve members' needs. In "late adulthood" and "old age," organizations experience diminished excitement, member complacency, and lack of zeal and sense of urgency, and they finally lose the ability to serve members' needs. Organizations need not follow this cyclical decline. To avoid it, organization leaders must be charismatic, visionary, and innovative, and remain engaged in the work of the organization (Shaver, 2004). Leaders must apply appropriate and innovative strategies to maintain organizational vitality and members' commitment. The vital, successful, and exciting organization is more likely to experience success, thereby providing members with a variety of opportunities to contribute to meaningful projects and services, mentor others, learn and practice new skills, have positive experiences, and most importantly, attract, nourish, and develop its next generation of leaders (Sherman, 2005).

## ORGANIZATIONAL LEADERSHIP AND POWER

There are many routes to achieving power and influence in contemporary nursing organizations. Certainly, members who have attained leadership roles in the organization have achieved some level of power and influence, as have highly placed staff members. General members can attain equally influential positions. Regardless of one's membership status, achieving power and influence requires knowledge and understanding, not only of the organization's structure, processes, and policies, but also of the personalities and priorities of key organizational staff and leaders.

Power is the ability to get things done through the attainment and mobilization of resources (Kantor, 1977). There are nurses who use coercion or fear to rule others, but this situation typifies powerless organizations in which oppression and deceit are used to meet goals (Carlson-Catalano, 1994) and typifies an organization in "old age" and on a path toward its demise (Tecker & Fidler, 1993). Clearly, an organization that evidences these traits is to be avoided if a prospective member hopes to be part of a respected, successful, and influential organization.

It can be useful to assess sources of power within the organization. The political interests of the organization's chief staff executive (executive director, chief executive officer), chief elected officer (e.g., president, board chairperson), and leaders in elected board roles will be mirrored in the organization's priorities. Do printed or spoken messages reflect an interest or priority in pertinent issues, or do the messages simply reflect a fleeting focus? These seemingly innocuous communiqués can be revealing with regard to the import leaders attached to a particular issue.

## ELECTED AND APPOINTED LEADERS

The possibilities for professional and personal growth that accompany service in leadership capacities are infinite. Organizations' elected leaders are offered unique experiences: opportunities to meet colleagues from a variety of settings at local, national, and international levels; the chance to explore concerns and goals and to work toward solutions to shared problems; and the capacity to interact with a host of leaders representing other disciplines who hold different, interesting, and challenging notions about addressing common concerns.

Many nurse leaders have parlayed organizational leadership skills into public policy roles, including election to national and state congressional seats, jobs as critical staff to elected leaders and policy-related agencies, and appointments to policymaking commissions (Feldman & Lewenson, 2000). Sheila Burke credits her active participation in the National Student Nurses Association as the catalyst that led to her policy-related achievements, including serving as former Senator Robert Dole's (R-KS) highly respected chief of staff; Burke is now the chief operating officer for the Smithsonian Institution in Washington, DC. Virginia Trotter Betts was elected president of the Tennessee State Nurses Association and was president of the American Nurses Association during the Clinton administration's attempts to reform the U.S. health care system. From there, Betts went on to become Senior Advisor on Nursing and Policy to the Secretary and Assistant Secretary of Health, U.S. Department of Health and Human Services, and the first nurse to be the Commissioner of Mental Health in the state of Tennessee. Elected members affect organizational direction and development of policy. A governing board or board of directors is accountable for the organization and exists on behalf of the larger group of members, who, in the case of nonprofit organizations, morally own the organization (Carver, 1997). This board is responsible for achieving what it should and avoiding the unacceptable. The board, acting as a body, defines, delegates, and monitors, but usually does not carry out, organizational work. Each governing board member holds a position that confers different responsibilities and expectations and requires mastery of a specific skill set in order to perform well in that role.

Organizations may differ in the use of titles, but generally, governing boards identify key officers— sometimes referred to as the "executive committee." Specific officers may be mandated by laws of the state where the organization is incorporated but usually consist of, at a minimum, the chief elected officer (e.g., president, board chairperson), a treasurer, and a secretary. The specific duties and powers of each officer are outlined in organizational bylaws. Depending on organizational bylaw and policy provisions, key officers or the executive committee may be conferred additional responsibilities not expected of other board members. For example, the executive committee might be called on to make decisions in lieu of a full board action. The executive committee may be expected to play active roles in evaluation of key staff members or lead important committees and other working group efforts. Finally, members of the executive committee could be in the direct line of leadership succession should another leader be unable to fulfill an elected role.

Additional governing roles are devised to meet the unique needs of the organization and are usually outlined in bylaws. So-called "at large" roles might serve organizational needs for geographic and constituency representation. Organizations that have an international focus might incorporate the international perspective within its board structure by allocating a board role specific to geographic constituencies. Some nursing organizations include laypersons who bring the consumer or patient perspective into governing structures. As leaders recognize a specific need not currently met by members, members with expertise in highly specialized areas such as fund-raising, health policy, international affairs, and organizational change may be appointed to specific roles that augment governing boards.

Although not explicit in legal or even organizational bylaws and policies, it is essential that organizational leaders convey commitment and passion, expressing that they care deeply about what the organization does (Bolman & Deal, 1997). Beyond this, and regardless of the elected or appointed position, governing board members have three general duties owed to the organization while serving in these roles: the duty of care, the duty of loyalty, and the duty of obedience (Yale, 1997). The duty of care implies that the responsibilities inherent in the role are accepted in good faith, with the care expected of a prudent person in a similar role, and in a manner that is in the best interests of the organization. The duty of loyalty suggests that the board member conducts himself or herself for the good of the organization and does not receive direct or indirect improper financial gain. Violation of this duty is referred to as a "conflict of interest." Elected and appointed organizational leaders are usually expected to sign agreements that identify potential conflicts of interest. Conflicts of interest might occur when a company or institution that, in some way, competes with or is in conflict with the organization employs a board member. Distribution of funding may pose dilemmas when a board member's employing agency, or a colleague in the same facility, has applied for project funding granted on the basis of a board vote. In these situations, board members might be asked to refrain from voting. The duty of obedience alludes to one's obligation to follow organizational documents and applicable laws.

## ORGANIZATIONAL ELECTIONS

Organizational elections, operating under a variety of more or less democratic principles, determine which members will be officially accountable for the organization's operation and direction. Organizations differ, to some extent, in the processes used to elect official leaders. Members who aspire to these roles, as well as general members who interact with elected leaders, should be fully informed about which positions are open on a given electoral slate; the qualifications, expectations, and time commitments of the various elected roles; the nomination and slating processes; campaign expectations and guidelines; and the voting process.

Some organizations elect leaders through a popular vote in which general members vote for candidates placed on a ballot through nomination and slating processes. Some might employ a system in which delegates are elected or appointed and are, in turn, charged with the responsibilities of voting. Other organizations select designated members of the governing board through a popular election, while the chief elected officer is determined by a vote of those serving on the board. Organizations, according to their bylaws, may hold elections in which each voting member must cast a ballot in person, whereas other organizations might allow voting to be done by postal mail and/or electronically via Internet and e-mail mechanisms.

A decision to pursue an elected leadership role in an organization should be made after very thoughtful consideration. Elected roles require a great deal of work. Nominees and candidates must make truly informed decisions about seeking elected office. The existence and level of staff support in the organization are important factors in the time commitment and expectations of volunteer leaders. Family members might be involved in a prospective candidate's decision to run for election, as normal family roles and routines are likely to be disrupted at least occasionally. Elected roles can consume significant amounts of time, work, and energy of members—time that may require absences from one's primary work role. Time away from a job can be a source of conflict for elected leaders and employers. Some organizations offer stipends to compensate elected leaders. A stipend may be offered to an employer in compensation for the elected employee's time away from the job or may be offered directly to the elected leader. Some organizations mandate evidence of commitment and support from employers.

Important prenomination considerations include the efforts and costs of mounting an election campaign. Knowledge of organizational policies and expectations with regard to campaigning is essential. Reflecting the debate surrounding national campaign finance reform, many organizations closely monitor candidates' campaign efforts with regard to truth and fairness. If organizational norms call for targeted member mailing, printing and postage costs can be substantial—so substantial, in fact, that qualified potential candidates may forgo the process. Candidates from less populous constituencies may lack the collegial and financial resources of candidates from urban or tertiary care settings.

Nurses often lack high-level organizational experience and are unprepared and naive as they enter association leadership roles. Many newly elected board members are shocked by the complexity of debate and decision-making that occurs at these governing levels. Few new board members are prepared to question or challenge the authority of highly placed staff members—the chief staff officer, for example (Ernstthal, 2001)—leaving the governing board somewhat weakened until new members gain confidence in their work. Annual turnover as a result of organizational elections results in some level of instability and inconsistency within the board. Most organizations attempt to compensate for personnel change by staggering board vacancies, leaving a majority of experienced members who can effectively orient and mentor newly elected members.

It is increasingly recognized that talent, experience, and leadership style—not tenure within the organization—matter most (Cufaude, 2001). A strong organization and wise, confident leaders will create and support processes that help members attain the talent, experience, and leadership needed to ensure the vitality and success of the organization. Box 30-1 identifies these basic talents and skills.

---

**BOX 30-1  Critical Skills for Organizational Leaders**

- Embrace and create chaos and change that stimulate creativity and innovation (Cufaude, 2001).
- Offer members exciting opportunities and projects that create personal connection, challenge, and professional development and provide members with a return on their investment of dues and commitment (Peters, 1994).
- Use facilitation behaviors to encourage others to bridge differences and focus on essentials.
- Collaborate with internal and external stakeholders.
- Act as talent scouts who recognize and nourish the development of members who contribute valuable interests, skills, and talents.
- Work toward building a "hierarchy of imagination," where an individual's imagination and passion, rather than position and political power, are the determinants of his or her voice in organizational strategy making and innovation (Hamel, 2000).
- Speculate *not* on what might happen but on what members can actually *make* happen (Hamel, 2000).
- Be prepared to champion the association's core values and ensure the preservation of the organization in an ever-changing environment (Collins & Porras, 1994).
- Be passionate about the role and contributions to the organization and to learning about the professional aspirations of other members.

---

## CHIEF EXECUTIVE

A nursing organization's elected leaders come and go. The chief staff executive—chief executive officer, chief staff officer, or executive director—is the one constant advocate for the mission and values of the organization. The chief executive reports to and receives executive authority from the governing board (Carver, 1997). The chief staff executive reflects and is the primary agent in shaping and sustaining the culture of the organization—the values, beliefs, rituals, and rules that are the unspoken assumptions about what matters and how things are done in the organization. Organizational leaders invest a great deal of trust in the chief executive, and consequently, this person assumes power that extends beyond administrative and program arenas (Albert, 1993). Organizations' governing boards hold the responsibility for monitoring the work, effectiveness, and outcomes of the chief staff executive (Tecker & Fidler, 1993).

## LEADERSHIP

Active participation in organizational work that comes to the attention of organizational leaders is a simple way to begin the process of developing influence and power in that organization—in short, to become an organizational leader. Here again, it is important to know and understand organizational norms, protocols, and expectations. Most organizations operate general member and governance board meetings according to bylaws provisions, usually under some version of *Robert's Rules of Order*, guidelines based on parliamentary practice. *Robert's Rules*, now in its 10th edition, was first published in 1876 by Army engineer Henry Martyn Robert as an attempt to bring order to the chaos of presiding over meetings *(www.robertsrules.com)*. *Robert's Rules* still affords order to leaders who are experienced in their use or have the wherewithal to use professional parliamentarians. Even in the absence of a handy copy of *Robert's Rules*, or when an organization uses alternative guidelines, "rules of order" are generally printed and stipulated as a first agenda item in any business meeting.

Other common group norms can affect one's organizational standing. Such conventions as arriving on time for meetings, arriving at meetings well prepared for discussion and debate, paying attention to implied or explicit dress codes, meeting the commitments inherent in the designated role, and going above and beyond role expectations are important to gaining the recognition and respect of organizational colleagues.

## BARGAINING AND NEGOTIATION: THE WIN-WIN APPROACH TO ORGANIZATIONAL CONFLICT

Large groups of people rarely achieve unanimous agreement on important issues. There is usually disagreement among members on which issues are considered important to an organization or how these issues ought to be addressed. Given the differences in values, beliefs, information, interests, and perceptions that exist among the organizational membership, disagreement and conflict should be accepted as the norm rather than the exception. In truth, conflict has costs and benefits (Bolman & Deal, 1997). Too much conflict or conflict that is poorly managed produces infighting and destructive power struggles. Alternatively, lack of conflict is symptomatic of an organization in which members and leaders are apathetic, uncreative, stagnant, and unresponsive. Conflict challenges the status quo and can stimulate new ideas and approaches to problems. It is key that leaders handle conflict well and achieve a balance that stimulates creativity and innovation.

Conflicts that emerge within an organization usually revolve around allocation of limited resources and prioritization of goals (Bolman & Deal, 1997), but issues that arise between volunteer members and the staff are another common source of conflict (Kincaide, 2001). A group of members may prefer that resources be used, for example, to influence a particular legislative issue, whereas another group desires the creation of an internal leadership development project. Staff and volunteer members, each group with its unique perspective, may differ on approaches to organizational concerns. How these differences of opinion play out can be the source of considerable conflict, or of innovative strategies that accommodate both sides.

Fisher, Ury, and Patton (1991), in *Getting to Yes*, recommend what they call "principled negotiation" to arrive at mutually acceptable agreements: Issues are decided on merits alone, as opposed to the personalities of those who raise the issues, and options are devised that satisfy groups on both "sides" of an issue. Strategies that "mine the talents" of member constituencies can be used to guide resolution of differences (Kincaide, 2001). A critical step in conflict resolution involves helping all parties agree on a philosophical framework. Gail Kincaide, executive director of the Association of Women's Health, Obstetric and Neonatal Nurses (AWHONN), credited the success of AWHONN's reorganization to a philosophical framework that focuses on commitment, trust, and consistency, a process that for many organizations is fraught with conflict.

Leaders must be sure that organizational policies and processes support the bargaining and negotiation processes that are the critical elements of conflict resolution. Each member is obligated to use organizational processes that are in place or else find ways to change processes through bylaw amendments, policy and procedural changes, position statements, and resolutions. Members acting in collaboration with other members are more likely to be viewed as having valid concerns than a member acting alone. An attempt to address an issue via an existing segment of the membership is generally a good starting place. For example, a clinical issue might be discussed among members of a clinical practice committee or relevant interest group. A policy issue might be discussed among members of a government relations committee or legislative task force. Shared concerns and suggestions are then brought forward to organizational leaders. Any member, leader or not, must have good supportive data in hand in order to influence change. Passion for an issue is important, but passion without solid information and effective communication is unlikely to change opinions or effect change. Relevant data include the scope of the problem, its relevance to the organization's mission and goals, the anticipated outcomes of nonaction versus the proposed action, a synopsis of proposed ways by which the issue could be addressed (including organizational costs), and the number of members who share this concern.

Box 30-2 identifies elements that are essential to managing organizational conflict.

## PROMOTING HEALTH POLICY FROM AN ORGANIZATIONAL PERSPECTIVE

Even though the necessity of nurses' political involvement is the premise for this book, it is still apparent that the majority of nurses remain politically apathetic (Boswell, Cannon, & Miller, 2005). However, active participation in nursing organizations, and opportunities to learn and practice political competencies, is believed to enhance

---

> **BOX 30-2   Resolving Organizational Conflict**
>
> - Examine and identify shared core values.
> - Frame the issue within the organization's mission, goals, and priorities.
> - Build and reinforce a shared philosophy of commitment, trust, and consistency among those on both sides of the conflict.
> - Use existing processes to address the issue.
> - Pick your battles and do not argue about everything; instead, take on only issues that are meaningful.
> - Be informed about the pros and cons of an issue or strategy to the extent possible.
> - Anticipate and be prepared to address opposing perspectives.
> - Act in collaboration. Look for and enlist like-minded colleagues, and find ways to get the attention and support of elected and appointed leaders.
> - Make sure every communication surrounding the issue is clear.
> - Look for the "win-win" scenario that characterizes a mutually acceptable agreement.

---

nursing political activism and efficacy (Beauregard et al., 2003; Boswell et al., 2005). Organizational involvement offers nurses various avenues to overcoming traditional barriers to political activism, including learning about political processes and tactics, establishing a network of role models and mentors, becoming involved in political activities, enhancing communication skills, and benefiting from peer support (Boswell et al., 2005). Within the organization, conflicts can arise concerning *which* issues and *which* policies organizational resources should be used to address, the level of resources to be expended on particular causes, and determination of acceptable end points. Individual nurses and professional nursing organizations have differed on critical and basic issues, such as access to care, Medicare, Medicaid and welfare reform, assisted suicide, a woman's right to abortion, unionization, the use of collective bargaining and strike actions, and the nursing profession's entry-level educational requirements. Specialty nursing organizations generally use their resources to address issues that primarily affect their specialty arena, diminishing nurses' potential for a cohesive approach to broader health policy and professional issues. The Nursing Organizations Alliance was formed to reduce divisiveness in the profession, thereby increasing nursing's impact on health and health care (Nursing Organizations Alliance, 2005).

## REFOCUSING ORGANIZATIONAL PRIORITIES

The distribution of an organization's resources reflects priorities given to its political and policy-related efforts. Appointment of identified staff roles—including the credentials, qualifications, and number of staff—that support political and policy efforts within the organization is evidence of support for policy-related work. Rather than hiring staff members whose roles are completely dedicated to policy work, many nursing organizations, especially those with smaller membership bases and limited fiscal and personnel resources, become associated with business entities that provide "health policy" consultants on a contractual basis. In this situation, the health policy consultant, sometimes referred to as a "lobbyist," may be contracted to work with several nursing organizations, providing expertise in the policymaking process. Legal firms with established bases in state capitals and/or Washington, DC, also offer lobbying services on a contractual basis. Because this contractual person or team of persons may or may not have expertise in the area of concern, it is critical that leaders and other experts provide solid direction in setting the organizations' policy-related priorities. Being among these recognized experts is a way in which an individual member can influence an organization's health policy agenda.

Organizational policies and processes offer the mechanisms through which any member or group of members can be a catalyst to changing the organization's focus, goals, and priorities. Usually, governing boards create a health policy agenda or governmental relations strategy, an established plan that is available to members, in which policy priorities are clearly identified. These priorities are influenced in the same way that other organizational priorities are, that is, by members who communicate with leaders about issues that are relevant to the profession, the organization, or its mission. Bylaws or mission statement changes, generated by members, can profoundly affect organizational direction. Resolutions and position statements, generated by members, can redirect organizational focus and allocation of resources. For example, an organization that creates a position on pain management is obligated to focus on effecting change according to action statements included in the position. Resolutions are equally binding. Many nursing organizations, for example, have passed resolutions that establish anti-tobacco activities among their priority issues.

## Key Points

- Professional nursing organizations offer one avenue through which individual nurses and the profession as a whole can achieve power and influence policy.
- For nurses who want to shape the work of a professional organization, it is essential to understand the organization's structure and policies for operating and decision-making and think strategically about moving an agenda forward.
- Holding an elective or appointed office in a professional organization provides opportunities for professional growth, influence within the organization, and moving nursing agendas externally through formal resolutions and position statements.

## Web Resources

**American Journal of Nursing Career Guide**
*www.nursingcenter.com/library/JournalArticle. asp?Article_ID=575885*
For a list of national nursing organizations:
**American Nurses Association**
*www.ANA.org*
**Nursing Organizations Alliance**
*www.nursing-alliance.org/*

## REFERENCES

Albert, S. (1993). *Hiring the chief executive: A practical guide to the search and selection process.* Washington, DC: National Center for Nonprofit Boards.

American Nurses Association (ANA). (2006). Mission statement. Retrieved March 22, 2006, from *www.nursingworld.org/about/mission1.htm.*

American Society for Pain Management Nursing. (2005). Mission statement. Retrieved August 14, 2005, from *www.aspmn.org.*

Association of Rehabilitation Nurses. (2005). Mission statement. Retrieved August 14, 2005, from *www.rehabnurse.org.*

Beauregard, M. A., Deck, D. S., Kay, K. C., Haynes, J., Inman, R., Perry, M., et al. (2003). Improving our image a nurse at a time. *Journal of Nursing Administration, 33,* 510-511.

Bolman, L. G., & Deal, T. E. (1997). *Reframing organizations: Artistry, choice, and leadership* (2nd ed.). San Francisco: Jossey-Bass.

Boswell, C., Cannon, S., & Miller, J. (2005). Nurses' political involvement: Responsibility versus privilege. *Journal of Professional Nursing, 21,* 5-8.

Burke, K. G., Mason, D. J., Alexander, M., Barnsteiner, J. H., & Rich, V. L. (2005). Making medication administration safe. *American Journal of Nursing, 3*(Suppl), 2-3.

Carlson-Catalano, J. (1994). Invest in yourself: Cultivating personal power. *Nursing Forum, 29*(2), 22-28.

Carver, J. (1997). *Boards that make a difference* (2nd ed.). San Francisco: Jossey Bass.

Carver, J., & Carver, M. (2006). Carver's policy governance model in nonprofit organizations. Retrieved April 3, 2006, from *www.carvergovernance.com/pg-np.htm.*

Collins, J., & Porras, J. (1994). *Built to last: Successful Habits of Visionary Companies.* New York: HarperCollins.

Cufaude, J. B. (2001). Telling a new leadership story. *Association Management, 53*(1), 43-50.

Cunningham, G., & Kitson, A. (2000). An evaluation of the RCN clinical leadership programme (Pts. 1 & 2). *Nursing Standard, 15*(12), 34-37; *15*(13), 34-40.

Ernstthal, H. L. (2001). Provocative questions for volunteer leaders. *Association Management, 53*(1), 60-62, 64.

Feldman, H. R., & Lewenson, S. B. (2000). *Nurses in the political arena: The public face of nursing.* New York: Springer.

Fisher, R., Ury, W., & Patton, B. (1991). *Getting to yes: Negotiating agreement without giving in* (2nd ed.). New York: Penguin.

Hamel, G. (2000). *Leading the revolution.* Boston: Harvard Business School Press.

Hughes, R. G. (2004). Avoiding the near misses. *American Journal of Nursing, 104,* 81-84.

Hummel, J. M. (1996). *Starting and running a nonprofit organization* (2nd ed.). Minneapolis: University of Minnesota Press.

Kantor, R. M. (1977). *Men and women of the corporation.* New York: Basic Books.

Kincaide, G. G. (2001). Planned partnership. *Association Management, 53*(1), 52-54, 56, 58-59.

Kitson, A. (2004). Drawing out leadership (Editorial). *Journal of Advanced Nursing, 48,* 211.

Mason, D. J. (2004). The Nursing Organizations Alliance: A new coalition provides hope for nurses' collective power. *American Journal of Nursing, 104,* 26.

Murphy, C. M., Ballon, L. G., Culhane, B., Mafrica, L., McCorkle, M., & Worrall, L. (2005). Oncology Nursing Society environmental scan 2004. *Oncology Nursing Forum—Online Exclusive, 32,* E76-E97.

Nanus, B. (1992). *Visionary leadership: Creating a compelling sense of direction for your organization.* San Francisco: Jossey-Bass.

National Gerontological Nursing Association. (2005). Mission statement. Retrieved August 14, 2005, from *www.1124.249.193.144/NGNA.*

Nursing Organizations Alliance. (2005). Retrieved August 14, 2005, from *www.nursing-alliance.org/about.cfm.*

Oncology Nursing Society. (2005). Mission statement. Retrieved August 14, 2005, from *www.ons.org.*

Peters, T. (1994). *The pursuit of wow!* New York: Vintage.

Phillips, S., & Lavin, R. (2004). Readiness and response to public health emergencies: Help needed now from professional nursing associations. *Journal of Professional Nursing, 20,* 279-280.

Robert, H. M., III, Evans, W. J., Honemann, D. H., Balch, T. J., & Robert, H. M. (Eds.). (2000). *Robert's rules of order* (10th ed., Newly revised). Cambridge, MA: Perseus.

Robinson, T. M. (2000). Mary Jane Ward. In V. Bullough & L. Sentz (Eds.), *American nursing: A biographical dictionary* (Vol. 3, p. 284). New York: Springer.

Sarna, L. & Bialous, S. A. (2004). Tobacco control policies of oncology nursing organizations. *Seminars in Oncology Nursing, 20,* 101-110.

Sharts-Hopko, N. C. (2005). Why every nurse should be concerned about prematurity. *American Journal of Nursing, 105,* 60.

Shaver, J. (2004). Envisioning novel and meaningful collaborations: Crucial leadership needed. *Nursing Outlook, 52,* 223-224.

Sherman, R. O. (2005). Growing our future nursing leaders. *Nursing Administration Quarterly, 29,* 125-132.

Sigma Theta Tau International. (1997). *The Woodhull Study on Nursing and the Media.* Indianapolis: Sigma Theta Tau International Honor Society of Nursing.

Sparks, J. D. (1997). *Lobbying, advocacy and nonprofit boards.* Washington, DC: National Center for Nonprofit Boards.

Tecker, G., & Fidler, M. (1993). *Successful association leadership: Dimensions of 21st century competency for the CEO.* Washington, DC: Foundation of the American Society of Association Executives.

Whalen, J. P. (2003). Health care in America: Lost opportunities amid plenty. *Qualitative Health Research, 13,* 857-870.

Yale, G. A. (1997). *Responsibilities and liabilities of Texas nonprofit organization directors.* San Antonio: Nonprofit Resource Center of Texas.

# chapter 31

# Nursing in Action: Policy Initiatives of Specialty Nursing Associations

Patricia W. Underwood

*"Great organizations demand a high level of commitment by the people involved."*

BILL GATES

The increasing success of nursing organizations in policy is a tribute to a growing maturity in the exercise of political influence and the ability to leverage the trust the public has for nurses. The following vignettes highlight the efforts of nine specialty nursing organizations in influencing public policy. These examples describe the groups' successes as well as the barriers they encountered so others can gain insight.

Due to limited resources, nursing organizations are prioritizing their policy initiatives around advocacy for the population groups served by their members and for their members. Specialty nursing organizations can play a particularly unique and important role in advocating on behalf of their clients. The efforts of the Association of Women's Health, Obstetric and Neonatal Nurses (AWHONN) to prevent birth defects by increasing the prepregnancy intake of folic acid reflect a focus on issues that are critical to the population they serve. The policy initiative of the American Nephrology Nurses Association (ANNA) is directed toward obtaining reimbursement for dialysis services; this, too, is a client-focused issue. Payment for dialysis significantly influences a patient's access to these services.

Three organizations have pursued policy that directly affects their members: The Association of periOperative Registered Nurses (AORN) has lobbied to obtain reimbursement for Registered Nurse (RN) First Assistants; the American Association of Occupational Health Nurses (AAOHN) is working to decrease violence in the workplace; and the American Association of Critical-Care Nurses (AACN) is promoting healthy work environments. The Emergency Nurses Association (ENA) is working to simultaneously influence the work environment of nurses and promote patient safety through their efforts to systematically achieve safe staffing levels in emergency departments.

The Oncology Nursing Society (ONS) has focused on an issue that is not specific to their members—increasing the funding for the Nurse Reinvestment Act—but has enlisted their patients as partners in the advocacy efforts. Passage and funding of the Nurse Reinvestment Act was part of the strategic political action undertaken by all the major nursing organizations to address the critical, impending shortage of nurses. This ONS initiative is an excellent illustration of collaboration between nurses and their clients and among nursing organizations.

Regardless of the focus—member or population served—the organization's members must collectively find the policy issue important in order to generate the commitment that is needed to sustain the efforts. Progress varies: It may come quickly, as seen with AACN's development of standards to transform the work environment, or it may be elusive for groups like the RN First Assistants who are seeking direct reimbursement.

## STRATEGIES FOR ACTION

### DEFINE THE PROBLEM AND EXAMINE THE POLITICAL FEASIBILITY

Reviewing the literature or analyzing data may not be as exciting as planning a media blitz or lobbying congress. But an in-depth understanding of the policy issue is critical to selecting strategies that are most likely to be successful. It is also important to identify the stakeholders and their stake in the issue, so that messages can capitalize on existing support and address the concerns of those who may be less enthusiastic. Important questions for an association to address include the following:

1. What is the actual problem that needs to be addressed?
2. What are the potential solutions and their advantages and disadvantages?
3. What evidence is there that the proposed solution will achieve the desired outcomes?
4. What are the financial implications?

AACN and ENA provide excellent examples of how specialty organizations began with an attempt to get as much information as possible about the issue as a basis for strategic planning. AAOHN showed how conducting a needs assessment survey could provide justification for the planned intervention.

### BUILD PARTNERSHIPS AND COALITIONS

Collaborating with others to advance a policy issue is evident in the actions of many of these specialty organizations. The focus of ONS' contribution to enhanced funding for the Nurse Reinvestment Act was on engaging patients as partners in advocating for funding. The effectiveness of ANNA's End Stage Renal Disease (ESRD) Education Week was enhanced by involving other dialysis organizations and Kidney Care Partners. In a similar manner, AWHONN collaborated with the National Council on Folic Acid to advance their work on that issue.

AAOHN used a two-pronged approach in their collaboration. They developed an alliance with a governmental agency—the Occupational Safety and Health Administration (OSHA)—and they collaborated with several universities to plan studies and conferences. The OSHA partnership provided access to broad resources and wide avenues for dissemination of information to employees and employers. The university partnership provided some of the knowledge and skill needed to undertake a particular action.

The National Association of Orthopaedic Nurses (NAON) used collaborative strategies to bring concerns about the safety of all-terrain vehicles to the attention of the public. First, they collaborated with a nursing organization that shared their interest—the Emergency Nurses Association—and then with the National Trails and Water Coalition. This latter collaboration enabled NAON to develop a Website through which they were able to reach a wider audience, especially other concerned parents. Website development can be a useful strategy when attempts to engage the traditional media have not been successful.

### INVOLVE THE BROADER NURSING COMMUNITY

A question that must be considered by specialty organizations when planning strategic action is "When is it appropriate to involve the broader nursing community"? That's easiest to answer when the issue involves all nurses. A reluctance to involve other organizations may occur because of concern about sharing credit for any outcomes achieved and a fear of losing control of the issue. However, the opportunity to share resources and maximize a power base, thus increasing the likelihood that the policy change will be successful, should outweigh these concerns. Careful preliminary discussions to assign responsibility for resources and strategies can overcome initial concerns. Nursing organizations do well to recognize that there are more than two options when confronting an issue (supporting or opposing). "Not opposing" is, in fact, politically positive and should be viewed as such.

## ENGAGE OTHER PROFESSIONAL OR LAY GROUPS

Developing or joining a coalition with professional or lay groups has disadvantages and advantages. Establishing and maintaining coalitions is time consuming and may require compromise and shared leadership. The significant advantage is that a coalition can often achieve what no single organization can accomplish on its own. Pooling resources and political capital heightens the potential for goal achievement. AACN used excellent initiative in building on their relationships with key physician organizations to encourage consideration of what doctors can contribute to produce healthier work environments.

When the focus of action is a selected health issue, establishing a coalition that includes those individuals who are most likely to experience that concern can be powerful in terms of the ownership of the issue by the health care consumer. Inclusion of those most directly affected by the policy change can enhance a commitment to the change in health behavior that the group is advocating. AWHONN described their collaboration with other groups to promote the increased intake of folic acid by women who are preparing for childbearing.

Collaboration and coalition building may bring unexpected dividends. ANNA's collaboration with other renal groups to initiate the ESRD Education Week has established them as leaders within the renal community. AWHONN's folic acid initiative has provided visibility for nurses as leaders addressing a significant public health issue. These efforts are particularly important in helping the public to view nurses as knowledgeable leaders within the health care community, not just trusted providers.

## FOCUS

Though most of the case studies presented here focus on education strategies and legislative activity, regulatory reform is another possible focus. AWHONN's efforts to lobby the Federal Drug Administration to increase the current fortification requirements to provide a more substantial amount of the recommended dietary allowance of folic acid per serving of enriched grain illustrates the opportunity to influence regulations.

## DETERMINE THE LEVEL OF INFLUENCE NEEDED: FEDERAL VERSUS STATE

Successful strategizing also demands that organizations consider to whom their lobbying should be directed. The decision about whether to seek legislative change at the state or federal level is not necessarily a simple one. If a federal law is passed, it has the potential to bring about the desired outcome in a more efficient manner. The political climate at the federal level may make passage of a particular bill more difficult. While state-by-state legislative success can take time, it is also true that passage of a specific piece of legislation by a few states may provide the momentum needed to encourage other states to follow.

Not all national nursing organizations have state counterparts. The nursing organizations most likely to have the political clout needed for achieving legislative change at the state level are the state nurses associations. AORN's attempts to attain reimbursement for RN First Assistants illustrates the considerations and challenges in attempting to pass legislation at both state and federal levels. In this situation, it was hoped that state-level legislation would prompt passage of legislation at the federal level. While this hope has not yet been realized, AORN's efforts are a sophisticated model.

## TARGET KEY POLICYMAKERS

Whether pursuing legislation at the state or federal level, it is essential to consider who can sponsor the legislation and to whom the lobbying efforts should be directed. Ideally, sponsors should come from both political parties because perceived bipartisan support will maximize the potential for success. Likewise, having many co-sponsors will facilitate passage. It is politically sound to target specific legislators who are on the committees that are most likely to have control over the intended bill. ANNA's work to educate lawmakers about the need for legislation to provide more comprehensive access to dialysis treatments is a wonderful illustration of strategically targeting legislators who sit on the congressional committees responsible for Medicare funding decisions. AORN targeted key legislators, but they also recognized that speaking with the legislators' aides who was equally important. The legislative staff will usually be the ones to draft the position statements that are promulgated by their boss.

## KEYS TO SUCCESS

Despite the fact that many of the policy initiatives discussed by the specialty organizations have not yet reached their desired conclusion, the work of these organizations illustrates strategies that are key to policy achievement. Four key strategies are evident: Be prepared, send a clear message, make the issue visible, and be persistent.

- *Be prepared.* In order for members of an organization to lobby effectively for policy change, they have to be well prepared. ENA's "Staffing Advocacy Packet" provides in-depth preparation to help members lobby effectively at the state and national levels. AORN described their initiative in preparing their members with talking points and scheduling appointments with their respective legislators.
- *Send a clear, consistent message.* Whatever form lobbying takes, a clear, consistent message is essential. "Speaking with one voice" must be the mantra of all nurses involved in a particular issue. This is especially critical when partnering with other organizations.
- *Make the issue visible to those in a position to create policy change.* The messages that nursing organizations convey not only have to be clear and consistent, they must make the issue visible. Policymakers are more likely to support changes when they can "see" the issue. ANNA's program to take legislators onto the dialysis units where they could talk with patients who needed dialysis and see the challenges that faced patients and staff was an effective way of making the problem real. The tours also helped to make the problem of the shortage of nurses visible and resulted in sponsorship of both the Kidney Care Quality and Improvement Act and the Nurse Reinvestment Act. AACN's carefully planned media event illustrates how an issue can be made visible to both policymakers and the wider public.

- *Be persistent.* Policy change occurs slowly, and tenacity in the pursuit of the desired outcome is essential. All of the case studies presented here reflect a commitment to action over the long term, none more clearly than AORN's pursuit of reimbursement for the RN First Assistants. It also is important that an organization remain optimistic and open to alternative strategies when the primary strategy is unsuccessful.

## FINAL THOUGHTS

While preparation, a clear consistent message, issue visibility, and persistence are key to the success in advancing any given policy change, there are a few general strategies that will enhance the political efforts of the organization. These include building political capital, considering unintended consequences, and celebrating small wins.

### BUILD POLITICAL CAPITAL

Often, specialty organizations do not have extensive resources for political action, so building political capital that can be drawn upon when the issue arises can be a wise investment of time. Political capital is built through development of relationships with legislators, and this cannot occur just at the time that something is wanted. It can be built by being involved in a legislator's campaign for election or re-election, endorsing a candidate, offering to provide information/data on a particular health issue, or connecting the legislator with a particular group of constituents. Building relationships by helping legislators does not mean that they will be obligated to honor requests, but it usually means that they will take a few minutes to listen to the organization's concern. It also may mean that when legislators are ready to develop legislation in a selected health area, members of the organization may be called upon to provide advice. Early involvement in policy development is ideal.

### CONSIDER UNINTENDED CONSEQUENCES

Unintended outcomes may occur with policy change. Consideration of potential unintended consequences generally occurs early in the planning process, and specialty organizations, as well as all organizations, would do well to discipline themselves to engage in this analysis.

## CELEBRATE EVEN SMALL WINS

Celebration can create or renew enthusiasm and energy that will sustain the organization's long-term efforts. Celebration is also critical to keeping a coalition together and focused on their collective goal.

The specialty organization case studies presented here illustrate the wonderful policy work that is being pursued on behalf of health care consumers and nurses. They demonstrate that policy outcomes may be achieved through means other than legislation. They also illustrate the value of preparation, formation of a clear, consistent message, and making the issue visible. Finally, these case studies show the importance not only of speaking with one voice but also of engaging the voices of other consumer and professional groups.

---

*Taking Action*  Kathleen M. McCauley, Connie Barden, Ramón Lavandero, & Dana Woods

## The American Association of Critical-Care Nurses: Establishing and Sustaining Healthy Work Environments

The American Association of Critical-Care Nurses (AACN) standards on healthy work environments are a bold policy initiative of the world's largest specialty nursing organization. AACN represents more than 400,000 critical care nurses in the United States with more than 100,000 member and non-member customers in a nationwide network of 240 chapters.

### WORK ENVIRONMENTS

#### Problems in Health Care Work Environments

In 2001, AACN's leaders identified the most significant issues facing the association and its constituents in order to best focus its resources. Creating healthy work environments emerged as a critical issue in terms of the nursing shortage and the challenges nurses face in clinical practice. Efforts to attract people into nursing careers have achieved some success, with nursing school enrollments increasing in 2004. However, if attention is not given to creating and sustaining healthy work environments, it will become increasingly difficult to retain nurses. Additionally, patient safety and the financial viability of health care organizations will continue to erode (McCauley, 2005).

#### Strategy for Transforming Work Environments

Intent on producing a white paper to draw attention to the issue, a task force led by AACN Past President Connie Barden reviewed the literature on the relationship between work environments and nurse recruitment and retention, patient safety and error prevention, and health care cost. The task force's analysis confirmed the need for immediate and definitive action to eliminate the factors that make work environments toxic for patients and professionals alike. The task force further confirmed that all parties in health care—nurses, physicians, administrators, clinical and academic leaders, and professional associations—must engage to make this transformation possible. To communicate a clear message, AACN developed and published standards to assist organizations to improve their environments: The *AACN Standards for Establishing and Sustaining Healthy Work Environments: A Journey to Excellence* (American Association of Critical-Care Nurses, 2005) (Box 31-1).

The standards prompt the thoughtful reflection and dialogue required to guide an organization in transforming its work environment. They bring into sharp focus the relationship-centered factors driving professional performance, support the achievement of the Institute of Medicine's core

competencies for professional practice, and are consistent with elements of a healthful work environment identified by the Nursing Organizations Alliance (Greiner & Knebel, 2004; Nursing Organizations Alliance, 2004).

Critical elements, those behaviors or processes necessary for each standard to be achieved, accompany each standard and paint the picture of what attainment of each standard requires.

## STANDARDS RELEASED AT MEDIA EVENT

The standards were released in January 2005 at a Washington, DC, news conference. More than 40 members of the media and health care institutions attended the news conference. Another 775 joined a simultaneous Webcast. Within four months of launch, the standards had been cited in more than 300 media articles with more than 45,000 copies downloaded.

### The Problem of Dysfunctional Work Environments

In a discussion moderated by AACN President Kathleen M. McCauley, Joint Commission on Accreditation of Healthcare Organizations' President Dr. Dennis O'Leary described the impact of dysfunctional work environments on patient safety and provider effectiveness. Joseph Grenny, president of the VitalSmarts consulting group, presented findings of his team's national study, *Silence Kills* (Maxfield, Grenny, McMillan, Patterson, & Switzler, 2005). Grenny noted that even when clinicians have witnessed a colleague taking dangerous shortcuts or displaying poor clinical judgment, only 10% confront the colleague. In this study, co-sponsored by AACN, unsafe practice, unsupportive behavior, and incompetence were found to be largely unchallenged.

### Influence of a Healthy Work Environment

Karlene Kerfoot, PhD, RN, CNAA, FAAN, senior vice president for patient care services and chief nurse executive at Indianapolis-based Clarian Health Partners, a 1200-bed multisite healthcare system, discussed how her organization's focus on improving workplace communication, several years ahead

---

**BOX 31-1   Summary of the AACN Standards for Establishing and Sustaining Healthy Work Environments**

Full downloadable text along with additional references, position statements, and resources to support work environment and practice improvement are available at *www.aacn.org/hwe*.

- Skilled Communication: Nurses must be as proficient in communication skills as they are in clinical skills.
- True Collaboration: Nurses must be relentless in pursuing and fostering true collaboration.
- Effective Decision-Making: Nurses must be valued and committed partners in making policy, directing and evaluating clinical care, and leading organizational operations.
- Appropriate Staffing: Staffing must ensure the effective match between patient needs and nurse competencies.
- Meaningful Recognition: Nurses must be recognized and must recognize others for the value each brings to the work of the organization.
- Authentic Leadership: Nurse leaders must fully embrace the imperative of a healthy work environment, authentically live it, and engage others in its achievement.

From American Association of Critical-Care Nurses. (2005). AACN standards for establishing and sustaining healthy work environments: A journey to excellence. *American Journal of Critical Care, 14*(3), 187-197. Retrieved July 25, 2005, from *www.aacn.org/hwe*.

of the standards, enhanced nurse recruitment and retention and reduced medical errors.

## NEXT STEPS

AACN is committed to ensuring that these standards will set the bar for transforming clinical environments throughout the United States. Its leaders are using the standards in their own workplaces and as a focus for regional and national presentations. AACN Standards Executive Editor Connie Barden is leading a work group to develop a guiding framework for development of practical implementation strategies.

### Collaboration for Change

The standards have prompted dialogues about improving patient safety with Joint Commission Resources and the Robert Wood Johnson Foundation. The partnership with VitalSmarts is educating strategic partners and constituents about the risks inherent in the current practice environment and effective solutions to mitigate those risks. AACN has a long history of effective collaboration with medical organizations. Those relationships have been used to increase awareness of the problems in the health care work environment and the need for commitment to solutions, with the standards as an achievable goal. Existing alliances with the American College of Chest Physicians, the Society of Critical Care Medicine, and the American Thoracic Society are educating physicians about the issue, prompting them to consider their own contributions to solutions.

### Communicating the Standards to a Broader Audience

Leaders of the collaborating organizations have conducted numerous presentations about the standards to showcase their resolve to collaborate in transforming health care work environments. At a leadership meeting of the American Lung Association, Dr. McCauley presented the standards, along with data on the negative consequences of poor collaboration and dysfunctional work environments.

## SUMMARY

AACN identified creation and sustainment of healthy work environments as a key strategic initiative. The association developed *AACN Standards for Establishing and Sustaining Healthy Work Environments: A Journey to Excellence* (American Association of Critical-Care Nurses, 2005). The association has used its influential alliances, within the profession and beyond, to focus much needed attention on the work environment changes that must occur to retain nurses and enable them to thrive in practice settings. The standards are a starting point for dialogue and will prompt development of strategies and tools to transform practice environments.

### *REFERENCES*

American Association of Critical-Care Nurses. (2005). AACN standards for establishing and sustaining healthy work environments: A journey to excellence. *American Journal of Critical Care, 14*(3), 187-197. Retrieved July 25, 2005, from *www.aacn.org/hwe.*

Greiner, A. C., & Knebel, E. (Eds.). (2004). *Health professions education: A bridge to quality.* Washington, DC: National Academy Press.

Maxfield, D., Grenny, J., McMillan, R. Patterson, K., & Switzler, A. (2005). *Silence kills: The seven crucial conversations for healthcare.* Provo, UT: VitalSmarts. Retrieved July 25, 2005, from *www.silencekills.com.*

McCauley, K. (2005). Guest editorial: A message from the American Association of Critical-Care Nurses. *American Journal of Critical Care, 14*(3), 186.

Nursing Organizations Alliance. (2004). Principles and elements of a healthful work environment. Retrieved July 25, 2005, from *www.nursing-alliance.org.*

## The Oncology Nursing Society: Engaging Support for the Nurse Reinvestment Act

The Oncology Nursing Society (ONS), the largest cancer-related specialty organization in the world, is composed of more than 33,000 nurses and other health professionals dedicated to ensuring access to quality care for people with cancer. Its health policy agenda prioritizes issues of importance to cancer patients and their families and to the nursing community as a whole.

### THE PROBLEM: THE NURSING SHORTAGE

A shortage of registered nurses (RNs) and nursing faculty threatens the health and well-being of U.S. citizens. In July 2002, the U.S. Department of Health and Human Services estimated that, by 2020, there will be a shortage of approximately 800,000 nurses nationwide (Health Resources and Services Administration, 2002). The Bureau of Labor Statistics, U.S. Department of Labor, reported in the February 2004 edition of the *Monthly Labor Review* that RNs will experience the largest job growth of all U.S. professions from 2002 to 2012 as health care facilities will need to fill more than 1.1 million nursing positions (Hecker, 2004). In the Institute of Medicine's (1999) report *To Err is Human: Building a Safer System,* the Institute found that as many as 98,000 hospitalized Americans die each year from treatment errors. Nursing shortages lead to increased nurse-patient ratios, which, in turn, increase patient morbidity and mortality.

### THE "PERFECT STORM"

The nursing workforce is aging. The average age of RNs is forecasted to be 45.4 years by 2010, with more than 40% of the workforce older than age 50 (Buerhaus, Staiger, & Auerbach, 2000), half of whom are expected to reach retirement age between the years 2010 and 2025. As the average age of current RN graduates is 31, these graduates will have fewer

years to work (Sigma Theta Tau, 2005). Nursing schools lack capacity due to faculty shortages. In 2003, Health Resources and Services Administration received more than 8300 applications for the Nurse Education Loan Repayment Program and more than 4500 applications for the Nurse Scholarship Program but could only fund 7% and 2%, respectively. In 2004, U.S. nursing schools turned away more than 32,000 qualified applicants for baccalaureate and graduate nursing programs, including 3000 students with the potential to fill faculty roles.

An aging population further strains the health care system. By 2030, the number of individuals in the United States older than age 65 years will double, and the number older than 85 years will quadruple. Age is the single greatest risk factor for developing cancer. Sixty percent of cancer cases and two thirds of cancer deaths occur in those older than 65. An overall nursing shortage predicts a commensurate decrease in trained oncology nurses. Oncology nursing care is rapidly changing, as targeted therapies, those agents that interfere with processes that support tumor growth and progression, display a different paradigm of side effects than traditional chemotherapeutic agents. The solution is two-fold: (a) a new cadre of nurses that require oncology-specific education, supervision, and mentoring by seasoned oncology nurses and (b) ongoing education for those nurses practicing in a multitude of care sites. Without an adequate supply of trained, educated, and experienced oncology nurses, the nation will falter in its delivery of the benefits derived from the federal investment in cancer research.

### THE NURSE REINVESTMENT ACT

Three years ago in response to the national nursing shortage, the Nurse Reinvestment Act (NRAct) of

2002 was signed into law with broad bipartisan support. It authorized new programs to increase the number of qualified nurses and the quality of nursing services in the United States. Although the enactment marked a significant moment for the American nursing community and the viability of the nation's health care safety net, authorizing statutes do not provide funding; separate appropriations measures must be enacted annually. Recently, serious budgetary constraints have limited Congress's ability to allocate sufficient resources for discretionary programs such as the NRAct. As such, whereas the NRAct has received increased funding each fiscal year since its enactment, annual congressional allocations for the NRAct have fallen far short of what the nursing community deems is necessary to stem the tide of the current and expected shortage.

## THE STRATEGIC POWER OF NUMBERS

According to a national poll released in February 2002 by the Vanderbilt University's School of Nursing and Center for Health Services Research in Nashville, Tennessee, 81% of Americans recognize there is a nursing shortage, and 65% believe it is either a major problem or a crisis. Ninety-three percent agree that the nursing shortage jeopardizes the quality of health care in the United States (American Nurses Association, 2002). ONS recognized that the nursing community could not be the sole voice advocating for funding for the NRAct to address the nursing shortage, and it made a strategic decision to educate cancer patients, affected families, and national cancer organizations about the nursing shortage and its potential to adversely affect access to quality cancer care and impede progress in cancer research. By educating and enlisting the cancer community in this regard, ONS helped create a "consumer movement" of patient advocacy organizations to increase congressional awareness of the nursing shortage and elicit support for increased funding. ONS regularly takes the lead in organizing cancer community letters to the House and Senate Labor Health and Human Services Appropriations Subcommittees that control funding for the NRAct. These efforts consistently net more than 45 cancer organizations

as signatories who join together in calling upon Congress for additional resources for the NRAct.

## THE OUTCOMES

Due to ONS's outreach and education efforts, two key cancer coalitions have added funding for the NRAct to their legislative agendas: One Voice Against Cancer, a collaboration of more than 45 voluntary health and advocacy organizations focused on increasing federal appropriations to fund cancer research and application programs and the National Coalition for Cancer Research, a nonprofit organization comprising 26 national organizations and dedicated to the eradication of cancer through a vigorous public and privately supported research effort. Many Capitol Hill staff have indicated that the cancer community sign-on letters, along with the cancer coalitions' support, have been critical in building the case for and securing increased funding for the NRAct. ONS maintains a commitment to working with the nursing and cancer communities to ensure that adequate resources continue to be allocated to the NRAct so that the nation has the nursing workforce necessary to care for the patients of today and tomorrow.

### REFERENCES

American Association of Colleges of Nursing. (2005). 2003-2004 enrollment and graduations in baccalaureate and graduate programs in nursing. Retrieved July 30, 2005, from *www.aacn.nche.edu*.

American Nurses Association. (2002). Poll, campaign address nursing shortage. Retrieved August 1, 2005, from *www.nursingworld.org/tan/marap02/inbrief.htm*.

Buerhaus, P. I., Staiger, D. O., & Auerbach, D. I. (2000). Policy responses to an aging registered nurse workforce. *Nursing Economics, 18*(6), 278-303.

Health Resources and Services Administration. (2002). Projected supply, demand and shortage of registered nurses, 2000-2020. Retrieved August 9, 2005, from *http://bhpr.hrsa.gov/healthworkforce/reports/rnproject*.

Hecker, D. E. (2004, February). Bureau of Labor Statistics. Occupational employment projections to 2012. *Monthly Labor Review*, pp. 80-105.

Institute of Medicine, Committee on Quality Health Care in America. (1999). *To err is human: Building a safer system.* Washington, DC: National Academy Press.

Sigma Theta Tau. (2005). Facts on the nursing shortage in North America. Retrieved July 30, 2005, from *www.nursingsociety.org/media/facts_nursingshortage.html*.

## *Taking Action*    Kathleen Kuchta & Nancy J. Sharp

# The American Nephrology Nurses' Association:
# A Grassroots Initiative to Educate Lawmakers

## THE ECONOMIC CONTEXT OF RENAL DISEASE

End stage renal disease (ESRD) affects 400,000 Americans whose lives depend upon renal dialysis or transplantation. In 1972, the U.S. Congress established Medicare coverage for the vast majority of these patients. In 1983, Congress approved reimbursement for dialysis providers under the first Medicare Prospective Payment System, which became known as the composite rate. Approximately 75% of all ESRD patients depend upon Medicare for some or all of their dialysis treatment reimbursement. State Medicaid programs pay for approximately 20% of the remaining ESRD reimbursement. More than 20 years after Congress approved the ESRD composite rate, it is still the only Medicare Prospective Payment System without an automatic annual update mechanism to adjust for inflation and changes in prices of dialysis services. Only Congress can approve changes in the ESRD composite rate and add an automatic increase based upon inflation.

## A PILOT INITIATIVE TO EDUCATE LAWMAKERS

In 2003, the American Nephrology Nurses' Association (ANNA), which has 115 chapters in 47 states and U.S. territories and whose membership is close to 12,000, piloted a grassroots advocacy project designed to educate lawmakers about ESRD, the need for a composite rate increase, and other issues facing the renal community, such as the nursing shortage. The pilot program had two component parts: a 16-page ESRD Briefing Book for State and Federal Policymakers and invitations to lawmakers to tour dialysis facilities in their home districts during their August summer recess. Thus was born the ESRD Education Day, first held on August 15, 2003.

ANNA chapter members were encouraged to participate in the pilot program, and a planning and orientation guide (P&OG) was developed to help members learn step by step how to participate in this new initiative. For easy access, both the briefing book and the planning and orientation guide were placed on the ANNA Website.

A list of key lawmakers was developed to include federal policymakers who sit on the three congressional committees responsible for ESRD Medicare funding decisions: the Senate Finance, the House Ways and Means, and the House Energy and Commerce Committees. The lawmaker list was then matched with corresponding ANNA chapters, and ANNA members were encouraged to invite their representatives to tour a dialysis facility in their area. Members were also encouraged to invite visits by state legislators, governors, Centers for Medicare and Medicaid Services personnel, state health department personnel, or other officials deemed important to the renal community.

ANNA members' enthusiasm for the pilot ESRD Education Day 2003 resulted in 62 lawmaker visits to 83 dialysis facilities in 30 states. These results convinced the ANNA Board of Directors to approve a resolution for an annual ESRD Education Day. The momentum from 2003 carried forward into 2004, during which 121 lawmakers visited 83 dialysis facilities in 33 states.

## BUILDING ON SUCCESS

In 2005, ANNA expanded the program to an entire week; the initiative was renamed ESRD Education Week and was held in early August 2005. Expansion of the program to a week provides more flexibility for lawmakers to tour facilities and makes it easier for elected officials to obtain state proclamations for ESRD Education Week.

Dialysis facility tours are an integral part of the ESRD education initiative. The tours allow policymakers to see the challenges facing patients and staff and learn firsthand about the issues in renal care. They begin to see the real need for an annual update mechanism for the composite rate and how the nursing shortage truly affects quality patient care. Lawmakers who toured dialysis facilities in 2005 remarked that it was time well spent and that they would return to Congress or their state legislatures with a much better appreciation of the issues facing the renal community. After touring dialysis facilities, several policymakers committed to supporting legislation that was enacted as the Title VIII Nursing Workforce Development Program.

## LESSONS LEARNED
### Follow Up
Pleasant but persistent follow-up by ANNA members is necessary to turn an invitation into an actual commitment by the lawmaker to tour a dialysis facility. The ANNA chapter members who excel in this area generally organize the most tours. Lawmakers are very busy, especially when they are on recess and in their home districts. They have many constituents who are asking for their time, and not every request can be honored. Therefore, we have learned to follow up, follow up, and follow up again. Sometimes, the sheer persistence of our members is the reason a lawmaker finally decides to tour a facility. Targeting specific members of Congress who sit on committees that regulate Medicare and Medicaid funding also results in more tours.

### Disseminate Information
Clearly defining the issues for the lawmaker is critical, and preparation of our members is key to their success. To help in this effort, ANNA members receive one-page informational documents designed to quickly educate them and lawmakers about key legislation such as the Kidney Care Quality and Improvement Act and the Nurse Reinvestment Act. We have also received excellent feedback from lawmakers regarding the ESRD Briefing Book for State and Federal Policymakers that we provide for them during their tour of a dialysis facility. The briefing book is designed to help laypersons understand the most common causes of ESRD and chronic kidney disease, different dialysis modalities, common complications of dialysis, vascular access, and composite rate information.

### Obtain Support from Other Interested Parties
The ANNA education initiative was supported by Kidney Care Partners. This is a coalition that includes large dialysis firms, pharmaceutical manufacturers, the National Renal Administrators Association, the Renal Physicians Association, and the National Kidney Foundation in addition to patient advocacy groups such as DaVita Patient Citizens and the Renal Support Network. Their support was critical in making it an effective means to communicate with key policymakers.

## OUTCOMES AND FUTURE PLANS
An unanticipated outcome of the ESRD Education Week was that ANNA received an award for this grassroots project. ANNA Past President Caroline Counts presented the project to the American Society of Association Executives, and ANNA received their 2004 Associations' Advance America Honor Roll award for the ESRD Education Day initiative. This award showcases organizations that help improve American society with innovative projects and inspire similar activities. The award provided visibility for the work ANNA has done in advancing policy changes.

The ESRD education initiative has also enabled ANNA members to assume a leadership role within the renal community. This grassroots advocacy project has not only led to significantly improved ESRD knowledge for lawmakers but has also given our membership an education in the political/legislative process with a hands-on fun and exciting initiative that they have truly embraced. Although the reimbursement legislation has not been modified, ANNA plans to continue to expand ESRD Education Week activities and is optimistic that changes will be achieved.

## Web Resources

**ANNA ESRD Briefing Book for State and
    Federal Policymakers**
*www.annanurse.org/download/reference/practice/
    legbrief.pdf*
**Centers for Medicare and Medicaid Services
    End Stage Renal Disease Information**
*www.cms.hhs.gov/ESRDGeneralInformation/*
**Kidney Care Partners**
*www.kidneycarepartners.com/about/index.html*
**Nursing Workforce Development
    Programs—Title VIII Public Health
    Service Act**
*www.bhpr.hrsa.gov/nursing/titleviii.htm*

## Taking Action    Rita L. Griffith

### The Association of periOperative Registered Nurses: Reimbursement Policy for Registered Nurse First Assistants

### THE ISSUE

A variety of individuals, with varying backgrounds and preparation, function as surgical first assistants, the individuals who provide direct support to surgeons during surgical procedures. Registered nurses, working under the professional name Registered Nurse First Assistant (RNFA), are one of the groups who serve in this capacity. But these nurses are not eligible to bill Medicare directly for reimbursement; instead, they are paid by the hospital or surgeon (Hackbarth, 2004).

The Association of periOperative Registered Nurses (AORN) has collaborated for years with RNFAs to promote legislation regarding state and Medicare reimbursement for RNFAs. These efforts include grassroots education, lobbying at the local and federal levels, contacts with state and federal lobbyists and strategists, the introduction of three House bills in Congress, and mandated reports by government agencies. It is AORN's belief that the RNFA is the most qualified provider of assistant-at-surgery services, and their reimbursement should be equitable with other non-physician providers.

### ROLE OF THE RNFA

A critical component of any effort to seek reimbursement for a category of provider is the clear definition of the provider's role and the establishment of credentials. The RNFA is a perioperative registered nurse who works in collaboration with the surgeon and health care team to achieve optimal patient outcomes. The RNFA must have acquired the necessary knowledge, judgment, and skills specific to the expanded role of RNFA clinical practice. Intra-operatively, the RNFA practices at the direction of the surgeon and does not concurrently function as a scrub nurse (AORN, 2005). There has been long-standing validation and support of the RNFA role:

1. The nurse practice acts in all 50 states recognize that the RNFA role is within the nursing scope of practice.
2. Professional associations, including AORN, the American Nurses Association, the National League for Nursing, and others, acknowledge the RNFA as a highly educated and qualified perioperative nurse, who assists the surgeon during an operation.
3. The AORN standards for RNFA programs (AORN, 2002b) provide the framework that registered nurses utilize to prepare for the role of the assistant-at-surgery in the operating room and other areas of surgical practice.
4. The RNFA Specialty Assembly, along with AORN, developed and published the RNFA competencies (AORN, 2002a). The competencies are a tool used to authenticate the level of RNFA clinical expertise when determining credentialing in facilities, job descriptions, and evaluations.
5. Individuals attain the RNFA credential by successfully completing an RNFA educational program.
6. Once eligibility criteria are met, board certification can be attained by successful completion of a national certification exam.

## ECONOMIC CONTEXT

The role of the RNFA in an expanded capacity within the operating room specialty is constantly evolving. RNFAs may be employed by hospitals or by surgeons, or they may act as independent practitioners.

Reimbursement has been pursued at the state level, and some gains have been made. Florida was the first state to pass legislation, in 1994, allowing direct reimbursement for the RNFA. By 2001, Kentucky, Maine, Minnesota, Rhode Island, and Washington had passed legislation allowing third-party RNFA reimbursement. As of 2005, there were 11 states, including Illinois, West Virginia, Texas, Louisiana, and Georgia, that had passed similar RNFA reimbursement legislation. Efforts to organize grassroots groups, educate hospital administrators, and lobby state legislators continue in all 50 states.

Medicare reimbursement is important to the marketability of the RNFA. Without it, the RNFA may experience limitations in employability. Surgeons and facility administrators do not always embrace the RNFA's value and training. Unfortunately, it is primarily a fiscal decision to hire and promote the federally reimbursed individual.

## INITIATIVES TO ACHIEVE REIMBURSEMENT

While RNFAs have pursued reimbursement for surgical assisting services at the state level, federal RNFA activity has also been under way. These initiatives have met with progress and defeat along the way. AORN has dedicated time and expertise to educating the RNFA membership to promote the RNFA's federal reimbursement initiatives. AORN has also supplied RNFAs with a dedicated health policy department, offered educational forums, and provided valuable resources in an attempt to move the RNFA Medicare reimbursement initiative. An annual "Lobby Day" in Washington, DC has provided opportunities to directly address congressional representatives and their health care aides. RNFAs are instructed on talking points and receive appointments with their respective senators and district representatives.

## OUTCOMES

### Bills Introduced in Congress

Three House bills, HR 1388 in the 108th Congress, HR 822 in the 107th Congress, and HR 3911 in the 106th Congress, were introduced to deal with the issue of RNFA reimbursement. The three bills were introduced by Representative Mac Collins (R-GA-3), had large bipartisan support, and were vetted by

AORN's lobbying firm but failed to gain a Senate sponsor and ultimately died without passage.

## Government Accountability Office Study on Registered Nurse First Assistants

On Dec 21, 2000, President Bill Clinton signed into law HR 4577, which included a provision that directed the Government Accounting Office (GAO) (renamed the Government Accountability Office in July of 2004) to conduct a study on the coverage of surgical first assisting services of certified RNFAs. The study was to focus on the impact of quality of care, appropriate education and training requirements, and appropriate rates of payment. The report by the GAO in January 2004, two years past due, did not meet the expectations of RNFAs. The report concentrated on all providers of surgical assisting services rather than focusing on RNFAs. The report stated the entire Medicare assisting services payment system needed an overhaul. It recommended that assisting service payments should be made from Medicare Part A rather than direct billing under Medicare part B (U.S. Government Accountability Office, 2004).

## A Medicare Payment Advisory Commission Study

A Medicare Payment Advisory Commission study on direct certified RNFA Medicare reimbursement was mandated by the Medicare Prescription Drug, Improvement and Modernization Act of 2003 (Medicare Payment Advisory Commission, 2004). The commission made a more positive statement, indicating that the RNFA is a qualified provider, but for an RNFA to become a Medicare provider, legislation would have to be passed by Congress.

## NEXT STEPS

RNFAs and AORN are actively pursuing the goal of achieving Medicare reimbursement for the RNFA. These efforts include the following:

1. Educating members of Congress
2. Seeking a legislative vehicle for possible amendment
3. Directing lobbying efforts toward obtaining sponsorship of members of House and Senate committees that influence Medicare spending decisions.

### REFERENCES

Association of periOperative Registered Nurses (AORN). (2002a). Registered nurse first assistant competencies. *AORN Journal, 76*, 671-679. Retrieved July 18, 2005, from *www.aorn.org/practice/pdf/rnfa_compet_8-02.pdf.*

Association of periOperative Registered Nurses (AORN). (2002b). Standards for first assistant programs. Retrieved July 8, 2005, from *www.aorn.org/practice/pdf/RNFAEdStand05.pdf.*

Association of periOperative Registered Nurses (AORN). (2005). AORN official statement on RN first assistants. Standards, recommended practices, and guidelines. Retrieved July 6, 2005, from *www.aorn.org/sa/RNFAbrochure3.pdf.*

Hackbarth, G. M. (2004). Letter to Honorable Richard B. Cheney, President of the Senate. Washington, DC: Medicare Payment Advisory Commission. Retrieved December 8, 2005, from *www.medpac.gov/publications/congressional_reports/Dec04_CRNFA.pdf.*

Medicare Payment Advisory Commission (MEDPAC). (2004). Report on the feasibility and advisability of paying certified registered nurse first assistants. Retrieved July 18, 2005, from *www.medpac.gov/publications/congressional_reports/Dec04_CRNFA.pdf.*

U.S. General Accounting Office. (2004). Medicare: Payment changes are needed for assistants-at-surgery. Retrieved July 18, 2005, from *www.gao.gov/new.items/d0497.pdf.*

# The American Association of Occupational Health Nurses: Policy Initiatives to Address Workplace Violence

## THE PROBLEM AND ECONOMIC CONTEXT

Workplace violence is a serious occupational risk for the U.S. workforce and a major public health problem. Wilkinson and Peek-Asa (2003) defined workplace violence as "any physical assault, threatening behavior, or verbal abuse that occurs in the workplace or arises because of an employment-based relationship" (p. xiii). Workplace violence occurs along a continuum ranging from psychological threats (threatening behavior, harassment, stalking, intimidation, and bullying) to physical assault (beating, shoving, biting, and slapping), to homicide. Approximately 2 million people in the United States are victims of workplace violence each year (Occupational Safety and Health Administration [OSHA], 2002). In 2002, homicide was the leading cause of workplace death for women and the second leading cause of death for men. Nearly one in five on-the-job fatalities results from homicide (Bureau of Labor Statistics, 2003). In 2000, 48% of all non-fatal injuries from occupational assaults and violent acts occurred in health care and social services. In fact, nurses had an incidence rate of 25.0 for injuries resulting from assaults and violent acts, compared to 9.3 for health service workers and 15.0 for social-service workers (OSHA, 2003). The impact of workplace violence on employers and employees is enormous. The combined costs of lost wages and lost productivity are estimated to be in the billions of dollars.

## SOLUTIONS

Recognizing this disturbing national trend, the American Association of Occupational Health Nurses (AAOHN) set out to raise awareness of workplace violence, influence public policy decisions on its prevention, and promote the role of occupational and environmental health nurses. Workplace violence prevention continues to be one of several key areas on the AAOHN annual public policy platform. With that serving as the driving force, the organization identified opportunities to create change and implemented a plan to move workplace violence prevention forward. This was accomplished through establishing a formal alliance with a federal government agency, partnering with universities for a pilot prevention program, conducting research into the scope of the problem, sponsoring educational conferences and providing speakers, and submitting comments on a proposed national workplace violence survey.

## STRATEGIES

On May 7, 2003, AAOHN and OSHA signed a formal alliance agreement to collaborate on workplace violence, one of three focus areas for both organizations. In the agreement, AAOHN and OSHA committed to the direct dissemination of workplace violence information and guidance to businesses and to the provision of information through meetings, conferences, events, and print and electronic media, including links from AAOHN's and OSHA's Websites. The organizations agreed to encourage AAOHN chapters to build relationships with OSHA's regional and area offices to address workplace violence. AAOHN and OSHA also agreed to develop electronic assistance tools for OSHA's webpage that address health and safety issues, including workplace violence.

Also in 2003, AAOHN developed a plan to create a series of workplace violence prevention programs at universities around the country. The programs would bring together health care providers, employers, community groups, and citizens to study, design, report, and disseminate research findings. AAOHN and Texas Woman's University partnered to secure a federal earmark for a pilot program that could be replicated at other colleges and universities. The pilot program will identify ways to improve an employer's ability to prevent violent incidents in the workplace and increase the number of workplace violence prevention programs across the country. Although the pilot program has not yet received funding, AAOHN and Texas Woman's University have actively lobbied Congress during 2004 and again in 2005 for funding of this critical information gathering and dissemination effort. This lobbying also included visits to the Georgia and Texas state delegations, stressing the importance of this program and how occupational and environmental health nurses help coordinate prevention efforts at worksites.

AAOHN designed and conducted a survey in October 2003 to gauge employee knowledge of the issue of workplace violence and demonstrate the need for violence prevention education. To help ensure survey accuracy, experts from the Federal Bureau of Investigation's National Center for Analysis and Violent Crime were consulted during the development of survey criteria. Respondents to AAOHN's survey were asked about their personal experiences, concerns, perceptions, and overall awareness of the issue. AAOHN's study found that nearly 20% of the entire workforce claimed they have experienced an episode of workplace violence firsthand, yet the majority still does not know what to look for when it comes to determining potential offender characteristics. The findings of the study were released in December 2003. The study results are being used to justify educational programs and how the occupational and environmental health nurse is critical to its success.

AAOHN also joined with the American Society of the University of Haifa to host an international conference titled "Living with Terrorism and Violence: Psychosocial Effects." The conference, hosted at the National Press Club in Washington, DC, in June of 2004, featured AAOHN members as speakers and panelists. Later in the year, AAOHN served on the planning committee for a workplace violence prevention conference hosted by the National Institute for Occupational Safety and Health.

## CONTINUING INITIATIVES

Committed to seeing progress and change on the issue of workplace violence, AAOHN has continued their work. In January of 2005, AAOHN reviewed and submitted comments on a proposed workplace violence survey being conducted by the Bureau of Labor Statistics and the National Institute for Occupational Safety and Health.

Through the survey work conducted by AAOHN and the relationships with other organizations interested in workplace violence prevention, AAOHN has identified the serious need for additional research of the causes, signs, and methods of preventing acts of workplace violence. AAOHN continues to identify areas of opportunities to promote workplace violence prevention and influence changes in public policy.

## *Lessons Learned*

- Workplace violence is a serious occupational risk affecting about 2 million people each year; however, the majority of people do not recognize signs or characteristics of workplace violence.
- Partnerships with businesses, governmental agencies, and universities are effective in the prevention of workplace violence.
- Occupational and environmental health nurses are instrumental in developing, managing, and implementing workplace violence programs in the workplace.

## *Web Resources*

**Federal Bureau of Investigation, Workplace Violence—Issues in Response**
*www.fbi.gov/publications/violence.pdf*
**Occupational Safety and Health Administration, Safety and Health Topics—Workplace Violence**
*www.osha.gov/SLTC/workplaceviolence/index.html*

*Continued*

*Web Resources — cont'd*

> **National Institute for Occupational Safety and Health, Violence in the Workplace— Risk Factors and Prevention Strategies**
> *www.cdc.gov/niosh/violcont.html*

### REFERENCES
Bureau of Labor Statistics. (2003). Regional variations in workplace homicide rates. Washington, DC: U.S. Department of Labor. Retrieved June 24, 2005, from *www.bls.gov/opub/cwc/sh20031119ar01p1.htm*.

Occupational Safety and Health Administration. (2002). Fact Sheet: Workplace violence. Washington, DC: U.S. Department of Labor. Retrieved June 24, 2005, from *www.osha.gov/OshDoc/data_General_Facts/factsheet-workplace-violence.pdf*.

Occupational Safety and Health Administration. (2003). Guidelines for preventing workplace violence for health-care and social-service workers (Publication No. 3148). Washington, DC: U.S. Department of Labor. Retrieved June 24, 2005, from *www.osha.gov/Publications/osha3148.pdf*.

Wilkinson, C., & Peek-Asa, C. (2003). Preface: Violence in the workplace. *Clinics in Occupational and Environmental Medicine, 3*(4), xiii-xiv.

# *Taking Action* Kathy Robinson

## The Emergency Nurses Association: Making the Case for Safe Staffing Systems

### THE PROBLEM

Several published studies have established what most nurses already know: there is a direct correlation between staffing and patient outcomes. One recent study conducted by researchers at the University of Pennsylvania found that higher nurse staffing levels, particularly with a greater number of registered nurses in the staffing mix, correlated with a 3% to 12% reduction in certain adverse outcomes, including urinary tract infection, pneumonia, shock, and upper gastrointestinal bleeding (Aiken, Clarke, Sloane, Sochalski, & Silber, 2002). Efforts focusing on quantifying the number of nurses needed to care for specific patient populations have identified thresholds at which certain patients are at a substantially increased risk of quality problems and, conversely, levels at which no additional improvements in quality are observed simply because the staffing level is increased. Although the lower threshold of staffing has tempted some activists to try to use them in terms of minimum "nurse-patient ratios," the concept of legislating ratios is complex, controversial, and a focus of the Emergency Nurses Association's (ENA) policy efforts.

### BACKGROUND

California was the first state to implement numeric staffing ratios for acute care hospitals in October 1999 when Governor Gray Davis signed AB394 into law. AB394 sets only the minimum number of nurse-to-patient ratios. Hailing this effort as a profound accomplishment, various labor groups have embarked on a mission to encourage similar legislation across the country. The problem is one size DOESN'T fit all.

An attempt to identify the appropriateness of establishing minimum staffing ratios in nursing homes was conducted by the U.S. Department of

Health and Human Services in 2000 (Feuerberg, 2000). However, this study does not fully address important related issues such as the following:

■ The relative importance of other factors, such as management, tenure, and training of staff, in determining nursing home quality
■ The reality of current nursing shortages
■ Other operational details, such as the difference between new nurses and experienced nurses, staff mix, retention and turnover rates, and staff organization

For these reasons and others, it would be improper to conclude that the staffing thresholds described in this study and its subsequent follow-up (Feuerberg, 2001) should be used as staffing standards. Most important, these studies do not provide enough information to address the question posed by Congress regarding the appropriateness of establishing minimum ratios. This opinion was seemingly supported by the Institute of Medicine; the institute was not prepared to recommend a minimum ratio, in part, because there was not sufficient knowledge to appropriately adjust any recommended ratio by the case mix of the patient population. Although the need for increased staff may seem intuitively obvious, the empirical evidence in support of this general position and in support of specific ratios is fragmentary.

A preliminary analysis by the Center for Medicare and Medicaid Service's Office of the Actuary indicated that the total national incremental cost of implementing the "preferred" minimum nurse staffing ratios identified in the phase 1 analysis is on the order of $7.6 billion for FY 2001. In spite of the lack of scientific merit for implementing mandated staffing ratios, labor organizations continue to aggressively advocate for them and challenge any countermeasures to their efforts as being driven by hospital administration to reduce costs at the expense of patient care.

## EMERGENCY NURSES ASSOCIATION'S RATIONALE FOR ACTION

With the implementation of staffing ratios in California, the realities, limitations, and drawbacks of this unilateral staffing measure have become apparent. Several emergency departments (EDs) have encountered a problem by achieving minimum staffing ratios but still not having enough nurses to properly care for patients, especially critical patients who are boarded in the ED. Some nurses believe that the law is too rigid, is difficult to follow at all times, and decreases the nurses' flexibility and choice in determining the best way to provide coverage for breaks and patient care.

To understand ENA's position on staffing ratios and its advocacy efforts to support safe staffing systems, it is important to understand the difference between benchmark staffing data and best practice staffing data, as this point illustrates our difference of opinion with the organizations who continue to advocate for mandated ratios.

Benchmarking is a common industry practice that facilities use to compare themselves to similar facilities with the common goal of achieving improvement. Currently, the most common administrative method for determining levels of nurse staffing in the ED is based on a productivity measure called "hours per patient visit" (HPPV). Using this method, the total number of paid nursing staff hours is divided by the total number of ED visits to yield a number in hours per patient visit. A critical limitation in the use of HPPV benchmarking data is that all patients are considered equal regardless of the nursing resources needed to provide care for the patient's condition. Neither nurse-to-patient ratios nor HPPV productivity benchmarks have been based on research or best practices regarding patient care and safety. Neither of them gives consideration to the key variables regarding ED patients. In other words, a patient requiring the administration of fibrinolytics for a myocardial infarction is considered the same as a patient with a sore throat, even though the resources needed to care for each patient are dramatically different. In its position statement on staffing and productivity in the ED, ENA rejects mandated ratios. ENA notes, "Staffing based solely on nurse to patient ratios or paid hours per visit is limited in scope without consideration of the variables that affect the consumption of nursing resources" (ENA, 2003a). Best practice staffing is defined by ENA as that which provides timely and efficient patient care and a safe environment for both patients and staff, while promoting an atmosphere of professional nursing satisfaction.

## STRATEGIES FOR SOLUTION

In 2001, ENA began researching new methodologies to assist EDs in determining best practice staffing. To identify safe, effective, realistic best practice staffing in EDs, the association developed the "ENA Guidelines for Emergency Department Nurse Staffing" (2003b), utilizing six key variables that were determined to be critical in the projection of staffing requirements, the development of staffing models, and accurate budget preparation. These guidelines calculate the number of patient care full-time equivalents (FTEs) needed to staff an ED based on its own unique patient population, nursing resources, and patient throughput in the ED. It assists managers and hospital administrators in analyzing census patterns in order to best plan for the distribution of appropriate nursing staff by patient volume trends. The guidelines were field tested over two years, utilizing data from 30 EDs of varied facility types, locations, and census across the country and included the use of computer simulation modeling. The six key variables are (1) patient census, (2), patient acuity, (3), patient length of stay, (4) nursing time for nursing interventions and activities by patient acuity (utilizing the Nursing Interventions Classification [NIC] system developed by the Center for Nursing Classification at the University of Iowa), (5) skill mix for providing patient care based on nursing interventions that can be delegated to a non-registered nurse, and (6) an adjustment factor for the nonpatient care time included in each FTE.

ENA strongly believes that the "appropriateness" of establishing minimum nurse staffing ratios cannot be inferred solely from empirical studies demonstrating a strong relationship between critical staffing ratio thresholds and patient outcomes. ENA's efforts in this regard are outlined in the association's current public policy agenda. An ED staffing advocacy packet was developed intended to educate members and to support member advocacy efforts at the state and federal levels to pass legislation that support safe staffing systems. The packet includes a how-to checklist, a template letter activating state ENA members, an issue brief on staffing in the ED, background articles and information, a template appointment letter to legislators, and a "leave behind" for legislators on staffing in the ED.

## ONGOING EFFORTS

Efforts with legislators and networking with other membership associations are ongoing, and the situation remains unresolved. Newer legislative efforts also include language that would require hospitals to prominently post their nurse staffing levels on a daily basis. Without clarification or guidance on interpreting such numbers and how they relate to patient census, acuity, and other related factors, one wonders if this strategy will be more successful in illustrating hospital shortfalls in staffing or encouraging frustrated patients and families to target nurses at a time when workforce shortages are affecting multiple health care disciplines and also the timeliness of patient care across the country.

### REFERENCES

Aiken, L. H., Clarke, S. P., Sloane, D. M., Sochalski, J., & Silber, J. H. (2002). Hospital nurse staffing and patient mortality, nurse burnout, and job dissatisfaction. *Journal of the American Medical Association, 288*, 1987-1993.

Emergency Nurses Association. (2003a). *ENA guidelines for emergency department nurse staffing*. Des Plaines, IL: Emergency Nurses Association.

Emergency Nurses Association. (2003b). *Position statement: Staffing and productivity in the emergency care setting*. Des Plaines, IL: Emergency Nurses Association.

Feuerberg, M. (2000, July 20). *Report to Congress: Appropriateness of minimum nurse staffing ratios in nursing homes*. Baltimore: Health Care Financing Administration.

Feuerberg, M. (2001, December). *Report To Congress: Appropriateness of minimum nurse staffing ratios in nursing homes: Phase II final*, Baltimore: Centers for Medicare and Medicaid Services.

*Taking Action* Karen G. Duderstadt, Richard Ricciardi,
& Mary Margaret Gottesman

## The National Association of Pediatric Nurse Practitioners: Taking Action on the Epidemic of Childhood Overweight

### COMMITMENT TO ADVOCACY

Since 1974, the National Association of Pediatric Nurse Practitioners (NAPNAP) has demonstrated a sustained commitment to advocacy on professional practice and child health policy issues. NAPNAP's efforts have contributed to securing prescriptive authority for nurse practitioners, obtaining federal funds for nurse practitioner educational programs, and ensuring nurse practitioners are eligible to be reimbursed for children's health services. NAPNAP's public policy agenda currently focuses on three areas of advocacy:

1. Promotion and protection of children's health
2. Access to comprehensive health care for all children
3. Promoting access to health care services provided by pediatric nurse practitioners

### THE EPIDEMIC OF CHILDHOOD OVERWEIGHT

Significant progress was made during the twentieth century on scope of practice issues for nurse practitioners and improvements in the health of children. However, we entered the twenty-first century with a growing health burden in the pediatric population: the epidemic of childhood overweight and obesity (Box 31-2).

Overweight/obesity is now the most common chronic condition in childhood, with its prevalence disproportionately affecting ethnically diverse children. Childhood overweight/obesity is associated with both immediate and long-term health risks. Children who are overweight are predisposed to type II diabetes, hypertension, dyslipidemia, and mental health problems (Barlow & Dietz, 2002; Strauss, 1999; Troiano & Flegal 1998). In addition to

health risks, there are considerable economic costs. The estimated annual cost of obesity and overweight in the United States in 2002 was $117 billion, accounting for an estimated 31% of the total direct costs of 15 comorbid conditions (Weschler, 2004).

### STRATEGY FOR ACTION

NAPNAP identified the prevention of childhood overweight/obesity as an issue of national priority and set a goal to significantly reduce this public

---

**BOX 31-2** How Are Obesity and Overweight Defined?

Overweight and obesity are labels for ranges of weight that are greater than what is considered healthy for a specific height. For adults, overweight and obesity ranges are determined by using weight and height to calculate the body mass index (BMI). However, for children and adolescents, gender and growth must be considered. Therefore, BMI for children is referred to as BMI-for-age and is gender and age specific (CDC, 2005).

The Centers for Disease Control and Prevention (CDC) provides BMI-for-age, gender-specific weight charts that contain specific percentiles. Health care professionals use these percentile cutoff points to assess underweight and overweight in children.

| WEIGHT STATUS | BMI-FOR-AGE |
|---|---|
| Underweight | < 5th percentile |
| Normal | 5th percentile to < 85th percentile |
| At risk of overweight | 85th percentile to < 95th percentile |
| Overweight | ≥ 95th percentile |

From Centers for Disease Control and Prevention. (2005). Body mass index for children and teens. Retrieved October 10, 2005, from *www.cdc.gov/nccdphp/dnpa/bmi/bmi-for-age.htm*.

health threat. The association is by no means alone in its advocacy efforts around childhood overweight. A challenge from the beginning was to distinguish NAPNAP's approach to the problem, to focus the initiative as clearly as possible so that a measurable difference in child health would be a realistic outcome, and to build collaborative relationships with other organizations whose goals were complementary to the NAPNAP initiative, Healthy Eating and Activity Together (HEAT).

While HEAT was initially conceived as an advocacy project enabling NAPNAP to assume a leadership role on an important pediatric health issue, association leaders quickly saw advocacy efforts needed to be joined to an active effort by the association to directly address the epidemic of childhood overweight. Without this substantial, parallel effort, the association risked appearing as only an audience for others. This proved an accurate prediction, as contact legislative aides on Capitol Hill inevitably posed the question, "What is NAPNAP doing to address the problem?"

A steering work group was convened in December 2003 by Past President Mary Margaret Gottesman to develop a plan for the HEAT initiative with four major strategic objectives: leadership, advocacy, practice, and education. The steering work group consisted of NAPNAP member leaders with expertise in infancy, early childhood, school age, adolescence, cultural diversity, advocacy, research/evaluation, and educational resources. The centerpiece of the initiative was to be the development of clinical practice guidelines focused on the prevention and early identification of childhood overweight for use by practitioners caring for children in a wide variety of community-based settings.

## CHALLENGES IN GUIDELINE DEVELOPMENT

The task of developing guidelines was daunting because of the enormous volume of literature regarding childhood overweight, the number of guidelines on the management of childhood overweight produced by other professional groups, and most important, the lack of a strong body of research on effective prevention strategies. The steering work group drew on the work and recommendations of

others, such as the U.S. Dairy Association Nutrition Guidelines for Americans, the Institute of Medicine report on prevention of childhood overweight (Koplan, Liverman, & Kraak, 2005), and the recommendations of the American Academy of Pediatrics, the American Dietetic Association, and the American Heart Association.

## WHAT WAS MISSING?

A review of existing guidelines showed they were narrowly focused on measures of height, weight, and body mass index; some laboratory values; and nutrition and physical activity for the individual child, without consideration of the context of the family and the parent-child relationship. The NAPNAP steering work group recognized feeding and physical activity are embedded in family lifestyle and shaped by parent preferences and experience, culture, and the changing demands of the growing and developing child. Further, there was recognition that child health is impacted by many environments outside the home, especially child care and school as well as the larger community and society in which children live. Critical elements of these larger environments shape access to, and quality of, resources for nutrition and physical activity. Finally, there was appreciation that the quality of the relationship between patients and providers is critical to effective health care provision. Therefore, a different type of guideline was conceived. The HEAT *Clinical Practice Guideline* includes recommendations addressing the contexts of family and community.

A review of the literature on clinical practice guidelines demonstrated that although great effort was expended in producing evidence-based guides to care, they were seldom implemented well in actual patient care. Some of the barriers identified included the lack of resources to make it easy to implement each aspect of a care guide, such as patient education materials; lack of consideration given to cultural appropriateness of recommendations or adaptations for care delivery with diverse populations; absence of guidance for implementation of the guidelines; and lack of buy-in from practitioners who were to use the guidelines. Therefore, the task of the steering work groups had to be focused not only on the content of the guideline but also on the identification and development of supporting resources and an effective strategy for implementation.

## FUNDING SUPPORT

The HEAT initiative received financial support from the Johnson & Johnson Pediatric Institute, the Gerber Foundation, and the Maternal-Child Health Bureau. The HEAT *Clinical Practice Guideline*, published in 2006, will be accompanied by a resource kit to support implementation.

Despite the significance of the epidemic of childhood overweight and the many organizations involved in addressing the issue, attracting the attention of legislators at the federal level to translate science into policy has proved difficult. Competing priorities have prevented this issue from gaining significant support on the federal agenda. NAPNAP's *Clinical Practice Guideline* includes an advocacy agenda for the local and state levels and several states have launched their own plans for encouraging healthier lifestyles for their citizens.

## THE ROAD AHEAD

An ambitious part of the dissemination plan of the NAPNAP guidelines focuses on the use of a "rapid cycle change" quality improvement strategy, coupled with the educational training sessions in the use of the guideline and resource kit materials. This effort to change practitioner practice has the ultimate goal of preventing movement of children from a normal weight status to an at-risk status or an actual overweight/obese status.

## SUMMARY

While the ultimate goal of the HEAT initiative is a measurable decrease in the rates of childhood overweight in all age groups, the NAPNAP steering work group recognizes that many complex factors, from the intrauterine environment to the home to the larger society, contribute to the epidemic of childhood overweight. Thus, a complex response is

needed to reverse the trend. This broad public health issue demonstrates the need for a multipronged approach that includes advocacy, educating policymakers and clinicians about the problem, and gaining the support of clinicians who can directly ameliorate the situation one patient at a time.

## REFERENCES

Barlow, S., & Dietz, W. (2002). Management of child and adolescent obesity. Summary and recommendations based on reports from pediatricians, pediatric nurse practitioners, and registered dieticians. *Pediatrics, 111,* 229-235.

Centers for Disease Control and Prevention. (2005). Body mass index for teens and children. Retrieved October 10, 2005, from *www.cdc.gov/nccdphp/dnpa/bmi/bmi-for-age.htm.*

Koplan, J. P., Liverman, C. T., & Kraak, V. A. (Eds.). (2005). Preventing childhood obesity: Health in the balance (Institute of Medicine report). Washington, DC: National Academies Press. Retrieved February 27, 2006, from *www.iom.edu/report.asp?id=22596.*

Strauss, R. S. (1999). Childhood obesity. *Current Problems in Pediatrics, 110,* 210-215.

Troiano R. P., & Flegal, M. D. (1998). Overweight children and adolescents: Description, epidemiology, and demographics. *Pediatrics, 101,* 497-504.

Wechsler, H. (2004, June 16). Testimony on "HHS efforts to combat the obesity epidemic among children and adolescents." Department of Health and Human Services. Retrieved March 26, 2006, from *www.hhs.gov/asl/testify/t040616.html.*

*Web Resources*

**Guide to Developing a School Wellness Program**
*www.schoolwellnesspolicies.org*
**NAPNAP's HEAT Initiative**
*www.napnap.org*
**National Institutes of Health—Childhood Obesity on the Rise**
*www.nih.gov/news/WordonHealth/jun2002/childhoodobesity.htm*
**2006 Trust for America's Health Report—F as in Fat: How Obesity Policies Are Failing in America**
*http://healthyamericans.org/reports/obesity2006*

*Taking Action*   Ann Walker-Jenkins

# The Association of Women's Health, Obstetric and Neonatal Nurses: Folic Acid Advocacy

## THE PROBLEM

It is estimated that more than 4000 pregnancies were affected by a neural tube defect (NTD) each year during the 1980s and for most of the 1990s in the United States (Centers for Disease Control and Prevention, 2004). The average lifetime cost of caring for a child afflicted with spina bifida, one of the most common NTDs, is $636,000, but many incur costs over $1,000,000 (Centers for Disease Control and Prevention [CDC], 2005a). Babies afflicted with anencephaly, another NTD, die before birth or shortly after birth. NTDs occur when the neural tube, which forms and closes between the 17th and 30th day of gestation, fails to do so properly, leaving the brain or part of the spine exposed to the amniotic fluid (CDC, 2005a). Most of these tragic cases can be prevented. Research shows that consuming 400 mcg of folic acid daily before pregnancy and early in pregnancy can prevent up to 70% of NTDs. How can this life-changing information get to people in a timely way? Will people change their behavior to better care for themselves and their babies if they get the information? These are some of the questions that motivated the Association of Women's Health, Obstetric and Neonatal Nurses (AWHONN) to utilize its position as a nursing organization to advocate for change that would improve the health of mothers and babies.

## THE HISTORY

A British study, which began in 1983, focused on women who had experienced a previous NTD-affected pregnancy and who were planning another pregnancy. The study was halted in 1991 when it became apparent that every woman in the study should be given folic acid because it drastically reduced the occurrence of having an NTD-affected pregnancy (MRC Vitamin Study, 1991). This study

moved the United States ahead on this issue and spurred debate over whether to fortify grains with folic acid and how much folic acid is safe to take. In 1998, after years of debate, the Food and Drug Administration (FDA) approved the fortification of enriched grains, and the National Council on Folic Acid (NCFA) was founded to respond to the educational and policy needs surrounding this issue. The fortification of enriched grains reduced the occurrence of NTDs in the United States each year from more than 4,000 to slightly more than 3,000 cases (CDC, 2004). This was a tremendous step forward in improving the health of babies, but fortification alone was not enough to save even the majority of pregnancies suffering from NTDs. An educational campaign was needed to tell women which foods to eat that were fortified, which foods had natural folate, and how taking a multivitamin every day could fill the gaps in diet, ensuring that even an unexpected pregnancy could be one free of an NTD.

## THE ADVOCACY

Nurses are the largest health care provider group in the United States. They care for women of all ages across the United States and have a vital role in promoting folic acid consumption that prevents NTD-affected pregnancies. Because NTDs can occur so soon into pregnancy and often before a woman knows she is pregnant, it is imperative to spread the word about folic acid consumption before pregnancy. Nurses, as patient-focused health care providers, are critical in communicating this prevention message. Influencing women to think about folic acid consumption has been particularly challenging because people think that care for a baby begins with pregnancy rather than before pregnancy. This shift in thought is key in the education about eating a healthy diet and is also critical in the continual debate over fortification and folic acid supplementation. AWHONN has been strategically involved in efforts to educate women about folic acid's benefits, by helping women's health, obstetric and neonatal nurses get the word out to those women they work with who might become pregnant. AWHONN has woven the folic acid message throughout all preconception care–related stories and publications and has advocated for federal funding for CDC programs, including the National Center on Birth Defects and Developmental Disabilities. Articles have been published in AWHONN's clinical journals and consumer magazines, and members are actively involved at the state level in raising awareness of these issues. According to a Gallup Organization poll commissioned by the March of Dimes, women are more likely to take a multivitamin if health care providers advise it (March of Dimes, 2005). So nurses keep educating in the face of challenges.

### THE CHALLENGE

Despite the progress that has been made through fortification and education about diet and multivitamin use, each year thousands of pregnancies are affected by these birth defects, and two thirds of women in the United States still do not get their recommended dietary allowance of folic acid. Many women choose not to take a multivitamin or forget to take a multivitamin. Furthermore, many women of child-bearing age are not thinking of getting pregnant; therefore, birth-defects prevention is not high on their list of priorities. However, because half of all pregnancies in the United States are unplanned, fortification and multivitamin use education is still essential, and nurses must continue their education efforts despite the challenges (Centers for Disease Control and Prevention, 2005b).

### THE TEAM EFFORT

AWHONN joined the National Council on Folic Acid (NCFA) with two goals in mind: to influence policy surrounding folic acid and to highlight nurses' invaluable role in patient advocacy. AWHONN's national leadership on the steering committee and co-chairing the legislative committee can ensure that nurses are seen as key providers of this public health message. In addition, progress can be made more effectively by harnessing the skills and knowledge of people from many organizations. As co-chair of NCFA's legislative committee, AWHONN has contributed to advocacy efforts that promote adequate folic acid consumption for the population. Some of the advocacy efforts have included discussion of a need for fortification of corn meal and birth control pills, discussion of the Women, Infants, and Children (WIC) food package to ensure that packages entitled Pregnant and Breastfeeding Women, Postpartum Women, and Breastfeeding Women have an adequate amount of folic acid, and comments on the Federal revision of dietary guidelines to include an emphasis on foods rich in folic acid. There has also been discussion about whether the science exists to begin talking to the FDA about an increase in the current fortification requirements to provide more of the recommended dietary allowance of folic acid per serving of enriched grain. It is important that, as a team, we continue to advocate for change that helps mothers and babies. Nurses must continue to lead the way in educating patients about the importance of folic acid for a healthy pregnancy and a healthy life.

*Web Resources*

**Association of Women's Health, Obstetric and Neonatal Nurses**
*www.awhonn.org/awhonn/?pg=872-16690*
**Centers for Disease Control (CDC) National Center on Birth Defects and Developmental Disabilities**
*www.cdc.gov/ncbddd*
**National Council on Folic Acid**
*www.folicacidinfo.org/index.php*
**National Folic Acid Awareness Week**
*www.folicacidinfo.org/campaign*

### REFERENCES

Centers for Disease Control and Prevention (CDC). (2004, May 7). Spina bifida and anencephaly before and after folic acid mandate—United States, 1995-1996 and 1999-2000. *Morbidity and Mortality Weekly Reports, 53*(17), 362-365. Retrieved July 26, 2005, from *www.cdc.gov/mmwr/preview/mmwrhtml/mm5317a3.htm.*

Centers for Disease Control and Prevention. (2005a). Frequently asked questions. National Center on Birth Defects and

Developmental Disabilities (NCBDDD). Retrieved August 12, 2005, from *www.cdc.gov/ncbddd/folicacid/faqs.htm.*

Centers for Disease Control and Prevention (CDC). (2005b). Having a healthy pregnancy. National Center on Birth Defects and Developmental Disabilities (NCBDDD). Retrieved July 26, 2005, from *www.cdc.gov/ncbddd/bd/abc.htm.*

March of Dimes. (2005). What providers can do. Retrieved July 26, 2005, from *www.marchofdimes.com/professionals/690_1401.asp.*

MRC Vitamin Study Research Group. (1991). Prevention of neural tube defects: Results of the Medical Research Council Vitamin Study. (1991, July 20). *Lancet, 338*(8760), 131-137.

# *Taking Action*   Linda Altizer, Cynthia M. Gonzalez, & Robin S. Voss

## The National Association of Orthopaedic Nurses: All-Terrain Vehicle (ATV) Safety Education and Legislation

### IDENTIFICATION OF THE PROBLEM

The National Association of Orthopaedic Nurses (NAON) began advocacy work in July of 2004 in the wake of an accident that involved a close friend of one of the association's directors. A friend's young son was killed while riding an all-terrain vehicle (ATV) in a field in western Maryland. He flew through the air and sustained a crushed trachea and severe head injuries. This young boy was but one of the many people who have died from injuries that occurred while riding an ATV. After much research, NAON found that regulations in relation to ATV riding are lax. NAON members are not strangers to witnessing different traumatic injuries, but as we looked more in depth at ATV issues, it became apparent that our members were all too familiar with these patients.

### STRATEGIES FOR ACTION

NAON initiated action on ATV safety by asking Linda Altizer, the executive board liaison, to develop a safety statement. This was approved by our board of directors and posted on NAON's Website and in the NAON newsletter. Much of the data input came from the Natural Trails and Waters Coalition, the Consumer Federation of America, and the U.S. Consumer Product Safety Commission (CPSC). The safety statement was also published by them, and NAON joined them in taking a stand to institute safety standards.

NAON President Cynthia M. Gonzalez contacted the Emergency Nurses Association to discuss partnering with them to support ATV safety. Because they had already supported this issue in the past, instead of working with NAON at this time, they extended an invitation for a NAON member to write an article for their journal discussing the actions that we were taking and the issues at hand.

### THE SCOPE OF THE PROBLEM

The CPSC's latest report states the following:

- Serious injuries requiring emergency room treatment increased 10%, from 113,900 in 2002 to 125,500 in 2003.
- The estimated number of ATV-related fatalities increased from 609 in 2001 to 621 in 2002.
- In 2003, ATVs killed at least 111 children younger than 16, accounting for 27% of all ATV-related fatalities.
- Children under 16 suffered 38,600 serious injuries in 2003, or 31% of all injuries.

Because of the increase in deaths, especially in the rural areas, several attempts were made to reach out to the media for exposure of the death and injury statistics. In western Maryland, after the death of two youths on an ATV, an article was written with current information and submitted to the newspaper editor. The article was refused. The following week, the front page of the newspaper had a large photo of an area resident bouncing through the fields on his ATV, with a statement about "now is the time for outdoor fun!"

Other, more successful attempts to expose the need for ATV safety were made by those in the health care field. Robert Demichelis, II, the legislative liaison for the Brain Injury Association of America (BIAA), helped get the NAON statement posted on the BIAA's Website. NAON also began sharing information and progressing forward with the BIAA as a team to make changes.

NAON's Pediatric Special Interest Group, led by a former NAON board member, Barbara Shoemaker, also supported the creation of a Website group by networking with the Natural Trails and Water Coalition and encouraging families dealing with injured children to reach out to each other. Contact was made with Carolyn Anderson from Massachusetts who had lost her son in an ATV accident. As we collaborated, the idea of organizing a group of suffering parents to support each other and join the march to make changes was implemented. Anderson accepted the task of coordinating the families. The group is called Concerned Families for ATV Safety (more information is available on their Website at *www.atvsafetynet.org/*). The Bone and Joint Decade, an initiative of a consortium of musculoskeletal organizations engaged in developing new research and education programs that will bring about significant advances in the knowledge, diagnosis, and treatment of musculoskeletal conditions, also has supported NAON's efforts to increase ATV safety. They published an article in their December 2004-January 2005 newsletter regarding the fact that health care providers are some of the most knowledgeable people of the devastating results of youth involved in ATV accidents.

NAON has encouraged nurses throughout the country to contact their local legislative representatives to discuss ATV safety with them. This has not been as successful as dealing with the medical professionals and those who have onsite recognition of the consequences of ATV-related accidents, such as the families.

## GAINING SUPPORT IN A STATE SENATE

One success we had occurred in 2005 when NAON President Robin Voss was able to contact a local television station in Winston-Salem, North Carolina,

and speak regarding ATV issues in the wake of the deaths of two children under age 5 who were killed when they were thrown from an ATV when riding with their 9-year-old brother. Ms. Voss was able to bring immediate attention to this issue and has worked successfully with State Senator Bill Purcell of North Carolina in recently passing the first ATV legislation in the state. She and current NAON President, Cynthia M. Gonzalez, also met with members of the legislative teams from North Carolina and Illinois to discuss ATV legislation in their respective states, as well as nationally, when in Washington, DC, for the National Orthopaedic Leadership Conference in 2005.

NAON's Pediatric Special Interest Group has contacted NAON members to inform them of NAON's efforts to encourage the CPSC to consider actions regarding the sale of ATVs for use by children under the age of 16. The letter sent to the CPSC had originally been sent in 2002, along with information that supported the benefits that a national safety standard imposed on ATV riders under age 16 could provide, but was tabled. This issue was revisited in February of 2005 with the recommendation from the CPSC not to support this.

In response, more than 140 people from more than 32 states, along with organizations such as NAON, sent a letter to the chairperson of the CPSC asking him to have his commission reconsider the ATV petition. At their meeting at the end of March 2005, the CPSC gave no indication of what action it was going to take. In June 2005, the chairman of the CPSC directed the commission to assess a range of ATV safety issues; no decision has yet been rendered.

Before 2004, it was difficult to find any information regarding the risks of ATV use with children. Now there are Websites, professional journals, newscasts, and educational brochures with information for the public. Some manufacturers are setting safety guidelines, but the goal is to implement laws to govern the activity, not just give suggestions. Most children that are killed on ATVs are ejected from the vehicle. The vehicles do not have roller bars or seat belts, and there are no laws enforcing age limitations. NAON, along with our partners, will strive to accomplish these goals, not for us but for the safety of children.

# chapter 32

# Where Policy Hits the Pavement: Contemporary Issues in Communities

Katherine N. Bent

*"I am of the opinion that my life belongs to the community, and as long as I live it is my privilege to do for it whatever I can."*

GEORGE BERNARD SHAW

Most people experience the effects of public policymaking in their communities. Not only is it in daily living that people feel the effect of policy and policy change, but it is in communities that individuals learn how to step up and take part in the policymaking process. In communities, nurses and other health professionals have immediate opportunities to advocate for policies that promote and protect health in multiple ways. Indeed, the Healthy People 2010 (United States Department of Health and Human Services [USDHHS], 2000) priorities to decrease disparities and emphasize health promotion place nursing in a key position to affect future health-related policies.

This chapter explores the nature of communities, prospects for health, and the health-related conditions that shape and are shaped by policy. It suggests how nurses, as they increasingly move outside institutional walls, can use their limited time and resources to support improvements in policies affecting health.

## WHAT IS A COMMUNITY?

Although community is a part of our daily life experiences, the idea of community is elusive and can mean many things, particularly in a health care context (Bent, 2003; Monroe, 1997; Peterson, 1997; Shields & Lindsey, 1998). The concept of community has broad appeal; attitudes about the role of community in health care and health policy differ when compared with attitudes about the role of community in other areas. For example, health care entrepreneurs view health care communities as a market where they are likely to find a concentration of persons to buy health care goods or services; however, public health professionals must be concerned about entire populations in a given area regardless of people's ability to buy, knowing that where economic market potential is lower, health risks and needs may actually be higher (Geronimus, 2000). In a politically charged environment, claims of community often become moral claims that may serve to divide people more than bring them together (Monroe, 1997). This effect has serious consequences for questions of public health and the policies that support or define public health, such as policies mandating reporting or treatment of communicable diseases.

A community is an environment with physical, social, political, and economic dimensions. Community is not the same as place, or neighborhood, or group, but has a specific ecologic balance that is sustained by many factors, including public policies (Wallace & Wallace, 1999). For example, differing neighborhoods within cities or towns may have competing interests for zoning regulations that affect traffic flow in and out of the community, local job opportunities, and health risks associated with production waste.

Milio (2002) has noted that the basis for health lies in communities, where we find homes, schools, recreation and entertainment centers, businesses, and governmental and voluntary organizations, including faith groups. These assets, along with means of communication and transportation, form a community's infrastructure. The quality, availability, and accessibility of the infrastructure make a difference in health prospects of the people who live in those communities. Infrastructure includes such elements as clean and pure water, air, and food; adequate housing, employment, childcare, health, education, police, and fire services; open media, civic opportunities, and social life; strong neighborhood, community, and labor groups; and a strong health care service safety net. In communities that have the resources, a sense of cohesion can bring about distribution of those resources to achieve sustainable health for the people who are part of those communities.

Communities must share both spirit and a sense of place in order to build, achieve, and sustain health and well-being. Through attachment to place, communities share attachment to social responsibility for creating healthy surroundings. This attachment does not exist among detached groups that may share other interests (Milio, 1996). Community and public responsibility for health, expressed in an environment that provides options for housing, education, work, health, and childcare, precedes self-responsibility for health and challenges most of our current health policy in its limited health services role (Citrin, 1998). Can you think about what kinds of actions or policies within your community may be affecting health or quality of life? How would you work within a multidisciplinary context

to promote health at the community level in these areas?

## HEALTHY COMMUNITIES

Late in the 1970s the World Health Organization (WHO) embraced the principles of social justice and equity and challenged nations to provide a basic level of health for all citizens. They called the principal means to this end *primary health care* (PHC) (WHO, 1978). PHC is essential, practical, scientific, socially accepted, universally accessible to all members of a community, affordable, and geared toward self-reliance and self-determination and involves multiple agencies and sectors in health. Although often used interchangeably with the term *primary care*, PHC is more global than is primary care. Generally, primary care means personal health care services provided in community rather than hospital settings as the first point of contact for a patient with a health concern. Primary care nursing activities are oriented toward assisting patients maintain and improve health and prevent future illness but generally exclude essential public health and environmental health services and are not inclusive of community participation in broad-scale health promotion activities.

This shift away from dependence on health professionals and toward personal and community involvement was echoed in the Ottawa Charter for Health Promotion with the establishment of Healthy Cities and Communities (WHO, 1986). The Ottawa Charter (WHO, 1986) recognized the relationship between health and broader political, economic, social, and environmental experiences, which happen in communities. The charter stressed again that to promote health, communities must have peace, shelter, education, food, income, a stable ecosystem, and social justice and equity. WHO reaffirmed its commitment to PHC and "Health for All" in the twenty-first century by issuing a new policy statement in which member states acknowledge that changes in the world health situation require relevant regional and national policies and strategies to support attaining health as a fundamental human right (WHO, 1998).

Some have critiqued the healthy communities and now the Health for All movements as trying to be all things to all people by making every issue in a community equally important. The risk, it is suggested, is that some of the very serious, underlying causes of ill health (e.g., poverty and its relationship to health issues such as incidence and prevalence of diabetes or hegemony in its many forms) will be obscured by the cacophony of needs in communities. The future of healthy cities and communities depends in large part on the extent to which those communities enact policies that create healthier living environments.

## A COMMUNITY IN ACTION: SAN JOSÉ

San José, an urban *barrio* (a Spanish-speaking neighborhood in a city or town in the United States, especially in the Southwest) in Albuquerque, New Mexico, is a community in which residents have responded to health threats posed by local environmental hazards with community-based environmental health policies and community-focused health and development strategies that have united diverse constituencies and generated sustained activity and impact over time.

This low-income, predominantly Hispanic (86%) community is geographically marked by the AT&SF (Atchison, Topeka & Santa Fe) railroad, one interstate highway, and the Rio Grande River. The community is also zoned for both residential and industrial use; oil refineries, tanneries, manufacturing plants, and salvage yards can be found alongside elementary schools and homes that frequently rely on private wells for water. As other established urban neighborhoods did, San José suffered a decline in services and development following the suburbanization of the United States that began after World War II (Morley, 1999). Despite this decline, families who had lived in San José for generations continued to stay, raise children, and age in the homes they owned with support from neighbors, church, and family.

As a result of a heavy concentration of toxic wastes sites, two locales in San José were listed on the Superfund National Priorities list in the late 1980s and 1990s. This was both practically and symbolically tragic to a community that was first developed and long defined by agriculture. In the early 1980s, during water testing conducted by the city of Albuquerque, the local aquifer was found to have a heavy concentration of petroleum and toxic solvents, which are known to endanger human health. In 1988, this formerly agricultural community on the banks of the Rio Grande River became New Mexico's first Superfund* site, the South Valley Superfund Site. In 1994 a second Superfund site (the AT&SF Site) was identified in San José where a wood treatment plant had contaminated soil and water over a 64-year period of treating railroad ties with creosote and oil.

The concentration of environmental pollutants and industrial contamination in San José caused a drop in property values as land use declined. Once a prosperous agricultural community, San José was zoned as a federal Pocket of Poverty.† Now, not only industrial emissions and toxic chemicals, but also the pervasive violence of street drugs, gang activity, crime, and urban decay pollute the community environment.

The Albuquerque San José Community Awareness Council (ASJCAC or Awareness Council) is a grassroots organization formed in 1988 in response to concerns about both the environmental health hazards in the community and concerns over how life might, or might not, change with the Superfund designation. After years of grassroots organizing, local efforts have brought about changes in crime rates, abandoned or derelict properties, and public services and made other improvements in quality of life for the people who live in San José.

As an urban, culturally and ethnically diverse community, San José embodies a key assumption of the Healthy Communities movement: When people have the opportunity to work out their own locally defined health problems, they will find

---

*Federal designation of industrial waste sites that are hazardous to human health and potentially eligible for federal funding for clean-up or remediation.

†Certification from the U.S. Department of Housing and Urban Development. Criteria include the following: 70% of residents have income below 80% of the median of the locality or state, whichever is lower; chronic abandonment or demolition of commercial or residential structures; and losses of jobs and business.

sustainable solutions (Flynn & Dennis, 1996). Although nurses have been involved in work at this level, they are not known for their efforts. This example illustrates the need for nurses to address broader health and social issues to improve the health of communities.

## PARTICIPATION AND PARTNERSHIPS FOR IMPROVING COMMUNITY HEALTH

Healthy communities may be achieved through truly active and collaborative partnerships among a broad representation of professional and lay community members, but it is important to examine all partnerships critically (Aronson, 1993). A sense of a larger good and public dialogue is necessary for successful, equitable, and effective partnerships. Partnerships may become a substitute for accountability in organizations or governments, as individuals or local communities are expected to assume labor and costs associated with initiatives to improve health. Roles for nurses in healthy community initiatives focus on community action, developing personal skills in community members, reorienting health care services, creating supportive environments, and creating healthy public policy.

Stevens (1989) noted that the more accurately and extensively individuals are able to perceive and reflect on social, political, and economic contexts, the more effective they are interacting with others. An effective nursing role is to foster such critical reflections among community members. The health change this supports includes not only health status of individuals, but also structures and processes that are the community-based determinants of health. Nurses cannot ignore political, social, or cultural structures, material conditions, or the play of power in relationships between and among individuals and groups in communities. We must continue to explore health policy in ways that make the relevance of community involvement in health development clear.

Nurses have a tradition of actively creating and fostering partnerships for health promotion and community health, and their role remains vitally important today, for they are named by WHO as the critical professional link to create communities that are healthier for both individuals and for the entire population (WHO, 2000). For example, in the Public Health Nursing Outreach for New Americans program (PHNONA) in Denver, Colorado, nurses partnered with the Catholic Church to create a health resource center for undocumented and transient migrants who couldn't access health care or meet other needs such as for food and clothing. This partnership further evolved into the Denver Refugee Center, which serves refugees and asylum seekers and has multiple roles for nurses, including provision of information and advocacy, health education, health assessment, and referral. Partnerships for health evolve on many levels, including the following:

- A single public health nurse who teaches groups of patients with diabetes how to read food labels
- Collaborations between public health providers and county commissioners to create environments that allow residents of a community to be healthy
- The partnerships necessary to pass national laws that may affect the delivery of health care services to seniors who have Medicare (Rodriquez, 1996).

A caring partnership between nurse and community is a collaboration that is an informed, flexible, and negotiated distribution and redistribution of power among the participants in the process of seeking change for improved community health status process and structure. Magilvy, Brown, and Moritz (1999) highlighted the "synergy of purpose" in community-focused efforts that lead to community-focused health strategies relevant to community needs. Ongoing challenges to successful community health partnerships include the assumption that nurses are necessary for community health or specifying partnerships as nursing "interventions" without attention to the dynamic process and philosophic underpinnings called for by true partnership. Partnerships may also suffer when they are rushed, for example, in the case of a health survey that is conducted by concerned professionals but remains unused because not all interest groups were involved in the planning of questions or the design of the survey.

## COMMUNITY HEALTH WORKERS

Known by various names, such as *lay health advisors* or *outreach workers,* Community Health Workers (CHWs) are trusted community members who establish vital links between the community and health providers. The CHW's purpose is to empower community members to identify their own needs, develop plans, and implement solutions that are appropriate for them (Nemcek & Sabatier, 2003). The federal government first endorsed the use of CHWs in the 1960s as a way to expand health access to underserved populations including migrant workers, African Americans, poor people, and Native Americans. Since that time the use of CHWs has been erratic. When used, CHWs are considered integral members of the health care workforce who expand access to and use of care, enhance therapeutic alliance between community members and providers, and help identify and reduce health risks among community members. They are considered insiders who possess language and cultural skills that contribute to an enhanced understanding of community health beliefs, health behaviors, and barriers to services.

Current national demand to eliminate health disparities has renewed attention on the use of CHWs to improve community health, yet a lack of evaluation literature and poor overall understanding of the CHW concept by the public as well as other health care providers contribute to underuse of CHWs and stagnant public policy regarding their use (Nemcek & Sabatier, 2003). The rationale for using CHWs to improve the delivery of community-based preventive care to diverse populations is strong, and the federal government continues to endorse their use. Yet they are often overlooked (Hill, Bone, & Butz, 1996) as members of a health care team who can advocate for individuals in communities and contribute to overall community health improvement. Nurses seeking ways to improve community health can become knowledgeable advocates for the use and evaluation of CHWs to address both individual and community-level health risks.

## HEALTHY PUBLIC POLICY

The term *healthy public policy* has evolved through widespread international discussion over the last quarter century. Healthy public policy is policy that is developed through a process of collaboration with those who are most affected by a policy. Some refer to this kind of policy as *health-making* or *health-sustaining* policy (Milio, 1981, 1996).

The goals and objectives of healthy public policy make two explicit assumptions:

- *Most people, most of the time, will make decisions and choices based on the options that are available.* The results are not exclusively personal, nor are they the result of totally free choices about lifestyle made in isolation from social, economic, cultural, and political contexts.
- *The options that are available, and from which people make choices, do not "just happen," but rather are the result of prior policy choices that represent the scope of health-sustaining policy,* including energy, technology, pollution, employment, income maintenance, taxation, prices, food, agriculture, transportation, housing, health care, child care, and other services.

A strategy for healthy public policy must eliminate, or increase the cost of, health-damaging options, while providing new options that are easier to access in areas that may lack health-promoting or health-sustaining resources. Specific objectives of healthy public policy would center on minimizing health-damaging environments. From the framework of healthy public policy, nurses eager to support health-related policies can eventually analyze the health impact of environments, ways of living that flow from them, and the effect of current policies on them.

Health policy will become healthy public policy and will best be able to serve the health interests of people when the focus becomes preventing illness in the primary sense, rather than treating illness in individuals, and fixing responsibility in a publicly accountable unit of government required to evaluate the impact of public policy on health and to design health-making policy options (Milio, 1981). The scope of such policy is broad and cuts across artificial boundaries between health and other types of policies and other policymaking bodies.

The effects of policies on community health cannot be estimated by trying to assess policies individually. Rather, the search for healthy public policy must include ways to conceptually and organizationally combine otherwise segregated types of policy, such as health and labor, which increasingly affect environments and community, and define individual experiences as health sustaining or not (Milio, 1981). Some communities are facing healthy public policy decisions as they consider including fast-food franchises in public school areas. Can you think of other examples of where multiple areas of public policy converge and have health-related outcomes?

There are conflicts within public policy arenas about the purpose of health policy: Is its primary purpose to deliver health services to or to improve the health and well-being of Americans? Although these goals are not mutually exclusive, the degree of emphasis on one or the other becomes more important as public policy is a highly influential force at all levels of health care in this country. Questions of emphasis remain relevant as national policies "decentralize," state policies "localize," and individuals and communities are told they hold more responsibility than ever for their own health experiences. This implies that the individual or the single community is responsible for the success (manifested through personal or population health measures) or failure (seen in ill health) of public health policy. Developing and championing healthy public policy is a vitally important part of nursing. In healthy public policy, we make visible our commitment to the total health experience of persons in expanding communities that are ecologically related.

## DETERMINANTS OF HEALTH IN COMMUNITIES

Social conditions are major determinants of health. Social determinants of health are factors in the social environment that contribute to or detract from the health of individuals and communities. These factors include, but are not limited to, income, education, occupation, transportation, sanitation, housing, access

to services and resources linked to health discrimination, social support, and environmental hazards. Social forces that act at a collective level, such as a community decision to build sidewalks to promote safe walking opportunities, shape individual biology, individual risk behaviors, environmental exposures, and access to resources that promote health. It is critical that nurses understand how the social determinants of health contribute to health disparities as well as how to advocate for policies that aim to lessen those forces that are associated with poor health outcomes.

Over the years, researchers have increasingly documented that the portion of population health status attributable to health care services is modest when compared with the contributions of other factors, including the social determinants of health. Indeed, Healthy People 2010, a federal effort to outline national public health objectives, identified access to health care as only one of 10 leading indicators that, in addition to income and education, could serve as measures for the health of the population. The other indicators are a combination of modifiable behavioral, social, and environmental factors known to affect health (USDHHS, 2000).

## SOCIOECONOMIC STATUS

Although the average life expectancy is improving in the United States (USDHHS, 2004a), there are differences in life expectancy and health among people with different levels of education, income, and types of jobs and among people who live in communities characterized by different levels of community wealth and infrastructure (Wilkinson & Marmot, 2003). Together, these characteristics measure socioeconomic position, and an extensive research literature documents the relationship between mortality and area-level socioeconomic factors, including income inequality, minority racial concentration, and various measures of social capital (Milyo & Mellor, 2003; Washington State Department of Health, 2002). One definition of social capital is the resources imbedded in social relations among people and organizations that facilitate cooperation and collaboration in communities (Gittell & Vidal, 1998). The American Public

Health Association (2001) has also called for monitoring the prevalence of low income as a health indicator and making its reduction a public health objective. Here are a few examples of how health is affected by socioeconomic status:

- In 2002 the overall percent of Americans living in poverty was 12.1%, up from 11.7% in 2001 and 11.3% in 2000, the first increase in the poverty rate since 1993 (USDHHS, 2004a).
- Infant mortality increases as mother's level of education decreases. In 2001 the mortality rate for mothers with less than 12 years of education was 49% higher than for infants of mothers with 13 or more years of education (USDHHS, 2004a).
- The age-adjusted death rate for persons 25 to 64 years of age with fewer than 12 years of education was 2.7 times the rate for persons with 13 or more years of education (USDHHS, 2004a).

Increasing levels of educational success and improving housing standards are policy examples of how nurses might focus their attention to improve health through its socioeconomic determinants.

## DIVERSITIES AND RELATIONSHIPS

By giving people the emotional and practical resources they need, strong social support is an important contributor to health. Not only is there a protective effect of feeling a sense of belonging, but supportive relationships may encourage healthier behavior patterns. The amount of emotional and practical social support people get varies by social and economic status, with poverty contributing to social exclusion and isolation. Although people of color in the United States have disproportionately high rates of poverty, poverty and its associated factors alone are not sufficient to explain all of the health disparities among people of different races. The USDHHS reports that people of color, particularly African Americans, have higher rates of death from homicide, human immunodeficiency virus (HIV) infection, infant mortality, diabetes, stroke, heart disease, cancer, and unintentional injury than whites (USDHHS, 2004b). In addition, race is a strong predictor of exposure to environmental toxins and hazardous waste sites (Brown, 1995).

- In 2002, more than half of African-American and Hispanic children under 18 years old and more than half of the African-American and Hispanic population age 65 years and older were either poor or near poor (USDHHS, 2004b).
- Homicide is the leading cause of death for young African-American men and the second leading cause for young Hispanic men (USDHHS, 2004b).
- Hispanic persons were more likely than non-Hispanic white and non-Hispanic black persons to have had no health care visits within the past 12 months (26% compared with 14% to 15%) (USDHHS, 2004b).
- The death rate for motor vehicle–related injury for young Native American men 15 to 24 years of age was almost 450% higher than the rate for young white men (USDHHS, 2004b).

Because the effect of race on health is controversial, particularly for its relationship to issues of poverty, further investigation is warranted to tease out contributions of each.

## ENVIRONMENTAL HEALTH AND ENVIRONMENTAL JUSTICE

People with lower socioeconomic status are more likely than people with higher socioeconomic status to live or work in environments that put them at risk of exposure to toxic substances. For example:

- People living in older, dilapidated housing are at risk for exposure to lead-based paints, which are especially hazardous for young children (Sargent, 1999; Washington State Department of Health, 2002).
- Members of lower socioeconomic groups are also more likely to work as manual laborers, thereby increasing their risk of occupational injury or death and their risk of exposure to toxic or carcinogenic substances (Rios, Poje, & Detels, 1993).
- Low socioeconomic neighborhoods are more likely than middle or higher socioeconomic neighborhoods to be situated near toxic waste sites and other potential environmental hazards (Mohai & Bryant, 1992).

Environmental health is an important and rich area for nurses seeking to use or affect public policy to improve health of communities. There is growing awareness that a view of the environment as a person's immediate circumstances or surroundings is limiting and limited. Rather, we need to view the environment as a network of relationships among social, political, economic, and cultural conditions that influence health and illness.

## FOOD

Healthy eating and an adequate supply of food are keys to promoting health and well-being. A shortage of food and lack of variety can cause malnutrition and deficiency diseases. Excess intake contributes to cardiovascular disease, diabetes, cancer, obesity, degenerative eye disease, and dental caries (Wilkinson & Marmot, 2003). The important community health policy issue is the availability and cost of healthy food, because access to affordable, good food makes a greater difference to what people eat than health education (Wilkinson & Marmot, 2003). Although expert committees all agree on dietary goals to prevent chronic diseases, social and economic conditions result in social differences in diet quality that contribute in turn to health inequalities (Wilkinson & Marmot, 2003). Policy implications for nurses in communities include:

- Advocating to integrate public health perspectives into the food production and distribution systems to provide affordable, nutritious fresh food for all, especially the most vulnerable. For example, the Supplemental Nutrition Program for Women, Infants, and Children (WIC) in many states has negotiated with farmers' markets to accept WIC vouchers for locally grown produce.
- Supporting sustainable agriculture and food production methods that conserve natural resources in communities.
- Assuring the availability of useful information about food, diet, and health—for example, about the risks of fast food and unhealthy vending machine choices offered in school cafeterias, especially for children.

## THE GLOBAL PERSPECTIVE

In other nations, such at the United Kingdom and Canada, broad, health-related social policies have been influenced by research on the social determinants of population health (Lurie, McLaughlin, & House, 2003). At the 2004 World Health Assembly, WHO Director-General Dr Lee Jong-Wook called for the formation of the Commission on Social Determinants of Health. Operating from 2005 to 2008, the Commission was charged with recommending interventions and policies to improve health and narrow health inequalities through action on social determinants. The Commission has worked to identify effective approaches and produce policy recommendations for overcoming the social barriers to health.

## NURSES AND COMMUNITIES

Many dimensions of community and community health suggest that there are policy needs and opportunities for nurses to be involved in setting the policy agenda to promote and sustain health. Identifying communities, advocating for health-promoting policies at all levels, and working to create and sustain partnerships with community members and organizations are all important features of the nursing role. The nurse who is concerned with policies that support health in communities finds that the role crosses areas of food and agricultural policy, housing policy, labor policy, aging policy, environmental policy, and social policy, among many others. Nurses today are better educated than ever before and well positioned to be involved in initiatives that extend the traditional boundaries of health policy to the creation of public policies that will truly support the health of communities.

## Key Points

- The health of communities derives more from the social determinants of health than from health care services.
- PHC focuses on self-reliance and self-determination of communities and requires collaborative partnerships between health care professionals and communities.
- Healthy public policies are those that are health promoting and sustaining and often address the

social determinants of health, such as socioeconomic factors, food, education, and environmental conditions.

■ Nurses are well positioned to form partnerships with communities to promote healthy public policies.

## *Web Resources*

**American Public Health Association**
*www.apha.org*
**Healthy Cities International**
*www.healthycities.org*
**Healthy People 2010**
*www.healthypeople.gov*
**World Health Organization (WHO)**
*www.who.int/en*

## REFERENCES

American Public Health Association. (2001). Resolution 200020: Raising income to protect health. *American Journal of Public Health, 91*(3), 504-505.

Aronson, J. (1993). Giving consumers a say in policy development: Influencing policy or just being heard? *Canadian Public Policy, 19*(4), 367-378.

Bent, K. N. (2003). The people know what they want: An empowerment process of sustainable, ecological community health. *Advances in Nursing Science, 26*(3), 215-226.

Brown, P. (1995). Race, class, and environmental health: A review and systematization of the literature. *Environmental Research, 69*(1), 15-30.

Citrin, T. (1998). Topics for our times: Public health—community or commodity? Reflections on healthy communities. *American Journal of Public Health, 88*(3), 351-352.

Flynn, B. C., & Dennis, L. (1996). Health promotion through Healthy Cities. In M. Stanhope & J. Lancaster, (Eds.), *Community health nursing: Promoting health of aggregates, families, and individuals* (4th ed.). St. Louis: Mosby.

Geronimus, A. (2000). To mitigate, resist, or undo: Addressing structural influences on the health of urban populations. *American Journal of Public Health, 90*(5), 762-767.

Gittell, R., & Vidal, A. (1998). *Community organizing: Building social capital as a development strategy.* Thousand Oaks, CA: Sage.

Hill, M. N., Bone, L. R., & Butz, A. M. (1996). Enhancing the role of community health workers in research. *Image: Journal of Nursing Scholarship, 28*(3), 221-226.

Lurie, N., McLaughlin, C., & House, J. S. (2003). In pursuit of the social determinants of health: The evolution of health services research. *Health Services Research,38*(6 Pt II), 1641-1643.

Magilvy, J. K., Brown, N. J., & Moritz, P. (1999). Community-focused interventions and outcomes strategies. In A. S. Hinshaw, S. Feetham, & J. Shaver (Eds.), *Handbook of clinical nursing research.* Thousand Oaks, CA: Sage.

Milio N. (1981). *Promoting health through public policy.* Philadelphia: F.A. Davis.

Milio, N. (1996). Linking health, communities, information technology and policy. In N. Milio, *Engines of empowerment: Using information technology to create healthy communities and challenge public policy.* Chicago: Health Administration Press.

Milio, N. (2002). Where policy hits the pavement: Contemporary issues in communities. In D. J. Mason, J. K. Leavitt, & M. W. Chaffee (Eds.), *Policy and politics in nursing and health care* (4th ed.) (pp. 659-668). St. Louis: Saunders.

Milyo, J., & Mellor, J. M. (2003). On the importance of age-adjustment methods in ecological studies of social determinants of mortality. *Health Services Research, 38*(6 Pt II), 1781-1790.

Mohai, P., & Bryant, B., (1992). Environmental racism: Reviewing the evidence. In B. Bryant & P. Mohai (Eds.), *Race and the incidence of environmental hazards.* Boulder, CO: Westview Press.

Monroe, J. A. (1997). Enemies of the people: The moral dimension to public health. *Journal of Health Politics, Policy and Law, 22*(4), 993-1020.

Morley, J. M. (1999). Albuquerque, New Mexico or Anywhere, USA?: Historical preservation and the construction of civic identity. *New Mexico Historical Review, 74*(2), 155-178.

Nemcek, M. A., & Sabatier, R. (2003). State of evaluation: Community health workers, *Public Health Nursing, 20*(4), 260-270.

Peterson, M. A. (1997). Community: Meaning and opportunity, and learning for the future. *Journal of Health Politics, Policy and Law, 22*(4), 933-936.

Rios, R., Poje, G. V., & Detels, R. (1993). Susceptibility to environmental pollutants among minorities. *Toxicology and Industrial Health, 10*, 797-820.

Rodriquez, R. (1996). Promoting healthy partnerships with migrant farm workers—Colorado. In E. T. Anderson & J. M. McFarlane (Eds.), *Community as partner: Theory and practice in nursing* (2nd ed.). Philadelphia: Lippincott.

Sargent, D. (1999). Child exposure to lead paint in two counties. *American Journal of Public Health, 89*(11), 1778-1783.

Shields, L. E., & Lindsey, A. E. (1998). Community health promotion nursing practice. *Advances in Nursing Science, 20*(4), 23-36.

Stevens, P. E. (1989). A critical social reconceptualization of environment in nursing: Implications for nursing. *Advances in Nursing Science, 11*(4), 58-68.

U.S. Department of Health and Human Services (USDHHS). (2000). Healthy People 2010. Retrieved March 24, 2005, from *www.healthypeople.gov.*

U.S. Department of Health and Human Services (USDHHS). (2004a). *Health, United States, 2004.* DHHS Publication No. 2004-1232 04-0068. Hyattsville, MD: USDHHS, Centers for Disease Control and Prevention, National Center for Health Statistics.

U.S. Department of Health and Human Services (USDHHS). (2004b). The initiative to eliminate racial and ethnic disparities in health: HHS fact sheet. Washington, DC: USDHHS Office of Minority Health. Retrieved April 14, 2005, from *www.omhrc.gov/rah/index.htm.*

Wallace, D., & Wallace, R. (1999). *A plague on your houses: How New York was burned down and national public health crumbled.* New York: Verso.

Washington State Department of Health. (2002). *Social determinants of health.* Retrieved March 22, 2005, from *www.doh.wa.gov/HWS/doc/RPF-Soc.doc.*

Wilkinson, R., & Marmot, M. (Eds.). (2003). *Social determinants of health: The solid facts.* Copenhagen, Denmark: World Health Organization.

World Health Organization (WHO). (1978). *Report of the International Conference on Primary Health Care,* (Alma Ata, USSR). Geneva, Switzerland: WHO.

World Health Organization (WHO). (1986) *Ottawa charter for health promotion, WHO Health promotion conference.* Ottawa, Canada: WHO.

World Health Organization (WHO). (1998). Health 21: Health for all in the 21st century. Retrieved March 22, 2005, from *www.euro.who.int/document/EHFA5-E.pdf.*

World Health Organization (WHO). (2000). Munich Declaration. Nurses and midwives: A force for health, 2000. Retrieved March 22, 2005, from *www.euro.who.int/aboutwho/policy/20010828_4.*

---

# *Vignette*   Becky Howard

## Homelessness and Health: Creating Lasting Solutions

*"Give a man a fish and he will eat for a day. Teach him how to fish and he will eat for a lifetime."*
CHINESE PROVERB

There are many reasons that people become homeless and, unfortunately, public policies often contribute to people becoming and remaining homeless*. Consider Denver, where there are people who have been homeless for 10 or more years. Federal, state, and local public policies have affected the availability of affordable housing. There is less money for housing provided by the Department of Housing and Urban Development as a result of federal policy changes. In Colorado, there is an allocation in the general fund for housing, but locally redevelopment or "gentrification" has changed the availability of affordable housing because there was no plan to replace low-income units.

The Colorado Coalition for the Homeless (CCH) and its health care clinic, the Stout Street Clinic

(SSC), were started by a nun who is a nurse and a small group of concerned citizens and local advocates who saw a need in the Denver metropolitan area for services specifically designed to provide to a growing population of homeless people, health care and housing opportunities. The clinic was started with a staff of six through a grant from the Robert Wood Johnson Foundation. CCH is currently funded by a combination of public and foundation grants.

CCH operates with a guiding mission of "creating lasting solutions" to the multifaceted and interrelated health and social problems of homelessness. SSC provides medical and mental health services to approximately 150 people a day. This is a story of how collaborative, creative thinking led to strategies for assisting our clients to become self sustaining and integrated into the community. These strategies include helping our clients access existing public support systems that constitute the country's "safety net."

### BART: PART OF THE "LASTING SOLUTION"

From the initial housing program and primary care health clinic, CCH has expanded and offers multiple

---

*Chronic homelessness is defined as being homeless for 1 year or having had many episodes of homelessness over several years.

programs for housing, case management for homeless persons with mental illness, and substance abuse treatment programs. A new program, the Benefits Acquisition and Retention Team (BART), is a multidisciplinary team that helps disabled homeless clients apply for and obtain Social Security benefits. Many people are homeless because they are disabled, have lost jobs, and lost their housing. Once awarded disability benefits, people are better able to secure and maintain housing and can then focus attention on health care needs that fell far lower on their list of priorities while they were homeless. Poverty is one of the causes of poor health and although receiving disability benefits does not provide an income much above the poverty level, they are eligible for additional benefits such as Section 8 housing, food stamps, Medicare and/or Medicaid, and discounted bus passes for transportation.

I am an Advanced Practice Nurse (APN) in psychiatry and the first full-time APN employed at SSC. I noticed that many of the obviously disabled clients were having difficulty negotiating the time-consuming and often overwhelming process of applying for disability benefits from the federal Social Security Administration (SSA) programs. Many who were clearly disabled and eligible were being denied benefits as a result of being unable to navigate a complex government process independently. There had not been a systematic way at SSC to identify those clients who were permanently disabled, and there was little understanding about how SSA worked and made decisions regarding disability determinations. The "system" was clearly failing homeless people and, unfortunately, so was the clinic is this regard. Initially, two APNs worked with the support of the vice president of operations for CCH and a staff member from Education and Advocacy to brainstorm about this problem and to identify solutions that would increase the number of medically and psychiatrically disabled homeless people who were awarded benefits.

The homeless population was growing, the national political climate had become less sympathetic to the plight of the homeless, and funding for "entitlement" programs was decreasing at an alarming rate. The state benefit for Colorado citizens, Aid to the Needy and Disabled (AND), was reduced in 2002 from $329 per month to $180 per month.

In keeping with the organizational philosophy of CCH of actively involving and enlisting the help and support of local business and political communities in developing sustainable resources for homeless people, we asked local representatives from SSA, the Colorado Disability Determination Services (DDS) and the Office of Hearing and Appeals (OHA) to problem solve with us. In engaging people from SSA and DDS at the local level, we were able to make a commitment on our part to approach applications for benefits differently, and they did so as well.

One of the new volunteers at CCH was an attorney who helped sort out the complexity of the disability application process, then helped to develop a streamlined process for CCH. He was available to clients and staff to assist in getting them to SSA appointments as well as translating the legal jargon contained in some of the correspondence that was coming to clients and the clinic from the SSA and DDS.

## SUPPORT FROM A FEDERAL AGENCY

I attended the 2002 annual national Conference on Homelessness and participated a workshop in which representatives of a program in the eastern United States presented a program they had implemented using the ideas and processes similar to those we were putting into place at CCH. We were having good results in some cases! A representative from the SSA was also in the audience so I took the opportunity to describe the problems we had identified and the initial solutions we had developed at CCH. The SSA representative was impressed, particularly with the idea of not only assisting in the initial application for benefits but also helping people retain those benefits. The SSA representative suggested that CCH apply for a new grant that would be coming out of the SSA in 2003 that was going to provide a 3-year funding opportunity for the selected organizations to implement a system for helping the disabled homeless navigate the SSA system and thereby increase the chance that they would be awarded benefits.

CCH was one of 53 sites awarded the grant, and we now have a team consisting of a case manager, an outreach worker, a Family Nurse Practitioner, a psychiatric APN, an occupational therapist, an attorney (who is now a paid employee), and a volunteer to take clients to appointments. We have a strong collaborative partnership with representatives from the local SSA, DDS, and OHA, as well as former clients who come quarterly to the BART team meeting in an advisory capacity. We have the respect of the collaborating agencies because they know that the clients for whom we advocate are truly disabled.

Part of the agreement and stipulation in the grant is that we help get people get housing and help them stay that way! Frequently CCH assumes the payeeship as a result of severity of the disability or lack of skills needed to maintain housing, with the goal of helping as many people as possible to eventually take over responsibility for their money.

## IMPACT

As of this writing the BART team has assisted 297 disabled homeless people apply for benefits. Of that number, 167 have been awarded benefits and approximately 135 have found permanent housing. Medicare is given 2 years after the award of benefits, and the recipients remain eligible for services at SCC until they receive Medicare, after which time the clinic staff makes referrals and helps to transition these clients to other providers in the community. Some are eligible for Medicaid and can be referred elsewhere in the community for services. We can now see the clinic as a transitional place for formally homeless people to engage with the larger community away from CCH and SSC. Financial resources and security give them access to many other resources outside of the CCH and SSC setting.

The APNs were able to "'think outside the box" and to conceptualize health and health care as more than just an office visit and perhaps a prescription for medication. With the help, support, and partnership of key individuals in large agencies, they were able to start a team that has had the effect of changing local implementation of state and national policies. Because of our success, we are offering workshops for other organizations in the Denver area, have been invited to present our work at national and international conferences, and have written a manual to be shared with and used by others. Perhaps most important, as more homeless individuals are getting housed through the efforts of the BART team, they are able to focus attention on being healthy, seeking health care appropriately, and truly integrating into the community.

## Lessons Learned

- Providing services to the homeless is not simply a matter of attending to medical care. And not simply finding a place for them to stay.
- The reasons for homelessness are varied and complex, and are sometimes a result of public and agency policies that may be short sited.
- At CCH, we have learned that in order to "create lasting solutions" we must also provide "wrap around" services, using a holistic approach to the immediate needs of the homeless and then to ongoing support and guidance until they are able to maintain housing and a place in a community on their own.

# SEX, SCIENCE, AND POLICY: APPROACHES TO ADOLESCENT SEXUAL HEALTH

Antonia M. Villarruel

*"Science cannot resolve moral conflicts, but it can help to more accurately frame the debates about those conflicts."*

HEINZ PAGELS

Parents, schools, health professionals, scientists, and policymakers have long been concerned with reducing adolescent pregnancy, sexually transmissible diseases (STDs), and in the past few decades, human immunodeficiency (HIV) infection. Yet despite shared concern, there is disagreement as to the type of strategies and policies needed to assist adolescents in making responsible sexual decisions. Furthermore, there is a disconnect between existing science and adolescent sexual health policies. In this section we describe existing policy approaches to sexual health domestically and abroad, discuss domestic and foreign policy, and present policy approaches to be considered for the future.

## SEX AND YOUTH

In 2003, 46.7% of teenagers in the United States reported having had sexual intercourse (Grunbaum et al., 2004). Risky behaviors such as unprotected sexual intercourse and multiple sex partners place young people at risk for HIV infection, other STDs, and pregnancy. Approximately 870,000 teens become pregnant each year, with 34% of girls becoming pregnant at least once before they reach the age of 20 (National Campaign to Prevent Teen Pregnancy, 2004).

In the past 10 years, however, the teen pregnancy rate has declined, with the highest decline (33%) occurring in 15- to 17-year-olds (Ventura, Abma, Mosher, & Henshaw, 2003). This all-time low has been attributed to delayed initiation of sexual intercourse and increased use of contraceptives (Santelli et al., 2004). However, these rates are still high when compared with those in other developed nations. Furthermore, there are also major differences between African-American or Hispanic youth compared with whites in pregnancy rates, which remain higher in the former groups, and contraceptive use, which is lower in these groups (Centers for Disease Control and Prevention [CDC], 2004b).

In addition to unintended pregnancies, sexually active teens are also at high risk for STDs. Each year approximately 19 million new cases of STDs are diagnosed in the United States, almost half of which occur in youth ages 15 to 24 (Weinstock, Berman, & Cates, 2004). Some of the highest STD rates in the country are among young people, especially among racial and ethnic minority adolescents (CDC, 2003b). In 2003, an estimated 3897 adolescents were diagnosed with HIV or acquired immunodeficiency syndrome (AIDS), approximately 12% of the total number of diagnoses that year (CDC, 2004a). African Americans were the largest group of young people affected by HIV, accounting for 56% of all HIV infections ever reported among those aged 13 to 24 (CDC, 2003a). Young women, especially African Americans and Hispanics, are increasingly at risk for HIV infection through heterosexual contact (CDC, 2004a).

## APPROACHES

The two predominant approaches that have been used for prevention of pregnancy and STDs, including HIV, are programs that emphasize abstinence and those that emphasize safer sex. Both approaches have similar aspects. For example, many abstinence and safer-sex curricula provide basic information about growth and development, pregnancy, STDs, and HIV. Many curricula also frame abstinence and safer sex in the context of being able to achieve later goals and dreams. Abstinence programs may focus on abstinence until marriage or delaying the onset of sexual intercourse. In contrast, although safer-sex curricula may also highlight abstinence as the only sure prevention against pregnancy and STDs, the focus of safer-sex program interventions centers on preventing the unintended consequences of sex. Curricular content may also include information about condoms and contraceptives, in addition to content related to developing technical skills associated with using contraceptive methods and negotiating with a partner to use them.

There is much debate as to what approach is best for adolescents. For example, some contend that an abstinence approach works best for younger adolescents whereas a safer-sex approach would work better for older adolescents. There is concern that, although many safer-sex approaches emphasize abstinence, adolescents may become confused by what some perceive as conflicting messages (i.e., "You should be abstinent—but if you are going to have sex, use contraceptives and condoms"). Others argue that this approach is similar to the widely accepted approach related to alcohol use (i.e., "Don't drink—but if you drink, don't drive"). In addition, there is concern that safer-sex approaches might actually promote sex; however, there is no evidence to support that such curricula increase the onset of sexual behavior, increase the frequency of sex, or promote multiple partners (Kirby, 2003). Conversely, there is concern that focusing only on abstinence will place adolescents at risk, as there have been some studies that indicate adolescents are more likely to have unprotected intercourse once abstainers become sexually active (Bruckner & Bearman, 2005).

## DOMESTIC AND FOREIGN POLICY

### U.S. Federal Policy

Currently there are no formal policy initiatives related to youth development and no major funding streams for safer-sex education. Federal support for pregnancy, HIV, and STD prevention centers on promoting abstinence, and section 510 of the 1996 Welfare Reform Act provides major funding for abstinence education. This law provided a federal matching grant to states of $25 million for over 5 years, which was later increased to $50 million per year in 2004.

In this legislation, detailed guidelines are provided for abstinence education. In the Personal Responsibility and Work Opportunity Reconciliation Act of 1996, abstinence education refers to programs that do the following (Personal Responsibility and Work Opportunity Reconciliation Act, 1996):

- Have as its exclusive purpose teaching the social, psychologic, and health gains to be realized by abstaining from sexual activity
- Teach abstinence from sexual activity outside marriage as the expected standard for all school-age children
- Teach that abstinence from sexual activity is the only certain way to avoid out-of-wedlock pregnancy, STDs, and other associated health problems
- Teach that a mutually faithful monogamous relationship in the context of marriage is the expected standard of human sexual activity
- Teach that sexual activity out of the context of marriage is likely to have harmful psychologic and physical effects
- Teach that bearing children out of wedlock is likely to have harmful consequences for the child, the child's parents, and society
- Teach young people how to reject sexual advances and how alcohol and drug use increases vulnerability to sexual advances
- Teach the importance of attaining self-sufficiency before engaging in sexual activity

There are several issues with an abstinence-only–based policy approach. First, there is not a scientific base that supports an abstinence-only policy. Few abstinence programs have been developed and rigorously tested. Those that have been tested do not indicate that these curricula delay the onset of sexual behavior. In fact, some studies indicate that once adolescents become sexually active, they are at risk because they do not use contraceptives or condoms (Bruckner & Bearman, 2005; Jemmott, Jemmott, & Fong, 1998).

Second, a congressional review of abstinence-only curricula used in funded state programs (U.S. Department of State, 2004) reported errors and distortions about the risk of sexual activity, contraceptive use, and abortion. For example, in some curricula, mental health issues such as depression were linked to sexual behavior. Inaccurate information was given related to the risk of abortion and contraceptive use. Furthermore, the report indicated that several abstinence-only curricula promoted stereotypes of males and females and blurred the line between religion and science. This is evident in information provided about abortion, but also in relation to addressing sex only in the context of marriage and only between a man and a woman. The policy does not address the issue of gay or bisexual youth, groups who are at high risk for HIV infection.

### U.S. International Policy

An abstinence focus is also a major component of President Bush's Emergency Plan for AIDS relief on a global level. The plan emphasizes curricula for adolescents of all ages that encourage youth to focus on their future, outlines the benefits of abstinence until marriage, and teaches refusal skills for sex, alcohol, and drugs. Condom use is recognized as an essential means of HIV prevention for high-risk populations, including prostitutes and substance abusers. Even in addressing condom use for high-risk populations, there is concern expressed by some policymakers and advocacy groups about confounding messages of abstinence, faithfulness, and partner reduction (U.S. Department of State, 2004). The issue of abstinence only in the United States is a challenge. This approach is increasingly complex in societies dissimilar to that of the United States, where the economic survival of women and their families may depend on their having sex regardless of personal risk or choice.

### Policies from Other Countries

When comparing adolescent pregnancy, STDs, and initiation of sexual intercourse in the United States with those in other countries, it is clear that our approaches to increase abstinence *or* contraceptive use are not effective. Other western countries, including France, Germany, the Netherlands, Sweden, and Great Britain, have a higher mean age of sexual initiation, fewer abortions, and lower rates of pregnancy and STDs among adolescents compared with U.S. adolescent (Lottes, 2002).

A major premise underlying policy in these European countries is that adolescents have a right to comprehensive and confidential sex education and services. The right to access contraceptive services—without parental permission—is also a part of this policy.

### FORECAST FOR THE FUTURE

While a European-type policy might be the ideal forecast for the future, it is not likely. The current religious ideology and values focused on marriage, heterosexual relationships, and monogamy are the major forces in directing health policy. Advocates for this perspective have been successful in shaping current health and science policy in the absence of evidence that supports an abstinence-only policy and despite evidence that safer-sex programs do protect adolescents without supporting promiscuity. The major block is that sound health policy is being guided not by science but by religious ideology and values. It is important to recognize that the abstinence and safer-sex education programs share a common goal of keeping adolescents healthy. There is a struggle to get both messages across despite media influences, which seem to promote both promiscuity and an absence of sexual responsibility.

Future research policy must support research to test effective interventions for both abstinence and safer sex. In particular, programs need to be tested through randomized controlled trials, programs need to be evaluated for at least 12 months, and outcomes should include some measure of behavior. This is especially true for abstinence interventions, given the lack of effective programs. It is important that "values"—promoting either abstinence or safer sex—be separated from evidenced-based prevention information. Values defining and promoting certain types of sexual behavior have a place in churches, in the home, and in other private arenas. However, sexual health education and policy should assume that adolescents can act responsibly both as adolescents and as adults. It is essential that adolescents be provided the information and opportunity to develop the skills necessary to make responsible decisions to maintain their health.

## Key Points

- The rates of teen pregnancy and STDs, including HIV, in the United States continue at unacceptable levels.
- A number of European countries have lower rates of teen pregnancy and STDs because of policies providing adolescents with comprehensive and confidential sex education and services, including the right to access contraception without parental permission.
- The scientific evidence does not support policies for abstinence—only approaches to reducing teen pregnancy and STDs. We do have evidence for comprehensive approaches that work and that include discussions of abstinence, but not exclusively. If we are to effectively reduce teen pregnancy and STDs, we must develop evidence-based public policies and programs.

## Web Resources

**Center for Reproductive Health Research and Policy, University of California at San Francisco**—promotes reproductive health, family planning, and the prevention of sexually transmitted infections, including HIV, worldwide through research, training, and policy analysis.
*http://crhrp.ucsf.edu/index.html*
**Centers for Disease Control and Prevention**
*www.cdc.gov*

**Contraception and Reproductive Health Branch of the National Institute of Child Health and Human Development, National Institutes of Health**
*www.nichd.nih.gov/cpr/crh/crh.htm*
**Healthy Teen Network**—national membership organization made up of practitioners, policymakers, and state and local coalitions concerned with adolescent pregnancy parenting and prevention
*www.noappp.org*
**National Library of Medicine and the National Institutes of Health**—reproductive health information
*www.nlm.nih.gov/medlineplus/reproductivehealth.html*

## REFERENCES

Bruckner, H., & Bearman, P. S. (2005). After the promise: The STD consequences of adolescent virginity pledges. *Journal of Adolescent Health, 36*, 271-278.

Centers for Disease Control and Prevention (CDC). (2004a). HIV/AIDS among Youth. National Center for HIV, STD and TB Prevention, Divisions of HIV/AIDS Prevention. Retrieved June 1, 2005, from *www.cdc.gov/hiv/pubs/facts/youth.htm*.

Centers for Disease Control and Prevention (CDC). (2004b). Teenagers in the United States: Sexual activity, contraceptive use, and childbearing, 2002. *Vital and Health Statistics, 23*(24). Retrieved June 13, 2005, from *www.cdc.gov/reproductivehealth/UnintendedPregnancy/Teen.htm*.

Centers for Disease Control and Prevention (CDC). (2003a). *HIV Prevention in the Third Decade*. Atlanta: U.S. Department of Health and Human Services. Retrieved June 1, 2005, from *www.cdc.gov/hiv/HIV_3rdDecade*.

Centers for Disease Control and Prevention (CDC). (2003b). Sexually transmitted disease surveillance, 2003. Atlanta: U.S. Department of Health and Human Services. Retrieved June 1, 2005, from *www.cdc.gov/std/stats*.

Grunbaum, J. A., Kann, L., Kinchen, S., Ross, J., Hawkins, J., et al. (2004). Youth risk behavior surveillance—United States, 2003. *MMWR Surveillance Summaries, 53*(SS-2). Retrieved June 1, 2005, from *www.cdc.gov/healthyyouth/yrbs*.

Jemmott, J. B., III, Jemmott, L. S., & Fong, G. T. (1998). Abstinence and safer sex HIV risk-reduction interventions for African American adolescents: A randomized controlled trial. *JAMA, 279*(19):1529-1536.

Kirby, D. (2003). Risk and protective factors affecting teen pregnancy and the effectiveness of programs designed to address them. In D. Romer (Ed.), *Reducing adolescent risk—Toward an Integrated Approach*. Thousand Oaks, CA: Sage.

Lottes, I. L. (2002). Sexual health policies in other industrialized countries: Are there lessons for the United States? *Journal of Sex Research, 39*, 79-83.

National Campaign to Prevent Teen Pregnancy. (2004). Factsheet: How is the 34% statistic calculated? Washington, DC. Retrieved March 22, 2006, from *www.teenpregnancy.org/resources/reading/pdf/35percent.pdf.*

Personal Responsibility and Work Opportunity Reconciliation Act. (1996). Public Law No. 104-193. Retrieved August 11, 2005, from *http://wdr.doleta.gov/readroom/legislation/pdf/104-193.pdf.*

Santelli, J. S., Abma, J., Ventura, S., Lindberg, L., Morrow, B., Anderson, J. E., et al. (2004). Can changes in sexual behaviors among high school students explain the decline in teen pregnancy rates in the 1990s? *Journal of Adolescent Health, 35,* 80-90.

U.S. Department of State. (2004). *The content of federally funded abstinence-only education programs.* Washington, DC: U.S. House of Representatives Committee on Government Reform—Minority Staff Special Investigations Division.

Ventura, S. J., Abma, J. C., Mosher, W. D., & Henshaw, S. (2003). Revised pregnancy rates, 1990-97, and new rates for 1998-99: United States. *National Vital Statistics Report, 52*(7), 1-16.

Weinstock, H., Berman, S., & Cates, W. (2004). Sexually transmitted diseases among American youth: Incidence and prevalence estimates, 2000. *Perspectives on Sexual and Reproductive Health, 36*(1), 6-10.

# **POLICY**SPOTLIGHT

## THE DEMISE OF AN ADOLESCENT SEXUALITY EDUCATION PROGRAM

Victoria J. Davey

*"Daring ideas are like chessmen moved forward; they may be beaten, but they may start a winning game."*

JOHANN WOLFGANG VON GOETHE

Montgomery County, Maryland wraps around the northeast and northwest quadrants of Washington, DC and serves as home to nearly a million highly educated federal government employees, professional and high-technology workers, a burgeoning Asian and Hispanic immigrant population, and their families. Voting resoundingly for John Kerry in the 2004 presidential election, it is diverse, affluent, and usually the bluest region of a blue state. The Montgomery County public school system serves nearly 135,000 children in 194 elementary, middle, and high schools (Montgomery Country Public Schools [MCPS], 2005a). Five of its 24 high schools were listed among *Newsweek*'s 100 top high schools for 2004 (Kantrowitz, 2005). The high schools graduate

over 90% of their students and pride themselves on sending graduates off to top colleges buoyed by high SAT scores and Advanced Placement credits (MCPS, 2005a). As the seventeenth largest school district in the nation, Montgomery County is a leader among public school systems because of its reputation for quality, innovation, and, usually, a balanced, fair, and broad-minded approach to the education of the county's children.

### A LONG-STANDING AND PROGRESSIVE SEXUAL HEALTH EDUCATION CURRICULUM

Montgomery County provides sex education as a part of a comprehensive health education curriculum that includes personal safety, drug and alcohol prevention, and lifestyle choices to help students "develop the life skills needed to enhance their potential for achieving academic success and healthier, happier, and more productive lives" (MCPS, 2005b). Sex education is delivered in age-appropriate units by teachers certified in the instruction of the content, and has contained material on contraception, including the use of condoms, for decades. The sexual health curriculum for eighth and tenth grades, which requires parental permission for students to attend, teaches abstinence as the absolute means of preventing pregnancy and sexually transmitted diseases (STDs), but also provides comprehensive information on contraception as well as multifaceted education on potential consequences of adolescent sexual activity, including teenage pregnancy and HIV/AIDS. For parents who prefer that their children not receive the comprehensive curriculum, alternative "abstinence only" or independent study on a health topic acceptable to the parents are offered (MCPS, 2005b). Montgomery County has had a long-standing, culturally sensitive, and organized approach to the teaching of human sexuality to its students.

## A BATTLE ERUPTS OVER SEX EDUCATION CURRICULUM CHANGES

Five years ago, county middle and high school teachers proposed changes in the health education curriculum based on their classroom teaching experiences. The requested changes were for instructional resources to discuss sexual orientation and better materials to illustrate proper condom use; teachers felt ill prepared to answer students' specific questions in these two areas. An advisory committee of county citizens worked for several years to draft and re-draft new materials, ultimately resulting in production of a new video illustrating correct condom use, entitled "Protect Yourself" (directed at tenth graders), and a respect- and tolerance-based curriculum for talking to eighth and tenth graders about sexual orientation. In November of 2004 the school board approved these new teaching materials and scheduled pilot implementation in five county schools for spring of 2005 (MCPS, 2005b).

Within weeks, county parents opposing the changes organized into a group called Citizens for a Responsible Curriculum (CRC), which objected to the new curriculum's "normalization" of nonheterosexual sexual behavior and the graphic instruction on condom use presented in the video, fearing that it would instigate sexual activity in teenagers.

Their opposition was assisted by a Virginia-based organization, Parents and Friends of ExGays and Lesbians (PFOX), which asserted that its viewpoint that homosexuality can be treated and surmounted was missing from the curriculum (CRC, 2004; PFOX, 2005). These opposing groups were countered by county parents organized under a group called TeachtheFacts.org, which encouraged the school board to continue its plan to present health education content based on peer-reviewed research and clinical evidence, and on tolerance and acceptance of multiple sexual orientations and their resulting family definitions (TeachtheFacts.org, 2005). The letter-writing and petition-signing campaigns that emerged were startling and polarizing for county citizens accustomed to the county's liberal-minded political identity and were carefully watched by other school systems facing similar curriculum battles in the teaching of human sexuality to adolescents.

The battle culminated in the May 2005 filing of a federal lawsuit by CRC and PFOX in federal court to block implementation of the new curriculum, citing First and Fourteenth Amendment violations. A federal judge granted a restraining order, based on concern that the teacher's instruction manual for the sexual orientation content specifically linked certain religious denominations to negative viewpoints on homosexuality and delved into theologic opinion on the morality of nonheterosexual orientations (*Citizens for a Responsible Curriculum et al. v. Montgomery County Public Schools et al.*, 2005). The County ultimately acknowledged that the teacher materials (which were never intended for the public's eyes) deemed certain religious denominations' views on homosexuality factually wrong and failed to list other existing viewpoints. This misstep and the court ruling caused the school board to cancel implementation of the sexual orientation content curriculum and the condom instruction video (Kaiser Daily Reproductive Health Report, 2005). The county later settled the lawsuit with CRC and PFOX, paying their legal costs. The advisory committee to the Montgomery County School Board that was originally responsible for drafting the new curriculum was reconstituted to include county residents who are CRC members and is engaged in writing new materials. As organizations, CRC and TeachtheFacts.org remain watchful and engaged on the sidelines in the crafting of the new curriculum (Fisher, 2005; Kennedy, 2005).

## THE POWER OF AN INFLUENTIAL MINORITY

Conservative political and religious groups, including the Alliance Defense Fund and the Culture and Family Institute, cheered the derailment of Montgomery County's updated sex education curriculum. Liberal groups, such as the Lesbian and Gay Rights Project of the American Civil Liberties Union, are concerned about potential wide-ranging repercussions in the United States (Janofsky, 2005). Montgomery County's path for sex education for its public school students was once clear and seemingly unassailable. It had adhered to a stated vision of health education content designed to provide balanced information, emphasizing safe choices for a healthy and productive adult life, and offered alternatives for families who desired them. The effort in 2005 to enhance and update its curriculum in a process guided by student needs and designed with community involvement failed. A minority political organization gained substantial influence and used it skillfully.

## REFERENCES

Citizens for a Responsible Curriculum (CRC). (2005). *Safe school, safe students.* Retrieved August 12, 2005, from *www.mcpscurriculum.com.*

*Citizens for a Responsible Curriculum et al. v. Montgomery Country Public Schools, et al.* Case 8:05-dv-01194-AW, Document 14. (United States District Court for the District of Maryland Southern Division. May 5, 2005). Retrieved August 12, 2005, from *www.mdd.uscourts.gov/Opinions152/Opinions/CRC050505.pdf.*

Fisher, S. A. (2005, August 25). A victory that protects values. *Washington Post, Montgomery Extra,* 13.

Janofsky, M. (2005, June 9). Gay rights battlefields spread to public schools. *New York Times.* Retrieved August 12, 2005, from *www.nytimes.com.*

Kaiser Daily Reproductive Health Report. (2005). Md. County school board votes to completely revise sex education curriculum, dissolve citizens advisory committee. Retrieved August 28, 2005, from *www.kaisernetwork.org/daily_reports/print_report.cfm?DR_ID=30304&dr_cat=2.*

Kantrowitz, B. (2005, May 16). The 100 best high schools in America. *Newsweek.* Retrieved August 12, 2005, from *www.msnbc.msn.com/id/7761678/sife/newsweek.*

Kennedy, J. (2005). A tolerant, scientific approach. *Washington Post, Montgomery Extra,* 13.

Montgomery County Public Schools (MCPS). (2005a). About us. Retrieved August 26, 2005, from *www.mcps.k12.md.us/about.*

Montgomery County Public Schools. (2005b). Health education. Retrieved August 12, 2005, from *www.mcps.k12.md.us/curriculum/health.*

Parents and Friends of ExGays and Gays (PFOX). (2004). Sexual orientation school curriculum for children. Retrieved August 12, 2005, from *www.pfox.org.*

TeachtheFacts.org. (2005). Retrieved August 12, 2005, from *www.teachthefacts.org.*

# THE POLITICS OF CHILDHOOD IMMUNIZATIONS

Mary Currier

*"The joy I felt at the prospect before me of being the instrument destined to take away from the world one of its greatest calamities [smallpox] was so excessive that I found myself in a kind of reverie."*

EDWARD JENNER

Vaccination is considered to be one of the great public health achievements of the twentieth century. The incidence of many childhood diseases, which routinely caused disability and death in children in the early 1900s, has declined to almost zero as a result of the development and use of effective and safe vaccines (Centers for Disease Control and Prevention [CDC], 1999). Today there are numerous issues surrounding vaccines that affect the intricate public-private partnerships that make up the vaccine delivery infrastructure in the United States. These include media publicity around perceived adverse events, liability for vaccine manufacturers and the resultant decrease in the number of manufacturers, decreasing perception of disease risk along with increasing perception of vaccine risk, loss of profit margin and increased cost to consumers, vaccine financing difficulties, and even bioterrorism. How these have affected current immunization policy is the focus of this discussion.

## PRINCIPLES OF VACCINE USE

Vaccines work by exposing a well individual to a substance so like the cause of a disease that the body produces immunity that protects against that disease. Usually this substance is a protein from the causative substance (bacteria), as with pertussis vaccine, or a weakened virus, as with the measles vaccine. Vaccines protect the immunized individual, and if enough of the population is immunized, they protect the community by providing a wall of immunity around those individuals who are unvaccinated (decreasing their likelihood of exposure). This is called *herd* or *community immunity*.

The incidence of nine infectious diseases, among which eight have vaccines that are universally recommended for use in children, has declined 100% (for smallpox) or nearly 100% (CDC, 1999) (Table 32-1). In addition to enormously decreasing morbidity and mortality from many infectious diseases, vaccines are cost effective. It is estimated that for every $1 spent on vaccination against these nine childhood diseases, $5.80 has been saved in direct medical costs (Zhou et al., 2005).

## LEGAL ISSUES

### Immunization Laws

There is no federal school immunization law; however, every state has laws requiring certain vaccines for school and licensed daycare center attendance. Some state laws specify which vaccines are required, and some leave that determination to an individual, such as the state health officer, or a group, such as the board of health (Malone & Hinman, 2003). In most places, nonvaccination results in not being allowed to attend school.

The constitutionality of mandated vaccinations was upheld in 1905, when the U.S. Supreme Court

**TABLE 32-1** Baseline Twentieth-Century Annual Morbidity and 2004 Provisional Morbidity from Nine Diseases with Vaccines Recommended before 1990 for Universal Use in Children, United States

| DISEASE | BASELINE TWENTIETH-CENTURY ANNUAL MORBIDITY | 2004 PROVISIONAL MORBIDITY | PERCENT DECREASE |
|---|---|---|---|
| Smallpox | 48,164[a] | 0 | 100% |
| Diphtheria | 175,885[b] | 0 | 100%[c] |
| Pertussis | 147,271[d] | 18,957 | 87.1% |
| Tetanus | 1314[e] | 26 | 98% |
| Poliomyelitis (paralytic) | 16,316[f, g] | 0 | 100% |
| Measles | 503,282[h] | 37 | 100%[c] |
| Mumps | 152,209[i] | 236 | 99.8% |
| Rubella | 47,745[j] | 12 | 100%[c] |
| Congenital rubella syndrome | 823[k] | 0 | 100% |
| Haemophilus influenzae type B | 20,000[l] | 172[m] | 99.1% |

Adapted from Centers for Disease Control and Prevention (CDC). (1999). Achievements in public health, 1900-1999. Impact of vaccines universally recommended for children—United States, 1900-1998. *MMWR Morbidity and Mortality Weekly Report, 48*(12), 243-248; provisional data (2004) supplied by Barry Sirotkin, National Immunization Program, CDC, personal communication, June 9, 2005.

[a]Average annual number of cases during 1900-1904.

[b]Average annual number of reported cases during 1920-1922, 3 years before vaccine development.

[c]Rounded to nearest tenth.

[d]Average annual number of reported cases during 1922-1925, 4 years before vaccine development.

[e]Estimated number of cases based on reported number of deaths during 1922-1926 assuming a case-fatality rate of 90%.

[f]Average annual number of reported cases during 1951-1954, 4 years before vaccine licensure.

[g]Excludes one case of vaccine-associated polio reported in 1998.

[h]Average annual number of reported cases during 1958-1962, 5 years before vaccine licensure.

[i]Number of reported cases in 1968, the first year reporting began and the first year after vaccine licensure.

[j]Average annual number of reported cases during 1966-1968, 3 years before vaccine licensure.

[k]Estimated number of cases based on seroprevalence data in the population and on the risk that women infected during a childbearing year would have a fetus with congenital rubella syndrome.

[l]Estimated number of cases from population-based surveillance studies before vaccine licensure in 1985.

[m]Excludes 71 cases of *Haemophilus influenzae* disease of unknown serotype.

issued its ruling in *Jacobson v. Massachusetts*, deciding that a health regulation requiring smallpox vaccination of the populace was within the rights of the state and did not violate the liberty of individuals: "...such reasonable regulations established directly by legislative enactment as will protect the public health and the public safety," were within the state's lawful authority (Hinman, Orenstein, Williamson, & Darrington, 2002; *Jacobson v. Massachusetts*, 1905; Malone & Hinman, 2003). Vaccination of the individual was seen as protecting society. In 1922 the U.S. Supreme Court upheld the constitutionality of school immunization laws in *Zucht v. King*, saying that city ordinances that excluded children from school attendance for failure to provide proof of immunization "confer...that broad discretion required for the protection of the public health" (*Zucht v. King*, 1922; Malone & Hinman, 2003). These legal decisions support the right of government to mandate vaccines for the public good over the individual's right to refuse, and recognize schools as a particularly important place for childhood diseases to be passed from person to person.

### Immunization Exemptions

All states allow individuals to be exempt from school and daycare vaccine requirements for medical reasons. The procedure for acquiring this exemption differs from state to state. All states but two

(Mississippi and West Virginia) allow exemption for religious reasons, and again, the procedure for obtaining this type of exemption differs by state. For example, some states require membership in a religion recognized not to allow vaccination, and others require only an assertion of religious opposition to immunization. However, in a study of exemptions nationwide, 32 of the 48 states that allow religious exemptions reported never denying an exemption request (i.e., all requests for exemptions were approved). An additional 20 states allow exemptions on the basis of personal philosophy (NCSL, 2004b). Required documentation and high complexity of steps necessary to obtain a religious or philosophic exemption have been found to be related to lower rates of exemptions (Rota et al., 2001). In other words, as the complexity of the procedure increases, the rate of exemptions decreases. In some states it is easier to acquire an exemption than it is to comply with vaccination requirements, which has led to a higher exemption rate. So, although laws mandate vaccination status for school and daycare center attendees, the interpretation of the law into regulation and procedure largely determines the difference among state rates of immunization exemptions.

### Immunization Recommendations

Written recommendations for the routine use and scheduling of vaccines for both children and adults are made by the Advisory Committee on Immunization Practices (ACIP), in collaboration with the American Academy of Pediatrics and the American Academy of Family Physicians (Orenstein, Douglas, Rodewald, & Hinman, 2005). The ACIP is a statutorily authorized advisory body to the Secretary of the U.S. Department of Health and Human Services (USDHHS), the Assistant Secretary for Health and the CDC, made up of experts in fields associated with immunization who are appointed by the Secretary of USDHHS (CDC, 2004a). ACIP recommendations are published by the CDC in the *Morbidity and Mortality Weekly Report* and are used by state health department immunization programs and by other health care providers to develop immunization policy and practice. Although these recommendations drive the policies

in individual clinics that determine vaccines given to each child at a particular visit, the final decision for vaccination is made between the health care provider—usually a nurse—and the parent. The nurse, being the primary executor of these recommendations and the primary educator concerning their value, has a huge amount of influence regarding whether or not the children she sees are appropriately vaccinated.

## SOCIOLOGIC ISSUES

### Media and Vaccine Risk

Although the media has publicized the suspected link between vaccine and several diseases, studies have found no association between measles vaccine and autism (Dales, Hammer, & Smith, 2001; Kaye, Melero-Montes, & Jick, 2001; Madsen et al., 2002); thimerosal and autism (Institute of Medicine [IOM], 2004); hepatitis B vaccine and multiple sclerosis; diphtheria, tetanus, pertussis vaccine and permanent neurologic disease; or Hib vaccine and diabetes (Dennehy, 2001). In several instances, however, the sensationalization of the possibility of a relationship has led to a decrease in immunization levels, with an accompanying increase in disease levels; for example, as publicity occurred surrounding suspected cases of encephalopathy and permanent neurologic damage following pertussis vaccination (although these are certainly consequences of pertussis disease itself), coverage declined in several countries, and pertussis rates became 10 to 100 times that of neighboring countries with continued high rates of immunizations (Gangarosa et al., 1998). In the United Kingdom alone, as vaccination levels dropped to 33%, three epidemics of pertussis occurred in the mid 1970s to the mid 1980s, resulting in hundreds of thousands of cases. Organized antivaccine groups used the media to further their cause, sensationalizing stories of children with neurologic disease, purported to be due to vaccine, with no scientific evidence for the relationship (Baker, 2003). In Japan, in response to the antivaccine publicity, the Ministry of Health and Welfare eliminated whole-cell pertussis vaccine use, later allowing it only for children over the age of 2 years. Pertussis coverage for infants fell to

10% in 1976. An epidemic of pertussis occurred in 1979, with more than 13,000 cases reported and 41 deaths. Although the whole-cell vaccine had a safety profile with a very low risk of serious side effects, it did cause fever and occasionally febrile seizures in some children. The development of acellular pertussis vaccine, with fewer of these side effects, improved the use of pertussis vaccine and was accompanied by a decline in pertussis cases (Gangarosa et al., 1998).

Vaccinations are given at regular frequent intervals during the first 2 years of a child's life, and many neurologic illnesses are manifested for the first time during the same time period. It is difficult for the public to differentiate between diseases associated with vaccination in time and a causal relationship. Anecdotal information, sensationalized by the media, can be associated with vast downturns in vaccination levels and the return of vaccine-preventable diseases on an epidemic level.

## The Controversy

As the incidence of vaccine-preventable diseases declines, it is easy to forget how deadly these diseases have been in the past. Parents of young children today have likely never seen someone in an iron lung because of polio infection or the effect of measles on a small child. There is little appreciation for the severity of these diseases, and an overestimation of the risks associated with the vaccines. Unlike other mandated preventive measures, such as seat belt laws or motorcycle helmet laws, and unlike other medications, which are usually given to an individual with an illness, vaccination requires the administration of a medical intervention to a healthy individual, making acceptance of any risk associated with vaccines more difficult (Isaacs, Kilhan, & Marshall, 2004; Malone & Hinman, 2003). However, studies have shown that even given the rarity of some of the vaccine-preventable diseases in the United States, persons who are unvaccinated are still at greater risk of disease and increase the risk of disease for those around them.

In a study of measles risk by Salmon and colleagues (1999), children with exemptions from immunizations were 35 times more likely to develop

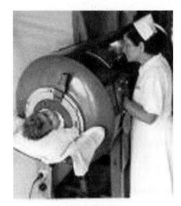

Patients whose respiratory muscles were affected were placed in an "iron lung" machine to enable them to breathe. (Courtesy of the World Health Organization. Retrieved from *www.vaccineinformation.org/photos/poliaap001.jpg*.)

measles than vaccinated children. In geographic areas with high exemption rates, the rate of measles among nonexempt children also increased by 5.5% to 30.8%, depending on the level of mixing between vaccinated and unvaccinated groups. Feiken and co-workers (2000) described the risk of developing measles or pertussis among children in Colorado by analyzing data on each case reported in the state over an 11-year period. Children with vaccine exemptions were 22 times more likely to develop measles and 5.9 times more likely to acquire pertussis than vaccinated children. In addition, in counties with higher exemption rates, rates of disease in vaccinated children were higher as well. Thirteen outbreaks of measles have been reported to the CDC among religious groups opposing vaccination during the 10-year period from 1985 though 1994. Outbreaks of polio (in the 1970s), pertussis, and rubella have been reported among the Amish (Hinman et al., 2002).

## Reality of Vaccine Adverse Events

The most-common side effects of vaccination are fever and pain at the site of the injection. Most people who get vaccinated experience no or mild side effects. However, as any medication, vaccines may rarely cause moderate to severe reactions, such as allergic reactions. Diphtheria, tetanus, acellular pertussis (DTaP) vaccine may cause a seizure (usually related to fever) in one child out of 14,000, and one in 1000 will cry inconsolably for 3 hours or more. Other more-severe, long-term events related in time to DTaP vaccination are so rare as to be unquantifiable, and it is difficult to determine if they are caused by the vaccine (CDC, 2004e).

There are vaccines that have rare but quantifiable serious side effects, such as the oral (live virus) polio vaccine (OPV). OPV causes an acute flaccid paralytic illness in one out of 2.4 million doses distributed. Because of that risk and the absence of wild poliovirus in the Western Hemisphere, the United States completely replaced OPV with an injectable inactivated virus vaccine in 2000. Because of increased intestinal immunity and increased population immunity resulting from secondary spread of the vaccine virus, OPV is still used in areas of the world where polio is still endemic (CDC, 2000). The rotavirus vaccine, which was recommended for use in mid 1998, was taken off the market by the manufacturer in October 1999, after use was suspended in July 1999 because of an excess number of cases of intussusception following vaccination reported to the Vaccine Adverse Events Reporting System. Further study found it likely that the excess risk of intussusception following vaccination was between one in 5000 and one in 11,000 vaccinees (CDC, 2004d).

Surveillance for vaccine injuries was improved through the establishment of the Vaccine Adverse Events Reporting System (VAERS) (42 U.S.C. §§ 300aa-25). This passive reporting system, administered by the U.S. Food and Drug Administration (FDA) and the CDC, provides postmarketing surveillance for adverse events, which allows rare events that can be detected only following the use of a vaccine in a large population to come to light. Physicians and other health care providers who provide immunizations are encouraged to report adverse events following vaccination, regardless of whether or not they think the event is related to the vaccine (Health Resources and Services Administration [HRSA], 2004). This system tracks adverse events and allows for the routine evaluation of and response to trends in side effects.

## ECONOMIC ISSUES

Vaccines are not inexpensive, and in 2005 private health providers paid approximately $790 per child for the vaccines included in the recommended school entry vaccination schedule. Vaccines purchased for public use through federally negotiated contracts cost about $500 per child (CDC, 2005a). The cost to private providers has increased from about $116 per child in 1987 because of an increased number of recommended vaccines (with newer vaccines being more costly) and increased price per dose.

Federal funding supports a large portion of childhood vaccine cost through two programs. The Immunization Grant Program (Section 317 of the Public Health Service Act), which operates through the CDC National Immunization Program, provides funding to state, local, and territorial public health agencies to support vaccine purchases and program operations for children vaccinated in public health clinics. This program awarded $418 million in 2003 and purchased about 11% of the pediatric vaccine used in this country (CDC, 2004b; Hinman, Orenstein, & Rodewald, 2004). The 317 program is subject to the yearly federal budget negotiations and therefore is influenced by the overall governmental budget situation and is largely inflexible outside the period of budget negotiation.

In 1993 the Vaccines for Children (VFC) program was established, which provides publicly purchased vaccines for participating providers (CDC, 2004c). The VFC program is an entitlement program that allows uninsured and Medicaid-eligible children, as well as American Indian and Alaskan Native children, to be immunized at their private provider's office for only an administrative cost. It also provides free vaccine at federally qualified health centers for children with insurance that does not cover immunizations (CDC, 2004c). When the ACIP adds vaccines to the recommendations for children, those vaccines are automatically covered by the VFC program. In 2003 the program awarded $975 million to state, local, and territorial public health agencies for program operation and vaccine purchase. It is estimated that in 2002 this program served about 41% of the childhood population (CDC, 2004c).

In addition, state funds are used to purchase about 5% of total pediatric vaccine doses (National Conference of State Legislatures [NCSL], 2004a). Each state health department has its own immunization program, through which the federal programs are operationalized. Eight states (Alaska, Idaho, Maine, Massachusetts, New Hampshire, New Mexico, Rhode Island, and Washington) have universal purchase programs, in which the states, using a combination of federal and state funding, purchase and distribute all vaccines to public and private immunization providers, allowing all children to receive the ACIP recommended vaccinations regardless of their insurance status (CDC, 2003).

The cost of vaccine administration is covered by insurance or the patient or is absorbed as a loss by the provider. Fifty-two percent of children under the age of 5 years have private insurance that covers immunization administration, 24% have public insurance (Medicaid or SCHIP), 14% have insurance that does not cover immunization, and 10% are uninsured (IOM, 2003). At least 28 states and the District of Columbia require insurance companies to cover childhood immunizations (NCSL, 2004a).

The funding for vaccine purchase and administration is through a patchwork of public and private sources. With no universal federal funding, as new vaccines are recommended and as costs of established vaccines increase, states struggle to provide this service for all their children.

## POLITICAL ISSUES

### National Response to Increased Costs

With the growing number of diseases for which vaccines are available, the decreasing number of companies producing vaccines, and the higher costs of producing safer and more effective vaccines, the National Immunization Program at CDC asked the IOM to assess current immunization financing and make recommendations to improve the way vaccines are purchased and

distributed in the United States. Their primary recommendations were as follows:

- Require insurance plans to cover recommended vaccines, establish a government subsidy to cover mandated vaccine costs and administration fees, and establish a voucher system for the uninsured.
- Change the membership and procedures of the ACIP so that its decisions regarding vaccine recommendations may include societal benefit and cost considerations (IOM, 2003).

The National Vaccine Program Office (NVPO, a coordinating office within USDHHS) and the National Vaccine Advisory Committee (NVAC, an advisory body to the NVPO) formed a Vaccine Financing Workgroup to respond to the IOM recommendations. This group met with stakeholders in 2004. Although it agreed with many of the observations and conclusions of the IOM report, the workgroup did not agree with the recommendations for action. The NVAC made responding recommendations based on the workgroup's activities; these consisted of more incremental changes, including expanding and stabilizing 317 funding to include support of infrastructure and operations and support of adolescent and adult immunization, as well as pediatric; rapidly approving increased 317 funds when new vaccines are recommended for universal use; including the underinsured in access to VFC vaccine at public health clinics; facilitating FDA approval of vaccines licensed in other countries; and several other changes that fix current administrative barriers that exist in insurance coverage for vaccine administration (Hinman, 2005). Neither set of recommendations has moved forward as of the publication of this text.

### Shortages: Role of the Federal Government

Vaccines are licensed by the FDA, which requires safety and efficacy studies before licensure, and continuing postlicensure surveillance. As the number of companies that produce vaccines declined in the 1980s, leading to sporadic shortages in several vaccines, the federal government approved the National Childhood Vaccine Injury Act, which established the National Vaccine Program within USDHHS to coordinate and oversee government-sponsored vaccine research and development, vaccine safety activities, and activities related to vaccination, and the National Vaccine Injury Compensation Program (VICP) to compensate for injuries associated with routinely administered childhood vaccine (P.L.99-660). The VICP is a no-fault program and was established to shift the monetary cost of rare vaccine injuries from the vaccinee and the vaccine manufacturers to a program funded by an excise tax on each vaccine dose (Malone & Hinman, 2003). Part of the cause of declining numbers of vaccine manufacturers was the cost of product liability. With the VICP in place, that cost decreased, and some pharmaceutical companies have returned to vaccine production and research (Malone & Hinman, 2003).

### Influenza Vaccine: An Example of Governmental Response to a Nationwide Shortage

Each year the viruses that are included in the influenza vaccine change, making last year's vaccine obsolete. The vaccine is tricky to make, requiring many time-consuming steps that include growing the vaccine viruses in eggs. Recent shortages of influenza vaccine have resulted from an unanticipated demand overwhelming the supply, production that was slower than anticipated, and production problems that led to a portion of the year's supply having to be withdrawn from the market. The decision of how much vaccine to produce is made by the manufacturer, based solely on the best estimate of demand, many months before the influenza season begins, and has very little cushion. These problems resulted in an increased involvement of the U.S. government in assuring adequate vaccine supplies and expanding the capacity to respond to an influenza crisis. Because of the shortages, USDHHS is developing financial incentives for manufacturers to enter the vaccine market. Additionally, Centers for Medicare and Medicaid Services has increased the administration fee to encourage providers to administer the vaccine. In addition to these policy changes, USDHHS is investing in new technologies to improve the timely production of vaccine and has created stockpiles of

influenza vaccine and antiviral medications (CDC, 2005b). The failure of a private portion of the public-private partnerships that make up the vaccine infrastructure to produce enough vaccine to meet the demand has led to more involvement of the government to assure continued access to the vaccine.

### ROLE OF THE HEALTH PROFESSIONAL

It is important that health professionals pay attention to the scientific data, which support immunizations as a very cost-effective and efficacious public health measure, and use their influence to assure this measure is supported in the future. Nurses, who in most cases educate the parents and deliver the vaccines, can have an impact at many levels. Nurses have the primary contact with the patient and parents at the time of vaccination, and daily can convey confidence in the vaccine if they have knowledge of the science supporting vaccines and of the history of vaccine-preventable diseases. Activism on a broader scope, through organized efforts at the state level to affect insurance coverage and state usage of federal vaccine funds and to support school immunization laws, plus at the federal level to affect national policy, can assure continuation of one of the most-effective public health measure we have.

## Key Points

- Mortality and morbidity from the nine diseases for which vaccines have been required among children since before 1990 have declined almost 100%.
- The vaccine development, distribution, and delivery infrastructure is a delicate, complicated combination of private-private partnerships that can be affected by many things that have little to do with science or health, such as vaccine production problems in a time of increased vaccine demand, media publicity about unproven side effects of vaccine, and funding issues.
- Health professionals can have a positive effect on policies that support a stronger immunization system.

## *Web Resources*

**General Vaccine Information**
*www.cdc.gov/node.do/id/0900f3ec8000e2f3*
*www.immunize.org*
**Anthrax Vaccine**—previously required for certain members of the armed services and currently offered but not mandated by court order.
*www.anthrax.mil/whatsnew/court.asp*
*www.cdc.gov/nip/vaccine/anthrax/default.htm*
**Smallpox Vaccine**—routinely used in the United States until 1972. The disease smallpox has been eradicated from the world, but the smallpox virus still exists in storage, and there is fear it will be used for bioterrorism. A smallpox vaccination program for public health and hospital response teams in each state was started in January of 2003, and over 39,000 persons have been vaccinated.
*www.bt.cdc.gov/agent/smallpox/*
*responseteams.asp*
*www.bt.cdc.gov/agent/smallpox/vaccination/vacc ine.asp*
**Influenza Vaccine**—influenza vaccine is a seasonal commodity, and there have been temporary shortages during influenza vaccination season as a result of fewer manufacturing companies making the vaccine and problems with vaccine manufacturing that slowed and/or decreased production, requiring new vaccine priority policies to be developed in the last several years. Pandemics of influenza have occurred throughout history, causing high mortality rates across the world. Pandemic preparedness depends on timely vaccine usage.
*www.cdc.gov/flu/pandemic/*
*www.cdc.gov/flu*
**Hepatitis B Vaccine**—currently recommended for all newborns. It is also recommended that persons at risk for hepatitis B exposure, including those health care workers who might contact blood or blood-containing

body fluids, in addition to persons at risk through sexual or IV drug-use behaviors, be vaccinated.
*www.osha.gov/pls/oshaweb/owadisp.show_docu ment?p_table=STANDARDS&p_id=10051*
*www.cdc.gov/nip/menus/vaccines.htm#hepb*
**HIV Vaccine**—there is ongoing HIV vaccine research, but development of a vaccine that prevents HIV infection has proved to be more difficult than expected.
*www.cdc.gov/hiv/vaccine.htm#vaccine*

## REFERENCES

Baker, J. P. (2003). The pertussis vaccine controversy in Great Britain, 1974-1986. *Vaccine, 21*, 4003-4010.

Centers for Disease Control and Prevention. (CDC). (1999). Achievements in public health, 1900-1999: Impact of vaccines universally recommended for children—United States, 1900-1998. *MMWR Morbidity and Mortality Weekly Report, 48*(12), 243-248.

Centers for Disease Control and Prevention (CDC). (2000). Poliomyelitis prevention in the United States. Updated recommendations of the Advisory Committee on Immunization Practices. *MMWR Recommendations and Reports, 49*(RR-5), 1-22.

Centers for Disease Control and Prevention (CDC). (2004a). ACIP charter: Advisory committee on immunization practices. CDC National Immunization Program. Retrieved June 2, 2005, from *www.cdc.gov/nip/ACIP/charter.htm*.

Centers for Disease Control and Prevention (CDC). (2004b). Program in brief: Immunization grant program (Section 317). Retrieved March 9, 2005, from *ww.cdc.gov/programs/immun04.htm*.

Centers for Disease Control and Prevention (CDC). (2004c). Program in brief: Vaccines for Children Program. Retrieved March 9, 2005, from *www.cdc.gov/programs/immun11.htm*.

Centers for Disease Control and Prevention (CDC). (2004d). Suspension of rotavirus vaccine after reports of intussusception—United States, 1999. *MMWR Morbidity and Mortality Weekly Report, 53*(34), 783-806.

Centers for Disease Control and Prevention (CDC). (2004e). Vaccine safety: Vaccine side effects. Retrieved June 1, 2005, from *www.cdc.gov/nip/vacsafe/concerns/side-effects.htm*.

Centers for Disease Control and Prevention (CDC). (2005a). CDC vaccine price list. Retrieved June 27, 2005, from *www.cdc.gov/nip/vfc/cdc_price_list.htm*.

Centers for Disease Control and Prevention (CDC). (2005b). Influenza: U.S. influenza supply and preparations for the future. Retrieved July 19, 2005, from *www.cdc.gov/washington/testimony/in02102005.htm*.

Centers for Disease Control and Prevention (CDC) National Immunization Program. (2003). Vaccines for children: Vaccine supply policy public. Retrieved June 23, 2005, from *www.cdc.gov/nip/vfc/st_immz_proj/data/vacc_supply_public_2002.htm*.

Dales, L., Hammer, S. J., & Smith, N. J. (2001). Time trends in autism and in MMR immunization coverage in California. *JAMA, 285*(9), 1183-1185.

Dennehy, P. H. (2001). Active immunization in the United States: Developments over the past decade. *Clinical Microbiology Reviews, 14*(4), 872-908.

Feiken, D. R., Lezotte, D. C., Hamman, R. G., Salmon, D. A., Chen, R. T., & Hoffman, R. E. (2000). Individual and community risks of measles and pertussis associated with personal exemptions to immunization. *Journal of the American Medical Association, 284*, 3145-3150.

Gangarosa, E. J., Galazka, A. M., Wolfe, C. R., Phillips, L. M., Gangarosa, R. E., et al. (1998). Impact of anti-vaccine movements on pertussis control: The untold story. *Lancet, 351*, 356-361.

Health Resources and Services Administration (HRSA). (2004). National Vaccine Injury Compensation Program: Fact sheet. Retrieved June 1, 2005, from *www.hrsa.gov/osp/vicp/fact_sheet.htm.*

Hinman, A. R. (2005). Perspective: Addressing the vaccine financing conundrum. The National Vaccine Advisory Committee weighs in with eight recommendations for more stable vaccine funding. *Health Affairs, 24*, 701-704.

Hinman, A. R., Orenstein, W. A., & Rodewald, L. (2004). Financing immunizations in the United States. *Clinical Infectious Diseases, 38*, 1440-1446.

Hinman, A. R., Orenstein, W. A., Williamson, D. E., & Darrington, D. (2002). Childhood immunization: Laws that work. *Journal of Law, Medicine & Ethics, 30*(Suppl 3), 122-127.

Institute of Medicine (IOM) Committee on Evaluation of Vaccine Purchase Financing in the United States. (2003). *Financing vaccines in the 21st century: Assuring access and availability.* Washington, DC: National Academies Press.

Institute of Medicine (IOM) Immunization Safety Review Committee. (2004). *Immunization safety review: Vaccines and autism.* Washington, DC: National Academies Press.

Isaacs, D., Kilhan, H. A., & Marshall, H. (2004). Should routine childhood immunizations be compulsory? *Journal of Paediatrics and Child Health, 40*, 392-396.

*Jacobson v. Massachusetts,* 197 U.S. 11 (1905).

Kaye, J. A., Melero-Montes, M. D., & Jick, H. (2001). Mumps, measles, and rubella vaccine and the incidence of autism recorded by general practitioners: A time trend analysis. *BMJ, 322*, 460-463.

Madsen, K. M., Hviid, A., Vestergaard, M., Schendel, D., Wohlfahrt, J., et al. (2002). A population-based study of measles, mumps, and rubella vaccination and autism. *New England Journal of Medicine, 347*(19), 1477-1482.

Malone, K. M., & Hinman, A. R. (2003). Vaccination mandates: The public health imperative and individual rights. (2003). In R. A. Goodman, M. A. Rothstein, R. E. Hoffman, et al. (Eds.), *Law in public health practice.* New York: Oxford University Press.

National Conference of State Legislatures (NCSL). (2004a). Financing childhood Immunizations. Retrieved February 9, 2005, from *www.ncsl.org/programs/health /imfinance.htm.*

National Conference of State Legislatures (NCSL). (2004b). States with philosophical exemptions from immunization school requirements. Retrieved July 19, 2005, from *www.ncsl.org/programs/health/2004ex/chart.htm.*

Orenstein, W. A., Douglas, R. G., Rodewald, L. E. & Hinman, A. R. (2005). Immunizations in the United States: Success, structure, and stress. *Health Affairs, 24*, 599-610.

Rota, J. S., Salmon, D. A., Rodewald, L. E., Chen, R. T., Hibbs, B. F., & Gangarosa, E. J. (2001). Processes for obtaining nonmedical exemptions to state immunization laws. *American Journal of Public Health, 91*, 645-648.

Salmon, D. A., Haver, M., Gangarosa, E. J., Phillips, L, Smith, N. J., & Chen, R. T. (1999). Health consequences of religious and philosophical exemptions from immunization laws: Individual and societal risk of measles. *JAMA, 281*, 47-53.

Zhou, F., Santoli, J., Messonnier, M. L., Yusuf, H. R., Shefer, A., et al. (2005). Economic evaluation of routine childhood immunization with DTaP, Td, Hib, IPV, MMR, HepB, and VAR vaccines in the United States, 2001. *Archives of Pediatrics & Adolescent Medicine, 159*, 1136-1144.

*Zucht v. King,* 260 U.S. 174. (1922). Pub. L. 99-660, title III, Nov. 14, 1986, 100 Stat. 3755, Retrieved March 28, 2006, from *http://uscode.house.gov/search/criteria.shtml.*

## WAKE-UP CALL: MOBILIZING COMMUNITIES TO IMPROVE HEALTH LITERACY

Veronica D. Feeg

*"[We] are coming to realize…that there is a certain sterility in economic monuments that stand alone in a sea of illiteracy. Conquest of illiteracy comes first."*

JOHN KENNETH GALBRAITH

*"Literacy is not a luxury, it is a right and a responsibility."*

PRESIDENT BILL CLINTON

Undeniably, although access to health care is a challenge that many U.S. citizens endure, understanding health care information presents a real and potential crisis for the public and puts many at risk for serious health consequences that are only recently gaining attention among policymakers. In fact, a growing number of physicians, volunteer health associations, universities, and health care companies describe low health literacy as a silent epidemic that affects approximately 90 million people; cannot be detected by physical examination, blood test, or diagnostic imaging system; and costs tens of billions of dollars per year (Pfizer Inc., 2003).

In 2004, the Committee on Health Literacy of the Institute of Medicine (IOM) released a report that documents the problem and describes its origins, consequences, and potential solutions in *Health Literacy: A Prescription to End Confusion* (IOM, 2004). It supported an earlier call from the Surgeon General and other health leaders: to mobilize professionals and policymakers around the priorities for health literacy as a goal central to the

efforts recommended by the IOM in its series of reports related to improving quality and safety in the health care system.

This policy spotlight describes the components that have shaped the recognition of health literacy as a public health problem and discusses its emergence in the health policy arena related to efforts toward improving quality in health care while protecting consumers from injury and untoward effects of misunderstanding health information. It addresses the safety concerns of patients' inability to interpret basic instructions such as prescriptions, medications, appointment slips, informed consent documents, and education materials. It also presents how policymakers and a variety of stakeholder groups have initiated action plans to mobilize professionals and consumer advocates. With the confluence of these activities, nurses and health professionals can recognize a variety of opportunities to engage with patients and organizations in community efforts that support the development of resources to enhance communication and improve health literacy.

### DEFINING HEALTH LITERACY AS A POLICY ISSUE

*Healthy People 2010* defines health literacy as "the degree to which individuals have the capacity to obtain, process, and understand basic health information and services needed to make appropriate health decisions" (USDHHS, 2000, pp. 11-20). Health literacy skills are needed for dialogue and discussion, reading health information, and interpreting tools. Such skills involve more than reading and include writing, numeracy, listening, speaking, and conceptual knowledge. Literacy is the foundation of health literacy, and health literacy is an active mediator between individuals and health contexts (IOM, 2004). Individuals bring specific sets of factors to the health context that include cognitive abilities, social skills, emotional state, and physical capacity such as visual and auditory acuity. Basic literacy is a complex function of educational, cultural, and psychosocial determinants. Literacy provides the skills that enable patients to understand and communicate health information to act in their own interest. With this perspective, the key sectors that are both contributors and potential intervention points include education systems, health systems, and societal factors (Figure 32-1). Although causal relationships between limited health literacy and health outcomes are not yet established, cumulative and consistent findings suggest such a causal connection (IOM, 2004).

In 2003, Surgeon General Richard Carmona called for a national effort to recognize that poor health literacy can be linked to health disparities and that it is particularly challenging because it is difficult for health care providers to recognize the problem when patients do not admit that it is a struggle to understand medical information

(Partnership for Clear Health Communication, 2003). He stated that a patient's ability to understand and act on medical information has tremendous impact on health outcomes. Research suggests that people with low health literacy are less likely to seek preventive treatments, make more medication or treatment errors, and are at a higher risk for hospitalization than people with adequate literacy skills.

With the release of a major report from the Agency for Healthcare Research and Quality (AHRQ) on literacy and health outcomes, director Carolyn Clancy called communication and information the "currency in health care" and added that "as the health care system struggles to address, in particular, the problem of chronic illness, the participation and engagement of the patient is not just a nice idea, it's required" (Vastag, 2004, p. 2181). Low literacy may impair functioning in the health care environment, affect patient-provider communication dynamics, and inadvertently lead to substandard medical care (American Medical Association [AMA], 1999). With the level of language used in consent forms, prescription drug directions, and oral instructions to patients more complex than the average comprehension level of adults, patients can make serious errors, take medicines on erratic schedules, miss follow-up appointments, and misunderstand procedural details (IOM, 2004; Vastag, 2004). These errors can result in adverse health outcomes with associated social and financial public health consequences.

## SCOPE OF THE PROBLEM

Nearly half of all American adults (47%)—90 million people—have difficulty understanding and acting on health information (Kirsch, Jungeblut, Jenkins, & Kolstad, 1993). In a recent report by Rudd, Kirsch, and Yamamoto (2004), health literacy was assessed to illuminate the relationship between literacy and health using data from large-scale surveys of adult literacy, the National Adult Literacy Survey (NALS) and the International Adult Literacy Survey (IALS), conducted by the Educational Testing Service for the U.S. Department of Education. Included in these assessments were a variety of health-related materials on topics such as drugs and alcohol, disease

*Health Literacy Framework*

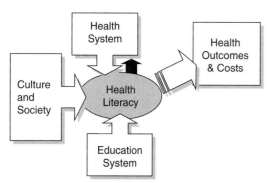

**Figure 32-1** Health literacy framework. (Reprinted with permission from *Health literacy: A prescription to end confusion.* Copyright 2004 by the National Academy of Sciences, courtesy of the National Academies Press, Washington, DC.)

prevention and treatment, safety and accident prevention, first aid, emergencies, and staying healthy. Survey respondents were asked to perform different literacy tasks based on these materials—for example, to read a medicine dosage chart and indicate the correct dose for a child of a particular weight and age. The survey also gathered extensive background demographic information. The researchers were able to create a new Health Activities Literacy Scale (HALS) linked to the NALS database and could create a similar progression of health-related literacy skills from low (Level 1) to high (Level 5). Data were analyzed for the population as well as for at-risk or vulnerable population groups.

For the total U.S. population, 12% is estimated to have skills in the lowest level (Level 1) on the HALS, and an additional 7% can be expected to have great difficulty performing even these simple tasks with a high degree of proficiency. Some 41% of those performing at Level 1 on the HALS report that they were born in a Spanish-speaking country, and roughly 51% report being born in the United States (Rudd et al., 2004).

For selected vulnerable or at-risk groups, performance on the HALS varies by respondents' level of education, race or ethnicity, country of birth, and age.

## Education

The average HALS score of adults who had not completed high school was far lower than that of individuals who had graduated from high school. Almost half (48%) did not score above Level 1, and slightly more than 80% did not exceed Level 2.

## Race and Ethnicity

The average proficiency of white adults on the HALS was significantly higher than the average proficiency of African American, Hispanic, and other adults. With the exception of white adults, more than 10% of each of the other racial or ethnic groups was estimated to be below Level 1. For Hispanic adults, 30% performed below Level 1.

## Country of Birth

The average HALS scores of foreign-born adults were significantly below those of the adults who were born in the United States.

## Age

The average HALS scores of younger adults were significantly higher than those of older adults. Almost half of the older adults in the United States performed at or below Level 1 on the HALS, and another 33% scored at Level 2.

The IOM report (2004) highlighted more than 300 peer-reviewed studies indicating that health-related materials for the mass culture far exceed the average reading level of adults. More importantly, the personal costs of limited health literacy also bear consideration: the committee concluded that the shame and stigma associated with limited literacy skills are major barriers to improving health literacy. Health illiteracy is a "silent epidemic": most professionals and policymakers lack understanding of the extent and effect of illiteracy and the individual shame associated with it that keeps it underappreciated and hidden. The IOM committee's findings related to the extent and associations of health literacy support the existence of links between education and health outcomes caused by a combination of poor literacy skills on one hand and complex health information materials on the other, resulting in a mismatch between the reading levels of materials and the reading skills of the intended audience. Of the 90 million adults who test below high school level, 40 to 44 million have difficulty finding information in unfamiliar or complex texts such as newspaper articles, editorials, medicine labels, forms, or charts. In one large public hospital study, 42% did not understand directions on a pill bottle for taking medication on an empty stomach, 43% did not understand the rights and responsibilities section of a Medicaid application, and 60% could not understand a standard informed consent form (Kirsch et al., 1993).

The committee also reported evidence of associations between limited health literacy and knowledge of disease management, health-promoting behaviors, poorer health status, and likelihood to use preventive services. In a recent study on the effectiveness of a primary care-based diabetes disease management program, 217 patients with type 2 diabetes and poor glycemic control were randomized and stratified by literacy status. After 12 months of follow-up for the control group and the comprehensive disease management intervention group, patients with higher literacy had similar odds of achieving good outcomes regardless of intervention status. Among patients with low literacy, intervention patients were more likely than control patients to achieve established goals. The authors concluded that literacy may be an important factor for predicting who will benefit from an intervention and who will not (Rothman et al., 2004).

In addition, the committee cited evidence of higher rates of hospitalization and use of emergency services among patients with limited literacy, suggesting that higher use can predict higher health care costs (Baker et al., 2002):

- Of 979 patients seen in an emergency department, statistical analysis showed that those with inadequate health literacy were more likely to be hospitalized (31.5%) than patients with adequate health literacy (14.9%).
- For the purpose of the IOM report, the committee commissioned an examination of the expenditure data collected on this study (Howard, 2004). Using econometric regression techniques, Howard found that predicted inpatient spending for patients with inadequate health literacy was $993 higher than that for persons with adequate health literacy. Emergency care costs incurred by individuals with inadequate health literacy scores were higher than in patients with adequate literacy, although pharmacy expenses were similar in both groups.
- In another study by the National Academy on an Aging Society, estimates of the costs of low health literacy to the health care system are between $30 billion and $73 billion annually (1998 dollars). Sixty-three percent of the additional costs attributed to low health literacy may be borne by public programs (Friedland, 1998).

### FROM PROBLEM TO POLICY PROCESS

Health literacy is a salient issue for health policy today, but it has been largely ignored in political dialogue (Rogers, Ratzan, & Payne, 2001). To achieve the goal of a health-literate America, we must acknowledge the severity of the problem and take steps to advance policies that address the issues.

Although low health literacy has been hidden, it is an emerging public issue that is often misunderstood as a condition that affects a specific portion of the population and that evokes shame. Its scope is broad, and its impact is severe. Although it can affect everyone regardless of background or educational level, studies show that limited literacy skills are a stronger predictor of an individual's health status than age, income, employment status, education level, and racial or ethnic group. It may play the pivotal role in health disparities among select, vulnerable citizens. Systemic changes are needed to counter the misinformation, miscommunication, and mistakes that characterize the health care experience of people with inadequate health literacy, and policy-oriented strategies are required (Parker, Ratzan, & Lurie, 2003). However, nurses and health providers calling for reform or orchestrating ambitious health policy efforts need to heed the political climate and policy streams to effectively move beyond the recognition of the problem of health literacy with its antecedents and consequences.

### POLITICAL CLIMATE AND POLICY CHALLENGE

Kingdon (2003) offers a framework for understanding the phrase "an idea whose time has come" in relation to what makes people in and around government attend, at any given time, to some issues and not to others. To promote understanding of the confluence of policymaking streams, Kingdon highlights the contributions of these streams from problem to the policy process. The streams include recognition of the problem, understanding the policy goals and ideas of those in policy subsystems, and sensing political factors that move or stall health agendas.

Recognizing the problem stream can be described as sorting through the complexities of health disparities and getting policymakers to focus on one problem associated with high out-of-pocket costs that also affects health. A problem such as health illiteracy is embedded in a larger problem such as social inequities and can be pulled out from the plethora of other problems. Although the evidence supports that poor literacy and low health literacy contribute to poor health and higher health care costs, the problems that contribute to poor literacy are fundamental, pervasive, and expensive to address.

Understanding the policy stream requires articulation of the policy goals, and matching ideas of those in policy subsystems such as researchers, congressional staff, agency officials, and interest groups or invested stakeholders. The strength of the evidence and the independence of the IOM committee give clout to the report and rationale to the policy recommendations. The timing, attention, and professional consensus of focusing on health literacy as a lynchpin for improving health quality and safety make the policy recommendations feasible and functional, even in these times of cautious spending initiatives. From federal to state and local governments, the health literacy chant plays well in public places.

Sensing the political stream requires skill in disentangling factors in the political environment that influence the policy agenda. Health literacy is ideologically neutral and politically feasible, with demonstrated good returns on investment. It makes it politically lightweight, without conflict in values or methods. Numerous initiatives from both political persuasions have emerged to stimulate initiatives to improve health literacy by decree or by funding. Kingdon sees policy streams as floating around and waiting for a "window of opportunity" to open through convergence and couplings of any two streams. It is apparent through the plethora of public and private programs and campaigns that health literacy has coupled a problem with potential solutions. It is an issue whose time has come. In the political climate of efforts to lower costs while improving quality and safety, initiatives to improve health literacy mobilize diverse communities with equal stakes in the outcome.

Making health literacy a priority, the office of the Surgeon General reports that low health literacy has gone largely unrecognized and untreated for too long. The task at hand is to learn the best ways to improve literacy. "Health literacy can save lives, save money, and improve the health and well being of millions of Americans...health literacy is the currency of success for everything I am doing as Surgeon General" (Carmona, 2003).

## GOVERNMENT ROLE IN ACHIEVING HEALTH LITERACY

The role of the government in addressing low health literacy includes functioning in a variety of roles in leadership, oversight, research, and education. Many of the federal health agencies have programs and activities for documenting and improving the health literacy of the public. These agencies can influence the health care and public health systems to develop and support integrated strategies addressing health literacy. They can also foster and support research to advance the state of the knowledge on effective interventions. In addition, the federal government is instrumental in producing and disseminating health-related information and the regulation of such information from other sources. Federal agencies that are part of these collective efforts include a number within USDHHS, such as the Food and Drug Administration (FDA) and the Centers for Disease Control and Prevention (CDC) (Box 32-1).

State governments have also identified health literacy as a critical issue. In addition to efforts to promote health literacy, states are intensively involved in running Medicaid, the health care assistance program for low-income individuals and families. With these costs rising rapidly, states have a vested interest in developing methods to address problems that contribute to health care inflation, such as the deleterious effects of low health literacy.

## COMMUNITY CALL TO ACTION

Parker, Ratzan, and Lurie (2003) call on a wide array of constituencies to take on health literacy as a policy challenge for advancing high-quality health care. They posit that creating a health-literate America may not be easy, but it is the right goal for health policy. Problems with health literacy are extremely common and costly, and the IOM report of its public health scale and impact has prompted a wake-up call for public and private stakeholders to take action. Many contemporary health policy debates that relate to government-financed Medicare and Medicaid, patients' rights, and privacy of health information rest on the assumption of adequate health literacy. The IOM listed health literacy as one of 20 priority areas in which quality

**BOX 32-1  Federal Agency Examples of Health Literacy Efforts**

Agencies within the U.S. Department of Health and Human Services (USDHHS) are involved in activities associated with health literacy.

- A Food and Drug Administration (FDA) regulation requires that over-the-counter medication labels be written such that an ordinary individual, including individuals of low comprehension, under customary conditions of purchase and use, can read and understand instructions.
- The Centers for Disease Control and Prevention (CDC) have a central role in successfully communicating information on health and illness to all members of the public and have focused efforts around use of plain language, including training, testing, and pretesting materials; conducting surveys; and providing health information to the media.
- The Centers for Medicare and Medicaid Services (CMS) run the Medicare program and are directly responsible for communication with people covered by Medicare.
- The National Institutes of Health (NIH) play a crucial role in determining federal funding for health literacy research.
- The Health Resources and Services Administration (HRSA) provides both service and educational programs intended to improve access to health care, the quality of health care, and health outcomes.
- The Agency for Healthcare Research and Quality (AHRQ) sponsors, carries out, and disseminates research on health care quality, medical errors and patient safety, health care costs, and health disparities.
- The lead agency for the health literacy objective of *Healthy People 2010* is the Office of the Secretary, Office of Disease Prevention and Health Promotion (ODPHP).

From Institute of Medicine (IOM). (2004). *Health literacy: A Prescription to end confusion.* Washington, DC: National Academies Press.

improvement could transform health care in America, based on the fact that communications between clinicians, patients, and families is fundamental to successful illness self-management (Adams & Corrigan, 2003).

## A VISION FOR HEALTH LITERACY

The IOM (2004) report on health literacy recommendations are built within a vision for an American health-literate society in which the following are true:

- Everyone has the opportunity to improve his or her health literacy.
- All people have the opportunity to use reliable, understandable information that could make a difference in their overall well-being, including everyday behaviors such as how they eat, whether they exercise, and whether they get checkups.
- Health and science content would be basic parts of K-12 curricula.
- People are able to accurately assess the credibility of health information presented by health advocate, commercial, and new media sources such as the Internet.
- There is monitoring and accountability for health literacy policies and practices. Public health alerts, vital to the health of the nation, are presented in everyday terms so that people can take needed action.
- The cultural contexts of diverse peoples, including those from various cultural groups and non–English-speaking peoples, are integrated into all health information.
- Health practitioners communicate clearly during all interactions with their patients, using everyday vocabulary.
- There is ample time for discussions between patients and health care providers.
- Patients feel free and comfortable to ask questions as part of the healing relationship.
- Rights and responsibilities in relation to health and health care are presented or written in clear, everyday terms so that people can take needed action.
- Informed consent documents used in health care are developed so that all people can give or withhold consent based on information they need and understand.

The IOM report concludes that health literacy can be improved, and these efforts must depend on efforts from all the sectors that contribute to the problem: government, schools, and the health care system. It calls on all stakeholders to mobilize their respective communities in order to reduce the effects of limited health literacy. These actions must be a combination of interventions directed at the roots of the problem through improved and earlier education in the schools, with simultaneous responsiveness from health service providers to modify their health information conversations and materials to address the fact that patients may not fully understand what they are being told. Specifically, the committee calls on government, providers, advocates, organizations, and the public to take action for promoting a health-literate America:

- USDHHS should take the lead in developing uniform standards for addressing literacy. In order to achieve meaningful research outcomes in all fields:
  - Investigators should involve patients in the research process to ensure that methods are valid and reliable and in a language easily understood.
  - The National Institutes of Health (NIH) should collaborate with appropriate federal agencies to formulate the policies and criteria to ensure that appropriate consideration of literacy is an integral part of the approval of research involving human subjects.
- Government and private funders should support the development and use of culturally appropriate new measures of health literacy, as well as multi-disciplinary research on the extent, associations, and consequences of limited health literacy.
- Educators should take advantage of opportunities to incorporate health-related tasks, materials, and examples into existing lesson plans.
- Professional schools and continuing education programs in the health fields should incorporate health literacy into their curricula and areas of competence.
- Health care systems should develop and support demonstration programs to establish effective approaches to reduce the negative effects of limited health literacy. These organizations should:
  - Engage consumers in the development of health communications and infuse insights gained from them into health messages

- Explore creative approaches to communicate health information using printed and electronic materials and media in appropriate and clear language—translated appropriately and interpreted for diverse audiences
- Establish methods for creating health information content in appropriate and clear language using relevant translations of health information
- Include cultural and linguistic competency as an essential measure of quality of care

## ACTION AGENDAS FOR HEALTH LITERACY

Numerous activities have flourished around health literacy from provider organizations, advocacy groups, insurers, businesses, and government agencies, producing numerous Internet Websites and resources for public use (see Web Resources). With the return of double-digit health care inflation, the continued difficulties many have with access to and affordability of basic health insurance, and alarming reports of widespread medical errors, policymakers and stakeholders in health care systems have focused their attention on a correctable obstacle in achieving a more informed and active health care consumer through health literacy initiatives.

The Council of State Governments (CSG) is active in analyzing states' roles in improving low health literacy and has made available to state government officials and staff a wide array of issue briefs, fact sheets, tools, and videos that support initiatives to improve health literacy. To assist state policymakers in addressing this problem, with funding from Pfizer, Inc., the CSG undertook a major national research project with goals of gathering data from research findings on health literacy, determining what states are doing to make it easier for someone with low health literacy to navigate the health care system, and reporting the information and tools necessary for state leaders to determine appropriate action (CSG, 2002). The guide is available with tools and resources for state officials to launch innovating programs for dealing with low health literacy (*www.csg.org/CSG/Policy/health/health+literacy/*

*default.htm).* Several promising state approaches include the following:

■ Virginia's Center for Primary Care and Rural Health established a Health Literacy Network to promote the use of plain language and to offer resources to health care providers, agency staff, and others wanting to assist specific populations access care. In 1999 the Center sponsored a health literacy conference for national, state, and local health care programs.

■ The Illinois Secretary of State's Literacy Office created a Health Literacy Task Force to spearhead "Health Literacy for All," a program designed to aid parents in understanding health information.

■ California approved its Health Framework for California's Public Schools, Kindergarten through Grade Twelve, a tool to aid health education curriculum development at the local level and to promote collaborations among schools, parents and the community.

■ Massachusetts' medical assistance programs have been at the forefront of providing multilingual assistance and videos in multiple languages and training staff to convey health care information in a way that is easy to understand. Massachusetts also has an Adult Basic Education Health Curriculum Framework for adult literacy classes.

■ Georgia's Department of Technical and Adult Education has hired a Health Literacy Coordinator to oversee the implementation of a series of health literacy classes throughout the state. Still in its early stages, this program has hosted classes in hospitals, senior centers, mental health facilities, and community health centers.

■ Alabama's Medicaid agency has done extensive pilot testing of materials for enrollees. Through this work the agency has learned that easy-to-read materials are preferred, even by those with proficiency in reading.

At a follow-up conference co-sponsored by the American College of Physicians Foundation (ACPF) and the IOM, "Moving Forward to Improve Health Literacy," the health literacy recommendations from the IOM report were advanced a notch with interactive discussions from a variety of perspectives: government, providers, foundations, insurers, businesses, and representatives from the nursing community. From the plenary sessions to the breakout sessions, participants engaged in discussions of concrete recommendations on steps toward the goal of health literacy (ACPF, 2004).

At the conference, for example, the AMA promoted its policy report that low health literacy is a barrier to effective medical diagnosis and treatment. Through its efforts to improve communication with patients with low health literacy, the AMA has developed an extensive Website and educational program with resources and materials in the health literacy kit. A health literacy curriculum was also designed, and 11 teams were trained from different state and specialty societies; the curriculum is currently being implemented throughout the country. From the foundations perspective, the Commonwealth Fund has supported several projects that promote communication and assist populations at risk for low health literacy through the use of new technologies. One such project is the Asthma Buddy Project, which makes use of a self-monitoring device for children who have poorly controlled asthma. Another project is called "Improving Diabetes Efforts across Language and Literacy," which tries to address the self-management challenge and patient education barriers posed by diabetic patients with low health literacy or poor English skills. From the insurance and business perspectives, speakers promoted that health literacy investments can reap benefits of cost savings, satisfied patients, and improved health outcomes. Suggestions for national protocols through collaboration among trade associations and medical specialty consortiums were made to promote programs that provide a health literacy standard (ACPF, 2004).

## PARTNERSHIPS FOR ACTION

The Partnership for Clear Health Communication, a coalition that includes the AMA, American Nurses Association (ANA), and American Public Health Association (APHA), has developed an action agenda and is actively developing tools to enable providers of information and providers of care to address the problem of low health literacy and improved health outcomes—one patient at a time.

The four-pronged action agenda of the Partnership is to do the following:

- Expand awareness and educate patients and providers about low health literacy.
- Develop and apply practical solutions to improve patient-provider communication and motivate the health care system to adopt them.
- Conduct an active advocacy program to increase support for health literacy policy and funding.
- Conduct nationally coordinated research to define the health literacy issue and evaluate solutions.

The Partnership for Clear Health Communication applauds the efforts of all groups to raise the visibility of low health literacy. The group's first campaign, called "Ask Me 3" *(www.askme3.org/PFCHC/)*, is geared at prompting patients to ask three questions: What is my main problem? What do I need to do? Why is it important for me to do this? Through a variety of voluntary efforts and campaigns such as this, patients and providers can be choreographed to take steps toward actualizing the vision of a health literate population.

The challenge of achieving a healthy nation faces health policymakers, providers, and numerous systems in our current health care environments. Achieving health literacy is a feasible policy goal that can be influenced by nursing research and practice.

## Key Points

- Health illiteracy is a public health issue. Studies show that almost half of all Americans have difficulty understanding and acting on health information.
- Health literacy skills involve basic literacy, numeracy, and health information knowledge that are necessary for consumers to make appropriate health decisions.
- Poor health literacy has been linked to health disparities and social inequities.
- Nurses and health professionals need to recognize that health illiteracy affects millions of citizens and results in billions of health care dollars lost per year.

- Professionals often lack understanding of the extent and effect of illiteracy and its social stigma, making it a "silent epidemic."
- Many federal, state, and local government health agencies have begun efforts to document and improve the health literacy of the public.
- Partnerships among professional, insurance, business, and advocacy groups have made health literacy a feasible action agenda that calls for improvements to educate patients and providers; nurses can play a major role in developing and implementing such agendas.

## Web Resources

**Centers for Disease Control and Prevention, Office of Communication—Beyond the Brochure** and **Scientific and Technical Information Simply Put**
*www.cdc.gov*

**FirstGov**—offers links to government agencies and departments, by keyword or agency name (e.g., Agency for Healthcare Research and Quality, Health Resources and Services Administration, National Institutes of Health, and Office of Minority Health)
*www.firstgov.gov*

**National Cancer Institute, Office of Communications—Clear and Simple: Developing Effective Health Materials for Low-Literate Readers and Making Health Communications Programs Work**
*www.nci.nih.gov*

**U.S. Food and Drug Administration, Office of Consumer Affairs**—includes brochures on breastfeeding and how to give medicines to children
*www.fda.gov*

**Education and Training Materials**
**American Medical Association Foundation—Health Literacy Introductory Kit**
*www.amafoundation.org/go/healthliteracy*

*Continued*

*Web Resources — cont'd*

**Diversity Rx**—provides information about meeting the health care needs of multicultural populations
*www.diversityrx.org*

**Harvard School of Public Health, Health and Literacy Studies Program**
*www.hsph.harvard.edu/healthliteracy*

**Health Literacy Center**—based at the University of New England, Biddeford, Maine, the Health Literacy Center offers a 4-day Health Literacy Institute on writing plain language health education materials
*www.une.edu/hlit*

## REFERENCES

Adams, K., & Corrigan, J. (Eds.). (2003). *Priority areas for national action: Transforming health care quality.* Washington, DC: Institute of Medicine (IOM), National Academies Press.

American College of Physicians Foundation (ACFP). (2004). Moving forward to improve health literacy (executive summary). October 26-27, 2004. Retrieved May, 2005, from *http://foundation.acponline.org/healthcom/hcc3_exsum.pdf.*

American Medical Association (AMA). (1999). Report: Ad Hoc Committee on Health Literacy for the Council on Scientific Affairs. *JAMA, 281,* 552-557.

Baker, D., Gazmararian, J., Williams, M., Scott, T., Parker, R., et al. (2002). Functional health literacy and the risk of hospital admission among Medicare managed care enrollees. *American Journal of Public Health, 92*(8), 1278-1283.

Carmona, R. (2003). Health literacy in America: The role of health care professionals. Prepared remarks given at the American Medical Association House of Delegates Meeting, Saturday, June 14, 2003. Retrieved May, 2005, from *www.surgeongeneral.gov/news/speeches/ama051403.htm.*

Council of State Governments (CSG). (2002). Executive summary: Excerpt from the CSG's state official's guide to health literacy. Retrieved May, 2005, from *www.csg.org/CSG/Policy/health/health+literacy/default.htm.*

Friedland, R. (1998). *New estimates of the high costs of inadequate health literacy. Conference proceedings report from Promoting Health Literacy: A Call to Action.* Washington, DC: Pfizer Inc.

Howard, D. (2004). The relationship between health literacy and medical costs (Appendix B). In Institute of Medicine (IOM), *Health literacy: A prescription to end confusion.* Washington, DC: National Academies Press.

Institute of Medicine (IOM). (2004). *Health literacy: A prescription to end confusion.* Washington DC: National Academies Press.

Kingdon, J. (2003). *Agendas, alternatives, and public policies* (2nd ed.). New York: Addison-Wesley Educational Publishers.

Kirsch, I., Jungeblut, A., Jenkins, L., & Kolstad, A. (1993). *Adult literacy in America: A first look at the National Adult Literacy Survey (NALS).* Washington, DC: National Center for Education Statistics, U.S. Department of Education.

Parker, R., Ratzan, S., & Lurie, N. (2003). Health literacy: A policy challenge for advancing high-quality health care. *Health Affairs, 22*(4), 147-153.

Partnership for Clear Health Communication. (2003). A day of understanding: Remarks from Richard Carmona, United States Surgeon General. Retrieved May 2005, from *www.askme3.org/surgeon_general.asp.*

Pfizer Inc. (2003). What is health literacy? Scope and impact. Retrieved May 5, 2005, from *www.pfizerhealthliteracy.com/whatis.html.*

Rogers, E., Ratzan, S., & Payne, J. (2001). Health literacy: A nonissue in the 2000 presidential election. *American Behavioral Scientist, 44*(12), 2172-2195.

Rothman, R., DeWalt, D., Malone, R., Bryant, B., Shintani, A., et al. (2004). Influence of patient literacy on the effectiveness of a primary care–based diabetes disease management program. *Journal of the American Medical Association, 292*(14), 1711-1716.

Rudd, R., Kirsch, I., & Yamamoto, K. (2004). *Literacy and health in America.* Princeton, NJ: Educational Testing Service (ETS). Retrieved May, 2005, from *www.ets.org/research/pic.*

U.S. Department of Health and Human Services (USDHHS). (2000). *Healthy People 2010: Understanding and improving health.* Washington, DC: USDHHS. Retrieved July 11, 2005, from *www.healthypeople.gov/document/pdf/Volume1/11HealthCom.pdf.*

Vastag, B. (2004). Low health literacy called a major problem. *Journal of the American Medical Association, 291*(18), 2181-2182.

# Childcare Policy: A Challenge for the Nation

Heather Lord & Sally Cohen

*"The greatest national resource that any country can have is its children."*

Danny Kaye

In recent years, childcare has emerged as one of the most important issues facing federal, state, and local policymakers (Cohen, 2001; Helburn & Bergmann, 2002). The best available estimates indicate that in fiscal year 2001 the federal government spent $16 billion and state and local governments spent a combined $9 billion on childcare (Barnett & Masse, 2002). Another $2.5 billion was spent by states on prekindergarten (PreK) initiatives in 2002-2003. The size of these investments is attributable, in part, to advocates' efforts to educate policymakers about key demographic, political, social, and economic trends that increase the needs of families and children for nonparental childcare and early education. Despite the large increase in public investments, it is estimated that only one in seven children eligible for federal childcare assistance actually receives a subsidy.

Nursing organizations have yet to take their place among the hundreds of groups that have been advocates for increasing the availability, accessibility, affordability, and quality of childcare. Furthermore, nurses, as providers of care to families with young children, have a huge and largely untapped potential to educate parents on how to identify high-quality care and the benefits of choosing such care for their children. This spotlight describes factors that shape childcare policymaking, highlights key issues facing policymakers, and identifies opportunities for nurses to assume leadership roles.

## DEFINING CHILDCARE AS A POLICY ISSUE

In a recent report issued by the Committee on Integrating the Science of Early Childhood Development, convened by the National Research Council and the Institute of Medicine, researchers concluded that, "second only to the immediate family, childcare is the context in which early development unfolds...for the vast majority of young children in the United States" (Shonkoff & Phillips, 2000, p. 297). One reason for this reliance on childcare is the dramatic rise in the proportion of mothers in the paid labor force, from 38% in 1970 to 68% in 2000 (Smolensky & Gootman, 2003). It is estimated that among children under age 6 with employed mothers, 80% are in nonparental childcare arrangements for almost 40 hours a week. Why the dramatic rise in maternal employment? The entry of women into the paid labor force is attributable in part to most families' economic need for two family incomes, reduced barriers to women's employment, and the rise of single-parent-households, largely headed by women. Single-mothers' labor force participation peaked in 2003 at 78%.

A fundamental challenge to policymaking in this area is the dual, and sometimes conflicting, roles of childcare as promoting child well-being and facilitating parental employment. An analogy used to distinguish these two purposes of care arrangements is the "kiddy container" model of care. At a most custodial level, childcare provides a "storage container" to keep children safe from harm while a parent is working. This type of childcare would match the hours of the workday and only meet children's basic health and safety needs. At the other end of the continuum from the "container" models of care are programs that focus on "early education." The latter include programs such as state funded PreK and Head Start. These programs have as their goal preparing preschool-age children for kindergarten and promoting early literacy and a child's cognitive, social, and emotional development through the implementation of developmentally appropriate curricula (Brauner, Gordic, & Zigler, 2004). Increasingly, policymakers have identified early education programs, including PreK and Head Start, as useful for preparing children for entry into kindergarten. For example, in 2002-2003, 38 states funded a state PreK initiative, serving nearly 740,000, or 10% of all 3- and 4-year-olds (Barnett, Hustedt, Robin, & Schulman, 2004). Head Start (Box 32-2) served 905,851 children in 2004. These programs, however, often require parental involvement and operate part-day during the school year and therefore are not necessarily conducive to parental employment.

Most childcare falls toward the center of this continuum and strives to meet the dual needs of parents and children. Childcare, as distinguished from early education programs (e.g., PreK, Head Start), falls into three basic categories: in-home care, family daycare, and center-based care. It should be noted, however, that the distinctions between childcare that facilitates parental employment and early education programs designed to serve children are often blurred, especially in center-based care, which can include a developmental curriculum. Regardless, the proportion of children in each arrangement varies as one considers infants, toddlers, preschoolers, and school-age children. In-home care is the smallest category and includes relative and nonrelative babysitters, au pairs, and nannies. Family daycare homes are a more-typical arrangement used by working mothers of infants, toddlers, and preschool-age children. Most often, this arrangement consists of a licensed or unlicensed provider caring for four to six children in her home. Although family daycare providers typically charge less than organized centers, they are largely unregulated and provide care of highly variable quality. Lastly, childcare centers are the most common form of nonparental care for children up to age 5. This type of arrangement operates under the auspices of various entities and includes religious

---

**BOX 32-2**   Head Start

Contrary to popular belief, Head Start is not a childcare program in the technical sense. It is a compensatory program that offers comprehensive services including referrals for health screenings, social services, and nutrition counseling to disadvantaged children and their families. Although Head Start offers many benefits to children from poor families, it cannot meet the childcare needs of most low-income working families. This is because Head Start programs typically are half-day programs, operate only during the school year, target very poor families, enroll mostly 3- and 4-year-olds, and require parental involvement. Therefore Head Start leaves gaps for parents who work full time, have infants and toddlers, or have incomes too high to qualify for the program.

Recent federal, state, and local initiatives aim to link Head Start with other early-education programs, such as school readiness initiatives and childcare, so as to enhance the availability of seamless, comprehensive services for young children. Each state has a Head Start collaboration grant from the federal government to promote such efforts. Early Start, an expansion of Head Start launched in the mid 1990s, extends Head Start services to infants and toddlers from eligible families.

Most recently there has been considerable debate at the federal level about the appropriate goals for Head Start and the level of administration. President Bush introduced new literacy goals and the National Reporting System, a highly controversial system of tests of Head Start children that links their performance on cognitive tasks to program funding. In addition, he proposed changing the funding structure from that of a federal to a local grant.

The per-pupil annual cost for Head Start ranges from $5021 for part-day, part-year services to $9811 for full-day, full-year services. In 2004, $6.8 billion was spent on Head Start. Expanding full-day, full-year services to all eligible children from birth to age 5 not currently served would cost approximately $25 billion (Smolensky, & Gootman, 2003).

---

organizations, public schools, private establishments, proprietary chains, and community-based agencies (Zigler & Hall, 2000).

One goal of childcare policymakers has been to integrate childcare into the provision of early education by providing "wrap around" care to better align the hours of operation with schedules of working parents. Some advocates and researchers have been urging policymakers to integrate childcare and early education into "early care and education" (ECE) that could be provided through the schools (Barnett et al., 2004). In the meantime, and in the absence of federal regulations for childcare, each state operates its own programs, with high variation in availability, accessibility, and quality (Kolker, Osborne, & Schnurer, 2004).

## Quality of Care

Childcare quality is a fundamental concern for researchers, advocates, and policymakers. Although good care can enhance a child's development, poor care, as evidenced by low staff-to-child ratios, lack of developmentally appropriate curricula and resources, and staff who do not nurture children's physical and emotional development, can be detrimental (Shonkoff & Phillips, 2000).

There is a wide and alarming range in the quality of care across the country, with much of it rated as poor to mediocre. The Cost, Quality, and Child Outcomes in Child Care Centers Study (Cost, Quality, and Child Outcomes Study Team, 1995) found that "fully 40 percent of the rooms serving infants...provided care that was of such poor quality as to jeopardize children's health, safety or development." Sharon L. Ramey, Director of the Georgetown Center on Health and Education, writes, "Positive care-giving by nonparents in childcare settings is rare...well over 50% of children receive care that is either 'very uncharacteristic' or 'somewhat uncharacteristic' of positive care (Box 32-3).

*Regulation of childcare quality.* One way to protect the well-being of children in childcare settings is to regulate childcare providers. Because of the lack of federal regulations, providers are required to adhere only to state regulations, which vary widely and are insufficient for ensuring adequate quality, especially in terms of staffing, curriculum, and provider qualifications. For example, 30 states do not require preservice training for teachers in childcare centers, 12 states exempt religious-based childcare centers, and 20 states exempt half-day nursery schools. As many as 50% of formal

**BOX 32-3** Overview of the National Institute of Child Health and Human Development Study of Early Child Care and Youth Development

In response to debate over the effects of childcare and need for authoritative information, the National Institute of Child Health and Human Development (NICHD) convened a group of experts, the Early Child Care Research Network, to design over 18 months the most ambitious and comprehensive longitudinal study of childcare and child development. The study follows a cohort of 1364 children born in 1991, begins in infancy, and collects information about the family, the child, childcare, and other aspects of developmental context (NICHD Early Child Care Research Network, 2005). Data collection efforts were originally concentrated in 10 sites across the United States, but as families relocate, researchers track these families and collect data in new geographic locations. Originally, children were assessed on school adjustment and family relationships, cognitive and language skills, school readiness, and physical health and well-being. As children age, new experts are brought in and age-appropriate measures are added to answer new research questions on the effects of childcare experiences on development in middle childhood and early adolescence. The Network provides training to others in the use of the datasets and in 2005 released a compilation of the most important findings for infants to 4½-year-olds, drawn from the over 100 scientific publications released to date. Further information on the study's methods, measures, reports, and available training is available at *http://secc.rti.org*.

childcare providers may be legally exempt from licensure because some states do not require childcare sponsored by religious agencies to be regulated in the same way as non–faith-based providers (Brauner, Gordic, & Zigler, 2004). Many providers choose to apply for and receive accreditation by private entities, such as the National Association for the Education of Young Children (NAEYC). Accreditation assures that programs have met standards beyond basic competency and offer high-quality care. It complements, rather than replaces, licensing.

***Childcare staff training and retention.*** One of the most important factors affecting overall quality is the quality of the staff. Turnover is a major problem, largely because of the woefully inadequate compensation for childcare staff. The average childcare provider salary was $17,310 in 2002. In 2003, the median American PreK teacher's salary was $22,190, nearly half of the median kindergarten teacher salary of $42,380 (U.S. Bureau of Labor Statistics, 2003). To give some perspective, the federal poverty threshold for a family of three was $15,020 in 2002. Furthermore, less than half of the estimated 2.3 million individuals in the childcare workforce receive health coverage from their employers (Whitebook & Sakai, 2003). Therefore it is no surprise that nationwide the annual childcare staff turnover rate is about 30%, surpassing that in almost all other occupations. Such a high turnover rate makes it difficult for centers to ensure good care, because having a consistent provider is crucial for children's sense of security, attachment, and other aspects of development.

Results of several recent national studies that have received wide media coverage have raised questions about the effect of childcare on child development (Belsky, 2001). However, the findings of these studies are often misreported, made sensationalistic, or do not account for care quality. In general, there are no conclusive studies demonstrating that high-quality childcare per se is harmful to children and a large body of evidence demonstrating that high-quality care can foster positive developmental outcomes (NICHD Early Child Care Research Network, 2005).

## NUANCES OF CHILDCARE POLICYMAKING

The growth in public spending on childcare is partly a result of the successful lobbying activities of state and national child advocacy organizations and recognition by policymakers that the provision of childcare was necessary to any successful effort to move families off welfare roles and into employment. These advocacy groups represent children, child health professionals, social service agencies, educators, public health administrators, state and local officials, labor unions, and women. These organizations have formed coalitions, testified before legislative committees, worked with government officials, collected and disseminated data on childcare and child development, and brought to the media's and the public's attention the importance of childcare for America's families. They have also argued that enhancing the availability of high-quality childcare can help employers reduce employee absenteeism, improve productivity, and foster long-term child development.

Despite the surge of interest in childcare policies, some public officials remain reluctant to support childcare, in particular for infants and toddlers. These individuals often have stereotypic images of childcare as only warehousing of children ("kiddy container") or think that working mothers of very young children have rejected their roles as maternal caregivers. Some of the same public officials find it easier to support programs for 3- and 4-year-olds framed as preschool or school-readiness initiatives than to support childcare proposals making care for very young children universally available.

But such views contradict the reality of family life in the twenty-first century. The nuclear family (married heterosexual parents, with the wife at home raising children), which flourished in the 1950s, has faded. Instead, children are being raised in a variety of family configurations, including the 12 million single parents in the United States today, 83% of whom are women. Single-parent families often lack the financial resources and social supports of two-parent families. Although men have begun to step up to the plate in assuming household responsibilities, the decisions about childrearing and housework in most families still fall to women. Therefore childcare plays a critical role in enabling women, including nurses, to pursue their career goals while providing for their families.

### Access to Childcare

Access to high-quality childcare depends on the availability and affordability of care within a community. The availability of childcare is affected by many factors. Shortages are most noticeable in rural areas, which typically lack community resources to support such programs. Furthermore, regardless of locale, transporting children to and from childcare can be a problem, especially when providers are located far from home or work and parents must rely on public transportation. In a strong economy, childcare workers, many of whom are women, can find work in more lucrative industries, which reduces the childcare workforce. Similarly, as families are forced to rely on two incomes to make ends meet, the availability of family members who might otherwise be available to help care for children has dwindled. Finally, many low-income families work minimum-wage jobs on evening or night shifts, during which childcare is typically unavailable. This is accentuated by welfare reform, which has led many women into service-sector jobs that require shift work. When evening or night care is available, it is too expensive for many families. The need for childcare during off hours is also a concern for nurses who provide 24-hour care for parents in a variety of settings.

Beyond availability, affordability of care is a powerful force in the childcare decision of many families. Childcare is expensive, with costs varying by location, child's age, and the extent to which government subsidies are available to a particular family. Generally, low-income families spend a larger portion of their annual household income on childcare than families in higher income brackets. About 60% of families earning less than $1200 a month pay out of pocket for their childcare. The cost accounts for 37% of their income. Care for a preschool age child averaged $4000 to $6000 per year in 2000. In urban areas in 48 states, childcare costs exceeded the cost of tuition at a public college (Children's Defense Fund, 2004). Families in rural areas also face high childcare costs, although rates are usually lower than in urban areas, and low supply of care (U.S. Census Bureau, 2003).

***Infants and toddlers.*** The problem of caring for infants and toddlers is especially challenging. The cost of this care is high because of low child-to-staff ratios and the limited availability of high-quality care. Survey data indicate the average cost of care for a 12-month-old was above $5750 per year in nearly 66% of cities surveyed and as high as $12,324 per year in Boston (Schulman, 2000).

***School-age children.*** Although most childcare policies focus on children below age 6, public and private leaders have recently taken a strong interest in before- and after-school programs for older children. Some of this interest was spurred by the rise in teen violence, dangers of self-care in the after-school hours, and impetus for improved academic outcomes under the federal No Child Left Behind legislation. The reasoning is that structured programs for school-age children can prevent risk-taking behaviors such as substance abuse, teen pregnancy, and crime and provide academic tutoring for struggling students. Some legislators find it easier to support care for older children than for infants and toddlers, because these programs do not evoke debates over the role of women, family, and child-rearing. However, the dramatic surge of spending on care for school-age children in the late 1990s and early 2000s was followed by a drop in such support under President George W. Bush and a highly controversial proposal to cut funding for the federal 21st Century Community Learning Center after-school programs (Mahoney & Zigler, 2006).

## PUBLIC POLICIES TO PROMOTE CHILDCARE

Unlike most European nations, in which the government heavily subsidizes the cost of childcare and early education, parents pay the largest share of the cost in the United States. Overall, parents pay well over half the costs, while the government and private sector (in particular) pay much less. Several provisions in the U.S. tax code are aimed at assisting parents and employers with these expenses.

### Using the Tax Code to Support Childcare

One of the major federal subsidies for childcare is the Credit for Child and Dependent Care Expenses. This allows taxpayers to claim a credit against income tax liability for a limited amount of employment-related dependent care expenses. (A qualifying dependent is a child under the age of 13 or a physically or mentally incapacitated dependent or spouse.) However, this credit is not refundable, making it of no value to families without any tax liability. Also, it has not been indexed to keep pace with inflation. As of 2003 the maximum amount of employment-related expenses a taxpayer could claim was $3000 for one dependent and $6000 for two or more dependents (Donahue & Campbell, 2002). In 2003, over $2.8 billion was paid out in tax benefits (U.S. House of Representatives Committee on Ways and Means, 2004). When the current expense limits were established in 1981, they reflected the average costs of childcare, but they are currently inadequate. Recent legislative proposals in Congress include making the credit refundable, extending it to families with stay-at-home parents, and adjusting it to reach more low-income families.

The IRS also allows employers to provide an employee with up to $5000 annually in childcare-related benefits, tax free. Although this program allows employers to provide reimbursements, on-site care, or vouchers tax free, it is generally administered as a salary-reduction plan by which employees set aside $5000 of their salary at the beginning of the year for childcare-related expenses. The benefit to employer and employee is that payroll taxes do not need to be paid for this money. The only downside is that any "leftover" money an employee sets aside but does not use for childcare expenses is lost (National Women's Law Center, 2004).

### Private Sector Support of Childcare

Another way of assisting parents with their childcare expenses is to increase the portion paid by the private sector while simultaneously providing incentives for employers to contribute to the costs of employee childcare. But such initiatives often fall short of need. According to a 1997 study, 13% of respondents had employers that offered direct financial assistance for childcare, and 29% had employers that put pretax dollars into an account to pay for care for a child or other dependent. Less than 3% of employers offered on-site childcare (Bond, Galinsky, & Swanberg, 1998).

Johnson & Johnson became a model corporation in this area after doing a "needs analysis" of its workforce of more than 42,000 employees in 1988. They found employees were suffering under the pressure of work-family conflicts; their number one issue was flexible work hours, and number two was childcare. Johnson & Johnson responded by hiring Bright Horizons Family Solution and established on-site childcare centers in New Jersey and Pennsylvania, landing them on Working Mother magazine's annual list of 100 Best Companies for Working Mothers for 17 years. Unfortunately, however, the availability of employer-sponsored childcare is generally limited to larger companies and targeted to highly skilled workers.

Bright Horizons Family Solutions found that 24% of nurses considered quitting their jobs because of difficulties finding affordable childcare. In response, nearly 20% of hospitals within the United States have taken steps to provide childcare to employees. This strategy appears to be successful, as the voluntary turnover among childcare center users was reduced by 89%, which translates into over $1 million in saved replacement costs alone (Bright Horizons Family Solutions, 2005).

### Child Care and Development Block Grant

The major source of federal and state childcare funding is the Child Care and Development Block Grant (CCDBG) (Box 32-4). The CCDBG is a block grant to states that subsidizes childcare for eligible low-income families with children under 13 years of age. The federal government distributed

---

**BOX 32-4**   Overview of the Child Care and Development Block Grant

The Child Care Bureau of the U.S. Department of Health and Human Services (USDHHS) is the agency responsible for implementing the Child Care and Development Block Grant (CCDBG) and coordinating federal childcare programs. One of the bureau's most important programs is Healthy Child Care America (HCCA). Its "Blueprint for Action" identifies 10 steps for communities to take to improve the health and safety of childcare. The American Academy of Pediatrics, with support from the Child Care Bureau and the federal Maternal and Child Health Bureau, has been coordinating the HCCA campaign since 1996. Many nurses have been leaders of state and national activities under HCCA. Extensive information about this program, including details about the program in each state, can be found online at *http://nccic. acf.hhs.gov/hcca.*

$4.7 billion to states in fiscal year (FY) 2004. States must spend at least 4% of their total expenditures on activities to improve the quality and availability of childcare.

The 1996 welfare reform law, the Personal Responsibility and Work Opportunity Reconciliation Act (PROWRA) (Public Law 106-193), authorized the CCDBG through 2002, and separate legislation extended appropriations at FY 2002 levels through 2005. Much of the recent debate about childcare policymaking focuses on the importance of childcare for welfare reform and the need to ensure that low-income families not on welfare also receive support.

Under the 1996 childcare block grant law, states may set income eligibility at no higher than 85% of the state's median income (SMI). Yet nearly all states have established lower limits, with the average between 55% and 60% SMI (Cohen & Lord, 2005). As a result, millions of children are eligible for but are not receiving childcare subsidies, and some estimates indicate that half a million children are on subsidy waiting lists (Children's Defense Fund, 2004).

The CCDBG has three funding streams—discretionary, mandatory, and matching—each with its own requirements and formulas. Each year Congress determines the exact amount of CCDBG discretionary funds that will be appropriated. Under mandatory funding, states are guaranteed to receive a fixed amount each year. States must spend at least 70% of their mandatory funding on welfare recipients. To receive federal matching funds, states must maintain childcare program spending at a specified level, referred to as a *state's maintenance of effort*. In addition, states must match the federal grant with some of their own funds.

Several provisions of the 1996 law are aimed at giving parents flexibility in their childcare options. For example, the 1996 law prohibits states from withholding or decreasing welfare assistance to mothers who cannot obtain childcare within a reasonable distance from their homes or jobs and who have children under age 6. Also, families who receive childcare subsidies under the CCDBG have the option of using a voucher, "which is a certificate assuring a provider that the state will pay a portion of the child care fee" (GAO, 2001, p. 9). Parents may also use a provider that has a contract with the state to render care for subsidized families. Most of the CCDBG care is delivered in centers and funded with vouchers (Cohen & Lord, 2005). It is interesting to note that the use of childcare vouchers, although somewhat controversial, has not been subject to the same criticism as school vouchers. This is partly because childcare vouchers have existed for decades under other federal programs and also because many policymakers consider childcare a social service not under the rubric of education. The CCDBG also subsidizes care offered by relatives and religious agencies, so that parents can choose the caregiver that best meets their needs and values.

## Linking Welfare Reform and Childcare Poses Policy Challenges

The 1996 welfare law revamped the welfare system. It ended the federal guarantee of cash assistance to all eligible low-income mothers and children and replaced it with Temporary Assistance to Needy Families (TANF) block grants that give states broad authority in administering their welfare programs. Under the 1996 reform, families are eligible to receive TANF benefits only for a limited amount of time. In particular, recipients are required to work within 2 years of receiving benefits and may receive TANF assistance only for a total of 5 years. During reauthorization, Congress can change this rule, however.

***Implications of welfare reform for childcare.*** Several aspects of the 1996 law have implications for childcare. For example, under the 1996 law, states may exempt mothers with children under age 1 from TANF work requirements. The block grant allows states to transfer up to 30% of their TANF block grant funds to the CCDBG, but funds used that way must adhere to CCDBG rules for percentage of funds devoted to quality and reporting requirements. The amount of TANF funds transferred to CCDBG peaked in FY 2000 at $2.3 billion. States have decreased the size of their transfers from TANF to CCDBG because of increasing welfare roles, state fiscal crises, and general decrease in availability of surplus TANF funds. States may also finance childcare directly out of their TANF grants and not be subject to CCDBG guidelines.

The need for publicly subsidized childcare has increased under the mandatory work participation requirements of the 1996 welfare reform law. The 1996 welfare reforms required parents enrolled in the TANF program to work or risk losing cash assistance. By 2002 states were required to have 50% of the TANF caseload engaged in work activities or else lose federal funds. The Congressional Budget Office recently estimated that over the next 5 years the cost of keeping pace with inflation for childcare services will be $4.8 billion, and the combined costs of keeping up with inflation and President Bush's proposed increased participation requirements would exceed $12 billion (Greenberg & Rahmanou, 2005).

In implementing the CCDBG, states need to balance the competing needs of various low-income families. This includes TANF recipients, families transitioning off TANF, teen parents, parents of children with special needs, low-income working families whose incomes are too high to qualify for TANF but who struggle to make ends meet, and middle-class families who also have difficulty arranging childcare. Many childcare advocates have pointed to the competing needs of other low-income families. Ironically, failure to help these families could result in many of them landing on welfare because of their inability to sustain work and afford childcare.

## CHILDCARE AS AN IMPORTANT POLICY ISSUE FOR NURSES

The interaction among federal, state, and local governments in administering and funding childcare, and the role of the private sector, make childcare an issue that offers many opportunities for nurse to become involved (Cohen, 2004; Cohen & Misuraca, 2001). The first step in doing so is to learn about the CCDBG and how it is implemented in one's own state. The federal Child Care Bureau and the Child Care and Early Education Research Connections Website *(www.childcareresearch.org)* provide extensive databases and lists of Websites relevant to childcare and early childhood education policies. The Children's Defense Fund *(www.childrensdefense.org)*,

National Women's Law Center *(www.nwlc.org)*, and NOW *(www.now.org)* all issue reports on the status of childcare and on early education policies in each state and legislative updates.

At the state level, nurses can connect with several important childcare organizations. Among them are the state childcare resource and referral agencies that are responsible for providing parents with information about how to locate care in their vicinity. Childcare resource and referral agencies also monitor state developments, including the relationship between childcare and child health. State affiliates of the NAEYC *(www.naeyc.org)* are open to any interested individual and offer ways for nurses to be involved. To understand how childcare is regulated, check with the agency responsible for such activities in your state. It is usually part of the department of public health or social services. Nurses might want to consider inviting representatives of these organizations as guest speakers at state and local nursing functions.

At the local level, nurses can check with their board of education, mayor's office, interfaith groups such as councils of churches and synagogues, and other community agencies to learn who runs childcare, Head Start, or other early-education programs. The administrators of those programs will often welcome nurses as paid or unpaid consultants who address health and safety issues. Nurses can advocate on their own behalf for employer-sponsored childcare.

Finally, nurses can communicate with federal, state, and local government officials about the role of childcare in building safe communities and the necessity of childcare for meeting their professional demands. The larger challenge facing childcare advocates is to ensure that the funding is adequate to reach all eligible children and that the quality of care will promote child development. These are issues well suited for nurses who work with families, young children, public health issues, and a host of community-based concerns. For example, a study of hospital preparedness plans for nurses acting as disaster responders during Hurricane Floyd in 1999 found that nurses voiced concerns about their families' welfare and childcare during the emergency (French, Sole, & Byers, 2002). Although all four hospitals in the study provided childcare, policies did not specify the location of the childcare. In focus groups, nurses commented, "If my family is secure, then I would come" and "I do not like leaving my family behind" (French et al., 2002, p. 5). (Also see *when a Hurricane Strikes: The Challenge of Crafting Workplace Policy following Chapter 16.*) Therefore childcare is important in these situations so that nurses can provide direct patient care without worrying about the safety of their children. With knowledge of the policy process and clinical insight into child development, health systems, and communities, nurses are well posed to assume leadership roles in policy development.

## Key Points

- The United States, unlike most European and developed countries, has no government subsidy for the cost of childcare and early education.
- Despite the need for childcare by the majority of nurses, nursing organizations have yet to take a major role as advocates for increasing the availability, accessibility, affordability, and quality of childcare.
- Nurses can take a leadership role in influencing both public and private childcare policies, particularly because of their expertise in health and their personal need for services.

## Web Resources

**Administration for Children and Families, Head Start Bureau**
*www.acf.hhs.gov/programs/hsb*
**Center for Law and Social Policy**
*www.clasp.org*
**Child Care Bureau**
*www.acf.hhs.gov/programs/ccb*
**Children's Defense Fund**
*www.childrensdefense.org*
**National Association for the Education of Young Children (NAEYC)**
*www.naeyc.org*

**National Center for Children in Poverty**
*www.nccp.org*
**National Child Care Information Center**
*www.nccic.org*
**National Women's Law Center**
*www.nwlc.org*
**NICHD Early Child Care Research Network**
*http://secc.rti.org*

## REFERENCES

Barnett, W. S., Hustedt, J. T., Robin, K. B., & Schulman, K. L. (2004). *The state of preschool: 2004 state preschool yearbook.* New Brunswick, NJ: National Institute for Early Education Research. Retrieved March 15, 2006, from *http://nieer.org/yearbook/pdf/yearbook.pdf.*

Barnett, W. S., & Masse, L. N. (2002). Funding issues for early childhood care and education programs. In C. Dryer, D. B. Bailey, & R. M. Clifford (Eds.), *Early childhood education and care in the USA.* Baltimore: Paul H. Brookes.

Belsky, J. (2001). Developmental risks (still) associated with early child care. *Journal of Child Psychology and Psychiatry, 42,* 845-859.

Bond, J. T., Galinsky, E., & Swanberg, J. E. (1998). *The 1997 national study of the workforce.* New York: Families and Work Institute.

Brauner, J., Gordic, B., & Zigler, E. (2004). Putting the child back into child care: Combining care and education for children ages 3-5. *Social Policy Report, XVIII*(III), 1-18.

Bright Horizons Family Solutions. (2005). The business impact of employee-sponsored child care in hospitals. Retrieved March 15, 2006, from *www.brighthorizons.com/site/pages/Hospital%20Study.FINAL.pdf.*

Children's Defense Fund. (2004). *Low-income children and families suffer as states continue to cut child care assistance programs.* Washington, DC: Children's Defense Fund.

Cohen, S. (2001). *Championing child care.* New York: Columbia University Press.

Cohen, S. S. (2004). Child care: A crucial legislative issue. *Journal of Pediatric Health Care, 18*(6), 312-314.

Cohen, S. S. & Lord, H. (2005). Implementation of the Child Care and Development Fund (CCDF): A research synthesis. *Nursing Outlook, 53*(5), 239-253.

Cohen, S. S., & Misuraca, B. L. (2001). PNPs as catalysts in child care policymaking. *Journal of Pediatric Health Care, 15*(2), 49-57.

Cost, Quality, and Child Outcomes Study Team (CQO). (1995). *Cost, quality and child outcomes in child care centers public report.* ED 386-297. Denver: Economics Department, University of Colorado-Denver.

Donahue, E. H., & Campbell, N. D. (2002). *Making care less taxing. Improving state child and dependent care tax provisions.* Washington, DC: National Women's Law Center.

French, E. D., Sole, M. L., & Byers, J. F. (2002). A comparison of nurses' needs/concerns and hospital disaster plans following Florida's hurricane Floyd. *Journal of Emergency Nursing, 28*(2), 111-117.

General Accounting Office (GAO). (2001). *Child care: States increased spending on low income families. Report No. 01-293.* Washington, DC: GAO.

Greenberg, M., & Rahmanou, R. (2005). *Administration's TANF proposal would not free up $2 billion for child care*. Washington, DC: Center for Law and Social Policy.

Helburn, S., & Bergmann, B. (2002). *America's child care problem*. New York: Palgrave.

Kolker, J., Osborne, D., & Schnurer, E. (2004). *Early care and education: The need for national policy*. Washington, DC: Center for National Policy.

Mahoney, J. L., & Zigler, E. G. (2006). Translating science to policy under the No Child Left Behind Act of 2001: Lessons from the national evaluation of the 21st Century Community Learning Centers. *Journal of Applied Developmental Psychology*.

National Institute of Child Health and Development (NICHD) Early Child Care Research Network. (2005). *Child care and child development: Results from the NICHD Study of Early Child Care and Youth Development*. New York: Guilford.

National Women's Law Center. (2004). Questions and answers about the dependent care assistance programs, tax year 2004. Retrieved March 25, 2006, from *www.nwlc.org/pdf/DCAP_Q&A_TY04.pdf*.

Schulman, K. (2000). *The high cost of child care puts quality care out of reach for many families*. Washington, DC: Children's Defense Fund.

Shonkoff, J. P., & Phillips, D. A. (Eds.). (2000). *From neurons to neighborhoods: The science of early childhood development*. Washington, DC: National Research Council & Institute of Medicine, Committee on the Science of Early Childhood Development, Board on Children, Youth, and Families, Division of Behavioral and Social Sciences and Education, National Academies Press.

Smolensky, E., & Gootman, J. A. (Eds.). (2003). *Working families and growing kids: Caring for children and adolescents*. Washington, DC: National Research Council & Institute of Medicine, Committee on Family and Work Policies, Board on Children, Youth, and Families, Division of Behavioral and Social Sciences and Education, National Academies Press.

U.S. Bureau of Labor Statistics. (2003). U.S. Department of Labor, occupational employment statistics. May 2003 national occupational employment and wage estimates. Retrieved March 25, 2006, from *www.bls.gov/oes/2003/may/oes_25Ed.htm*.

U.S. Census Bureau. (2003). *Who's minding the kids? Child care arrangements: Spring 1999*. Washington, DC: U.S. Census Bureau, Population Division, Fertility and Family Statistics Branch.

U.S. House of Representatives Committee on Ways and Means. (2004). 2004 Green book: Background material and data on programs within the jurisdiction of the Committee on Ways and Means. (108th Congress, 2nd Session, WMCP: 108-6). Washington, DC: U.S. Government Printing Office.

Whitebook, M., & Sakai, L. M. (2003). Turnover begets turnover: An examination of job and occupation instability among child care center staff. *Early Childhood Research Quarterly, 18*, 273-293.

Zigler, E. F., & Hall, N. W. (2000). *Child development and social policy*. Theory and applications. Boston: McGraw-Hill.

*chapter*

# 33

# Working with the Community for Change

Mary Ann Christopher, Theresa L. Beck, & Eileen H. Toughill*

*"What you leave behind is not what is engraved in stone monuments, but what is woven into the lives of others."*

PERICLES

Comprehensive family-service programs, development of water systems, neighborhood school-based health centers, nurse-managed community health centers, faith-based initiatives, community-conducted health fairs, and revitalization of an urban school—such have been the community collaborations facilitated by registered nurses. In the current climate there are several imperatives that make the ability of nurses to collaborate with communities a particularly relevant and marketable skill. Shrinking revenues for acute care hospitalization, third-party payers concerned with meeting the needs of populations, and reduced reimbursement for services are the variables driving the health care industry to redefine itself. Compounding the issue is a global nursing shortage (Armstrong, 2001; Boyle, 2001; Caro & Kaffenberger, 2001; Smith, Inoue, Ushikubo, & Amano, 2001). The nursing shortage heralds the need to re-look at the health care delivery system and underscores the

need to work with communities if societal health is to be realized.

An emphasis on population-based and community-based prevention of disease, injury, disability, and premature death will force a realignment of the role and responsibility of the public health sector. Indeed, states have already begun to redefine the role of the public health sector, placing increased emphasis on effective community collaboration. Increasingly, funders are incentivizing organizations to collaborate as a condition for grant awards. The only way that total health care system costs will be controlled is to focus significantly on the prevention of illness conditions, which will improve the collective state of health (Gebbie, 1999). Nursing is at the core of this shift to community collaboration.

Implementation of the *Healthy People 2010* health objectives is tied to effective community collaboration at the local level (U.S. Department of Health and Human Services [USDHHS], 2000). Any risk-reduction program or health care service must reflect a community-based response that incorporates the behavioral norms within groups (Rawlings-Anderson, 2001).

## FRAMEWORK FOR WORKING WITH COMMUNITIES

What framework should nurses use to build on their strong tradition of community-based leadership? The ability to work effectively with communities is

---

*The authors wish to acknowledge the contribution of Judith Miller, MS, RN, to the original version of this chapter, which was first published in the third edition (1998) of the book.

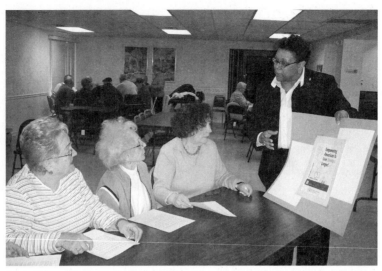

**Figure 33-1** Older adults are helped to understand their health risks through education by a VNACJ community health nurse.

tied to the mastery of three basic concepts: the differentiation between community and population, a broad conceptualization of health, and a methodology that fosters participation.

## COMMUNITY AND POPULATION

Understanding the differential concepts of community and population is critical to effective community collaboration. *Population* refers to a collective of individuals with common properties, whereas *community* exists when individuals share a locale and engage in patterns of social interactions, share a common identity and participate in interdependent activities, and work toward shared goals and collective activities. It is this concept of community, grounded in locality development, that has been the hallmark of effective community collaboration. This model has its emphasis on problem-solving by a cross-section of community members in a geographic area (Kang, 1995). "Community is a group of people with diverse characteristics who are linked by social ties, share common perspectives and engage in joint action in geographical locations or setting" (MacQueen et al., 2001). The failure of managed care to have an impact on the immunization rates of children is due in part to managed care organizations' focus on population rather

than community. In other words, within a given geographic area, a managed care organization would focus on the needs of its beneficiaries only; uninsured or underinsured children within that community would not have the benefit of outreach. This has become a critical issue among new immigrant populations living within given geographic areas. The issue of childhood immunization when parents are distrustful of the system, combined with the emergence of communicable diseases such as tuberculosis and pneumonia, has prompted the Visiting Nurse Association of Central Jersey (VNACJ) to partner with local health departments to address these unmet needs (Figure 33-1).

At VNACJ, an effort to establish board presence across a 550-square-mile area was unsuccessful. The board included 40 people, most of whom were concentrated near the organization's headquarters. This resulted in impaired visibility in the northern county, which negatively affected market share and local funding support. Because of the diversity of socioeconomic, ethnic, and cultural needs of the populations served across the service area, people's unwillingness to serve on a centrally located board indicated that people identify with neighborhood-specific issues rather than regional ones. Recognizing that decisions about community-based care are, for the most part locally determined, the organization established a second board in the northern county. The impact has been an enhanced visibility among new immigrant populations, improved recruitment of staff, and an increase in local funding support. Furthermore, the board has been effective in guiding staff to more effectively locate and serve hard-to-reach, disenfranchised populations.

The same phenomenon is evidenced in public policy approaches to major health and human services issues. The child welfare system in New Jersey is being realigned in accordance with the neighborhood-based partnership model. Recognizing that the needs of children at risk for abuse and neglect are best addressed at a local level, the entire child welfare system is being restructured to include the development of community collaboratives in at-risk areas. Funding will be directed from state government to local community organizations. This policy shift is based on the premise that "Children and families do not exist in isolation. They live in overlapping circles of extended family, block associations, neighborhood groups, community organizations, schools, workplaces and businesses, religious and civic organizations, and much more" (New Jersey Department of Human Services, 2004, p. 6).

The national demonstration project of the W.K. Kellogg Foundation and the Robert Wood Johnson Foundation (RWJF), Turning Point, was founded on the idea that diverse groups working together can better identify and influence health determinants. It starts at the local level and builds broad community support and participation. It is "anchored in two convictions: communities have strength and everyone has a stake in public health" (Oklahoma Turning Point, 2005, p. 1).

## CONCEPTUALIZATION OF HEALTH

Another critical skill in working with communities successfully is to conceptualize and define health broadly. Nurses who are the most effective with community collaboration are those who have a comfort level with program designs that define roles in nontraditional ways. A broad conceptualization of health is based on a definition that encompasses physical, emotional, social, and spiritual dimensions of well-being. A healthy community is defined as more than merely the absence of disease; it includes those elements that help people live productive lives (USDHHS, 2000).

**Environmental Health.** An example of this focus on social and living conditions is the Harlem Children's Zone Asthma Initiative. Developed in response to the fact that 25% of the children in the Zone had asthma, a registered nurse (RN) worked within a consortium model to diagnose and intervene with at-risk families. Of nearly 2000 children screened, 580 were found to have asthma. Consortium interventions were holistic, with a significant focus on environmental triggers. Toward that end, project staff made comprehensive home visits aimed at environmental interventions such as the distribution of HEPA cleaners, mite-proof bedding covers, and vacuum cleaner filters and home renovation and repair ("Treating asthma in the zone," 2003).

In yet another example, residents in an urban blighted community undergoing revitalization were asked to participate in the identification of future health and human services needs. Although providers were focused on the issue of neighborhood-based service delivery, the residents expressed concern about housing and jobs, with the recommendation that housing and commercial development be developed in tandem.

A community needs assessment conducted in a local suburban community resulted in the issue of physical inactivity being raised as a high-priority concern. As a result, VNACJ and a local health department are engaged in sponsoring a year-long series of weekend walks, with health presentations being a component. In yet another example, the staff of the VNACJ Community Health Center was asked to participate with community residents in a "Walkability Tour" to evaluate the degree to which a local community facilitated walking.

Another example, the Rural Elderly Enhancement Project, was a nurse-initiated grant funded by the W.K. Kellogg Foundation (Faulk, Coker, & Farley, 2001). The major purpose was to develop a model of community participation and empowerment. Leadership development of citizens increased their capacity to organize volunteer coalitions, secure funding, implement projects, and affect public policy. Accomplishments included the establishment of volunteer coalitions to assist the elderly with housekeeping and structural repairs and the development of two water systems serving over 500 families.

**Psychosocial and Mental Health.** Since 1984 the VNACJ's Mobile Outreach Clinic Program (MOCP) nurses have delivered on-site health assessment and case management for more than 2000 deinstitutionalized mentally ill residents living in single-room occupancies and boarding homes. Understanding that meaningful work is a vital health component for all adults, the MOCP has undertaken a collaborative initiative with the county division of social services to help identify clients in the community who are appropriate candidates for work rehabilitation. Based on a complete biopsychosocial and skills assessment, these nurses are linking clients to necessary health services, which facilitates improvement in overall functioning and reentry into the workforce.

When communities indicated that the needs of the community were better met by relocating selected numbers of deinstitutionalized mentally ill persons to other counties, the nurses' role again changed from a traditional health focus. A nurse actually accompanied the residents on a van throughout the state as they sought new housing, easing the anxiety that accompanied their relocation and assisting them in the process of selecting a new home. The nurses' presence fostered the residents' ability to make an informed choice. In addition, it demonstrated to communities at large and to policymakers that anticipatory planning must accompany any major policy shift.

The conceptualization of health as encompassing hope is never more evident than with children who have experienced severe loss through the death of a parent, sibling, or friend. The VNACJ Hospice Program began a bereavement program, Children Adjusting to New Situations (CANS) (Aldrich, 1989), for children of the agency's Hospice Program patients. Groups meet weekly for 6 consecutive weeks to discuss the effect of death and loss and to reinforce with participants that they are not the only ones experiencing sadness. This message of hope was brought to the larger community by a VNACJ nurse practitioner working in a school-based program at a local high school. Understanding that loss can have many precipitous effects, she introduced CANS into the high school to enable the children to cope with the anger that comes from the loss of income, health, family stability, and housing.

**Family-Centered Health.** To strengthen the preventive health care of childbearing families, a prenatal and postpartum culturally competent program was developed for Hawaiian, Filipino, and Japanese women on the Island of Hawaii. It was built, mindful of the importance of family and community to the women. Coordinated by public health nurses, the program is designed to complement, not duplicate, prenatal care from medical practitioners. The goal is to help women enter prenatal care early and remain in care until 3 months postpartum. Visits are scheduled for participant convenience, at locations including the workplace, a McDonald's restaurant, and the favorite gathering place, the beach (Mayberry, Affonso, Shibuya, & Clemmens, 1999).

As part of the Kellogg and RWJF initiative, Turning Point, the city of Sitka, Alaska established a partnership to "actively engage the residents of Sitka and…create a new approach to community health" (Cavanaugh & Cheney, 2002, p. 14). At one monthly meeting it was noted that one of the projects, a playtime program for mothers and toddlers, was on hold because of building construction. Another member immediately offered her site, the Sitka Pioneer Home for seniors. This afforded the regular interaction of children and seniors, and the intergenerational program was so successful that the program remained housed at the senior site.

Another example of family-centered care involved nursing care of a 75-year-old woman residing in an area motel with two developmentally disabled adult sons. When the VNACJ nurse arrived to attend to the woman's health care needs, she was forced to wait outside while the adult sons determined whether they were comfortable letting her in. When the nurse gained entry, she found the woman suffering from heat exhaustion, diabetes, and hypertension. Afraid of the dripping water from the air conditioner outside their motel, the sons were fearful of allowing it to be turned on. Through months of neglect, debris had been piled up in the shower, which interfered with the family's attention to personal hygiene. In addition to attending to the mother's physical health problems, the nurse walked the brothers around the motel, past the other units, to prove that the leaking fluid was benign. A local cleaning service was mobilized for the immediate environmental needs. The nurse then engaged the local housing authority, who located an available subsidized apartment for the family. Finally, through her extensive community network, the nurse arranged for a day vocational-rehabilitation program for the sons. This case underscores the degree to which intergenerational issues must be addressed within the context of community caregiving.

**Holistic Health.** Literacy is a critical component of health. The nurses of the VNACJ's MOCP identified this need while addressing the complex needs of homeless families living in motels in various communities. After years of moving from motel to motel to escape a battering father, a 7-year-old child was illiterate and starting her third year of kindergarten. Alarmed at the social and psychologic implications of this, the nurses initiated a reading program at the motel. The goal was to demonstrate to mothers, overwhelmed by life demands, how to use reading as a tool to help their children learn and to reinforce bonding among parent, child, and siblings.

Not long after this project began, the primary care providers at the VNACJ primary care centers became involved in the national Reach Out and Read program (ROR). Under the ROR program the primary care centers receive grants to purchase children's books. When a child comes for a wellness visit, the nurse practitioner writes a special "prescription" for an age-appropriate book, and the child is allowed to choose a book to take home. ROR has the double effect of promoting both literacy and preventive health by rewarding parents who maintain their schedule of follow-up visits.

## PARTICIPATION METHODS

The third competency that has implications for effective community collaboration is the development of the collective mindset. The two dimensions of that changed mindset are the focus on aggregate needs and participative interventions. It is often in ministering to individuals that nurses have the ability to mobilize and facilitate community involvement that contributes to the health of the aggregate (Drevdahl, 1995). The goal of building community collaboration is achieved because barriers are reduced, trust is increased, and common goals are identified. The participative model in action was evidenced by the interventions of a nurse who was caring for community-based clients in a motel. Called by a local motel owner to minister to one of his tenants, the nurse determined that the patient had scabies. In addition to administering the treatment to him, the nurse went from motel room to motel room to assess the conditions of the other residents. What resulted was the identification of a widespread outbreak of scabies throughout the site. The nurse called on many community providers to treat this community. She asked a VNACJ nurse practitioner to visit the residents and write a prescription for medications. She worked with a local pharmacy that was willing to order the medications required. Because none of the tenants had insurance, she worked with the board of social services and acquired a voucher to purchase the medications. Initially unwilling to be involved, the motel owner was educated on the need to decontaminate the facility. He eventually agreed to help, and even had all the mattresses replaced. This nurse's unwillingness to focus her assessment on her one client and her ability to mobilize many community providers had a positive impact on the health status of all motel residents.

**Community Collaboration.** The VNACJ spent several years developing a neighborhood nursing philosophy of care, which is built on exactly this premise of community collaboration (Reinhard et al., 1996). As an example, one nurse found that in her caseload significant numbers of elderly persons were malnourished, which resulted in frequent hospital readmissions. This observation, based on her care of individual patients, led her to work with the community and local churches to develop an extensive program of home-delivered meals for patients who did not meet the eligibility requirements of the federal entitlement program for senior citizens. Staff members working with individuals in communities have the opportunity and responsibility to act on trends that are individually manifested but geographically significant. For example, a community health nurse, having witnessed the social isolation and depression of seniors living in the only unlocked housing facility in a high-crime area, petitioned the town council and the county to secure the building.

**The Power of Partnerships.** The second dimension of the collective mindset is a true belief in the power of partnerships and participation. Participatory approaches are most effective because they increase interpersonal relationships and feelings of personal and political confidence. For example, in addition to attending traditional health-related community events such as health fairs, neighborhood nurses at VNACJ participate in town parades, Parent-Teacher Association (PTA) meetings, and city celebration days, often in the evenings, on weekends, and on holidays. These activities further validate for the community that the organization is a partner and that the nurse is engaged in the fabric of community.

**Trust and Mutuality.** Courtney and co-workers (1996) defined the partnership model as the negotiated sharing of power between health professionals and community members. The basic condition of partnership is trust, whereby members become confident that other participants will uphold formal and informal agreements. The mutuality in contributions to the partnership means that the professional does not take on all the responsibility, accountability, or authority. Partners play a mutual role in determining goals and actions, with the ultimate goal being to enhance the capacity of communities to act more effectively on their own behalf (Kang, 1995). For the partnership to be truly reflective of the community we serve means we must

seek "not only the usual voices heard in the discussions of health, but actively seek out unusual voices such as business owners, faith representatives, youth, and other minority groups...to identify individuals who had credibility and respect among those missing at our meetings and those who were willing to communicate the partnership business on a regular basis to them and ask for input from them" (Cavanaugh & Cheney, 2002, p. 17).

**Outreach.** VNACJ employs these principles in an attempt to reduce the rate of human immunodeficiency virus (HIV) infection in a city with one of the highest infection rates in the nation. Through a faith-based model, The Balm in Gilead, the program manager involves members of the clergy as partners in the outreach project. The kick-off involved a dinner, hosted in the community and attended by over 100 people, many of them members of the clergy. From this resulted a modification of the outreach methodology. Outreach was scheduled at the churches, a natural and comfortable meeting place for the at-risk population; however, the stigma attached to HIV and acquired immunodeficiency syndrome (AIDS) was so strong that it was seen as a barrier to participation. To address this, a method known as the "tent event" was developed. In addition to serving refreshments, the program manager sets up a little portable cubicle at the church that the attendees can visit for education about a variety of health issues including hypertension, diabetes, and breast and cervical cancer as well as HIV and AIDS. By framing HIV outreach in a venue and within a program that are comfortable for the at-risk populations, optimal outreach benchmarks have been achieved.

**Issues.** Gauthier and Metteson (1995) noted that the issues that must be resolved for community collaboration to work are power and control, protection of turf, competition among partners, and challenges of sustainability. An example of negotiating power for the purpose of facilitating partnership involves the Roman Catholic Diocese in central New Jersey and its efforts to establish a network of parish nursing programs. With over 126 parishes in a four-county area, only nine parish nursing programs existed. A centralized steering committee with representatives from each of the counties developed the mission and protocol for the programs. Through a series of lectures and meetings to which each parish was requested to send a representative, and cognizant of the fact that parish structures are vastly different, parish liaisons contributed input to a model that was flexible to their needs. The diocesan department served as a centralized resource to parishes in various stages of evolution with their programs, with 72 parish nursing programs being established or expanded. Another technique was the use of quarterly roundtables in which parish nurses shared best practices. The tremendous success of this program has to do with the fact that it was a bottom-up approach, which was nurtured rather than dictated. As a result, more-experienced parish nurses were able to meet on common ground with new parish nurses just starting their work. New programs were nurtured by the mentoring of experienced program members.

## COLLABORATIVE PARTNERSHIPS IN ACTION

The movement toward collaboration among equals and away from victimization was evidenced recently during strategic planning in a blighted urban municipality. Community members insisted on the inclusion of strengths—not just the traditional problem list and negative statistics. Programs flowing from these assessments were built on strengths rather than being focused solely on need.

Another example occurred in a small South Dakota city where adolescent pregnancy with subsequent dropping out of high school was a major health concern (Fahrenwald et al., 1999). Four nursing students studied the problem, bringing together information from teens and key informants, such as the director of an alternative school. Based on this information, the students developed a Mentor-Mom parenting program for area adolescents and presented it to a local teen pregnancy task force, which secured funding for the project. The program matches pregnant and parenting adolescents one on one with experienced mentor mothers. The mentors provide friendship, support, advocacy, resources, and education to assist the pregnant and parenting teens to finish school.

It is critical that nurses involved in effective community collaboration guard against the trap of falling into the rhetoric of empowerment. This rhetoric just reinforces the power of the professional and strengthens the view that the professional knows best. The rhetoric of empowerment has caused competent communities to be invaded, captured, and weakened by mottoes that speak of collaboration and empowerment but actually reinforce feelings of powerlessness (Courtney et al., 1996). In these cases, needs of organizations are met, rather than the needs of communities.

An example of collaborative partnership is the Escalante Health Partnerships, a community-based, nurse-managed program for older adults in an Arizona community. Initiated in 1991 by the state university school of nursing, the local health department, and the community action committee, the program quickly expanded to include the community hospital, the city community council, local businesses, law enforcement, and other senior services such as daycare and the office on aging. Coalition members have pulled limited resources together to provide a full spectrum of care. The health outcomes of the participating 1400 seniors compared with national norms demonstrate the effectiveness of the partnership, with seniors reporting better general health, role performance, and social functioning with fewer medical visits (Nunez, Armbruster, Phillips, & Gale, 2003).

Yet another example of transforming the professional role into a partnership role occurred with a local community collaborative formed for the purpose of reducing the incidence of child abuse and neglect in a small community on the Jersey Shore. Members of the collaborative represented the local school district, child abuse advocates, VNACJ, municipal and county government, religious organizations, mental health organizations, local hospitals, and community members. One result was that a community member was selected as the chairperson; and, in addition to traditional programs such as school-based advanced practice nurse (APN) programs, the collaborative developed innovative programs including a resource center open to the community, with programs and services provided by many organizations.

Mutuality among partners and patients was highlighted, in yet another example, when VNACJ and five other service providers were approached by a regional funder to identify a community project. Sensitive to the community's spoken concern that funded activities should be "of the people," the service providers engaged the community in the development of a community leadership program. Applications were distributed throughout the city of Asbury Park, New Jersey, inviting residents to be leaders with an idea to benefit the community. Enthusiasm abounded and many applied, with 10 leaders being selected. After a weekend retreat the leaders met weekly for 12 weeks to learn about the history and resources of the city, community development, and leadership skills. The provider agencies, which serve as repositories of the funding, provide a project site and mentorship for the leaders. Among the community projects that the leaders launched were the following: senior citizen women working with young, school-aged girls in a program called "Be Yourself, Support Yourself"; a creative cultural arts program for elementary school children; a "fun to fitness" group for girls aged 5 to 14 years to learn about their bodies and minds; a Haitian program for children aged 14 to 18 years to encourage them in the development of greater cultural understanding and to teach them how to interact within the community; an entrepreneurial training course for older youth, aged 18 to 21 years, to teach them how to set up their own vendor business; a read-aloud group for children aged 6 to 12 years; a performance art program; and an environmental program titled "We Sea," in which children aged 7 to 12 years are exposed to hands-on activities along the beach. The outcomes of this project were threefold: resolution of community need, development of community pride and well-being, and development of future community leaders.

## COMMUNITY ORGANIZING

A community-organizing approach, rather than a traditional medical or health-planning model, supports community collaboration and participation.

In the medical model, community participation is minimal and the health professional maintains control. Community participation is greater in the health-planning model; however, the intent is to maximize the resources of the professionally defined program, not those of the community itself. In contrast, in the community-organizing approach, the community is mobilized through community participation and control, and the professional is the resource and catalyst for change. The program and direction come from the community itself (Flick, Reese, Rogers, Fletcher, & Sonn, 1994). As an example of this, city administrators in an urban at-risk community became concerned about the number of calls to local police, fire, and first aid departments by the large number of deinstitutionalized mentally ill and elderly residing in the community. In response, they formulated a strategy that involved providing funding for VNACJ to provide a "city nurse" to address these concerns.

An example of the community-organizing approach is a community health center launched in a medically underserved area by VNACJ. The center is a freestanding organization with a board of trustees derived from local community-based organizations and the community itself. The role of the nurse practitioners in the center has taken on a form much different from that in other community health centers in similar geographic locales. For instance, one of the nurse practitioners spends time at the boys' and girls' club, the center recently hosted an art contest for another youth group in the city, and staff served as "guest readers" for their literacy program. Each year the nurse practitioners provide free physicals for over 100 Pop Warner football players and cheerleaders. In yet another example, a nurse practitioner provides outreach to senior citizens on the issues of substance abuse, medication compliance, and social isolation. This center has truly taken the form of the community it serves because of a board structure that provides the community a forum for input and control (Figure 33-2).

A VNACJ nurse practitioner recognized the lack of attention being paid to the emergent issue of neglected adolescent health. Collaboration between the VNACJ Community Health Center and the local

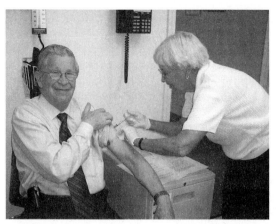

**Figure 33-2** Immunizations are not just for kids! A VNACJ nurse administers the influenza vaccine to a senior.

school district enabled the VNACJ to secure a 3-year demonstration grant from the RWJF to augment traditional school nurse services with nurse practitioner services at the middle school. In addition, the VNACJ's grant writer worked with the district's high school and other community providers to secure funding from the New Jersey Department of Human Services for the School-Based Youth Services Program.

**Hiring from Within.** Another method of ensuring that program and direction come from the community itself is to hire from the community in which an organization operates. This is the basic reason for the success of the peer worker programs that have been so effective with hard-to-reach groups such as youth (Sanders, 2001).

The 125 Flower Estate health project in Sheffield, England has worked to improve the health of people under age 18 since 1998. After identifying that young adults were not using available health services, the group initiated education workshops in which teenagers explore a variety of health topics (e.g., smoking, substance abuse, sex, relationships). The involvement of peer educators using young people with a lot of street credibility proved to be an effective way to discuss risk-taking behaviors and explore ways for youth to resist pressure from peers (Sanders, 2001).

The nurse practitioner at the RWJF-funded middle-school program realized that the children were at very high risk for HIV and AIDS because of their environment, lack of knowledge, and lack of social supports. With another community agency she developed a peer education program through which seventh grade volunteers were educated on HIV and AIDS and role-modeling interventions. These peer workers were able to have a positive impact at school and at social events and to support their peers in healthy behaviors.

**Phases of Development.** Community organizing and participation require three phases of development: locality development, social planning, and social action. In the locality development phase, "local communities are empowered to create change," and the outcome is the cultivation of community capacity to provide self-help, with the professional assuming the role of coordinator and enabler. Social planning involves data collection, with the professional assuming the role of fact gatherer and facilitator. During the social action component "disadvantaged and marginalized groups organize to make demands from the larger society," and there is a shift in the relationship in an attempt to address social injustices and to create institutional change, with the health care professional assuming the role of activist. Community collaboration thus becomes a self-perpetuating process in which residents initiate future activity after the organization's formal role has been completed (Drevdahl, 1995, 2002).

Throughout this process, several action steps must be initiated. It is critical that an exploration of environmental conditions that contribute to illness or interfere with wellness be undertaken. Coalitions must be formed to engage the community in the process. Critical dialogue must be facilitated with community members, and conditions that interfere with full participation must be changed. Finally, because of the interrelationships among local issues and national and international trends, the global environment must be evaluated relative to the grassroots problem that has been identified. Critical discussions focusing on methods available to change larger sociopolitical structures must be conducted (Drevdahl, 1995).

For instance, the economic situation in a locality, state, or nation has a significant impact on how people live and feel. Changing demographics in the community heightened the need for community organization and action in a community served by the VNACJ nurses. Concurrent gentrification and immigration of non–English-speaking residents had taxed health care providers, schools, and churches. Initiated by the School-Based Youth Services Program at the high school, a "unity day" brought the community together.

Another example of the relationship among issues is the Welfare to Work initiative occurring nationally. In New Jersey the process for rolling out the Welfare to Work initiative is overseen on a local level by workforce investment boards composed of welfare beneficiaries and the private and public sectors. A critical issue now being raised is how self-sufficiency will be sustained in the face of large-scale gentrification of neighborhoods that traditionally offered the availability of low-income housing. Community partners are addressing the issue of the diminishing affordable housing stock at local, county, state, and federal levels.

These are the kinds of discussions in which nurses must meaningfully participate.

## VISIONARY LEADERSHIP

Visionary leadership is imperative in effective community collaboration. The visionary leader is one who remains simultaneously tenacious and decisive, as well as caring and flexible. The group is best served when the leader helps the followers to develop their own initiative. Visionary leadership strengthens individuals in the use of their own judgment and allows them to grow and become better contributors. The shift must be from the health care providers to the community for visionary direction (USDHHS, 2000).

An example at VNACJ involved a collaborative venture with a local Hispanic church. Church leaders and a local physician had identified the need for an on-site primary care center to be situated in a trailer in the church's parking lot. Inquiries by VNACJ about the possibility of collaboration resulted in the organization's management being sought for a consultation role. Initially the VNACJ

manager assumed the role of directing the group, designing a nurse practitioner–physician collaborative model, and preparing proposals to foundations. What quickly became apparent was that the physician and the church leaders felt threatened by what they perceived to be a control issue by the manager.

In a meeting between church leaders and VNACJ administration, the administration asked a simple question: "What would you like us to do?" That simple question, aimed at returning the locus of control to church leaders, resulted in VNACJ's role being defined by the group to be more consultative.

In yet another example, VNACJ approached a local school system about the possibility of having an on-site nurse practitioner at the school. The goal was to afford children without adequate parental and social supports with accessible primary care services. Although this was the initial foray into wellness, the school and parents went on to expand and fund the program to include a mental health component and an attendance officer.

Increasingly, the leader is a gatherer of people and a facilitator of processes to help reach agreement (Porter-O'Grady, 1997). Success demands that attention be paid to the external environment. Bennis (1991) identified four basic dimensions as contributing to visionary leadership: management of attention, of meaning, of trust, and of self.

*Management of attention* is defined as the ability to focus on the vision, even in times of uncertainty and chaos. The critical vision that must underlie any community partnership is the fact that professional-citizen mutuality can be sustained even during the transition process. In fact, professional-citizen mutuality must be maintained not only to sustain partnership but also to achieve the ultimate vision. VNACJ, in response to community need, developed and began to implement plans for a nurse-managed, community-based primary care center in a high-risk, isolated urban municipality. Stresses within the community were such that political uncertainty existed: controversy among agencies, residents, and city government was the norm. Fourteen city and school elections and reelections had taken place in less than 4 years. In response to the challenge, the VNACJ leadership met frequently with both elected officials and city management. However, the players and the agenda often changed from meeting to meeting. Management focused on repeating the same message of our vision and mission. In addition, management joined with residents and colleagues at meetings to state the vision and mission. Foremost in those statements were family and community needs as the core reason for the proposal. The vision prevailed, and the center was awarded a certificate of occupancy by the city and a designation as a Federally Qualified Health Center (FQHC) Look-Alike by the federal government. Keeping mission and community partnership foremost, VNACJ then invited the local health department and the area hospital into partnership, a significant gesture because both had been opponents during the competitive process. A sustained commitment to purpose has resulted in the center's receiving full FQHC designation and funding.

*Management of meaning* has to do with the ability to communicate. Continuous communication is critical so that professional and citizen participants understand and have input into the direction of the program. For nearly 20 years a VNACJ manager had served on the boards and committees of three counties, as well as at the state level. Recognized as an expert in the management of services for persons and families with HIV and AIDS, she achieved success in creating partnerships among fiercely competitive organizations as a direct result of her communication style. Through discussion, negotiation, caring, and understanding, the VNACJ manager exhibited active listening, which created a constant feedback loop for participants. She also extended her communication outreach to the grassroots county- and state-level constituencies. As a result of her management of meaning, this regional HIV and AIDS consortium is recognized as a model in the state.

An additional aspect in managing meaning is to use the appropriate communication vehicles. A case in point is an Alaskan public health nurse who traveled to her patients via plane, jeep, and snowmobile. A major concern for her was the age-appropriate immunizations of toddlers. She initiated the "I Did it by Two" program, promoting it through one of

Alaska's most famous events, the Iditarod dogsled race. Volunteers at the event were engaged to spread the message about immunizations to parents. In addition, sled dogs wore vests highlighting the message, and husky dog toys were distributed to reinforce the education (Roberts, 2003).

*Management of trust* is facilitated by ensuring that all stakeholders have a place at the table and that these collaborators stay involved over time. Over the years, VNACJ has been involved in responding to a variety of natural disasters including nor'easters, floods, explosions, and fires. Staff has participated in Red Cross training, and close relationships have been established with the emergency management systems throughout the service area. As a result the organization has come to be recognized as a key participant and decision-maker. These relationships fostered over time have enabled the organization to staff shelters and rely on a local network of thrift shops for clothing, restaurants for food, and pharmacies for medication deliveries for affected and displaced residents. The relationships fostered at these tables positioned VNACJ to respond effectively and competently to the needs of the hundreds of area residents and families affected by 9/11. VNACJ's involvement included collaboration with the Red Cross and United Way in the distribution of funds for living expenses, offering of support groups to survivors and bereavement intervention to spouses and children of the victims, provision of wound care and rehabilitation intervention to the injured, and participation in the planning, development, and implementation of a Family Resource Center. That work and the relationships established through it have further enabled the organization to participate fully, as a partner, in local, state, and national emergency preparedness planning and programs.

*Management of self* revolves around the leader's understanding of and sensitivity to her own strengths and weaknesses. If the nurse leader is particularly adept at managing and responding to the global environment but is less adept at managing operational details, she must pair her own abilities with the abilities of the group. The leader must always be sensitive to enhancing the visibility and accomplishments of the entire group. Successful organizers are those able to enjoy the reflective glow of others' successes.

A program launched by a VNACJ nurse provides intensive home visiting to vulnerable new patients. Although the nurse brought extensive clinical, managerial, and public health experience to the program, she was not a layperson living in a low-income, blighted urban area. She recruited community members, training them to provide ongoing support and anticipatory guidance. At state and county meetings the nurse described the success of the program in terms of the peer worker and family accomplishments.

Management of self can also draw on the collective strengths of organizations. VNACJ is partnering with a local United Way in the Nurse Family Partnership. This is a research-based model of nursing intervention focused on addressing the health care needs of teen mothers and their babies through the second year of life. The partnership builds on the strength of each organization, with the United Way providing leadership, community, and corporate visibility and funding, and VNACJ the grassroots connections, professional competency, and operational oversight (Figure 33-3).

## NURSING'S ROLE IN THE COMMUNITY

Working with communities provides the most fertile opportunity for the nursing profession in the new millennium. Key competencies that health

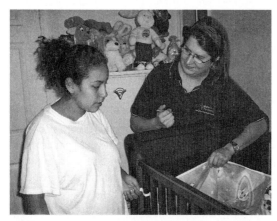

**Figure 33-3** A staff member of the Nurse Family Partnership mentors a young mother to improve her childcare skills

care professionals will need in the future include expertise in healthy lifestyles, preventive and primary care, improved communication skills, and enhanced community health and partnership abilities involving complex negotiations. According to Gebbie (1999), public health focuses on populations, communities, and building coalitions. It is key to the community infrastructure and must continually ensure that essential services are available when needed.

Nurses' assumption of leadership roles is paramount to solving the health disparities problem that exists today, particularly that found in minority populations. Nurses are entrenched in all services and service components of health care and receive education that should position them as leaders; yet "proportionately few nurses emerge as recognized leaders in healthcare" (Keltner, Kelley, & Smith, 2004, p. 182). To capture the opportunity to make changes in the health care system and reduce disparities of care, nursing leaders are needed now (Keltner, Kelley, & Smith, 2004).

Cognizant of the changing state of health care systems, the University of Delaware and the Delaware Division of Public Health created an academic–public health partnership (Partners in Action) to provide undergraduate public health nursing clinical experience for bachelor of science students. Students developed competencies in public health functions addressing population-based health and prevention in a variety of sites in medically underserved areas. Importantly, students were assisted to become active in grant writing, marketing, and the political process as preparation for leadership roles in the future (Hall-Long, 2004).

To establish cultural competence by RNs, Washington State University College of Nursing Vancouver and Southwest Washington Health District collaborated on a project for RNs who are seeking a baccalaureate degree. Among its primary objectives were to identify strategies to improve understanding and role performance and identify barriers to improving performance, and to enhance curriculum and faculty ability to respond to changing trends. The project resulted in academic changes, including an interactive manual for mentors and students, and development of a collaborative relationship between faculty and public health mentors (Doutrich & Storey, 2004).

In 1996, Erickson urged that the concepts of poverty, caring, and activism be included as building blocks of nursing curricula, with home visits and health strategies the teaching tools employed to reinforce these core competencies. That position has been reinforced in the American Nurses Association Social Policy Statement (2003), which emphasizes the relationship between caring and health and healing. In addition, the Pew Health Professions Commission (1998) highlighted community-based service learning as essential to health professional curricula. Kemsley and Riegle (2004) note that the American Association of Colleges of Nursing has recommended since 1996 that service learning be integrated into the mission statement of schools of learning. These principles have been integrated beyond the academic arena into the staff-development programs of health care providers. The Rural Alabama Health Professional Training Consortium provided interdisciplinary training for nurses and other health professionals from 1990 to 1996 in impoverished rural areas (Leeper, Hullett, & Wang, 2001). There was a significant increase in clinical practice, with over 80% of students considering employment in a rural area after graduation. The VNACJ, with funding from the W.K. Kellogg Foundation, developed a competency-based practice model based on the novice-to-expert continuum. Among the skills required for the expert community health nurse are networking, critical thinking, community development, assessment (of individual, family, and community), care planning, leadership, caseload management, clinical and intervention skills, teaching, case finding, and screening.

At the foundation of effective community collaboration is clinical competence. Mentoring is more important than ever because of the demands made on nurses. Mentors provide career guidance, role modeling, intellectual stimulation, inspiration, advice, and emotional support. Mentoring entails collaboration versus competition and makes nurses deliberately establish relationships and caring that will guide, protect, and instruct other nurses. The role of mentorship becomes increasingly critical as society expects nurses not only to master the art of nursing but also to establish networks and foster collaboration. Mentoring is reciprocal; thus it strengthens the profession and enhances leadership role preparation (Vance, 2001; Vance, 2002; Vance & Olson, 1998).

Because of the changing imperatives in the health care delivery system, nurses are uniquely positioned to build on their strong tradition of community-based partnerships. As a society, we must be committed to maintaining the well-being of communities—the infrastructure of our culture.

## Key Points

- Three concepts that require mastery by nurses are a keen understanding of the differentiation between community and population, a broad conceptualization of health, and the development of a collective mindset.
- Nurses must seek and understand aggregate data and the community-organizing approach.
- A sensitivity to the larger sociopolitical environment is critical.
- Strategies that are essential to working with communities include drawing partners from the grassroots community itself, addressing the needs of the community *with* the community (not *for* the community), facilitating community members' ability to be advocates for themselves, and maintaining relationships with stakeholders through time.

## Web Resources

**Building Community Collaboration and Consensus**
*www.communitycollaboration.net*
**Comm-Org**—online conference on community organizing and development
*http://comm-org.wisc.edu*
**Public Health Nursing Section of the American Public Health Association**
*www.csuchico.edu/~horst*
**Visiting Nurse Associations of America**
*www.vnaa.org*

## REFERENCES

Aldrich, L. (1989). *Children adjusting to new situations.* Moorestown, NJ: Samaritan Hospice.

American Nurses Association (ANA). (2003). *Social policy statement.* Washington, DC: ANA.

Armstrong, F. (2001). Addressing workforce issues. *Australian Nursing Journal, 9*(1), 28-30.

Bennis, W. (1991, Winter). Learning some basic truisms about leadership. *Phi Kappa Phi Journal,* 13.

Boyle, A. (2001, August 13). Wanted: More than a few good nurses. *New York Times,* 14CN-3.

Caro, F. G., & Kaffenberger, K. R. (2001). The impact of financing on workforce recruitment and retention. *Generation, 25*(1), 17-22.

Cavanaugh, N., & Cheney, K. (2002). Community collaboration—a weaving. *Journal of Public Health Management Practice, 8*(1), 13-20.

Courtney, R., Ballard, E., Fauver, S., Gariota, M., & Holland, L. (1996). The partnership model: Working with individuals, families, and communities toward a new vision of health. *Public Health Nursing, 13*(3), 177-186.

Doutrich, D., & Storey, M. (2004). Education and practice: Dynamic partners for improving cultural competence in public health. *Family & Community Health, 27*(4), 298-307.

Drevdahl, D. (1995). Coming to voice: The power of emancipatory community interventions. *Advances in Nursing Science, 18*(2), 13-24.

Drevdahl, D. (2002). Social justice or market justice? The paradox of public health partnerships with managed care. *Public Health Nursing, 19*(3), 161-169.

Erickson, G. P. (1996). To pauperize or empower: Public health nursing at the turn of the 20th and 21st centuries. *Public Health Nursing, 13*(3), 163-169.

Fahrenwald, N., Fischer, C., Boysen, R., & Maurer, R. (1999). Population-based clinical projects: Bridging community-based and public health concepts. *Nurse Educator, 24*(6), 28-32.

Faulk, D., Coker, R., & Farley, S. (2001). After the funding is gone. *Nursing and Health Care Perspectives, 22*(4), 184-186.

Flick, L., Reese, C., Rogers, G., Fletcher, P., & Sonn, J. (1994). Building community for health: Lessons from a seven-year old neighborhood/university partnership. *Health Education Quarterly, 21*(3), 369-380.

Gauthier, M. A., & Metteson, P. (1995). The role of empowerment in neighborhood-based nursing education. *Journal of Nursing Education, 34*(8), 390-395.

Gebbie, K. M. (1999). The public health workforce: Key to public health infrastructure. *American Journal of Public Health, 89*(5), 660-661.

Hall-Long, B. (2004). Partners in action, a public health program for baccalaureate nursing students. *Family & Community Health, 27*(4), 338-345.

Kang, R. (1995). Building community capacity for health promotion: A challenge for public health nurses. *Public Health Nursing, 21*(5), 312-318.

Keltner, B., Kelley, F. J., & Smith, D. (2004). Leadership to reduce health disparities: A model for nursing leadership in American Indian communities. *Nursing Administration Quarterly, 28*(3), 181-190.

Kemsley, M., & Riegle, E. (2004). A community-campus partnership: Influenza prevention campaign. *Nurse Educator, 29*(3), 126-129.

Leeper, J., Hullett, S., & Wang, L. (2001). Rural Alabama health professional training consortium: Six-year evaluation results. *Family & Community Health, 24*(2), 28-26.

MacQueen, K., McLellan, E., Metzger, D., Kegeles, S., Strauss, R., et al. (2001). What is community: An evidenced-based definition for participatory public health. *American Journal of Public Health, 91*(12), 1929-1938.

Mayberry, L., Affonso, D., Shibuya, J, & Clemmens, D. (1999). Integrating cultural values, beliefs and customs into pregnancy and postpartum care: Lessons learned from a Hawaiian public health nursing project. *Journal of Perinatal & Neonatal Nursing, 13*(1), 15-26.

New Jersey Department of Human Services. (2004). *A new beginning: The future of child welfare in New Jersey.* Retrieved April 10, 2006, from *www.state.nj.us/humanservices/CWA/ A%20New%20Begining/A_New_Begining.pdf.*

Nunez, D., Armbruster, C., Phillips, W. T., & Gale, B. J. (2003). Community-based senior health promotion program using a collaborative practice model: The Escalante Health Partnership. *Public Health Nursing, 20*(1), 25-31.

Oklahoma Turning Point. (2005). Turning point: Building healthy communities in Oklahoma through partnerships. Retrieved March 14, 2005, from *www.health.state.ok.us/partners/ whatis.html.*

Pew Health Professions Commission. (1998). *Recreating health professional practice for a new century: The fourth report of the Pew Health Professions Commission.* Retrieved April 20, 2005, from *www.futurehealth.ucsf.edu/pdf_files/recreate.pdf.*

Porter-O'Grady, T. (1997). Quantum mechanics and the future of healthcare leadership. *Journal of Nursing Administration, 27*(10), 15-20.

Rawlings-Anderson, K. (2001). Working with older people from minority ethnic groups. *Nursing Older People, 13*(5), 21-25.

Reinhard, S., Christopher, M. A., Mason, D. J., McConnell, K., Toughill, E., & Rusca, P. (1996). Promoting healthy communities through neighborhood nursing. *Nursing Outlook, 44*(5), 223-228.

Roberts, K. (2003), Going the distance: An itinerant nurse takes health care to the corners of Alaska. *American Journal of Nursing, 103*(12), 102-103.

Sanders, K. (2001). Three of the best. *Community Practitioner, 74*(7), 253-255.

Smith, R. D., Inoue, T., Ushikubo, M., & Amano, S. (2001). Nursing in Japan. *Australian Nursing Journal, 9*(1), 39-40.

Treating asthma in the zone: Nursing with the Harlem Children's Zone Asthma Initiative. (2003). *American Journal of Nursing, 103*(11), 118-119.

U.S. Department of Health and Human Services (USDHHS). *Healthy People 2010: Understanding and improving health* (2nd ed.). (2000). Washington, DC: USDHHS.

Vance, C. (2001, February/March). The value of mentoring. *Imprint,* 38-41.

Vance, C. (2002). Mentoring at the edge of chaos. *Creative Nursing, 8*(3), 7, 14.

Vance, C., & Olson, R. K. (1998). *The mentor connection in nursing.* New York: Springer.

## REGULATING INDUSTRIAL CHEMICALS TO PROTECT THE ENVIRONMENT AND HUMAN HEALTH

Charlotte Brody

*"Only within the moment of time represented by the present century has one species—man—acquired significant power to alter the nature of his world."*

RACHEL CARSON

### HISTORY OF FOOD AND DRUG REGULATION

In 1785 the lawmakers of Massachusetts added a preamble to explain the purpose of the new law they were putting into place:

Whereas some evilly disposed persons, from motives of avarice and filthy lucre, have been induced to sell diseased, corrupted, contagious or unwholesome provisions, to the great nuisance of public health and peace. (Swann, 2001)

The Massachusetts Act Against Selling Unwholesome Provisions is one of the first examples of a law aimed at protecting the health of the American public from contaminated products and the "avarice-motivated" people who sell them.

As industrialization increased in the United States, so did the distance between commodity producers and the consumers of those foods and products. This increased distance heightened concerns about chemicals and other suspect additives in commercially available food and drugs. In 1862, President Abraham Lincoln added a chemist to the staff of the U.S. Department of Agriculture (USDA) to investigate the safety of chemical preservatives and the adulteration and mislabeling of drugs and foods. This Bureau of Chemistry eventually became the U.S. Food and Drug Administration (FDA).

In the late 1800s the USDA's Bureau of Chemistry had too little power and authority to properly safeguard commercially available products. The states responded by passing their own pure food and dairy laws. But these laws were difficult to enforce, according to a 1900-1901 U.S. Senate Investigation (Law & Libecap, 2003). Continuing health concerns led progressive women's clubs, the home economics movement, muckraking journalists, and public health advocates to lobby Congress for more protections. In 1885 the floor debate on the bill included this explanation of the necessity for more federal government involvement:

In ordinary cases the consumer may be left to his own intelligence to protect himself against impositions. By the exercise of a reasonable degree of caution, he can protect himself from frauds in under-weight and in under-measure. If he cannot detect a paper-soled shoe on inspection, he detects it in the wearing of it, and in one way or another he can impose a penalty upon the fraudulent vendor. As a general rule the doctrine of laissez faire can be applied. Not so with many of the adulterations of food. Scientific inspection is needed to detect the fraud, and scientific inspection is beyond the reach of the ordinary consumer. In such cases the Government should intervene. (Congressional Record, 49th Congress, 1st Session, p. 5043)

In 1906 the U.S. Congress passed the Food and Drug Act. In the hundred years since, consumers have come to expect that the federal government's laws and enforcement mechanisms provide the scientific inspections that are beyond our reach as ordinary consumers. The public believes that, given the existence of the FDA and the Consumer Products Safety Commission, the products we use every day have gone through safety and health testing and official review of these tests before they can be sold.

This is the path for new drugs. Before a new drug can be marketed, the FDA reviews animal tests on the substance and the protocol for testing on human subjects. A local institutional review board must also approve the human study design. Then three rounds of human studies are done: The first phase of studies determines the safety of the drug in healthy human subjects. If the drug is shown to not be toxic to healthy people, then the second phase of studies is done for efficacy on people who are sick. Typically these studies are done with a control group of patients with the same disease. If this round of studies is successful, then a third phase begins with more study participants, more variation in dose and population, and more attention paid to side effects and the interaction of the studied drug with other medications. Only then does the FDA allow a new drug to be offered for sale, requiring a fourth phase of review after a drug is on the market and extensive labeling on the ingredients, the recommended dose, the possible side effects, interactions, and contraindications (Meadows, 2002).

Recent headlines have shown that this four-step process isn't enough to fully protect the public from unnecessarily dangerous prescription drugs. But lurking below the headlines is the larger story of industrial chemicals that work like drugs but are put on the market without any FDA-like approval or labeling requirements.

## HISTORY OF CHEMICALS CAUSING DISEASE AND THE LACK OF REGULATION

Mercury provides one example of how long science has recognized that chemicals can harm health. Galen, born in 129 AD, described mercury as "a cold poison." In 1860, *Transactions of the Medical Society of New Jersey* published a clinical description of "mecurialism" among workers who used mercury to make fur hats (Hightower, 2004). The Mad Hatter

in Lewis Carroll's 1865 classic Alice in Wonderland exhibited the most visible of these symptoms of "tremor, psychic disturbances such as irritability, timidity, irascibility and difficulty in getting along with people, headaches, drowsiness, gastrointestinal disturbances, sore mouth, insomnia and weakness."

Our early knowledge about the hazards of mercury and other chemicals was mostly ignored as the twentieth-century economy built itself on the use of thousands of chemicals. These chemicals were introduced into the marketplace without any government-required premarket studies of possible health effects. Only when people in certain occupations with certain exposures started developing certain diseases did the health professions and the public learn of a chemical's danger. In the 1920s the press covered the story of the 11 men who died and the 149 more who were poisoned by the tetraethyl lead being added to gasoline (Rosner & Markowitz, 2002). In 1928 a medical journal published the first finding of benzene-related leukemia, and reports of lung cancer associated with asbestos exposure started showing up in the medical literature in the 1930s and 1940s (Gee et al., 2001). In 1970 animal studies were published that showed that exposure to vinyl chloride, the basic component of vinyl or PVC, resulted in angiosarcoma, a cancer of the blood vessels in the brain or liver at half the exposure level that workers were being told was safe (Rosner & Markowitz, 2002).

These stories of workers, exposure, and disease share a plotline. First, the studies showing harm are ignored. Then they are disputed, usually by the industry that employs the affected workers. When those positions are overwhelmingly challenged by the scientific evidence and political will, the argument shifts to how much exposure to that chemical is necessary before workers start getting a specific disease. Instead of focusing on finding safer alternative materials or processes that would eliminate the exposure problem, scientists and policymakers review the animal and human studies on exposure to a certain industrial chemical, decide the amount of exposure that the studies show will cause a health problem, add a safety factor, and set a limit for exposure.

This policy option, most often called *risk assessment*, is used to set limits on exposure not only to substances present in factories but also to chemicals added to personal care products, contaminants in drinking water, toxic contaminants in food, outdoor air pollution from vehicles, factories, and power plants, and indoor air pollution from building materials and furnishings. Risk assessment is based on the following assumptions:

- That we have the information we need to make good decisions
- That most chemicals are benign
- That although chemicals may cause harm when workers are overdosed, there is a safe level for even the most dangerous chemicals
- That exposure to the less-benign chemicals will result in unique disease that can be tied to the exposure to a single chemical
- That it is morally acceptable to wait and see what disease manifests itself in exposed workers and, since Love Canal, exposed communities before taking action

The Toxic Substances Control Act of 1976, or TSCA (pronounced "toska"), enshrines this set of assumptions. TSCA finds all chemicals in use before 1976 to be safe unless the government can prove that their use poses "an unreasonable risk." More than 99% of the volume of chemicals on the market today is part of the TSCA inventory list of "innocent until proven guilty" chemicals. There are additional requirements for new chemicals under TSCA. This higher standard for chemicals created after 1976 has limited innovation by promoting the continued use of chemicals that were grandfathered in at a lower standard (Tickner, Geiser, & Coffin, 2005).

Drugs must be shown to be safe, but chemicals must be shown to be guilty. Federal law requires rigorous reviews of the animal and human data by the FDA before a drug can be commercially sold, but the U.S. Environmental Protection Agency (EPA) has to gather the evidence to prove that a chemical "will present an unreasonable risk," that the regulation it proposes to reduce the risk to "an acceptable level" is the least burdensome to industry, and that the benefit of the regulation outweighs the cost to industry.

The numbers reveal the level of protection that results from these two very different regulatory methodologies:

- According to the Tufts Center for the Study of Drug Development, about one in five drugs that enter clinical testing ultimately is approved by the FDA (Meadows, 2002).
- According to the U.S. Government Accountability Office (GAO) June 2005 report, of the 60,000 chemicals on the TSCA inventory, EPA has successfully restricted five.
- A coarse mathematic comparison yields this statistic: 80% of new drugs never get to market, but only 0.008% of TSCA-listed chemicals have been restricted by government action.

## EMERGING FIELD OF ENVIRONMENTAL HEALTH

The 10,000-fold difference in the restrictions of the EPA on chemicals and approvals by the FDA on prescription drugs suggests that they are entirely different societal issues that affect public health in entirely different ways. But over the last 20 years, the emerging field of environmental health has demonstrated that in some very important ways, chemicals work very much like pharmaceutical drugs.

Specifically, for both chemicals and drugs:

- The size of the patient matters, especially when the patient is still in utero.
- The unique sensitivities of the patient matter.
- Interactions, synergies, and cumulative effects matter.

### Size Matters

Prescribing the correct dose, depending on the size and age of the patient, is a standard part of the practice of medicine. If a drug is considered safe for children, the appropriate dose is much smaller than the adult amount. And many drugs that are approved for adult use are restricted for pregnant women because of the potential impact on the developing child.

An exposure to chemicals from a product or a food, or from air, water, or soil pollution, takes place without modification in dose. A 1-inch human embryo can get the same dose as a 6-foot tall man. So when a 6-foot man eats mercury-contaminated tuna with his newly pregnant wife, the mercury in the fish may not harm either adult but can profoundly affect the brain and nervous system development of a fetus. When human populations have been poisoned by mercury in environmental accidents, exposed pregnant women who reported few or no symptoms have given birth to children who had severe brain and nervous system damage (National Research Council Commission on Life Sciences, 2000).

### Sensitivity Matters

Asking a patient if he or she is allergic to any food or drug is essential to the delivery of any health service. And warning of side effects, even if they are unlikely to occur in most patients receiving a particular medication or treatment, is routine.

Just as with drugs, some people can be harmed by chemical exposures that do not seem to affect other people. New studies are suggesting that genetic differences are at least partly responsible for these differences. A 2004 study of women in Connecticut, for example, showed that women with a particular variation of a gene that helps metabolize toxic substances have a greater risk for breast cancer if they are exposed to PCBs (Zhang et al., 2004). The correlation between childhood vaccines containing mercury as a preservative and the onset of autism may be explained by a genetic variation in the affected children that leaves them unable to safely metabolize the mercury (Environmental Working Group, 2004).

### Interactions Matter

Why do we ask patients about the medications they are currently taking? One important answer is so we don't prescribe another medication that might create a dangerous drug interaction.

New studies are suggesting that interactions, synergies, and cumulative effects also take place between chemicals. In 1997, *Lancet* published a study by Rothman and colleagues that shows that people exposed to the Epstein-Barr virus and PCBs had a higher risk of non-Hodgkin's lymphoma than people exposed to only one risk factor.

Cumulative effects can also make tiny doses add up to harm. Rajapakse, Silva, and Kortenkamp (2002)

are among the scientists who have noted how chemicals that work like estrogens can mix with natural hormones in the body and double the effect of natural estrogen. What's safe one at a time isn't so safe in combination (e.g., a patient who takes three cold medicines in one swallow and experiences undesirable results).

### REGULATING CHEMICALS LIKE WE'RE SUPPOSED TO REGULATE DRUGS

As the emerging field of environmental health teaches us that chemicals work like drugs, we can also be learning from the history of drug regulation about how we might regulate chemicals.

- Use carefully constructed animal studies to predict human effects.
- Heed early warnings. When good science shows that a chemical is causing harm to animals or humans, mandate the move to safer substitutes.
- Good policies are built on good data and the government's ability to act on the findings.

### Animal Studies Matter

For pharmaceuticals, animal studies are always done first to predict human impacts. Only after laboratory animal studies have predicted the success of a new drug will manufacturers prepare to spend millions of dollars on human trials, if the FDA gives permission. Similarly, well-crafted and replicable animal studies of chemicals should be recognized as predictive of human impact.

An important difference between chemicals and drugs makes the recognition of animal studies even more important: Because chemical exposures in humans do not cure disease or alleviate pain, it is not ethical for society to engage in the types of human studies that we use for pharmaceuticals. Studies have repeatedly demonstrated, for example, that the male reproductive system of laboratory animals can be harmed by exposure to the phthalate DEHP in utero or before puberty (Center for the Evaluation of Risks to Human Reproduction, 2005). Studies have also shown that male infants receiving treatment in a neonatal intensive care unit (NICU) can be exposed to DEHP in PVC medical devices at levels higher than those that cause harm in animal studies (Green et al., 2005). Is it ethically appropriate to purposefully expose baby boys in NICUs to DEHP and then follow them to adulthood to determine if the animal studies accurately predict that their reproductive capacities are harmed?

## Early Warnings Matter

After Vioxx and Bextra, two pain-relieving prescription drugs, were pulled off the market over an 8-month period in 2004 and 2005, the FDA's top officials acknowledged that their Adverse Event Reporting System (AERS) was flawed and called together experts to determine how to improve the system (American Journal of Health-System Pharmacy, 2005). The holes in the FDA's safety net have been attributed to understaffing, underfunding, and low morale at FDA's Office of Drug Safety; the underreporting by physicians of their patients' drug reactions; internal FDA pressures to keep a drug that has been approved on the market; and the influence of the drug industry and its lobbyists.

The AERS process and its flaws underscore the importance of taking action based on the timely recognition of a problem by well-resourced, independent reviewers who are fed information from a broad and diverse group of trained observers and who are protected from inappropriate industry influence. Early warnings are supposed to matter.

Because most chemicals are on the market without any government review or permission, public policy that requires premarket and postmarket health testing of chemicals and that adequately collects and acts on adverse chemical events are even more important. This improved FDA-like approach would replace the failed EPA TSCA system, which has led to federal action only a handful of times.

## ABSENCE OF INFORMATION IS NOT THE SAME AS ABSENCE OF HARM

Because there is no law requiring that more than 99% of the volume of chemicals on the market be tested for their health impacts and because the EPA does not have the FDA-like authority to require the recall of a chemical based on adverse reports, we know very little about the chemicals in use. When the Canadian government legislated a comprehensive review of chemicals in commerce in 1999, the

resulting findings showed that the government had no toxicity data for more than 90% of chemicals.

We are in the dark about the toxic effects of most chemicals. In that darkness, public and corporate policy should be based on knowing that what we can't see can still hurt us and that when something is so big and glaring that we can see it in the darkness, we had better pay close attention.

## Number and Quality of the Stressors on the Patient Matter

Not every person who is exposed to a virus will get sick. The strength of the immune system, access to health care services, family support, the existence of other disease, age, weight, alcohol or tobacco use, mental state, and other risk factors can all make a difference.

Biomonitoring studies of human blood and urine by the U.S. Centers for Disease Control (CDC), the Environmental Working Group, and Commonwealth have demonstrated that every person has a body burden of toxic chemicals. But for communities bordering polluting industries, for children growing up in neighborhoods full of diesel engine fumes, for farm workers working in fields sprayed with toxic pesticides, the impacts of toxic chemicals can be much worse. In 1991, recognition of this disparity or environmental racism led to a national conference, the First National People of Color Environmental Justice Leadership Summit. The summit defined environmental justice as the antidote to environmental racism and created the Principles of Environmental Justice based on the shared recognition that social justice issues like race, class, income status, and political power were inextricably linked to environmental justice issues like the proximity of polluting industries and hazardous waste sites.

President Clinton acknowledged the importance of environmental justice in issuing Executive Order 12898 on February 11, 1994. The order, entitled "Federal Actions to Address Environmental Justice in Minority Populations and Low-Income Populations," established environmental justice as a national priority (EPA, 2004).

As Clark Atlanta University Professor Robert D. Bullard (2001) explains in his essay "Environmental

Justice in the 21st Century," environmental justice links the issues of "public health, worker safety, land use, transportation, housing, resource allocation and community empowerment."

The linked problems that make up environmental racism can be thought of as health stressors; lack of community power, inadequate housing, unsafe jobs, racism, and lack of resources can all multiply the effects of toxic chemicals.

### Any Stressors You Can Remove Matter

In Lisbeth B. Schorr's 1988 book *Within Our Reach—Breaking the Cycle of Disadvantage*, she describes the stressors or risk factors for "rotten outcomes" for America's disadvantaged children and the elements of successful programs to prevent those rotten outcomes.

Schorr explains that "it takes multiple and interacting risk factors to produce damaging outcomes... Lasting damage occurs when the elements of a child's environment—at home, at school, in the neighborhood—multiply each other's destructive effect."

But just as the adding on of risk factors can multiply harm, the removal of risk factors can divide the negative impact. Schorr explains:

The implication is clear: The prevention of rotten outcomes is not a matter of all or nothing...It will be of value if we can eliminate one risk factor or two, even if others remain. By distinguishing between those factors we can do something about and those we can't, the problem becomes less intractable.

There are many environmental health factors we can do something about. From transforming our personal habits to transforming global chemicals policy, we can make the problem of chemicals less intractable.

### CHANGING POLICIES

#### In Our Communities

Some cities have taken their cues from the environmental health work of hospitals and have banned the sale of mercury-containing thermometers. Other municipalities have made it illegal to use lawn pesticides for cosmetic purposes. San Francisco and other Bay Area governments have passed the

precautionary principle ordinances that require their purchasing departments to select products and services that minimize negative impacts to human health and the environment, thereby driving manufacturers to engage in research and development toward the production of additional innovative alternative products. The District of Columbia passed an ordinance forbidding the rail shipment of toxic chemicals through the heart of that city.

Many communities have also adopted environmentally preferable purchasing policies that encourage public expenditure on products that are more protective of public health.

### In Legislatures

In Maine, Washington, and other states, new laws are being passed that phase out the use and the production processes that produce certain toxic chemicals. As their predecessors did more than 100 years ago, state legislators are trying to protect their constituents in the absence of federal law. But just like 100 years ago, we need a federal solution.

The European Union is working to create such a law for their continent. The proposal, called REACH (Registration, Evaluation and Authorization and

---

**Taking Action: At Home**

On the personal level, we can send a signal to manufacturers and retailers about the kinds of products we want to be available and affordable for everyone. Buy organic food when you can, use nontoxic alternatives to pesticides and herbicides, and choose cosmetics and other personal care products from companies that have pledged to reduce their use of toxic chemicals.

These signal-sending activities are also safer for you and your family. When we avoid spreading pesticides on our lawns, we reduce the chance of bringing those chemicals into our homes, where they can build up inside carpets or dust. When the shower curtain is made from nylon or cotton instead of vinyl, when nail polish is made without the phthalate DBP, when the number on the bottom of the shampoo bottle shows it's made from a soft plastic instead of #3 PVC, we are doing what we can to decrease the phthalates in our bodies.

Restriction of Chemicals), would over time require chemical companies that sell to the European market to provide health studies that show that a chemical is safe or take the chemical off the market. This "no data, no market" approach to chemicals would move us toward a chemical regulation system like the drug-approval system of the FDA. Coupled with an adverse event reporting and action program that recalls chemicals from the market that are strongly linked to disease, the United States could begin to heal the harm created by the use of chemicals. And if these chemical policy reform efforts are linked with the reduction of other stressors like racism, inadequate housing, unsafe working conditions, and limited access to health care services, we will have affirmed the aspirations of the 1785 Massachusetts legislature in reducing a "great nuisance of public health and peace."

## *Key Points*

- Industrial chemicals affect human health and functioning as drugs do, but are put on the market without any FDA-like approval or labeling requirements.
- Fetal exposure to industrial chemicals can be particularly harmful.
- Chemicals can interact and accumulate to produce toxic effects.
- Chemicals are assumed to be safe unless evidence suggests otherwise.
- Federal policy should embrace the concepts of social justice and harm reduction to reduce the risk of chemical exposures to individuals and communities.

## *Web Resources*

**Health Care Without Harm**
*www.noharm.org*
**Hospitals for a Healthy Environment**
*www.h2e-online.org*
**Luminary Project**
*www.theluminaryproject.org*

## REFERENCES

American Journal of Health-System Pharmacy. (2005). FDA's adverse-event surveillance needs improvement, advisers say. Retrieved May 29, 2005, from *www.ajhp.org/cgi/content/full/62/13/1336.*

Bullard, R. (2001). Environmental justice in the 21st century. United Nations Racism and Public Policy Conference, September 3-5, 2001, Durban, South Africa.

Center for the Evaluation of Risks to Human Reproduction. (2005). Draft NTP-CERHR expert panel update on the reproductive and developmental toxicity of di(2-ethylhexyl) phthalate. Retrieved April 14, 2005, from *http://cerhr.niehs.nih.gov/news/dehp/DEHP-Update-Report-08-08-05.pdf.*

Environmental Working Group. (2004). Overloaded: New science, new insights about mercury and autism in susceptible children. Retrieved December 26, 2004, from *www.ewg.org/reports/autism.*

Gee, D., Vaz, S. G., Harremoes, P., MacGarvin, M., Stirling, A., et al. (2001). Late lessons from early warnings: The precautionary principle, 1896-2000. Retrieved July 15, 2004, from *http://reports.eea.eu.int/environmental_issue_report_2001_22/en.*

Green, R., Hauser, R., Calafat, A. M., Weuve, J., Schettler, T., et al. (2005). Use of di(2-ethylhexyl) phthalate-containing medical products and urinary levels of mono(2-ethylhexyl) phthalate in neonatal intensive care unit infants. Retrieved May 29, 2005, from *http://ehp.niehs.nih.gov/docs/2005/7932/abstract.html.*

Hightower, J. (2004). Environmental health, mercury and human health: A case study in science and politics. *San Francisco Medicine, 77*(4). Retrieved June 6, 2005, from *www.sfms.org/sfm/sfm404e.htm.*

Law, M. T., & Libecap, M. T. (2003). Corruption and reform? The emergence of the 1906 pure food and drug act. Retrieved June 6, 2005, from *http://ideas.repec.org/p/icr/wpicer/20-2003.html.*

Meadows, M. (2002). The FDA's drug review process: Ensuring drugs are safe and effective. Retrieved June 8, 2005, from *www.fda.gov/fdac/features/2002/402_drug.html.*

National Research Council Commission on Life Sciences. (2000). Toxicological effects of methylmercury. Retrieved November 1, 2004, from *www.nap.edu/books/0309071402/html/R1.html.*

Rajapakse, N., Silva, E., & Kortenkamp, A. (2002) Combining xenoestrogens at levels below individual no-observed-effect concentrations dramatically enhances steroid hormone action. *Environmental Health Perspectives, 110*, 917-921.

Rosner, D., & Markowitz, G. (2002). Industry challenges to the principle of prevention in public health: The precautionary principle in historical perspective. Retrieved June 6, 2005, from *www.publichealthreports.org/userfiles/117_6/117501.pdf.*

Rothman, N., Cantor, K. P., Blair, A., Bush, D., Brock, J. W., et al. (1997, July 26). A nested case-control study of non-Hodgkin lymphoma and serum organochlorine residues. *Lancet, 350*, 240-244.

Schorr, L. (1988). Within our reach: Breaking the cycle of disadvantage. New York: Anchor Press.

Swann, J. P. (2001). History of the FDA. Retrieved June 6, 2005, from *www.fda.gov/oc/history/historyoffda/default.htm.*

Tickner, J. A., Geiser, K., & Coffin, M. (2005). The U.S. experience in promoting sustainable chemistry. Retrieved June 6, 2005, from *www.springerlink.com/app/home/contribution.asp?wasp=52a196a5053d4a739a8b2b4896f11a2a&referrer=parent&backto=issue,10,11;journal,3,4;linkingpublicationresults,1:112851,1.*

U.S. Environmental Protection Agency (EPA). (2004). Environmental justice fact sheet: National Environmental Justice Advisory Council (NEJAC). Retrieved May 29, 2005, from *www.epa.gov/compliance/resources/publications/ej/factsheets/fact_sheet_nejac.pdf.*

U.S. Government Accountability Office (GAO). (2005). Report to congressional requesters, chemical regulation: Options exist to improve EPA's ability to assess health risks and manage its chemical review. Retrieved August 11, 2005, from *www.gao.gov/new.items/d05458.pdf.*

Zhang, Y, Wise, J. P., Holford, T. R., Xie, H., Boyle, P., et al. (2004). Serum polychlorinated biphenyls, cytochrome P-450 1A1 polymorphisms and risk of breast cancer in Connecticut women. *American Journal of Epidemiology 160*, 1177-1183.

# Taking Action
Christine N. Stainton

## The Condom Lady

*"The most important political office is that of private citizen."*

JUSTICE LOUIS DEMBITZ BRANDEIS

I'm a nurse and a problem solver. When I've encountered public health policy issues, I've taken the bull by the horns and have tried to make a difference in people's lives. The recipe for change isn't always the same, and it isn't always easy. But it is always worth it.

### MY PUBLIC HEALTH ROOTS

For a long time I knew nursing was the profession for me; it just took awhile to make it official. I come from a family of seven nurses; all were involved in public health. My mother attended nursing school but had to leave because of illness. She worked in public health, though, as a women's health activist and counseled young women at Planned Parenthood Federation in Niagara Falls, New York. She helped women with little access to health services obtain care. Her activities led to our house being picketed in the 1960s. That raised my awareness about the importance of political action and advocacy.

My aunt Elisabeth was a public health nurse in Philadelphia in the 1930s. She worked with new mothers, most of whom were very poor and had little support. Aunt Elisabeth contracted tuberculosis and was committed to a tuberculosis sanitarium for 6 months (the standard of care at the time). When she was released from the sanitarium, my aunt returned to her inner city nursing outreach. The work I saw my mother and my aunt do with the underserved fostered my sense of duty and social responsibility. Their work in reproductive health and parenting, topics not generally discussed at the time, sparked my interest and steered me toward a nursing career and advocating for safe-sex measures.

### A PATH LESS TRAVELED INTO NURSING

My nursing education was done later than that of many people, but I learned a lot on the way there. Before I entered nursing, I raised three children, taught fifth grade to hearing-impaired children, did social work, and raised money for several health care charities including the United Way, the American Red Cross, the American Heart Association, and the Planned Parenthood Federation. I served on school boards, where I advocated for human sexuality education; this was important at home, too. When our son was a teenager, we had lots of his friends at our house. I took the opportunity to talk with him and his friends about safe sex—and they seemed to welcome the information and open discussion. During this time I decorated our Christmas tree with gold-wrapped condoms—which increased the teenaged visits to look at our "golden tree"!

I was a member of the Board of Directors of Planned Parenthood of Southeastern Pennsylvania (PPSP) for many years, and I worked to expand safe-sex education in Planned Parenthood's seven clinics in my area. Although I hadn't yet been able to begin my nursing education, all of this work taught me about advocacy, empowerment through community building, and health education. I also began to realize the interplay among politics, access to care, and choices. I had no idea at the time how these skills, learned through a variety of life experiences, would affect my future career as a nurse.

#### Better Late Than Never

Finally, in my fifties, I embarked on a nursing career. I graduated with an associate's degree in nursing from Gwynedd-Mercy College near Philadelphia. I then moved to Baltimore to attend Johns Hopkins University for my bachelor's degree because of its strong public health programs. I completed a master's degree in community health at Hopkins in 2001.

**955**

## PUTTING MY NURSING KNOWLEDGE TO WORK

### A New Definition of "Working Vacation"

When I earned my nursing degrees, I decided it was time to put my knowledge to work in the Caribbean. My husband, our three children, and I often vacationed on Antigua in the British Virgin Islands. I grew concerned about Antigua's proximity to Haiti, where there had been a dramatic increase in the incidence of human immunodeficiency virus (HIV) infection and acquired immunodeficiency syndrome (AIDS). Haiti and the Dominican Republic account for 85% of all AIDS cases in the region. Heterosexual transmission is the most common source of infection, followed by mother-to-child transmission (Centers for Disease Control and Prevention [CDC], 2005). I wanted to help establish a safe-sex and disease-prevention program in Antigua using a curriculum I had written. It was critical to work closely with Antiguan community leaders. I contacted the Antigua Planned Parenthood Director, Inez Stevens, and AIDS Secretariat, Janet Weston, to offer my assistance. I wanted to build on and strengthen any efforts they had in place, and I did not want to "step on any toes." It took time to develop their trust and create a collaborative relationship.

### Family Advocacy

I told local Antiguan leaders that I wanted to help them financially. This would be our family-funded volunteer project; we wanted to supply condoms, educate people, and address other needs. My daughter, Lucia St. George, is a doctoral student in sexuality education. Since 2000 she and I have visited about six communities in Antigua in an effort to prevent sexually transmitted disease by supplying condoms by the thousands and providing reproductive health education in small groups. We've presented education programs at hotels, schools, and villages. At one high school there were over 900 students in attendance. We demonstrate proper use of condoms with a wooden penis and build attendees' confidence in their ability to use condoms effectively. Lucia does the practical aspects of sexuality education, and I discuss how

infections are transmitted. With all of our efforts, we worked very closely with Planned Parenthood of Antigua and the AIDS Secretariat. Our curriculum is based on the health beliefs model. We believe that through self-empowerment, the adolescent and adult will develop the knowledge, confidence, and skills needed to reduce their risk of HIV and sexually transmitted infection through abstinence or using condoms.

To test whether we have delivered our message clearly, Lucia and I do role-playing in front of small groups of women. We pretend to be amorous men and ask the women, "What do you do if a man wants to have sex without a condom?" They usually respond with a chorus of "No sex without a condom!" We reward this mantra by handing out extra condoms! Empowering women to make wise choices about their sexual and reproductive life is a vital message in this male-dominated culture.

### The Condom Wish List

Several times a year, our family ships thousands of condoms to Antigua. To increase use, I get a condom

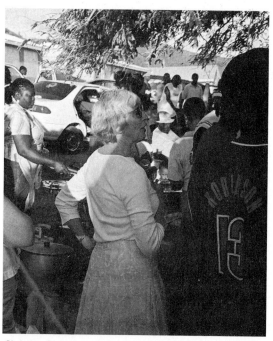

Christine Stainton in Antigua. (Courtesy of Evelyn Hockstain)

"wish list" from the five community health workers with whom we work closely. We provide the flavors and colors of the condoms our populations prefer. In Thailand, the use of colored condoms and access to condoms has been credited with an increase in condom use among commercial sex workers to close to 100%. This is largely because of the work of AIDS crusader Mechai Viravaidya (Sternberg, 2004).

## Celebrating Success

On my arrival at the airport in Antigua during one family trip, I was called by one of the most active community health workers, Althea Marshall, and invited to lecture on safe sex at the Easter Carnival Cricket Match. Their scheduled speaker had cancelled at the last minute, and a program of safe-sex education had been advertised on television and radio for a week. When we arrived at the Easter Carnival, beer had been flowing freely to the cricket players and audience. The crowd was quite glad to learn about our condom distribution mission—the "Condom Lady" had arrived! Music was playing, and eventually we realized that the lyrics included, "Wear your condoms." Our family of four handed out 3000 condoms that day. One of the Antiguans wore the colored condoms hanging from his belt and said "I am wearing *my* condoms."

## MATCHING THE POLITICAL STRATEGY TO THE PROBLEM

Handing out condoms is not all I do. Some other issues I've tackled include the ones discussed in the following sections.

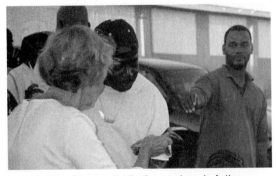

Christine Stainton distributing condoms in Antigua.

## Get out the Vote

Voting is the backbone of a democracy, so I've chosen to help with a number of voter initiatives. During the 2004 presidential race I helped Planned Parenthood to "get out the vote." I worked with Gloria Steinem, feminist and founder of *Ms. Magazine*; Gloria Feldt, former President of Planned Parenthood Federation of America; and other outreach workers. We went door to door, targeting a specific suburban area of Philadelphia. This work to "get out the vote" occurred over 3 days. Busloads of workers came from New York, New Jersey, and areas around Philadelphia to launch this effort.

## Dining for Dollars

In order to raise funds for the Planned Parenthood "Get out the Vote" initiative I had a dinner party fundraiser for 70 guests. Dinner parties with well-known, interesting guests are a very effective strategy to encourage political donations. The potential donors spent the evening with Gloria Steinem and Gloria Feldt—both of whom explained the importance of "getting the vote out."

## Partnering

I got permission to put voter registration forms in some Starbucks coffee shops. We worked with Planned Parenthood of Southeastern Pennsylvania; the agency encouraged their patients to vote and distributed voter registration forms. We believe our efforts in Pennsylvania fostered a large voter turnout, and we raised significant funds.

## Collaborating

I have been a volunteer with the Trust for America's Health (TFAH) in Washington, DC, a nonprofit organization working to protect the health of communities through awareness about the impact of epidemics. TFAH graded the states on their ability to handle a public health emergency, with the highest score being a 10. My home state of Pennsylvania received a 3, meaning it was not well prepared. That got my attention. I joined forces with Shelley Hearne, the chief executive of TFAH, and Ernesta Ballard, former president of the National Abortion Rights Action League (NARAL).

We organized health experts from the University of Pennsylvania School of Medicine and Children's Hospital of Pennsylvania (CHOP) to meet with the Pennsylvania Secretary of Health, Dr. Calvin Johnson. The purpose of the first meeting, led by Shelley Hearne of TFAH, was to address the state of Pennsylvania's emergency preparedness. The meeting was a catalyst for action. Shelly Hearne was invited to speak to the Pennsylvania state legislature on disaster preparedness. In 2006, I was selected to serve on the Mayor of Philadelphia's Disaster Preparedness Focus Group, where I am on the Health and Human Services Subcommittee. Our goal is to make sure the health system can meet the community's needs in a disaster.

### Gaining Credibility

I've worked to obtain funding to purchase a health van to bring health services to underserved adolescents in Philadelphia. To strengthen our proposal, I connected with Bridgitte Patterson, a family nurse practitioner on the faculty of the University of Maryland. She has been involved with mobile health vans that the University of Maryland School of Nursing uses to extend care to remote areas of the state and underserved areas in Baltimore. We are collaborating with a number of agencies to develop this important activity. With Bridgitte's help we received a grant from the state of Pennsylvania to receive funding in 2006.

There are public health needs everywhere in our environment. I believe one person, one family, or one small group can make a difference. I saw my mother and the nurses in my family make a difference in people's lives. I've learned as a nurse that I can have a powerful influence, too. I can't fix every problem, but I can sure take a shot at eliminating a few!

## *Web Resources*

**Planned Parenthood Federation of America**
*www.plannedparenthood.org*
**Trust for America's Health** (TFAH)
*www.healthyamericans.org*

### REFERENCES

Centers for Disease Control and Prevention (CDC). (2005). GAP in Haiti. Retrieved September 1, 2005, from *www.cdc.gov/nchstp/od/gap/countries/haiti.htm.*

Sternberg, S. (2004, July 12). Condoms and comedy to the rescue in Thailand; AIDS crusader's model program holds nothing back. *USA Today*, D-1.

# *Taking Action*  Terry Fulmer & Vernice Ferguson

## *Influencing the Community by Serving on a Board*

*"A generous heart, kind speech, and a life of service and compassion are the things which renew humanity."*

BUDDHA

There is an enormous rush of excitement when one is invited to participate on a board. It is a heady feeling to be invited, and in most cases that feeling is well founded. There are myriad board-room experiences in which nurses can participate. We'll talk about some of these, drawing examples from our own service on boards, and discuss the do's and don't's for participating on such boards.

### SERVING ON BOARDS: NEW VOICES FOR NEW PLACES

Volunteerism is engrained in the American experience. Long before the emergence of the large number of two-career families, mothers and wives as well as single women were heavily engaged in volunteer activities. This remains so today. Just as white males continue to dominate the corporate boards, women continue to devote their talent, time, and fund-raising ability to nonprofit organizations as they bring higher levels of service to their constituents. Their well-known and successful activities have stood in the way of a larger presence of women on corporate boards. How often does a corporate woman seek out women as appropriate candidates for board seats? How many of them know where to turn to get the necessary information?

Fortunately, groups of women in some major cities such as Philadelphia, Atlanta, and Chicago are conducting annual surveys about women serving on boards of nonprofit and for-profit organizations and corporations and are heavily involved in providing information to those seeking it (Women on Boards, 2004). Because of these data, the voices of more women leaders are being heard and opportunities for board service are being provided. An untapped pool of women chief financial officers, women running major divisions of larger companies, women partners in law and accounting firms, and women running their businesses and major nonprofit organizations is being identified, and the women are serving as mentors to younger women as they advance in their careers. Nurse leaders should be considered in this pool, as well. The ability to manage large departmental budgets and personnel to assure acceptable patient outcomes or student success in academia are valuable assets that nurse leaders would bring to the corporate table.

In the post-Enron world, where a higher standard of ethical conduct is expected, corporate America, their stockholders, the public at large, and government would do well to advance the cause of gender parity in the corporate world. National polls continue to reveal the public's high regard for nurses, the majority of whom are women, as ethical professionals, outranking members of other well-known groups. In these polls the public cites the nursing profession as one that puts the interest of others ahead of its own, unlike all other groups cited. A large presence of nurse leaders on corporate boards would serve corporate America well as confidence is restored in ethical behavior and concern for others.

Nationally, according to Catalyst, a nonprofit organization that focuses on women in the workplace, women hold just 12.4% of the board seats in the Fortune 500 companies and 8.9% of all seats in the Fortune 501 to 1000 companies (Catalyst, 2002). Only 15.7% of corporate officers in Fortune 500 companies are women. Women of color hold only 2% of the 8941 board seats in the 839 companies for which Catalyst could confirm race and ethnicity; they hold corporate office in a mere 1.6% of corporate offices in the Fortune 500 companies and 1.3% in the Fortune 501 to 1000 companies (Catalyst, 2001). Change must come, for women make up approximately half of the work force and make 85% of all consumer decisions every year.

There is a major pipeline problem that must be addressed. More champions for the advancement of women are needed—particularly male champions. Thirty years ago there were few women in medicine, law, and pharmacy. Few served as presidents of coeducational colleges and universities. Today there are increasing numbers of women in these fields, as well as foundation presidents, chancellors and provosts in academic institutions, and deans who are women beyond the nursing school. There is no need to continually recycle the women who are well known, for there are many talented women who are out there, unheralded and unknown.

The emergence of more women as chief executive officers and in other corporate leadership positions must be actively nurtured to assure a larger pool of talented women for corporate board seats, as they add value to the deliberations. There is research evidence that the representation of women in leadership positions has a positive correlation with economic performance measured in tangible terms such as organizational growth, increased market share, and return on investment (Rhode, 2003). The Women's Executive Groups in Philadelphia and Chicago, as well as the Board of Directors Network in Georgia, have also found a correlation between the presence of women in leadership positions and corporate financial performance. Why fight success? Embrace it!

*Vernice Ferguson has been involved with these women's executive groups to bring women's voices to corporate boardrooms. In the process she is advocating for nurses to be included, in particular.*

## BOARD PARTICIPATION

Board participation is both exciting and rewarding. The opportunity to help shape governance and provide oversight to an organization that you feel has an important mission is very satisfying. Dimma (2002) has noted a set of overarching premises related to boards that help provide insight into the anticipated role:

- Boards don't manage—they govern. With management, a board helps develop a vision for long-term

---

### Ten Basic Responsibilities of Nonprofit Boards

1. Determine the organization's mission and purpose. It is the board's responsibility to create and review a statement of mission and purpose that articulates the organization's goals, means, and primary constituents served.

2. Select the chief executive. Boards must reach consensus on the chief executive's responsibilities and undertake a careful search to find the most-qualified individual for the position.

3. Provide proper financial oversight. The board must assist in developing the annual budget and ensuring that proper financial controls are in place.

4. Ensure adequate resources. One of the board's foremost responsibilities is to provide adequate resources for the organization to fulfill its mission.

5. Ensure legal and ethical integrity, and maintain accountability. The board is ultimately responsible for ensuring adherence to legal standards and ethical norms.

6. Ensure effective organizational planning. Boards must actively participate in an overall planning process and assist in implementing and monitoring the plan's goals.

7. Recruit and orient new board members and assess board performance. All boards have a responsibility to articulate prerequisites for candidates, to orient new members, and periodically and comprehensively to evaluate their own performance.

8. Enhance the organization's public standing. The board should clearly articulate the organization's mission, accomplishments, and goals to the public and garner support from the community.

9. Determine, monitor, and strengthen the organization's programs and services. The board's responsibility is to determine which programs are consistent with the organization's mission and to monitor their effectiveness.

10. Support the chief executive and assess his or her performance. The board should ensure that the chief executive has the moral and professional support he or she needs to further the goals of the organization.

strategy. Management is responsible for carrying out the vision-driven strategy and reports to a board and a chairman. Boards are trustees of the vision, mission, and goals of an organization. Carver and Carver (1996) refer to this as "moral ownership" (p. 15).

■ The relationship between a board and management should be characterized by "creative tension." There should be neither an adversarial relationship nor one that is blatantly uncritical. Mutual trust and respect are key to good working relationships between boards and management.

■ Markers of success of any organization should be clearly understood.

There are several books that outline ideal boards and the way they should be measured (Carver, 1997; Carver & Carver, 1996; Chait, Ryan, & Taylor 2005; Houle, 1997). Of course, boards vary widely from family member boards to large corporate boards. Nursing benefits when members of our profession are invited to prestigious boards, and similarly, boards benefit from the broad range of experience and knowledge that our profession brings to the table. Board membership can be voluntary or very well compensated, and in each case the nurse considering the role needs to contemplate what will be gained (e.g., new knowledge) and what will be given up (e.g., time) by agreeing to participate.

## GETTING ONTO A BOARD

How does one go about getting onto a board? For the most part, you have to make your interest in

---

### Types of Boards

**NONPROFIT BOARD**

A board that serves a nonprofit organization and is responsible for oversight of the executive director as the mission of the organization is carried out (e.g., school boards, nursing home boards, alumni boards)

**CORPORATE BOARD**

A board that provides oversight of a specific corporation that is for profit (e.g., banks, companies such as Avon)

---

serving on a board known to individuals who can forward your name to those making the appointment. To be selected for board participation, you must be qualified for the role. Your resume must support that you have something to offer the specific organization you have in mind. If it is not readily apparent, you have to make the case in a cover letter or interview. Being extremely well-versed in the organization you hope to join is obviously necessary.

Persistence is important. You should not give up if you are not selected on the first round. Ask for feedback if you are not selected the first time.

Once you're appointed to a board, it's essential that you become savvy about how to make the most of this opportunity and contribute significantly to the organization's mission. *In the following section, Terry Fulmer describes her own experiences to illustrate and share the lessons we've learned as members of different kinds of boards.*

## BOARD EXPERIENCES

### My First Board: When the College Calls

As a new nurse the first board on which I was invited to participate was my college alumni board of trustees. You can imagine the excitement I felt in being included in Skidmore College's enterprise, for which I had such high regard. My 3-year experience on that board provided deep insight into the academic framework of colleges and universities. I served as secretary, and in that 3-year term I was included in important deliberations related to goals and strategies for Skidmore College in the twentieth century. The experience was one of engaging social exchange. There was always a dinner the evening before the board meeting, then a subsequent day that was carefully orchestrated by the staff of the college, followed by a summary of the meeting and anticipated next steps.

My primary role as secretary was to write letters to families who had had a recent bereavement. As a nurse I certainly was familiar with thinking about the words I would use with individuals who had had a loss, and I found it to be a comfortable role. (The staff of the college took the actual minutes of the board meetings.) My experience created an enormous bond with the college, and to this day I am devoted to the institution, even though the school of nursing was closed in 1985. I serve as an area alumni coordinator and as a "fund chair" for the class of 1975. I am active in alumni events and keep in regular contact with the president of the college. Many of my dear friends who attended the college are far less enthusiastic about participating, given their dismay at the closing of the school. But my experience was different because of my board experience.

This experience illustrates various functions of boards; ways that people participate on boards; and ways that the experience affects future relationships. My initial board experience was one that was very positive and relatively lacking in any controversy. My next board engagement would be less positive.

### Learning the Hard Way: Troubled Boards

As a practicing nurse, I was already passionate about my area of geriatric nursing and began addressing clinical practice and policy issues related to elder abuse and neglect. Because of this interest and my involvement related to mandatory reporting of elder abuse in the state of Massachusetts, I was invited to serve on the board of a nonprofit organization that provided legal research and services for the elderly. This board experience was a nightmare. Here, also, I was very pleased and honored to be invited to participate and felt that this board experience would be good for my career and informative.

The executive director of this organization was passionate about his work and his commitment to the elderly. The work of the organization, as can be inferred by its label, was to help older individuals who might need aid; and, in particular, a goal was to service elder abuse and neglect cases for which guardianship might be required. Those of us serving on that board were knowledgeable clinicians, lawyers, and policymakers and had a deep commitment to the topic.

As it turned out, the board members had very little experience with the nature and fundamental underpinnings of nonprofits and boards. We knew that the organization was on a very tight budget

and, in fact, struggling to meet the challenges of providing services for indigent clients, but none of us had the savvy to carefully review the business plan and note that the federal taxes were being withheld but were not paid in a timely manner to the internal revenue service. My first inkling of this came with a shocking phone call that indicated that I would need a lawyer, that the internal revenue service might well put a lien on my home, and that I was to be sued for $110,000 as a board member for this egregious decision by the executive director. Imagine the conversation between my husband and me, given that our condominium in metropolitan Boston was worth $60,000 at that time.

Of my many mistakes, I naïvely never asked the question, "Is there board insurance for board members?" Another question should have been, "What is my liability in the event that there is a financial problem with this private 501(c)(3) organization?" You can rest assured that that question has always been asked early in any subsequent discussions of board participation. In this case, it turned out that there was board insurance and that the IRS settled with the organization. My husband never let me forget the experience and urged me never to serve on a board again. I love my husband of 30 years but did not listen to him, and my subsequent board experiences have been much more positive.

### Leading a Board

The next board I participated on was nursery school board in my community. In this voluntary parent board—another 501(c)(3) organization—I learned quickly that there was board insurance and understood that my responsibility was to oversee the role of the executive director as she managed a really large, bustling, and high-visibility nursery school program in a suburban community. The role of board members was to ensure that there was an appropriate vision that fit well with the community. The board met monthly in the evenings as we assisted the director with her decisions related to appropriate staffing, accreditations, safety for the children, physical space, and fund-raising activities. I served two consecutive 3-year terms, and in the second term, was board president before leaving the board.

Certainly this type of experience translates into a number of important skills for leadership. Fairness in salaries, regular evaluation of the executive director, and communication with the local community all fall to board members. As with most boards, we had monthly meetings and we were expected to serve on subcommittees as appropriate. Dimma (2002) has outlined "ideal processes" for boards, and the way subcommittees should be set up for optimal function. He notes that subcommittees should be small—three to five people, depending on the scope of the work. Compensation committees and fund-raising committees are two examples. Carver does an excellent job of outlining the board's responsibility for itself, with emphasis on "moral ownership," obligation for board performance including preparation for meetings and attendance, and attention to diversity and the dynamics of the interplay between the board and staff that creates the positive tension already mentioned.

This board was an extremely positive experience, although time consuming. The benefit to my professional life as an academic dean has been notable. I learned a great deal about fiscal accountability, goal setting, and the positive tension role between the executive director and board members. As president of that board, I was responsible for the performance review of the executive director for annual raises as well as for commenting on the progress and outcomes of the program. This board experience gave me a view into the way boards of nonprofits balance goals and resources and provided me with a solid background for my next board invitation.

### When the Mission Changes

In 1990 I was invited to be interviewed for consideration for a position on the board of a nursing home in my community. This long-term care facility, with a $30 million endowment at that time, was in the midst of a strategic process (called Pathway 2000) and was at a crossroads in terms of keeping the nursing home of 110 beds at its current state or making a bold innovative investment that would transform the nursing home into a continuing care community for 400 residents with a new 84-bed, state-of-the-art nursing home. After reviewing the

charter of the nursing home and checking board insurance, I joined that board and served for the next 8 years. This was a tension-filled, high-activity board because of the high-stake decisions that were underway. The retirement community executive management knew that in the absence of investing adequate funds for upgrading the facility, the corpus of the endowment would ultimately be needed to run the facility. It was estimated that the facility would close in the next two decades without action.

Board members for this long-term care facility included individuals who were partners at large investment firms, a former mayor of the city, and a dean from a very prestigious university. I was inspired by their presence and quickly understood my role: The business of the organization was nursing care, and I was the only nurse in the room. What I did not anticipate, as I agreed to serve on this board, were the time commitment, hard work, and presence that would need to be invested to participate adequately. I was on the health care and homecare committees, which each met approximately four times a year. It was absolutely expected that every member would attend every board meeting unless there was a very good excuse. There was no compensation for this board, but the activity fulfilled the role of "community service" for academics.

I stepped down from the board at a time when I felt I was losing interest in the role and there were competing demands for my time. We had met the goals of Pathway 2000. The organization seemed in a steady state, and although there had been some disappointing lawsuits with contractors, the new facility was fabulous, and I felt like I had played an important role in helping the organization think about care of older individuals. However, my interest waned when I felt that the board activities were more focused on the hotel management side of the equation rather than on the unique programs that could be developed for care of older individuals. When I stepped down from the board, it was likely to the relief of the executive director, whom I perceived to be mildly amused and vaguely annoyed with my regular harping about high-quality nursing care. After 1 year elapsed, I received a phone call inviting me to the board to resume the "nursing voice." I have done so and recognize that I have a varied role on that board.

## Advising Industry

I have served in other advisory board roles such as the geriatric advisory panel for a medication containment company. The company is responsible for mail order pharmacy benefits. This activity required twice-a-year advisory board meetings that usually occurred in major cities, and the compensation was approximately $5000 per year. My responsibilities were to read board materials related to the programs of the company, including mail order distribution of medications, and to comment on the program from my perspective as a geriatric expert.

This board required a great deal of preparation and reading. When I discuss boards with individuals who have far more experience than I have, it is clear that any board member needs to come very carefully prepared, having read the materials in advance, with additional reviews of what a member considers to be pertinent materials (which should be brought to the meeting, as well).

In this case one needs to be very careful with allocating time and balancing it with faculty or organizational employment. Faculty bylaws clearly state that all of us need to balance our external advisory activity and compensation carefully with our primary role as acting members. This type of activity needs to be judiciously documented in disclosure forms on an annual basis to the university, and any conflict of interest must be carefully considered.

The medication containment company board experience was extremely educational for me in that the board members were highly respected health care practitioners and scholars. The dialogue was always at an extremely high level, with the geriatric mission first and the older person's best interests in mind. I am pleased to have had the ability to serve in that role.

## Current Service

My current role as an advisory role member at a pharmaceutical committee that evaluates vaccines for herpes zoster and older adults is similarly intellectually challenging and educational, and the compensation here is what I deem generous ($5000).

The boards that I have outlined are voluntary with modest compensation (stipends) and are at a far different level than health insurance boards, for which the compensation is as generous as $200,000 per year. On those boards there is an annual review for effectiveness of the board member, and his or her term is discontinued if it is found that he or she does not add value or does not come adequately prepared. It would not be at all acceptable to be absent from any board meeting at this level.

## Lessons Learned

Nurse experts who play an active role in the oversight of hospitals, nursing homes, and related health care organizations are good for public relations, can have a positive influence on board members, can have great influence in the community, and provide great stature for all of us in the profession. As a profession, we need to accelerate our rate of participation on corporate boards in order to educate the professional "public" as well as the public at large regarding what nurses offer nonprofits as well as large for-profit companies. We believe the next decade will see an era of increased participation for nurses, with positive and exciting results.

As you contemplate volunteering for a board, keep in mind the following lessons that we have learned and share with you:

- Board work is labor intensive. Plan your time carefully in order to do the job well. Very few boards are honorific, and organizations will expect you to come prepared to meetings and to participate.
- Few boards have any idea what a nurse can offer to a discussion of issues related to an organization. It is for us to translate our background knowledge and skills for the benefit of the organization being served. This also serves our profession. Be aggressive about conveying your interest in serving and articulating what you believe you can offer. Membership is very gratifying and an important civic contribution.

■ Be a savvy board member. Know what the liabilities are, and anticipate where you might need legal counsel before you commit. Ask current members about the organization and any information they think you should know.

## Web Resources

**BoardSource**—formerly the National Center for Nonprofit Boards; a resource for practical information, tools and best practices, training, and leadership development for board members of nonprofit organizations
*www.boardsource.org*

**Corporate Board Member Magazine**—resource for officers and directors of publicly traded corporations, top private companies, and Global 1000 firms
*www.boardmember.com*

## REFERENCES

Carver, J. (1997). *Boards that make a difference: A new design for leadership in nonprofit and public organizations* (2nd ed.). San Francisco: Jossey-Bass.

Carver, J., & Carver, M. M. (1996). *Your roles and responsibilities as a board member: The CarverGuide series on effective board governance*. San Francisco: Jossey-Bass.

Catalyst. (2001). Women of color in corporate management: Three years later. Retrieved December 4, 2005, from *www.catalyst.org/knowledge/titles/title.php?page=woc_corpmngt3yrs_01*.

Catalyst. (2002). 2002 Catalyst census of women corporate officers and top earners in the Fortune 500. Retrieved December 4, 2005, from *www.catalyst.org/files/fact/COTE%20Factsheet% 202002updated.pdf*.

Chait, R. P., Ryan, W. P., & Taylor, B. E. (2005). *Governance as leadership: Reframing the work of nonprofit boards*. Hoboken, NJ: John Wiley & Sons.

Dimma, W. A. (2002). *Excellence in the boardroom: Best practices in corporate directorship*. Etobicoke, Ontario: John Wiley & Sons.

Houle, C. O. (1997). *Governing boards: Their nature and nurture*. San Francisco: Jossey-Bass.

Klenke, K. (1996). *Women and leadership: A contextual perspective*. New York: Springer.

Rhode, D. (Ed.). (2003). The *difference "difference" makes: women and leadership*. Stanford, CA: Stanford University Press.

*Women on Boards*. (2004). Fort Washington, PA: Forum of Executive Women.

# 34

# Nursing in the International Community: A Broader View of Nursing Issues

Judith A. Oulton

*"We cannot live for ourselves alone. Our lives are connected by a thousand invisible threads…our actions run as causes and return to us as results."*

HERMAN MELVILLE

In the late 1960s, Marshall McLuhan coined the term *global village*. McLuhan was referring to the fact that through advances in communications, time and space have vanished. Not only was there a new, multisensory view of the world in 1967, but people from around the world could communicate as if they lived in the same village. Yet when McLuhan outlined his vision nearly 40 years ago, the Internet did not exist, nor did the World Trade Organization (WTO) and its Global Agreement on Trade in Services (GATS). Acquired immuno-deficiency syndrome (AIDS) was a little-known wasting disease in Africa, and the world was celebrating its first heart transplant and bypass operations.

During the past 30-odd years, we have witnessed the increased globalization of commerce, travel, information, trade, and disease. In 1955 there were

51 million airline passengers and in 2004 there were 1.8 billion, despite 3 years' lost growth after 9/11 (International Air Transport Association [IATA], 2005).

Today, people, images, and messages move around the world with ease, and we truly have a sense of being a global village. Today we have a professional obligation to understand the village-world in its broader context and to base our decision-making on a broader understanding of ourselves, our clients, and our circumstances. By having a global view, we are capable of synthesizing a broad range of information to make informed decisions. It begins with understanding the policies and politics of globalization and of other key international health and nursing issues.

## GLOBALIZATION

Globalization is the growing interdependence of the world's people, integrating economy, culture, technology, and governance. Globalization changes the way nations and communities work, shrinking time, space, and borders. It means that national policy and action are increasingly shaped by international forces.

Globalization creates new economic and cultural zones, such as Silicon Valley, and it brings new people to our countries and communities. The increase in international travel means the ready spread of disease and threat to security as people move freely across borders and continents. SARS and avian flu are two examples of global health risks and helped prompt IATA to create the post of Medical Director in 2004 to liaise with the World Health Organization (WHO) on issues of global public health crises (IATA, 2004). Today, nations and health professionals must learn to care for new illnesses, deal with the added risks of exposure, and handle acts of terrorism (United Nations [UN] Development Programme, 1999).

With GATS and the general globalization of trade, health services and the health professions are increasingly seen as commodities. Health tourism is gaining in popularity as nations vie for patients interested in traveling to another state for health care. As well, many countries are expressing interest in mutual recognition agreements that lower barriers for health professionals to practice in other countries. Increased communication, easier air travel, and the easing of trade restrictions have made mobility and migration easier (Figure 34-1).

## MIGRATION: A CASE IN POINT

Migration is a key issue for nursing. According to the International Organization on Migration (IOM), there were 175 million international migrants in 2000, meaning one in every 35 persons was an international migrant. In 2005, the number was estimated to increase to 185 to 192 million, nearly half of whom were women (IOM, 2005).

People move around for many reasons: to work; to study; to have fun; to receive health care; or to escape violence, poverty, and famine in their native countries. This movement brings with it the problems of unemployment, discrimination, racial tensions, and harmful cultural practices, such as female genital mutilation. Today's nurses must understand health, illness, and coping mechanisms from the perspectives of many cultures. Equally important is the need for

the profession to be an advocate for sound health and nursing policy that considers the well-being of the client along with that of the profession and its practitioners.

Governments—bilaterally, regionally, or through the WTO—negotiate terms for the movement of goods and people for economic gain. With the growing shortage of health professionals, particularly nurses, in many parts of the world, individuals and institutions at all levels—governments, employers, policymakers, the public, the professions, and professionals—are interested in the movement of nurses (Box 34-1).

Substantial numbers of nurses are on the move. Nurses may leave one country to work in a second, then either return to their home country, or move on to a third. They may live in one country and cross a national border on a regular basis to work in another (International Council of Nurses [ICN], 2000). For

---

**BOX 34-1** World Trade Organization

Established in 1995, the World Trade Organization (WTO) is the successor to the General Agreement on Tariffs and Trade (GATT). Its mandate is to ensure that trade in goods and services flows as smoothly, predictably, and freely as possible. It does so by:

- Administering trade agreements
- Acting as a forum for trade negotiations
- Settling trade disputes and reviewing national trade policies
- Assisting developing countries in trade policy issues through technical assistance and training programs
- Cooperating with other international organizations

Multilateral trade agreements are the legal ground rules for international commerce that countries trade rights to and that bind governments to keep their trade policies within agreed limits. The General Agreement on Trade in Services (GATS) is a multilateral agreement to reduce barriers to international trade in services. It seeks to improve trade in services and investment conditions through a set of mutually agreed on rules, including a dispute settlement system.

Headquartered in Geneva, WTO today includes nearly 150 countries, accounting for 97% of world trade (WTO, 2001; WTO, 2005).

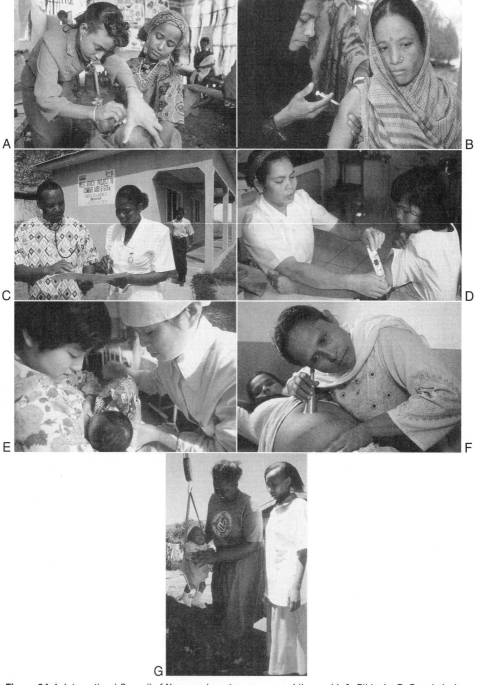

**Figure 34-1** International Council of Nurses advocates: nurses and the world. **A,** Ethiopia; **B,** Bangladesh; **C,** Ghana; **D,** Indonesia; **E,** China; **F,** Pakistan; and **G,** Kenya. (Courtesy of David Barbour [A], Nancy Durrell McKenna [B, D, and F], Pierre St. Jacques [C], Roger Lemoyne [E], and Stephanie Colvey [G], as well as ACDI/CIDA.)

example, although the data are poor, we know that about 85% of employed Filipino nurses (some 150,000) are working abroad (Lorenzo, 2002).

Nurses from the Caribbean are moving to North America and the United Kingdom, as are nurses from the Philippines. A significant number of Indian nurses and doctors are migrating to the Gulf states. There is also considerable movement in Africa as nurses leave Zimbabwe, Ghana, and other countries to work in South Africa, and as South African nurses migrate to the United Kingdom, the United States, Canada, Australia, and New Zealand.

Migration enables nurses to earn a living, continue their education, experience other cultures, or expand their professional experience. Most nurses searching for work abroad do so because of poor salaries and working conditions in their home countries. In many countries, employers have failed to address long-standing deficiencies related to hours of work, salary, continuing education, staffing levels, security, housing, and daycare facilities. For example, nurses in several countries—Trinidad and Tobago, Zambia, Malawi—tell the ICN that they often work alone at night caring for 50 to 60 patients.

Nurses in Ghana are pushed to consider migration because of low salary and remuneration, limited career prospects, lack of respect or value for their work, concern about management of the health care system, and poor retirement benefits. For nurses in South Africa the main factors are lack of competitive incentives in the public sector, work pressures (long hours, high patient loads and poor resources), limited opportunities for career development, and escalating crime, and the increase in human immunodeficiency virus (HIV) infection and AIDS (Buchan, Kingman, & Lorenzo, 2005).

Nurses also choose to migrate as a means to learn new knowledge and skills or to practice more autonomously in innovative environments. Others move for new cultural experiences, to be with families, or for personal safety and political reasons (Oulton, 1998). A 1999 study by ICN, the World Medical Association (WMA), and WHO of migration patterns of nurses and physicians showed the same incentives for migration. The study also found differences in language and culture were strong disincentives (ICN, 2000) (Box 34-2).

---

**BOX 34-2** World Health Organization

The World Health Organization (WHO), established in 1948, is governed by 192 member countries through the World Health Assembly. Its objective is the attainment by all peoples of the highest possible level of health. Through six regional offices, a Geneva-based secretariat, and offices in many countries, the organization promotes technical cooperation for health among nations, carries out programs to control and eradicate disease, and strives to improve the quality of human life.

WHO has four main functions:
- To give worldwide guidance in the field of health
- To set global standards for health
- To cooperate with governments in strengthening national health programs
- To develop and transfer appropriate health technology, information, and standards

WHO defines *health* as "a state of complete physical, mental and social well-being and not merely the absence of disease or infirmity" (WHO, 2001a; WHO, 2005a).

---

The nursing community has been vocal nationally and internationally in addressing migration policy and practice.
- In 2001, ICN issued its policy on Ethical Recruitment, which supports the right of nurses to migrate but denounces unethical recruitment and condemns the practice of recruiting nurses to countries where authorities have failed to implement sound human resource planning. ICN has called for regulated recruitment and implementation of thirteen principles to support recruitment and retention (ICN, 2001). These are:
  - Effective human resources planning and development
  - Credible nursing regulation
  - Access to full employment
  - Freedom of movement
  - Freedom from discrimination
  - Good faith contracting
  - Equal pay for work of equal value
  - Access to grievance procedures
  - Safe work environment
  - Effective orientation, mentoring, and supervision

- Employment trial periods
- Freedom of association
- Regulation of recruitment
- Many national nurses associations have actively lobbied their governments for ethical recruitment of nurses. In line with the ICN position on nurse retention, transfer, and migration and its position on ethical recruitment, nurses have condemned the practice of recruiting offshore rather than effectively addressing human resource planning (including the problems that cause nurses to leave the profession and discourage them from returning to nursing) (ICN, 1999a, 2001).
- National nurses associations are monitoring employers to ensure that the rights of the new nurses are upheld and are helping to ensure that immigrating nurses have adequate support systems in place.
- Some governments (such as those of the United Kingdom, the Netherlands, New Zealand, and Canada) are responding to pressure from the nursing profession by issuing recruitment guidelines for employers, launching studies of working conditions, and reviewing nursing resource plans.
- In 2003 the Commonwealth Ministers of Health agreed on a Commonwealth Code of Practice for the International Recruitment of Health Care Workers. The code has three guiding principles (transparency, fairness, and mutuality of benefit). However, it also has the same weaknesses as other recruitment codes in that it lacks incentives, sanctions, and monitoring systems and applies only to the public sector (Commonwealth Code of Practice for the International Recruitment of Health Care Workers, 2003).
- At the 2005 World Health Assembly, Ministers of Health adopted a resolution calling for WHO to strengthen its program on health and human resources and to report back to the Assembly in 2006. It was also agreed in 2005 that HRH would be the theme of the World Health Report and World Health Day 2006 (WHO, 2005b).
- The global nursing shortage and lack of focus on nursing prompted ICN to undertake a global study in 2004 focusing in particular on migration, incentives, characteristics of good employers, regulation, policy and planning, and case studies featuring Latin America and sub-Saharan Africa. The papers are available online at *www.icn.ch.*
- One outcome of the 2004 ICN study was the decision to create an International Centre on Nurse Migration in partnership with the Commission on Graduates of Foreign Schools of Nursing. Launched in May 2005, the Centre is designed to serve as a global resource for the development, promotion, and dissemination of research, policy, and information on nurse migration. It will:
  - Promote, collect, create, and disseminate data and information on nurse migration
  - Act as a resource center for nurse migration
  - Track trends and patterns of global health care workforce migration
  - Analyze current policy, generate policy options, and advocate for sound policy concerning nurse migration
  - Promote, undertake, and disseminate research on nurse migration, particularly concerning the immigrant nurse workforce
  - Provide consultation and expert advice on nurse migration
  - Offer continuing education about migration

## THE MILLENNIUM DEVELOPMENT GOALS

With the advent of the new millennium the UN adopted the Millennium Declaration and introduced the Millennium Development Goals (MDGs), addressing peace, security, human rights, development, and fundamental freedoms. With a target date of 2015 the eight MDGs address poverty, education, women, child mortality, maternal health, HIV and malaria, the environment, and a global social compact (UN, 2005). Achieving the MDGs ultimately affects the health and well-being of the world's 6.5 billion people.

These ambitious goals will not be met unless governments seriously address two issues: Africa and the global health human resource crisis, particularly the nursing shortage. Today nearly all nations face a growing shortage of nurses brought about by increasing demand and diminishing supply. In many countries there is an ageing nursing workforce, a shortage of other professional and ancillary staff, increasing acuity of illness, a poor image of nursing, and continuing health sector reform. For Africa, HIV and AIDS further complicate the shortage.

Although shortages vary by field of nursing, geography, level of care, sector, and organization, one commonality exists: there are both a real shortage and a pseudoshortage. Pseudoshortages exist primarily when there are enough nurses in the country but not enough willing to work under the conditions available. This is the case in both developed and developing nations. Ireland is a case in point. In 2004 the Irish Nurses Organization, in a study of nurse availability, found there were 15,000 nurses in Ireland who would not work in the system as it exists. In South Africa there are 31,000 vacant public sector nursing posts and 35,000 unemployed nurses. Although some want nursing work, others say the system must first change. The lack of a positive practice environment (low salaries, poor benefit packages, lack of supplies and equipment, inadequate nurse/patient ratios, unsatisfactory patient and staff safety, lack of access to professional development and promotions, lack of family-friendly policies, and lack of decision-making input) remains the most critical element in all countries.

Africa is in dire straits. As Tony Blair noted to Parliament, "Africa is the only continent which, without change, will not meet any of the Millennium Development Goals. Although there are success stories in Africa, four million children under five die in Africa every year. Three thousand children die a day from malaria. Fifty million Africa children don't go to primary school. Life expectancy is plummeting—by 2010 it will be down to just 27 years in some countries" (Blair, 2005). The Blair government's Commission for Africa called for an initial increase in donor funding of US$10 billion a year up to 2010 and, subject to review, a further increase to US$20 billion a year in the subsequent 5 years (Department for International Development [DFID], 2005). The G8, made up of the heads of state of Canada, France, Germany, Italy, Japan, Russia, the United Kingdom, and the United States, who meet annually to deal with major national and international economic and political issues, agreed to doubling of aid for Africa by $25 billion a year by 2010. The G8 recently put particular emphasis on health and education, agreeing to free primary education and basic health care for all (Blair, 2005). It will be important that nurses and other stakeholders monitor and lobby national governments to keep these commitments. Ultimately we need to decrease poverty and increase health for all nations.

## POVERTY

Today poverty is the world's most devastating scourge. The World Bank estimates that there are about 1.3 billion extremely poor people in the world, with women representing 70% of the absolute poor (UN Development Programme, 1997). Although the numbers have dropped in Asia and Latin America in the past decade, they have continued to rise in Africa (UN, 2005). One third of the world's children are hungry and undernourished, and about 2.5 million annually die of malnutrition (WHO, 1998). More than 80 countries have lower income per capita than they did 10 years ago. To put it in context, the assets of the world's top three billionaires in 1999 was greater than the combined gross national product of the 49 least-developed countries and their 600 million people (UN Development Programme, 1999). Unequal distribution of wealth and of health services has dire consequences for the poor, whether in developing countries or in the United States. The poor have a greater burden of ill health and disability, attributable in large part to infectious diseases, malnutrition, and the complications of childbirth. Children living in absolute poverty are five times more likely to die before the age of 5 than children who are not poor (WHO, 1999).

Poor countries have few public services, and these are of poor quality. This means longer travel and waiting times for care, fewer drugs, shared beds, and more corruption and graft. Often it means user fees and out-of-pocket payments at a time when people are ill and most in need of care. Although user fees may bring in money to buy more supplies, they often create unanticipated problems. For example, they may keep the working poor from seeking care, leading to enhanced chronicity and disability. A 1997 survey in Nigeria showed that user fees deterred at-risk women from seeking antenatal care, thereby increasing the number of emergency admissions and accounting for 70% of maternal mortality (Kelsey & Harrison, 1997). Furthermore, in places where crime and hunger are rampant, user fees leave the nurse, who handles the money, vulnerable to attack. The World Bank continues to support user fees. Noting that they pose a potential barrier to accessing health services for the very poor, however, the Bank asserts that a system of waivers and exemptions can offset this (Bitran & Giedon, 2003).

Health care has deteriorated in numerous countries, and previous gains are being lost as decision-makers reduce resources for health, education, and social services. However, our increasing ability to demonstrate the economic advantage of good health is beginning to be heard. Although the conclusions remain suggestive rather than definitive, studies show that healthier people are more productive. Preliminary results from a study in Latin America and the Caribbean show that growth in gross domestic product (GDP) is statistically associated with increased life expectancy. Mexican data suggest that every added year of male life expectancy means an added 1% increase in GDP 15 years later (WHO, 1999).

This growing body of evidence has added weight to calls by the UN organizations and nongovernmental groups (NGOs) such as ICN for a concerted attack on poverty. As a result the G8 countries (Canada, France, Germany, Japan, Italy, Russia, the United Kingdom, and the United States) have committed billions of dollars to a massive effort to fight the diseases of poverty. These diseases—primarily tuberculosis, HIV and AIDS, malaria, childhood diseases (such as measles and diarrheal conditions), and the complications associated with pregnancy and delivery—inflict a terrible and disproportionate toll of death and disability on the world's poorest people. A coordinated approach is needed and desperately lacking. For example, the Global Fund to Fight AIDS, Tuberculosis and Malaria (GFATM) was created by the G8 in 2002 to scale up global effort and pool resources to fight these diseases. Yet today the Fund is facing a budget shortfall of $1.6 billion (U.S. dollars [USD]) to meet the anticipated need. Funding is decreasing, and a number of countries and private sector organizations are funding separate initiatives for which there is little if any communication, let alone coordination (Boxes 34-3 and 34-4).

ICN believes nurses have a vital role in reducing poverty and its impact on health and well-being, including the following (ICN, 1999b):

■ Involving the family and community in defining their problems and seeking solutions

---

**BOX 34-3 International Council of Nurses**

The International Council of Nurses is a federation of national nurses associations (NNAs) representing nurses in more than 125 countries. Founded in 1899, the ICN is the world's first and widest-reaching international organization for health professionals. Operated by nurses for nurses, the ICN works to ensure high-quality nursing care for all, sound health policies globally, the advancement of nursing knowledge, and the presence worldwide of a respected nursing profession and a competent and satisfied nursing workforce.

The ICN advances nursing, nurses, and health through its policies, partnerships, advocacy, leadership development, networks, congresses, and special projects and its work in the arenas of professional practice, regulation, and socioeconomic welfare. The ICN is particularly active in ethics, AIDS, advanced practice, research, leadership development, the international classification of nursing practice, women's health, regulation, human resources development, occupational health and safety, conditions of work, career development, and human rights.

The ICN works with agencies of the United Nations (UN) system, such as WHO, UNAIDS, UNICEF, UNESCO, UNCTAD, and ILO; other intergovernmental organizations such as the World Bank, WTO, and the International Organization on Migration; and international, regional, and national nongovernmental organizations.

---

**BOX 34-4** World Bank Group

The World Bank, established in 1944, is composed of the International Bank for Reconstruction and Development, the International Development Association, the International Finance Corporation, the Multilateral Investment Guaranty Agency, and the International Centre for Settlement of Investment Disputes. The World Bank Group is owned by its member countries, whose numbers vary according to the agency. The International Bank for Reconstruction and Development (IBRD) is the largest, with 184 member countries. The World Bank Group is staffed by 9300 employees from 160 countries.

The Bank's mission is to fight poverty and improve the living standards of people in the developing world. It is a development Bank that provides loans, policy advice, technical assistance, and knowledge-sharing services to low- and middle-income countries to reduce poverty.

The World Bank is the world's largest source of development assistance and works with governments, nongovernmental organizations, and the private sector and within more than 100 developing economies, bringing a mix of finance and ideas to improve living standards and eliminate the worst forms of poverty.

To become a member of the World Bank a country must first join the International Monetary Fund (IMF) (World Bank Group, 2005) (Box 34-5).

---

**BOX 34-5** International Monetary Fund

The International Monetary Fund (IMF) is an international organization of 184 member countries, with its headquarters in Washington, DC. IMF was established in 1945 to promote international monetary cooperation; secure financial stability; facilitate international trade; promote high employment and sustainable economic growth; assist in the establishment of a multilateral system of payments; make its general resources temporarily available to its members experiencing balance of payment difficulties under adequate safeguards; and shorten the duration and lessen the degree of disequilibrium in the international balances of payments of members.

Its operations involve surveillance, financial assistance, and technical assistance. Financial assistance includes credits and loans extended by the IMF to member countries with balance of payment problems to support policies of adjustment and reform.

The bulk of the IMF's resources derive from members' subscriptions (called *quotas*) that are broadly based on each member's relative size in the world economy (IMF, 2005).

---

- Lobbying for antipoverty measures such as access to credits, job creation, income supplements, nutrition gardens, and self-help initiatives
- Supporting the shift to community-based care and a household approach
- Lobbying for equity in health care and social services
- Working to initiate pro-poor social and health policy
- Focusing attention on the impact of poverty on women and other vulnerable groups

Education, particularly education of females, plays a key role in poverty reduction. It leads to lower fertility and infant mortality rates, better health and nutrition, higher productivity, better gender equity, and improved chances that the next generation will in turn be educated. However, because of poverty, illness, cultural practices, fear, and violence, girls are less likely than boys

to be educated. In fact, girls account for 60% of the estimated 113 million out-of-school children. Most of these children live in sub-Saharan Africa (Florence Nightingale International Foundation [FNIF], 2005).

Given the value of education to health and poverty reduction, the ICN and its sister organization, FNIF, have launched the *Girl Child Education Fund* to support the primary and secondary schooling of orphaned daughters of nurses, beginning in sub-Saharan Africa, where there are an estimated 16 million AIDS orphans (Box 34-6).

## HIV AND AIDS

If poverty is the world's greatest scourge, then AIDS is surely second. AIDS has penetrated every nation of the world. Globally there are 39 million people living with HIV or AIDS, and more than 20 million people have died since the disease was first reported 25 years ago (UN, 2005). In the United States at the end of 2003, an estimated 1,039,000 to 1,185,000

---

**BOX 34-6** The Girl Child Education Fund: A Nursing Initiative for Orphaned Girls

**THE NEED**

Orphaned children, particularly girls, often have no access to schooling despite our understanding that education plays an enormously important role in improving health and reducing poverty. Educating females in particular plays a key role in poverty reduction, leading to lower fertility and infant mortality rates, better health and nutrition, higher productivity, better gender equity, and improved chances that the next generation will in turn be educated. Today, because of poverty, illness, cultural practices, fear, and violence, girls are less likely than boys to be educated, and account for 60% of out-of-school children. Most out of school children (113 million) and most orphans (e.g., 16 million AIDS orphans) live in sub-Saharan Africa, where less than 4% of orphans are receiving any kind of support.

**THE FUND**

ICN and FNIF aim to support the primary and secondary schooling of orphaned daughters of nurses, beginning in sub-Saharan Africa. The fund will provide for the cost of fees, uniforms, and books. An annual donation of $200 covers the costs of primary education, and $500 annually means an African colleague's orphaned daughter can attend secondary school.

For more information on this initiative, visit *www.fnif.org.*

---

persons were living with HIV or AIDS, with an estimated 43,171 persons having been newly diagnosed with AIDS. Although the estimated number of HIV cases is greatest in the white non-Hispanic community, the black non-Hispanic group had the largest estimated number of diagnosed AIDS cases in 2003 (Centers for Disease Control and Prevention [CDC], 2005b). According to the CDC, HIV and AIDS were among the top three causes of death for African-American men aged 25 to 54 years in 2001 and among the top four causes of death for African-American women aged 20 to 54 years. Although they make up only 12.3% of the population, they account for 40% of the

infections since the epidemic began (Herbert, 2001; CDC, 2005a).

HIV infections in Russia are increasing at an alarming rate. By the end of 2002 a total of 246,285 people had been diagnosed, with more than a fifth (50,529) of that total added in 2003 alone (AVERT, 2005a). Similarly, in India, HIV infection rates are increasing rapidly, with 5.1 million people affected in 2003. As in China, where only 840,000 infections were known in 2003, it would be easy to under estimate the extent of the disease (AVERT, 2005b). In sub-Saharan Africa, an estimated 3.8 million adults and children became infected with HIV during 2000, bringing the total number of sub-Saharans with HIV and AIDS to 25.3 million. In India, roughly 3.7 million people have been infected with HIV (UNAIDS, 2000; UNAIDS & WHO, 2000).

In Africa the disease is devastating communities and nations and creating a generation of AIDS orphans. It is also taking its toll among the nurses who care for the ill, and who may be infected themselves. According to UNAIDS, sub-Saharan Africa is home to more than 60% of all people living with HIV and AIDS, which is the leading cause of premature death there and with which 25 million people are infected. In 2004 an estimated 3.1 million people became newly infected and 2.3 million died of AIDS. Women and girls make up 57% of HIV infections in the region, and 16 million children have lost one or both parents to the epidemic (UNAIDS, 2005).

In late 2003, the newly appointed WHO Director-General announced the "3×5" strategy, committing to supplying 3 million people living with HIV and AIDS in developing countries access to antiretroviral treatment (ART) by the end of 2005. By June 2005 the numbers had reached 1 million. The goal was not reached by the end of 2005, although the numbers in treatment have more than doubled since the initiative was launched. The fact remains there are still 5 million people in developing countries infected and in need of ART.

Nurses could be the key to success if permitted to work to their full potential. Nurses have been at the forefront of care, management, research, education, and politics. In more than 30 countries, nurses have formed special interest groups to advance their knowledge of the disease and of care, to support nurses in their roles as providers and persons living with HIV or AIDS, and to lobby governments for increased funding for research, education, treatment, and care. Nurses form the core of care in most countries, particularly in the developing world, where money and drugs are scarce, beds are full, and myths flourish. Nurses, working alone or in collaboration with other sectors, continue to develop and deliver educational programs and to counsel individuals, families, and groups worldwide. In addition to convincing adolescents of their vulnerability, the biggest problem for nurses in African countries is changing the social attitudes toward sex, including the myth that having intercourse with a virgin can rid a man of HIV. Nurses in Africa are also advocating for better home care and self-care and are carrying out research in these areas.

AIDS increases nursing workloads and fuels burnout and frustration, thereby contributing to absenteeism, attrition, and migration. In addition to caring for HIV and AIDS patients at work, nurses often also care for family and friends after hours and many are themselves ill. Estimates are that absenteeism can take up 50% of the work time of a health worker living with AIDS in his or her final year of life. In Malawi it is estimated that 25% of public health workers (including nurses) will be dead of AIDS by 2009 (*New York Times,* 2004).

Fear of occupational exposure may be reducing entrants into the workforce, as well as encouraging current members to leave. Nurses and midwives face a high risk of being exposed to infected blood and body fluids during work. Unpublished reports from the East Central and Southern Africa College of Nursing (ECSACON) in 1999 and 2000 revealed lack of infection prevention and control policies and guidelines or their enforcement where they existed (Munjanja, Kibuka, & Dovlo, 2005).

Few sub-Saharan countries offer health workers counseling, support, or ART. In 2003, ICN began advocating free ART for health care workers and their families and began working with Boeringer-Inglehelm, the Norwegian Nurses Association, and the Zambian Nurses Association

to provide free nevirapine to pregnant health care workers. Nevirapine is used to decrease the potential mother-to-child transmission of HIV. In 2004, ICN began working with Zambia and Swaziland to develop proposals for providing ART and community-based care to health care workers and their families.

Care has been the missing piece in much of the UN's work, and nurses have yet to be used to their full potential within the UN system. As recently as 2000, WHO appointed a physician to head its HIV/AIDS Care Services, over the objections of nurses, and UNAIDS eliminated its nursing position and appointed a physician to head care and prevention services. This example illustrates the policy and personnel imbalance within the UN and many national health systems, where nurses play a minor role in health policy development. It also illustrates the prevalent UN notion that "care" is equivalent to "medical care."

## NURSING'S POLICY VOICE

Achieving nursing's policy potential is perhaps the greatest challenge facing the profession in the twenty-first century. Nursing's success in shaping policy is variable, depending on the country, the issue, and the group under consideration. On the other hand, the limiting factors are fairly universal and include nursing's image, perceived value, and social status, educational requirements, gender issues, and numbers. The ratio of nurses to other health workers, the scope of practice, legislation, and cultural norms affect the influence of nurses, as does the presence of strong national nursing associations. Equally important is the extent to which nurses are perceived to be interested in improving health for all, versus being interested in only personal and professional gains.

There is no doubt that policy influence is an uphill battle for many. In some newly independent countries, nurses are engaged in learning about nursing autonomy and lobbying for the right to chart their own actions. Nursing groups are lobbying in several countries to create a government Chief Nurse, to maintain the position, or to reinstate it. Nursing too often lacks a single senior nurse, let alone a cadre of influential nurses, within the health department.

Without nurses in key positions in international health departments, there is little or no focus on nursing or the effects of decisions on nursing. For example, new technologies and programs may be introduced without any assessment of their impact on the current deployment of nurses. This problem is compounded when there is no strong national nursing organization to monitor the quality of care or human resource issues.

# NURSING WITHIN GOVERNMENTS AND THE WORLD HEALTH ORGANIZATION

## THE WORLD HEALTH ORGANIZATION

The lack of influential nurses within WHO and governments has handicapped nursing, particularly compared with the influence of physicians. In 2000, of the number of WHO professional posts in the category that includes dental, medical, nursing, and veterinary staff, 90.8% were medical specialists and 2.9% nurses (WHO, 2001b). In the report to the Assembly in 2005, 91.7% were medical specialists and 2.1% nurses.

WHO has one nurse scientist within its Geneva-based secretariat, and the same secretariat is unable to state the numbers of nurses in other positions, despite repeated requests by the ICN. Only five of the six WHO regional offices have designated Regional Nurse Advisors. The Pan-American Health Organization (PAHO), the regional office of the Americas, has none, although there is one designated nursing post.

Nurses occupy non-nursing posts in program areas at headquarters, regional, and country levels. As well there are now two nurses who are WHO Country Representatives, the highest country level WHO post.

Physicians are the most numerous professional personnel within WHO. Mostly from the "old school" of health care, WHO physicians are inclined to overlook the potential roles nurses could play. Most see the general practitioner as the pivotal professional in health care and do not see the need to address nursing issues. Repeatedly, with senior staff changes at WHO, the question arises as to why WHO needs a Nurse Scientist.

The current nursing shortage and the global health care reform movement offer an opportunity to change the influence of nurses within WHO and nationally. Most countries have a growing disease burden along with shrinking health resources, including personnel. Strengthening nursing is seen as a means to address health care problems, and the World Health Assembly, made up of representatives of ministries of health from nearly 200 countries, has resolved to address nursing issues. The resolution, passed by the assembly in May 2001, acknowledges the nursing shortage; recognizes that nurses and midwives play a crucial and cost-effective role in promoting healthy lifestyles and reducing excess mortality, morbidity, and disability; and concludes that further action is needed to maximize the contribution of nurses and midwives. Among a series of actions, the resolution urges governments to do the following: (1) involve nurses and midwives in health policy development, planning, and implementation at all levels; (2) establish comprehensive human resource development programs that support the recruitment and retention of a skilled and motivated nursing and midwifery workforce within health services; (3) develop and implement policies and programs that ensure healthy workplaces and high-quality work environments for nurses and midwives; and (4) develop and enhance nursing's evidence base (WHO, 2001c). The WHO Secretariat is to provide the Assembly with a progress report in 2006.

Nursing has been on the WHO agenda periodically for more than 40 years, placed there through the lobbying of groups such as the ICN and interested governments. Skeptics might say that this resolution represents more of the same. However, there is a difference this time as a result of the pervasiveness of the nursing shortage, the bleakness of nursing recruitment, the new challenges of an aging population, the double burden of chronic and infectious diseases that most nations face, and the rising costs of health care.

## NATIONAL GOVERNMENTS

Nurses hold staff, appointed, and elected posts in small numbers within national governments. And although the number of nurses in Chief Nurse posts is not increasing overall, there is an increase in the number of nurse politicians, particularly nurses holding cabinet positions. ICN has recently established a network for Nurse Politicians.

Governments now have increasing evidence of the impact nurses can have. This is clear in the new Family Health Nurse initiative underway in WHO's European region. For Europe the Family Health Nurse concept is based on a professional nurse whose work focuses on prevention and providing care. The nurse is trained to detect early signs of emerging problems, make appropriate referrals to other health professionals and other services within the system, and give family members advice suited to their age, lifestyle, and gender. The Family Health Nurse is also an active member of local community health programs. Nurses are skilled in community development and are able to translate experience with families into programs for the community. The nurse is, in other words, an effective agent for community-based care. Today there are 18 pilot sites throughout Europe, several of them in countries where nursing traditionally has enjoyed no autonomy or recognition of the profession's potential.

There is increased interest in the nurse practitioner movement in several countries, and a number of countries are implementing nurse prescribing. The United Kingdom has introduced the consultant nurse, and in the United States there is growing acceptance that nurse anesthetists need not work directly under the supervision of an anesthesiologist. Telecommunications is offering new alternatives, and countries such as the United States, the United Kingdom, Japan, Canada, Portugal, Australia, and Norway are using telecommunications for education, consultation, and treatment. Telenursing, particularly telephone triage by nurses, is the fastest-growing new nursing-related initiative by governments in many years.

Overall we are not making much headway with respect to government chief nurse posts. The number of chief nurses is growing in Europe and in Central and Eastern Europe and the former Soviet Union. Lobbying for positions in South America continues; the Caribbean and some African countries have lost posts as part of health care reform. There is little activity in the French-speaking states in Africa or Europe, where there is no history of the position and little call for it. The lack of a strong united nongovernmental nursing voice in many of these countries means that nursing continues to be disadvantaged in the policy arena.

In South America a number of strong national and regional nursing groups have had some policy success, particularly in raising the level of nursing education. In English-speaking Africa, as in most other Anglophonic countries, nursing has a long tradition of influence, often holding high nonnursing government posts, and such countries remain staunch supporters of the profession. However, this appears to be waning with the latest round of reform as physicians vie for these posts.

Nursing has a growing policy and political voice in Asia through both the nurses associations and nurses in parliament. Finally, the Middle East and South Pacific are also seeing the rise of a stronger nursing voice, particularly through the professional association.

Nursing's policy influence in this century will require more nurse politicians, more unity of voice, and more strategic alliances, along with leadership development and added political and policy skills for all new graduates. Currently, a real danger in many countries is the potential split in the external nursing voice as more specialty organizations develop, particularly outside the umbrella of the national nurses association. The United States has felt the impact of divided nursing interests for many years and has developed mechanisms, such as forums and issue-specific lobbies, to bring the nursing voice together on key issues. Such strategic alliances are part of today's socioeconomic and political fabric. Touted first by management gurus and then applied to industry, strategic alliances have come to the fore in international health.

# PARTNERSHIPS AND STRATEGIC ALLIANCES: A WAY FORWARD

There has been a long tradition of partnership between NGOs and the UN agencies, such as WHO. The ICN was the first health professional group to attain official relations status with WHO in 1948. Since then, about 60 UN and inter-governmental agencies have been created, and more of them have begun to address health care issues. Many regional intergovernmental groups and regional NGOs have been created, including regional nursing groups such as the Northern Nurses Federation, the Caribbean Nurses Organi-zation, the European Union Permanent Committee on Nursing, and the Commonwealth Nurses Federation. Today there is more collaboration among intergovernmental agencies themselves, among NGOs, and between UN agencies and NGOs. In 1996 the European Region of WHO created the European Forum of National Nursing and Midwifery Associations and WHO in order to accomplish the following (WHO, 1996):

- Inform the debate of improving health and quality of care in Europe
- Promote the exchange of information, ideas, and policies between nursing and midwifery and WHO
- Support the integration of appropriate policies for health for all into nursing practice as well as education
- Formulate consensus and policy statements and recommendations on health-, nursing-, and midwifery-related issues

The ICN works with the European Forum and with other regional and international groups, includ-ing the WMA; the International Pharmaceutical Federation (FIP), representing pharmacists; the International Confederation of Midwives (ICM); and the World Dental Federation, the International Hospital Federation, and so on. In 1999 the ICN, WMA, and FIP created the World Health Professions Alliance, launched publicly during the World Health Assembly. In 2005 the World Dental Federation became a member. Through pooled resources, the alliance not only strengthens collaboration among

the four professions but also addresses key health issues, such as health resources planning, human rights, tobacco addiction, antimicrobial resistance, AIDS, and ethics.

The ICN is party to a number of other strategic alliances. Some involve nursing groups only and really are joint ventures to deliver services. Examples of these include a joint venture with the East, Central, and Southern African College of Nurses to deliver the ICN's Leadership for Change program to nurses in 14 African countries. Others involve UN agencies, donor agencies, private sector companies, and NGOs.

A new twist to strategic alliances within the UN system has been the addition of the corporate sector as partner. Recently, several new initiatives have involved key UN agencies, the World Bank, foundations, transnational corporations, and NGOs. Operating under the direction of one of the agencies or through creation of a new third-party vehicle, such as a management board, these new issue-specific entities address key public health issues. The Global Alliance for Vaccines and Immunization (GAVI) is a case in point.

Established in 2000, GAVI represents an historic alliance of public- and private-sector partners assem-bled in a worldwide network. The partners are the Bill and Melinda Gates Children's Vaccine Program, the International Federation of Pharmaceutical Manufacturers Associations (IFPMA), public health and research institutions, national governments, the Rockefeller Foundation, UNICEF, the World Bank Group, and WHO. GAVI's mission is to protect children of all nations and of all socioeco-nomic levels against vaccine-preventable diseases. The alliance addresses its objectives by working to secure adequate funds, improve donor collaboration, strengthen national immunization services, enhance coordination among governments and development partners, and enhance collaboration with global vaccine industry partners to provide the highest-quality vaccines at the lowest appropriate pricing (GAVI, 2001).

By the end of 2004, GAVI had secured dona-tions and commitments of $1.3 billion USD as well as another $1.9 billion in pledges. Seventy-one countries have benefited through increased access to vaccines, increased vaccine coverage, and strengthening of immunization systems and safety. The impact in terms of lives saved and illnesses avoided has been enormous (GAVI, 2005).

## GETTING INVOLVED

Shared goals, vision, and values are key ingredients to policy and program initiatives such as GAVI. The same is true for nursing. Any significant advancement toward realizing nursing's policy potential nationally, regionally, and internationally will require multiple strategies and joint efforts on many fronts. Ultimately it means the commitment of individual nurses who share a vision and values and believe that nurses can make a difference for themselves and, most of all, for the people they serve. There are many ways to participate:

- Begin at home—get involved. Know the issues and values. Support organized nursing initiatives. This may mean working on issues and policy papers, engaging in lobbying activities, or running for public or nursing office.
- Think globally, act locally. Cultivate a worldview when addressing local nursing and health issues. Be sensitive to the cultural aspects of policy and practice.
- Commit to learning more about trade agreements and how they affect your practice and your potential. Although some aspects are positive, there are pitfalls too. Health services are now part of the WTO agenda. Ministries of trade and foreign affairs have already consulted nursing representatives in some countries. Make sure yours is one of them.
- Through the association or your workplace, help colleagues in other countries as they work to strengthen nursing and health care. Nurses in many countries are working against incredible odds and would welcome help at work and in their associations. Remember, the developing world carries 90% of the disease burden yet enjoys only 10% of health resources.
- Undertake research to build evidence of nursing effectiveness in areas key to nursing's progress. Pilot new nursing roles, such as the Family Nurse.

- Advocate, initiate, and document nursing's role in policy.
- Know where your government stands on key international health and nursing matters, and lobby the government to support the initiative. Lobby governments to urge them to pay their UN dues if they are lagging behind. Without funds, it is impossible to accomplish much.
- Join others in ensuring that national and local structures are in place so that nursing's voice is heard in policy and practice.
- Ensure that new graduates know about policy and politics, how to analyze the environment, how to develop strategy, and how to work together.
- Get involved in international issues and team up with like-minded groups and individuals at home and internationally.
- Know the stance taken by regional and international organizations, such as the ICN, on key nursing and health issues.
- Share your ideas and achievements through publications and the Internet and papers presented at international conferences.

Nursing remains the backbone of health systems worldwide. If we are to achieve better health for all people, it will be through evidence that we are a strong profession, committed to sound nursing and health policies and practices, and skilled in policy, politics, and care. One of the key tenets of primary health care is that communities should participate in decisions affecting them. It follows, then, that nursing, as a community and as part of the global society, needs to be engaged in all aspects of health policy.

## *Key Points*

- We need to engage beyond our jobs and daily practice; doing so enriches our lives and those of others.
- Migration is a fact of life. Although we need to aim for domestic self-sufficiency, we also need to treat new workers fairly and respectfully, promoting mutual gain.
- Poverty and AIDS are every nurse's business.
- Strengthening nursing's policy voice benefits patients, the public, employers, and nursing; get involved, and make your voice heard.

## *Web Resources*

**Centers for Disease Control and Prevention (CDC)**—agency of the U.S. Department of Health and Human Services; principal U.S. agency addressing health protection and safety; globally recognized for its public health initiatives
*www.cdc.gov*

**Florence Nightingale International Foundation (FNIF)**
*www.fnif.org*

**International Council of Nurses (ICN)**
*www.icn.ch*

**International Monetary Fund**
*www.Imf.org*

**International Organization for Migration (IOM)**—works with migrants and governments to provide humane responses to migration challenges; like the WTO, not a UN agency, but works closely with the UN system, countries, and NGOs
*www.iom.int*

**UNAIDS**—Joint United Nations Programme on HIV and AIDS; created to coordinate, lead, and support the response to HIV and AIDS through leadership and advocacy, information and technical support, partnerships, and resource mobilization
*www.unaids.org*

**United Nations Development Programme**—UN's global development network; helps developing countries attract and use aid effectively and produces the annual *Human Development Report*, focusing on key development issues
*www.undp.org*

**World Bank**
*www.worldbank.org*

**World Health Organization (WHO)**
*www.who.int*

**World Trade Organization (WTO)**
*www.wto.org*

## REFERENCES

AVERT. (2005a). HIV/AIDS in Russia, Eastern Europe and Central Asia. Retrieved August 12, 2005, from *www.avert.org/ecstatee.htm*.

AVERT. (2005b). HIV and AIDS in India. Retrieved August 12, 2005, from *www.avert.org/aidsindia.htm*.

Bitran, R., & Giedon, U. (2003). *Careful design of waiver systems makes access to health services more equitable*. Washington, DC: World Bank.

Blair, T. (2005). Statement to Parliament on the G8 Summit. Retrieved August 20, 2005, from *www.g8.gov.uk/servlet/Front?pagename=OpenMarket/Xcelerate/ShowPage&c=Page&cid=1078995903270&a=KArticle&aid=1119521193501*.

Buchan, J., Kingman, M., & Lorenzo, M. (2005). *Issue paper 5. International migration of nurses: Trends and policy implications*. Geneva: International Council of Nurses (ICN).

Centers for Disease Control and Prevention (CDC). (2005a). HIV/AIDS among African Americans. CDC Fact Sheet. Retrieved August 20, 2005, from *www.cdc.gov/hiv/pubs/facts/afam.htm*.

Centers for Disease Control and Prevention (CDC). (2005b). HIV/AIDS surveillance report 2003. Retrieved August 20, 2005, from *www.cdc.gov/hiv/stats.htm#hivest*.

Commonwealth Code of Practice for the International Recruitment of Health Care Workers. (2003). Adopted at the preWHA Meeting of Commonwealth Ministers of Health, May 18, 2003, Geneva. Retrieved August 12, 2005, from *www.thecommonwealth.org*.

Department for International Development (DFID). (2005). Commission for Africa. Our common interest. Retrieved August 12, 2005, from *www.dfid.gov.uk/news/files/cfa-executivesummary.pdf*.

Florence Nightingale International Foundation (FNIF). (2005). *The Girl Child Education Fund: A nursing initiative for orphaned girls*. Retrieved October 30, 2005, from *www.fnif.org/girlfund.htm*.

Global Alliance for Vaccines and Immunization (GAVI). (2001). More about GAVI. Retrieved March 18, 2001, from *www.vaccinealliance.com/reference/moreabout.html*.

Global Alliance for Vaccines and Immunization (GAVI). (2005). *GAVI/The Vaccine Fund—Progress and Achievements. Fact Sheet*. Retrieved August 12, 2005, from *www.vaccinealliance.org*.

Herbert, B. (2001). In America: The quiet scourge. *New York Times*. Retrieved April 15, 2001, from *www.nytimes.com/pages/opinion/index.html*.

International Air Transport Association (IATA). (2004). Activity report 2004. Retrieved August 12, 2005, from *www.iata.org/NR/ContentConnector/CS2000/Siteinterface/sites/whatwedo/file/activity_report-2004.pdf*.

International Air Transport Association (IATA). (2005). Annual report 2005. Retrieved August 12, 2005, from *www.iata.org/iata/Sites/agm/file/2005/file/Annual_report_2005.pdf*.

International Council of Nurses (ICN). (1999a). *Nurse retention, transfer and migration. ICN position statement*. Geneva: ICN.

International Council of Nurses (ICN). (1999b) *ICN on poverty and health: Breaking the link*. Nursing Matters Fact Sheet. Geneva: ICN.

International Council of Nurses (ICN). (2000). *ICN/WMA/WHO mobility survey* (internal correspondence). Geneva: ICN.

International Council of Nurses (ICN). (2001). *Ethical nurse recruitment: ICN position statement*. Geneva: ICN.

International Monetary Fund (IMF). (2005). About the IMF. Retrieved August 21, 2005, from *www.imf.org/external/pubs/ft/ar/2004/eng/index.htm.*

International Organization on Migration (IOM). (2005). World migration 2005: Costs and benefits of international migration. Retrieved August 12, 2005, from *www.iom.int//DOCUMENTS/PUBLICATION/wmr_sec03.pdf.*

Kelsey, & Harrison. (1997, March). Maternal mortality in Nigeria: The real issue. *African Journal of Reproductive Health.* 8.

Lorenzo, F. (2002). *Nurse supply and demand in the Philippines.* Manila, Philippines: Institute of Health Policy and Development Studies, University of the Philippines.

Munjanja, O., Kibuka, S., & Dovlo, D. (2005). *Issue paper 7. The nursing workforce in sub-Saharan Africa.* Geneva: International Council of Nurses.

New York Times. (2004, August 13). Africa's health care brain drain. *New York Times,* section A, 20.

Oulton, J. A. (1998). International trade and the nursing profession. In *International trade in health services: A development perspective.* Geneva: United Nations Conference on Trade and Development.

UNAIDS. (2000, December). AIDS epidemic update 2000. Retrieved March 18, 2001, from *www.unaids.org/wac/2000/wad00/files/WAD_epidemic_report.htm.*

UNAIDS. (2005). Africa fact sheet. Retrieved August 22, 2005, from *www.unaids.org/NetTools/Misc/DocInfo.aspx?LANG=en&href=http://gva-doc-owl/WEBcontent/Documents/pub/Publications/Fact-Sheets04/FS_SSAfrica_en.pdf.*

UNAIDS, & World Health Organization (WHO). (2000). India: Epidemiological fact sheet on HIV/AIDS and sexually transmitted infections: 2000 Update. Retrieved June 26, 2001 from the *www.unaids.org/hivaidsinfo/statistics/june00/fact_sheets/pdfs/india.pdf.*

United Nations (UN). (2005). *The Millennium Development Goals report.* New York. United Nations Department of Public Information.

United Nations Development Programme. (1997). *Human development to eradicate poverty: The human development report 1997.* New York: Oxford University Press.

United Nations Development Programme. (1999). *Globalization with a human face: The human development report 1999.* New York: Oxford University Press.

World Bank Group. (2005). About us. Retrieved August 21, 2005, from *http://web.worldbank.org/WBSITE/EXTERNAL/EXTABOUTUS/0,,contentMDK:50004946~menuPK:271153~pagePK:34542~piPK:329829~theSitePK:29708,00.html.*

World Health Organization (WHO). (1996, November). *European Forum of Nursing and Midwifery Associations and WHO established "a formidable force for change."* (Press Release EURO/07/96.) Copenhagen: WHO Regional Office for Europe.

World Health Organization (WHO). (1998). *Life in the 21st century: A vision for all. The World Health Report 1998.* Geneva: WHO.

World Health Organization (WHO). (1999). *Making a difference. The World Health Report 1999.* Geneva: WHO.

World Health Organization (WHO). (2001a). About WHO. Retrieved March 15, 2001, from *www.who.int/aboutwho/en/mission.htm.*

World Health Organization (WHO). (2001b). *Human resources: Annual report, 2000. Report by the Secretariat* (107th Executive Board, Doc EB107/14, 11 January 2001). Geneva: WHO.

World Health Organization (WHO). (2001c). *Strengthening nursing and midwifery.* (54th World Health Assembly, Doc WHA 54.12. 21, May 2001.) Geneva: WHO.

World Health Organization (WHO). (2005a). About WHO. Retrieved August 21, 2005, from *www.who.int/about/en.*

World Health Organization (WHO). (2005b). *Human resources: Annual report, 2004. Report by the Secretariat* (World Health Assembly, Doc A58/34, 28 April 2005). Geneva: WHO.

World Trade Organization (WTO). (2001). *The WTO.* Retrieved March 25, 2001, from *www.wto.org/english/thewto_e/thewto_e.htm.*

World Trade Organization (WTO). (2005). The World Trade Organization in brief. Retrieved August 21, 2005 from *www.wto.org/english/res_e/doload_e/inbr_e.pdf.*

# GLOBAL MIGRATION OF NURSES: MANAGING A SCARCE RESOURCE

Marla E. Salmon & Victoria Guisinger

*"We have to choose between a global market driven only by calculations of short-term profit, and one which has a human face."*

KOFI ANNAN

The migration of nurses has become the subject of increasing awareness and concern in every region of the world. Rich and resource-poor countries alike are involved in and affected by the movement of nurses within and among countries. The increasing numbers of such nurses and the impact of their movement on both home and receiving countries have generated serious questions about the costs and benefits of such migration. The fundamental question is whether or not strategies can be developed to reduce the negative impact of nurse migration and optimize the positive gains for the individuals and countries involved.

## MIGRATION AS A GLOBAL PHENOMENON

The history of humankind is essentially about the movement of people. Whether geographically, culturally, socially, economically, or biologically, the desire and need to move are part of the human condition. The physical movement of people from place to place is intrinsically connected to the basic human drive to seek better lives and reflected in an ever-increasing number of people who not only move within their own countries but who move across borders and beyond their home continents. Movement is so fundamental to the well-being of people, it is recognized in the Universal Declaration

of Human Rights as a separate article (General Assembly Resolution 217 A [III], 1948).

As the movement of people worldwide has increased, so has its impact on those who migrate as well as on those who remain and those who receive them. In 2005 there were an estimated 185 to 192 million migrants worldwide (United Nations, 2003), almost 3% of the world's population (International Organization for Migration, 2005a) and nearly double the number of migrants just 25 years ago (United Nations Population Division, 2002). Migration is increasingly associated with the search for better employment opportunities outside one's homeland. Among migrants, women are ever more prominent both in numbers (48.6% [International Organization for Migration, 2005a]) and in all types of job categories. And, because labor markets have become global, there are extremely serious implications for these migrants, their families, and the countries from which they have come and in which they seek and engage in work.

The increasing numbers of women who are represented in work-related migration are evident in the ranks of health workers, particularly within nursing. In 2002 the United Kingdom's National Health Service (NHS) employed 30,000 foreign workers, and it plans to hire an additional 25,000 by 2008 (International Organization for Migration, 2005b). Because of widespread growing shortages of nurses in the developed world, migration of nurses to these countries from less-developed nations is having a profoundly damaging affect on the health and well-being of people in countries from which the nurses emigrate. A 2004 study

(Anand & Barnighausen, 2004) identified that a decrease in nursing density is directly related to an increase in maternal mortality. This is a daunting finding when matched with migration statistics. In 2001, 923 Ghanaian nurses sought verification of nursing credentials for emigration (Buchan & Dovlo, 2004); in the same year 382 Zimbabwean nurses were registered in the United Kingdom, but the number of nurses who graduated in Zimbabwe between 1998 and 2000 was just 340 (Stilwell et al., 2003). The result can be witnessed at the main labor ward in Lilongwe, Malawi where 10 nurse-midwives deliver over 10,000 babies a year (Dugger, 2004).

The purpose of this section is to discuss the migration of nurses in the context of a global health labor market. Specifically, the current dynamics and factors involved in migration of nurses are addressed, along with an exploration of the important roles and responsibilities of all parties involved in the international migration of nurses. Possible strategies for reducing the negative impact on "sending" countries will be explored using the Caribbean regional model of "Managed Migration." The chapter closes with recommendations for action by individuals, the profession of nursing, policymakers, and others to address the negative impact of migration on individuals, families, communities, and countries.

## GLOBAL MIGRATION OF NURSES

### Popularized Perspectives

Migration of nurses among countries has been underway for more than a century. Common languages, familiar customs, and travel back and forth among countries with shared colonial heritages or trade connections provided links that enabled early nurses to move back and forth among countries. In some instances these nurses left their own countries to pursue training in another country and ultimately returned to their own countries or, even migrated back and forth between their homelands and the countries in which they were trained. This arrangement was particularly true in the English-speaking countries with shared histories and established a pattern that remains to this day.

Although the migration of nurses among countries is a long-standing practice, the intensity of migration has increased dramatically with respect to numbers of nurses, distance traveled to migrate, and cultural differences. For example, in the late 1990s, approximately 4000 Filipino nurses emigrated each year, but the numbers started to rise in 1999, and in 2001 over 13,500 nurses emigrated to countries as near as Singapore but as far away as the United States, Ireland, and Saudi Arabia (Buchan & Calman, 2004). Clearly, globalization has played a major role in this upswing in migration, as ease in communication, travel, and acculturation has increased dramatically over the last two decades. Increasingly nurses see themselves as members of a global professional workforce as they engage across borders in their education, professional organizations, and professional literature. In addition, family members and friends who have migrated before them provide natural communities and networks for nurses when they go to other countries.

The actual choice to leave one's homeland for work in another country, however, reflects a complex set of decisions influenced by many variables. These variables have been loosely classified into two categories: "push" factors, those conditions that are seen to "drive" nurses away from their current situations, and "pull" factors, conditions that attract nurses to either a different situation or keep them in their current one. Push and pull factors exist within institutions, communities, and countries and among countries.

As Table 34-1 illustrates, there are numerous specific conditions that fall into these two categories. Push factors are generally those that cause nurses to look for options to leave their current circumstances. Among these are compensation; work conditions; lack of employment and professional opportunities; social, economic, and political conditions; and fear of harm to self or family. In resource-poor countries virtually every one of these conditions may influence decisions on migration. For example, in some of the countries of sub-Saharan Africa, poorly paid nurses may be called on to work extra hours with little or no compensation, have no opportunities for advancement, live in

**TABLE 34-1**   Push Pull Factors

| PUSH | PULL |
|------|------|
| ■ Low wages | ■ Training opportunities |
| ■ Lack of benefits (pension, housing, etc.) | ■ Shortage of health personnel in developed countries |
| ■ Fear of occupational infection | ■ Better standard of living for self and family |
| ■ Occupational stress | ■ Prestige |
| ■ Dysfunctional health system (lack of equipment, supplies, drugs, etc.) | ■ Personal network of friends and family |
| ■ Gender-based discrimination | |
| ■ Poor leadership | |
| ■ Limited career prospects | |
| ■ Political instability | |
| ■ Poor economic conditions (lack of good schools and employment opportunities for family members) | |

From Buchan, J., & Calman, L. (2004). *The global shortage of registered nurses: An overview of issues and actions.* Geneva: International Council of Nurses; Physicians for Human Rights. (2004). *An action plan to prevent brain drain: Building equitable health systems in Africa.* Boston: Physicians for Human Rights; Stilwell, B., Diallo, K., Zurn, P., Dal Poz, M. R., Adams, O., & Buchan, J. (2003). Developing evidence-based ethical policies on the migration of health workers: Conceptual and practical challenges. *Human Resources for Health,* 1(1), 8.

difficult and dangerous social circumstances, and fear for their own safety because of human immunodeficiency virus (HIV) and acquired immunodeficiency syndrome (AIDS), civil unrest, and other, related concerns. In fact, significant increases in salary may have little impact on retaining nurses given the strength of other push factors (Dovlo, 2003). Pull factors, on the other hand, are those that outweigh the push factors and cause nurses to stay in their current circumstance or attract them to other situations. The subcategories are quite similar to those falling within the push category, but they reflect more-favorable rather than less-favorable circumstances.

As one might imagine, pull factors and push factors reflect a dynamic that compels an individual to make a choice at some point either to stay or to leave, particularly in the face of their perceived inability to change the conditions that they currently face. The powerlessness to change the status quo is a major factor in moving one from contemplating options to actually making a conscious choice.

It is important to note that nurses in resource-poor countries are not alone in facing push factors. In fact, the inadequate supply of nurses in the developed world reflects a highly complex set of conditions that have either made retention of

nurses difficult or made nursing a relatively unattractive profession to young people. In these countries, the ever-increasing complexity of care in hospitals, draconian cost-containment and "reform" strategies, issues relating to work conditions and career opportunities, and public devaluing of the profession have had a major impact on nurses' decisions to stay or leave the profession and on the ability to replace them with young people choosing first-time career training.

The decision to migrate to another country is one that is not made in isolation from the influences of others. In fact, increasingly the migration of nurses has been influenced by aggressive marketing opportunities and recruitment by paid recruiters who offer services that facilitate movement to other countries. Marketing and recruiting practices associated with institutions and systems in developed countries have met major criticisms relating to insensitivity to the needs of poorer countries and the ethics surrounding their actual practices. Concerns regarding recruiting practices led to the establishment of the "Code of Practice for the International Recruitment of Healthcare Professionals: December 2004" for recruiting practices in the United Kingdom. However, other countries have been slow in adopting similar frameworks, standards, or regulations.

It is useful to examine the case example of one country relative to the complexity of dynamics associated with the migration of nurses. The United States is, by far, the largest consumer of nurses when compared with any other country. Clearly, the health system of the United States has placed a very strong emphasis on institutionally based, technologically intense care. Hospitals are the primary focus for this care. And, because of cost-driven reduction of patients' length of stay in these hospitals, the intensity and complexity of their care is greater than ever. As a result, of the 2,201,800 employed nurses in the United States, 59.1% work in the hospital sector (U.S. Department of Health and Human Services, 2000). To meet the nursing demand, the U.S. Bureau of Labor Statistics estimates that 1,000,000 new and replacement nurses will be needed by 2012 (Occupational Outlook Quarterly, 2004), this at a time with a decrease of United States–trained nurses entering the profession (American Association of Colleges of Nursing, 2005). The inflow of newly licensed foreign-trained nurses is rapidly increasing, and approximately one third of the increase in nurses in the United States from 2001 to 2003 represented foreign-born nurses (Aiken, 2005). Currently, foreign-born nurses account for 11% of the U.S. nursing stock, and the labor market would be able to absorb significantly more foreign-born nurses without affecting the shortage (Aiken, 2005).

The United States is not alone in its seemingly unquenchable thirst for foreign-born nurses, 80% of who come from the developing world (Aiken, 2005). The United Kingdom, Australia, and Canada have had similar experiences, although of smaller magnitude.

## Controversy and Complexity

The recent history of global migration of nurses has brought fundamental questions about the rights of individuals and the well-being of nations to the forefront of public attention. Headlines about unethical recruiters "poaching" desperately needed nurses from the world's poorest countries appear in mainstream national newspaper worldwide. The media tell stories about nurses being wooed from countries in which the serious needs of patients and communities are being left unmet, resulting in even worsening conditions within these countries. These stories also speak to the developed world's seemingly endless appetite for nurses.

Within resource-poor countries, the complexity of the situation becomes quite clear when one attempts to catalogue the varying perspectives. For health institutions and systems the loss of nurses is devastating, and there are few, if any, solutions in sight. For the nurses who leave, there are opportunities to better their own lives and those of their families as they seek higher salaries, more education, and better, safer work conditions. For the families left behind, there is the cost of the missing family member, but at the same time, the benefit of remittances (the portion of workers' earnings from employment abroad that is saved and sent home) that promise to improve their lives. A nurse in Kenya is paid about $70 a month (Physicians for Human Rights, 2004), so working in a developed country can significantly increase family income. Government officials in sending countries who are outside of the health sectors are also conflicted in their views of migration. On the one hand, they may see remittances as money that benefits the community and country (remittances from Filipinos equaled 9.45% of the Philippines' gross domestic product [GDP] in 2002 [International Organization for Migration, 2005b), yet they are also aware of the great cost incurred by their country when a nurse leaves. Governments are also caught in the human rights dilemma of trying to preserve vital health resources while protecting the individual rights of the nurses involved.

Although the complexities surrounding migration have been in place for decades, recent important global developments have introduced new concerns and possibilities. Specifically, governments have begun to negotiate agreements with another country (bilateral) or more than one other country (multilateral) that structure frameworks for nurse migration. The most simple of these are straightforward agreements that involve the "sending" or exportation of a specific number of nurses over a specified period of time, with some sort of compensation or assistance provided by the receiving country to the sending country. Such agreements have been in place for a number of years, particularly in regions with close cultural and geographic proximity (Aiken, Buchan, Sochalski, Nichols, & Powell, 2004). One such area is the Caribbean region, in which there have been bilateral and multilateral agreements in place that relate to both the training and service of nurses (Reid, 2000).

Another type of agreement that has emerged relates to promises by developed countries to recruit only in certain circumstances. "The Code of Practice for the International Recruitment of Healthcare Professionals: December 2004" (Eastwood et al., 2005) was developed by the U.K.'s Department for Health to specifically address concerns about unethical recruiting practices and the perception of "poaching" nurses in the developing world. This agreement has been heralded as a model for other developed countries to adopt as one way of addressing poor recruiting practices.

Recent agreements among governments are also beginning to incorporate the private sector as well. For example, smaller countries may seek to develop a relationship with a major health system in a developed country. Also, bilateral and regional multilateral agreements are becoming overshadowed by the establishment of global trade agreements that include health and other services. The most comprehensive and controversial of all of these is the General Agreement on Trade in Services (GATS), adopted in 1995 by some 140 countries (Adlung & Carzaniga, 2001). GATS allows countries to make commitments to particular sectors, including health services, and GATS specifically incorporates the services of health professionals into the agreement, which opens up even greater possibilities for migration of nurses.

The movement of nurse migration into the domain of global trade introduces an enormous number of new forces and factors that need to be addressed if resource-poor countries are to be served. For example, ministries of health are seldom if ever involved in the development and negotiation of trade agreements. This means that decisions relating to nurse migration may be made apart from public health concerns. Issues of human

rights and the vulnerability of the developing world are not always fully considered in global trade agreements. And, of course, trade agreements are generally not at all associated with the need to improve work conditions in resource-poor countries as part of retention strategies.

The growing importance of trade agreements as factors in enabling and shaping global nurse migration is reflective of the reality of a global health marketplace. Increasingly, services, goods, and information relating to health and health care are crossing national borders. As this occurs, these forces inevitably shape the actions of individuals, institutions, and nations. One recent example is the growing interest in offering actual U.S. nursing licensure examinations in other countries. Unfortunately, most of the forces at work appear to move in the direction of enabling migration from resource-poor countries to the wealthier developed countries.

## BALANCING THE EQUATION: STRATEGIES FOR MANAGING MIGRATION

Until early 2000 the migration of nurses was generally not seen as a major concern requiring government intervention or management. This reflected both the invisibility of nurses as an important part of delivering health services and the migration of people as a common experience for these countries. However, as the enormous appetite for nurses in developed countries began to seriously deplete the population of nurses, and as health crises such as HIV and AIDS became more widespread, governments, the private sector, and professional groups began to try to find ways to respond differently.

In some countries, such as the Philippines, there was recognition that production of nurses for import could have a positive economic impact on both the private sector and the overall economy. Although no specific governmental plan was implemented, there was general support for the development of educational capacity to train nurses for export. In other countries, efforts were made to restrict or discourage migration through punitive measures such as bonds or other "taxes" on nurses leaving the country. Zimbabwe "bonds" nurses for 3 years before they are allowed to leave the country. Ghana and Lesotho have similar schemes but these can be difficult to enforce and often result in new graduates staying whereas more-experienced nurses are free to leave (Physicians for Human Rights, 2004). Furthermore, some countries even make it difficult for nurses returning to their home countries to resume their careers in nursing and often require these experienced nurses to begin in the lowest-paid, starting positions. What has become apparent is that none of these individual single-country strategies has really succeeded in actually assuring an adequate nursing workforce. Piecemeal strategies within individual countries have simply not worked well.

## The Caribbean Experience—Managed Migration

The failure of single-country, scattered efforts to address migration was noted within a number of countries in the Caribbean. Because the region has a history of collaboration within nursing among a number of Caribbean countries, there was a natural opportunity to consider a markedly different approach to address the crisis of nurses leaving the region. And a true crisis it was and continues to be. Each year, Jamaica loses around 8% of its registered nurses and over 20% of its specialist nurses (*Gleaner,* 2002); roughly two thirds of the nurse population of Jamaica has already emigrated (Lowell & Findlay, 2001). In 2003 the average vacancy rate in the countries of the Caribbean Community (CARICOM) was 40%, with individual country rates ranging from 10% to over 50% (Pan-American Health Organization [PAHO], 2003).

The loss of nurses in the Caribbean has had a devastating effect for several reasons. These include the relative numbers of nurses who leave the region coupled with the unrelieved loss of these nurses. The loss of the most experienced nurses and tutors in nursing schools has been crippling. Furthermore, the inability to assimilate nurses when they return has been a deterrent to returnees. The Caribbean has also been particularly targeted by aggressive recruitment from developed countries and, at the same time, faces increased demand for and complexity of care within the region.

In 2001 the PAHO Office of Caribbean Program Coordination initiated a review of the scope and impact of nurses' migration in the Caribbean. This review resulted in the creation of a steering committee to lead in the development of an overall strategy for the region. Building on the concept of Managed Migration originally developed in Jamaica, the Steering Committee defined the Managed Migration Program of the Caribbean as "…a regional strategy for retaining an adequate number of competent nursing personnel to deliver health programs and services to the Caribbean

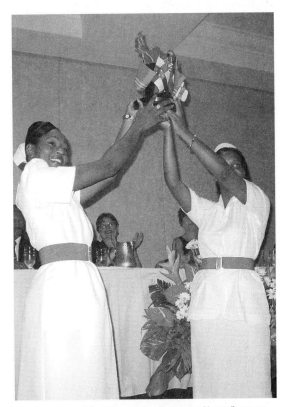

In celebration of the "Year of the Caribbean Nurse," nurses hold aloft a special Caribbean nursing symbol featuring a lighted lamp against a backdrop of all the region's flags, highlighting the theme of "Nurses Lighting the Way to Professional Excellence." Observed from May of 2003 to August of 2004, the celebration of nursing and nurses focused on increasing recruitment and retention, strengthening nursing and midwifery services, and recognizing the best of nursing and nurses in the region.

nationals at the highest level of quality" (Deyal, 2003). They identified two foundational values: nurses have the right as individuals to freedom of movement within and beyond the region, and all people have the right of access to high-quality health services and programs. They articulated an overall proactive approach encouraging governments and other stakeholders to play a more-active role in the migration of health workers.

Ultimately, these concepts were incorporated into the formal Managed Migration Program of Work through identification of six critical areas: terms and conditions of work; recruitment, retention, and training; value of nursing; utilization

and deployment; management practices; and policy development. To move the Program of Work forward, a Managed Migration Implementation Team was created in 2001 and included representatives from ministries of health (Regional Nursing Board), professional organizations (Chief Nursing Officers), training institutions, regulatory bodies, labor unions, and regional agencies (PAHO, CARICOM, and the University of the West Indies). Table 34-2 identifies the programs and partners associated with each of the Critical Areas within the Managed Migration Program of Work.

The Managed Migration Program continues to evolve. Individual countries have adopted strategies

**TABLE 34-2**  Caribbean Managed Migration Implementation Plan—Partnership Matrix

| CRITICAL AREAS | PROGRAMS | PARTNERS |
|---|---|---|
| Terms and conditions of work | Convention on Nursing | RNB, PAHO, ILO |
| | Training Program (SOLVE) | RNB, PAHO, ILO |
| | Health Workplace | RNB, PAHO, UK Department of Health |
| Recruitment, retention, and training | Caribbean Nursing Campaign | RNB, CNO, PAHO, LCCIN, J&J RNB, PAHO |
| | Study on Training Capacity in Nursing | DANE, UWI, PAHO, Health Canada |
| | Distance Education Program in Nursing (BSc and Masters) | RNB, COMSEC |
| | Mentorship Program | |
| Value of nursing | Social Marketing | RNB, COMSEC |
| | Caribbean Nursing Website | RNB, CNO, PAHO, LCCIN |
| | Year of the Caribbean Nurse | RNB, CNO, PAHO, UWI, LCCIN, J&J, UK Department of Health, Health Canada, LIAT |
| Utilization and deployment | Workload Measurement System | RNB, PAHO, BVI Department of Health Services (for regional license), GRASP Inc. |
| Management practices | Magnet Program | RNB, PAHO, ANCC, LCCIN |
| | Leadership for Change Program | RNB, ICN |
| Policy and health service research | Regional Managed Migration Plan | RNB, PAHO, CARICOM Regional Negotiating Machinery |
| | Attachment and Exchange Programs | RNB, LCCIN, Health Canada |

ANCC—American Nurses Credentialing Center, *www.nursingworld.org/ancc*
BVI—British Virgin Islands, *www.bvi.gov.vg/template.php?main=atbvi&section=health*
Caricom—Caribbean Community, *www.caricom.org*
COMSEC—Commonwealth Secretariat, *www.thecommonwealth.org*
DANE—Department of Advance Nursing Education, UWI, *www.mona.uwi.edu/fms/index.htm*
GRASP Inc.—*www.graspinc.com*
Health Canada—*www.hc-sc.gc.ca/*
ICN—International Council of Nurses, *www.icn.ch*
ILO—International Labor Organization, *www.ilo.org*
J&J—Johnson and Johnson, *www.discovernursing.com*
LCCIN—Lillian Carter Center for International Nursing, *www.nursing.emory.edu/lccin*
LIAT—LIAT Airlines, *www.liatairline.com*
PAHO—Pan American Health Organization, *www.paho.org*
RNB—Regional Nursing Body, *www.nursing.emory.edu/lccin/rnb*
UK Department of Health—*www.dh.gov.uk*
UWI—University of West Indies, *www.uwi.edu*

aimed at managing migration in their own contexts, and the focus of discussion and vision for Managed Migration has begun to identify potential opportunities for macromanagement of migration through trade and multilateral agreements relating to nursing service and education. Within the region a number of interesting initiatives are being developed to maximize the benefits and minimize the costs to the countries and to the professionals. Examples of these arrangements are as follows:

- Grenada has opened up its excess training capacity to neighboring Antigua.
- The Caribbean Canadian Proposal allows temporary movement of skilled nursing professionals but involves creating incentives for nurses to return to the Caribbean and disincentives to overstay in Canada.
- Temporary migration of Jamaican nurses, who spend 2 weeks working in Miami and the remainder of the month working in Jamaica.

The Managed Migration Program as a strategy shows that governments and stakeholders can work together in developing interventions to ensure that migration is managed and moderated. It is a good example of a coordinated intervention that minimizes the impact of migration while securing some benefits from the process.

## THE UNITED STATES: PROFESSIONAL RESPONSIBILITY AND GLOBAL CITIZENSHIP

The United States occupies a particularly important place in the myriad of forces that shape the global migration of nurses. As the single largest consumer of foreign nurses and one of the world's leading nations, the United States has the potential to make the greatest contributions to assuring the balanced development of nursing capacity around the world.

The single most significant action that the United States could take is to solve its own nursing workforce shortage. Although there is growing awareness of the impact of the U.S. nursing shortage on the health of its own citizens, there has been little concern nationally about the devastation that our shortage is having on other countries as the United States aggressively consumes resources abroad. Unless the United States actually solves or at least reduces its shortage of U.S. born nurses, the likelihood of resource-poor countries being able to address their shortages is extremely small.

### Action at the National Level

Until the U.S. shortage is solved, a number of actions can be taken by both the U.S. government and the nursing profession. Because global trade policies are heavily driven by U.S. interests, it is very important that issues of global nursing shortages be part of trade discussions and negotiations. Congress and government trade representatives should be made aware of the challenges and influenced to adopt trade positions that are of benefit to the resource-poor countries. This will mean that nursing leaders and others in the health arena will need to become informed and able to navigate the complexities of trade policies and practices.

It is also very important that U.S. foreign aid, regardless of source, be aimed at building health-related human resources capacity within all countries receiving aid. Increasingly it is becoming apparent that programs aimed at global health issues, such as HIV and AIDS, are facing major challenges on the ground because of the lack of health workers to implement them. A recent estimate shows that sub-Saharan Africa has a shortfall of over 600,000 nurses needed to meet the Millennium Development Goals (Buchan & Calman, 2004). As well, the success of other types of aid programs, such as those aimed at education and agriculture, is being threatened by the serious health problems facing poorer nations—the same nations whose health workforces are eroding through migration.

The United States can also help resource-poor countries address factors that will recruit and retain nurses, including improved work conditions, education, and status of nursing within society at large. Technical assistance, targeted funding, performance requirements for loans, and other types of mechanisms can be used by both public and nongovernmental organizations to help these countries address their ongoing workforce capacity needs. Again, this means that U.S. agencies need to become better informed and more involved in these types of strategies. This also means that nurses in the United States need to be active in these arenas and become able to discuss and shape this important work.

### Action at the Individual Level

The profession of nursing and all of its members must take responsibility for making positive contributions to the problems associated with the migration of nurses. Individual nurses can engage in a vast array of activities ranging from those in the work setting to global policy. On a very simple, everyday level, U.S.-born nurses can be professionally and personally supportive of foreign-born nurses to assure their safe practice and fair treatment. It is truly possible for every U.S.-born nurse today to be a responsible, global citizen here in our work settings. The more that we learn about the cultures, values, interests, experiences, and capacities of foreign-born nurses, the better care becomes and the more enriched we are as individuals and professionals.

The professional responsibility of U.S.-born nurses also includes activism through our professional organizations. It is crucial that these associations weigh in on matters of trade, foreign aid, immigration policy, regulation, and standards relating to recruitment and the treatment of foreign-born nurses in the United States. This requires a much different knowledge and skill set than most of us have developed; however, without the ability to act, the problems will only be exacerbated. And, again, U.S. nurses need to continue to press for solutions to our own shortage.

There are many other things that U.S. nurses can do to improve the global nurse migration situation. Nurses who volunteer to serve in resource-poor countries, working through reputable agencies and programs, can help to educate nurses, improve work conditions, and build important networks that transcend boundaries. When U.S. nurses see themselves as global citizens and interface with global professional, mission, relief, and other health-related organizations, such as the International Council of Nurses and the World Health Organization, significant improvements can be realized in the lives of nurses and those they serve worldwide.

## Key Points

- The migration of nurses is increasing and must be recognized and responded to at the global level by policymakers, health ministers, finance ministers, international organizations, and others. With a global shortfall of nurses, attempts to address shortages in one country by hiring foreign-born nurses often leads to shortages in other countries.
- The United States and other developed nations need to solve their nursing shortages within national borders rather than relying on hiring nurses away from resource-poor countries.
- Governments need to address the "push factors" that lead to shortages by improving work conditions for nurses (e.g., wages commensurate with skills and responsibilities, training and advancement opportunities, safe work environments) and social conditions (e.g., standard of living, access to education, political stability).
- Nurses as individuals have the right to migrate. Programs that facilitate the movement of nurses to and from host countries and that also benefit the countries from which the nurses depart can be developed. The Caribbean has adopted the Managed Migration Program to minimize the impact of "out" migration while securing some benefits from the process.

## Web Resources

**Commission on Graduates of Foreign Nursing Schools**
*www.cgfns.org*
**Global Health Trust**
*www.globalhealthtrust.org*
**International Council of Nurses**
*www.icn.ch*
**International Organization for Migration**
*www.iom.int*
**U.K. Department of Health**
*www.dh.gov.uk/Home/fs/en*
**U.S. Health Resources and Services Administration**
*http://bhpr.hrsa.gov*
**World Health Organization**
*www.who.int*

## REFERENCES

Adlung, R., & Carzaniga, A. (2001). Health services under the General Agreement on Trade in Services. *Bulletin of the World Health Organization, 79*(4), 352-364.

Aiken, L. H. (2005). Bellagio Conference on International Nurse Migration. Retrieved September 1, 2005, from *www.academyhealth.org/international/nursemigration/aiken.pdf.*

Aiken, L. H., Buchan, J., Sochalski, J., Nichols, B., & Powell, M. (2004). Trends in international nurse migration. *Health Affairs, 23*(3), 69-77.

American Association of Colleges of Nursing. (2005). Nursing shortage fact sheet. Retrieved August 31, 2005, from *www.aacn.nche.edu/Media/pdf/NursingShortageFactSheet.pdf.*

Anand, S., & Barnighausen, T. (2004). Human resources and health outcomes: Cross-country econometric study. *Lancet, 5*(364), 1603-1609.

Buchan, J., & Calman, L. (2004). *The global shortage of registered nurses: An overview of issues and actions.* Geneva: International Council of Nurses.

Buchan, J., & Dovlo, D. (2004). International recruitment of health workers to the UK: A report for DFID. Retrieved August 31, 2005, from *www.dfidhealthrc.org/shared/publications/reports/int_rec/int-rec-main.pdf.*

Deyal, T. (2003). Hasta la vista, paradise! Retrieved October 12, 2005, from *www.paho.org/English/DD/PIN/Number17_article5_4.htm.*

Dovlo, D. (2003). The brain drain and retention of health professionals in Africa. Retrieved August 31, 2005, from *www.worldbank.org/afr/teia/conf_0903/dela_dovlo.pdf.*

Dugger, C. W. (2004, July 12). An exodus of African nurses puts infants and the ill in peril. *New York Times,* A1, A6-A7.

Eastwood, J., Conroy, R., Naicker, S., West, P., Tutt, R., & Plange-Rhule, J. (2005). Loss of health professionals from sub-Saharan Africa: The pivotal role of the UK. *Lancet, 365,* 1893-1900.

General Assembly Resolution 217 A (III). (1948). Universal Declaration of Human Rights. Retrieved August 25, 2005, from *www.un.org/rights/50/decla.htm.*

*Gleaner.* (2002, May 20). US, UK seeking more local nurses. *Gleaner.* Retrieved April 9, 2006, from *www.jamaica-gleaner.com/gleaner/20020520/lead/lead6.html.*

International Organization for Migration. (2005a). *International migration: Facts and figures.* Retrieved August 29, 2005, from *www.iom.int.*

International Organization for Migration. (2005b). *World migration 2005: Costs and benefits of international migration.* Geneva: International Organization for Migration.

Lowell, B. L., & Findlay, A. M. (2001). *Migration of highly skilled persons from developing countries: Impact and policy responses.* Geneva: International Labour Organization.

Occupational Outlook Quarterly. (2004). High-paying occupations with many openings, projected 2002-12. Retrieved October 11, 2005, from *www.bls.gov/opub/ooq/2004/spring/oochart.pdf.*

Pan American Health Organization (PAHO). (2003). Country Profiles: Guyana. *Epidemiological Bulletin, 24*(1), 9-13.

Physicians for Human Rights. (2004). *An action plan to prevent brain drain: Building equitable health systems in Africa.* Boston: Physicians for Human Rights.

Reid, U. V. (2000). Regional Examination for Nurse Registration, Commonwealth Caribbean. *International Nursing Review, 47,* 174-183.

Stilwell, B., Diallo, K., Zurn, P., Dal Poz, M. R., Adams, O., & Buchan, J. (2003). Developing evidence-based ethical policies on the migration of health workers: Conceptual and practical challenges. *Human Resources for Health, 1*(1), 8.

United Nations. (2003). *Trends in migrant stock: The 2003 revision.* New York: Department of Economic and Social Affairs, Population Division.

United Nations Population Division. (2002). The international migrant stock: A global view. Retrieved August 31, 2005, from *www.iom.int/DOCUMENTS/OFFICIALTXT/EN/UNPD_Handout.pdf.*

U.S. Department of Health and Human Services. (2000). The registered nurse population: Findings from the National Sample Survey of Registered Nurses. Retrieved August 31, 2005, from *ftp://ftp.hrsa.gov/bhpr/rnsurvey2000/rnsurvey00.pdf.*

# Infectious Disease: A Global Health Care Challenge

Felissa R. Lashley

*"I skate to where the puck is going to be, not to where it has been."*

WAYNE GRETZKY

As we begin the twenty-first century, the problem of infectious diseases, especially those considered to be emerging, continues to demand new attention, cooperation, collaboration, and resources. Throughout history various authors and historians have documented the relationship between infectious disease and political, economic, and social instability. These events serve dual roles as both causative factors and outcomes.

## BACKGROUND

In the mid-twentieth century it was widely believed that infectious diseases could be controlled by hygienic and sanitary practices, antibiotics, and immunizations and therefore did not present a meaningful threat to public health. The well-known immunologist and Nobel laureate Sir MacFarlane Burnet wrote in 1962 that one could think of the middle of the twentieth century as the end of one of the most important social revolutions in history, the virtual elimination of infectious disease as a significant factor in social life (Burnet, 1962, p. 3). Indeed, the number of deaths resulting from infectious diseases in the United States had decreased significantly for a number of reasons. These included the discovery and use of antibiotics, widespread immunization programs, and strong public health infrastructure and surveillance systems.

## Emergence of Drug-Resistant Microorganisms

Between 1980 and 1992 this changed, and the death rate from infectious diseases increased 58% (Centers for Disease Control and Prevention [CDC], 1999). The most famous emerging infectious disease contributing to significant morbidity and mortality worldwide was, and still is, human immunodeficiency virus (HIV) infection and acquired immunodeficiency syndrome (AIDS), along with associated sequelae such as multidrug-resistant tuberculosis. Among the reasons for the increased emergence of certain infectious agents and drug-resistant organisms has been a prevalent complacency that infectious diseases are no longer a threat, particularly in developed countries.

## Protecting the Public versus Individual Rights

Another trend that eventually shaped policies in a negative way for public health (although in a positive way for patient rights) is the emphasis on individual rights over the needs and greater good of the community and population (Richards, 2001). From this perspective, Nobel laureate Joshua Lederberg noted that today restraining the rights and freedoms of individuals is a far greater sin than allowing the infection of others, and went on to say that the restraints placed on Typhoid Mary might not be acceptable today, when some would prefer to give her unlimited rein to infect others, with litigation their only recourse (Lederberg, 1997). Typhoid Mary (Mary Mallon) was a cook who was an asymptomatic typhoid carrier. She infected numerous families for whom she worked in New York with typhoid during the period of 1906 to 1915.

She was isolated twice—an early isolation period, from which she was released, only to infect more people, and a second, permanent confinement to North Brother Island from 1915 until her death in 1938. Discussion of the U.S. Supreme Court case of *Jacobson v. Massachusetts* in 1905 has brought attention to the need for preserving respect for individual liberty while protecting the public health. In this case, Jacobson (a private citizen) challenged the Cambridge, Massachusetts Board of Health's authority to require smallpox vaccination during an epidemic. The state's power for specific, mandatory action to protect the public by compulsory vaccination was upheld (Gostin, 2005; Mariner, Annas, & Glantz, 2005).

### Defining Emerging and Reemerging Infections

In 1992, a report was released by the Institute of Medicine (IOM) that called attention to the global problem of emerging infectious diseases (Lederberg, Shope, & Oaks, 1992). This was followed by two reports from the CDC (CDC, 1994, 1998). *Emerging infectious diseases* were defined as new, reemerging, or drug-resistant infections whose incidence in humans has increased within the past two decades or whose incidence threatens to increase in the near future. *Reemerging diseases* refers to the reappearance of a known disease after a decline in incidence (Lederberg et al., 1992). This has been elaborated on to include not only newly recognized organisms and new diseases caused by known organisms, but also an extension of the geographic range of an organism or one causing infection in a new host, such as a disease that has moved from animals to humans (Lashley, 2003, 2004; Lashley & Durham, 2002). The emergence or reemergence of infectious diseases may result from a variety of factors, alone or in combination. Thirteen factors were identified in a 2003 report from the IOM updating the 1992 report (Lederberg et al., 1992; Smolinski, Hamburg, & Lederberg, 2003). These factors include the following (Cohen & Larson, 1996; Lashley, 2003, 2004; Lashley & Durham, 2002; Lederberg et al., 1992; Smolinski et al., 2003):

- Social and behavioral changes, including increased use of childcare

- Increased use of antimicrobial agents, including those used in animal feed
- Globalization of travel and trade, and demands for exotic and imported foodstuffs
- Increased eating in restaurants and fast-food establishments, combined with greater popularity of buffets
- Widespread travel and recreational pursuits, bringing animals and people into closer contact
- Demographic factors such as population growth, migration, population demographics, and housing density
- Socioeconomic factors such as poverty and crowded conditions
- Environmental alterations and ecosystem changes, such as land use development, irrigation, deforestation, and natural disasters
- Climatic and weather changes such as global warming and increased rainfall
- Disasters (e.g., earthquakes) and wars and conflicts, resulting in stress, crowding, and declines in disease control and preventive health practices such as immunizations
- Decline in the public health infrastructure, resulting in deficiencies in communication and information, fewer and less-prepared staff, and limited public health laboratory capacity
- Microbial evolution such as mutation, new tissue specificities, and cross-species transmission
- Health care and technology advances such as iatrogenic immunosuppression, increases in organ transplantation, and use of medical devices
- Human immunocompromise from iatrogenic and developmental causes and from malnutrition resulting from famine and poverty
- Lack of political will to address needed health measures
- Deliberate dissemination of microbial agents for political and social purposes

### Bioterrorism

The actual and potential role of emerging infectious diseases in the national security of the United States and of other countries is well recognized (National Intelligence Council, 2000). Certain microorganisms remain potential agents for bioterrorist activities, especially those causing anthrax, smallpox, plague, and botulism, as well as more sophisticated approaches such as genetically altered influenza viruses. A troubling recent example was the deliberate dissemination of *Bacillus anthracis*, the bacteria causing anthrax, in parts of the United States beginning in September 2001. In late 2000, additional provisions for public health emergencies were signed into law as part of the Public Health Improvement Act (Public Law [PL] 106-505). This allowed an immediate response to public health emergencies, including infectious disease outbreaks or bioterrorist attacks.

## A GLOBAL CONCERN

Today, emerging infectious diseases are truly global, as one can travel around the world in only 30 hours, and can no longer be considered as only internal or domestic. For example:

- The West Nile virus was recognized in the Western hemisphere only in 1999, yet it was recognized earlier as a cause of encephalitis in Africa, the Middle East, and parts of Europe (Hughes, 2001). In only a few short years, West Nile virus spread across the Western hemisphere, with a high potential for becoming endemic (Granwehr et al., 2004).

- The coronavirus associated with severe acute respiratory syndrome (SARS) first emerged in southern China in late 2002. A traveler who was incubating SARS traveled from Guangdong province to Hong Kong. In the course of his activities he infected fellow hotel guests in Hong Kong, who then returned to their own countries, seeding SARS outbreaks in at least 26 countries (Christian, Poutanen, Loutfy, Muller, & Low, 2004; Skowronski et al., 2005). In February of 2003 the World Health Organization (WHO) first reported an outbreak of "acute respiratory syndrome" in China (WHO, 2003). This outbreak, with the accompanying global pandemic alert by WHO, resulted in severe economic effects from loss of tourism in various cities including Toronto, Canada. The outbreak was considered contained in July of 2003 (Christian et al., 2004; Poon, Guan, Nichols, Yuen, & Peiris, 2004).

- The epidemiologic link between certain animals such as palm civets in China that become close to

humans in situations such as wet markets (where live animals are sold) has called attention to the legal and illegal trade in domestic and exotic animals. In the United States, an example was the human monkeypox outbreak that occurred in the midwestern United States in 2003. This outbreak was found to have been caused by contact with affected prairie dogs that had been housed during transport with an infected Gambian giant rat (CDC, 2003b), and an embargo on the import, sale, and transport of rodents from Africa and the sale or movement of prairie dogs was announced in June 2003 (CDC, 2003a).

- The avian influenza H5N1 outbreak, in which there has been transmission from infected birds to humans, began in 1997 in Hong Kong with what was thought to be limited human-to-human transmission (Bridges et al., 2002). A more recent outbreak beginning in 2004 with human-to-human transmission has caused concern about the possibility of a pandemic. By April 12, 2006, 194 confirmed human cases of avian influenza had been reported to WHO, and 109 people had died (WHO, 2006).

These outbreaks have sparked various conferences and documents addressing international cooperation for surveillance, prevention, epidemiologic investigation, rapid diagnosis, and research across disciplines including among those who focus on animals and insects and those who focus on humans (WHO, 2005a; Knobler, Mack, Mahmoud, & Lemon, 2005).

The major policies associated with emerging and reemerging global infectious disease outbreaks are communicable disease surveillance and reporting, immunization, quarantine, travel and immigration restrictions, the use of antimicrobial agents, good sanitation, vector control, access to clean drinking water and food, and restrictions related to import and export of goods and animals. This policy spotlight concentrates on the first five of these.

## SURVEILLANCE AND REPORTING POLICIES

For the most part, policies that address emerging infectious disease threats take place on the national, state, or local level rather than in the international arena. There is, however, a legal treaty known as the

*International Health Regulations*, which was adopted in 1971 and amended in the 1980s, long before epidemics of the viral hemorrhagic diseases such as Ebola were known. New regulations were adopted by the World Health Assembly on May 23, 2005 and will come into effect in June 2007. The purpose and scope is to prevent, protect against, control, and provide a public health response to the international spread of disease in ways that are commensurate with and restricted to public health risks, and which avoid unnecessary interference with international traffic and trade (WHO, 2005b). A public health emergency of international concern refers to an extraordinary public health event determined to constitute a public health risk to other states through the international spread of disease and to potentially require a coordinated international response (WHO, 2005b). This broadens the scope from the original three specified diseases (cholera, plague, and yellow fever) to include a spectrum of diseases and emergencies. Coordination with other groups such as the World Trade Organization and the Food and Agriculture Organization will be important because of measures related to food safety and standards and because of the trade in animals.

## Surveillance and Reporting Systems

Surveillance and reporting for infectious diseases relies on both formal and informal systems and may be broad or narrowed to one or few specific organisms or settings. Examples of these systems include the following:

- In the United States the CDC has mandated reporting from the states for certain nationally notifiable diseases such as AIDS through the National Notifiable Disease Surveillance System (NNDSS); reports are transmitted through the National Electronic Telecommunications System for Surveillance (NETSS).
- The CDC also has other surveillance activities, including syndromic surveillance; sentinel surveillance; an eight-city enhanced terrorism surveillance project; an Emerging Infections Program Network that includes an Active Bacterial Core Surveillance program; the National Malaria Surveillance System; the Health Alert Network; the National Respiratory and Enteric Virus Surveillance System; the National West Nile Virus Surveillance System; the National Tuberculosis Genotyping and Surveillance Network; and others. Certain data analysis can be applied to syndromic surveillance systems for early detection of outbreaks, especially those that might be part of a terrorist event, such as the Enhanced Surveillance Project, which monitors sentinel hospital emergency rooms when high-profile events such as the Super Bowl take place, and the Early Aberration Reporting System, which is another syndromic surveillance tool.
- FoodNet (Foodborne Diseases Active Surveillance Network) is a collaborative project including cooperation among the CDC, Emerging Infections Program sites, the U.S. Department of Agriculture, and the U.S. Food and Drug Administration. The focus is on active surveillance for foodborne diseases.
- GeoSentinel (Global Emerging Infections Sentinel Network) is funded through an agreement with CDC and consists of travel and tropical medicine clinics around the world that monitor trends in morbidity among travelers through the International Society of Travel Medicine.
- The National Nosocomial Infections Surveillance System (NNIS) is under the Hospital Infections Program of the CDC, which also cooperates with Emory University in Project ICARE (Intensive Care Antimicrobial Resistance Epidemiology), providing data on antimicrobial resistance and use in U.S. health care agencies. The Gonococcal Isolate Surveillance Project monitors antimicrobial resistance in *Neisseria gonorrhoeae*, and Surveillance of Emerging Antimicrobial Resistance Connected to Healthcare (SEARCH) specifically reports on the isolation of *Staphylococcus aureus* with reduced susceptibility to vancomycin in a network of hospitals, health departments, and others.
- The Border Infectious Disease Surveillance (BIDS) project is an example of an interregional system that has been developed along the U.S.–Mexican border with the cooperation of the Mexican Secretariat of Health, CDC, certain

state and Mexican border health departments, and the Pan American Health Organization (PAHO). BIDS focuses on surveillance in sister cities, such as Nuevo Laredo, Mexico, and Laredo, Texas. An example of the fruits of these efforts in detecting emerging infectious diseases has been the detection of dengue fever at the U.S.–Mexican border.

- WHO has a variety of global and regional surveillance activities. Under the overall umbrella of Communicable Disease Surveillance and Response (SCR) is the Global Outbreak Alert and Response Network (GOARN), which consists of a variety of ministries of health, WHO regional and country offices, nongovernmental agencies, and more. It monitors communicable diseases and related conditions such as chemical events and food and water safety. WHO also has specific outbreak verification lists and surveillance networks such as the WHO Influenza Surveillance Network and the Mediterranean Zoonoses Control Programme.
- Specific regional endeavors exist, such as the Integrated Disease Surveillance and Response (IDSR), which is a strategy of the WHO African Regional Office with technical assistance by the CDC and others.
- ProMED *(www.promedmail.org)* is an online information system and discussion forum for infectious disease professionals worldwide.
- The Global Public Health Intelligence Network is an early warning system through the Public Health Agency of Canada for chemical, biologic, radiologic, and nuclear public health threats throughout the world.
- Cell for Epidemic Alert and Response (CARE) is a program of the Institut Pasteur in France that recognizes that a public health problem has appeared and that can provide assistance.

Many other country-specific networks exist. Despite these networks, many of the laws governing the reporting of communicable diseases became somewhat weakened in the period of time when the public health infrastructure was not well funded and began to deteriorate. However, the potential for infectious disease agents to be used as weapons has renewed detection and response networks.

## IMMUNIZATION POLICY

Immunization laws are specific for school entry, children, and immigrants. They spell out the types of vaccinations that are needed in various circumstances as well as the information on the risks and benefits of vaccination that must be given to parents and guardians before their child is immunized. School immunization laws in the United States are state mandated, and exemptions, such as for religious reasons, are specified. At this time, immunizations for travel and for adults (except for military personnel) are recommended but not mandated. As of July 1997, all individuals seeking permanent entry to the United States must prove that they have been inoculated against all vaccine-preventable diseases (CDC, 2005). This includes infants or children entering as part of international adoption.

Among the recommendations from an IOM report on immunization practices and policies were calls for strengthening federal and state immunization partnerships, developing a strategy for increasing financial support, and ensuring that immunization policy be national in scope (Guyer, Smith, & Chalk, 2000). In the United States in 2002, preemptive mass public vaccination against smallpox was debated but not implemented. Arguments for it included protection against the release of the variola virus by terrorists; arguments against it included possible vaccine-related illness and the possible deaths of immunosuppressed persons (Fauci, 2002). Voluntary smallpox vaccination programs for hospital and public health workers recruited many fewer volunteers than anticipated.

## QUARANTINE POLICY

Quarantine is a major tool to contain contagious diseases. The United States maintains a Division of Global Migration and Quarantine within the CDC's National Center for Infectious Diseases. In 1967, when it moved from the Department of Health, Education, and Welfare, it had more than 500 staff members and 55 quarantine stations at every port, international airport, and major border crossing. The staff had had a marked decrease in recent years, and the number of quarantine stations was decreased. In response to concerns about bioterrorism and the importation of disease, the number of facilities was increased from eight in 2004 to 18 in 2005. The facilities have authority to detain, medically examine, and conditionally release individuals and wildlife suspected of carrying a communicable disease. The Division of Global Migration and Quarantine works in cooperation with other agencies, such as state and local health departments, the U.S. Customs Service, the Immigration and Naturalization Service (INS), the U.S. Fish and Wildlife Service, and the U.S. Department of Agriculture.

A list of quarantinable diseases is found in an Executive Order of the President. It includes such diseases as cholera, plague, infectious tuberculosis, yellow fever, and viral hemorrhagic fevers, and in 2005 an executive order added "influenza caused by novel or reemergent influenza viruses that are causing, or have the potential to cause, a pandemic" (CDC, National Center for Infectious Diseases, Division of Global Migration and Quarantine, 2000; Bush, 2005). Special quarantine policies may apply in wartime.

## TRAVEL AND IMMIGRATION POLICY

The movement of people for travel or migration has had effects on communicable diseases, both for the travelers and for natives of recipient nations. As the pandemic of HIV and AIDS grew, a movement began in the mid 1980s to secure national boundaries against travelers, migrants, refugees, and immigrants with AIDS (Gellert, 1993). Immigration laws in the United States have excluded aliens (defined as any person not a citizen or national) for health-related reasons since 1879, when such legislation was first enacted. Distinction may be made among immigrants, long-term and short-term travelers, temporary residents, and refugees seeking political asylum. Since then, modifications have been added, and several U.S. agencies have become involved with immigration laws. One of these is the Public Health Service, a branch of the Department of Health and Human Services; another is the aforementioned Division of Global Migration and Quarantine. Among the health-related criteria for exclusion of aliens is infection with any dangerous contagious disease (CDC, 2004b).

Quarantine and exclusion had rarely been used in the United States before 1994. In 1994, however, an outbreak of plague was reported from a region in India, and several countries closed their borders to travelers from India and discontinued air flights to and from India. Some countries behaved irrationally, banning such items as Indian postage stamps (Garrett, 2000). Under the International Health Regulations described earlier, plague is quarantinable, and vehicles and passengers may be detained or inspected. The CDC worked with airline employees and representatives of the INS and U.S. Customs in recognizing symptoms of plague. Heightened surveillance in place in the United States detected 13 persons with suspected plague identified in airports, and seven who had reached private physicians. None actually had the plague (Fritz et al., 1996). However, Garrett (2000) points out that the majority had already left their planes. Therefore if they had been ill with plague, they would have allowed exposure to many more contacts, including their fellow passengers.

In the late 1980s and early 1990s, amid a political storm, more than 50 countries instituted mandatory HIV testing for aliens despite appeals of various organizations, including WHO. An HIV test may be an entry requirement even for travelers staying in a given country for as little as 2 weeks. Some countries accept certification from the person's health care provider in his or her own country, whereas others do not. A major impetus behind this type of testing was supposedly to prevent HIV-infected persons from becoming an economic burden to the country they were entering, yet many viewed this as discrimination. In the United States, someone who is HIV positive can obtain a waiver for a maximum of 30 days.

Another example of the widespread effects of an infectious disease outbreak is the foot-and-mouth disease outbreak that began in England in February of 2001. Early responses were not forthcoming from the European Union, and countries responded individually to the threat. Responses included the banning of the importation of livestock, milk, and other bovine products first from Britain and then, as disease spread, from other countries affected. Other responses included the incineration of nearly 3 million farm animals in Great Britain, mass immunization, compensation to farmers whose animals were destroyed, and increased restriction of access of tourists and travelers to agricultural areas in affected countries. In some cases, returning travelers not only were questioned about whether they had visited farms, but had their shoes sprayed with disinfectants. The tires of vehicles returning from the United Kingdom were disinfected. There were severe economic consequences that extended to tourism and other seemingly unrelated industries, such as the scarcity of meat for zoo animals (BBC News, 2001).

This outbreak points out the need for quick and cooperative global response to emerging infectious disease threats in order to provide effective containment. For the United States it has pointed out another vulnerable area for a bioterrorist attack. In the wake of the 2001 SARS outbreak described previously, as part of the protection program, the CDC Division of Global Migration and Quarantine boarded airplanes to assess any ill travelers and facilitated their transport to medical treatment facilities (CDC, 2004a).

### SUMMARY

In the last few decades, health care and medicine have focused on cures. As we move further into the new millennium, preventive health, along with appropriate policies, must receive new attention, not only from the government and health professionals, but from the public with enthusiasm for a full partnership in this essential endeavor. Research, education, and funding must be directed to shape policies that will rebuild the public health infrastructure and ensure readiness to deal with future public health emergencies in the area of emerging infectious diseases. Furthermore, the reality that global connections are only hours away is permeating health policies. Fears of an influenza pandemic are fueling global cooperation efforts among various agencies, governments, and private enterprises.

The current climate in the United States, and indeed in the entire world, has been molded by the terrorist attacks of September 11, 2001, and the aftermath has resulted in shifts in public policy initiatives related to infectious diseases. These shifts may result in stronger legislation to protect the greater public, with a lessening of emphasis on individual rights and considerations. There has been increased funding to support additional surveillance and protective initiatives. It is hoped that the financial resources long sought by the public health community not only to maintain programs but to recruit needed experts will be sustained and increased. Greater speed and efficiency of reporting unusual symptoms or circumstances to central points (such as the CDC) by electronic surveillance means has become the norm across the country after the inadequacy of the present systems became apparent during the anthrax episodes of October 2001. Greater restrictions with regard to travel and immigration can also be expected. Nurses will be involved not only in their professional roles but also in their roles as citizens.

## Key Points

- Serious infectious disease outbreaks occurring anywhere in the world can be easily transmitted globally within hours.
- Reasons for the emergence of infectious disease involve complex demographic, social, and political factors.
- Global infectious disease surveillance and control affects many policies in the United States and globally, including immigration, quarantine, and immunization.

## Web Resources

**Centers for Disease Control and Prevention**
*www.cdc.gov*
**ProMed**
*www.promedmail.org*
**World Health Organization**
*www.who.int*

# REFERENCES

Avian influenza—Eastern Asia (64): FAO/OIE/WHO. *ProMed 2005 (No. 285)*, July 6, 2005, unpaginated.

BBC News. (2001, June 4). Foot-and-mouth in Europe. Retrieved August 5, 2001, from *http://news.bbc.co.uk/hi/english/world/ europenewsid_1191000/1191046.stm*.

Bridges, C. B., Lim, W., Hu-Primmer, J., Sims, L., Fukuda, K., et al. (2002). Risk of influenza A (H5N1) infection among poultry workers, Hong Kong, 1997-1998. *Journal of Infectious Diseases, 185*, 1005-1010.

Burnet, F. M. (1962). *Natural history of infectious disease* (3rd ed.). Cambridge, England: Cambridge University Press.

Bush, G. W. (2005). Executive order: Amendment to E. O. 13295 relating to certain influenza viruses and quarantinable communicable diseases. The White House, April 1, 2005. Retrieved August 2, 2005, from *www.whitehouse.gov/news/releases/2005/04/20050401-6.html*.

Centers for Disease Control and Prevention (CDC). (1994). *Addressing emerging infectious disease threats: A prevention strategy for the United States*. Atlanta: U.S. Department of Health and Human Services, Public Health Service.

Centers for Disease Control and Prevention (CDC). (1998). *Preventing emerging infectious diseases: A strategy for the 21st century*. Atlanta: U.S. Department of Health and Human Services.

Centers for Disease Control and Prevention (CDC). (1999). Control of infectious diseases. *MMWR. Morbidity and Mortality Weekly Report, 48*, 621-628.

Centers for Disease Control and Prevention (CDC). (2003a). Multistate outbreak of monkeypox—Illinois, Indiana, and Wisconsin, 2003. *MMWR. Morbidity and Mortality Weekly Report, 52*, 537-540.

Centers for Disease Control and Prevention (CDC). (2003b). Update: Multistate outbreak of monkeypox—Illinois, Indiana, Kansas, Missouri, Ohio, and Wisconsin, 2003. *MMWR. Morbidity and Mortality Weekly Report, 52*, 642-646.

Centers for Disease Control and Prevention. (2004a). The U.S. response to SARS: Role of CDC's Division of Global Migration and Quarantine. National Center for Infectious Diseases, Division of Global Migration and Quarantine. Retrieved August 2, 2005, from *www.cdc.gov/ncidod/dq/roleofdq.htm*.

Centers for Disease Control and Prevention (CDC). (2004b). History of quarantine. National Center for Infectious Diseases, Division of Global Migration and Quarantine. Retrieved August 2, 2005, from *www.cdc.gov/ncidod/dq/history.htm*.

Centers for Disease Control and Prevention (CDC). (2005). Immunization laws. National Vaccine Program Office. Retrieved August 2, 2005, from *www.cdc.gov/od/nipo/law.htm*.

Centers for Disease Control and Prevention (CDC), National Center for Infectious Diseases, Division of Global Migration and Quarantine. (2000, May). History of quarantine. Accessed July 5, 2001, at *www.cdc.gov/ncidod/dq/history.htm*.

Centers for Disease Control and Prevention (CDC), National Vaccine Program Office. (2001, July 14). Immunization laws. Accessed online, August 1, 2001, at *www.cdc.gov/od/nipo/law.htm*.

Christian, M. D., Poutanen, S. M., Loutfy, M. R., Muller, M. P., & Low, D. E. (2004). Severe acute respiratory syndrome. *Clinical Infectious Diseases, 38*, 1420-1427.

Cohen, F. L., & Larson, E. (1996). Emerging infectious diseases: Nursing responses. *Nursing Outlook, 44*, 164-168.

Fauci, A. S. (2002). Smallpox vaccination policy: The need for dialogue. *New England Journal of Medicine, 346*(17), 1319-1390.

Fritz, C. L., Dennis, D. T., Tipple, M. A., Campbell, G. L., McCance, C. R., & Gubler, D. J. (1996). Surveillance for pneumonic plague in the United States during an international emergency: A model for control of imported emerging diseases. *Emerging Infectious Diseases, 2*, 30-36.

Garrett, L. (2000). *Betrayal of trust: The collapse of global public health*. New York: Hyperion.

Gellert, G. A. (1993). International migration and control of communicable disease. *Social Science & Medicine, 37*, 1489-1499.

Gostin, L. O. (2005). *Jacobson v. Massachusetts* at 100 years: Police power and civil liberties in tension. *American Journal of Public Health, 95*, 576-581.

Granwehr, B. P., Lillibridges, K. M., Higgs, S., Mason, P. W., Aronson, J. F., et al. (2004). West Nile virus: Where are we now? *Lancet 9*, 547-556.

Guyer, B., Smith, D. R., & Chalk, R. (2000). Calling the shots: Immunization finance policies and practices. Executive summary of the report of the Institute of Medicine. *American Journal of Preventive Medicine, 19*(3S), 4-12.

Hughes, J. M. (2001). Emerging infectious diseases: A CDC perspective. *Emerging Infectious Diseases, 7*(Suppl 3), 494-496.

Knobler, S. L., Mack, A., Mahmoud, A., & Lemon, S. M. (Eds.). (2005). *The threat of pandemic influenza: Are we ready?* Washington, DC: National Academies Press.

Lashley, F. R. (2003). Factors contributing to the occurrence of emerging infectious diseases. *Biological Research for Nursing, 4*, 258-267.

Lashley, F. R. (2004). Emerging infectious diseases: Vulnerabilities, contributing factors and approaches. *Expert Review of Anti-infective Therapy, 2*, 299-316.

Lashley, F. R., & Durham, J. D. (2002). *Emerging infectious diseases: Trends and issues*. New York: Springer.

Lederberg, J. (1997). Infectious disease as an evolutionary paradigm. *Emerging Infectious Diseases, 3*, 417-423.

Lederberg, J., Shope, R. E., & Oaks, S. C., Jr. (Eds.). (1992). *Emerging infections: Microbial threats to health in the United States*. Washington, DC: National Academies Press.

Mariner, W. K., Annas, G. J., & Glantz, L. H. (2005). *Jacobson v. Massachusetts:* It's not your great-great-grandfather's public health law. *American Journal of Public Health, 95*, 581-590.

National Intelligence Council. (2000). *The global infectious disease threat and its implications for the United States* (National Intelligence Estimate 99-17D). Washington, DC: National Intelligence Council.

Poon, L. L. M., Guan, Y., Nichols, J. M., Yuen, K. T., & Peiris, J. S. M. (2004). The aetiology, origins, and diagnosis of severe acute respiratory syndrome. *Lancet Infectious Diseases, 4*, 663-671.

Richards, E. P. (2001). Emerging infectious diseases and the law. *Emerging Infectious Diseases, 7*(suppl 3), 543.

Skowronski, D. M., Astell, C., Brunham, R. C., Low, D. E., Petric, M., et al. (2005). *Annual Review of Medicine, 56*, 357-381.

Smolinski, M. S., Hamburg, M. A., & Lederberg, J. (Eds.). (2003). *Microbial threats to health: Emergence, detection, and response*. Washington, DC: Institute of Medicine, National Academies Press.

World Health Organization (WHO). (2003). Acute respiratory syndrome, China. *Weekly Epidemiological Record, 78,* 41-48.

World Health Organization (WHO). (2005). *Avian influenza: Assessing the pandemic threat.* Geneva, Switzerland: WHO.

World Health Organization (WHO). (2005).*Epidemic and Pandemic Alert and Response (EPR). Frequently asked questions about the international health regulations.* Geneva: WHO. Retrieved on April 12, 2006, from *www.who.int/est/ihr/en.*

World Health Organization (WHO). (2006). Cumulative number of confirmed human cases of avian influenza A/(H5N1) reported to WHO. Retrieved on April 12, 2006, from *www.who.int.esr.disease/avian_influenza/country/cases. table_2006_04_12/en/index.html.*

# **POLICY**SPOTLIGHT

## THE GLOBAL HIV/AIDS CRISIS: POLICY RESPONSES IN THE FACE OF LIMITED RESOURCES

Helen M. Miramontes, Deborah von Zinkernagel, & Donna Gallagher

*"How wonderful it is that nobody need wait a single moment before starting to improve the world."*

ANNE FRANK

### HIV/AIDS PANDEMIC IN LOW-RESOURCE SETTINGS

The human immunodeficiency virus/acquired immunodeficiency syndrome (HIV/AIDS) global pandemic has had a profound impact on many regions of the world. It is both an immediate and devastating crisis for whole populations and the health and socioeconomic systems that serve them. Since the first AIDS diagnosis in 1981 there have been 20 million deaths worldwide from AIDS. According to the United Nations (UN) AIDS Program (UNAIDS) there are approximately 40 million people currently living with HIV/AIDS, with the majority, 25.4 million, living in Africa (UNAIDS, 2004). Some regions of the world, such as the sub-Saharan region of Africa, have older epidemics of HIV/AIDS with increasing rates of infection; other regions, such as Southern Africa, Eastern Europe, the Caribbean, Asia, and Southeast Asia have newer epidemics that are rapidly expanding. Globally UNAIDS (2004)

estimates that 14,000 people are newly infected every day. Most of the infections occur in people 15 to 49 years of age, with the 15- to 24-year-olds accounting for nearly half of all new infections (UNAIDS, 2004). Life expectancy in many of the African countries has decreased by 10 to 20 years.

Effective care and treatment, including antiretroviral (ARV) medications, are desperately needed in low-resource countries. However, few of the people who need these drugs have access to them, in spite of increased global investment in AIDS, decreases in the price of medications, and pressure on high-resource countries to expand access to the life-prolonging medications. At the end of 2003, only 7% of the people in low-resource settings in need of the ARVs were actually receiving these therapies (UNAIDS, 2004). The continued expansion of this pandemic has already reversed many of the public health achievements in low-resource countries, and threatens to give rise to long-term political and social instability that undercuts achievement of the UN Millennium Development Goals by 2015 (Joint Learning Initiative, 2004; UN, 2000).

## DESCRIPTION OF THE POLICY PROBLEM

There are numerous, complex policy and program issues associated with the delivery of consistently high-quality HIV/AIDS care in those low-resource countries heavily burdened by HIV. These include, but are not limited to, inadequate health system infrastructure, massive debt obligations, economic restrictions in the health sector, political instability, lack of access to affordable ARV drugs, and a shortage of qualified professional health care providers. An added challenge in establishing effective HIV/AIDS programs is the mismatch between Western models of care advanced by the donor community and the reality of how health care is delivered in many poor countries. The unquestioning emphasis on a medical care model without addressing the realities of what is occurring in the provision of care and treatment contributes to the difficulties of meeting the health care needs of people, including people living with HIV disease. As will be discussed in this policy spotlight, there is an urgent need to adapt existing models of primary care in low-resource settings to treat and monitor large numbers of HIV-positive individuals.

## HEALTH CARE DELIVERY SYSTEMS IN LOW-RESOURCE SETTINGS

According to the report by the International Council of Nurses (ICN) on the global shortage of nurses, many health care delivery systems have collapsed because of the extensive and prolonged HIV/AIDS pandemic (Buchan & Calman, 2004). In addition, health sector reform and organizational restructuring have not always been successful in low-resource countries (Buchan & Calman, 2004; Joint Learning Initiative, 2004). Many reforms have been driven by external donors, such as the World Bank and the International Monetary Fund, and may be based on models and experiences from more highly resourced countries. Also, many reforms were initiated during the 1980s with the goal of achieving sustained growth by controlling wages and public expenditures through structured adjustment programs. Unfortunately, little attention was given to the impact on the health sector (Buchan & Calman, 2004). As a result national health systems were weakened and, consequently

national health programs could not be sustained (Buchan & Calman, 2004; Joint Learning Initiative, 2004).

## HEALTH CARE PROVIDERS DELIVERING HIV/AIDS CARE IN LOW-RESOURCE SETTINGS

In most low-resource countries, public health services are organized around maternal-child health and primary care, relying heavily on nurses, midwives, and health workers, as well as unpaid volunteers, at the village and community level. Nurses are often the only trained professional providers a patient will see. Care is episodic, with individuals seeking curative services only when symptoms are advanced and have not been resolved by traditional healers who are usually the first point of contact when a person seeks treatment. The shortage and maldistribution of physicians and the expense of medical care limits how often individuals can see these providers for care and treatment.

## GOALS OF SCALING UP CARE AND TREATMENT

On World AIDS Day 2003, the World Health Organization (WHO) and UNAIDS announced the 3×5 Initiative. The goal of the initiative was to have 3 million people living with AIDS on ARV treatment by the end of 2005. The target settings were 50 low-resource countries in which 6 million infected people were in need of ARV treatment. At the time of the announcement the two agencies released a comprehensive plan targeting five critical areas: delivery of ARVs, reliable supply of drugs and diagnostics, rapid dissemination of new knowledge, sustained support for country efforts, and global leadership. To accomplish this goal, 100,000 health workers were projected to need training, and health systems and infrastructures needed to be developed and built (WHO, 2003).

In January of 2005, WHO and UNAIDS released a progress report stating that by the end of 2004, 700,000 people worldwide were receiving ARV treatment (WHO, 2005). The number of Africans on these ARV medications is 310,000, but there are still almost 4 million people who need treatment. In addition, the report identifies significant deficits in both funding and health system capacity needed to provide treatment in order to reach the goal of 3 million people by the end of the year (AfricaFocus Bulletin, 2005).

## INTRODUCTION TO THE WORKFORCE ISSUES

The capacity to provide access to preventive and curative health services in much of the developing world is directly related to addressing the crisis in human resources for health (Joint Learning Initiative, 2004). The HIV/AIDS epidemic has both starkly highlighted and contributed to the widening gap between available human capacity and the urgent need for caregivers in those countries most highly affected by the epidemic. A recent report issued by the Office of the United States Global AIDS Coordinator (OGAC) identified the lack of human resource capacity as a fundamental limitation to expanding access to ARV therapies and care and treatment for HIV, as a result of both absolute shortages and maldistribution and inefficient use of available personnel (OGAC, 2005). Because nurses are the backbone of and frontline staff in most health delivery systems, new approaches and policies are needed to respond to these challenges if global goals for HIV treatment are to be realized (Buchan & Calman, 2004).

## SHORTAGE OF TRAINED PROFESSIONALS

The global shortage of skilled nurses and doctors is most acute in many countries also shouldering the full force of the HIV/AIDS epidemic. Sub-Saharan Africa bears over 60% of the world's burden of HIV infections (UNAIDS, 2004) and has only 1.3% of the global health workforce (Mullan, Panosian, & Cuff, 2005). Mozambique, a country of 18 million people, has roughly one tenth the number of physicians and nurses needed to meet the WHO's minimum recommended standard to meet basic health needs (WHO, 2004b). Similar patterns of severe undersupply of skilled workers can be seen in Ethiopia (one nurse per 4900 population), Rwanda, Malawi, and many other countries with heavy burdens of disease, as shown in Table 34-3. About 38 of 47 countries in sub-Saharan Africa do not meet the WHO's recommended minimum for physicians, with 13 having five or fewer doctors per 100,000 population (Friedman, 2004). Moreover, the ratio of physicians to the population, already low in many places, does not represent the number of providers delivering care in the public sector, as these doctors may be engaged in the private sector or serving in governmental administrative positions. Throughout the developing world, delivery of health care is heavily reliant on nurses and uncounted numbers of informal, traditional, community, and allied health workers (Joint Learning Initiative, 2004).

A number of recent reports have examined the issues of health worker shortages and in particular those dynamics affecting the global supply of nurses (Buchan & Calman, 2004; Joint Learning Initiative, 2004; Friedman, 2004; Mullan et al.,

**TABLE 34-3**  Nurses and Physicians per 100,000 Population by Country

| COUNTRY | NURSES | | DOCTORS | |
| --- | --- | --- | --- | --- |
| | NO. | PER 100,000 | NO. | PER 100,000 |
| Uganda | 2200 | 8.8 | 1175 | 4.7 |
| Ethiopia | 13,018 | 18.9 | 1971 | 2.9 |
| Mozambique | 3664 | 20.5 | 435 | 2.4 |
| Rwanda | 1735 | 21.0 | 155 | 1.9 |
| Malawi | 3094 | 25.5 | 137 | 1.1 |
| Cote d'Ivoire | 4582 | 31.2 | 1322 | 9.0 |
| Kenya | 24,679 | 90.1 | 3616 | 13.2 |
| Zambia | 10,598 | 113.1 | 647 | 6.9 |

From World Health Organization (WHO). (2004b). Global atlas of the health workforce. Retrieved July 31, 2005, from *www.who.int/GlobalAtlas/DataQuery/default.asp*.
WHO Recommended Minimum Standard: Nurses, 1:500 population (200 per 100,000); doctors: 1:5000 population (20 per 100,000).

**BOX 34-7**  Major Factors Leading to Health Workforce Shortages

- Chronic underinvestment in human resources, as economic and sectoral reforms have capped expenditures, frozen salaries, and restricted public budgets for health
- Accelerating international migration of health workers, depleting nurses and doctors from countries that can least afford the loss of skilled providers
- Inadequate numbers of new providers being trained each year, with underinvestment in professional schools and shortages of qualified faculty
- HIV-related morbidity and mortality among health workers, as rising numbers of HIV-positive providers become ill and die; those not absent for their own health reasons must often take time away to care for sick relatives; others leave work in response to psychosocial stress and burnout. Between 18% and 41% of the workforce in many sub-Saharan countries is estimated to be HIV positive (Friedman, 2004)
- Poor work environment with low salaries and benefits, poor working conditions and lack of supplies, and lack of career opportunities all serving as disincentives to enter or remain in the nursing workforce

2005; OGAC, 2005). Key factors contributing to profound shortages across sub-Saharan Africa are summarized in Box 34-7.

The shortage of skilled professionals is further compounded by inequitable distribution of doctors and nurses within countries, with a greater concentration of health workers in urban settings, while rural and marginal communities, where large segments of the population reside, may have few or no health workers at all (Table 34-4).

## POLICY AND PROGRAM IMPLICATIONS FOR MODELS OF CARE

Within this context of acute shortages of physicians and nurses in low-resource settings and an expanding HIV epidemic, there is an urgent need to employ and deploy available professionals (human resources) as effectively as possible to urgently scale access to care and treatment. The Joint Learning Initiative (Joint Learning Initiative, 2004) has called for a massive mobilization of the workforce in countries facing a health emergency from HIV/AIDS. This has implications for the three major programs funding HIV prevention, care, and treatment programs in highly affected countries: the

**TABLE 34-4**  Urban-Rural Distribution of Health Workers in Selected Countries

| COUNTRY | POPULATION | RURAL POPULATION (%) | PROVIDER DISTRIBUTION |
|---|---|---|---|
| Malawi | 12,158,929* | 87%[†] | 96.6% of clinical officers are in urban health facilities<br>25% of nurses and half of physicians are in four central hospitals[‡] |
| South Africa | 44,415,866[†] | 46%[†] | 12% of physicians practice in rural areas<br>19% of nurses practice in rural areas[‡] |
| Kenya | 27,390,339[†] | 67%[†] | Urban: (Nairobi) 688 health workers per 100,000<br>Rural: North-Eastern Province, 138 health workers per 100,000[‡] |
| Ghana | 20,471,206[†] | 56%[§] | Urban: Greater Accra Region, 0.3 doctors and 1.20 nurses per 1000 population<br>Rural: Northern Region, 0.01 doctors and 0.34 nurses per 1000 population[ǁ] |

*From Central Intelligence Agency (CIA). (2005). The world fact book. Washington DC: CIA. Retrieved September 30, 2005, from *www.cia.gov/cia/publications/factbook/geos/mi.html.*

[†]From World Health Organization (WHO). (2004b). Global atlas of the health workforce. Retrieved July 31, 2005, from *www.who.int/GlobalAtlas/DataQuery/default.asp.*

[‡]From Friedman, E. (2004). *An action plan to prevent brain drain: Building equitable health systems in Africa.* Boston: Physicians for Human Rights.

[§]From Boakye-Yiadom, L. (2004). Paper prepared for the International Conference on Ghana's Economy at the Half Century, July 18-20. Accra, Ghana. Retrieved September 30, 2005, from *www.isser.org/Evolution%20of%20Welfare%20in%20Gh.pdf.*

[ǁ]From AntwiBoasiako, Y. (2005). Oslo Consultation on Human Resources for Health. Oslo, Norway, February 24-25. Retrieved September 30, 2005, from *www.norad.no/default.asp?FILE=items/3070/108/Oslopresentation2.ppt.*

President's Emergency Plan for AIDS Relief (PEPFAR), the UN Global Fund to Fight AIDS, Tuberculosis and Malaria (Global Fund), and the Multi-Country HIV/AIDS Program for Africa, sponsored by the World Bank (Mullan et al., 2005). At the outset of each program, technical review panels evaluating grant applications drew heavily on Western experts in HIV/AIDS treatment, and physicians were designated as the primary clinicians for ARV treatment. More recently, innovative models have been piloted to safely extend life-saving treatment to more people.

### Processes to Strengthen the Care System

Five steps to address workforce shortages and expand access to HIV treatment are discussed here as a guide for planners, policymakers, and funders.

*Health workforce assessment.* Expanding access to care must start with accurate information on the available workforce and patterns of care (Joint Learning Initiative, 2004; Friedman, 2004; Mullan et al., 2005). A needs assessment should include the number, skill mix, and functional roles of health providers, their geographic distribution, and their participation in public or private sector care. It is also important to identify those factors affecting recruitment and the retention of workers in order to stabilize and build the supply of health workers. In most rural villages and small towns in sub-Saharan African countries, the nurses are the only trained professionals providing health services. Understanding who is providing care, and how they are interfaced with the target population and broader medical systems, lays the foundation for effective planning of rapid scale-up of care.

*Development of care networks.* A fundamental strategy to rapidly scale up access to ARVs and HIV primary care is development of networks that link community- and clinic-based providers with more highly trained clinicians at district or tertiary care facilities. The WHO model promoted in the 3×5 Initiative uses first-level health workers, following clear treatment guidelines and linking them with a progressive ladder of medical expertise, consultation, and referral backup (Joint

Learning Initiative, 2004; WHO, 2004a). The PEPFAR programs have also adopted a network-based approach to building capacity and expanding access to treatment, linking satellite clinics, mobile units, and health centers with district hospitals and regional expertise (OGAC, 2005). Effective models have been developed and tested using nurses as the primary professional providers of ARV treatment and care, overseeing the work of larger numbers of community health workers, while scarce physician resources are strategically leveraged.

*Match training with care model.* Knowledge of who is providing care and what models of care are proposed informs the training needs in a given area. Many countries have now developed standards of care that guide routine evaluation for HIV disease progression, diagnosis and treatment of opportunistic infections (OIs), criteria for initiating ARVs, and appropriate laboratory and clinical follow-up. Other components of care include psychosocial and practical support, symptom management, and compassionate end-of-life care. Many training programs to prepare nurses and community health workers as primary providers of HIV treatment have been developed, with careful attention to indications for consultation and referral to more expert providers with practical skills in physical assessment. For nurses taking on expanded roles and responsibilities for HIV care, mentoring support has been important to sustain the benefits of training.

*Policy barriers.* National policies may restrict the ability of nurses to carry out important care activities, such as prescribing medications to prevent and treat OIs or to control symptoms and pain (Buchan & Calman, 2004; Joint Learning Initiative, 2004). Nurses may also be restricted in carrying out basic physical assessments, which markedly narrows the scope of primary HIV/AIDS care services they can provide. Regulations or legislations, including Nurse Practice Acts, that prevent nurses from being effective as frontline providers of HIV treatment need to be considered by policymakers and revised in concert with training or certification requirements that ensure nurses are well prepared and protected in assuming more clinical responsibilities.

***Funding investment in human resources.*** Decades of underinvestment in human resources and related health sector spending may be the underlying cause of health worker shortages and weak public health systems in low-resource countries. As the global investment in HIV/AIDS increases, new policy choices to invest in human resources are back on the table as part of the overall approach to expanding care. The Global Fund permits resources to be used for health system strengthening, including human resources for health, as part of a country plan to combat HIV, tuberculosis, or malaria (Friedman, 2004). Following early concerns that a relative underemphasis on infrastructure and human capital threatened achievement of the program's goals, PEPFAR has supported greater focus on funding human capacity development as part of the country operating plans (Mullan et al., 2005). Many possible approaches may be employed to increase direct investment in health workers, such as incentives, bonuses, enhanced career opportunities, and workplace improvements that help to attract and retain valuable workers.

## NURSE-DIRECTED MODELS OF CARE AND TREATMENT

Nurse-directed models of care are quite prevalent in the countries most affected by HIV. However, explicit recognition of these models is infrequent, making the successful outcomes of these models a well-kept secret. The perception of nursing is dependent on the view of nursing within the health care hierarchy and the way nurses view themselves. For example, in rural Cambodia, efforts to provide intensive HIV training programs have been rejected by nurses who do not have the interest in becoming HIV specialized. In other places, nurses have been trained to provide one specific component of nursing care and do not have the desire to increase their skills. Commonly, the relationship between physicians and nurses reflects a more traditional model that puts a negative light on nurses who "know too much and overstep their boundaries," even where

the physician supply is near nonexistent. Efforts by donor programs and international nurse colleagues to provide assistance and support for successful nurse-directed systems of care must respect the unique situations and differences in nurses' practice environments within each country.

In South Africa, well-educated and well-motivated nurses have risen to the challenge of providing high-quality, creative care to people living with HIV. The successes reported in South Africa are directly related to the amount of educational support, the availability of trained nurses, and affordable medications. However, the real backbone of these successful programs is the multicomponent models that include nurses in all areas of the health care hierarchy. The involvement of nursing educators, physicians, nursing unions, and licensure bodies has facilitated the expanding roles of nurses in a variety of practices throughout South Africa. This, too, was not without controversy, but a persistent effort from the nurses in the field and partnerships from abroad that were designed to support in-country efforts have moved this effort toward fruition. In this case, American nurses were able to serve as facilitators and partners who provided information, training, and support for the efforts initiated by the South African nurses.

One model will not fit all in our sister countries, as one model has not fit all here in the United States. Successful partnerships will include knowledge of the current nursing policies in the specific country and the ability of American nurses to facilitate the tailoring of programs to fit the individual needs of the countries in which they are working. However, under conditions of acute worker shortages, substantial international attention should be directed toward expanding nurse-directed systems of care in order to meet the urgent demands for treatment.

The following are examples of nurse-directed models of care and treatment in the Caribbean and Africa.

### Bahamas

A nursing colleague from the Bahamas related to us that among the Bahamas, 29 inhabited islands, the government has systematically and strategically established health clinics covering both urban and rural settings. Over 90% of these clinics are managed by public health nurses or nurse midwives. A physician is attached to the clinic, but in rural settings the physician may actually be at the clinic only once a week or once a month (personal communication, Shane Neely-Smith, July 1, 2005). As the Bahamas scale up the national HIV treatment plan, these nurses will be the first line of care in monitoring and routinely following up patients and coordinating their care with several tertiary facilities.

## South Africa

Nurses are responding to the HIV epidemic in South Africa by providing leadership and creative models to meet the overwhelming task of "rolling out" ARV therapy to millions of people currently in need of treatment. The health care landscape in South Africa consists of many hospital-based clinics in the urban areas and scattered rural clinics in the poor remote rural areas that surround the urban centers. The largest number of people living with HIV is heavily concentrated in the townships (densely populated areas of intense poverty where black South Africans were relocated during the apartheid era) that surround the urban areas such as the KwaZulu-Natal (KZN) province. Many lessons have been learned in the course of supporting nurse colleagues in this challenging work, some of which are offered here (Box 34-8).

*Inthemba clinic.* Three years ago a creative program was developed at the Inthemba Clinic on the grounds of St. Mary's Hospital, located outside of Durban, KZN, alongside a large township. Nurses participated in an intensive training program to become experts on ARVs, including management of side effects and adherence counseling. This nurse-directed program provides each patient with a 2-week orientation before the start of ARV treatment. Nurses meet with the patients to provide education about the medications and side effects, along with in-depth education about the virus and strategies to reduce the risk of transmission. Patients are started on medication when the nurses feel they are ready. Presently, the clinic physician prescribes the ARVs and the patient is

---

**BOX 34-8**    Building Effective Nurse Models: Lessons from the Field

**IN-COUNTRY PARTNERSHIPS**

In-country partnerships are an essential first step. A successful example is the ongoing "think tank" operating in the KwaZuluNatal area of South Africa. This group was formed to identify the needs of nurses in the region and includes representation from hospitals, administrators, educators, home care nurses, union leaders, and occasionally physicians from the Health Ministry. The goal of this group is to facilitate needs assessment and planning and to bring all the voices of in-country nurses to the table along with U.S. nurse partners to identify a roadmap for change. Over the course of 2 years, plans for human resource development and retention of the current workforce, as well as strategies to reach all practicing nurses with education and training in HIV/AIDS, have been developed and are being implemented.

**ONGOING SUPPORT AND NETWORKING**

Development of a plan for ongoing support is critical as partnerships are formed. Goals that are identified usually require time for implementation. Opportunities to make return visits to country colleagues, to support their efforts, and to help strategize adjustments to plans are critical to program success.

**EVALUATION**

Evaluation is essential. An evaluation plan, and mechanisms to adjust programs based on findings, can also strengthen networking relationships between in-country and international nurse colleagues. Trust is the benefit that is realized over time; as these relationships mature, many of the "unspoken issues" will surface, giving the whole group an opportunity to problem-solve together.

**INDIVIDUALIZED PARTNERSHIPS**

Partnerships between host-country nurses and international colleagues may have a different look in each setting, requiring flexibility and openness on the part of out-of-country partners.

carefully monitored by the nursing staff on a regular schedule, with documentation of patient progress maintained. This program has over 300 patients successfully taking ARVs, with an adherence rate over 95%. Nurses have become so skilled in this program that they play a key role in identifying which patient should be considered for ARV treatment. A Boston-Durban nurses-to-nurse partnership has evolved over the course of educational exchanges, supporting nurses in their expanded roles in the clinic and surrounding community.

*Vulindlela township.* Another successful program is in Vulindlela, a township area located in the KZN capital of Pietermaritzburg. Vulindlela is an extremely rural, poverty-stricken area where patients may have to travel 30 to 50 miles to reach the nearest hospital-based site offering ARV treatment. In the rural areas transportation is a challenge even when available. Hospital-based clinics have long ARV waiting lists, and reliance on these can discourage patients and increase feelings of desperation as well as depression.

In rural areas most of the primary care clinics are run by nurses. Rural clinic models may have a physician on site, or a physician may be available only one or two times per week. In either case the nurses are the anchor for the clinic, providing continuity for patients who come for care. The ARV clinic has four nurses, a physician, a pharmacist, and several counselors, but "more than two-thirds of the patient visits are handled by the nurses," as reported by Terence Moodley, a research clinician who is evaluating the program for the Centre for the AIDS Programme of Research in South Africa (allAfrica.com, 2005). Patients are followed frequently by the nurses and are seen on a quarterly basis by the physician (more often if necessary). Adherence training, risk reduction counseling, and all other aspects of HIV care are available through nurses in the clinic. Similar to the success of the Inthemba clinic, Vulindlela has almost 200 patients on ARVs, with a drug adherence rate of greater than 90%. Both of these nurse-directed clinics have a higher success rate with adherence than programs in the United States, where adherence rates are generally below 90% (Bangsberg, et al., 2003).

### Ethiopian Nursing Clinics

A major challenge to scaling up the national ARV program in Ethiopia is the limited number of health care workers, specifically nurses, to provide HIV care and treatment for people living with HIV/AIDS. Moving from a "physician-centered" model to a "nurse-intensive" model is an essential first step toward developing alternative staffing patterns without depleting the number of physicians available for other health services. To accomplish this, the Ministry of Health and the Ethiopia Nurses Association have been working together to develop intensive and comprehensive HIV care trainings and a nationally supported expanded role for nurses at the hospital and health-center levels.

Several different models of health care delivery are present throughout Ethiopia. Over 85% of health care is delivered in the rural areas, where the majority of the population lives, by approximately 15% of the health care workforce. This disparity has resulted in an expanded role for the nurse in the rural health care settings and district hospitals, where physicians and other essential members of the multidisciplinary team may be absent. Nurses provide primary care to patients, diagnosing, treating, and prescribing. In some rural areas nurses are functioning as pharmacists and dentists with minimal, if any, additional education and training. Recently a rural clinic was set to provide ARVs

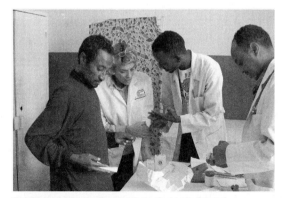

Pat Daoust, a consultant with the federally funded International Training and Education Center of HIV/AIDS (also known as *I-TECH*), conducts a clinical mentoring session with Ethiopian male nurses in Mekele, Ethiopia.

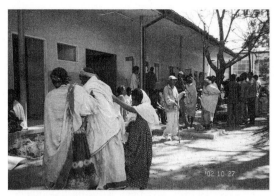

People in Gondar, Ethiopia, wait in an outdoor area for emergency services.

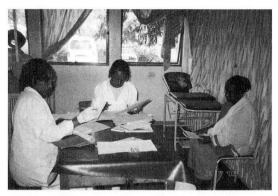

Nurses charting on a medical unit in a facility in Addis Ababa, Ethiopia.

for patients, many of whom traveled long distances to reach care. On opening day, there was one nurse for 300 patients lined up outside the clinic. This example of overwhelming demand is disheartening, but with support nurses can and do manage as the frontline providers of care in the rural areas.

The urgency to scale up HIV care and ARV treatment in Ethiopia has provided the opportunity to evaluate the existing nursing models of care and initiate training and advocacy for needed changes in the nurse practice act. The success of nurse-directed models in underserved rural communities has triggered a national assessment and response to strengthen capacity building within the nursing workforce, along with an assessment of preservice training to expand the future supply of nurses (personal communication, MaryAnn Vitiello, July 31, 2005).

## IMPLICATIONS FOR FUTURE POLICY CONSIDERATIONS

### Implications for Funding Sources

Funding sources, such as PEPFAR, the Global Fund, and other national and international funders, should consider the following issues:

- Investment in capacity development of nursing workforce is an effective method to rapidly scale up HIV/AIDS care and treatment, particularly in rural areas, where nurses may be the only providers. Funding strategies to improve retention and recruitment of nurses, and appropriate

training to match skills with clinical responsibilities, can rapidly extend the effectiveness of the existing workforce.
- A health workforce assessment is the essential first step to using existing capacity and planning to match worker supply and training with the need for care and treatment.
- Donors should work closely with national governments to support increased capacity and management of human resources for health, including addressing policy barriers that limit effective use of existing resources.

### Implications for Domestic Nursing Organizations

U.S. domestic nursing organizations should seek out opportunities to work with colleagues in low-resource settings by developing collaborative, professional relationships. Some of the strategies to be considered are as follows:

- Support nursing colleagues in low-resource counties by establishing equitable partnerships in education and training projects, research studies, and clinical practice.
- Seek identification by colleagues in low-resource countries of the issues and resources that would most support them in their settings.
- Provide mentorship opportunities to colleagues in low-resource settings.
- Work with colleagues in low-resource settings to develop leadership roles that foster and advance capacity-building among nurses within their specific countries.

## Implications for International Nursing Organizations

International nursing organizations should work with nursing colleagues in low-resource settings to facilitate the long-term expansion of professional nursing by highlighting and addressing broader policy issues and goals. Some of the policy issues to be considered are as follows:

- Issues of scope of nursing practice within the specific countries. It is important to support country-level nursing associations in their policy work to strengthen the practice of nursing, as well as redefine their practice legislation to reflect the evolving, expanding scope of practice that is the actual reality occurring on the ground at country-level.
- Provide guidance and leadership in facilitating the expansion of nursing leadership at the country level.
- Assist in research and documentation of the evolving nursing roles and nurse-directed models of care. Provide assistance and resources in the dissemination of information on successful evolving practices and nurse-directed models of care.

Nurses represent one of the largest workforces in the world and have provided leadership throughout the HIV epidemic as providers and policymakers. The needs of our international colleagues are extensive but not unfamiliar to nurses who have worked to solve the same issues in the United States. The evidence shows that nurses are highly effective but heavily burdened in countries most devastated by HIV/AIDS. The opportunity to provide professional and moral support and mentorship are privileges that we should embrace. The future of 44 million people with HIV/AIDS in need of care is in our hands.

- The most appropriate response, at this time, is to provide immediate and life-long comprehensive care and treatment, including ARV medications and drugs for OIs, for individuals who are HIV infected and effective, sustainable prevention programs for those who are not infected. In addition, the issues of poverty, political instability, and scare resources, which significantly increase the vulnerability of communities and individuals to the risk of becoming HIV infected, must be addressed.
- The health workforce issues must be identified and addressed in order to provide the comprehensive care and treatment that are required. National and international organizations and funders must be willing to explore, develop, implement, and fund different models of care and treatment, such as nurse-directed models of care. It is essential that the existing systems of care, including nursing models, be rapidly scaled up to provide care and treatment.

## *Web Resources*

**International Council of Nurses (ICN)**
*http://icn.ch*
**Joint Learning Initiative, Harvard University—Lincoln Chen, Director**
*www.globalhealthtrust.org*
**UNAIDS**—Joint United Nations Programme on AIDS that leads and strengthens an expanded response to the epidemic
*www.unaids.org*
**World Health Organization (WHO)**
*http://who.int*

## *Key Points*

- The HIV/AIDS pandemic is having a profound and devastating impact on many countries of the world, thereby creating development problems affecting the long-term stability and viability of entire global regions.

## REFERENCES

AfricaFocus Bulletin. (2005). Africa: AIDS progress real but limited. Retrieved January 31, 2005, from *procaare@healthnet.org*.

allAfrica.com. (2005). South Africa: Nurses to fill the gaps. Retrieved July 27, 2005, from *http://allafrica.com/stories/printable/200507120751.html*.

AntwiBoasiako, Y. (2005). Oslo Consultation on Human Resources for Health. Oslo, Norway, February 24-25.

Retrieved September 30, 2005, from *www.norad.no/default.asp?FILE=items/3070/108/Oslopresentation2.ppt.*

Bangsberg, D. R., Charlebois, E. D., Grant, R. M., Holodniy, M., Deeks, S., et al. (2003). High levels of adherence do not prevent accumulation of HIV drug resistance mutations. *AIDS, 17*(13), 1925-1932. Retrieved August 14, 2005, from *http:aidsetc.org/aidsetc?page=et-40-00&post=1&pid=1catid=arvtadher&pmid=12960825.*

Boakye-Yiadom, L. (2004). Paper prepared for the International Conference on Ghana's Economy at the Half Century, July 18-20. Accra, Ghana. Retrieved September 30, 2005, from *www.isser.org/Evolution%20of%20Welfare%20in%20Gh.pdf.*

Buchan, J., & Calman, L. (2004). The global shortage of nurses: Issues and actions. Retrieved May 20, 2005, from *www.icn.ch/global/shortage.pdf.*

Central Intelligence Agency (CIA). (2005). The world fact book. Washington DC: CIA. Retrieved September 30, 2005, from *www.cia.gov/cia/publications/factbook/geos/mi.html.*

Friedman, E. (2004). *An action plan to prevent brain drain: Building equitable health systems in Africa.* Boston: Physicians for Human Rights.

Joint Learning Initiative. (2004). *Human resources for health: Overcoming the crisis.* Cambridge, MA: Harvard University Press.

Mullan, F., Panosian, C., & Cuff, P. (Eds.). (2005). *Healers abroad: Americans responding to the human resource crisis in HIV/AIDS.* Washington, DC: National Academies Press.

Neely-Smith, S. (2005, July 1). Personal communication.

Office of United States Global AIDS Coordinator (OGAC). (2005). *Engendering bold leadership: The president's emergency plan for AIDS relief. First annual report to Congress.* Washington, DC: U.S. Government Printing Office.

United Nations (UN). (2000). United Nations millennium declaration. Retrieved May 1, 2005, from *www.un.org/millenium/declaration/ares552e.pdf.*

UNAIDS. (2004). Global summary of the HIV and AIDS epidemic, December, 2004. Retrieved July 1, 2005, from *www.unaids.org/wad2004/EPI_1204_pdf_en/Chapter/_intro_en.pdf.*

Vitiello, M. (2005, July 31). Personal communication.

World Health Organization (WHO). (2003). The 3 by 5 Initiative. Retrieved August 8, 2005, from *www.int/3by5/about/initiative/en/print.html/en/.*

World Health Organization (WHO). (2004a). *Chronic HIV care with ARV therapy, interim management of adolescent and adult illness: Interim guidelines of first level facility health workers.* Geneva, Switzerland: WHO.

World Health Organization (WHO). (2004b). Global atlas of the health workforce. Retrieved July 31, 2005, from *www.who.int/GlobalAtlas/DataQuery/default.asp.*

World Health Organization (WHO). (2005). The 3 by 5 Initiative. Retrieved August 1, 2005, from *www.who.int/3by5/progressreportJune2005/en/printr.html/en/.*

# **POLICY**SPOTLIGHT

# Conflict and War: Impact on the Health of Societies

Richard Garfield

*"War may sometimes be a necessary evil. But no matter how necessary, it is always an evil, never a good. We will not learn how to live together in peace by killing each other's children."*

JIMMY CARTER

## TRENDS IN GLOBAL CONFLICT

The World Health Organization (WHO) estimates that about 588,000 people died in wars in 1998 (Krug, 2002), and 310,000 people died from war-related injuries in 2000. That made war the fourth most common type of injury death in 1998, after unintended injuries, suicides, and homicides. These deaths are categorized according to the International Classification of Disease (ICD) codes for injuries resulting from operations of war (ICD-91 E990-E999 or ICD-102 Y36) (WHO, 1992, 1993, 1994). Rates of war-related deaths varied from less than 1 per 100,000 population in high-income countries to 6.2 per 100,000 in low-income and middle-income countries. Worldwide, the highest rates of war-related deaths were found in the WHO African Region (32 per 100,000), followed by low-income and middle-income countries in the WHO Eastern Mediterranean Region (8.2 per 100,000) and WHO European Region (7.6 per 100,000), respectively. Across the globe, war ranked as the thirteenth most common cause of death for 0- to 1-year-olds, fifth for 5- to 14-year-olds, and fifth for 15- to 44-year-olds in 1998.

Between the sixteenth and twentieth centuries, the estimated totals of conflict-related deaths per century were, respectively, 1.6 million, 6.1 million, 7.0 million, 19.4 million, and 109.7 million (Garfield & Nuegut, 1991). Such figures naturally conceal the circumstances in which people died. Six million people, for instance, are estimated to have lost their lives in the capture and transport of slaves over four centuries, and 10 million indigenous people in the Americas died at the hands of European colonists.

According to one estimate, some 191 million people lost their lives directly or indirectly in the 25 largest instances of collective violence in the twentieth century (Garfield & Nuegut, 1991). Conflict-related deaths in the 25 largest events included 39 million soldiers and 33 million civilians. Aside from the First and Second World Wars, the Stalinist reign of terror in Russia (1930s to 1950s) and the Great Leap Forward period in China (1958 to 1960) caused the most catastrophic loss of life. Both events are still surrounded by uncertainty over the scale of human losses. Famine directly related to conflict or genocide in the twentieth century killed a further 40 million people.

There have been a number of violent deaths of civilian United Nations (UN) employees and workers from nongovernmental organizations (NGOs) in conflict zones. In 1985 to 1998, over 380 deaths occurred among humanitarian workers, with more UN civilian personnel than UN peacekeeping troops being killed (Sheik, Gutierrez, & Bolton, 2000). Torture and humiliation are common practices in many conflicts. Because many victims are inclined to hide the trauma they have suffered

(Weinstein, Dansky, & Iacopino, 1996), and because there are also political pressures to conceal the use of torture, it is difficult to estimate how widespread it is.

Most recent conflicts are within rather than between states. Since the Second World War, there have been a total of 190 armed conflicts, only a quarter of which were between states. Most of the armed conflicts since the Second World War have been shorter than 6 months in duration. Those that lasted longer often went on for many years. For example, in Viet Nam, violent conflict spanned more than two decades. Other examples include the conflicts in Afghanistan and Angola, which lasted for decades. The total number of armed conflicts in progress was less than 20 in the 1950s, exceeded 30 in both the 1960s and 1970s, and rose to over 50 during the late 1980s. Although there were fewer armed conflicts in progress after 1992, those that took place were, on average, of longer duration. An estimated 17 million people have died from direct and 34 million people from indirect causes related to conflicts since World War II (White, 2005).

While conflicts within states are most common, conflicts between states still occur. The war between Iraq and the Islamic Republic of Iran in 1980-1988 is estimated to have left 450,000 soldiers and 50,000 civilians dead (White, 2005). The conflicts between Eritrea and Ethiopia in the last decade were fought between two conventional armies using heavy weaponry and trench warfare and claimed tens of thousands of lives. There have also been multinational forces engaged in conflict by means of massive air attacks, as in the Gulf War against Iraq in 1991 and in the North Atlantic Treaty Organization (NATO) campaign against the Federal Republic of Yugoslavia in 1999.

An estimated 5% of all deaths during the twentieth century were a result of the immediate or secondary impact of such collective violence. This was higher than in the seventeenth through the nineteenth centuries, in which 2% of deaths are estimated to have resulted from collective violence. The 40-fold rise in the number of deaths among soldiers in the twentieth century greatly exceeded a doubling of the globe's midcentury population. Military deaths per million population rose 18-fold

**TABLE 34-5** Estimated Average Annual Military Deaths in Wars, Worldwide, by Century

| CENTURY | AVERAGE ANNUAL MILITARY DEATHS | WORLD MIDCENTURY POPULATION IN MILLIONS | AVERAGE ANNUAL MILITARY DEATHS PER MILLION POPULATION |
|---|---|---|---|
| Seventeenth | 9,500 | 500 | 19.0 |
| Eighteenth | 15,000 | 800 | 18.8 |
| Nineteenth | 13,000 | 1,200 | 10.8 |
| Twentieth | 458,000 | 2,500 | 183.2 |

From White, M. (2005). Twentieth century atlas. Death tolls for the major wars and atrocities of the twentieth century. Retrieved March 28, 2006, from *http://users.erols.com/mwhite28/warstat2.htm.*

from the nineteenth to the twentieth century (Table 34-5). Deaths related to genocide and democide (the mass killing of people of the same ethnic or national group) also rose in the twentieth century as the centralization of large political and economic systems and the emergence of new technologies made mass killings possible (Rummel, 1994).

The number of direct deaths in war peaked in 1994 (Figure 34-2). Indirectly caused deaths, however, are claiming a growing proportion of all conflict-related deaths. There may have been an average of about 300,000 people dying per year as a result of wars in the last decade. However, this number has dropped rapidly and may have been under 100,000 in 2005.

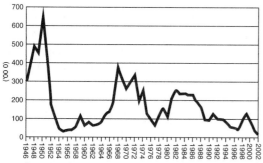

**Figure 34-2** Battle deaths by year, 1946-2002. (From Marshall, M., & Gurr, T. [2005]. *Peace and conflict 2005: A global survey of armed conflicts, self-determination movements, and democracy.* College Park: University of Maryland, Center for International Development and Conflict Management.)

Laying siege, destroying essential goods and services, poisoning water supplies, or enslaving a losing enemy often accompanied warfare in premodern times (Keegan, 1982). In European war since the establishment of nation-states in the seventeenth century, soldiers of one nation engaged in direct battle almost exclusively with soldiers of a rival nation. Anticolonial wars, often based on guerilla warfare, further blurred the distinction between the military and civilians. This distinction has been further eroded with the breakdown of national states since the end of the Cold War. Most conflicts are now internal to a country. In many internal conflicts that often pit the state against a section of the civilian population, torture, disappearances, and other forms of repression have been practiced in pursuit of political and ideologic objectives. These tactics extend the impact of conflict to a much larger, noncombatant population (Garfield, 2002).

More and more, troops are irregular, representing a political faction or social group rather than a national army with an accountability structure. Their targets, also, are more frequently civilians, who may be irregular troops or simply the "other" social group. Targeting civilians or the infrastructure on which their daily lives depend has become more common, and leverage points to redress this have been lost (Machel, 2001; Rhodes, 1988; Sivard, 1996).

A lack of a common definition of terrorism haunts international affairs; one group's terrorist is another's freedom fighter. Among all definitions, terrorism is defined as an act of violence employed by clandestine individuals. The purpose is not to target people but to disrupt "life as usual" among the resident population (Cornish, 2001; Goodhand & Hulme, 1999). Terrorism is sometimes referred to as the peacetime equivalent of a war crime, as the targets of terrorist acts are most often neither combatants nor political leaders of the opposition.

Under the Geneva Conventions of 1949, the rules of war require the application of principles of proportionality and distinction in the choice of targets. Proportionality involves an assessment of ways to minimize likely civilian casualties when a military objective involves targeting that is not exclusively military. Distinction focuses on avoiding civilian targets whenever possible. Attempts to regulate the brutality of conflicts have not kept pace with the evolving forms of conflict (Robertson, 1999). Most importantly, international humanitarian law and the Geneva Conventions are focused on states waging war and therefore fail to deal adequately with conflicts within states or among multinational coalitions against a single state.

The chance of injury or death among large groups of the population increases with the use of depersonalized high-tech weaponry; fighting among informal, non-state actors; and the use of indiscriminant weapons in terror attacks. Along with an increasing number of natural disasters and economic disruptions around the world, the number and severity of humanitarian crises and the populations affected by them have risen. Globalization has also contributed to economic disruption since the end of the Cold War. For the first time in the modern era, some states are experiencing sustained economic declines. Of the 10 countries with the highest under-5 mortality rates in the world, seven have experienced recent civil conflict (Black, Morris, & Bryce, 2003).

The majority of new wars and economic declines are in Africa, but every continent is affected by them except for North America, which after the September 11 attacks can no longer be comforted by the belief that it is immune from conflict. Indeed, the disruptions caused by those terror attacks, the arbitrary nature of civilian victims, and the lasting impact on vulnerable groups—including women and children, family members, those with heightened anxiety, and those who lost employment—is part of a worldwide trend toward the increasing impact of conflict on everyday life.

## IMPACT OF CONFLICT ON HEALTH

Wars and deaths from conflict have been concentrated in poor parts of the world since the end of World War II (Figure 34-3). Per capita income alone is not the best measure of social development. The Human Development Index (HDI) combines information on income, education, mortality, and life expectancy to characterize both the productivity of a society and the use of that productivity in health and education. High-HDI countries have no conflict deaths, and most deaths occur in countries with low-HDI levels.

The number and distribution of disasters such as earthquakes and floods in the world does not follow the same pattern (International Federation of Red Cross and Red Crescent Societies, 1999). Disasters are concentrated in neither the high-HDI nor the low-HDI countries. Midlevel-development countries experience the most, and an increasing number of, disasters. Actually, the process of development is a cause of the increasing number of disasters, as rapid urbanization, lack of safety infrastructure, and environmental degradation conspire in these areas.

For each person killed in conflict, there may be 10 injured and 100 displaced. Disasters, wars, and the economic challenges underlying both have uprooted more people than at any time since the end of World War II. The small number who become refugees outside their native lands are mainly in the high- and mid-level-HDI countries (such as the United States and Iran, respectively). Most remain in their home countries, becoming displaced internally to camps, to periurban settlements, or to other family homesteads or migrating throughout the country. In these ways, conflict can have widespread effects on health, well-being, and social development (Centers for Disease Control and Prevention [CDC], 1992; Harris & Telfer, 2001; Toole & Waldman, 1990, 1993). This is especially the case when one combatant death is associated with 10 noncombatant deaths, as noted for many recent conflicts.

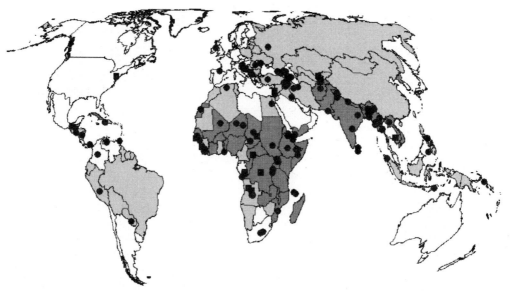

**Figure 34-3**  Per capita income and distribution of conflicts, 1946-2002. Darker areas have lower average incomes. It can be seen that most wars in the last 50 years occurred in, or between, these countries. (From Marshall, M., & Gurr, T. [2005]. *Peace and conflict 2005: A global survey of armed conflicts, self-determination movements, and democracy.* College Park: University of Maryland, Center for International Development and Conflict Management.)

Historically, most international conflicts resulted in an end to hostilities when one side was defeated. There were almost no casualties among military or civilians during U.S.- or NATO-led occupations from World War II until the war on terror. This pattern has changed in recent wars. Not only were there more than 20 times more deaths among noncombatants, but for the first time in the history of the United States there were more military casualties after the overthrow of the regime in Iraq than during the period of major hostilities associated with the invasion.

Conflict is one form of intentional injury. Suicide and homicide are the others. It is notable that there are more deaths resulting from the last two causes, and also less difference between poor and rich countries in the rates of death from these causes (Figure 34-4) (Murray, King, Lopez, Tomijima & Krug, 2002). Deaths resulting from the most common cause of unintentional injury—motor vehicle accidents—number even higher in both poor and rich countries.

A small group of countries have experienced the majority of deaths and displacement caused by armed conflict or disasters since 1991. Data sources on the numbers of people killed or affected vary widely, as few of these countries have adequate vital registration systems and conflict deaths are seldom

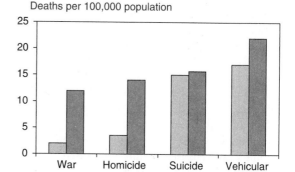

**Figure 34-4**  Death rates by type: 1998. (Data from *World Report on Violence and Health,* World Health Organization.)

recorded by neutral agencies. In nearly all of these countries there are many more refugees or displaced people than conflict deaths, and many more living people affected by disasters than killed by disasters.

Conflict was responsible for the death of more than 10% of the national populations in three areas: East Timor, Angola, and Rwanda. Over the last decade, the Democratic Republic of Congo, Afghanistan, and Iraq each experienced uniquely high rates of infant mortality at greater than 10% (100 per 1000 live births). See additional resources at the end of the chapter for data and discussion of individual country situations.

## CONFLICT PREVENTION AND REDUCTION OF HARM FROM INTENTIONAL INJURIES

Good health practice requires identifying risk factors and determinants of collective violence and developing approaches to resolve conflicts without resorting to violence. A range of risk factors for major political conflicts has been identified (Box 34-9) (Carnegie Commission on Preventing Deadly Conflict, 1997; Stewart, 2000; Stewart & Fitzgerald, 2001). In combination, these factors interact with one another to create conditions for violent conflict. On their own,

none of them may be sufficient to lead to violence or disintegration of a state.

The strongest predictor of violence is stagnation in economic and social development. Where the distribution of goods and services in a society is becoming more equitable, productivity growth will generally result in improved access to goods and services needed for human well-being. Manifestations of such improvement include a decline in child malnutrition, an increase in the proportion of all births to occur in health institutions, reduced mortality among infants and young children, an increase in schooling, and increased access of women to health services and education (Commission of the UN Secretariat, 2006). These are at the heart of the Millennium Development Goals (MDGs), established by the nations of the world via the UN in 2000 as key monitoring and action indicators for the world for the next 15 years. In 2005, one third of the way into the grand challenge presented by the MDGs, there was progress in some health indicators, but the world is doing poorly overall in the areas of women's health and girls' education. Conflict gets in the way of achieving all of these goals (Tables 34-6 and 34-7).

Achieving the MDGs is likely the best way to reduce political violence, and strengthening nursing in poor countries is one of the best way to achieve the MDGs. Nursing has a critical role to play in addressing the harm caused via conflict. Nursing is the first and major profession for women in many developing countries. Employment as a nurse can provide economic relief and mobility to a family. A robust and empowered nursing workforce can also be the least-expensive and most cost-effective way to improve the health of malnourished children and birthing mothers. Nursing is unique in its ability to raise community and public health standards and practices, improve the care and treatment of civilian populations injured and affected by conflict, and reduce morbidity and mortality among women and children. No other profession has as much to offer, in so many different areas, toward the achievement of the MDGs.

Even without economic growth, social development can occur and can result in reduced violence. It also reduces mortality rates and increases

---

**BOX 34-9    Risk Factors for Violent Conflicts**

**POLITICAL FACTORS**
- A lack of democratic processes
- Unequal access to power

**ECONOMIC FACTORS**
- Grossly unequal distribution of resources
- Unequal access to resources
- Control over key natural resources
- Control over drug production or trading

**SOCIETAL AND COMMUNITY FACTORS**
- Inequality among groups
- The fueling of group fanaticism along ethnic, national, or religious lines
- The ready availability of small arms and other weapons

**DEMOGRAPHIC FACTORS**
- Rapid demographic change

**TABLE 34-6** Examples of the Direct Impact of Conflict on Health

| HEALTH IMPACT | CAUSES |
|---|---|
| Increased mortality | External causes, mainly related to weapons |
| | Infectious diseases (such as measles, poliomyelitis, tetanus, and malaria) |
| | Noncommunicable diseases, as well as deaths otherwise avoidable through medical care (including asthma, diabetes, and emergency surgery) |
| Increased morbidity | Injuries from external causes, such as those from weapons, mutilation, antipersonnel landmines, burns, and poisoning |
| | Morbidity associated with other external causes, including sexual violence |
| | Infectious diseases: |
| |     Water-related (such as cholera, typhoid, and dysentery) |
| |     Vector-borne (such as malaria and onchocerciasis) |
| |     Other communicable diseases (such as tuberculosis, acute respiratory infections, human immunodeficiency virus [HIV] infection, and other sexually transmitted diseases) |
| | Reproductive health: |
| |     A greater number of stillbirths and premature births, more cases of low birth weight, and more delivery complications |
| | Nutrition: |
| |     Acute and chronic malnutrition and a variety of deficiency disorders |
| | Mental health: |
| |     Anxiety |
| |     Depression |
| |     Posttraumatic stress disorder |
| |     Suicidal behavior |
| | Increased disability: |
| |     Physical, psychological, social |

people's participation in determining their destinies. The Central Intelligence Agency identified a lack of decline in the rate of infant mortality as the strongest predictor of social disruption and conflict. Moreover, rapid infant mortality decline seems to provide social peace even when other conditions could encourage violence.

In Cuba, for example, despite profound economic setbacks, infant, child, and maternal health outcomes have continued to improve (Garfield, 2000). Infant deaths reached an all time low of 7.1 per 1000 live births in 1998. Despite a shortage of available calories, the percentage of all newborns that were below 2500 g reached an all time low of 6.7% in that same year. More than 99% of all births occurred in health institutions, and an all-time low of 47 maternal deaths occurred per 100,000 births. The infant mortality in Cuba is about as low, and life expectancy at birth is nearly as high, as in developed countries despite per capita

incomes 90% to 95% lower. Similarly, the countries of Central Europe, which enjoyed the least violence during the 1990s were those that experienced rapid infant mortality declines *even when* the economies stagnated or declined. Those with the most violence have stagnant, high rates of infant mortality, with or without economic growth.

In these countries, limited resources were used more carefully, and with more popular participation, to derive social benefit. Nurses are key to encouraging such activities as boiling water when sanitation cannot be assured, encouraging breastfeeding, and encouraging families to feed pregnant women and children first. Even in poor countries, there are usually enough resources available to improve health and education. Education and health promotion in communities are needed to improve the use of these latent resources. Nurses, on the front lines of community health, are able to identify the dynamics of families and participants

**TABLE 34-7** Impact of Conflict on Health Care Services

| OBJECT OF IMPACT | MANIFESTATION OF IMPACT |
|---|---|
| Access to services | Reduced security (e.g., through factors such as landmines and curfews) |
| | Reduced geographic access (e.g., through poor transport) |
| | Reduced economic access (e.g., because of increased charges for health services) |
| Service infrastructure | Destruction of clinics |
| | Disrupted referral systems |
| | Damage to vehicles and equipment |
| | Poor logistics and communication |
| Human resources | Injury, disappearance, and death of health workers |
| | Displacement and exile of people |
| | Low moral |
| | Difficulty in retaining health workers in insecure areas |
| | Disrupted training and supervision |
| Equipment and supplies | Lack of drugs |
| | Lack of maintenance |
| | Poor access to new technologies |
| | Inability to maintain cold chain for vaccines |
| Health care activity | Shift from primary to tertiary care |
| | Increased urbanization |
| | Reduction in community-based activities |
| | Reduced outreach, prevention |
| | Disrupted health information systems |
| | Compromised vector control programs |
| Health policy | Weakened national capacity |
| | Inability to coordinate |
| | Less engagement in policy debates locally and internationally |
| | Weakened community structures and reduced participation |
| Relief activities | Limited access to certain areas |
| | Increased cost of delivering services |
| | Increased pressure on host communities, systems, and services |
| | Greater insecurity for relief personnel |
| | Weakened coordination and communication among agencies |

From Zwi, A., Ugalde, A., & Richards, P. (1999). The effects of war and political violence on health services. In L. Kurtz (Ed.), *Encyclopedia of violence, peace and conflict*. San Diego: Academic Press.

in their communities and communicate good public health practices in a way that most other health or development workers cannot.

Economic growth alone will not bring peace. When economies grow but the benefits of this growth remain in few hands, the seeds of conflict grow even if infant mortality declines. The economies of Cuba, Nicaragua, and Liberia grew rapidly in the 1950s or 1960s. This growth sharpened conflict between the "haves" and the "have-nots." Government in these countries grew more rigid in limiting options to redress inequities, creating a type of social pressure cooker. This led to subsequent decades of internal fighting in these countries.

Expectations of levels and processes to create equity are culture bound. Acceptable levels of inequity in Costa Rica are very different from those in neighboring Panama, or in Canada compared with the United States, or in Serbia compared with Austria. But acceptable levels and processes may change in a society in a short time. Equity, for example, is seen very differently in China today compared with two decades ago.

Similarly, acceptable levels of malnutrition or infant mortality are very different in Cuba compared with the Dominican Republic, in Costa Rica compared with Nicaragua, and in Afghanistan compared with Pakistan. Assessment of these variables depends on rates of change more than on interstate comparisons.

Social equity is more than the distribution of social benefits. A strong state can sometimes organize beneficial handouts efficiently, but it cannot make its people feel that the state's destiny is theirs. Exclusion from political participation, as happened, for example, to the Kosovars in Yugoslavia around 1990, the Tutsis in Rwanda in 1990, and the Kurds in Northern Iraq in the 1980s, is an incubator for violence. Subsequent reverse-exclusion when the first group seizes control is a formula for continued violence, as has occurred in Kosovo, Burundi, Iraq, and the Congo.

## HEALTH PROMOTION IN AREAS OF CONFLICT—A KEY ROLE FOR NURSES

### Service Provision during Conflicts

Common problems confronting humanitarian operations during periods of conflict include the following (Leaning, Briggs, & Chen, 1999):

- How best to upgrade health care services for the host population in parallel with providing services for refugees
- How to provide high-quality services humanely and efficiently
- How to involve communities in determining priorities and the way in which services are provided
- How to create sustainable mechanisms through which experience from the field is used in formulating policy

Refugees fleeing their countries across borders lose their usual sources of health care. They then become dependent on whatever is available in the host country or can be provided in additional services by international agencies and NGOs. The services of the host government may be overwhelmed if large numbers of refugees suddenly move into an area and seek to use local health services. This can be a source of antagonism between the refugees and the population of the host country, which may spill over into new violence. Such antagonism may be aggravated if refugees are offered services, including health services, that are more easily obtained or are cheaper than what is available to the local population, or if the host country does not receive

resources from outside to cope with its greatly increased burden. When ethnic Albanians from Kosovo fled into Albania and the former Yugoslav Republic of Macedonia during the conflict in 1999, WHO and other agencies tried to help the existing health and welfare systems of these host countries to deal with the added load, rather than simply allowing a parallel system to be imported through the aid agencies.

### Service Provision after Conflicts

There has been considerable discussion about how best to reestablish services as countries emerge from major periods of conflict (Kumar, 1997). When inaccessible areas open up in the aftermath of complex emergencies, they release a backlog of public health needs that have long previously been unattended to, typically flagged by epidemics of measles. In addition, ceasefire arrangements, even if precarious, need to include special health support for demobilizing soldiers, plans for demining, and arrangements for refugees and internally displaced people to return. All these demands are likely to occur at a time when the infrastructure of the local health system is seriously weakened and when other economic resources are depleted. More precise information is needed on interventions in various places, the conditions under which they take place, and their effects and limitations (Banatvala & Zwi, 2000). Usually, the boundary between the end of a conflict and the beginning of the postconflict period is far from clear-cut, as significant levels of insecurity and instability often persist for a considerable time. The provision of health services can significantly reduce this period, reestablishing normalcy and contributing to development. This is especially true for mental health–related services (Bracken, Giller, & Summerfield, 1995; Quirk & Casco, 1994; Summerfield, 1991).

## FOLLOWING IN NIGHTINGALE'S FOOTSTEPS

Nursing's involvement in war is a double-edged sword, one which ultimately threatens the heart of humanitarianism. Nursing is often identified with national, patriotic interests of each warring power.

These are nurses who serve in a nation's armed forces. Nursing's other character is humanist, with a non-nationalistic ethic of social reform, represented by nursing leaders Lavinia Dock of the American Nurses Association and Ethel Fenwick of the International Council of Nurses (Garfield, Dresden, & Rafferty, 2003). These are nurses who make up the majority of professional staff in humanitarian and development organizations like Doctors Without Borders, CARE, and International Medical Corp and in UN agencies like WHO and UNICEF.

Both threads were represented by Florence Nightingale, who worked to improve the fighting capacity of the British army. At the same time, she opposed the formation of the International Committee of the Red Cross, as she feared it would relieve individual governments of the responsibility to protect noncombatants (Garfield, 2005). (Ironically, national Red Cross associations may have done more to advance the role of nursing in the public's eyes than professional nursing organizations.) Throughout the history of nursing's involvement in conflict, there are contradictions and tensions in our own understanding of a nurse's role:

■ Ethically in favor of care for all, but demonstrating patriotism for one's own country and its interests

■ Trying to promote humanism in the care of all while strengthening the fighting capacity of one's army

■ Struggling to strengthen professionalism in nursing while acting docile under the command of doctors and political leaders

The profession of nursing is well placed to contribute to the global arena of humanitarian policy and research. Nurses bring a wealth of experience and a strong historical grounding in situations of conflict and crisis. To fulfill our potential, nursing must include, but go beyond, a clinical response to the individual patient.

The strength of nursing lies in our accessibility and ability to engage in advocacy in the public's interests. Both in and outside areas of conflict, in most countries, there are more nurses than any other kind of health professional. Nurses are accessible because they work everywhere and in close proximity to those in need. In both times of stability and times of conflict, nurses are prepared to provide care. From our close relations with individuals, families, and communities, we become aware of the strengths and needs of our clients. This privileged glimpse into others' realities allows us to holistically assess and respond. After the September 11 attack on the World Trade Center, for example, nurses led community-based activities to reestablish community psychologic health, provided assistance to harmed individuals in recovery, and dealt with many other "alterations in daily function" that did not generate a physician encounter or hospital visit.

Funds in the United States are now being directed to readiness, training for emergency response, improved communications, and upgrading of biologic detection capacity. Important as these foci are, they fail to pull in the full range of nursing capacities. With a humanist perspective and a presence in key environments, nurses can do more. For example, early detection of many biologic threats may occur among young people in schools. There is a long way to go to fully incorporate school nurses into systems for early detection and public health promotion. Nurses are frequently involved in assisting survivors to grieve and recover; far more preparation needs to go into developing their skill base to do this well.

To do population-oriented work, nurses need further integration into mass emergency response systems. They need training and practice to apply their logistic and organizational skills as well as their clinical skills. Communications strategies for nurses to serve in situations with mass casualties need to be developed. There is a need for evaluation tools and templates with which we can learn and improve our systems. Each new mass casualty experience is an opportunity for systems development and improvement.

Research is needed to identify characteristic patterns for the different kinds of collective violence and their implications and trends for affected population groups. Conflicts within or between states, using high- or low-technology weapons, and in countries of different resource bases will have markedly different patterns.

The impact of conflict on families and communities, and the resources they can draw on for resiliency and recovery, are key topics for nursing research.

## IMPLICATIONS FOR NURSING

These observations suggest the following actions for nurses:

- Identify and serve those affected by conflict with clinical health services, whether they are in poor countries or our neighbors, refugees or displaced
- Train all professional nursing students in emergency care and disaster preparedness, to better serve in a world experiencing changing and less-predictable patterns of violence
- Assess and support communities affected by conflict to organize to support health and well-being
- Strengthen the training and employment of nurses in poor countries, who can help improve health and social equity and thereby help achieve the MDGs, thus reducing conflict
- Highlight the roles, already extensive and deeply embedded in our history, of nurses who serve with humanitarian international organizations in their own countries or internationally
- Concentrate evaluation and research on indicators that are sensitive to changes in well-being of individuals and groups, rather than reporting only on clinical health or nutrition measures
- Move from a focus on national income to the use of resources for improved health and education outcomes and enhancement of the social and political roles of women

*Web Resources*

**Care**
*www.care.org*
**Doctors Without Borders (Médecins Sans Frontières)**
*www.doctorswithoutborders.org*
**International Committee of the Red Cross**
*www.icrc.org*
**International Rescue Committee**
*www.theirc.org*

## REFERENCES

Banatvala, N., & Zwi, A. (2000). Public health and humanitarian interventions: Improving the evidence base. *BMJ, 321,* 101-105.

Black, R., Morris, S., & Bryce, J. (2003). Where and why are 10 million children dying every year? *Lancet, 361,* 2226-2234.

Bracken, P. J., Giller, J. E., & Summerfield, D. (1995). Psychological responses to war and atrocity: The limitations of current concepts. *Social Science & Medicine, 40,* 1073-1082.

Carnegie Commission on Preventing Deadly Conflict. (1997). *Preventing deadly conflict: Final report.* New York: Carnegie Corporation.

Centers for Disease Control and Prevention (CDC). (1992). Famine affected, refugee, and displaced populations: Recommendations for public health issues. *MMWR. Morbidity and Mortality Weekly Report, 41*(RR-13), 1-76.

Commission of the UN Secretariat. (2006). Investing in development: A practical plan to achieve the Millennium Development Goals. Retrieved April 2, 2006 from *www.unmillenniumproject.org/reports/index.htm.*

Cornish, P. (2001). Terrorism, insecurity and underdevelopment. *Conflict, Security & Development, 1,* 147-151.

Garfield, R. (2000). The public health impact of sanctions: Contrasting responses of Iraq and Cuba. *Middle East Report, 215,* 16-19.

Garfield, R. (2005). Nightingale in Iraq. *American Journal of Nursing, 105*(2), 69-72.

Garfield, R., Dresden, E., & Rafferty, A. M. (2003). Commentary: The evolving role of nurses in terrorism and war. *American Journal of Infection Control, 31,* 163-167.

Garfield, R. M. (2002). Economic sanctions, humanitarianism, and conflict after the Cold War. *Social Justice, 29*(3), 94-107.

Garfield, R. M., & Nuegut, A. (1991). Epidemiologic analysis of warfare: A historical review. *JAMA, 266*(5), 688-692.

Goodhand, J., & Hulme, D. (1999). From wars to complex political emergencies: Understanding conflict and peace-building in the new world disorder. *Third World Quarterly, 20,* 13-26.

Harris, M. F., & Telfer, B. L. (2001). The health needs of asylum seekers living in the community. *Medical Journal of Australia, 175,* 589-592.

International Federation of Red Cross and Red Crescent Societies. (1999). *World disasters report 1999.* Dordrecht: Martinus Nijhoff.

Keegan, J. (1982). *The face of battle.* New York: Penguin.

Krug, E. (Ed.). (2002). *World report on violence and health.* Geneva: World Health Organization.

Kumar, K. (Ed.). (1997). *Rebuilding societies after civil war.* Boulder, CO: Lynne Rienner.

Leaning, J., Briggs, S. M., & Chen, L. C. (Eds.). (1999). *Humanitarian crises: The medical and public health response.* Cambridge: Harvard University Press.

Machel, G. (2001). *The impact of war on children.* London: Hurst and Company.

Marshall, M., & Gurr, T. (2005). *Peace and conflict 2005: A global survey of armed conflicts, self-determination movements, and democracy.* College Park: University of Maryland, Center for International Development and Conflict Management.

Murray, C. J. L., King, G., Lopez, A. D., Tomijima, N., & Krug, E. G. (2002). Armed conflict as a public health problem. *BMJ, 324,* 324-349.

Quirk, G. J., & Casco, L. (1994). Stress disorders of families of the disappeared: A controlled study in Honduras. *Social Science & Medicine, 39,* 1675-1679.

Rhodes, R. (1988). Man-made death: A neglected mortality. *Journal of the American Medical Association, 260,* 686-687.

Robertson, G. (1999). *Crimes against humanity. The struggle for global justice.* Harmondsworth: Penguin.

Rummel, R. J. (1994). *Death by government: Genocide and mass murder since 1900.* New Brunswick: Transaction Publications.

Sheik, M., Gutierrez, M. I. & Bolton, P. (2000, July 15). Deaths among humanitarian workers. Education and debate. *British Medical Journal, 321,* 166-168.

Sivard, R. A. (1996). World military and social expenditures. *The Ploughshares Monitor, 17*(3), 1-20. Retrieved April 2, 2006 from *http://www.ploughshares.ca/libraries/monitor/mons96c.html.*

Stewart, F. (2000). The root causes of humanitarian emergencies. In E. W. Nafziger, F. Stewart, & R. Varynen (Eds.), *War, hunger and displacement: The origin of humanitarian emergencies.* Oxford: Oxford University Press.

Stewart, F., & Fitzgerald, V., (Eds.) (2001). *War and underdevelopment.* Oxford: Oxford University Press.

Summerfield, D. (1991). The psychosocial effects of conflict in the Third World. *Development in Practice, 1,* 159-173.

Toole, M. J, & Waldman, R. J. (1990). Prevention of excess mortality in refugee and displaced populations in developing countries. *JAMA, 263,* 3296-3302.

Toole, M. J., & Waldman, R. J. (1993). Refugees and displaced persons: War, hunger and public health. *JAMA, 270,* 600-605.

Weinstein, H. M., Dansky, L., & Iacopino, V. (1996). Torture and war trauma in primary care practice. *Western Journal of Medicine, 165*(3), 112-117.

White, M. (2005). Death tolls for the major wars and atrocities of the twentieth century. Retrieved on April 2, 2006, from *http://users.erols.com/mwhite28/warstat2.htm.*

World Health Organization (WHO). (1992). *International statistical classification of diseases and related health problems, tenth revision. Volume 1: Tabular list.* Geneva: WHO.

World Health Organization (WHO). (1993). *International statistical classification of diseases and related health problems, tenth revision. Volume 2: Instruction manual.* Geneva: WHO.

World Health Organization (WHO). (1994). *International statistical classification of diseases and related health problems, tenth revision. Volume 3: Index.* Geneva: WHO.

Zwi, A., Ugalde, A., & Richards, P. (1999). The effects of war and political violence on health services. In L. Kurtz (Ed.), *Encyclopedia of violence, peace and conflict.* San Diego: Academic Press,

## ADDITIONAL RESOURCES

Cliff, J., & Noormahomed, A. R. (1988). Health as a target: South Africa's destabilization of Mozambique. *Social Science & Medicine, 27,* 717-722.

Garfield, R. (2001). Health and well-being in Iraq: Sanctions and the impact of the oil for food program. *Transnational Law & Contemporary Problems, 11*(2), 278-297.

Garfield, R. M., Frieden, T., & Vermund, S. H. (1987). Health related outcomes of war in Nicaragua. *American Journal of Public Health, 77,* 615-618.

Goma Epidemiology Group. (1995). Public health impact of Rwandan refugee crisis: What happened in Goma, Zaire, in July 1994? *Lancet, 345,* 339-344.

Kloos, H. (1992). Health impacts of war in Ethiopia. *Disasters, 16,* 347-354.

Prunier, G. (1995). *The Rwanda crisis: History of a genocide.* New York: Columbia University Press.

Roberts, L., & Zantop, M. (2003). Elevated mortality associated with armed conflict—Democratic Republic of Congo, 2002. *MMWR. Morbidity and Mortality Weekly Report, 52*(20), 469-471.

Smallman-Raynor, M., & Cliff, A. (1991). Civil war and the spread of AIDS in central Africa. *Epidemiology of Infectious Diseases, 107,* 69-80.

Spiegel, P. B., & Salama, P. (2000). War and mortality in Kosovo, 1998-1999: An epidemiological testimony. *Lancet, 355,* 2204-2209.

Steering Committee of the Joint Evaluation of the Emergency Assistance to Rwanda. (1996). *The international response to conflict and genocide: Lessons from the Rwanda experience.* Odense: Strandberg Grafisk.

Taylor, W. R., Chahnazarian, A., Weinman, J., Wernette, M., Roy, J., et al. (1993). Mortality and use of health services surveys in rural Zaire. *International Journal of Epidemiology, 22*(Suppl 1), S15-S19.

Ugalde, A., Selva-Sutter, E., Castillo, C. Paz, C., & Canas, S. (2000). The health costs of war: Can they be measured? Lessons from El Salvador. *British Medical Journal, 321,* 169-172.

Welch, M. (2002). The politics of dead children. *Reason, 33*(10), 52-59.

# *Vignette*   Laura B. Cobey & James C. Cobey

## *International Emergencies: Health Care and Human Rights*

*"There are risks and costs to action. But they are far less than the long range risks of comfortable inaction."*

JOHN FITZGERALD KENNEDY

Over the last few decades the world has seen an explosion of civil, ethnic, and religious conflicts. Over 50 million people have become refugees or are internally displaced. Wars, famines, and genocide have destroyed societies. As the late Senator Moynihan observed, the world is "in a state of pandaemonium" as groups work for the undefined term of "self-determination" (Moynihan, 1993). Complex humanitarian emergencies have been magnified by the proliferation of arms and forced migration. Many international organizations, United Nations (UN) agencies, and nongovernmental agencies (NGOs) are mobilized to assist in these crises.

In any disaster, those giving aid must understand the roles of the three major players. First are the displaced victims, who may be refugees if they have crossed an international border or internally displaced people (IDPs) if they have stayed in their own country. Second is the government of the victims, either the victim's home government or the government of a neighboring country. Third are the international caregivers—international organizations, UN agencies, or NGOs.

In the last decade, displaced victims are IDPs who have been forced to move by their governments or militias seeking land or trying to purify their perceived ethnic culture. Sometimes groups are persecuted because they are perceived as doing economically better than the rest of society. For example, in Darfur the roving bands of militia called the *Janjaweed* have been trying to get more grazing land and water for their animals by forcing farmers off their own land. Struggles between herdsmen and farmers go back centuries, especially when water is scare. The displaced farmers have become IDPs and do not have the protection of their own government. The government, in fact, has tried to hide the problems and has impeded international relief efforts by claiming these issues are purely domestic and that international sovereignty does not allow foreign intervention.

If the victims have crossed an international border, they are designated as refugees by the 1951 UN Convention on Refugees and become eligible for help from the UN High Commissioner for Refugees (UNHCR) (Brownlie, 1971). Although other organizations can also provide aide, all are considered guests of the host or recipient country. Assisting organizations must abide by the rules and immediate relief needs of the host country if they want to be permitted to stay and help. The host county can demand help for its citizens, who often may be worse off than the refugees.

It is essential that all international organizations understand the host government's position on the crisis. Jumping in and giving relief without the permission of the local government is an effort doomed to failure. These emergencies are complex, each side claiming the need for "self-determination" as a necessary goal.

Relief agencies have their own constraints. Their boards may have different specific goals, and they may have different funding priorities. Some may be emphasizing religious issues, whereas others may be more concerned with feeding or vaccinating people. Often each wants to appear as the lead agency to assure maximum ability to raise funds (Box 34-10).

Each agency has its own mission and purpose in providing help. It is important that volunteers from

**BOX 34-10** Relief Agencies

**UNITED NATIONS AGENCIES**

UNHCR (UN High Commission for Refugees)
*www.unhcr.org*
UNRWA (UN Relief and Works Agency)—for
   Palestine refugees
*www.unrwa.org*
WFP (World Food Program)
*www.wfp.org*
UNICEF (United Nation International Children's
   Emergency Fund)
*www.unicef.org*
OCHA (Office of Civil and Humanitarian Affairs)
*http://ochaonline.un.org*
Or *www.reliefweb.int*
WHO (World Health Organization)
*www.who.org*

**RED CROSS ORGANIZATIONS**

ICRC (International Committee of the Red Cross)
*www.icrc.org*
IFRC (International Federation of Red Cross and
   Red Crescent Societies)
*www.ifrc.org*

**NONGOVERNMENTAL ORGANIZATIONS (NGOs)
(PARTIAL LISTING)**

IRC (International Rescue Committee)
*www.theirc.org*
MSF (Médecins Sans Frontières/Doctors Without
   Borders)
*www.msf.org*
PHR (Physicians for Human Rights)
*www.phrusa.org*
CARE (Committee for Relief Everywhere)
*www.care.org*
CRS (Catholic Relief Service)
*www.catholicrelief.org*

the different groups understand each other's constraints. There is always a need to work cooperatively and collaboratively in the field, although it is often hard to do so.

The UNHCR will be the overall coordinator in a refugee action. It will call on the assistance of the World Food Program (WFP) to obtain food, which will be distributed by different aide organizations.

The United Nations International Children's Emergency Fund (UNICEF) will be involved in the food and water distribution, often the most difficult problem. Getting clean or chlorinated water

to desperate people is often the most expensive and pressing need. The Office of Civil and Humanitarian Affairs (OCHA) will try to work as the lead agency or at least be the agent of collaboration for IDPs.

The Red Cross takes a special role in disasters. The International Committee of the Red Cross (ICRC) is a private Swiss organization that is specifically mentioned in the Geneva Conventions to be authorized to give relief. Their actions are neutral. The ICRC works on both sides of a war conflict. It receives funds from many governments and uses those relief funds to help all people affected by the disaster. The organization's neutrality enables it to have access to the various people in need. It handles massive relief programs with well-organized logistic capacity.

The other part of the Red Cross is the Federation. The Federation is made up of nearly 180 National Red Cross societies. It handles natural disasters, whereas the ICRC handles manmade or war disasters. The Federation works to coordinate the relief efforts of the many national societies that arrive in a disaster. It sets standards for appropriate response through such efforts as the "Sphere" programs, which define the parameters of effective disaster relief.

There are thousands of NGOs that do excellent work. However, each new disaster creates new NGOs, which try to fill what they perceive to be an unmet need. The new NGOs often make the mistake of accepting and distributing "goods in kind," such as clothing, mattresses, or sample drugs. Experienced NGOs realize that the greatest need is always cash because it is cheaper to purchase goods locally than to send large material donations from outside the country. The workers on the ground best determine local needs. Some NGOs are religious, some are not. Most disaster relief workers feel that religious organizations can do great work as long as there is no proselytizing in the field.

Many NGOs do human rights work and use the media to broadcast the human rights abuses they see. This function is very important, but often these groups are asked to leave the country by the host government. The Red Cross usually can stay, because their neutrality allows them access to victims. In Ethiopia in the 1980s, Médecins Sans

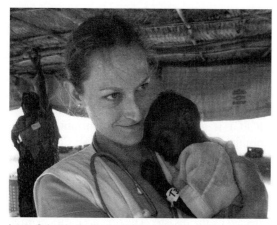

Laura Cobey in the Darfur Region of Sudan while serving with Médecins Sans Frontières (MSF) Holland.

Frontières (MSF) told the world about abuses of displaced peoples by the government. They were forced to leave the country. The ICRC kept quiet about what its representatives saw and was allowed to stay to continue helping the IDPs. Often it is best that human rights work be done by those who are not actually giving aid, such as Human Rights Watch, Physicians for Human Rights (PHR), and Refugees International. These groups are expert at researching problems, collecting data, and publicizing it. Others may want to tell the world what they see, but they risk expulsion.

## OUR HUMANITARIAN EXPERIENCES

### The Thai-Cambodian Border: Direct Care

One of my (JCC) first experiences with disaster relief was at the Thai-Cambodian border in 1979. I was from the American Red Cross assigned as an ICRC medical delegate. The Cambodian refugees had come pouring across the Thai border, running from the Vietnamese. The Vietnamese had invaded the country to drive out the Khmer Rouge, who had killed more than a quarter of the population in an effort to make a new agrarian society and to discredit the intellectual leaders. The result was massive illiteracy. The world, tired of the Vietnam War, had done nothing for 2 years as the Khmer Rouge used genocide to try to kill those whom they considered to be intellectual or who were literate. My mission, with the ICRC, was a chance to

bring aid to both the Khmer Rouge and the Khmer Serei (free Cambodians) who were fleeing the advancing army.

Though I am an orthopaedist, I was one of the few physicians with a public health background and previous experience in developing countries. As a result, I became the medical coordinator of a refugee camp of over 60,000 people. We were on the Cambodian side of the border, although no one knew where the border actually was. Only the ICRC was able to get into Cambodia. The other 40 NGOs were inside of Thailand, working in a large and more stable camp under the protection of the Thai government.

After constructing simple roads, we worked with UNICEF to bring in food and tankers of chlorinated water. A challenge was how to distribute food equitably and not allow it to be diverted to the Cambodian army. We had to design water tanks that forced people to use spigots rather than contaminating the water with buckets.

One of our first errors was setting up clinics. We quickly learned that the healthy ones come to the clinics, while the sick children with diarrhea and cerebral malaria died in their huts. We set up protocols for what conditions we would treat and what we would not treat. During a disaster is not the time to raise the level of medical care above what it had been before the disaster. I had an ophthalmologist who wanted to operate on cataracts, but what I needed was staff to debride wounds from landmines and run a feeding program. CARE staff assisted in establishing intensive feeding centers for dehydrated children and supplementary feeding centers for underweight children and lactating mothers.

One of my greatest problems was handling truckloads of donated drugs. The ICRC and the World Health Organization (WHO) have developed essential drug lists for use in disasters. WHO rarely gets involved in direct relief but does excellent work setting standards. The international organizations can buy large quantities of drugs at very low prices. In spite of this, people collect sample drugs from doctors and hospitals and send them abroad, with the cost of transportation being far more than the value of the drugs. I had an epidemic of injection abscesses from people inject-ing each other with injectable vitamins. Soon I real-ized it was better to burn these shipments before they reached the refugees and caused more damage. In spite of this, certain NGOs tried to circumvent our supply system and send us antibiotics that we did not need.

We know that the greatest needs of displaced people are for water, food, and shelter. These needs take precedence over any medical effort. We learned that the first action in a disaster is assessment before treatment. We started by taking a census of the refugees in the camp in our first month. The second effort must be to secure plenty of clean water, then food appropriate for the local diet. Last, there must be shelter, which may be protection from armed militia. After these three needs are attended to, measles vaccination must be started, because measles is the greatest killer of malnour-ished people. Vitamin A must be given to the children, not just to protect their eyes, but to dramatically decrease their death rate from diarrhea.

After these priorities are met, curative care can start on the most prevalent diseases. To decide which diseases to treat, one must make house-to-house visits, not wait for the sick to come to a clinic.

Many international agencies and NGOs were created during the Cambodian experience and learned to incorporate public health and epidemio-logic methodology in later disasters.

### Cambodia: Human Rights Work

The second type of international work that I (JCC) have been involved with is human rights work. This is a different type of international effort. I have worked primarily with PHR and Human Rights Watch. In human rights work the focus is to gather data about abuses and disseminate it. As one would expect, the country's government may not want the world to know the information. This is very differ-ent from the work the Red Cross does but is essen-tial to stop abuse.

My first assignment was to study the epidemiol-ogy of land mines in Cambodia. PHR is an organi-zation that quantifies human rights abuses. Our team was asked to measure the severity of the appar-ent landmine epidemic in Cambodia. We discretely

entered the country and surveyed hospital and operative records throughout the country. In most hospitals of developing countries in which I have worked, the medical records are useless. Every surgical facility, however, has a surgical log. In 1991, we counted all the surgical cases that had been treated at six surgical facilities. We then estimated the population of the country and came up with the figure that one out of every 236 Cambodians had stepped on a land mine. We now know that half of those who step on mines never make it to a hospital, so the injury rate is actually much higher.

Our team and PHR staff then wrote a book: *Landmines in Cambodia—*
*The Coward's War* (Asia Watch & PHR, 1991). PHR distributed the text to the White House, to all members of Congress, and to the members of the UN. That effort resulted in the launch of the International Campaign to Ban Landmines (ICBL). The ICBL and its members spent the next 6 years pushing to ban landmines as a weapon. We believed that putting an explosive in the ground and walk-ing away from it for any reason is immoral. The ICBL received the Nobel Peace Prize in 1997 for developing a new method for making international arms-control law. Usually superpowers debate for decades to make arms-control treaties. In this case small countries, with the help of NGOs, drafted and initiated the signature and ratification process of a new treaty in 14 months.

### Congo-Rwandan Border: Direct Care

In 2002, I (LBC) was asked by the International Rescue Committee (IRC) to work at the Congo-Rwandan border, where there was a long-standing armed conflict among many groups. I had just been working in Kosovo with sexually abused women in an area that was still under a lot of tension, with NATO troops trying to maintain peace. In the Democratic Republic of Congo (DRC) there was no international police force. Ugandan, Congolese, Rwandan, and Angolan forces controlled the area, and the situation was worsened by roving militias of the Interahamwe. The Interahamwe are the mili-tant Hutu that had fled Rwanda after they had participated in genocide against the Tutsi.

I was asked to assist in administering 32 clinics that were staffed by 65 Congolese doctors and nurses—all men. The Office of Disaster Assistance (OFDA), part of the U.S. Agency for International Development (USAID), funded this IRC mission.

When I arrived I realized I had a choice of two languages, French or Swahili. English was not an option except when talking to other expatriates. On my first day I found myself in front of a meeting of some 60 health workers who were demanding money. The complaint was that the IRC had not sent money in the last 3 months. I reminded them that the clinics were to be one third financed by the local government, although I knew there was no functioning local government with a tax base to finance anything. One third was supposed to be collected from fees from the patients, but they had no money. The last third was from the OFDA through the IRC. The IRC could not release the funds, because the clincs had not kept an account of finances for the last 6 months. The local doctors tried to tell me not to worry about the lack of accounting; they knew how to spend the money. We were at a stalemate until I clarified that I was not their leader, but their coach. Empowering local staff is key for development. The medical staff accepted this approach and developed an accounting system. After 3 months they were making their own budgets and doing all the ordering of supplies.

Besides handling the administration of the clinics, I became involved in a large bed net program to prevent malaria. Bed nets are still the least expensive and most effective way to prevent malaria, because most mosquitoes bite in the evening. I worked with local women's groups to develop systems for them to order and distribute the nets. However, we had a major practical problem that affected our program outcome. I discovered that the small villages were often raided at night by the Interahamwe militias, which forced the local people to flee to the jungle in the evening. As a result we were thwarted in controlling malaria.

I worked on a major epidemiologic project to determine the overall death rate in the area. In our well-distributed study (Roberts et al., 2001), we showed that at that time there were 1 million excess deaths resulting from the ongoing conflict. The data

were collected by going hut to hut (cluster sampling) to talk with people directly about the deaths in their families. We compared the death rate in areas of conflict with that in areas of no conflict. There are now up to 3 million deaths, and the war continues. Excess deaths are determined by the increased death rate in the areas of war conflict compared to similar demographic areas in the DRC with no conflict. This number continues to rise, even though there is now a UN-sponsored multinational peace-keeping force present.

### Darfur, Sudan: Relief Work

In 2004, I (LBC) was asked by MSF Holland to go to Darfur in Sudan. In Darfur the local community of farmers was being driven out by the Janjaweed, Some of the inhabitants of the Sudan went to Chad and became refugees who could be protected by the UNHCR.

The government of Sudan did not want the world to know about the problems of the displaced people and made it very hard for outside groups to get entry visas. Literally tons of food and medicine were sitting either in Khartoum or in Port Sudan while the government took its time to "clear" the goods. This meant that when the medicines did arrive at the camp, over 70% had been destroyed by the extreme heat. We also were not allowed to use VHF hand-held radios, so communication depended on erratic mobile telephone connections.

A major effort of MSF was to set up a feeding center for children in one of the larger IDP camps. In spite of our efforts, one or two babies died at the center each day. I worked with other NGOs responsible for food distribution to make sure that the mothers obtained the food rations for the rest of their families. Even this very simple effort was difficult to coordinate and execute.

One of the first projects we undertook was a measles vaccination campaign in the camp. In three days time, we immunized a total of 9050 children aged 6 months to 15 years. We were also concerned about cholera outbreaks because of the lack of sanitation and clean water in the camp. Overnight the camp grew from approximately 15,000 people to over 40,000, and the camp flooded during the rainy season.

The community health workers who were the eyes and ears of the camp would visit the huts and tents where people lived to find sick children and bring them to our center. They were essential in doing a head count to determine the basic demographics of the camp. Population counts are often politically difficult because the results often vary with NGO data versus government data. We have both found in our travels that government census data may be wrong and is used by the government to misrepresent a local population's size for political gain. Our study, however, showed 47,000 in the camp. Without this extensive outreach, we could never have reached most of the children. These workers were trained to identify infectious disease outbreaks and to identify families that needed special assistance and emotional support. They taught families how to cook with the supplemental foods we distributed and started a handwashing campaign by distributing soap.

Several times the expatriate aid community was not allowed into the camp, making it even more critical for the IDPs to be trained to manage the feeding centers and other programs on their own. For example, when the UN Security Council considered sanctions against Sudan, anti-Western sentiment started brewing in the town where the aid staff stayed. We were told to stay in our houses because government officials suspected the NGO staff of reporting atrocities in the field to the press. At other times the police or other government officials would try to force the IDPs back to their villages, making it unsafe for us to be in the camp.

## SUMMARY

In international relief work it is essential to understand the motivation of all the groups involved and to set priorities early to prevent wasting precious resources and time. Besides giving direct relief aid, it is critical to assess the overall health problems in the host country to be sure your intervention is appropriate.

If one wants to do more than give neutral impartial assistance, one must accept the consequences. Many NGOs get involved in trying to change the political situation on the ground or publicize their findings and are forced out.

Clinics may help, but the first priority is to stop the wars. In order to improve the health care of a community, economic development must be the priority. Without economic development, the health care from externally supported NGO clinics will have minimal effect. Only by improving the economy of the country can we hope to decrease the mortality rate and provide access for much-needed health care to impoverished people.

### REFERENCES

Asia Watch & Physicians for Human Rights (PHR). (1991). *Land mines in Cambodia—The Coward's War.* New York: Asia Watch.

Brownlie, I. (1971). *Basic documents on human rights.* Oxford: Clarendon Press.

Moynihan, D. P. (1993). *Pandaemonium: Ethnicity in international politics.* New York: Oxford University Press.

Roberts, L., Hale, C., Belyakdoumi, F., Cobey, L., Ondeko, R., & Despines., M. (2001). *Mortality in the eastern Democratic Republic of Congo.* New York: International Rescue Committee.

# Index

Page numbers followed by *b*, *t*, or *f* indicate boxes, tables, or figures, respectively. Italicized numbers indicate photos.

# Vignettes

# POLICY SPOTLIGHT